Handbook of
Substance Abuse
Neurobehavioral Pharmacology

Handbook of Substance Abuse
Neurobehavioral Pharmacology

Edited by

RALPH E. TARTER

University of Pittsburgh Medical Center
Pittsburgh, Pennsylvania

ROBERT T. AMMERMAN

Allegheny University of the Health Sciences
Pittsburgh, Pennsylvania

and

PEGGY J. OTT

University of Pittsburgh Medical Center
Pittsburgh, Pennsylvania

Plenum Press • New York and London

Library of Congress Cataloging-in-Publication Data

Handbook of substance abuse : neurobehavioral pharmacology / edited by
  Ralph E. Tarter, Robert T. Ammerman, and Peggy J. Ott.
      p.   cm.
    Includes bibliographical references and index.
    ISBN 0-306-45884-5
    1. Substance abuse--Treatment--Handbooks, manuals, etc.
  2. Neuropsychopharmacology--Handbooks, manuals, etc.   I. Tarter,
  Ralph E.   II. Ammerman, Robert T.   III. Ott, Peggy J.
  RC564.15.H36   1998
  616.86'06--dc21   98-36286
                                                             CIP

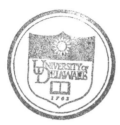

ISBN 0-306-45884-5

© 1998 Plenum Press, New York
A Division of Plenum Publishing Corporation
233 Spring Street, New York, N.Y. 10013

http://www.plenum.com

10 9 8 7 6 5 4 3 2 1

Printed in the United States of America

Contributors

Shana Bacal • UCLA-VAMC Laboratory for the Study of Addictions, Los Angeles, California 90073

Marsha E. Bates • Center of Alcohol Studies, Rutgers University, Piscataway, New Jersey 08855

Ann Bordwine Beeder • Cornell University Medical College, New York, New York 10036

Neal L. Benowitz • Departments of Medicine, Psychiatry, and Biopharmaceutical Science, University of California at San Francisco, San Francisco, California 94143

Lisa Borg • Laboratory on the Biology of Addictive Diseases, The Rockefeller University, New York, New York 10021

Janet Brigham • SRI International, Menlo Park, California 94025

Marilyn E. Carroll • Department of Psychiatry, University of Minnesota, Minneapolis, Minnesota 55455

Erminio Costa • Department of Psychiatry, The University of Illinois at Chicago, Chicago, Illinois 60612

John W. Daly • National Institutes of Health, Bethesda, Maryland 20892

Harriet de Wit • Department of Psychiatry, University of Chicago, Chicago, Illinois 60637

M. Elena Denison • UCLA-VAMC Laboratory for the Study of Addictions, Los Angeles, California 90073

Stephen H. Dinwiddie • Department of Psychiatry, Finch University of Health Sciences, The Chicago Medical School, North Chicago, Illinois 60064

Mauro G. Di Pasquale • Department of Physical and Health Education, University of Toronto, Toronto, Canada K0K 3K0

Eric B. Evans • National Starch and Chemical Company, Bridgewater, New Jersey 08807

Suzette M. Evans • The New York State Psychiatric Institute, New York, New York 10032

Forrest J. Files • Department of Physiology and Pharmacology, Wake Forest University School of Medicine, Winston-Salem, North Carolina 27157

Joanna S. Fowler • Chemistry Department, Brookhaven National Laboratory, Upton, New York 11973

S. John Gatley • Medical Department, Brookhaven National Laboratory, Upton, New York 11973

Frank H. Gawin • UCLA-VAMC Laboratory for the Study of Addictions, Los Angeles, California 90073

A. James Giannini • Department of Psychiatry, The Ohio State University, Columbus, Ohio 43210

Andrew N. Gifford • Medical Department, Brookhaven National Laboratory, Upton, New York 11973

Richard A. Glennon • Department of Medicinal Chemistry, Virginia Commonwealth University, Richmond, Virginia 23298

Mark S. Gold • University of Florida Brain Institute, Gainesville, Florida 32610

David E. Hartman • Isaac Ray Center, Rush Presbyterian St. Luke's Hospital, Chicago, Illinois 60612

Catherine A. Hayes • Department of Psychiatry and Human Behavior, The University of Mississippi Medical Center, Jackson, Mississippi 39216

Stephen T. Higgins • Departments of Psychiatry and Psychology, University of Vermont, Burlington, Vermont 05401

Allyn C. Howlett • Saint Louis University School of Medicine, St. Louis, Missouri 63104

Walter A. Hunt • National Institute on Alcohol Abuse and Alcoholism, Neurosciences and Behavioral Research Branch, Bethesda, Maryland 20892-7003

Christopher R. Johnson • Department of Psychiatry, Baylor University, Houston, Texas 77030

Angela Justice • Department of Psychiatry, University of Chicago, Chicago, Illinios 60637

Andrea C. King • Laboratory of the Biology of Addictive Diseases, The Rockefeller University, New York, New York 10021; *present address:* Department of Psychiatry, The University of Chicago, Chicago, Illinois 60637

Jeffrey M. Kirk • Department of Psychiatry, University of Chicago, Chicago, Illinois 60637

Debra L. Klamen • Department of Psychiatry, The University of Illinois at Chicago, Chicago, Illinois 60612

Mary Jeanne Kreek • Laboratory on the Biology of Addictive Diseases, The Rockefeller University, New York, New York 10021

Christopher S. Martin • University of Pittsburgh Medical Center, Pittsburgh, Pennsylvania 15213

Una D. McCann • National Institute of Mental Health, Bethesda, Maryland 20892

Melissa Mertl • National Institute of Mental Health, Bethesda, Maryland 20892

Norman S. Miller • Department of Psychiatry, The University of Illinois at Chicago, Chicago, Illinois 60612

Robert B. Millman • Cornell University Medical College, New York, New York 10036

Nancy K. Morrison • Department of Psychiatry, The University of New Mexico, Albuquerque, New Mexico 87131

Alfonso Paredes • UCLA-VAMC Laboratory for the Study of Addictions, Los Angeles, California 90073

Kenneth A. Perkins • Department of Psychiatry, University of Pittsburgh School of Medicine, Pittsburgh, Pennsylvania 15213

Bruce Phariss • Cornell University Medical College, New York, New York 10036

George V. Rebec • Program in Neural Science, Department of Psychology, Indiana University, Bloomington, Indiana 47405

George A. Ricaurte • Department of Neurology, The Johns Hopkins Bayview Medical Center, Baltimore, Maryland 21224

Craig R. Rush • Department of Pharmacology and Toxicology, The University of Mississippi Medical Center, Jackson, Mississippi 39216

Herman H. Samson • Department of Physiology and Pharmacology, Wake Forest University School of Medicine, Winston-Salem, North Carolina 27157

Richard B. Seymour • Haight-Ashbury Free Medical Clinic, San Francisco, California 94117

Jewell W. Sloan • Department of Anesthesiology, University of Kentucky College of Medicine, Lexington, Kentucky 40536

David E. Smith • Haight-Ashbury Free Medical Clinic, San Francisco, California 94117

Wesley Sowers • Center for Addictions Services, St. Francis Medical Center, and Department of Psychiatry, University of Pittsburgh Medical Center, Pittsburgh, Pennsylvania 15201

Thomas J. Spencer • Psychopharmacology Unit, Massachusetts General Hospital, Boston, Massachusetts 02114; and Department of Psychiatry, Harvard Medical School, Boston, Massachusetts 02114

Maxine Stitzer • Department of Psychiatry, Division of Behavioral Biology, Johns Hopkins University, Baltimore, Maryland 21224

Ralph E. Tarter • Western Psychiatric Institute and Clinic and Department of Psychiatry, University of Pittsburgh Medical School and Center for Education and Drug Abuse Research, Pittsburgh, Pennsylvania 15213-2593

Nora D. Volkow • Medical Department, Brookhaven National Laboratory, Upton, New York 11973

Elzbieta P. Wala • Department of Anesthesiology, University of Kentucky College of Medicine, Lexington, Kentucky 40536

Ellen A. Walker • Department of Psychology, University of North Carolina at Chapel Hill, Chapel Hill, North Carolina 27599

Sharon L. Walsh • Behavioral Pharmacology Research Unit, Department of Psychiatry and Behavioral Sciences, Johns Hopkins University School of Medicine, Baltimore, Maryland 21224

Timothy E. Wilens • Psychopharmacology Unit, Massachusetts General Hospital, Boston, Massachusetts 02114; and Department of Psychiatry, Harvard Medical School, Boston, Massachusetts 02114

Stephen A. Wyatt • Department of Psychiatry, Yale University School of Medicine, New Haven, Connecticut 06519

James P. Zacny • Department of Anesthesia and Critical Care, The University of Chicago, Chicago, Illinois 60637

Douglas Ziedonis • Department of Psychiatry, Yale University School of Medicine, New Haven, Connecticut 06519

Preface

The manifold problems caused by addictive drugs are ubiquitous in society. Violence, infection, suicide, chronic diseases, crime, traumatic injury, psychosocial maladjustment, and fetal injury are well-recognized sequelae of habitual drug use. These outcomes are the culmination of a host of complex interacting factors that predispose to and are concomitant with drug consumption. Marijuana hybrids, purified cocaine, synthetically manufactured "designer" drugs, and novel drug combinations comprise an ever expanding pharmacopoeia of increasingly potent licit and illicit compounds that have addictive potential.

To discern the etiological factors underlying the substance use disorders and their associated health and psychosocial outcomes, it is necessary to understand the biobehavioral actions and clinical correlates of psychoactive drugs that have abuse and addiction potential. Pharmacological research provides the foundation for delineating the causes and natural history of the substance use disorders. This book reviews the neuropharmacology, behavioral pharmacology, and clinical pharmacology of the compounds that are recognized to induce an abuse or dependence disorder. Each of the sections of this book corresponds to a drug class featured in the fourth edition of the *Diagnostic and Statistical Manual of Mental Disorders* (American Psychiatric Association, 1994). This format enables the book to be used as a reference for practitioners and clinical researchers in substance abuse and provides in one volume a comprehensive updating of knowledge of substance abuse pharmacology for basic science researchers.

Numerous reasons point to the need for a volume linking pharmacology and clinical research in the substance use disorders. For example, widening acceptance of pharmacotherapy for the treatment of addiction underscores the importance of comprehending the actions of abusable drugs in clinical practice. Pharmacological research also has important social policy ramifications, as illustrated most poignantly by research on the addictive properties of nicotine. We hope that this compendium will further catalyze investigations directed at integrating pharmacological and psychosocial processes for understanding the etiology and treatment of the substance use disorders.

The editors express their appreciation to the contributors for their timely and authoritative articles. Patricia Park's dedication and initiative in assisting in all phases of this effort are gratefully recognized.

Finally, we wish to acknowledge our colleagues at the Center for Education and Drug Abuse Research (CEDAR), a NIDA-funded center on the etiology of adolescent substance abuse. Indeed, this volume was, in part, an outgrowth of the stimulating interchanges among CEDAR faculty.

Ralph E. Tarter, Ph.D.
Robert T. Ammerman, Ph.D.
Peggy J. Ott, Ph.D.

Contents

IV. Cocaine

V. Hallucinogens

VI. Inhalants

VII. Nicotine

VIII. Opiates

IX. Sedatives, Hypnotics, and Anxiolytics

X. Amphetamines

XI. Other Substances of Abuse

Introduction

Defining Drugs of Abuse

RALPH E. TARTER

Pharmacology is the scientific discipline concerned with determining the biochemical actions and behavioral effects of drugs. Understanding the pharmacological actions of drugs on brain and behavior is thus the cornerstone of basic research directed at elucidating etiology of the substance use disorders (American Psychiatric Association, 1994). Although etiology of the substance use disorders involves manifold factors, including genetic predisposition, social context (family, peers, societal norms, demography), psychological disposition (temperament, personality, cognition), as well as regulations and legal controls determining drug cost and availability, the complex causal variables resulting in these clinical disorders originate from pharmacology.

The fourth edition of the *Diagnostic and Statistical Manual of Mental Disorders* (*DSM-IV;* American Psychiatric Association, 1994) recognizes 11 classes of compounds that induce substance use disorder. The compounds are alcohol, amphetamines, caffeine, cannabis, cocaine, hallucinogens, inhalants, nicotine, opioids, phencyclidine, and sedatives. This book consists of 11 sections which map to these compounds by providing comprehensive reviews of the pharmacological basis of the corresponding substance use disorders. In addition, this volume reviews the literature pertaining to two specific compounds that are increasingly recognized as having abuse potential, namely, anabolic steroids and ecstasy. As a companion to the *DSM-IV,* this book provides up-to-date information about the pharmacological actions of abusable compounds from both neurobiological and behavioral perspectives in conjunction with discussions of their clinical correlates and consequences.

A book on drug abuse pharmacology is timely and important for several reasons. The substance use disorders are among the most prevalent of all psychiatric disorders, with a lifetime prevalence rate of up to 25% (Regier *et al.,* 1991). The cost to society directly attributable to the treatment of substance use disorders combined with costs associated with lost wages, crime, infection, and traumatic injuries is billions of dollars annually. Violence during acute drug exposure and from chronic usage additionally has a persistent unsettling effect on society. Elucidating how abusable drugs affect brain and behavior is thus the essential starting point for understanding the factors associated with the risk for developing a substance use disorder.

RALPH E. TARTER • Western Psychiatric Institute and Clinic and Department of Psychiatry, University of Pittsburgh Medical School and Center for Education and Drug Abuse Research, Pittsburgh, Pennsylvania 15213-2593.

Handbook of Substance Abuse: Neurobehavioral Pharmacology, edited by Tarter *et al.* Plenum Press, New York, 1998.

A defining feature encompassing all drugs that produce a substance use disorder (abuse or dependence) has yet to be identified. Wide variation is observed with respect to their capacity to induce intoxication, produce tolerance, and establish physical dependence. The severity of withdrawal symptoms following cessation is also extremely variable. Although drugs with abuse liability share the property of altering emotional, cognitive, or behavioral functioning, this property is not unique to abusable drugs.

Drugs having abuse liability may be positively reinforcing such that the motivation to consume is directed at achieving an enhanced state of energy, arousal, or euphoria. Alternatively, consumption can be negatively reinforcing by relieving an aversive emotional or motivational state (e.g., fatigue, stress, depression). To fully explain the link between pharmacology and substance use disorder, it is necessary to understand the motivational underpinnings of drug-seeking behavior. That is, the factors predisposing to first exposure and the factors sustaining habitual consumption need to be considered in relation to pharmacology for understanding substance use etiology. This task is especially challenging because abusable drugs differ greatly with respect to their reinforcing properties.

Most drugs in the *DSM-IV* system that have abuse liability produce dependence following chronic exposure. Dependence is most starkly demonstrated by withdrawal symptoms on cessation of drug intake. However, the strength of the link between dependence and withdrawal is variable across drugs. Severity of withdrawal can range from mild craving for the drug to a life-threatening neuropsychiatric syndrome depending on the drug type, the person's drug consumption history, and circumstances surrounding drug termination. For example, withdrawal symptoms other than mildly dysphoric mood are either absent or transitory following cessation of cannabis consumption. Withdrawal symptoms are not observed following chronic PCP, inhalant and hallucinogen consumption even though these latter compounds produce dependence.

Another factor invoked to classify compounds according to whether or not they have abuse liability pertains to whether intoxication can be induced. This criterion, however, excludes nicotine, which is perhaps the most commonly ingested compound producing dependence.

There is thus substantial variation among the 11 classes of drugs that produce a substance use disorder. These compounds share the feature of adversely affecting health and social adjustment; however, from the pharmacological perspective, no single unifying attribute has been revealed.

Apart from classification issues, it is also noteworthy that terminology is not consistent. The terms *abuse* and *dependence* can be applied to characterize the properties of the drug (e.g., "abuse liability") or the clinical diagnosis of the person ("substance use disorder—abuse"). The diagnosis of *abuse* is essentially a residual category, reflecting persistent drug use in hazardous situations in conjunction with adverse interpersonal and legal consequences. The diagnosis of *dependence* is subdivided according to whether there is dependence (tolerance and withdrawal symptoms) or the less severe variant in which there is compulsive use without tolerance or withdrawal symptoms. With the exception of nicotine, which produces dependence but not abuse, and caffeine, which produces neither abuse nor dependence, the drug classes are associated with both abuse and dependence disorders.

The term *liability* also has been differently employed by the various disciplines. Among pharmacologists, the term generally describes the efficacy of a compound in inducing habitual consumption, as, for example, selection of one compound instead of another. The term, as used by etiology researchers, denotes the likelihood or risk that a person will develop a substance use disorder.

Table 1 summarizes the *DSM-IV* criteria for diagnosing the disorders of abuse and dependence. A diagnosis of "substance use disorder—abuse" is assigned if the person qualifies for at least one of four criteria within the prior 12-month period. The diagnosis of "substance use disorder—dependence" is assigned if the

TABLE 1. DSM-IV Criteria for Diagnosis of Abuse and Dependence

Abuse	Failure to maintain role expectations at school, home, or work
	Consumption in situations that are dangerous
	Legal problems caused by substance use
	Continued consumption despite interpersonal problems caused by drug use
Dependence	Tolerance
	Withdrawal
	Longer duration or larger amount of drug use than intended
	Inability to reduce or control drug use
	Extensive effort to procure, consume, or recover from drug use
	Relinquishing of personal or social obligations and roles
	Continued use despite knowledge of having a problem with the drug

person qualifies for at least 3 of 7 symptoms within the prior 12 months. Depending on the particular configuration of symptoms, dependence is specified as either having or not having a physiological substrate.

Assigning a substance use disorder diagnosis serves the societal need of identifying persons whose consumption behavior presents a risk to themselves or others. For example, using a drug in itself may not be problematic (at least initially); however, self-administration with infected needles poses imminent dangers. Thus, from the pharmacological perspective the defining attribute of all drugs that are considered to have abuse liability may be elusive, but consensus can be approached when the focus is on potential or current adverse health or social adjustment consequences.

In considering whether a drug is potentially abusable, it is essential to recognize the critical importance of individual differences. Significantly, only a small proportion of individuals develop a dependence disorder following drug exposure. There is a dearth of empirical information pertaining to person–drug interactions with respect to the induction of a substance use disorder. Clearly, individual differences in biobehavioral makeup contribute to the risk for a substance use disorder. Research thus needs to address the specific characteristics of individuals whose risk is augmented for a substance use disorder following repeated or even

single drug exposure across the range of abusable drugs, recognizing their widely disparate pharmacologic actions on the brain and their effects on behavior.

An overarching research goal pertains to determining how the particular pharmacological properties contribute to the person's risk for developing a substance use disorder. The pharmacological actions of drugs, in conjunction with genetic, developmental, neurobiological, behavioral, and social policy factors, are undoubtedly involved, and contribute to the risk for developing a substance use disorder. This book coalesces the literature pertinent to the neurobehavioral pharmacology of the 11 classes of compounds that have the potential to induce a substance use disorder. It is intended to catalyze comprehensive and multidisciplinary research on the etiology of the substance use disorders and inform about the biological and behavioral processes of the specific drugs comprising the *DSM-IV* taxonomic system.

References

American Psychiatric Association. (1994). *Diagnostic and statistical manual of mental disorders* (4th ed.). Washington, DC: Author.

Regier, D., Farmer, M., Rae, D., Locke, B., Keith, S., Judd, L., & Goodwin, F. (1991). Comorbidity of mental disorders with alcohol and other drug abuse. Results from the Epidemiologic Catchment Area Study. *Journal of the American Medical Association, 264,* 2511–2518.

I

Alcohol

1

Pharmacology of Alcohol

WALTER A. HUNT

Introduction

Ethanol is the most abused substance in the world today. In the United States, roughly two thirds of the population drinks alcoholic beverages without ill effects. However, over 7% of adults, based on a 1992 survey, are considered alcoholic, with many more classified as alcohol abusers (B. F. Grant *et al.*, 1994). Excessive ethanol consumption accounts for 3% of all deaths, including 50% of traffic fatalities, 38% of drowning deaths, 50% of homicides, 30% of suicides, most cases of cirrhosis of the liver, and fetal alcohol syndrome, the leading cause of mental retardation. This chapter provides the essential pharmacology of ethanol, including its basic properties, how the body processes it when ingested, its behavioral effects, and its possible mechanisms of action.

Ethanol, because of its simple molecular structure and its actions on multiple targets, has diverse effects on the body and brain. It is distributed quickly throughout the body and is metabolized primarily by the liver. Behavioral effects of ethanol range from sociability and euphoria to coma and death. Tolerance and dependence as well as brain damage can develop after chronic ethanol ingestion. The mechanisms of action of ethanol involve many inter-

cellular and intracellular processes responsible for synaptic transmission, including neurotransmitters and their receptors, second messengers, and other regulatory proteins. Because of this assortment of actions, a variety of potential therapeutic targets could be exploited for medications development.

Chemical Properties, Absorption, Distribution, Metabolism, and Elimination

Considering the multitude of problems caused by ethanol consumption, it is not surprising that ethanol is a simple molecule with many diverse actions. Ethanol is a member of a class of organic compounds known as short-chain aliphatic alcohols. These alcohols consist of a hydrocarbon chain with a hydroxy group attached to one carbon. Ethanol is a two-carbon alcohol with the structure CH_3CH_2OH that has properties in common with other short-chain aliphatic alcohols. The major property is their ability to dissolve in both lipids and water, making them amphiphilic. This property allows not only easy distribution into tissue water but also the ability to act on functional elements in membranes of all cell types including neurons.

Because of its high water solubility, ethanol is quickly absorbed from the gastrointestinal system. The rate of absorption is determined by the quantity of ethanol consumed, the concentration of ethanol in the beverage, the rate of consumption, and the composition of gastric contents. The type of food consumed can

WALTER A. HUNT • National Institute on Alcohol Abuse and Alcoholism, Neurosciences and Behavioral Research Branch, Bethesda, Maryland 20892-7003.

Handbook of Substance Abuse: Neurobehavioral Pharmacology, edited by Tarter *et al.* Plenum Press, New York, 1998.

affect the rate of absorption, especially if the food has a high fat content, which reduces absorption of ethanol.

Ethanol is quickly distributed throughout the body, the rate to different organs depending on the degree of vascularization. In organs such as the brain, ethanol concentrations equilibrate rapidly with blood concentrations. However, estimating brain ethanol concentrations by determining blood ethanol concentrations can be erroneous when the latter is rising; that is, brain ethanol concentrations are underestimated and can complicate legal determinations of intoxication.

The metabolism and elimination of ethanol are primarily accomplished by the liver, although some is lost in the urine and expired air. Two enzymatic oxidative steps are involved in this process. Ethanol is first converted to acetaldehyde by alcohol dehydrogenase, then to acetate by aldehyde dehydrogenase. Various enzymes further metabolize acetate to water and carbon dioxide. At low blood ethanol concentrations (<50 mg/dl), the rate at which alcohol dehydrogenase metabolizes ethanol is concentration-dependent: the higher the concentration, the higher the rate. At higher blood ethanol concentrations, the enzyme cannot operate any faster and ethanol is converted to acetaldehyde at a fixed rate of about 10–15 g/hr in an average-size person. Other enzymes contributing to the oxidation of ethanol include cytochrome P450IIEI and catalase. However, their contribution is considered minor (Damgaard, 1982; Inatomi, Kato, Ito, & Lieber, 1989). Acetaldehyde does not usually accumulate in the blood. However, in Asian populations, some individuals have a nonfunctional form of acetaldehyde dehydrogenase and acetaldehyde accumulates, contributing to the resulting flushing response. This response may account in part for lower alcohol consumption in some Asians (Chao, 1995).

Behavioral Effects: Intoxication, Tolerance, and Dependence

Ethanol has a well-known depressant effect on the brain and behavior, although at low blood ethanol concentrations, forms of activation are experienced (Hunt, 1994). At concentrations below 50 mg/dl, drinkers are more sociable and possibly euphoric. They are often more talkative, but sometimes aggressive, even violent. This level of intoxication is sometimes called disinhibition. At blood ethanol concentrations of 50–100 mg/dl, depression progressively dominates, reflected as disturbances in gait, lack of concentration, and increased reaction times. In most states, concentrations of 80–100 mg/dl are the limits at which an automobile can be driven legally. Ataxia, slurred speech, and impaired mental and motor function, including short-term memory problems, are present at concentrations of 100–150 mg/dl. Higher blood concentrations lead progressively to a lack of response to sensory stimuli, coma, and death from respiratory arrest.

The effects of blood ethanol levels stated above reflect those of low to moderate social drinkers. Those individuals who drink heavily or frequently can develop tolerance to the effects of ethanol. Tolerance is a condition in which the effect of a given amount of a drug declines with continued use, or more drug is needed to attain the same effect. There are two general forms of tolerance to ethanol: metabolic tolerance and functional tolerance.

Metabolic tolerance occurs when enzymes that convert ethanol to acetaldehyde are induced, thereby elevating the metabolism and elimination of ethanol. The activity of cytochrome P450IIEI, a mixed-function oxidase, increases with chronic ethanol exposure, whereas alcohol dehydrogenase does not (Lieber, 1988). A major concern of metabolic tolerance to ethanol is its modification of the metabolism of other drugs transformed in the liver by cytochrome P450IIEI, including barbiturates, coumarins, and anticonvulsants, thereby reducing their effectiveness. With barbiturates, metabolic tolerance can lead to increasing use and the risk of abuse.

Functional tolerance to ethanol occurs when the body adapts to its effects by reducing the response to ethanol (Tabakoff, Cornell, & Hoffman, 1986). A major problem with developing ethanol tolerance is the possibility of consuming increasing amounts of ethanol, leading to dependence and organ damage. Tolerance developing to the aversive effects of ethanol but not the pleasurable ones would aggravate this problem. In addition, ethanol tolerance can develop at varying rates on different tasks, allowing a person to adequately perform some tasks but not others.

Several forms of functional tolerance to ethanol exist and are characterized by their time-course of development and the influence of environmental stimuli. One form of tolerance, called acute tolerance, occurs after a single drinking session. Acute tolerance is expressed when an effect of ethanol declines over time, even at constant or higher blood ethanol concentrations (Bennett, Cherek, & Spiga, 1993). This form of tolerance occurs primarily to the aversive effects of ethanol and may lead to further ethanol consumption (Vogel-Sprott, 1992).

When ethanol tolerance develops over several periods of exposure, it is known as chronic tolerance. This form of tolerance occurs more rapidly when ethanol consumption takes place in the same or similar environment and is called environment-dependent tolerance. Social drinkers performing a hand–eye coordination task in either an office- or a bar-like setting perform the task better in the latter setting. This observation suggests that cues found in bars are associated with ethanol consumption and can promote this form of tolerance (McCusker & Brown, 1990). Chronic tolerance can develop without environmental influences, but greater doses of ethanol are required than needed for developing environment-dependent tolerance (Melchior & Tabakoff, 1981). Finally, ethanol tolerance can be augmented when a task is practiced under the influence of ethanol, during which tolerance develops more quickly (Vogel-Sprott, Rawana, & Webster, 1984). The expectation of reward can also contribute to such learned tolerance (Sdao-Jarvie & Vogel-Sprott, 1991).

Acute tolerance may play a role in the risk for developing alcoholism in those with a family history of the disease. Experiments with ethanol-preferring and -nonpreferring rats demonstrated that the ethanol-preferring ones rapidly develop tolerance to the effects of ethanol, whereas the nonpreferring ones do not (Waller, McBride, Lumeng, & Li, 1983). Sons of alcoholics were less affected by ethanol in some studies than sons of nonalcoholics (Schuckit, 1985; Schuckit & Gold, 1988). In another study, sons of alcoholics experienced a greater effect initially but developed tolerance later in the drinking session (Newlin & Thomson, 1990). These results suggest that when subjects perceive the pleasurable effects of ethanol more strongly at the beginning of a drinking session and fewer aversive effects later in the session, the stage is set for higher ethanol consumption. Indeed, nonalcoholic subjects experiencing reduced behavioral or physiological responses after ethanol exposure have a much higher incidence of alcoholism years later at follow-up, especially if they have a family history of the disease (Berman, Whipple, Fitch, & Noble, 1993; Hill, Steinhauer, Lowers, & Locke, 1995; Schuckit, 1994; Schuckit & Smith, 1996). However, whether reduced sensitivity to ethanol actually causes a predisposition to alcoholism or is merely correlated with it is presently unclear.

Similarly to other abused drugs, ethanol can be addictive. Chronic misuse of ethanol can lead to psychological and physical dependence, which presumably results from the readjustment of homeostatic mechanisms adapting to the continued presence of ethanol (O'Brien, 1996). Psychological dependence based on *DSM-IV* criteria (Hasin & Grant, 1994) is expressed as uncontrolled ethanol consumption, whereby large quantities are consumed even in the face of negative consequences. Upon withdrawal, craving for or a strong desire to drink ethanol occurs. In cases where physical dependence is present, various signs and symptoms of the ethanol withdrawal syndrome develop, characterized by tremors, hallucinations, seizures, and delirium tremens (Victor & Adams, 1953).

Mechanisms of Action

The mechanism of any drug is determined largely by its molecular structure and its specificity toward a receptor. However, the simple molecular structure of ethanol does not have sufficient complexity to act on a specific receptor. Thus, it can be expected to have a multitude of actions. Early studies of these actions centered on ethanol as an anesthetic.

Membrane Effects

Around the turn of the twentieth century, one site of action of alcohol was postulated to be the membrane surrounding cells. This idea was based on findings that the more lipid soluble the alcohol, the more potent it was in inducing anesthesia. Known as the Meyer–Overton Principle, the theory stated that the potency of straight, short-chain aliphatic alcohols related directly to their degree of partitioning between a lipid phase and a water phase (Meyer, 1899; Overton, 1896). As the partition coefficient increased, the potency of the alcohol also increased. Although the theory has been refined over the years (Hunt, 1985), the basic concept of ethanol acting on biological membranes remains dominant.

The importance of lipid solubility in inducing intoxication extended to other alcohols and even other classes of substances, except that the relation between potency and lipid solubility had limits (McCreery & Hunt, 1978). Using a broad range of compounds including short- and long-chain, straight and branched, aliphatic and aromatic mono- and polyhydroxyalcohols, alkyl halides and thiols, and hydrocarbons, those that had partition coefficients within a certain range induced intoxication qualitatively similar to ethanol, both in time to onset and duration. Those substances with very low or very high lipid solubility were less effective.

Using molecular probes to study the microenvironment in which ethanol resides in membranes, investigators found that ethanol fluidized or disordered membranes in a concentration-dependent manner (Chin & Goldstein, 1977b; Harris & Schroeder, 1981). Short-chain alcohols had effects similar to those of ethanol and had potencies proportional to their lipid solubility (Lyon, McComb, Schreurs, & Goldstein, 1981). In addition, chronic ethanol exposure resulted in tolerance to this disordering effect (Chin & Goldstein, 1977a). Although the data were consistently showing evidence of the membrane being a site of action of ethanol, they did not explain how ethanol acts to alter the activity of neurons. Changes in the properties of bulk lipids per se do not necessarily explain how ethanol impairs functional elements in the membrane regulating electrical activity.

Research over the last 15 years has focused more on the effects of ethanol on specific neurotransmitters, the receptors on which they act, ion channels, and second messengers; the functions of all of these are disrupted by ethanol. The effects of ethanol on neurotransmission have been extensively studied (Hunt, 1985, 1993). Although many neurotransmitters have been examined, recent basic research has focused on the biogenic amines dopamine and serotonin, opioid peptides, and the amino acids γ-aminobutyric acid (GABA) and glutamate.

Neurotransmitters

Dopamine and Serotonin

A crucial question in alcohol research is why some people are unable to control their intake of ethanol. To address this question, we need knowledge about the biological basis of the reinforcing qualities of ethanol. Dopamine and serotonin have been implicated in ethanol reinforcement using different approaches. One approach uses animal models in which rats are trained to self-administer quantities of ethanol sufficient to produce measurable blood ethanol concentrations. For example, rats, which normally find the taste of ethanol aversive, can be conditioned to self-administer ethanol by initially hiding its taste with a normally liked substance such as sucrose, then reducing the amount of sucrose over time until only ethanol solutions are consumed (Samson, 1986). Known as the sucrose-fading procedure, this approach has proven exceptionally useful in studying the reinforcing properties of ethanol.

Another approach uses selectively bred lines of rats that either prefer to drink large quantities of ethanol instead of water or prefer to drink little ethanol at all (Li, 1991). Typically, measurements are performed on both lines of rats, bred from a common heterogeneous stock, to learn whether differences exist between the lines that would explain the differences in their ethanol preference. Many pairs of selected lines have been developed in several laboratories, and some lines have suggested a role of dopamine and serotonin in ethanol preference.

Several laboratories have reported that ethanol injections or ethanol self-administration increases dopamine and serotonin release in the nucleus accumbens, striatum, and frontal cortex, areas of the brain involved in behavioral reinforcement (Darden & Hunt, 1977; Imperato & DiChiara, 1986; Kiianmaa, Nurmi, Nykanen, & Sinclair, 1995; McBride et al., 1993; Portas, Devoto, & Gessa, 1994; Rossetti, Melis, Carboni, Diana, & Gessa, 1992; Weiss, Lorang, Bloom, & Koob, 1993; Weiss et al., 1996; Yoshimoto, McBride, Lumeng, & Li, 1992). The effect on dopamine release is presumably due to an activation of dopaminergic neurons originating in the ventral tegmental area and synapsing in the nucleus accumbens (Gessa, Muntoni, Vargui, & Mereu, 1985).

With chronic exposure to ethanol, tolerance develops. However, dopamine and serotonin release decreases below preexposure levels after withdrawal (Darden & Hunt, 1977; Rossetti et al., 1992; Weiss et al., 1996). In addition, the dependent rats will drink more ethanol than the nondependent ones (Schulteis, Hyytiä, Heinrichs, & Koob, 1996) and in sufficient amounts to restore dopamine and serotonin release to preexposure levels (Weiss et al., 1996). These responses after withdrawal correspond to an increased threshold for intracranial self-stimulation, having a similar time-course to overt signs of a withdrawal syndrome (Schulteis, Markou, Cole, & Koob, 1995). Since these latter two responses are associated with negative affective states, increased ethanol consumption observed during this period may be an attempt to relieve dysphoria occurring after withdrawal and partially

explain the basis for psychological dependence on ethanol (Weiss et al., 1996).

Consistent with the hypothesis that functional dopamine or serotonin deficiencies can contribute to ethanol consumption, the ethanol-preferring (P) rats have lower concentrations of dopamine and serotonin and their major metabolites in the nucleus accumbens, compared to ethanol-nonpreferring (NP) rats (McBride, Murphy, Lumeng, & Li, 1990; Murphy, McBride, Lumeng, & Li, 1987). In addition, dopaminergic and serotonergic agonists reduce ethanol consumption of P rats (McBride et al., 1990) and of rats self-administering ethanol (Haraguchi, Samson, & Tolliver, 1990; Koob & Weiss, 1990; Samson, Tolliver, & Schwartz-Stevens, 1990).

Although deficiencies in neurotransmission at dopaminergic and serotonergic synapses at critical synapses have been correlated to high ethanol consumption, increases in transmitter release per se may not tell the whole story. Such increases are not necessarily greater in rodent strains that naturally consume more ethanol than others. The degree of dopamine release is greater at the same blood ethanol concentrations in P rats, compared with ethanol-nonpreferring Wistar rats (Weiss et al., 1993). However, ethanol-induced increases in dopamine or serotonin release do not differ between ethanol-preferring HAD and -nonpreferring LAD rats (Yoshimoto et al., 1992), ethanol-preferring AA and ethanol-avoiding ANA rats (Kiianmaa et al., 1995), and Sardinian ethanol-preferring and nonpreferring rats (Portas et al., 1994).

The hypothesis that a dopamine and/or serotonin deficiency contributes to the development of alcoholism has support in a study with humans. This study examined the concentrations of 5-hydroxyindoleacetic acid (5-HIAA), the major metabolite of serotonin, in the cerebral spinal fluid of early-onset alcoholics (i.e., less than 25 years of age), and found that 5-HIAA was reduced compared to late-onset alcoholics (Fils-Aime et al., 1996). In addition, those alcoholics reporting that both parents were alcoholics had particularly low 5-HIAA concentrations, as well as low tryptophan (a precursor of serotonin) and homovanillic acid (a metabolite of dopamine) concentrations.

Opioid Peptides

Opioids have gained the increasing attention of alcohol researchers, in part because of recent FDA approval of naltrexone, an opioid antagonist, for the treatment of alcoholism. Studies in animals have suggested a reciprocal relationship between opioid receptor activity and ethanol consumption. Various studies have reported that low doses of morphine resulted in increased ethanol consumption, whereas injections of naltrexone reduced consumption (Froehlich & Li, 1993; Gianoulakis, 1993). However, morphine does not alter self-administration of ethanol, but naltrexone will suppress it (Schwartz-Stevens, Files, & Samson, 1992). This latter effect was not specific for ethanol responding but was also observed in sucrose responding. Thus, opioids may play a general role in consummatory behavior (Koob, 1992).

Further insights into the role of opioids in ethanol consumption may be gained by observing what happens after morphine is administered concurrently with ethanol, then withdrawn. Rats given morphine for seven days reduced their consumption of ethanol, but increased it after morphine administrations ceased (Volpicelli, Ulm, & Hopson, 1991). This latter effect suggests that if a certain level of endogenous opioid activity is considered normal, a deficiency of such activity may lead to relapse in alcohol abusers. Indeed, preventing relapse is the basis for naltrexone therapy (O'Malley et al., 1992; Volpicelli, Alterman, Hayashida, & O'Brien, 1992).

How naltrexone works in alcoholics is not known. One explanation derives from a theory designed to understand opiate dependence (Kosterlitz & Hughes, 1975). When opiates are taken in large doses, an excessive stimulation of opioid receptors occurs. In an effort to adapt to this effect, opioid synthesis, the number of opioid receptors, or both decline. With the withdrawal of the exogenous opiates, a deficiency in endogenous opioid activity induces a dysphoria that an addict discovers can be re-

lieved by ingesting more opiates. With ethanol consumption, some evidence supports a similar mechanism involving endogenous opioids.

Acute ethanol exposure stimulates the activity of opioid receptors, making them more sensitive to endogenous opioids (Tabakoff & Hoffman, 1983). With chronic ethanol administration, opioid receptors become hypoactive (Hoffman, Urwyler, & Tabakoff, 1982; Lucchi, Bosio, Spano, & Trabucchi, 1981). Brain concentrations of met-enkephalin, an endogenous opioid peptide, are also reduced (Hong, Majchrowicz, Hunt, & Gillin, 1981; Przewlocki et al., 1979; Schulz, Wüster, Duka, & Herz, 1980). However, this reduction occurs only during an ethanol withdrawal syndrome and not while animals are intoxicated (Hong et al., 1981). Furthermore, administration of opiate antagonists do not result in ethanol withdrawal (Goldstein & Judson, 1971). These findings suggest that opioid peptides are not involved in physical dependence per se but may still underlie a compulsion to drink ethanol after withdrawal.

Another possible explanation of how naltrexone reduces the incidence of relapse has been proposed by Froehlich and Li (1994). They suggest that ethanol exposure releases endogenous opioid peptides, thereby priming the subject to continue drinking. When naltrexone is administered, this priming effect is inhibited. Thus, little incentive exists to consume more ethanol. Indeed, recent clinical studies support the rodent studies. Both alcoholics and nonalcoholics given naltrexone report being less high when they consume ethanol (Swift, Whelihan, Kuznetsov, Buongiorno, & Hsuing, 1994; Volpicelli, Watson, King, Sherman, & O'Brien, 1995). These data suggest that abstinent alcoholics have fewer relapses because they are not obtaining the positive reinforcement they expect from ingesting ethanol. This effect can persist during the first 6 months after therapy is discontinued (O'Malley et al., 1996).

GABA

Over the past 15 years, research supports an action of ethanol on GABA receptors. GABA is the major inhibitory transmitter in the brain, and two types of GABA receptors have been identified: the $GABA_A$ and $GABA_B$ receptors. The $GABA_B$ receptor is coupled to calcium or potassium channels through a G-protein–mediated mechanism. G-proteins couple some receptors to second messenger systems to complete synaptic transmission. The $GABA_A$ receptor is a macromolecular protein complex composed of various subunits forming an ion channel to specifically move chloride ions through the neuronal membrane (Lüddens & Korpi, 1996; Macdonald & Olsen, 1994). The $GABA_A$ receptor contains specific binding sites for a variety of substances, including GABA, picrotoxin, barbiturates, benzodiazepines, and anesthetic steroids. The non-GABA binding sites modify the binding of GABA to the receptor. At least 15 different subunits of the $GABA_A$ receptor have been identified. Thus, various combinations of these subunits when assembled can provide diverse structures to confer specificity to these drug classes.

Ethanol enhances the ability of GABA to promote the movement of chloride ions through the membrane, especially in the cerebellum (Suzdak, Schwartz, Skolnick, & Paul, 1986). This action is more pronounced in mice bred for high sensitivity for ethanol compared with those bred for low sensitivity (Allan, Spuhler, & Harris, 1988). Since activating inhibitory neurons in the brain leads to a reduction in neuronal firing, the action of ethanol on $GABA_A$ receptors may underlie the depressant effects of ethanol on behavior.

Not all $GABA_A$ receptors are sensitive to ethanol. The effectiveness of ethanol in enhancing GABAergic function varies by brain area. Electrophysiological studies show that $GABA_A$ receptors are sensitive to ethanol in the medial septum, substantia nigra reticulata, inferior colliculus, globus pallidus, red nucleus, and ventral pallium, whereas they are not sensitive in the lateral septum, ventral tegmental area, and hippocampus (Criswell et al., 1993). The sensitivity of the GABA receptor to ethanol corresponds to the degree of binding of zolpidem, a benzodiazepine. Thus, the density of zolpidem binding sites may predict ethanol sensitivity to-

ward the $GABA_A$ receptor (Criswell et al., 1995). Given the complexity of the $GABA_A$ receptor, the effectiveness of ethanol may depend on the specific subunit composition in a given area of the brain (Duncan et al., 1995).

As with many actions of ethanol, chronic exposure results in the development of tolerance to the GABA enhancement of chloride movements (Allan et al., 1988; Morrow, Suzdak, Karanian, & Paul, 1988). In addition, molecular changes in the receptor subunit composition may occur that are relevant to physical dependence on ethanol (Mhatre & Ticku, 1992; Morrow, Devaud, Bucci, & Smith, 1994). One change may be responsible for the increased binding of benzodiazepine inverse agonists, drugs with proconvulsant and anxiogenic properties, to the $GABA_A$ receptor and the enhanced ability of GABA to promote chloride ion influx after chronic ethanol exposure (Buck & Harris, 1990; Mhatre & Ticku, 1989). The concentration of the $GABA_A$ receptor subunit mRNA that encodes the binding site for benzodiazepine inverse agonists is substantially elevated in the cerebellum after chronic ethanol exposure (Mhatre & Ticku, 1992). This effect, along with an apparent reduction in GABA release after withdrawal (Wixon & Hunt, 1980), may provide a partial molecular mechanism for the convulsions and anxiety that appear during an ethanol withdrawal syndrome. Such effects would reduce normal inhibitory control of electrical activity.

A hypoactive GABAergic system after withdrawal from chronic ethanol exposure provides a target for therapeutic intervention. In fact, benzodiazepine administration is the treatment of choice for an ethanol withdrawal syndrome (Sellers & Kalant, 1976). Benzodiazepines can control anxiety, restlessness, tremor, seizures, and delirium tremens observed during withdrawal. However, they can induce sedation, enhance the actions of any ethanol still present in the body, disturb sleep, and may maintain ethanol consumption (Hunt, 1985).

Since benzodiazepines are agonists of the $GABA_A$ receptor, another option might be benzodiazepine antagonists, which have no intrinsic activity of their own. One antagonist, flumazenil, has been tested in rats and in humans with mixed results. Overall, flumazenil reduced withdrawal scores in rats but increased the tendency for audiogenic seizures (Uzbay, Akarsu, & Kayaalp, 1995). In humans, 2 of 8 patients showed marked improvement, but the subjects reported a short-lived anxiogenic effect (Nutt *et al.*, 1993).

Glutamate

The major excitatory neurotransmitter in the brain is the amino acid glutamate. The glutamate receptor has several types that may be involved in different functions (Hollmann & Heinemann, 1994; Kalb, 1995). The types of glutamate receptors discussed here facilitate the movement of ions into the neuron. Three ionotropic types of glutamate receptors are called, based on the glutamate analogs used to characterize the types, kainic acid, α-amino-3-hydroxy-5-methyl-4-isoxazolepropionic acid (AMPA), and N-methyl-D-aspartate (NMDA) receptors. The kainic acid and AMPA receptors mediate fast, excitatory responses by moving sodium and potassium ions through the neuronal membrane, whereas NMDA receptors mediate slow excitatory responses by moving calcium ions in addition to sodium and potassium ions. NMDA receptors are activated when glutamate binds to it, and the membrane concurrently depolarizes to overcome NMDA receptor blockade by magnesium ions. Like GABA receptors, NMDA receptors have multiple subunits. The NMDA receptors are believed to be involved in learning and memory, seizure production, and neurotoxicity.

During the past 5 years, ethanol has been reported, using both electrophysiological and neurochemical techniques, to inhibit NMDA receptors and the movement of calcium ions mediated by these receptors (Dildy-Mayfield, Machu, & Leslie, 1991; Hoffman, Rabe, Moses, & Tabakoff, 1989; Lovinger, White, & Weight, 1989). As with the $GABA_A$ receptor, not all NMDA receptors are sensitive to ethanol. NMDA receptors are sensitive in the medial septum, inferior colliculus, hippocampus, cerebellum, and ventral tegmental area but not in the lateral septum or caudate nucleus (Simson, Criswell, & Breese, 1993; Yang, Criswell, Simson, Moy, & Breese, 1996). Furthermore, in those areas where ethanol is effective, not all NMDA neurons respond to ethanol. Ethanol sensitivity correlates with the ability of ifenprodil, an NMDA receptor antagonist, to inhibit NMDA receptors (Yang *et al.*, 1996). Thus, ethanol and ifenprodil may act on a common subtype of the NMDA receptor. Finally, the inhibition of NMDA receptors by ethanol mediates the attenuation of long-term potentiation in the hippocampus induced by ethanol (Morrisett & Swartzwelder, 1993). Because long-term potentiation may be one of the electrical events leading to learning and memory (Cotman *et al.*, 1989), ethanol-mediated disruption of NMDA receptor function may underlie memory disturbances induced by ethanol (Alkana & Malcolm, 1980).

After chronic exposure to ethanol, the number of binding sites for glutamate and NMDA (K. A. Grant, Valverius, Hudspith, & Tabakoff, 1990; Michaelis, Mulvaney, & Freed, 1978) and intracellular calcium concentrations increase, compared with controls (Iorio, Reinlib, Tabakoff, & Hoffman, 1992). Since the binding of all ligands to the NMDA receptor is not enhanced, chronic ethanol exposure may alter the subunit composition of the receptor (Snell, Tabakoff, & Hoffman, 1993; Trevisan *et al.*, 1994).

Because NMDA receptors play a role in seizure production (Dingledine, Hynes, & King, 1986), they may play a role in ethanol withdrawal-induced seizures. Electrophysiological studies indicate that NMDA-mediated synaptic excitation and after discharges in the hippocampus evoked by high-frequency stimuli and associated calcium spikes are augmented during ethanol withdrawal hyperexcitability (Morrisett, 1994; Whittington, Lambert, & Little, 1995). The NMDA and glutamate antagonists suppress withdrawal seizures (Freed & Michaelis, 1978; K. A. Grant *et al.*, 1990; Ripley & Little, 1995). In addition, injections of NMDA antagonists into the inferior colliculus or pontine reticular formation block auditory seizures (Riaz & Faingold, 1994).

Consequences of long-term ethanol consumption are cognitive deficits and brain damage (Hunt & Nixon, 1993). A mechanism underlying ethanol-induced brain damage involves the NMDA receptor (Crews and Chandler, 1993). Brain damage through NMDA receptors begins with excessive influx of calcium into neurons and is followed by a cascade of neurodegenerative processes leading to cell death. As discussed earlier, acute ethanol exposure inhibits NMDA receptors and associated calcium influx. This action also retards NMDA-mediated neurotoxicity (Chandler, Sumners, & Crews, 1993; Lustig, Chan, & Greenberg, 1992). However, after chronic ethanol exposure, the increased number of NMDA receptors and associated calcium influx accelerates the rate of neuronal death (Chandler, Newsom, Sumners, & Crews, 1993; Iorio, Tabakoff, & Hoffman, 1993). Moreover, intracellular calcium concentrations directly correlate with neuronal toxicity (Ahern, Lustig, & Greenberg, 1994). The ethanol withdrawal-induced neurotoxicity can be reduced with NMDA antagonists (Iorio *et al.,* 1993). Thus, NMDA antagonists may be useful not only in treating withdrawal-induced seizures but also in reducing withdrawal-associated neurotoxicity (Hoffman, Iorio, Snell, & Tabakoff, 1995).

Second Messengers

Many neurotransmitter receptors, including dopamine, norepinephrine, and adenosine, are coupled to second messenger systems that involve a series of reactions leading to changes in ion movements across the neuronal membrane. The one most extensively studied in ethanol research is adenosine-3′,5′-cyclic monophosphate (cAMP). cAMP is synthesized by the enzyme adenylate cyclase by converting adenosine triphosphate to cAMP, which in turn is degraded by phosphodiesterase to adenosine monophosphate. Regulatory proteins couple the receptor to this reaction and can be either stimulatory or inhibitory, depending on the ultimate physiological response. This response often involves phosphorylation of proteins that in turn leads to changes of ion movements

across the neuronal membrane. Alterations in the functioning of these regulatory proteins can modify the intensity of responses evoked by a given degree of receptor occupancy. Other intracellular proteins further contribute to the physiological response by altering the activity of ion channels or other functional proteins by phosphorylating them.

The major effect of ethanol on the cAMP system is stimulation of adenylate cyclase (Diamond & Gordon, 1994; Hoffman & Tabakoff, 1990). Stimulation of the enzyme by ethanol, whether its rodent brain tissue or neural cell cultures, occurs when activated by dopamine, norepinephrine, or adenosine (Bode & Molinoff, 1988; Gordon, Collier, & Diamond, 1986; Rabin & Molinoff, 1981). A mechanism of this response is a direct activation of a regulatory protein called a G-protein (Luthin & Tabakoff, 1984; Rabin & Molinoff, 1983; Saito, Lee, & Tabakoff, 1985). G-proteins couple the receptor to adenylate cyclase with energy supplied by guanosine triphosphate hydrolysis.

Using cultured neural cells, researchers have suggested other mechanisms underlying ethanol-induced stimulation of adenylate cyclase by adenosine. Ethanol inhibits the uptake of adenosine into cells by interacting with a nucleoside transporter (Nagy, Diamond, Casso, Franklin, & Gordon, 1990). This effect in turn elevates extracellular concentrations of adenosine and activates adenosine$_2$ (A$_2$) receptors, thereby increasing intracellular cAMP concentrations (Krauss, Ghirnikar, Diamond, & Gordon, 1993). Inhibition of the nucleoside transporter by ethanol depends on its phosphorylation state, regulated by cAMP-dependent protein kinase. Adenosine uptake is unaffected by ethanol in cells lacking cAMP-dependent protein kinase (Nagy, Diamond, & Gordon, 1991). Thus, unless the transporter is phosphorylated, ethanol does not inhibit adenosine uptake.

With chronic ethanol exposure, adaptive mechanisms reduce or eliminate the stimulatory effect of ethanol on neurotransmitter-activated adenylate cyclase. Since this effect is observed with several transmitters, it is called heterologous desensitization (Gordon *et al.,*

1986). Several mechanisms may be involved (Gordon *et al.*, 1986; Tabakoff *et al.*, 1995). A reduction in responsiveness or amount of G-proteins mediating stimulatory responses has been reported in studies using cell cultures (Mochly-Rosen *et al.*, 1988; Saito, Lee, Hoffman, & Tabakoff, 1987) but not with rat brain preparations (Tabakoff *et al.*, 1995; Wand, Diehl, Levine, Wolfgang, & Samy, 1993). Desensitization to adenosine involves tolerance to ethanol-induced inhibition of adenosine uptake. This tolerance results from excess stimulation of adenosine receptors, since adenosine deaminase, which degrades extracellular adenosine, and adenosine receptor antagonists block tolerance (Krauss *et al.*, 1993; Nagy *et al.*, 1989). Since the adenosine transporter must be phosphorylated to be inhibited by ethanol, desensitization may also be due to a reduction in cAMP-dependent protein kinase (Sapru, Diamond, & Gordon, 1994).

Neurotransmitter/Effector Interactions and Implications for Treatment

The transmission of information throughout the brain and long-term adaptive processes, such as learning and memory and drug addiction, involve a myriad of reactions that include stimulation of receptors by neurotransmitters and mediators, activation of second messengers and ion channels, phosphorylation of proteins, and gene expression (Nestler, 1995). Many of these processes can be influenced by the presence of ethanol. Not only does ethanol alter the release of key neurotransmitters and the functioning of the receptors on which they act, it also interferes with the processing of receptor-activated reactions that ultimately control the various activities of neurons, including ion movements and gene expression. Such complexity in the actions of ethanol provides a diversity of potential targets for therapeutic intervention.

General agonists and antagonists of neurotransmitters alter the actions of ethanol. Naltrexone is certainly a success story in how a generic antagonist of opioid receptors can have beneficial effects in treating alcoholism. Furthermore, the various subtypes of neurotransmitter receptors present an opportunity to develop medications with more precise outcomes and fewer side effects. For example, because the actions of ethanol on $GABA_A$ and NMDA receptors may depend on their subunit composition in areas of the brain important in the expression of ethanol-induced behaviors, new drugs with specific actions on a particular subunit assembly of the receptor could provide more effective treatment.

The second messenger system is sensitive to both acute and chronic ethanol exposure. Part of the response to chronic exposure includes adaptive responses that may contribute to the development of drug dependence. For example, for cocaine and heroin, blocking the activation of stimulatory G-proteins in the nucleus accumbens increases drug self-administration (Self, Terwilliger, Nestler, & Stein, 1994). Since chronic ethanol exposure also leads to a reduced amount of these G-proteins, at least in neuronal cell lines, such an effect could contribute to the development of ethanol dependence. Restoring the activity of G-proteins and kinases involved in protein phosphorylation could be another therapeutic strategy for treating alcoholism.

Finally, long-term changes associated with the development of ethanol dependence may involve changes in gene expression. Although chronic ethanol exposure can alter gene expression (Miles, Diaz, & DeGuzman, 1992), it is not known whether or how the induced genes contribute to ethanol-induced changes in neuronal function. Isolating these genes, understanding the function of the gene products and the mechanism of regulation of the expression of these genes could provide important clues to other potential therapeutic targets.

References

Ahern, K. B., Lustig, H. S., & Greenberg, D. A. (1994). Enhancement of NMDA toxicity and calcium responses by chronic exposure of cultured neurons to ethanol. *Neuroscience Letters, 165,* 211–214.

Alkana, R. L., & Malcolm, R. D. (1980). Comparison of the effects of acute alcohol intoxication on behavior in humans and other animals. In K. Eriksson, J. D. Sinclair, & K. Kiianmaa (Eds.), *Animal models in alcohol research* (pp. 193–269). London: Academic Press.

Allan, A. M., Spuhler, K. P., & Harris, R. A. (1988). Gamma aminobutyric acid–activated chloride channels: Relationships in ethanol sensitivity. *Journal of Pharmacology and Experimental Therapeutics, 244,* 866–870.

Bennett, R. H., Cherek, D. R., & Spiga, R. (1993). Acute and chronic alcohol tolerance in humans: Effects of dose and consecutive days of exposure. *Alcoholism: Clinical and Experimental Research, 17,* 740–745.

Berman, S. M., Whipple, S. C., Fitch, R. J., & Noble, E. P. (1993). P3 in young boys as a predictor of adolescent substance use. *Alcohol, 10,* 69–76.

Bode, D. C., & Molinoff, P. B. (1988). Effects of ethanol in vitro on the beta-adrenergic receptor-coupled adenylate cyclase system. *Journal of Pharmacology and Experimental Therapeutics, 246,* 1040–1047.

Buck, K. J., & Harris, R. A. (1990). Benzodiazepine agonist and inverse agonist actions on $GABA_A$ receptor-operated chloride channels. II. Chronic effects of ethanol. *Journal of Pharmacology and Experimental Therapeutics, 253,* 713–719.

Chandler, L. J., Newson, H., Sumners, C., & Crews, F. T. (1993). Chronic ethanol exposure potentiates NMDA excitotoxicity in cerebral cortical neurons. *Journal of Neurochemistry, 60,* 1578–1581.

Chandler, L. J., Sumners, C., & Crews, F. T. (1993). Ethanol inhibits NMDA receptor-mediated excitotoxicity in rat primary neuronal cultures. *Alcoholism: Clinical and Experimental Research, 17,* 54–60.

Chao, H. M. (1995). Alcohol and the mystique of flushing. *Alcoholism: Clinical and Experimental Research, 19,* 104–109.

Chin, J. H., & Goldstein, D. B. (1977a). Drug tolerance in biomembranes: A spin label study of the effects of ethanol. *Science, 196,* 684–685.

Chin, J. H., & Goldstein, D. B. (1977b). Effects of low concentrations of ethanol on the fluidity off spin-labeled erythrocyte and brain membranes. *Molecular Pharmacology, 13,* 435–441.

Cotman, C. W., Bridges, R. J., Taube, J. S., Clark, A. S., Geddes, J. W., & Monaghan, D. T. (1989). The role of the NMDA receptor in central nervous system plasticity and pathology. *Journal of NIH Research, 1,* 65–74.

Crews, F. T., & Chandler, L. J. (1993). Excitotoxicity and the neuropathology of ethanol. In W. A. Hunt & S. J. Nixon (Eds.), *Alcohol-induced brain damage* (pp. 355–371). Bethesda, MD: National Institutes of Health.

Criswell, H. E., Simson, P. E., Duncan, G. E., McCown, T. J., Herbert, J. S., Morrow, A. L., & Breese, G. R. (1993). Molecular basis for regionally specific action of ethanol on γ-aminobutyric acid$_A$ receptors: generalization to other ligand-gated ion channels. *Journal of Pharmacology and Experimental Therapeutics, 267,* 522–537.

Criswell, H. E., Simson, P. E., Knapp, D. J., Devaud, L. L., McCown, T. J., Duncan, G. E., Morrow, A. L., & Breese, G. R. (1995). Effect of Zolpidem on γ-aminobutyric acid (GABA)-induced inhibition predicts the interaction of ethanol with GABA on individual neurons in several rat brain regions. *Journal of Pharmacology and Experimental Therapeutics, 273,* 526–536.

Damgaard, S. E. (1982). The D(VK) isotope effect of the cytochrome P-450–mediated oxidation of ethanol and its biological applications. *European Journal of Biochemistry, 125,* 593–603.

Darden, J. H., & Hunt, W. A. (1977). Reduction of striatal dopamine release during an ethanol withdrawal syndrome. *Journal of Neurochemistry, 29,* 1143–1145.

Diamond, I., & Gordon, A. S. (1994). Role of adenosine in mediating cellular and molecular responses to ethanol. In B. Jansson, H. Jornvall, U. Rydberg, L. Terenius, & B. L. Vallee (Eds.), *Toward a molecular basis of alcohol use and abuse* (pp. 175–183). Boston: Birkhauser Verlag.

Dildy-Mayfield, J. E., Machu, T., & Leslie, S. W. (1991). Ethanol and voltage- or receptor-mediated increases in cytosolic Ca^{2+} in brain cells. *Alcohol, 9,* 63–69.

Dingledine, R., Hynes, M. A., & King, G. L. (1986). Involvement of N-methyl-D-aspartate receptors in epileptiform bursting in the rat hippocampal slice. *Journal of Physiology, 380,* 175–189.

Duncan, G. E., Breese, G. R., Criswell, H. E., McCown, T. J., Herbert, J. S., Devaud, L. L., & Morrow, A. L. (1995). Distribution of [^{3}H]zolpidem binding sites in relation to messenger RNA encoding the α1, β2, and γ2 subunits of $GABA_A$ receptors in rat brain. *Neuroscience, 64,* 1113–1128.

Fils-Aime, M. L., Eckardt, M. J., George, D. T., Brown, G. L., Mefford, I., & Linnoila, M. (1996). Early-onset alcoholics have lower cerebrospinal fluid 5-hydroxyindoleacetic acid levels than late-onset alcoholics. *Archives of General Psychiatry, 53,* 211–216.

Freed, W. J., & Michaelis, E. K. (1978). Glutamic acid and ethanol dependence. *Pharmacology, Biochemistry, and Behavior, 5,* 509–514.

Froehlich, J. C., & Li, T-K. (1993). Opioid peptides. In M. Galanter (Ed.), *Recent developments in alcoholism* (Vol. 11, pp. 187–205). New York: Plenum.

Froehlich, J. C., & Li, T-K. (1994). Opioid involvement in alcohol drinking. *Annuals of the New York Academy of Sciences, 739,* 156–167.

Gessa, G. L., Muntoni, F., Vargui, L., & Mereu, G. (1985). Low doses of ethanol activate dopaminergic neurons in the ventral tegmental area. *Brain Research, 348,* 201–203.

Gianoulakis, C. (1993). Endogenous opioids and excessive alcohol consumption. *Journal of Psychiatry and Neuroscience, 18,* 148–156.

Goldstein, A., & Judson, B. A. (1971). Alcohol dependence and opiate dependence: Lack of relationship in mice. *Science, 172,* 290–292.

Gordon, A. S., Collier, K., & Diamond, I. (1986). Ethanol regulation of adenosine receptor-dependent cAMP levels in a clonal neural cell line: An in vitro model of cellular tolerance to ethanol. *Proceedings of the National Academy of Sciences* (USA), *53,* 2105–2108. .

Grant, B. F., Harford, T. C., Dawson, D. A., Chou, P., Dufour, M., & Pickering, R. (1994). Prevalence of DSM-IV alcohol abuse and dependence: United States, 1992. *Alcohol Health & Research World, 18,* 243–248.

Grant, K. A., Valverius, P., Hudspith, M., & Tabakoff, B. (1990). Ethanol withdrawal seizures and the NMDA receptor complex. *European Journal of Pharmacology, 176,* 289–296.

Haraguchi, M., Samson, H. H., & Tolliver, G. A. (1990). Reduction in oral ethanol self-administration in the rat by the 5-HT uptake blocker fluoxetine. *Pharmacology, Biochemistry, and Behavior, 35,* 259–262.

Harris, R. A., & Schroeder, F. (1981). Ethanol and the physical properties of brain membranes: Fluorescence studies. *Molecular Pharmacology, 20,* 128–137.

Hasin, D., & Grant, B. (1994). 1994 draft DSM-IV criteria for alcohol use disorders: Comparison to DSM-III-R and implications. *Alcoholism: Clinical and Experimental Research, 18,* 1348–1353.

Hill, S. Y., Steinhauer, S., Lowers, L., & Locke, J. (1995). Eight-year longitudinal follow-up of P300 and clinical outcome in children from high-risk for alcoholism families. *Biological Psychiatry, 37,* 823–827.

Hoffman, P. L., & Tabakoff, B. (1990). Ethanol and guanine nucleotide binding proteins: A selective interaction. *FASEB Journal, 4,* 2612–2622.

Hoffman, P. L., Urwyler, S., & Tabakoff, B. (1982). Alterations in opiate receptor function after chronic ethanol exposure. *Journal of Pharmacology and Experimental Therapeutics, 222,* 182–189.

Hoffman, P. L., Rabe, C. S., Moses, F., & Tabakoff, B. (1989). N-methyl-D-aspartate receptors and ethanol: Inhibition of calcium flux and cyclic GMP production. *Journal of Neurochemistry, 52,* 1937–1940.

Hoffman, P. L., Iorio, K. R., Snell, L. D., & Tabakoff, B. (1995). Attenuation of glutamate-induced neurotoxicity in chronically ethanol-exposed cerebellar granule cells by NMDA receptor antagonists and ganglioside GM_1. *Alcoholism: Clinical and Experimental Research, 19,* 721–726.

Hollmann, M., & Heinemann, S. (1994). Cloned glutamate receptors. *Annual Review of Neuroscience, 17,* 31–108.

Hong, J. S., Majchrowicz, E., Hunt, W. A., & Gillin, J. C. (1981). Reduction in cerebral methionine-enkephalin content during the ethanol withdrawal syndrome. *Substance and Alcohol Actions/Misuse, 2,* 233–240.

Hunt, W. A. (1985). *Alcohol and biological membranes.* New York: Guilford.

Hunt, W. A. (1993). Neuroscience research: How has it contributed to our understanding of alcohol abuse and alcoholism?—A review. *Alcoholism: Clinical and Experimental Research, 17,* 1055–1065.

Hunt, W. A. (1994). Ethanol and other aliphatic alcohols. In C. R. Craig & R. E. Stitzel (Eds.), *Modern pharmacology* (4th ed., pp. 451–457). Boston: Little, Brown.

Hunt, W. A., & Nixon, S. J. (1993). *Alcohol-induced brain damage.* Bethesda, MD: National Institutes of Health.

Imperato, A., & DeChiara, G. (1986). Preferential stimulation of dopamine release in the nucleus accumbens of freely moving rats. *Journal of Pharmacology and Experimental Therapeutics, 239,* 219–228.

Inatomi, N., Kato, S., Ito, D., & Lieber, C. S. (1989). Role of peroxisomal fatty acid beta-oxidation in ethanol metabolism. *Biochemical and Biophysical Research Communications, 163,* 418–423.

Iorio, K. R., Reinlib, L., Tabakoff, B., & Hoffman, P. L. (1992). Chronic exposure of cerebellar granule cells to ethanol results in increased N-methyl-D-aspartate receptor function. *Molecular Pharmacology, 41,* 1142–1148.

Iorio, K. R., Tabakoff, B., & Hoffman, P. L. (1993). Glutamate-induced neurotoxicity is increased in cerebellar granule cells exposed chronically to ethanol. *European Journal of Pharmacology, 248,* 209–212.

Kalb, R. G. (1995). Current excitement about the glutamate receptor. *The Neuroscientist, 1,* 60–63.

Kiianmaa, K., Nurmi, M., Nykanen, I., & Sinclair, J. D. (1995). Effect of ethanol on extracellular dopamine in the nucleus accumbens of alcohol-preferring AA and alcohol-avoiding ANA rats. *Pharmacology, Biochemistry, and Behavior, 52,* 29–34.

Koob, G. F. (1992). Neural mechanisms of drug reinforcement. *Annals of the New York Academy of Sciences, 654,* 171–191.

Koob, G. F., & Weiss, F. (1990). Pharmacology of drug self-administration. *Alcohol, 7,* 193–197.

Kosterlitz, H. L., & Hughes, J. (1975). Some thoughts on the significance of enkephalin, the endogenous ligand. *Life Sciences, 17,* 91–96.

Krauss, S. W., Ghirnikar, R. B., Diamond, I., & Gordon, A. S. (1993). Inhibition of adenosine uptake by ethanol is specific for one class of nucleotide transporters. *Molecular Pharmacology, 44,* 1021–1026.

Li, T-K. (1991). What can we expect from models in alcohol research? Limitations and relevance to the human condition. In T. N. Palmer (Ed.), *Alcoholism: A molecular perspective* (pp. 323–332). New York: Plenum (NATO ASI Series).

Lieber, C. S. (1988). The microsomal ethanol oxidizing system: Its role in ethanol and xenobiotic metabolism. *Biochemical Society Transactions, 16,* 232–239.

Lovinger, D. M., White, G., & Weight, F. F. (1989). Ethanol inhibits NMDA-activated ion current in hippocampal neurons. *Science, 243,* 1721–1724.

Lucchi, L., Bosio, A., Spano, P. F., & Trabucchi, M. (1981). Action of ethanol and salsolinol on opiate receptor function. *Brain Research, 232,* 506–510.

Lüddens, H., & Korpi, E. R. (1996). GABA_A receptors: pharmacology, behavioral roles, and motor disorders. *Neuroscientist, 2,* 15–23.

Lustig, H. S., Chan, J., & Greenberg, D. A. (1992). Ethanol inhibits excitotoxicity in cerebral cortical cultures. *Neuroscience Letters, 135,* 259–261.

Luthin, G. R., & Tabakoff, B. (1984). Activation of adenylate cyclase by alcohols requires the nucleotide-binding protein. *Journal of Pharmacology and Experimental Therapeutics, 228,* 579–587.

Lyon, R. C., McComb, J. A., Schreurs, J., & Goldstein, D. H. (1981). A relationship between alcohol intoxication and the disordering of brain membranes by a series of short-chain alcohols. *Journal of Pharmacology and Experimental Therapeutics, 218,* 669–675.

Macdonald, R. L., & Olsen, R. W. (1994). GABA_A receptor channels. *Annual Review of Neuroscience, 17,* 569–602.

McBride, W. J., Murphy, J. M., Lumeng, L., & Li, T-K. (1990). Serotonin, dopamine and GABA involvement in alcohol drinking of selectively bred rats. *Alcohol, 7,* 199–205.

McBride, W. J., Murphy, J. M., Gatto, G. J., Levy, A. D., Yoshimoto, K., Lumeng, L., & Li, T-K. (1993). CNS mechanisms of alcohol self-administration. *Alcohol and Alcoholism, 2* (Suppl.), 463–467.

McCreery, M. J., & Hunt, W. A. (1978). Physico-chemical correlates of alcohol intoxication. *Neuropharmacology, 17,* 451–461.

McCusker, C. G., & Brown, K. (1990). Alcohol-predictive cues enhance tolerance to and precipitate "craving" for alcohol in social drinkers. *Journal of Studies on Alcohol, 51,* 494–499.

Melchior, C. L., & Tabakoff, B. (1981). Modification of environmentally cued tolerance to ethanol in mice. *Journal of Pharmacology and Experimental Therapeutics, 219,* 175–180.

Meyer, H. (1899). Welche Eigenschaft der Anasthetica bedingt ihre narkitische Wirkung? *Naunyn-Schmiedebergs Archiv für Experimentelle Pathologie und Pharmakologie, 42,* 109–118.

Mhatre, M., & Ticku, M. J. (1989). Chronic ethanol treatment selectively increases the binding of inverse agonists for benzodiazepine binding sites in cultured spinal cord neurons. *Journal of Pharmacology and Experimental Therapeutics, 251,* 164–168.

Mhatre, M., & Ticku, M. J. (1992). Chronic ethanol administration alters γ-aminobutyric acid_A receptor gene expression. *Molecular Pharmacology, 42,* 415–422.

Michaelis, E. K., Mulvaney, M. J., & Freed, W. J. (1978). Effects of acute and chronic ethanol intake on synaptosomal glutamate binding activity. *Biochemical Pharmacology, 27,* 1685–1691.

Miles, M. F., Diaz, J. E., & DeGuzman, V. (1992). Ethanol-responsive gene expression in neural cell cultures. *Biochimica et Biophysica Acta, 1138,* 268–274.

Mochly-Rosen, D., Chang, L., Cheever, L., Kim, M., Diamond, I., & Gordon, A. S. (1988). Chronic ethanol causes heterologous desensitization by reducing α_s mRNA. *Nature* (London), *333,* 848–850.

Morrisett, R. A. (1994). Potentiation of N-methyl-D-aspartate receptor-dependent afterdischarges in rat dentate gyrus following in vitro ethanol withdrawal. *Neuroscience Letters, 167,* 175–178.

Morrisett, R. A., & Swartzwelder, H. S. (1993). Attenuation of hippocampal long-term potentiation by ethanol: A patch-clamp analysis of glutamatergic and GABAergic mechanisms. *Journal of Neuroscience, 13,* 2254–2272.

Morrow, A. L., Suzdak, P. D., Karanian, J. W., & Paul, S. M. (1988). Chronic ethanol administration alters gamma aminobutyric acid, pentobarbital and ethanol-mediated ³⁶Cl⁻ uptake in cerebral cortical synaptoneurosomes. *Journal of Pharmacology and Experimental Therapeutics, 246,* 158–164.

Morrow, A. L., Devaud, L. L., Bucci, D., & Smith, F. D. (1994). GABA_A and NMDA receptor subunit mRNA expression in ethanol dependent rats. *Alcohol and Alcoholism, 2* (Suppl.), 91–97.

Murphy, J. M., McBride, W. J., Lumeng, L., & Li, T-K. (1987). Contents of monoamines in forebrain regions of alcohol-preferring (P) and -nonpreferring (NP) lines of rats. *Pharmacology, Biochemistry, and Behavior, 26,* 389–392.

Nagy, L. E., Diamond, I., Collier, K., Lopez, L., Ullman, B., & Gordon, A. S. (1989). Adenosine is required for ethanol-induced heterologous desensitization. *Molecular Pharmacology, 36,* 744–748.

Nagy, L. E., Diamond, I., Casso, D. J., Franklin, C., & Gordon, A. S. (1990). Ethanol increases extracellular adenosine by inhibiting adenosine uptake via the nucleotide transporter. *Journal of Biological Chemistry, 265,* 1946–1951.

Nagy, L. E., Diamond, I., & Gordon, A. S. (1991). cAMP-dependent protein kinase regulates inhibition of adenosine transport by ethanol. *Molecular Pharmacology, 40,* 812–817.

Nestler, E. J. (1995). Molecular basis of addictive states. *Neuroscientist, 1,* 212–220.

Newlin, D. B., & Thomson, J. B. (1990). Alcohol challenge with sons of alcoholics: A critical review and analysis. *Psychological Bulletin, 108,* 383–402.

Nutt, D., Glue, P., Wilson, S., Groves, S., Coupland, N., & Bailey, J. (1993). Flumazenil in alcohol withdrawal. *Alcohol and Alcoholism 2* (Suppl.), 337–341.

O'Brien, C. P. (1996). Drug addiction and drug abuse. In J. G. Hardman, L. E. Limbird, P. B. Molinoff, R. W. Ruddon, & A. G. Gilman (Eds.), *Goodman & Gilman's The pharmacological basis of therapeutics* (9th ed., pp. 557–577). New York: McGraw-Hill.

O'Malley, S. S., Jaffe, A. J., Chang, G., Schottenfeld, R. S., Meyer, R. E., & Rounsaville, B. (1992). Naltrexone and coping skills, therapy for alcohol dependence. A controlled study. *Archives of General Psychiatry, 49*, 881–887.

O'Malley, S. S., Jaffe, A. J., Chang, G., Rode, S., Schottenfeld, R. S., Meyer, R. E., & Rounsaville, B. (1996). Six-month follow-up of naltrexone and psychotherapy for alcohol dependence. *Archives of General Psychiatry, 53*, 217–224.

Overton, E. (1896). Über die osmotischen Eigenschaften der Zelle in ihrer Betdeutung für die Toxikologie und Pharmakologie. *Zeitschrift für physikalishe Chemie, 22*, 189–209.

Portas, C. M., Devoto, P., & Gessa, G. L. (1994). Effect of ethanol on extracellular 5-hydroxytryptamine output in rat frontal cortex. *European Journal of Pharmacology, 270*, 123–125.

Przewlocki, R., Hollt, V., Duka, T. H., Kleber, G., Gramsch, C. H., Haarmann, I., & Herz, A. (1979). Long-term morphine treatment decreases endorphin levels in rat brain and pituitary. *Brain Research, 174*, 357–361.

Rabin, R., & Molinoff, P. B. (1981). Activation of adenylate cyclase by ethanol in mouse striatal tissue. *Journal of Pharmacology and Experimental Therapeutics, 216*, 129–134.

Rabin, R., & Molinoff, P. B. (1983). Multiple sites of action of ethanol on adenylate cyclase. *Journal of Pharmacology and Experimental Therapeutics, 227*, 551–556.

Riaz, A., & Faingold, C. L. (1994). Seizures during ethanol withdrawal are blocked by focal microinjection of excitant amino acid antagonists into the inferior colliculus and pontine reticular formation. *Alcoholism: Clinical and Experimental Research, 18*, 1456–1462.

Ripley, T. L., & Little, H. J. (1995). Effects on ethanol withdrawal hyperexcitability of chronic treatment with a competitive N-methyl-D-aspartate receptor antagonist. *Journal of Pharmacology and Experimental Therapeutics, 272*, 112–118.

Rossetti, Z. L., Melis, F., Carboni, S., Diana, M., & Gessa, G. L. (1992). Alcohol withdrawal in rats is associated with a marked fall in extraneuronal dopamine. *Alcoholism: Clinical and Experimental Research, 16*, 529–532.

Saito, T., Lee, J. M., & Tabakoff, B. (1985). Ethanol's effects on cortical adenylate cyclase activity. *Journal of Neurochemistry, 44*, 1037–1044.

Saito, T., Lee, J. M., Hoffman, P. L., & Tabakoff, B. (1987). Effects of chronic ethanol treatment on the β-adrenergic receptor-coupled adenylate cyclase system of mouse cerebral cortex. *Journal of Neuroscience, 48*, 1817–1822.

Samson, H. H. (1986). Initiation of ethanol reinforcement using a sucrose-substitution procedure in food- and water-sated rats. *Alcoholism: Clinical and Experimental Research, 10*, 436–442.

Samson, H. H., Tolliver, G. A., & Schwartz-Stevens, K. (1990). Oral ethanol self-administration: A behavioral pharmacological approach to CNS control mechanisms. *Alcohol, 7*, 187–191.

Sapru, M. K., Diamond, I., & Gordon, A. S. (1994). Adenosine receptors mediate cellular adaptation to ethanol in NG108-15 cells. *Journal of Pharmacology and Experimental Therapeutics, 271*, 542–548.

Schuckit, M. A. (1985). Ethanol-induced changes in body sway in men at high alcoholism risk. *Archives of General Psychiatry, 42*, 375–379.

Schuckit, M. A. (1994). Low level response to alcohol as a predictor of future alcoholism. *American Journal of Psychiatry, 151*, 184–189.

Schuckit, M. A., & Gold, E. O. (1988). A simultaneous evaluation of multiple markers of ethanol/placebo challenges in sons of alcoholics and controls. *Archives of General Psychiatry, 45*, 211–216.

Schuckit, M. A., & Smith, T. L. (1996). An 8-year follow-up of 450 sons of alcoholic and control subjects. *Archives of General Psychiatry, 53*, 202–210.

Schulteis, G., Markou, A., Cole, M., & Koob, G. F. (1995). Decreased brain reward produced by ethanol withdrawal. *Proceedings of the National Academy of Sciences* (USA), *92*, 5880–5884.

Schulteis, G., Hyytiä, P., Heinrichs, S. C., & Koob, G. F. (1996). Effects of chronic ethanol exposure on oral self-administration of ethanol or saccharin by Wistar rat. *Alcoholism: Clinical and Experimental Research, 20*, 164–171.

Schulz, R., Wüster, M., Duka, T., & Herz, A. (1980). Acute and chronic ethanol treatment changes endorphin levels in brain and pituitary. *Psychopharmacology, 68*, 221–227.

Schwartz-Stevens, K. S., Files, F. J., & Samson, H. H. (1992). Effects of morphine and naloxone on ethanol- and sucrose-reinforced responding in nondeprived rats. *Alcoholism: Clinical and Experimental Research, 16*, 822–832.

Sdao-Jarvie, K., & Vogel-Sprott, M. D. (1991). Response expectancies affect acquisition and display of behavioral tolerance to alcohol. *Alcohol, 8*, 491–498.

Self, D. W., Terwilliger, R. Z., Nestler, E. J., & Stein, L. (1994). Inactivation of G_i and $G_{(o)}$ proteins in nucleus accumbens reduces both cocaine and heroin reinforcement. *Journal of Neuroscience, 14*, 6239–6247.

Sellers, E. M., & Kalant, H. (1976). Alcohol intoxication and withdrawal. *New England Journal of Medicine, 294*, 757–762.

Simson, P. E., Criswell, H. E., & Breese, G. R. (1993). Inhibition of NMDA-evoked electrophysiological activity by ethanol in selected brain regions: Evidence for ethanol-sensitive and ethanol-insensitive NMDA-evoked responses. *Brain Research, 607*, 9–16.

Snell, L. D., Tabakoff, B., & Hoffman, P. L. (1993). Radioligand binding to the N-methyl-D-aspartate receptor/ionophore complex: Alterations by ethanol in vitro and by chronic in vivo ethanol ingestion. *Brain Research, 602,* 91–98.

Suzdak, P. D., Schwartz, R. D., Skolnick, P., & Paul, S. M. (1986). Ethanol-stimulates gamma-aminobutyric acid receptor mediated chloride transport in rat brain synaptoneurosomes. *Proceedings of the National Academy of Sciences* (USA), *47,* 1942–1947.

Swift, R. M., Whelihan, W., Kuznetsov, O., Buongiorno, G., & Hsuing, H. (1994). Naltrexone-induced alterations in human ethanol intoxication. *American Journal of Psychiatry, 151,* 1463–1467.

Tabakoff, B., & Hoffman, P. L. (1983). Alcohol interactions with brain opiate receptors. *Life Sciences, 32,* 197–204.

Tabakoff, B., Cornell, N, & Hoffman, P. L. (1986). Alcohol tolerance. *Annals of Emergency Medicine, 15,* 1005–1012.

Tabakoff, B., Whelan, J. P., Ovchinikova, L., Nhamburo, P., Yoshimura, M., & Hoffman, P. L. (1995). Quantitative changes in G proteins do not mediate ethanol-induced downregulation of adenylyl cyclase in mouse cortical cortex. *Alcoholism: Experimental and Clinical Research, 19,* 187–194.

Trevisan, L., Fitzgerald, L. W., Brose, N., Gasic, G. P., Heinemann, S. F., Duman, R. S., & Nestler, E. J. (1994). Chronic ingestion of ethanol up-regulates NMDAR1 receptor subunit immunoreactivity in rat hippocampus. *Journal of Neurochemistry, 62,* 1635–1638.

Uzbay, T. T., Akarsu, E. S., & Kapaalp, S. O. (1995). Effects of flumazenil on ethanol withdrawal syndrome in rats. *Arzneimittelforschung, 45,* 120–124.

Victor, M., & Adams, R. D. (1953). The effect of alcohol on the nervous system. In H. H. Merritt & C. C. Hare (Eds.), *Metabolic and toxic diseases of the nervous system* (pp. 526–573). Baltimore: Williams & Wilkins.

Vogel-Sprott, M. D. (1992). Acute recovery and tolerance to low doses of alcohol: Differences in cognitive and motor skill performance. *Psychopharmacology, 61,* 287–291.

Vogel-Sprott, M. D., Rawana, E., & Webster, R. (1984). Mental rehearsal of a task under ethanol facilitates tolerance. *Pharmacology, Biochemistry, and Behavior, 21,* 329–331.

Volpicelli, J. R., Ulm, R. R., & Hopson, N. (1991). Alcohol drinking in rats during and following morphine injections. *Alcohol, 8,* 289–292.

Volpicelli, J. R., Alterman, A. I., Hayashida, M., & O'Brien, C. P. (1992). Naltrexone in the treatment of alcohol dependence. *Archives of General Psychiatry, 49,* 876–880.

Volpicelli, J. R., Watson, N. T., King, A. C., Sherman, C. E., & O'Brien, C. P. (1995). Effect of naltrexone on alcohol high in alcoholics. *American Journal of Psychiatry, 152,* 613–615.

Waller, M. B., McBride, W. J., Lumeng, L., & Li, T-K. (1983). Initial sensitivity and acute tolerance to ethanol in P and NP lines of rats. *Pharmacology, Biochemistry and Behavior, 19,* 683–686.

Wand, G. S., Diehl, A. M., Levine, M. A., Wolfgang, D., & Samy, S. (1993). Chronic ethanol treatment on the beta-adrenergic receptor-coupled adenylate cyclase activity in the central nervous system on two lines of ethanol-sensitive mice. *Journal of Biological Chemistry, 268,* 2595–2601.

Weiss, F., Lorang, M. T., Bloom, F. E., & Koob, G. F. (1993). Oral alcohol self-administration stimulates dopamine release in the rat nucleus accumbens: Genetic and motivational determinants. *Journal of Pharmacology and Experimental Therapeutics, 267,* 250–258.

Weiss, F., Parsons, L. H., Hyytiä, P., Schulteis, G., Lorang, M. T., Bloom, F. E., & Koob, G. F. (1996). Ethanol self-administration restores withdrawal-associated deficiencies in accumbal dopamine and 5-hydroxytryptamine release in dependent rats. *Journal of Neuroscience, 16,* 3474–3485.

Whittington, M. A., Lambert, J. D., & Little, H. J. (1995). Increased NMDA receptor and calcium channel activity underlying ethanol withdrawal hyperexcitability. *Alcohol and Alcoholism, 30,* 105–114.

Wixon, H. N., & Hunt, W. A. (1980). Effect of acute and chronic ethanol treatment on gamma-aminobutyric acid levels and on aminooxyacetic acid-induced GABA accumulation. *Substance and Alcohol Actions/Misuse, 1,* 481–491.

Yang, X., Criswell, H. E., Simson, P., Moy, S, & Breese, G. R. (1996). Evidence for a selective effect of ethanol on NMDA responses: Ethanol affects a subtype of the ifenprodil-sensitive NMDA receptor. *Journal of Pharmacology of Experimental Therapeutics, 178,* 114–124.

Yoshimoto, K., McBride, W. J., Lumeng, L., & Li, T-K. (1992). Ethanol enhances the release of dopamine and serotonin in the nucleus accumbens of HAD and LAD lines of rats. *Alcoholism: Clinical and Experimental Research, 16,* 781–785.

2

Behavioral Pharmacology of Alcohol

HERMAN H. SAMSON AND FORREST J. FILES

The actions of ethyl alcohol (ethanol) on behavior are diverse and depend on amount of ethanol administered, the time-course of administration, route of administration, and particularly blood ethanol level. Blood ethanol level is determined by the administration parameters, exposure history (both long term and recent), and environmental context. A wide spectrum of behavioral effects have been studied, particularly positive reinforcing actions maintaining self-administration and aversive effects observed in conditioned taste aversion. This chapter reviews the behavior pharmacology of ethanol.

Behavioral Effects of Ethanol

Operant Behavior

Operant behavior refers to behavior that is maintained, or suppressed, by its consequences. The consequence can either increase the probability that the behavior will occur again (reinforcement) or decrease the probability that the behavior will occur again (pun-

HERMAN H. SAMSON AND FORREST J. FILES • Department of Physiology and Pharmacology, Wake Forest University School of Medicine, Winston-Salem, North Carolina 27157.

Handbook of Substance Abuse: Neurobehavioral Pharmacology, edited by Tarter *et al.* Plenum Press, New York, 1998.

ishment). *Positive reinforcement* occurs when an appetitive stimulus is presented contingent on a response. A common example is when a rat presses a response lever and a food pellet is presented. *Negative reinforcement* occurs when an aversive stimulus is removed contingent on the response. An example would be when an electric shock is turned off when a rat presses a lever. Each of these consequences, the presentation of a food pellet and the termination of the shock, would be likely to increase the probability of the occurrence of the behavior that produced them.

Positive punishment occurs when an aversive stimulus is presented contingent on the response. An example would be when an electric shock is presented when a rat presses a lever. In operant punishment procedures, responding is typically maintained by food reinforcement. Electric shock is then superimposed and a suppression of the food maintained behavior occurs. *Negative punishment* occurs when an appetitive stimulus is removed following a response. These consequences decrease the probability of the behavior that produced them.

Each type of consequences can be scheduled in a variety of ways based on the number of responses made since the last presentation of the reinforcer or punisher (*fixed ratio* [FR] or *variable ratio* [VR] schedules), or on the amount of time that has elapsed since the presentation of the last reinforcer or punisher (*fixed interval*

[FI] or *variable interval* [VI] schedules). Note that interval schedules are response dependent. That is, the reinforcer (or punisher) is presented contingent on the first response that is emitted *after* the interval elapses.

Reinforcement or punishment can also be scheduled based on the rate of ongoing behavior. For example, a food pellet can be delivered following every response that is emitted at least 60 sec after the preceding response. This type of schedule is referred to as a *differential reinforcement of low rates* (DRL) schedule and produces very low rates of responding because pausing between responses is reinforced. High rates of responding can likewise be reinforced. This type of schedule is called a *differential reinforcement of high rates* (DRH) schedule.

Each of these schedule types results in highly stable and reproducible patterns of responding (Ferster & Skinner, 1957). This feature is critical since the study of drug effects is so heavily dependent on the use of sensitive and stable baselines. The effects of ethanol on responding maintained by positive reinforcement are generally to reduce rates of responding. Responding under FR schedules of reinforcement has been observed to increase at low doses and then decrease at higher doses in pigeons (Katz & Barrett, 1978) and decrease with increasing doses in rats (F. A. Holloway, King, Michaelis, Harland, & Bird, 1989). Under FI schedules, ethanol has been shown to produce dose-related decreases in responding in pigeons (Katz & Barrett, 1978). Ethanol has been observed to decrease high rates of responding in rats just before reinforcement, while the lower rates of responding observed during the initial portion of the interval were less affected (Crow & Hart, 1983). Under DRL schedules of reinforcement, low doses of ethanol have been shown to produce increases in responding while higher doses decreased responding (Bird & Holloway, 1989). This pattern produced a decrease in reinforced responses at the lower doses and an increase in reinforced responses at higher doses. Thus, ethanol disrupts behavior maintained by positive reinforcement under a variety of situations.

Ethanol typically reduces rates of responding maintained by negative reinforcement. This reduction can result in less efficient avoidance behavior leading to an increased frequency of presentation of the aversive stimulus. For example, Galizio, Hale, Liborio, and Miller (1993), and Galizio, Perone, and Spencer (1986) studied the effects of ethanol on two types of negatively reinforced behavior. In a two-lever experimental apparatus, responses on one lever postponed the delivery of a scheduled electric shock. Responding on the second lever produced a 2-min time-out period during which the shock avoidance schedule was suspended. Ethanol produced decreases in shock avoidance responding and an increase in time-out–reinforced responding at low doses followed by a decrease at high doses.

As with other anxiolytic drugs, ethanol generally increases behavior that has been suppressed by punishment. That is, ethanol has an antipunishment effect. For example, Koob and colleagues (1989) found, in rats, that ethanol produced a significant increase in responses that produced both a food pellet and an electric shock. Glowa and Barrett (1976) found that ethanol increased responding in squirrel monkeys on a FI 5-min schedule of food presentation that also produced an electric shock every 30th response (FR 30 punishment). They also found that ethanol produced decreases in responding on a FI 5-min schedule of food reinforcement alone. Others have found, however, that the antipunishment effects of ethanol are attenuated when response and reinforcement rates are equated under punished and nonpunished conditions (Pitts, Lewis, & Dworkin, 1993).

Another way that ethanol can be studied using operant procedures is the *drug discrimination* paradigm (see Barry, 1991; K. A. Grant, 1994; Winter, 1978 for general reviews and Stolerman, Samele, Kanien, Mariathasan, & Hague, 1995 for a recent bibliography). Drug discrimination refers to a condition in which animals are trained to respond differentially depending on whether the drug (in this case ethanol) has been administered. In the typical paradigm, experimental sessions are conducted in an operant chamber that contains two response levers (lever A and lever B). On alternate days, the animals are administered either the training dose of ethanol or the drug vehicle (typically water or saline). When ethanol is administered, only responding on lever A is reinforced. Likewise, when the vehicle is administered, only responding on lever B is reinforced. After many training sessions, animals typically respond with greater than 80% accuracy on the drug- or vehicle-associated lever. That is, the training dose of ethanol and the vehicle come to function as *discriminative stimuli* that set the occasion for responding on a particular lever. Once the discriminative performance is established, other doses of ethanol, or other drugs, can be substituted for the training dose or drug to determine the degree to which their effects are similar or dissimilar to those of the training dose or drug. For example, when animals trained to discriminate ethanol from water are given pentobarbital (Shelton & Balster, 1994) or diazepam (Lytle, Egilmez, Rocha, & Emmett-Oglesby, 1994) instead of ethanol, substantial drug-appropriate responding has been observed. Similarly, the discriminative stimulus functions of ethanol have been shown to be antagonized by d-amphetamine (Schecter, 1974) and by 5-HT$_3$ antagonists (K. A. Grant & Barrett, 1991). Drugs found not to substitute for the ethanol discriminative stimulus have included muscimol and baclofen (Shelton & Balster, 1994).

Respondent Behavior

Respondent behavior refers to the relationship between an *unconditioned response* (UR) and the *unconditioned stimulus* (US) that elicits it (i.e., a reflex). A common example is the knee jerk following a tap to the patellar tendon. Respondent conditioning usually results when a stimulus that is initially neutral in effect is paired in time with the presentation of the unconditioned stimulus. Following a number of pairings, the previously neutral stimulus can elicit a response in the absence of the unconditioned stimulus. Once conditioning has taken place, the previously neutral stimulus is re-

ferred to as a *conditioned stimulus* (CS) and the behavior that it elicits is called a *conditioned response* (CR). The conditioned response can take the same form as the unconditioned response, or it can be quite different from the unconditioned response. This type of behavior has been used for many years to study the behavioral effects of drugs, including ethanol.

Conditioned taste aversion occurs when a flavor is paired with an aversive bodily state. For example, if the taste of a sweet solution (the CS) is paired with the injection of something that will make the animal sick (the US), the animal will avoid the sweet solution when given a choice between it and another fluid. Ethanol has been shown to act as both a US (Berman & Cannon, 1974) and as a CS (Nachman, Larue, & LeMagnen, 1971) in this paradigm.

Another application of respondent conditioning is the place conditioning paradigm (see Swerdlow, Gilbert, & Koob, 1989 for a general review). In this procedure, the injection of a drug (the US) is paired with a certain novel environment (the CS, for example, a chamber painted black). On alternate days, injections of the drug vehicle are paired with a second novel environment (a chamber painted white). After several pairings of each, the animal is given a choice between the two environments. Conditioned place preference is said to have occurred if the animal enters and stays in the environment that was paired with the drug injection. If the animal enters and stays in the environment paired with vehicle injections, a conditioned place aversion is said to have developed. This technique has been used to assess the appetitive or aversive properties of ethanol, which can produce both place preferences (Cunningham & Prather, 1992; Stewart & Grupp, 1981) and place aversions (Cunningham, 1979, 1980).

Self-Administration of Ethanol

A variety of procedures have been used to investigate ethanol self-administration in a variety of animal species. While the majority of studies have employed either rats or mice, studies using nonhuman primates have provided valuable comparative data (Meisch &

Stewart, 1994). In some studies, ethanol is available for only a limited time period each day (the limited access paradigm). In others, ethanol is available continuously during the day (the continuous access paradigm).

Most ethanol self-administration studies have used the oral route. However, both intragastric (IG) (Altschuler, Weaver, & Phillips, 1975) and intravenous (IV) (Winger & Woods, 1973) self-administration routes have been utilized and provide for important comparisons with data obtained using the oral route. The IG and IV route obviously bypass any contributions the taste of the ethanol beverage might have on consumption, a factor known to influence oral self-administration (Files, Samson, & Brice, 1995; Samson, Files, & Brice, 1996).

Many studies of self-administration have focused on determining the amounts and patterns of ethanol consumption in various conditions while others have examined primarily the ability of ethanol to function as a reinforcing stimulus. In the first case, procedures such as home-cage two-bottle choice procedures are perhaps the most common (Li & Lumeng, 1984). In studies of the reinforcing functions of ethanol, operant paradigms have been extensively employed (Samson, 1987; Samson, Pfeffer, & Tolliver, 1988). Since operant procedures require the animal to make some response (at least in most cases) in addition to licking a drinking spout, measures of response rate and number, along with the effects of schedules of reinforcement, provide for a detailed examination of the ability of ethanol to maintain self-administration. With the use of drinkometer circuits, however, licking patterns have been used to quantify oral self-administration patterns (Dole, Ho, & Gentry, 1983; Gill & Amit, 1987). Without the additional response requirement present in the operant paradigm, the assumed ability of oral ethanol to function as a reinforcer as measured in the two-bottle type procedure remains problematic (George, 1988a, 1988b).

Home-Cage Procedures

In two-bottle home-cage procedures it is possible to generate home-cage 24-hr intakes which suggest that ethanol's reinforcing properties are controlling drinking. However, after most home-cage procedures, if a second, new response is required to obtain access to ethanol, animals often fail to learn the new response. Since learning a new response is one criterion for determining the ability of a stimulus to function as a reinforcer, it appears that ethanol consumption from a drinking tube may not be sufficient to result in ethanol being able to function as a reinforcing stimulus. Thus, various ethanol initiation procedures appear to be required to effectively demonstrate that ethanol can function as a reinforcing stimulus.

The acclimation procedure (Linseman, 1987; Sinclair & Senter, 1967; Veale, 1973; Wayner et al., 1972) involves slowly increasing over days the ethanol concentration presented to the animal. In some cases, the presentation of ethanol is made during limited daily access periods, with water available at other times. In other procedures, it is the only fluid available continuously. In all of the procedures, intakes of ethanol at concentrations of 10% ethanol or greater can be achieved. In 24-hr access situations in rats, intakes as high as 4–5 g/kg have been noted following acclimation, while in limited-access conditions, intakes between 0.5 and 1.0 g/kg in 1–3 hr have been observed. Depending on the protocol used, choice of ethanol over water has been demonstrated in a two-bottle choice situation following acclimation. Little success in training ethanol-reinforced operant responding following these acclimation procedures, however, has been reported.

Another procedure used to study home-cage ethanol consumption is the use of solutions that have a tastant added. The most common substance used to adulterate ethanol has been some type of sweet-tasting substance (e.g., sucrose or saccharin) (Gilbert, 1974). Beer and wine have also been employed (Lancaster, Spiegal, & Zaman, 1987; Samson, Denning, & Chappelle, 1996). Substantial increases in home-cage ethanol consumption are observed in these procedures (as high as 8 g/kg/day). However, when the sweetener is removed, intakes have been found to decrease dramatically, even when the sweetener is slowly reduced over days. In addition, if the animal is given a choice between the sweetened solution alone and the sweetened ethanol solution, in most cases, the sweetened solution alone is chosen.

A concern with two-bottle choice procedures is the use of the ethanol "preference" measure as a method to determine the reinforcing capability of the ethanol solution. The preference ratio (ethanol intake expressed as a percentage of total fluid intake), has been used by some to indicate the reinforcing capacity of ethanol. Unfortunately, this measure has not been related systematically to operant behavior maintained by ethanol reinforcement (George, 1988a, 1988b; Ritz, George, & Meisch, 1989; Tolliver, Sadeghi, & Samson, 1988). Thus, caution must be taken when using this preference ratio as a measure of ethanol's reinforcing efficacy.

Schedule Induction

The use of schedule-induced polydipsia (Falk, 1961) has been used to induce substantial ethanol self-administration (Falk & Tang, 1988). In this procedure, small amounts of food are presented periodically (on a FI or VI schedule) to a food-deprived animal. Following each food presentation, the animal will, over sessions, begin to consume excessively whatever fluid is available. When ethanol is the only fluid available, intakes approaching the daily limits of ethanol metabolism have been reported (Falk, Samson, & Winger, 1972). The use of these procedures has been employed to initiate ethanol self-administration in limited-access operant situations (Meisch, 1976). When the food restriction required to maintain schedule induction is removed, however, the amount of ethanol self-administered in these paradigms is substantially decreased (Meisch & Thompson, 1973).

Sucrose Substitution/ Secondary Conditioning

In attempts to develop additional animal models of operant ethanol self-administration, a combination of the use of sweet fluids and operant techniques has been employed (for a review, see Samson, Pfeffer, & Tolliver, 1988). By utilizing the reinforcing capability of sweet fluids with animals that are neither food nor water restricted, these models have demonstrated that ethanol self-administration can be initiated and ethanol can function as an effective reinforcing stimulus. In the sucrose substitution procedure, responding is first reinforced by the presentation of a sucrose solution. Then over sessions, ethanol is added at increasing concentrations while the concentration of sucrose is decreased. After 20–30 sessions, responding is maintained with 10% or higher ethanol concentrations, with no sucrose added to the solution (Samson, 1986, 1987).

In the secondary conditioning model of initiation, licking a tube containing ethanol is reinforced by the presentation of a sucrose solution (Grant & Samson, 1985). After a series of sessions in which the animals drink 10% ethanol maintained by sucrose reinforcement, the drinking tube is removed from the chamber and a lever inserted. Lever pressing can then be trained using 10% ethanol reinforcement.

Using these techniques, researchers have explored a variety of variables related to the control of ethanol self-administration (for reviews see Samson, Pfeffer, & Tolliver, 1988; Samson, Schwarz-Stevens, Tolliver, Andrews, & Files, 1992). The techniques have also been employed to determine the effects of initiation on continuous access ethanol consumption (Samson, Tolliver, Pfeffer, Sadeghi, & Haraguchi, 1988; Tolliver & Samson, 1989). In both limited and continuous access conditions, variables known to affect the delivery of many reinforcers, including the magnitude of the reinforcer and the schedule of reinforcement, have been shown to influence ethanol self-administration.

In a series of recent studies, the role of an added sweetener in the ethanol solution has been investigated (Files *et al.*, 1995; Heyman & Oldfather, 1992; Samson, Files, & Brice, 1996). From these studies it appears clear that an ethanol-sucrose mixture has a different reinforcing efficacy than either the sucrose or ethanol solutions alone. Since humans tend to drink flavored ethanol beverages, these studies, and those described earlier employing beer, suggest that animal models using flavored ethanol beverages may be appropriate in examining the variables that control ethanol self-administration. Clearly, the taste of the beverage consumed plays an important role in the amount consumed.

Tolerance and Dependence

Major effort has been directed to examining tolerance to ethanol (see Wolgin, 1989). Studies on tolerance have concentrated on the use of unconditioned responses to ethanol (e.g., hyperthermia, sleep time, motor responses) (Kalant, LaBlanc, & Gibbins, 1971; Samson & Falk, 1974; Wenger, Tiffany, Bombardier, Nicholls, & Woods, 1981) and the response-reducing effects of ethanol on operant behavior. Most studies have demonstrated that major components of the observed tolerance following repeated exposure to ethanol are related to the existing environment present during exposure, the learning of a new response while in the intoxicated state, the loss of reinforcement due to ethanol's response-reducing effects, or a combination of these factors. Thus, animals that may show tolerance to the hypothermic effect of ethanol in one experimental setting will fail to show tolerance in a novel setting (Mansfield & Cunningham, 1980). Also, animals that receive ethanol after the daily experimental session fail to demonstrate tolerance while those animals that receive ethanol prior to the daily session show tolerance (Chen, 1968; F. A. Holloway, Bird, Holloway, & Michaelis, 1988). These studies indicate that exposure to ethanol alone is not sufficient to produce tolerance and the occurrence of a counterconditioned response can play an important role in the expression of tolerance. The importance of environmental and behavioral factors in the development of tolerance must be considered, therefore, when interpreting the effects of multiple exposures to ethanol.

Cunningham and colleagues have examined the role of tolerance to the hypothermic effects

of ethanol on several behaviors. They have shown that while tolerance to the hypothermic effects of ethanol can enhance ethanol self-administration, this occurs only in situations in which a CS has been paired with the ethanol effect during the development of tolerance (Cunningham, 1994; Cunningham & Niehus, 1989). In addition, context-specific tolerance can be shown to influence ethanol's disruption of operant behavior (Cunningham, Losli, & Risinger, 1992).

Several researchers have suggested that withdrawal symptoms associated with dependence on ethanol could result in increased ethanol self-administration. Until recently, however, data to support this hypothesis has been scant. Most early studies failed to show increased ethanol consumption during withdrawal. However, recent data suggest that withdrawal effects may affect subsequent ethanol consumption.

Acute withdrawal effects (i.e., hangover) have been studied by Gauvin, Holloway, and colleagues (Gauvin, Goulden, & Holloway, 1993; Gauvin, Youngbood, & Holloway, 1992; F. Holloway, Michaelis, Hartland, Criado, & Gauvin, 1992). They found that the effects of a large acute dose of ethanol administered 24 hr previously can function as a discriminative stimulus and alter operant responding maintained by food reinforcement. While tolerance to disruptive effects was observed when ethanol was given prior to the daily operant session, less tolerance was observed and hangover effects continued when ethanol was administered after the daily operant session.

Using animals that had first been initiated to self-administer ethanol by the sweetened-solution substitution procedure, Koob and colleagues (Roberts & Koob, 1996; Schulteis, Hyytia, Heinrichs, & Koob, 1996) have recently demonstrated that during ethanol withdrawal following high involuntary chronic ethanol exposure (liquid diet and inhalation), ethanol self-administration increases. This is the first set of studies that provides evidence for withdrawal-enhanced ethanol reinforcement in an animal model.

Aggression/Stress/Social Interaction

The behavioral effects of ethanol on aggression, stress, and social interaction in both rodents and primates have been examined in various paradigms. The studies have led to conflicting results and have failed to provide convincing support for the popular hypothesis that ethanol consumption leads to increased aggression and that stress reduction is a factor in controlling ethanol consumption (for reviews see Pohorecky, 1990; Tornatzky & Miczek, 1995). More recent data indicate, however, that when individual differences are taken into consideration, increased aggressive behaviors are apparent in a subset of animals when low to moderate doses of ethanol are administered (Miczek, DeBold, & van Erp, 1994). These increases have been observed in animals that self-administer ethanol (van Erp & Miczek, 1995; van Erp, Samson, & Miczek, 1994), indicating that in social interactions in rodents, the amount and distribution of ethanol consumption contribute to aggressive behavior. A compendium of papers on this topic has been published by Hunt and Zakhari (1995).

In nonhuman primates, Higley and colleagues have examined social factors involved in ethanol consumption. Depending on social rank and gender, alcohol consumption impacts differentially on behavior (Higley, Hasert, Suomi, & Linnoila, 1991; Linnoila, Virkkunen, George, & Higley, 1993). These authors also note the similarity between their data in nonhuman primates and deficits in impulse control in humans (Linnoila *et al.*, 1993).

Final Considerations

The scientific examination of the behavioral effects of ethanol has a long and diverse history. While disparate results have been reported for many of ethanol's actions, a reasonable generalization that can be drawn from this literature is that ethanol has a disruptive effect on many types of behavior. On operant behavior maintained by positive and negative reinforcement, ethanol decreases rates of responding. These decreases result in loss of positive reinforcement or an increase of the presentation of aversive events in negative reinforcement studies. These data suggest, therefore, that ethanol produces effects that are disadvantageous to the animal in that behaviors essential for the animal's survival (i.e., the procurement of food or the avoidance of potentially harmful events) are disrupted. In punishment studies, it appears on the surface that ethanol produces a beneficial effect because it results in an increase in the presentation of positive reinforcement. However, ethanol is disruptive in this case to the extent that the usual behavioral process of suppression by the presentation of an aversive stimulus is altered. Such disruption can result in behavior that is potentially dangerous to an organism. This sort of "disinhibiting" effect in humans could lead to an increased likelihood of behavior that is normally suppressed, such as that which could lead to severe physical or social consequences. Social behavior and aggression are also altered by ethanol. Administration of ethanol can change the normal social interactions in animal groups and can, under certain circumstances, lead to aggression that might not occur normally. Thus, the administration of ethanol can have a negative effect on the normal functioning of animals in a variety of circumstances. These effects in many cases model those observed in humans.

A further generalization that can be made from the literature is that ethanol can and does function as a stimulus in ways similar to other stimuli. Studies of the stimulus properties of ethanol have helped to elucidate behavioral processes and pharmacological mechanisms responsible for ethanol's effects. Ethanol self-administration studies have demonstrated that ethanol can function as a positive reinforcer in animal models, allowing for the manipulation of variables that might be impossible to study with humans. Ethanol discrimination studies have provided data that have helped researchers investigate the interaction of ethanol and neurotransmitter systems. Finally, studies using respondent conditioning procedures have pointed to the importance of the environmental context in which ethanol exposure occurs. The present challenge to behavioral pharmacologists interested in the effects of ethanol is to explore these areas further in order to discover the functional relations controlling ethanol's various effects. With this knowledge, the development of better treatment and prevention programs for alcohol abuse and alcoholism will be possible.

ACKNOWLEDGMENTS

The preparation of this chapter was supported in part by grants AA00142 and AA06845 from the National Institute on Alcohol Abuse and Alcoholism to HSS.

References

Altschuler, H., Weaver, S., & Phillips, P. (1975). Intragastric self-administration of psychoactive drugs by Rhesus monkeys. *Life Science, 17*, 883–890.

Barry, H. (1991). Distinctive discriminative effects of ethanol. In R. A. Glennon, T. U. C. Jarbe, & J. Frankenheim (Eds.), *Drug discrimination: Application to drug abuse research* (NIDA Research Monograph No. 116, pp. 131–144). Washington, DC: U.S. Government Printing Office.

Berman, R. F., & Cannon, D. S. (1974). The effect of prior ethanol experience on ethanol-induced saccharin aversions. *Physiology and Behavior, 12*, 1041–1044.

Bird, D. C., & Holloway, F. A. (1989). Development and loss of tolerance to the effects of ethanol on DRL performance of rats. *Psychopharmacology, 97*, 45–50.

Chen, C. S. (1968) A study of the alcohol-tolerance effect and an introduction of a new behavioral technique. *Psychopharmacologia, 12*, 433–440.

Crow, L. T., & Hart, P. J. (1983). Alcohol and behavioral variability with fixed-interval reinforcement. *Bulletin of the Psychomonic Society, 21*, 483–484.

Cunningham, C. L. (1979). Flavor and location aversions produced by ethanol. *Behavioral and Neural Biology, 27*, 362–367.

Cunningham, C. L. (1980). Spatial aversion conditioning with ethanol. *Pharmacology, Biochemistry and Behavior, 14*, 263–264.

Cunningham, C. L. (1994). Modulation of ethanol reinforcement by conditioned hypothermia. *Psychopharmacology, 115*, 79–85.

Cunningham, C. L., & Niehus, D. (1989). Effects of ingestion-contingent hypothermia on ethanol self-administration. *Alcohol, 6*, 337–380.

Cunningham, C. L., & Prather, L. K. (1992). Conditioning trial duration affects ethanol-induced conditioned place preference in mice. *Animal Learning and Behavior, 20*, 187–194.

Cunningham, C. L., Losli, S., & Risinger, F. (1992). Context-drug pairings enhance tolerance to ethanol-induced

disruption of operant responding. *Psychopharmacology, 109*, 217–222.

Dole, V., Ho, A., & Gentry, R. (1983). An improved technique for monitoring the drinking behavior of mice. *Physiology and Behavior, 30*, 971–974.

Falk, J. (1961). Production of polydipsia in normal rats by an intermittent food schedule. *Science, 133*, 195–196.

Falk, J., & Tang, M. (1988). What schedule-induced polydipsia can tell us about alcoholism. *Alcoholism: Clinical and Experimental Research, 12*, 577–584.

Falk, J., Samson, H., & Winger, G. (1972). Behavioral maintenance of high concentrations of blood ethanol and physical dependence in the rat. *Science, 177*, 811–813.

Ferster, C. B., & Skinner, B. F. (1957). *Schedules of reinforcement.* Englewood Cliffs, NJ: Prentice-Hall.

Files, F. J., Samson, H., & Brice G. (1995). Sucrose, ethanol, and sucrose-ethanol reinforced responding under variable-interval schedules of reinforcement. *Alcoholism: Clinical and Experimental Research, 19*, 1271–1278.

Galizio, M., Perone, M., & Spencer, B. A. (1986). Variable interval schedules of timeout from avoidance: Effects of ethanol, naltrexone and CGS 8218. *Pharmacology, Biochemistry and Behavior, 25*, 439–448.

Galizio, M., Hale, K. L., Liborio, M. O., & Miller, M. (1993). Variable-ratio schedules of timeout from avoidance: Effects of anxiolytic drugs. *Behavioral Pharmacology, 4*, 487–493.

Gauvin, D., Youngblood, B., & Holloway, F. (1992). The discriminative stimulus properties of acute ethanol withdrawal (hangover) in rats. *Alcoholism: Clinical and Experimental Research, 16*, 336–341.

Gauvin, D., Goulden, K., & Holloway, F. (1993). State-dependent stimulus control: Cueing attributes of ethanol "hangover" in rats. *Alcoholism: Clinical and Experimental Research, 17*, 1210–1214.

George, F. (1988a). Genetic and environmental factors in ethanol self-administration. *Pharmacology, Biochemistry and Behavior, 27*, 379–384.

George, F. (1988b). Genetic tools in the study of drug self-administration. *Alcoholism: Clinical and Experimental Research, 12*, 586–590.

Gilbert, R. (1974). Effects of food deprivation and fluid sweetening on alcohol consumption by rats. *Quarterly Journal of Alcohol Studies, 35*, 42–47.

Gill, K., & Amit Z. (1987). Effects of serotonin uptake blockade on food, water and ethanol consumption in rats. *Alcoholism: Clinical and Experimental Research, 11*, 444–449.

Glowa, J. R., & Barrett, J. E. (1976). Effects of alcohol on punished and unpunished responding of squirrel monkeys. *Pharmacology, Biochemistry and Behavior, 4*, 169–173.

Grant, K., & Samson, H. (1985). Induction and maintenance of ethanol self-administration without food deprivation in the rat. *Psychopharmacology, 86*, 475–479.

Grant, K. A. (1994). Emerging neurochemical concepts in the actions of ethanol at ligand-gated ion channels. *Behavioral Pharmacology, 5,* 383–404.

Grant, K. A., & Barrett, J. E. (1991). Blockade of the discriminative stimulus effects of ethanol with 5-HT3 receptor antagonists. *Psychopharmacology, 104,* 451–456.

Heyman, G., & Oldfather, C. (1992). Inelastic preference for ethanol in rats: An analysis of ethanol's reinforcing effects. *Psychological Sciences, 3,* 122–130.

Higley, J., Hasert, M., Suomi, S., & Linnoila, M. (1991). Nonhuman primate model of alcohol abuse: Effects of early experience, personality, and stress on alcohol consumption. *Proceedings of the National Academy of Science of the USA, 88,* 7261–7265.

Holloway, F., Michaelis, R., Hartland, R., Criado, J., & Gauvin, D. (1992). Tolerance to ethanol's effects on operant performance in rats: Role of number and pattern of intoxicated practice opportunities. *Psychopharmacology, 109,* 112–120.

Holloway, F. A., Bird, D. C., Holloway, J. A., & Michaelis, R. C. (1988). Behavioral factors in development of tolerance to ethanol's effects. *Pharmacology, Biochemistry and Behavior, 29,* 105–113.

Holloway, F. A., King, D. A., Michaelis, R. C., Harland, R. D., & Bird, D. C. (1989). Tolerance to ethanol's disruptive effects on operant behavior in rats. *Psychopharmacology, 99,* 479–485.

Hunt, W., & Zakhari, S. (1995). *Stress, gender, and alcohol-seeking behavior* (NIAAA Research Monograph No. 29). Washington, DC: U.S. Government Printing Office.

Kalant, H., LeBlanc, A., & Gibbins, R. (1971). Tolerance to, and dependence on some non-opiate psychotropic drugs. *Pharmacological Reviews, 23,* 135–191.

Katz, J. L., & Barrett, J. E. (1978). Effects of ethanol on behavior under fixed-ratio, fixed interval, and multiple fixed-ratio fixed-interval schedules in the pigeon. *Archives Internationales de Pharmacodynamie et de Therapie, 234,* 88–96.

Koob, G. F., Mendelson, W. B., Schafer, J., Wall, T. L., Britton, K. T., & Bloom, F. E. (1989). Picrotoxinin receptor ligand blocks anti-punishment effects of alcohol. *Alcohol, 5,* 437–443.

Lancaster, F., Spiegal, K. S., & Zaman, M. (1987). Voluntary beer drinking in rats. *Alcohol and Drug Research, 7,* 393–403.

Li, T.-K., & Lumeng, L. (1984). Alcohol preference and voluntary alcohol intakes of inbred rat strains and the National Institutes of Health heterogeneous stock of rats. *Alcoholism: Clinical and Experimental Research, 8,* 485–486.

Linnoila, M., Virkkunen, M., George, T., & Higley, D. (1993). Impulse control disorders. *International Clinical Psychopharmacology, 8,* 53–56.

Linseman, M. (1987). Alcohol consumption in free-feeding rats: Procedural, genetic and pharmacokinetic factors. *Psychopharmacology, 92,* 254–261.

Lytle, D. A., Egilmez, Y., Rocha, B. A., & Emmett-Oglesby, M. W. (1994). Discrimination of ethanol and diazepam: Differential cross-tolerance. *Behavioral Pharmacology, 5,* 451–460.

Mansfield, J., & Cunningham, C. (1980). Conditioning and extinction of tolerance to the hypothermic effect of ethanol in rats. *Journal of Comparative and Physiological Psychology, 94,* 962–969.

Meisch, R. (1976). The function of schedule-induced polydipsia in establishing ethanol as a positive reinforcer. *Pharmacological Reviews, 27,* 465–473.

Meisch, R., & Stewart, R. (1994). Ethanol as a reinforcer: A review of laboratory studies with non-human primates. *Behavioral Pharmacology, 5,* 425–440.

Meisch, R., & Thompson, T. (1973). Ethanol as a reinforcer: Effects of fixed ratio size and food deprivation. *Psychopharmacologia, 28,* 171–183.

Miczek, K., DeBold, J., & van Erp, A. (1994). Neuropharmacological characteristics of individual differences in alcohol effects on aggression in rodents and primates. *Behavioral Pharmacology, 5,* 407–421.

Nachman, M., Larue, C., & LeMagnen, J. (1971). The role of olfactory and orosensory factors in the alcohol preference of inbred strains of mice. *Physiology and Behavior, 6,* 53–95.

Pitts, R. C., Lewis, M. J., & Dworkin, S. I. (1993). Effects of ethanol on punished and nonpunished responding under conditions of equated reinforcement rates and similar response rates. *Life Sciences, 52,* PL1–PL6.

Pohorecky, L. (1990). Interaction of ethanol and stress: Research with experimental animals—An update. *Alcohol and Alcoholism, 25,* 263–276.

Ritz, M., George, F., & Meisch, R. (1989). Ethanol self-administration in ALKO rats: I. Effects of selection and concentration. *Alcohol, 6,* 227–233.

Roberts, A., & Koob, G. (1996). *Intra-amygdala muscimol decreases operant self-administration in dependent rats.* Manuscript under review.

Samson, H. (1986). Initiation of ethanol reinforcement using a sucrose-substitution procedure in food- and fluid-sated rats. *Alcoholism: Clinical and Experimental Research, 10,* 436–442.

Samson, H. (1987). Initiation of ethanol-maintained behavior: A comparison of animal models and their implication to human drinking. In T. Thompson, P. Dews, & J. Barrett (Eds.), *Neurobehavioral pharmacology: Advances in behavioral pharmacology* (Vol. 6, pp. 221–248). Hillsdale, NJ: Erlbaum.

Samson, H., & Falk, J. (1974). Ethanol and discriminative motor control: Effects on normal and dependent animals. *Pharmacology, Biochemistry and Behavior, 2,* 791–801.

Samson, H., Pfeffer, A., & Tolliver G. (1988). Oral ethanol self-administration in rats: Models of alcohol-seeking behavior. *Alcoholism: Clinical and Experimental Research, 12,* 591–598.

Samson, H., Tolliver, G., Pfeffer, A., Sadeghi, K., & Haraguchi, M. (1988). Relation of ethanol self-administration to feeding and drinking in a non-restricted access situation in rats initiated to self-administer ethanol using the sucrose-fading technique. *Alcohol, 5*, 375–385.

Samson, H., Tolliver, G., & Schwarz-Stevens, K. (1991). Ethanol self-administration in a non-restricted access situation: Effect of ethanol initiation. *Alcohol, 8,* 43–53.

Samson, H., Schwarz-Stevens, K., Tolliver, G., Andrews, C., & Files, F. (1992). Ethanol drinking patterns in a continuous access operant situation: Effects of ethanol concentration and response requirement. *Alcohol, 9,* 409–414.

Samson, H., Denning, C., & Chappelle, A. (1996). The use of non-alcoholic beer as the vehicle for ethanol consumption in rats. *Alcohol, 13,* 365–368.

Samson, H., Files, F., & Brice G. (1996). Patterns of ethanol consumption in a continuous access situation: The effect of adding a sweetener to the ethanol solution. *Alcoholism: Clinical and Experimental Research, 20,* 101–109.

Schecter, M. D. (1974). Effects of propranolol, d-amphetamine and caffeine on ethanol as a discriminative cue. *European Journal of Pharmacology, 29,* 52–57.

Schulteis, G., Hyytia, P., Heinrichs, S., & Koob, G. (1996). Effects of chronic ethanol exposure on oral self-administration of ethanol or saccharin by Wistar rats. *Alcoholism: Clinical and Experimental Research, 20,* 164–171.

Shelton, K. L., & Balster, R. L. (1994). Ethanol drug discrimination in rats: Substitution with GABA agonists and NMDA antagonists. *Behavioral Pharmacology, 5,* 441–450.

Sinclair, J. D., & Senter, R. J. (1967). Increased preference for ethanol in rats following alcohol deprivation. *Phychonomic Science, 8,* 11–12.

Stewart, R. B., & Grupp, L. A. (1981). An investigation of the interaction between the reinforcing properties of food and ethanol using the place preference paradigm. *Progress in Neuropsychopharmacology, 5,* 609–613.

Stolerman, I. P., Samele, C., Kanien, J. B., Mariathasan, E. A., & Hague, D. S. (1995). A bibliography of drug discrimination research, 1992–1994. *Behavioral Pharmacology, 6,* 642–668.

Swerdlow, N. R., Gilbert, D., & Koob, G. F. (1989). Conditioned drug effects on spatial preference: Critical evaluation. In A. A. Boulton, G. B. Baker, & A. J. Greenshaw (Eds.), *Neuromethods: Volume 13. Psychopharmacology* (pp. 399–446). Clifton, NJ: Humana.

Tolliver, G., & Samson, H. (1989). Oral ethanol self-administration in a continuous access situation: Relation to food response requirements. *Alcohol, 6,* 381–387.

Tolliver, G., Sadeghi, K., & Samson, H. (1988). Ethanol preference following the sucrose-fading initiation procedure. *Alcohol, 5,* 9–13.

Tornatzky, W., & Miczek, K. (1995) Alcohol, anxiolytics and social stress in rats. *Psychopharmacology, 121,* 135–144.

van Erp, A., & Miczek, K. (1995). Alcohol self-administration and aggression in rats: Dopamine and serotonin in n. accumbens. *Society for Neuroscience Abstracts, 21,* 1702.

van Erp, A., Samson, H., & Miczek, K. (1994). Alcohol self-administration, dopamine and aggression in rats. *Society for Neuroscience Abstracts, 20,* 1614.

Veale, W. (1973). Ethanol selection in the rat following forced acclimation. *Pharmacology, Biochemistry and Behavior, 1,* 233–235.

Wayner, M., Greenberg, I., Tartaglione R., Nolley, D., Fraley, S., & Cott, A. (1972). A new factor affecting the consumption of ethyl alcohol and other sapid fluids. *Physiology and Behavior, 9,* 737–740.

Wenger, J., Tiffany, T., Bombardier, C., Nicholls, K., & Woods, S. (1981). Ethanol tolerance in the rat is learned. *Science, 213,* 575–577.

Winger, G., & Woods, J. H. (1973). The reinforcing property of ethanol in the Rhesus monkey: Initiation, maintenance and termination of intravenous ethanol-reinforced responding. *Annals of the New York Academy of Sciences, 215,* 162–175.

Winter, J. C. (1978). Drug-induced stimulus control. In D. E. Blackman & D. J. Sanger (Eds.), *Contemporary research in behavioral pharmacology* (pp. 209–237). New York: Plenum.

Wolgin, D. L. (1989). The role of instrumental learning in behavioral tolerance to drugs. In A. J. Goudie & M. W. Emmett-Oglesby (Eds.), *Psychoactive drugs: Tolerance and sensitization* (pp. 17–114). Clifton, NJ: Humana.

3

Psychological and Psychiatric Consequences of Alcohol

CHRISTOPHER S. MARTIN AND MARSHA E. BATES

Introduction

This chapter reviews the effects of chronic heavy alcohol consumption on psychiatric, neuropsychological, and psychological functioning. Most research reviewed herein was conducted with samples of "alcoholics," defined variously by participation in inpatient or outpatient treatment, the presence of alcohol problems, or a diagnosis of alcohol dependence. We use the broad phrase "chronic heavy drinkers" to capture the heterogeneous nature of the samples studied in this research area.

The definitions of psychiatric, neuropsychological, and psychological consequences are broad and overlapping. Psychiatric consequences include specific psychiatric disorders and psychiatric symptoms that are caused or exacerbated by chronic heavy drinking. These symptoms include psychological, social, interpersonal, and physical problems that affect a person's functioning in a clinically significant manner. Psychological consequences of chronic heavy drinking can be defined by the broad domains of affective, cognitive, motivational, and behavioral problems. Some psychological consequences serve as symptoms of alcohol abuse and dependence and other psychiatric disorders. Neuropsychological consequences are defined by direct and indirect effects of chronic heavy drinking on the brain that influence human behavior and functioning. The inclusion of neuropsychological consequences in this chapter highlights their functional connections to psychological and psychiatric consequences. Much of what we know about psychological and psychiatric consequences of excessive alcohol consumption (e.g., memory impairment, dementia) has come from the neuropsychology literature. Psychiatric, neuropsychological, and psychological consequences are best seen as complementary domains that describe a range of alcohol's effects on human functioning.

Psychiatric, neuropsychological, and psychological consequences are reviewed below in separate sections. The first section reviews psychiatric presentation during alcohol withdrawal, and the effects of chronic heavy drinking on anxiety disorders, mood and affective disorders, other psychiatric disorders, and suicide. The second section describes specific neuropsychological syndromes associated with chronic heavy drinking. Other neuropsychological impairment due to chronic heavy drinking is described, as are individual differences in vulnerability to these effects and recovery of

CHRISTOPHER S. MARTIN • University of Pittsburgh Medical Center, Pittsburgh, Pennsylvania 15213. MARSHA E. BATES • Center of Alcohol Studies, Rutgers University, Piscataway, New Jersey 08855.

Handbook of Substance Abuse: Neurobehavioral Pharmacology, edited by Tarter *et al.* Plenum Press, New York, 1998.

function with abstinence. The third section reviews the psychological topics of craving, increases in the motivational significance of alcohol consumption, and impaired control over drinking behavior.

The topics covered in this chapter are very broad, and a great deal of research has been conducted in each of them. Space limitations preclude a comprehensive review of the relevant literatures. Instead, areas of inquiry are briefly overviewed, with the goal of introducing the reader to the literature and the current state of knowledge in these areas. In each section, we provide references to more comprehensive reviews and volumes and to key papers in the primary literature.

Psychiatric Consequences

Clinical and epidemiological studies indicate that alcohol use disorders and many other psychiatric disorders are highly comorbid. However, the field is only beginning to understand the extent to which alcohol problems and heavy drinking are cause or consequent to specific types of psychiatric disturbance. There are numerous specific ways in which chronic heavy drinking and other psychiatric disturbance could influence each other. Tracy, Josiassen, and Bellack (1995) outlined a number of potential frameworks for understanding such etiologic relations. In the *shared vulnerability* framework, associations are determined by shared premorbid genetic or environmental risk factors or both. In the *early potentiation* framework, those who are vulnerable to a psychiatric disorder increase the likelihood of onset of this disorder via heavy substance use. In the *exacerbation* framework, substance use increases the severity of symptomatology among those already affected by a disorder. In the *sensitivity* framework, a psychiatric disorder produces increased sensitivity to cognitive or behavioral consequences of chronic heavy substance use. In the *interactive* framework, central nervous system (CNS) effects from substance use and psychiatric disturbance interact to produce a particular pattern of deficits not found in persons with either problem alone. In the *enhancement* framework, psychiatric problems may be attenuated (albeit temporarily) by substance use. That is, substance use is driven by the self-medication of psychiatric symptoms.

While chronic heavy alcohol use does not appear to be a direct etiological agent for most psychiatric disorders, it often plays a role in potentiating or exacerbating the clinical course of these disorders. Heavy drinking and psychiatric symptomatology often show reciprocal influences over time that can affect the course and treatment of both types of problem. This section focuses on psychiatric presentation during alcohol withdrawal, and the effects of chronic heavy drinking on anxiety disorders, suicide, affective disorders, and other psychiatric disorders.

Psychiatric Symptomatology during Alcohol Withdrawal

The clinical presentation of the alcohol withdrawal syndrome is well established. In the *DSM-IV* (American Psychiatric Association, 1994), the withdrawal syndrome is defined by two of the following eight symptoms: autonomic hyperactivity, increased hand tremor, insomnia, nausea, psychomotor agitation, anxiety, transient hallucinations, and grand mal seizures. Alcohol withdrawal occurs on a continuum of severity, and varies with the amount of consumption and duration of a drinking episode (Sellars & Kalant, 1976). Different symptoms tend to present in two distinct phases of the alcohol withdrawal syndrome. In the first phase, early symptoms are tremor, insomnia, anxiety, and motor and autonomic hyperexcitability (Kalant, 1977). Several of these symptoms are similar to those in anxiety syndromes, particularly generalized anxiety disorder and panic disorder. In some cases, seizures also appear in this first phase. These symptoms typically peak in intensity during the first 2 days following cessation of drinking.

In more severe cases, another phase of the withdrawal reaction occurs 2 to 3 days after the end of drinking. Delirium tremens, known as Alcohol Withdrawal Delirium in the *DSM-IV*, is characterized by disorientation, reduced awareness of surroundings, hallucinations, and cognitive deficits in memory or language. Alcohol Withdrawal Delirium may indicate the presence of co-factors that influence cognitive status, including liver dysfunction, malnutrition, or head trauma. In most cases, psychotic symptoms associated with delirium tremens (e.g., hallucinations) subside within several days after they appear (Castaneda & Cushman, 1989; Sellars & Kalant, 1976).

While acute withdrawal usually remits within a week of abstinence, anxiety, insomnia, and autonomic dysfunction sometimes persist for several months at lower levels of intensity (Satel, Kosten, Schuckit, & Fischman, 1993). This period has been described as "protracted withdrawal," and is accompanied by craving, mood disturbance, and a high risk of relapse (G. A. Marlatt, 1985). However, there is no accepted definition of protracted withdrawal, and little controlled research; it is not yet clear whether a specific syndrome exists (Satel *et al.*, 1993).

Anxiety and Anxiety Disorders

Acute and chronic alcohol consumption can increase levels of self-reported anxiety in some persons (e.g., Freed, 1978; Mendelson & Mello, 1979; Nathan, Titler, Lowenstein, Solomon, & Rossi, 1970). Prolonged bouts of heavy drinking appear to increase anxiety (Stockwell, Hodgson, & Rankin, 1982). It has been speculated that the legal, interpersonal, and occupational dysfunction caused by excessive drinking leads to increased levels of anxiety and stress (e.g., Vaillant, 1980). Following the initiation of abstinence, patients in alcohol treatment have shown improvements in anxiety self-reports and symptom ratings (Brown, Irwin, & Schuckit, 1991; Ludenia, Conham, Holzer, & Sands, 1984). These findings suggest that anxiety can be caused or exacerbated by chronic heavy drinking in some persons.

The associations between alcohol and anxiety disorders have been reviewed by Kushner, Sher, and Beitman (1990) and Clark and Sayette (1993). Alcohol disorders and anxiety disorders are associated in epidemiological studies at levels well beyond those expected by base rates. In the Epidemiological Catchment Area study (Robins & Reiger, 1991) men and women with alcohol abuse or dependence had increased rates of phobic disorders, obsessive-compulsive disorder, and particularly panic disorder. Rates of alcohol disorders are similarly elevated among individuals with agoraphobia and social phobia. In contrast, simple phobias and alcohol disorders do not co-occur above the level expected from their base rates.

The nature of the relation between alcohol disorders and anxiety disorders depends on the type of anxiety disorder (Kushner *et al.*, 1990). Available data suggest that agoraphobia and social phobia tend to precede alcohol problems in most persons (e.g., Chambless, Cherney, Caputo, & Rheinstein, 1987; Hesselbrock, Meyer, & Keene, 1985; Mullaney & Tripett, 1979). Further, in many cases it appears that alcohol problems develop in part from attempts at self-medication of symptoms (Bibb & Chambless, 1986). Kushner and colleagues conclude that agoraphobia and social phobia are not caused by chronic heavy drinking. Similarly, it appears that Post-Traumatic Stress Disorder is also not a consequence of chronic heavy drinking (Clark & Sayette, 1993). Rather, it appears that these anxiety disorders can initially cause an increase in alcohol consumption and related problems. Subsequently, however, heavy drinking and these anxiety disorders can show reciprocal negative influences (Bibb & Chambless, 1986).

Kushner and colleagues (1990) conclude that panic disorder and generalized anxiety disorder, in contrast to other anxiety disorders, often follow from chronic heavy alcohol consumption (Breier, Charney, & Heninger, 1986; Ross, Glasser, & Germanson, 1988). These effects may be specific to anxiety states produced during alcohol withdrawal (Stockwell *et al.*, 1982). Some symptoms of acute alcohol withdrawal mimic those of panic attacks and generalized anxiety disorder (Roelofs, 1985), and anxiety levels decrease in days or weeks following alcohol treatment. These findings may explain the high rates of these anxiety disorders reported in many alcohol treatment samples. The *DSM-IV* contains the category of "Alcohol-Induced Anxiety Disorder," defined by occurrence of anxiety only during intoxication or withdrawal, and remission upon abstinence. Chronic drinking also may increase the likelihood of developing panic and generalized anxiety disorder through other mechanisms; more research is needed to address this issue.

Affective Disorders

In both clinical and community samples, alcohol disorders are highly comorbid with depression (Regier *et al.,* 1990; Weissman, Meyers, & Harding, 1980) and with bipolar disorder (Helzer & Pryzbeck, 1988; Winokur *et al.,* 1995). There is evidence that in some cases, excessive drinking can cause or exacerbate affective disturbance. Acute and chronic alcohol consumption can produce labile euphoric and dysphoric mood (Freed, 1978). A high proportion of alcoholics presenting for treatment have depressive symptomatology, with many qualifying for a diagnosis of affective disorder (Schuckit, 1983, 1985). Depressive symptoms tend to remit over several weeks of abstinence in most alcoholics (e.g., Dakis, Gold, Pottash, & Sweeney, 1986; Nakamura, Overall, Hollister, & Radcliffe, 1983; Schuckit, 1983). Reflecting these findings, the *DSM-IV* contains a category of "Alcohol-Induced Mood Disorder," defined by occurrence of depression symptoms only during intoxication or withdrawal, and remission with continued abstinence.

Researchers have adopted a primary–secondary distinction, typically defined by order of onset, when examining those who meet criteria for both an alcohol disorder and an affective disorder (Schuckit, 1985; Winokur, 1990). The primary–secondary distinction has been heuristic in understanding differences in the course of affective symptoms among alcoholics. Brown and colleagues (1995) found that among dually diagnosed males, those with primary alcohol dependence showed greater improvements in depressive symptoms over time compared with those with a primary affective disorder. Three weeks of abstinence were needed to differentiate these groups. These findings suggest that disturbances in mood can be caused or exacerbated by chronic heavy drinking among individuals with primary alcoholism and secondary depression.

Winokur and colleagues (1995) used the primary–secondary classification to study the clinical course among inpatients presenting with both alcohol dependence and bipolar disorder. Those with primary alcohol dependence had fewer episodes of affective illness during a 5-year follow-up, compared with those with primary bipolar disorder. The authors concluded that individuals with primary alcohol dependence and secondary bipolar disorder may have a decreased vulnerability for bipolar illness, and that chronic heavy drinking is required for an affective disturbance to be manifest. Excessive alcohol use plays a role in a large proportion of hospitalizations for mania, even when an affective disturbance is the primary complaint or predates heavy drinking (Winokur, Clayton, & Reich, 1969). This may be a case of excessive drinking being caused by, and in turn exacerbating, psychopathology. The role of heavy drinking and drug use in the pathogenesis and presentation of manic episodes is an interesting area that awaits detailed empirical study.

Suicide and Suicidal Ideation

Evidence suggests that chronic heavy drinking increases the likelihood of suicidal ideation and suicide attempts. Among persons who attempt suicide, the presence of alcoholism confers a greatly increased risk for repeated future attempts (Hawton, Fogg, & McKeown, 1989). Major depression, followed by alcohol dependence, are the most common psychiatric disorders among persons who commit suicide (Henriksson *et al.,* 1993; Rudd, Dahm, & Rajab, 1993; Winokur & Black, 1987). Furthermore, there is disproportionate suicidal ideation among treatment samples with both alcoholism and an affective disorder, compared to either disorder alone (Cornelius *et al.,* 1995). Recent interpersonal loss distinguishes alcoholic suicides from suicides among those with affective disorder and no alcohol disorder (Murphy, 1992). In adolescents, mood disorders and substance abuse (including alcohol) have been found to independently and interactively predict increased suicidal ideation and suicide attempts (Levy & Deykin, 1989).

While the etiology of suicide is not well established, low levels of serotonergic functioning have been found in suicide victims (J. J. Mann, Stanley, McBride, & McEwen, 1986), and chronic heavy drinkers (e.g., Ballenger, Goodwin, Major, & Brown, 1979; Banki, Arato, Papp, & Kurca, 1984), and are associated with impulsivity (Moss, 1987). It appears that the majority of alcoholic suicides occur during or shortly after a drinking episode (Murphy, 1992), and acute intoxication is known to increase impulsive behaviors.

Other Psychiatric Disorders

There is little evidence to suggest that chronic heavy drinking or alcohol dependence is a direct etiologic agent for other types of psychiatric disorder. Alcohol use does not appear to be a direct causal factor for schizophrenic disorders. Some persons with a primary diagnosis of alcohol dependence show psychotic symptoms during withdrawal states, particularly hallucinations. These psychotic symptoms tend to remit soon after abstinence. Individuals with psychotic features during alcohol withdrawal have a future illness course that is similar to that of other alcoholics, and dissimilar from that of schizophrenics (Schuckit, 1982). Rates of alcohol problems are elevated among schizophrenics and may sometimes play a role in precipitating and exacerbating psychotic episodes among vulnerable individuals with a personal or family history of psychotic disorder (Milin, 1996). Persons with comorbid schizophrenia and substance use disorders tend to show increased morbidity, treatment noncompliance, and a more severe course of illness compared with schizophrenics without a substance use disorder (Milin, 1996; Tracy *et al.,* 1995).

Most other psychiatric disorders tend to antedate chronic heavy drinking, or are not associated with heavy drinking beyond levels expected from population base rates. While heavy drinking may be an important subtyping feature for bulimics, it does not typically antedate the onset of eating disorders. Anorectic populations have rates of substance abuse far lower than the general population (Holderness, Brooks-Gunn, & Warren, 1994). While highly comorbid with alcohol use disorders, Antisocial Personality Disorder (ASPD) is thought to involve etiologic factors that precede chronic heavy alcohol use. It has been postulated that ASPD and some forms of alcoholism share common genetic risk factors (Cloninger, 1987). Among those engaging in heavy drinking, a greater proportion of antisocial persons progress to the full alcohol dependence syndrome compared with other populations (Lewis, Rice, & Helzer, 1983).

The literature on the psychiatric consequences of heavy drinking suggests the importance of assessment and treatment of excessive alcohol use even in those whose sole diagnosis or primary complaint involves another form of psychopathology. Similarly, careful assessment of psychiatric symptomatology during alcohol treatment provides information that is directly relevant for treatment decisions. Differential psychiatric diagnoses and related decisions concerning psychiatric medication should be made after acute withdrawal subsides. The order of onset of multiple diagnoses, and their apparent role in exacerbating each other, should be carefully assessed.

Neuropsychological Consequences

This section overviews major neuropsychological disorders and nonspecific impairment resulting directly or indirectly from chronic heavy alcohol use. The pathological effects of alcohol use that are relevant to cognitive status and mental functioning have been described by a number of researchers (e.g., Ryan & Butters, 1986; Victor, 1992). A comprehensive review of alcohol-associated impairment can be found in Knight and Longmore (1994). This chapter reviews impairment mediated by nutritional disturbance, followed by impairment mediated by hepatic disturbance, often known as hepatic encephalopathy. Next, conditions of multiple or uncertain etiology are discussed. Finally, other effects of chronic heavy drinking on neuropsychological functioning are described, as is improvement of cognitive functioning following abstinence.

Impairment Mediated by Nutritional or Metabolic Disturbances

The prevalence of malnutrition in chronic heavy drinkers is difficult to estimate due to confounding factors (Marsano, 1994). Deficiencies in vitamins such as thiamine and minerals are common in alcoholics and may contribute to neuropsychological impairment (Lehman, Pilich, & Andrews, 1993).

Wernicke–Korsakoff Syndrome

Wernicke–Korsakoff syndrome is one of the most familiar neurological disorders associated with chronic, excessive alcohol use (Butters & Cermack, 1980). During the acute phase, Wernicke's encephalopathy is characterized by ataxia, disordered eye movements, and confusion (Walton, 1994). Most of those who survive this acute phase develop Korsakoff amnesic syndrome marked by a profound anterograde amnesia, that is, an inability to learn new information (Butters & Cermack, 1980). Despite both anterograde and retrograde memory deficits, crystallized verbal abilities often remain relatively intact (Ryan & Butters, 1986), as do implicit memory processes (Jernigan & Ostergaard, 1995).

There is a well-documented causative role of thiamine deficiency in precipitating Wernicke–Korsakoff syndrome. In alcoholics, thiamine deficiency can occur via a variety of mechanisms, including inadequate dietary intake, reduced gastrointestinal absorption, decreased hepatic storage, and impaired utilization (Charness, 1993). Acute thiamine deficiency produces damage to diencephalic structures in the brain. Neuroanatomical studies show characteristic symmetrical lesions in diencephalic structures, with damage to the medial dorsal nuclei of the thalamus thought to be most crucial to the characteristic memory disorder associated with this syndrome (Victor, 1992). Significant lesions in diencephalon structures, marked passivity and emotional blunting, confabulation, and profound memory

deficit are thought to be distinguishing features of the Korsakoff syndrome (Lezak, 1995). Onset may be sudden or slow (Bowden, 1990; Charness, 1993).

The extent to which thiamine and other nutritional and metabolic deficiencies explain all alcohol-related impairment in this disorder is still not clear. Bowden (1990) provided substantial evidence that Korsakoff alcoholics appear to be much more heterogeneous than previously suspected with respect to extent of neuropsychological and functional impairment. Alcohol-induced damage to structures other than the diencephalon also may be important factors in the expression of Wernicke–Korsakoff syndrome. There are graded decrements in visuoperceptive and problem-solving impairment from Korsakoff alcoholics to non-Korsakoff alcoholics to controls, suggesting a dual etiology of thiamine deficiency and direct neurotoxic effects of alcohol on the frontal lobes (Butters & Salmon, 1986; Jacobson, Acker, & Lishman, 1990).

Alcohol-Related Cerebellar Degeneration

Cerebellar damage occurs after an extended history of heavy drinking and impaired nutrition, with about half of the cases also showing liver disease (Victor, 1992). Abnormalities of stance and gait are often notable, but atrophy or shrinkage of the cerebellum may be present in the absence of these symptoms (Sullivan, Rosenbloom, Deshmukh, Desmond, & Pfefferbaum, 1995). Both rapid and slow progression over weeks or months may occur. Abstinence and correction of vitamin B deficiency may partially reverse symptoms (Lehman *et al.,* 1993). Victor (1992) suggests that the pathological cerebellar changes do not differ from those observed in Wernicke syndrome, and that these two syndromes may represent the same disease process.

Impairment Mediated by Hepatic Disturbance (Hepatic Encephalopathy)

The liver performs numerous metabolic functions vital to the integrity of the CNS. Liver disease, particularly hepatitis and cirrhosis, may cause cognitive impairment through disruptions of these functions. Hepatic en-cephalopathy is a general term for disorders in which the liver lacks the capacity to degrade neurotoxic substances in the circulation due to scarring (cirrhosis) and associated cholestasis. Hepatic encephalopathy is generally progres-sive without treatment, from a subclinical level of disturbance to hepatic coma (Butterworth, 1995).

In chronic heavy drinkers, alcoholic hepati-tis and alcoholic cirrhosis are thought to be characterized by two different inflammatory processes in the liver occurring in response to alcohol or its metabolites (Adams, 1994). He-patic encephalopathy, which sometimes devel-ops in alcoholics with liver disease (Charness, 1993), is characterized by cognitive deficits and motor dysfunction. Abstracting abilities, learning, memory, and visuospatial and psy-chomotor skills are often impaired, but verbal abilities may not be affected (Tarter, Arria, & Van Thiel, 1993). Brain atrophy (Harper & Kril, 1991) and cognitive impairment (Arria, Tarter, Kabene, et al., 1991) have been found to be greater in alcoholics with liver disease than in alcoholics without liver disease. Sever-ity of liver disease is correlated with neuropsy-chological performance in alcoholic patients at various stages of cirrhosis (Pomier, Nguyen, Faucher, Giguere, & Butterworth, 1991). Par-tial recovery of cognitive functions has been observed in alcoholics following liver trans-plantation (Arria, Tarter, Starzl, & Van Thiel, 1991). Alcohol and advanced liver disease have both been found to contribute to memory deficits observed in alcoholics (Arria, Tarter, Kabene, et al., 1991). However, the pattern of findings regarding memory functions is com-plex, and differences in abstracting abilities between cirrhotic and noncirrhotic alcoholics have not always been found (Tarter, Switala, Lu, & Van Thiel, 1995).

Neuropsychological Syndromes of Multiple or Uncertain Etiology

Marchiafava–Bignami Disease

This disorder is characterized by degenera-tion or demyelination of the corpus callosum.

It is a rare complication of alcoholism seen primarily in males ages 45–60. Due to varia-tion in clinical presentation, ranging from stu-por or coma to a slowly progressive dementia, it is difficult to diagnose antemortem. How-ever, neuroimaging techniques can now iden-tify lesions (Charness, 1993). It is uncertain whether this disorder is caused by a metabolic abnormality, malnutrition associated with chronic alcohol consumption, or the direct neurotoxic effects of alcohol (Charness, 1993; Victor, 1994).

Central Pontine Myelinosis

This rare disorder of cerebral white matter involves a characteristic lesion in the base of the pons. It is often caused by a too rapid med-ical correction of low levels of sodium circula-tion in alcoholics (Charness, 1993; Charness, Simon, & Greenburg, 1989). Symptoms may be absent, obscured by other conditions, or in-clude lethargy, confusion, and coma. Lesions in the striatum, thalamus, cerebellum, and cerebral white matter are sometimes present (Wright, Laureno, & Victor, 1979). More than half the cases have been reported in late-stage alcoholics, often in conjunction with Wer-nicke–Korsakoff syndrome (Victor, 1992).

Alcohol Dementia

Alcohol Dementia was first proposed as a taxonomic category in the *DSM-III-R* (Ameri-can Psychiatric Association, 1987), and is clas-sified as Alcohol-Induced Persisting Amnestic Disorder in the *DSM-IV.* However, it is not clear whether it represents a specific disorder. This putative dementia category involves widespread, generalized cognitive deficits typ-ically following many years of excessive alco-hol use, occurring most often in older persons. In addition to impaired abstract reasoning and visuospatial skills, patients show deficits in vi-suomotor coordination and verbal functions such as vocabulary and information. Memory impairments also are notable (Ryan & Butters, 1986).

Victor (1992, 1994) suggests that data have not clearly demonstrated that Alcohol Demen-tia results from a direct toxic effect of alcohol on the brain, and that this condition has not been differentiated from established dementias secondary to alcoholism or aging (e.g., Wernicke–Korsakoff syndrome, Alzheimer's disease), or from other pathologies primarily mediated through liver dysfunction, malnutrition, or metabolic disturbance. Postmortem studies found that a diagnosis of alcohol dementia was often given to patients who actually had Wernicke–Korsakoff syndrome (Harper, Giles, & Finlay-Jones, 1986). More research is needed on the degree of specificity in the etiology and presentation of the putative syndrome of Alcohol Dementia.

Other Alcohol-Related Neuropsychological Impairment

There has been sustained interest in determining whether there are specific neurotoxic effects of chronic alcohol ingestion apart from those mediated through hepatic, nutritional, or metabolic abnormalities, and whether specific brain areas are particularly susceptible to neurotoxic alcohol effects (Evert & Oscar-Berman, 1995; Nixon, 1993). Even in the absence of significant nutritional, metabolic, or hepatic impairment, chronic excessive alcohol use has been consistently associated with neuropsychological impairment. The proportion of alcoholics exhibiting some form of mild to moderate neuropsychological dysfunction is much larger than the proportion found to have any of the specific syndromes discussed above (Parsons, 1993). About 50% to 70% of alcoholics entering treatment have been found to show some form of clinically significant neuropsychological impairment (Martin, Adinoff, Weingartner, Mukherjee, & Eckardt, 1986). These rates appear to be representative of alcoholics in the general population (Loberg & Miller, 1986). Chronic heavy drinkers often show morphological brain abnormalities such as sulcal widening and ventricular enlargement, and functional abnormalities in brain blood flow and glucose utilization. However, it is difficult to determine whether alcohol's apparent neurotoxic effects are due to common coexisting conditions in chronic heavy drinkers, including polydrug use, head trauma, hepatic dysfunction, and malnutrition.

The most consistent evidence of behavioral impairment consequent to chronic heavy drinking has been found on tasks requiring fluid cognitive abilities: visuospatial and visuomotor skills, abstract reasoning, new learning, attention, and certain forms of memory (Bates, 1993; Knight & Longmore, 1994). Overlearned or crystallized verbal skills, such as vocabulary and general information, are less affected (Barron & Russell, 1992). Effects of chronic heavy drinking are more likely on controlled, analytic, and effortful information processing involving attentional resources (Smith & Oscar-Berman, 1992). Alcohol's chronic effects on controlled, effortful, and attention-demanding information processing operations may underlie performance decrements across a variety of demanding neuropsychological tasks (Goldman, 1995; Ingle & Weingartner, 1995; Tracy et al., 1995).

A number of recent reviews (e.g., Bowden, 1990; Nixon, 1993) have discussed theories of selective brain vulnerability in alcoholics. These theories include disruption of right hemisphere functions, damage to frontal-diencephalic regions, diffuse cortical damage, and premature aging of the brain. The evidence for each selective brain vulnerability hypothesis has been equivocal, highlighting the heterogeneity of observed deficits and the difficulty in adequately specifying and controlling the multitude of potentially confounding factors. At present, a diffuse model most adequately predicts the range of observed impairment in alcoholics, although the frontal-diencephalic systems seem particularly susceptible (Nixon, 1993; Oscar-Berman & Hutner, 1993). The most apparent weakness of the diffuse model is its inability to be disproved because it accommodates all varieties and patterns of deficits (Nixon, 1993). It is also possible that the tendency of researchers to report group averages has tended to obscure the identification of subtypes of alcoholics having more specific deficits.

Although alcohol-related brain damage is often diffusely distributed, interest in frontal lobe deficits has increased in recent years, due in part to renewed interest in the importance of "executive functions" responsible for behavioral control (Benton, 1994). The prefrontal cortex is functionally specialized for strategic planning, use of environmental feedback, working memory, goal selection, and response inhibition. Executive deficits present functionally as poor planning ability, response sequencing difficulties, impairment to working memory, inflexibility of thought processes, and difficulty orienting behavior toward future goals (Lezak, 1995). These functions are of special relevance to understanding the development of alcohol use behaviors and risk of relapse following treatment.

Gender

Neuropsychological research generally suggests that male and female alcoholics tend to exhibit similar patterns and severity of deficit (e.g., Glenn & Parsons, 1992; K. Mann, Batra, Gunthner, & Schroth, 1992; Nixon, Tivis, & Parsons, 1995), although among those females with deficits typically shorter and less severe drinking histories are reported than in males. Data also suggest that on average females develop liver disease with lower daily alcohol intake and shorter drinking histories than males (Lancaster, 1994). Thus, women may be at heightened risk for hepatically mediated cognitive dysfunction.

Recovery of Function

Neuropsychological impairments tend to be most severe for 1 to 4 weeks following cessation of drinking (Goldman, 1987). Different neurocognitive abilities show varying degrees and rates of spontaneous, time-dependent recovery (Goldman, 1987; Muuronen, Bergman, & Hindmarsh, 1989). Verbal deficits tend to recover within the first few weeks of abstinence; while memory and visuospatial abilities show partial recovery during the first month (Parsons & Leber, 1982). New learning, complex or novel problem solving, and speeded information processing tasks require the longest recovery time (Goldman, 1987, 1995). Neuroimaging studies have confirmed

that alcohol-related brain damage is often partially or fully reversible (Bates & Convit, in press).

Little is known about the mediators of individual differences in recovery, with the exception of age and drinking behavior. Younger alcoholics (Goldman, 1983; Parsons & Leber, 1982), and those who stop or greatly reduce drinking (Guthrie & Elliott, 1980; Muuronen et al., 1989) are more likely to experience faster and more complete improvements in cognitive functioning, although performance may still not reach normal levels. Decreases in depression and recovery of liver function (Schafer, Butters, & Smith, 1991) may moderate improvement in abstinent alcoholics.

Psychological Consequences

Many consequences of chronic heavy drinking that could be described as psychological have already been covered in this chapter's sections on psychiatric and neuropsychological consequences, highlighting the conceptual overlaps between these areas of research. This section of the chapter reviews psychological consequences of chronic heavy drinking not covered in the previous sections. These consequences are craving, increases in the salience of alcohol use, and impaired control over drinking behavior. Research on each of these topics has increased our knowledge of the psychological processes involved in addiction.

Almost all clinical descriptions and theoretical conceptualizations of alcohol dependence have invoked psychological features, rather than merely the physiological dependence processes of tolerance and withdrawal (e.g., Cloninger, 1987; Jellinek, 1955). Craving, increased salience of alcohol, and impaired control over drinking behavior are core features of the alcohol dependence syndrome described by Edwards and Gross (1976) and Edwards (1986). In this syndrome, psychological processes are viewed as essential component features of alcohol dependence. Like many other psychological constructs, the psychological aspects of alcohol dependence clearly have a physiological basis. Nevertheless, their description at a psychological level has been heuristic in understanding addictive behavior.

Craving

Craving has been defined and conceptualized in numerous ways (Kassel & Shiffman, 1992; Kozlowski & Wilkinson, 1987; Tiffany, 1990). Improved understanding of the craving construct is essential for clarifying its role in addiction (Pickens & Johanson, 1992). The primary nature of craving has been variously described as subjective, cognitive, affective, or motivational. Craving is often described as a state that reflects withdrawal from, or appetitive responses to, alcohol and drugs. In some theories, craving reflects conditioned responses to cues previously associated with drug administration. Several negative reinforcement theories of addiction view craving as an aversive state, the alleviation of which motivates drug use (e.g., Siegel, 1983; Solomon & Corbit, 1973). Alternatively, positive reinforcement models of drug use and addiction have viewed craving as an appetitive motivational process, in which anticipation of positively rewarding drug effects drives drug seeking and drug taking (e.g., Stewart, de Wit, & Eikelboom, 1984; Wise, 1988). Certainly these views are not mutually exclusive, but they emphasize that "craving" may be quite different depending on the operation of appetitive or withdrawal-relief mechanisms.

Numerous authors have described pathological levels of craving for alcohol as a central feature of addiction (Jellinek, 1955). But the relationship of craving to addiction, and its very utility as a construct, have been controversial (e.g., Kozlowski & Wilkinson, 1987). Investigation of craving has been hampered by the fact that researchers have used different definitions and measures. Further, many studies have used only one craving measure (typically self-report), so that the convergence of multiple measures under different conditions has received little attention. Nevertheless, self-reports of craving predict relapse (Brandon, Tiffany, & Baker, 1985; Killen, Fortmann, Kraemer, Varady, & Newman, 1992; Shiffman, Paty, Gnys, Kassel, & Elash, 1995; West,

Hajek, & Belcher, 1989). Recent efforts to reduce craving during treatment with cue exposure procedures have been promising (Drummond & Glautier, 1994; Monti et al., 1993).

A motivational model of craving was detailed by Baker, Morse, and Sherman (1987). Craving is defined by a set of motivational-affective states that produce subjective, cognitive, and behavioral changes that increase the propensity to consume a drug. The authors posit two distinct craving networks: the positive affect network, which is appetitive, and the negative affect network, which increases the withdrawal-relief incentive for drug use. Both the positive and negative craving networks become more articulated with increased drug use, and each involves cognitive, subjective, and behavioral craving responses. Environmental and personal factors, such as positive and negative mood, drug deprivation state, and drug availability, increase the relative likelihood of activation of one of the two networks (Zinser, Baker, Sherman, & Cannon, 1992).

Using a motivational framework, some research has begun to examine craving response systems (Rankin, Hodgson, & Stockwell, 1979), as has been done with fear (Lang, 1968). Using a cue exposure paradigm with alcoholics in treatment, Sayette and colleagues (1994) found that during exposure to alcohol cues, but not control cues, reaction times on a secondary task increased, and this effect was correlated with self-reported urge to drink. This result suggests that craving may involve the assignment of limited-capacity cognitive resources to alcohol cues. Findings of this sort suggest the utility of conceptualizing craving as a motivational construct that affects multiple response systems, as suggested by Baker and colleagues (1987) and others (e.g., Kassell & Shiffman, 1992).

Increased Salience (Motivational Significance) of Alcohol Consumption

Clinical descriptions of alcohol dependence have long included the psychological construct of increased salience of alcohol use. Salience refers to the motivational significance of alcohol use relative to other reinforcing activities and behaviors. Increased salience of drinking is one of the fundamental features of the alcohol dependence syndrome. Persons with alcohol dependence often neglect previously reinforcing activities in favor of drinking (Edwards & Gross, 1976). Symptoms related to increased salience of drinking are contained in the psychiatric nomenclatures of the *DSM-IV* and the *International Classification of Diseases,* 10th edition (*ICD-10*) (World Health Organization, 1993). In the *DSM-IV,* alcohol dependence symptoms related to "much time spent drinking" and "important social, occupational, or recreational activities given up or reduced because of drinking" are both conceptually related to increased salience.

One framework for understanding how the salience of alcohol consumption may increase is Robinson and Berridge's (1993) incentive sensitization theory of addiction. These authors review substantial evidence suggesting that increases in the salience of drug use (i.e., incentive sensitization) occur after chronic heavy use, and are central to the neurobiology and psychology of addiction. According to the incentive sensitization theory, addictive drugs such as alcohol enhance neurotransmission in mesencephalic dopaminergic brain systems. One psychological function of activation of this neural system is to attribute incentive salience to stimuli, imbuing them with appetitive motivational significance. Repeated drug use (including alcohol) causes long-term increases (sensitization) in the incentive salience accorded to drugs and associated cues. The sensitization of the system transforms ordinary drug wanting into pathological levels of drug craving in the addict. Robinson and Berridge (1993) further postulate that the neural systems that underlie incentive salience are independent of the neural systems that underlie drug pleasure. The salience accorded to a drug can sensitize even when a person develops tolerance to the pleasurable effects of that drug. That is, drug "wanting" or craving can increase even while drug "liking" decreases in the chronic heavy user. This may help explain why craving and compulsive use patterns can persist even when pleasurable drug effects are greatly diminished, and even in the face of extreme negative consequences.

The incentive sensitization theory may help explain several aspects of addiction to alcohol and drugs that are not well understood. First, it provides a view of craving that integrates psychological and neurobiological functioning. Second, it can explain the well-known phenomenon that drug cravings often persist after months or years of abstinence. Finally, it provides a framework for examining why compulsive drug use often persists in the face of devastating physical, psychological, occupational, legal, and social problems. Regardless of the ultimate status of Robinson and Berridge's (1993) model, the notion of increased incentive salience for alcohol with continued heavy drinking is powerful and may help explain many aspects of alcohol dependence, including craving and impaired control phenomena. The concept of increased incentive salience of alcohol use helps provide a motivational framework for conceptualizing addiction to alcohol.

Impaired Control over Drinking Behavior

Impaired control over drinking behavior, sometimes described as pathological or compulsive alcohol use, has long been considered a cardinal feature of alcohol dependence (Jellinek, 1952, 1960). Impaired control is an important aspect of the alcohol dependence syndrome; this syndrome has been described as "marked by impaired capacity to control alcohol intake" (Edwards, Gross, Keller, Moser, & Room, 1977). Several *DSM-IV* symptoms of alcohol dependence reflect undercontrolled drinking behavior: "drinking more or longer than intended," "repeated unsuccessful attempts to abstain or cut down on drinking," and "continued use despite knowledge of physical or psychological problems caused or exacerbated by drinking." Impaired control also may be reflected in the *DSM-IV* abuse symptom "continued use despite knowledge of social or interpersonal problems caused or exacerbated by alcohol use."

Some have described compulsive drinking behavior in terms of *loss* of control, but such terminology does not reflect the control shown by former problem drinkers who achieve abstinence or low levels of consumption (Miller, 1993). Control over drinking seems better described on a continuum (Ludwig & Wikler, 1974). The popular adage "one drink, then drunk" suggests that an initial dose of alcohol necessarily primes a binge reflecting loss of control in the alcoholic. However, data suggest that cognitive variables play a role in the self-regulation of intake, even in heavy users (Wilson, 1987). G. Marlatt, Demming, and Reid (1973) found that in both social drinkers and alcoholics, the belief that one has consumed a small amount of alcohol, rather than the actual drinking of this small amount, produced the greatest amount of ad lib drinking. Nevertheless, priming doses of alcohol do increase self-reported desire to drink and ad lib consumption among heavier drinkers, especially when the priming dose is large and when it is the person's preferred beverage (Stockwell, 1991). Greater amounts of alcohol consumption may cause fewer attentional resources to be devoted to the self-regulation of drinking behavior, leading to excessive intake (Steele & Josephs, 1990; Tiffany, 1990).

Behavior reflecting impaired control may reflect, in part, psychological processes of craving and increased incentive salience attributed to alcohol and alcohol cues. "Undercontrol" may actually reflect the output of motivational systems in which drinking has much more incentive salience than other reinforcers and consequences. Of course, such a motivational analysis of impaired control needs to consider the relative salience of drinking compared to other reinforcers available in a person's environment. Another approach to impaired control over drinking relates addictive behaviors to dyscontrol in general self-regulatory processes (Baumeister, Tice, & Heatherton, 1994; Heather, Miller, & Greeley, 1991). More research is needed to determine the psychological processes involved in impaired control over drinking.

Conclusions

Alcohol's effects on psychiatric, neuropsychological, and psychological functioning are important domains of alcohol problems. Research on the psychiatric consequences of chronic heavy drinking has informed the psychiatric taxonomy literature on comorbidity, particularly in terms of the clinical utility of the primary–secondary distinction of alcohol and other disorders. The literature on the medical and psychiatric management of alcohol withdrawal provides a good example of research directly informing diagnosis and treatment decisions and benefiting the care of patients.

There are numerous areas in need of research regarding the role that heavy drinking plays in the pathogenesis and presentation of psychiatric disorders in those at risk for, or who are already affected by, these disorders. Available data suggest that chronic heavy drinking and other psychopathology often show reciprocal negative influences over time. However, it has not been established that chronic heavy drinking is a direct etiological agent for psychiatric disorders. It is possible that excessive alcohol use is directly involved in the etiology of some types of panic disorder and generalized anxiety disorder, and some forms of secondary affective disorder, such that alcohol's effects are a necessary condition for expression of the pathology. While consistent with the literature, this remains highly speculative, and conclusions must await further research.

Much of our knowledge of alcohol's chronic effects on cognitive functioning comes from the literature on neuropsychological consequences. The neuropsychology literature has been successful in identifying brain syndromes and delineating some of the mechanisms by which chronic drinking exerts its effects on information processing. Neuropsychology has begun to articulate many of the mechanisms of alcohol's chronic effects on the brain at anatomical, functional, and behavioral levels. As knowledge of these mechanisms advances, this area promises to tell us much more about individual and group differences in the vulnerability to neuropsychological effects, and how negative consequences can be prevented or treated.

With regard to psychological consequences, research on craving, increased salience of alcohol consumption, and impaired control over drinking behavior have increased our understanding of the psychological processes involved in addiction, dependence, and relapse. Future research should focus on how these consequences develop, to better understand individual differences in risk for addiction. Research on psychological aspects of addiction provides a means to effectively target key variables during assessment and treatment and to better understand motivational aspects of behavior during times of high risk for relapse.

Alcohol's psychological consequences (i.e., effects on affective, cognitive, and motivational functioning) are arguably as important in alcohol dependence as is physiological tolerance and withdrawal. Research on physiological and psychological processes in alcohol addiction are mutually beneficial. Psychological research can help the field synthesize physiological processes and explain the mechanisms by which they produce their observable effects. Future research promises to tell us much more about the neurobiological basis of psychological processes in addictive behavior, including compulsive use, craving, and incentive motivational processes. Efforts to integrate psychological and physical aspects of alcohol dependence promise to increase our understanding of the nature of this disorder.

It should be noted that there are important limitations in the populations to which conclusions can be firmly generalized. Most of the research reviewed in this chapter was conducted on samples that were entirely or predominantly male. While research on gender differences has expanded, in many cases basic research with females still remains to be conducted. Many studies, especially those conducted in VA hospitals, were characterized by older subjects with relatively severe and chronic problems. A general limitation of the literatures reviewed in this chapter is that most research was conducted only on persons presenting for alcohol treatment.

An overarching issue that clearly emerges in this chapter is that neither psychiatric, neuropsychological, nor psychological consequences are uniform across persons. There is a great deal of heterogeneity in the type of consequences that occur and in the amount and pattern of alcohol consumption that precipitates such problems. Many consequences occur in only a small proportion of chronic heavy drinkers. Clearly, the expression of alcohol-related psychological and psychiatric problems is highly dependent on individual differences in vulnerabilities to such problems. In some cases, key diatheses have been identified, such as the role of thiamine deficiency in Wernicke–Korsakoff's syndrome and the increase in suicide risk among those with both alcohol dependence and major affective disorder. Nevertheless, much more remains to be learned about individual vulnerabilities that interact with excessive drinking to produce particular psychiatric, neuropsychological, and psychological consequences. Increased knowledge of individual vulnerabilities will lead to improvements in the prevention and treatment of the consequences of chronic heavy drinking.

References

Adams, D. H. (1994). Leucocyte adhesion molecules and alcoholic liver disease. *Alcohol and Alcoholism, 29,* 249–260.

American Psychiatric Association. (1987). *Diagnostic and statistical manual of mental disorders* (3rd ed., rev.). Washington, DC: Author.

American Psychiatric Association. (1994). *Diagnostic and statistical manual of mental disorders* (4th ed.). Washington, DC: Author.

Arria, A. M., Tarter, R. E., Kabene, M. E., Laird, S. B., Moss, H., & Van Thiel, D. H. (1991). The role of cirrhosis in memory functioning of alcoholics. *Alcoholism: Clinical and Experimental Research, 15,* 932–937.

Arria, A. M., Tarter, R. E., Starzl, T. E., & Van Thiel, D. H. (1991). Improvement in cognitive functioning of alcoholics following orthotopic liver transplantation. *Alcoholism: Clinical and Experimental Research, 15,* 956–962.

Baker, T.B., Morse, E., & Sherman (1987). The motivation to use drugs: A psychobiological analysis of urges. In

C. Rivers (Ed.), *The Nebraska Symposium on Motivation: Alcohol use and abuse* (pp. 257–323). Lincoln: University of Nebraska Press.

Ballenger, J. C., Goodwin, F. K., Major, L. F., & Brown, G. L. (1979). Alcohol and central serotonin metabolism in man. *Archives of General Psychiatry, 36,* 224–227.

Banki, C. M., Arato, M., Papp, Z., & Kurca, M. (1984). Biochemical markers in suicidal patients. *Journal of Affective Disorders, 6,* 341–350.

Barron, J. H., & Russell, E. W. (1992). Fluidity theory and neuropsychological impairment in alcoholism. *Archives of Clinical Neuropsychology, 7,* 175–188.

Bates, M. E. (1993). Psychology. In M. Galanter (Ed.), *Recent developments in alcoholism* (Vol. 11, pp. 45–72). New York: Plenum.

Bates, M. E., & Convit, A. (in press). Neuropsychological functions affected by alcohol and drug abuse. In A. Calev (Ed.), *Neuropsychological functions in psychiatric disorders.* Washington, DC: American Psychiatric Press.

Baumeister, R. F., Tice, D. M., & Heatherton, T. F. (1994). *Losing control: How and why people fail at self-regulation.* San Diego, CA: Academic Press.

Benton, A. L. (1994). Neuropsychological assessment. *Annual Review of Psychology, 45,* 1–23.

Bibb, J. L., & Chambless, D. L. (1986). Alcohol use and abuse among diagnosed agoraphobics. *Behavior Research and Therapy, 24,* 49–58.

Bowden, S. C. (1990). Separating cognitive impairment in neurologically asymptomatic alcoholism from Wernicke–Korsakoff syndrome: Is the neuropsychological distinction justified? *Psychological Bulletin, 107,* 355–366.

Brandon, T. H., Tiffany, S., & Baker, T. B. (1985). The process of smoking relapse. In F. M. Tims & C. G. Leukefeld (Eds.), *Relapse and recovery in drug abuse* (National Institute of Drug Abuse Research Monograph No. 72, pp. 104–117). Washington, DC: U.S. Government Printing Office.

Breier, A. L., Charney, D. S., & Heninger, G. R. (1986). Agoraphobia with panic attacks: Development, diagnostic stability, and course of illness. *Archives of General Psychiatry, 43,* 1029–1036.

Brown, S. A., Irwin, M., & Schuckit, M. A. (1991). Changes in anxiety among abstinent male alcoholics. *Journal of Studies on Alcohol, 52,* 55–61.

Brown, S. A., Inaba, R. K., Fillin, J. C., Schuckit, M. A., Stewart, M. A., & Irwin, M. R. (1995). Alcoholism and affective disorder: Clinical course of depressive symptoms. *American Journal of Psychiatry, 152,* 45–52.

Butters, N., & Cermak, L. S. (1980). *Alcoholic Korsakoff's Syndrome: An information processing approach to amnesia.* New York: Harcourt Brace Jovanovich.

Butters, N., & Salmon, D. (1986). Etiology and neuropathology of alcoholic Korsakoff's Syndrome: New findings and speculations. In I. Grant (Ed.), *Neuropsychiatric correlates of alcoholism* (pp. 61–108).

Monograph Series of the American Psychiatric Press. Washington, DC: American Psychiatric Press.

Butterworth, R. F. (1995). The role of liver disease in alcohol-induced cognitive deficits. *Alcohol Health and Research World, 19,* 122–129.

Castaneda, R., & Cushman, P. (1989). Alcohol withdrawal: A review of clinical management. *Journal of Clinical Psychiatry, 50,* 278–284.

Chambless, D. L., Cherney, J., Caputo, C., & Rheinstein, B. (1987). Anxiety disorders and alcoholism: A study with inpatient alcoholics. *Journal of Anxiety Disorders, 1,* 29–40.

Charness, M. E. (1993). Brain lesions in alcoholics. *Alcoholism: Clinical and Experimental Research, 17,* 2–11.

Charness, M. E., Simon, R. P., & Greenberg, D. A. (1989). Ethanol and the nervous system. *New England Journal of Medicine, 321,* 442–454.

Clark, D. B., & Sayette, M. A. (1993). Anxiety and the development of alcoholism: Clinical and scientific issues. *American Journal on Addictions, 2,* 59–76.

Cloninger, C. R. (1987). Neurogenetic mechanisms in alcoholism. *Science, 236,* 410–416.

Cornelius, J. R., Salloum, I. M., Mezzich, J., Cornelius, M. D., Fabrega, H., Ehler, J. G., Ulrich, R. F., Thase, M. E., & Mann, J. J. (1995). Disproportionate suicidality in patients with comorbid major depression and alcoholism. *American Journal of Psychiatry, 152,* 358–364.

Dakis, C. A., Gold, M. S., Pottash, A. L., & Sweeney, D. R. (1986). Evaluating depression in alcoholics. *Psychiatry Research, 17,* 105–109.

Drummond, C. D., & Glautier, S. P. (1994). A controlled trial of cue exposure treatment in alcohol dependence. *Journal of Consulting and Clinical Psychology, 62,* 809–817.

Edwards, G. (1986). The Alcohol Dependence Syndrome: Concept as a stimulus to enquiry. *British Journal of Addiction, 81,* 171–183.

Edwards, G., & Gross, M. M. (1976). Alcohol dependence: Provisional description of a clinical syndrome. *British Medical Journal, 1,* 1058–1061.

Edwards, G., Gross, M. M., Keller, M., Moser, J., & Room, R. (1977). *Alcohol-related disabilities* (WHO Offset publication No. 32). Geneva, Switzerland: World Health Organization.

Evert, D. L., & Oscar-Berman, M. (1995). Alcohol-related cognitive impairments: An overview of how alcoholism may affect the workings of the brain. *Alcohol Health and Research World, 19,* 89–96.

Freed, E. X. (1978). Alcohol and mood: An updated review. *International Journal of the Addictions, 13,* 173–200.

Glenn, S. W., & Parsons, O. A. (1992). Efficiency measures in male and female alcoholics. *Journal of Studies on Alcohol, 53,* 546–552.

Goldman, M. S. (1983). Cognitive impairment in chronic alcoholics: Some cause for optimism. *American Psychologist, 38,* 1045–1054.

Goldman, M. S. (1987). The role of time and practice in the recovery of function in alcoholics. In O. A. Parsons, N. Butters, & P. E. Nathan (Eds.), *Neuropsychology of alcoholism: Implications for diagnosis and treatment* (pp. 291–321). New York: Guilford.

Goldman, M. S. (1995). Recovery of cognitive functioning in alcoholics: The relationship to treatment. *Alcohol Health and Research World, 19,* 148–154.

Guthrie, A., & Elliot, W. A. (1980). The nature and recoverability of cerebral impairment in alcoholism: Treatment implications. *Journal of Studies on Alcohol, 41,* 147–155.

Harper, C. G., & Kril, J. (1991). If you drink your brain will shrink: Neuropathological considerations. *Alcohol and Alcoholism 1* (Suppl.), 375–380.

Harper, C. G., Giles, M., & Finlay-Jones, R. (1986). Clinical signs in the Wernicke–Korsakoff complex: A retrospective analysis of 131 cases diagnosed at necropsy. *Journal of Neurology Neurosurgery and Psychiatry, 49,* 341–345.

Hawton, K., Fogg, J., & McKeown, S. (1989). Alcoholism, alcohol and attempted suicide. *Alcohol and Alcoholism, 24,* 3–9.

Heather, N., Miller, W. R., & Greeley, J. (Eds.). (1991). *Self-control and the addictive behaviors.* Sydney, Australia: Maxwell Macmillan.

Helzer, J., & Pryzbeck, T. (1988). The co-occurrence of alcoholism with other psychiatric disorders in the general population and its impact on treatment. *Journal of Studies on Alcohol, 49,* 219–224.

Henriksson, M. M., Aro, H. M., Marttunen, M. J., Heikkinen, M. E., Isometsa, E. T., Kuppasalmi, K. I., & Lonnqvist, J. K. (1993). Mental disorders and comorbidity in suicide. *American Journal of Psychiatry, 150,* 935–940.

Hesselbrock, M. N., Meyer, R. E., & Keene, J. J. (1985). Psychopathology in hospitalized alcoholics. *Archives of General Psychiatry, 42,* 1050–1055.

Holderness, C. C., Brooks-Gunn, J., & Warren, M. P. (1994). Co-morbidity of eating disorders and substance abuse review of the literature. *International Journal of Eating Disorders, 16,* 1–34.

Ingle, K. G., & Weingartner, H. J. (1995). Cognitive deficits in alcoholism: Approaches to theoretical modeling. *Alcohol Health and Research World, 19,* 155–158.

Jacobson, R. R., Acker, C. F., & Lishman, W. A. (1990). Patterns of neuropsychological deficit in alcoholic Korsakoff's syndrome. *Psychological Medicine, 20,* 321–334.

Jellinek, E. M. (1952). Phases of alcohol addiction. *Quarterly Journal of Studies on Alcohol, 13,* 673–684.

Jellinek, E. M. (1955). The "craving" for alcohol. *Quarterly Journal of Studies on Alcohol, 16,* 35–38.

Jellinek, E. M. (1960). *The disease concept of alcoholism.* New Brunswick, NJ: Rutgers Center of Alcohol Studies.

Jernigan, T. L., & Ostergaard, A. L. (1995). When alcoholism affects memory functions: MRI of the brain. *Alcohol Health and Research World, 19,* 104–107.

Kalant, H. (1977). Alcohol withdrawal syndromes in the human: Comparison with animal models. In M. W. Gross (Ed.). *Alcohol intoxication and withdrawal,* (3rd ed.) New York: Plenum.

Kassel, J. D. & Shiffman, S. (1992). What can hunger teach us about drug craving? A comparative analysis of the two constructs. *Advances in Behaviour Research and Therapy, 14,* 141–167.

Killen, J., Fortmann, S., Kraemer, H., Varady, A., & Newman, B. (1992). Who will relapse? Symptoms of nicotine dependence predict long-term relapse after smoking cessation. *Journal of Consulting and Clinical Psychology, 60,* 797–801.

Knight, R. G., & Longmore, B. E. (1994). *Clinical neuropsychology of alcoholism.* Hillsdale, NJ: Erlbaum.

Kozlowski, L. T., & Wilkinson, D. A. (1987). Use and misuse of the concept of craving by alcohol, tobacco, and drug researchers. *British Journal of Addiction, 82,* 31–36.

Kushner, M. E., Sher, K. J., & Beitman, B. D. (1990). The relation between alcohol problems and the anxiety disorders. *American Journal of Psychiatry, 147,* 685–695.

Lancaster, F. E. (1994). Gender differences in the brain: Implications for the study of human alcoholism. *Alcoholism: Clinical and Experimental Research, 18,* 740–746.

Lang, P. J. (1968). Fear reduction and fear behavior: Problems in treating a construct. In J. M. Schlien (Ed.), *Research in psychotherapy* (Vol. 3, pp. 90–103). Washington, DC: American Psychological Association.

Lehman, L. B., Pilich, A., & Andrews, N. (1993). Neurological disorders resulting from alcoholism. *Alcohol Health and Research World, 17,* 305–309.

Levy, J. C., & Deykin, E. Y. (1989). Suicidality, depression, and substance abuse in adolescence. *American Journal of Psychiatry, 146,* 1462–1467.

Lewis, C. E., Rice, J., & Helzer, J. E. (1983). Diagnostic interactions: Alcoholism and antisocial personality. *Journal of Nervous and Mental Disease, 171,* 105–112.

Lezak, M. D. (1995). *Neuropsychological assessment* (3rd ed.). New York: Oxford University Press.

Lishman, W. A. (1990). Alcohol and the brain. *British Journal of Psychiatry, 156,* 635–644.

Loberg, T., & Miller, W. R. (1986). Personality, cognitive, and neuropsychological correlates of harmful alcohol consumption: A cross-national comparison of clinical samples. *Annals of the New York Academy of Sciences, 472,* 75–97.

Ludenia, K., Conham, G. W., Holzer, P. D., & Sands, M. (1984). Anxiety in an alcoholic population: A normative study. *Journal of Clinical Psychology, 40,* 356–358.

Ludwig, A. M., & Wikler, A (1974). "Craving" and relapse to drink. *Quarterly Journal of Studies on Alcohol, 35,* 108–130.

Mann, J. J., Stanley, M., McBride, P. A., & McEwen, B. S. (1986). Increased serotonin₂ and beta-adrenergic binding in frontal cortices of suicide victims. *Archives of General Psychiatry, 43,* 954–959.

Mann, K., Batra, A., Gunthner, A., & Schroth, G. (1992). Do women develop alcoholic brain damage more readily than men? *Alcoholism: Clinical and Experimental Research, 16,* 1052–1056.

Marlatt, G., Demming, B., & Reid, J. (1973). Loss of control drinking in alcoholics: An experimental analogue. *Journal of Abnormal Psychology, 81,* 233–241.

Marlatt, G. A. (1985). Relapse prevention: Theoretical rationale and overview of the model. In G. A. Marlatt & J. G. Gordon (Eds.), *Relapse prevention* (pp. 3–70). New York: Guilford.

Marsano, L. (1994). Alcohol and malnutrition. *Addictions Nursing, 6,* 62–71.

Martin, P. R., Adinoff, B., Weingartner, H., Mukherjee, A. B., & Eckardt, M. J. (1986). Alcoholic organic brain disease: Nosology and pathophysiologic mechanism. *Progress in Neuro-Psychopharmacology and Biological Psychiatry, 10,* 113–242.

Mendelson, J. H., & Mello, N. K. (1979). *The diagnosis and treatment of alcoholism.* New York: McGraw-Hill.

Milin, R. P. (1996). Comorbidity of substance abuse and psychotic disorders: Focus on adolescents and young adults. *Child and Adolescent Psychiatric Clinics of North America, 5,* 111–121.

Miller, W. R. (1993). Alcoholism: Toward a better disease model. *Psychology of Addictive Behaviors, 7,* 129–136.

Monti, P. M., Rohsenow, D. J., Rubonis, A. V., Niaura, R. S., Sirota, A. S., Colby, S. M., Goddard, P., & Abrams, D. B. (1993). Cue exposure with coping skills treatment for male alcoholics: A preliminary investigation. *Journal of Consulting and Clinical Psychology, 61,* 1011–1019.

Moss, H. B. (1987). Serotonergic activity and disinhibitory psychopathology in alcoholism. *Medical Hypotheses, 23,* 353–361.

Mullaney, J. A., & Trippett, C. J. (1979). Alcohol dependence and phobias: Clinical description and relevance. *British Journal of Psychiatry, 135,* 565–573.

Murphy, G. E. (1992). *Suicide in alcoholism.* New York: Oxford University Press.

Muuronen, A., Bergman, H., & Hindmarsh, T. (1989). Influence of improved drinking habits on brain atrophy and cognitive performance in alcoholic patients: A 5-year follow-up study. *Alcoholism: Clinical and Experimental Research, 13,* 137–141.

Nakamura, M. M., Overall, J. E., Hollister, L. E., & Radcliffe, E. (1983). Factors affecting outcome of depressive symptoms in alcoholics. *Alcoholism: Clinical and Experimental Research, 7,* 188–193.

Nathan, P. E., Titler, N. A., Lowenstein, L. M., Solomon, P., & Rossi, A. M. (1970). Behavioral analysis of chronic alcoholism: Interaction of alcohol and human contact. *Archives of General Psychiatry, 22,* 419–430.

Nixon, S. J. (1993). Application of theoretical models to the study of alcohol-induced brain damage. In W. A. Hunt & S. J. Nixon (Eds.), *Alcohol-induced brain damage* (NIH Publication No. 93-3549, pp. 213–228; NIAA Research Monograph No. 22). Bethesda, MD: National Institute of Alcohol Abuse and Alcoholism.

Nixon, S. J., Tivis, R., & Parsons, O. A. (1995). Behavioral dysfunction and cognitive efficiency in male and female alcoholics. *Alcoholism: Clinical and Experimental Research, 19,* 577–581.

Oscar-Berman, M., & Hutner, N. (1993). Frontal lobe changes after chronic alcohol ingestion. In W. A. Hunt & S. J. Nixon (Eds.), *Alcohol-induced brain damage* (NIH Publication No. 93-3549, pp. 121–156; NIAA Research Monograph No. 22). Rockville, MD: National Institute of Alcohol Abuse and Alcoholism.

Parsons, O. A. (1993). Impaired neuropsychological functioning in sober alcoholics. In W. A. Hunt & S. J. Nixon (Eds.), *Alcohol-induced brain damage* (NIH Publication No. 93-3549, pp. 173–194; NIAA Research Monograph No. 22). Rockville, MD: U.S. Department of Health and Human Services, National Institute on Alcohol Abuse and Alcoholism.

Parsons, O. A., & Leber, W. R. (1982). Alcohol, cognitive dysfunction and brain damage. In *Biomedical processes and consequences of alcohol use* (Alcohol and Health Monograph No. 2, pp. 213–253). Rockville, MD: National Institute on Alcohol Abuse and Alcoholism.

Pickens, R., & Johanson, C. (1992). Craving: Consensus of status and agenda for future research. *Drug and Alcohol Dependence, 30,* 127–131.

Pomier, L. G., Nguyen, N. H., Faucher, C., Giguere, J. F., & Butterworth, R. F. (1991). Subclinical hepatic encephalopathy in cirrhotic patients: Prevalence and relationship to liver function. *Canadian Journal of Gastroenterology, 5,* 121–125.

Rankin, H., Hodgson, R., & Stockwell, T. (1979). The concept of craving and its measurement. *Behaviour Research and Therapy, 17,* 389–396.

Regier, D. A., Farmer, M. E., Rae, D. S., Locke, B. Z., Keith, S. J., Judd, L. L., & Goodwin, F. K. (1990). Comorbidity of mental disorders with alcohol and other drug abuse. *Journal of the American Medical Association, 264,* 2511–2518.

Robins, L., & Reiger, D. (Eds.). (1991). *Psychiatric disorders in America: The epidemiologic catchment area study.* New York: Macmillan.

Robinson, T., & Berridge, K. (1993). The neural basis of craving: An incentive-sensitization theory of addiction. *Brain Research Reviews, 18,* 247–291.

Roelofs, S. M. (1985). Hyperventilation, anxiety, craving for alcohol: A subacute alcohol withdrawal syndrome. *Alcohol* (Oxford), *2,* 501–505.

Ross, H. E., Glasser, F. B., & Germanson, T. (1988). The prevalence of psychiatric disorders in patients with alcohol and other drug problems. *Archives of General Psychiatry, 45,* 1023–1031.

Rudd, M. D., Dahm, P. F., & Rajab, M. H. (1993). Diagnostic comorbidity in persons with suicidal ideation and behavior. *American Journal of Psychiatry, 150,* 928–934.

Ryan, C., & Butters, N. (1986). Neuropsychology of alcoholism. In T. D. Wedding, A. M. Horton, & J. S. Webster (Eds.), *The neuropsychology handbook* (pp. 376–409). New York: Springer.

Satel, S. L., Kosten, T. R., Schuckit, M. A., & Fischman, M. W. (1993). Should protracted withdrawal from drugs be included in DSM-IV? *American Journal of Psychiatry, 150,* 695–704.

Sayette, M. A., Monti, P. M., Rohsenow, D. J., Bird-Gulliver, S., Colby, S., Sirota, A., Niaura, R. S., & Abrams, D. B. (1994). The effects of cue exposure on attention in male alcoholics. *Journal of Studies on Alcohol, 55,* 629–634.

Schafer, K., Butters, N., & Smith, T. (1991). Cognitive performance of alcoholics: A longitudinal evaluation of the role of drinking history, depression, liver function, nutrition, and family history. *Alcoholism: Clinical and Experimental Research, 15,* 653–660.

Schuckit, M. A. (1982). The history of psychotic symptoms in alcoholics. *Journal of Clinical Psychiatry, 43,* 53–57.

Schuckit, M. A. (1983). Alcoholic patients with secondary depression. *American Journal of Psychiatry, 140,* 711–714.

Schuckit, M. A. (1985). The clinical implications of primary diagnostic groups among alcoholics. *Archives of General Psychiatry, 42,* 1043–1049.

Sellars, E. M., & Kalant, H. (1976). Alcohol intoxication and withdrawal. *Medical Intelligence, 294,* 757–762.

Shiffman, S., Paty, J., Gnys, M., Kassel, J., & Elash, C. (1995). Nicotine withdrawal in chippers and regular smokers: Subjective and cognitive effects. *Health Psychology, 14,* 301–309.

Siegel, S. (1983). Classical conditioning, drug tolerance, and drug dependence. In Y. Israel, F. Glaser, H. Kalant, R. Popham, W. Schmidt, & R. Smart (Eds.), *Research advances in alcohol and drug problems* (Vol. 7, pp. 207–246). New York: Plenum.

Smith, M. E., & Oscar-Berman, M. (1992). Resource-limited information processing in alcoholism. *Journal of Studies on Alcohol, 53,* 514–518.

Solomon, R., & Corbit, J. (1973). An opponent process theory of motivation: 2. Cigarette addiction. *Journal of Abnormal Psychology, 81,* 158–171.

Steele, C., & Josephs, R. (1990). Alcohol myopia: Its prized and dangerous effects. *American Psychologist, 45,* 921–933.

Stewart, J., de Wit, H., & Eikelboom, R. (1984). Role of unconditioned and conditioned drug effects in the self-administration of opiates and stimulants. *Psychological Review, 91,* 251–268.

Stockwell, T. (1991). Experimental analogues of loss of control: A review of human drinking studies. In N. Heather, W. R. Miller, & J. Greeley (Eds.), *Self-control and the addictive behaviors* (pp. 180–197). Botany, Australia: Maxwell Macmillan.

Stockwell, T., Hodgson, R., & Rankin, H. (1982). Tension reduction and the effects of prolonged alcohol consumption. *British Journal of Addiction, 77,* 65–73.

Sullivan, E. V., Rosenbloom, M. J., Deshmukh, A., Desmond, J. E., & Pfefferbaum, A. (1995). Alcohol and the cerebellum: Effects on balance, motor coordination, and cognition. *Alcohol Health and Research World, 19,* 138–141.

Tarter, R. E., Arria, A., & Van Thiel, D. H. (1993). Liver–brain interactions in alcoholism. In W. A. Hunt & S. J. Nixon (Eds.), *Alcohol-induced brain damage* (NIH Publication No. 93-3549, pp. 415–430; NIAA Research Monograph No. 22). Rockville, MD: National Institute of Alcohol Abuse and Alcoholism.

Tarter, R. E., Switala, J., Lu, S., & Van Thiel, D. (1995). Abstracting capacity in cirrhotic alcoholics: Negative findings. *Journal of Studies on Alcohol, 56,* 99–103.

Tiffany, S.T. (1990) A cognitive model of drug urges and drug-use behavior: Role of automatic and nonautomatic processes. *Psychological Review, 97,* 147–168.

Tracy, J. I., Josiassen, R. C., & Bellack, A. S. (1995). Neuropsychology of dual diagnosis: Understanding the combined effects of schizophrenia and substance use disorders. *Clinical Psychology Review, 15,* 67–97.

Vaillant, G. E. (1980). Natural history of male psychological health: 8. Antecedents of alcoholism and "orality." *American Journal of Psychiatry, 137,* 181–186.

Victor, M. (1992). The effects of alcohol on the nervous system. In C. S. Lieber (Ed.), *Medical and nutritional complications of alcoholism: Mechanisms and management* (pp. 413–457). New York: Plenum Medical Book Company.

Victor, M. (1994). Alcoholic dementia. *Canadian Journal of Neurological Science, 21,* 88–99.

Walton, J. N. (1994). *Brain's diseases of the nervous system* (10th ed.). Oxford, England: Oxford University Press.

Weissman, M. M., Meyers, J. K., & Harding, P. S. (1980). Prevalence and psychiatric heterogeneity of alcoholism in a United States urban community. *Journal of Studies on Alcohol, 41,* 672–681.

West, R., Hajek, P., & Belcher, M. (1989). Severity of withdrawal symptoms as a predictor of outcome of an attempt to quit smoking. *Psychological Medicine, 19,* 981–985.

Wilson, G. T. (1987). Cognitive processes in addiction. *British Journal of Addiction, 82,* 343–353.

Winukor, G. (1990). The concept of secondary depression and its relationship to comorbidity. *Psychiatric Clinics of North America, 13,* 567–583.

Winokur, G., & Black, D. W. (1987). Psychiatric and medical diagnoses as risk factors for mortality in psychiatric patients: A case-control study. *American Journal of Psychiatry, 144,* 208–211.

Winokur, G., Clayton, P. J., & Reich, T. (1969). *Manic depressive illness.* St. Louis, MO: Mosby.

Winokur, G., Coryell, W., Akiskal, H. S., Maser, J. D., Keller, M. B., Endicott, J., & Mueller, T. (1995). Alcoholism in manic-depressive (bipolar) illness: Familial illness, course of illness, and the primary-secondary distinction. *American Journal of Psychiatry, 152,* 365–372.

Wise, R. (1988). The neurobiology of craving: Implications for understanding and treatment of addiction. *Journal of Abnormal Psychology, 97,* 118–132.

World Health Organization. (1993). *International classification of diseases* (10th ed.). Geneva, Switzerland: Author.

Wright, D. G., Laureno, R., & Victor, M. (1979). Pontine and extrapontine myelinolysis. *Brain, 102,* 361–385.

Zinser, M., Baker, T., Sherman, J., & Cannon, D. (1992). Relation between self-reported affect and drug urges and cravings in continuing and withdrawing smokers. *Journal of Abnormal Psychology, 101,* 617–629.

II

Caffeine

4

Pharmacology of Caffeine

JOHN W. DALY

Introduction

The widespread societal use of caffeine-containing beverages has engendered extensive interest in the pharmacological mechanisms underlying the *in vivo* effects of caffeine, and to a lesser extent the other naturally occurring methylxanthines, namely, theophylline and theobromine. Caffeine is ingested primarily because of mild central stimulant properties, whereby it tends to increase vigilance and defer sleep. Research, therefore, has focused primarily on the pharmacological effects of caffeine relevant to the central nervous system. The pharmacology of methylxanthines, in particular caffeine, has been reviewed in detail (Daly, 1993; Fredholm, Arslan, Johansson, Kull, & Svenningsson, 1997; Nehlig, 1994) and the present chapter will attempt only a succinct overview without extensive citations of the literature covered in those reviews.

Caffeine is a remarkable drug, whose diuretic and respiratory and central stimulant properties were exhaustively studied for decades before clues as to possible pharmacological sites of action were uncovered. In the late 1950s, caffeine was found to affect calcium-dependent processes (Axelsson & Thesleff, 1958; Bianchi, 1961; Frank, 1960)

and to inhibit cyclic AMP phosphodiesterases (Rall & Sutherland, 1958). About 10 years later, caffeine was found to block adenosine receptors (Sattin & Rall, 1970), and in 1979 it was found that caffeine interacted with $GABA_A$-receptors (Marangos *et al.*, 1979). These four sites of action remain the most relevant to the pharmacology of caffeine.

Caffeine readily equilibrates throughout the body, including the brain, and has a half-life to 3 to 5 hr in humans. Plasma levels attained in humans after moderate to high consumption of caffeine-containing beverages (100–300 mg/day) are estimated to range from 5 to 20 μM. In addition to its societal use in beverages, caffeine and also theophylline have been used to treat bronchial asthma and neonatal apnea. In such treatments, plasma levels of 50 μM or more are reached. Caffeine at high doses is less likely than theophylline to cause tachycardia, but both are cardiotonic and both increase coronary flow. Both also have diuretic activity and stimulate gastric secretion. Both stimulate lipolysis and inhibit platelet aggregation. The well-recognized somnolytic properties of caffeine led to its former use in the treatment of narcolepsy. Caffeine is used as a flavor enhancer in carbonated beverages and as an adjunct in certain analgetics, diuretics and cold-allergy remedies. Although caffeine and theophylline can induce or exacerbate tremors, theophylline has been proposed for treatment of essential tremor. Caffeine increases duration in electroconvulsive therapy and has been used clinically (Francis &

JOHN W. DALY • National Institutes of Health, Bethesda, Maryland 20892.

Handbook of Substance Abuse: Neurobehavioral Pharmacology, edited by Tarter *et al.* Plenum Press, New York, 1998.

Fochtmann, 1994). Theobromine, the third naturally occurring methylxanthine, is relatively ineffective as a central stimulant, but has been used in treatment of asthma and as a vasodilator, cardiotonic, and diuretic. There is a wide range of reported interactions of caffeine with other centrally active drugs, in particular those affecting dopamine (amphetamine, cocaine), acetylcholine (nicotine) and GABA (diazepam) receptors or function.

The central activity of caffeine could be termed biphasic. At low doses the effects of caffeine are positive in nature, enhancing alertness, combating fatigue, and improving mood. However, at high doses, caffeine can cause restlessness and anxiety in humans. For humans caffeine consumption ranges between 1 and 5 mg/kg/day, while pharmacological studies in animals usually employ dosages of 5 to 20 mg/kg. In rodents, high doses (>30 mg/kg) of caffeine and theophylline can cause choreiform (dancelike) movements (Nikodijević, Jacobson, & Daly, 1993a), automutilation, and aggressiveness (Mueller, Saboda, Palmour, & Nyhan, 1982). Convulsions occur at dosages of 200 mg/kg or more. Undoubtedly because of the biphasic action of caffeine, humans tend to titrate consumption only to levels at which the negative effects are not yet manifest, and individuals sensitive to the negative effects avoid caffeine-containing beverages. The term "caffeinism" has been used to describe the symptoms of agitation, anxiety, and insomnia associated with excessive consumption of caffeine. Caffeine in some paradigms appears to have reinforcing effects on self-administration in animals, and reinforcing effects are manifest in humans (Griffiths & Mumford, 1996). Tolerance develops to caffeine, both in humans and animals. A withdrawal syndrome that occurs within the first 24 hours of withdrawal is well documented in humans and usually includes headache, listlessness, irritability, and nervousness.

The mechanisms underlying the pharmacological effects of caffeine remain controversial. Four major hypotheses have been advanced: (1) the mobilization of calcium, (2) the inhibition of phosphodiesterases, (3) the competitive antagonism of adenosine receptors, and (4) effects on $GABA_A$-receptors. The release of catecholamines has also been invoked. Caffeine clearly is a drug with multiple sites of action, some of which may still remain undiscovered.

Mobilization of Calcium

Discovery of the ability of caffeine to mobilize intracellular calcium stemmed from studies in the late 1950s on caffeine-induced contractures of striatal muscle (Axelsson & Thesleff, 1958; Bianchi, 1961; Frank, 1960). The release of catecholamines by caffeine from adrenal medulla also appears due to mobilization of intracellular calcium (Poisner, 1973). Such effects require millimolar concentrations of caffeine. It is now known that caffeine binds to a site on a cyclic ADP ribose-sensitive calcium channel and thereby enhances calcium-dependent activation of the channel, resulting in a release of calcium from intracellular storage sites in the sarcoplasmic and endoplasmic reticulum. Caffeine is widely used as a research tool for the study of the functional importance of this calcium pool (Ehrlich, Kaftan, Bezprozvannayan, & Bezprozvanny, 1994). From the standpoint of relevance to the *in vivo* pharmacology of caffeine, it should be stressed that caffeine has a very low potency at such calcium channels with thresholds for effects being about 250 mM, while 2 to 20 mM concentrations are required for robust effects. Such a threshold concentration is in the range in which caffeine is a convulsant and even lethal drug. Thus, it seems unlikely that the stimulatory effects of caffeine on calcium release play a major *in vivo* role in the pharmacology of caffeine.

Phosphodiesterase Inhibition

In the late 1950s, the inhibition of phosphodiesterases by caffeine and theophylline was discovered through studies on cyclic AMP systems (Rall & Sutherland, 1958). However, both caffeine and theophylline have proven to be very weak inhibitors of all of the principal phosphodiesterases having IC_{50} values of > 100 μM (Ukena, Schudt, & Sybrecht, 1993).

Thus, near-convulsant doses of caffeine would be required to cause effective inhibition of phosphodiesterases *in vivo*. It would appear that inhibition of phosphodiesterases by caffeine is unlikely to significantly contribute to the *in vivo* pharmacology of moderate doses of caffeine. However, there are systems in which phosphodiesterase inhibition may be involved in the pharmacological effects of high doses of caffeine and theophylline. Thus, in the cardiovascular system, cardiac stimulation, relaxation of vascular smooth muscle and vasodilation do occur with certain inhibitors of phosphodiesterases and with caffeine. Since high doses of caffeine and theophylline do cause tachycardia and vasodilation, inhibition of phosphodiesterases may play a role. It should be noted that caffeine and theophylline have vasoconstrictive effects on the cerebrovascular system, whereby blood flow is decreased in particular to certain brain regions (Nehlig, 1994; Nehlig, Daval, & Debry, 1992). However, it seems unlikely that inhibition of phosphodiesterases is involved in such effects, which are more likely due to blockade of vasodilatory action of endogenous adenosine. Caffeine increases glucose utilization in areas of rat brain rich in norepinephrine, dopamine, and serotonin (Nehlig, Daval, Boyet, & Vert, 1986). Such effects probably reflect, in part, alterations in cerebral blood flow. Tolerance to these effects of caffeine does not develop. In the respiratory system, relaxation of bronchioles and trachea does appear correlated with the potencies of xanthines as phosphodiesterase inhibitors (Brackett, Shamim, & Daly, 1990; Miyamoto *et al.*, 1994). Caffeine and theophylline do cause such relaxations and such effects probably underlie the antiasthmatic effects of caffeine and theophylline. It has been suggested that in the central nervous system, the behavioral depressant effects seen in rodents at high doses of caffeine and theophylline are due to inhibition of phosphodiesterases (Choi, Shamim, Padgett, & Daly, 1988). It is of interest that papaverine, a nonspecific phosphodiesterase inhibitor, partly generalizes to high doses of caffeine in drug-discrimination studies (Holloway, Modrow, &

Michaelis, 1985). Hypothermic effects of high doses of caffeine and other xanthines appear due to inhibition of phosphodiesterases (M. J. Durcan & Morgan, 1991; M. T. Lin, Chandra, & Lui, 1980) and perhaps in part due to release of catecholamines. Such high doses of caffeine also increase blood levels of ACTH, corticosterone, and glucose (LeBlanc, Richard, & Racotta, 1995).

Antagonism of Adenosine Receptors

In the late 1960s, caffeine and theophylline were discovered to block adenosine-mediated stimulation of cyclic AMP formation (Sattin & Rall, 1970). It now appears that the major site of action for low to moderate doses of caffeine are the A_1- and A_2-adenosine receptors. Such receptors modulate adenylate cyclase and other effector systems. The A_1-adenosine receptors are inhibitory to adenylate cyclase and can also be inhibitory to calcium channels, stimulatory to potassium channels, and stimulatory to phosphoinositide breakdown. The A_2-adenosine receptors of which there are two subtypes, the A_{2A} and A_{2B}, are stimulatory to adenylate cyclase. Caffeine and theophylline represent the classical antagonists for such adenosine receptors, but compared with the many other xanthines that have been developed as potent and selective antagonists, caffeine and theophylline have low potency and no selectivity. Nonetheless, with an inhibitory constant (K_i) in the 30–50 μM range, caffeine at moderate doses will presumably cause significant inhibition of tonic adenosine-mediated activation of A_1- and A_{2A}-adenosine receptors. Theophylline is more potent with a K_i of 10–15 μM. There is a third adenosine receptor, the A_3-receptor, that is relatively insensitive to blockade by xanthines. Evidence for a key role for blockade of adenosine receptors in the central stimulatory action of caffeine comes from correlative behavioral and biochemical studies with caffeine, theophylline, and other xanthines. In the first such study, an excellent correlation was found between the affinities of xanthines for brain A_1-adenosine receptors and the threshold dosages for stimulation of locomotor activity in mice (Snyder, Katims, Annau, Bruns, & Daly, 1981). The major exception was an isobutylmethylxanthine, which was found to be a behavioral depressant. Isobutylmethylxanthine is a very potent phosphodiesterase inhibitor and later studies demonstrated that xanthines that are potent phosphodiesterase inhibitors are behavioral depressants, even though they have affinities for adenosine receptors greater than those of caffeine and theophylline (Choi *et al.,* 1988). The third naturally occurring methylxanthine theobromine is both a weak phosphodiesterase inhibitor and a very weak adenosine receptor antagonist. It is also very weak as a behavioral stimulant (Kuribara & Tadokoro, 1992). The correlation of phosphodiesterase inhibition with behavioral depression provides one plausible explanation for the biphasic effects of caffeine and theophylline on behavior. The stimulatory phase at lower doses of the methylxanthine is proposed to be linked to blockade of adenosine receptors, while the subsequent inhibitory phase, seen as the dose of the xanthine is increased, is proposed to be due to inhibition of phosphodiesterases (Choi *et al.,* 1988). The relative role of blockade of A_1- and/or A_{2A}-adenosine receptors in the stimulation of locomotor activity of rodents by caffeine and other xanthines has proven difficult to define; some studies implicate A_1-receptors (Kaplan *et al.,* 1992; Kaplan, Greenblatt, Kent, & Cotreau-Bibbo, 1993) and others implicate A_{2A}-receptors (M. Durcan & Morgan, 1989). It now appears, based on recent studies, that A_{2A}-receptors, which through tonic activation by endogenous adenosine enhance the activity of GABAergic neurons involved in the dopaminergic arousal–reward system, are the major target involved in the behavioral stimulation elicited by caffeine (Fredholm *et al.,* 1997). Somnolytic effects of caffeine and other xanthines had been proposed to be linked to blockade of adenosine receptors (Virus, Ticho, Pildtich, & Radulovacki, 1990). Even the epileptogenic effects of caffeine and other xanthines appear correlated with affinities for adenosine receptors (Moraidis & Bingmann, 1994).

Consonant with the proposal that the pharmacological effects of caffeine and theophylline are in part due to blockade of adenosine receptors are the observations that the effects of adenosine analogs on the cardiovascular, respiratory, renal, and central nervous systems are opposite to those of caffeine and theophylline and can be reversed by caffeine, theophylline, and other xanthines (Daly, 1993). Not only do caffeine and theophylline reverse the behavioral depressant effects of adenosine analogs, but they are more potent in reversing such behavioral depression than in causing stimulation when administered alone (Katims, Annau, & Snyder, 1983; Snyder *et al.,* 1981). The behavioral depression elicited by adenosine analogs may be due in part to hypothermia, which is readily reversed by caffeine and other xanthines (Anderson, Sheehan, & Strong, 1994; Mehta & Kulkarni, 1983; Seale, Abla, Shamim, Carney, & Daly, 1988). To what extent central or peripheral sites are involved in adenosine analog–elicited hypothermia is unclear. Remarkably, caffeine and other xanthines can cause a greater stimulation of behavioral activity when combined with a depressant dose of an adenosine analog than they cause when administered alone (Barraco, Coffin, Altman, & Phillis, 1983; Coffin, Taylor, Phillis, Altman, & Barraco, 1984; Katims *et al.,* 1983; Snyder *et al.,* 1981). Even a depressant xanthine, such as isobutylmethylxanthine, can be a behavioral stimulant when combined with an adenosine analog. An explanation for the augmentation of behavioral stimulation by combinations of caffeine or other xanthines with an adenosine analog has not been forthcoming (Nikodijević, Jacobson, & Daly, 1993b). However, it should be stressed that the adenosine analogs will activate not only central adenosine receptors already tonically activated by endogenous adenosine but also other adenosine receptors. The pharmacology of caffeine as an antagonist, when administered alone, will reflect blockade only of central adenosine receptors that are constitutively activated under normal physiological conditions, while the pharmacology of caffeine administered with adenosine analogs will also involve blockade of other adenosine receptors. The anxiogenic effects of caffeine are not reversed by adenosine analogs (Baldwin & File, 1989). However, a recent study did report reversal of anxiogenic effects of caffeine by an A_1-selective adenosine analog (Jain, Kemp, Adeyemo, Buchanan, & Stone, 1995), and another study reported reversal by an A_{2A}-selective adenosine analog (Imaizumi, Miyazaki, & Onodera, 1994). Studies with xanthines and adenosine analogs that are highly selective for A_1-adenosine or A_{2A}-adenosine receptors provide tentative evidence that behavioral stimulation by xanthines requires blockade of both A_1- or A_{2A}-adenosine receptors (Daly, Shi, Nikodijević, & Jacobson, 1994) and that behavioral depression by adenosine analogs is maximal when both A_1- and A_{2A}-adenosine receptors are activated (Nikodijević, Sarges, Daly, & Jacobson, 1991). Activation of A_{2A}-adenosine receptors in striatum has recently been reported to desensitize A_1-adenosine receptors (Dixon, Widdowson, & Richardson, 1997). Caffeine and theophylline, both of which are nonselective toward A_1- and A_{2A}-adenosine receptors and both of which readily penetrate into the brain, are the prototypic behavioral stimulants among the many xanthines that have been synthesized as adenosine antagonists and phosphodiesterase inhibitors. Xanthines, such as 8-p-sulfophenyltheophylline, which do not penetrate into the central nervous system and hence will block adenosine receptors only outside the brain (Daly, Padgett, Shamim, Butts-Lamb, & Waters, 1985), and xanthines that selectively block A_1- or A_{2A}-adenosine receptors without effects on calcium mobilization or phosphodiesterases (Brackett *et al.*, 1990; Daly & Jacobson, 1995; Müller & Daly, 1993) have been developed and have proven useful research tools for investigating the pharmacology of caffeine.

Interactions with GABA Receptors

Effects on the $GABA_A$-receptor-channel may be relevant to the pharmacology of caffeine even though caffeine is very weak with an affinity (Ki) of about 300 µM versus [^{3}]di-azepam binding (Marangos *et al.*, 1979). While perhaps relevant to the anxiogenic effects at moderate to high doses of caffeine, benzodiazepine site of action probably becomes truly important only at convulsant and toxic doses of caffeine. However, caffeine both *in vivo* at 20 and 40 mg/kg and *in vitro* at 50 µM has been reported to affect GABA receptor-channel function and binding of a channel blocker (Lopez, Miller, Greenblatt, Kaplan, & Shader, 1989). Caffeine at 30 mg/kg in mice increased uptake and binding of a benzodiazepine-antagonist (Kaplan, Greenblatt, Leduc, Thompson, & Shader, 1989). Benzodiazepines do antagonize caffeine-induced seizures (Marangos, Martino, Paul, & Skolnick, 1981), but whether this is due to direct competition at the GABA receptor-channel is not known.

Other Biochemical Effects

Caffeine and theophylline have a number of other effects on enzymes, receptors, ion channels, and uptake systems (Daly, 1993; Ehrlich *et al.*, 1994). Caffeine and theophylline are, however, in all cases relatively weak inhibitors at such sites with affinities (IC_{50} or K_I values) greater than 100 µM. Inhibitory effects of caffeine and other xanthines on 5'-nucleotidases (Fredholm & Lindgren, 1983) might lead to increases in adenosine levels, an effect that would be counteracted through blockade at adenosine receptors by the xanthine. Caffeine has recently been reported to increase plasma levels of adenosine in rats (Conlay, Conant, deBros, & Wurtman, 1997). High doses of caffeine (> 50 mg/kg) can enhance early gene (c-fos) expression in certain central neurons, a phenomenon correlated with the degree of neuronal activation (Svenningsson, Strom, Johansson, & Fredholm, 1995). In contrast, caffeine at the lower doses that stimulate locomotor activity causes a reduction in expression of early genes in certain striatal neurons (Svenningsson *et al.*, 1997). Such striatal GABAergic neurons coexpress both A_{2A}-adenosine receptors and D_2-dopamine receptors, which have opposing effects on activity of these inhibitory GABAergic neurons, with A_{2A}-receptors being stimulatory and D_2-receptors being inhibitory (Fredholm *et al.*, 1997). These and other results strongly suggest that the A_{2A}-receptors are tonically activated and that caffeine, by blockade of such receptors, enhances the inhibitory effects of activation of the D_2-dopamine receptors.

Effects on Central Neurotransmitters

Many of the *in vivo* effects of caffeine are probably due to the blockade by caffeine of a tonic inhibitory input by endogenous adenosine through A_1-adenosine receptors in various tissues and organs. Examples include the lipolytic effects of xanthines linked to blockade of A_1-adenosine receptors on adipocytes and the diuretic effects of xanthines linked to blockade of A_1-adenosine receptors in the kidney. In the central nervous system activation of A_1-adenosine receptors located on synaptic terminals by endogenous adenosine can result in an inhibition of release of neurotransmitters, including norepinephrine, dopamine, serotonin, acetylcholine, GABA, glutamate, and probably neuropeptides. Blockade of tonic inhibitory effects of endogenous adenosine on such neurotransmitter release by caffeine would have effects on the activity of the target postsynaptic neurons, resulting either in enhanced activity, if release of an excitatory neurotransmitter is augmented by caffeine, or in reduced activity, if release of an inhibitory transmitter is augmented by caffeine. Thus, it is not surprising that turnover and levels of neurotransmitters, in particular biogenic amines, and acetylcholine, can be affected by caffeine (Daly, 1993).

Release of norepinephrine by caffeine or theophylline has been invoked as a major contributor to the pharmacology of such xanthines (Berkowitz, Tarver, & Spector, 1970). Whether this is a direct effect linked to calcium mobilization or to phosphodiesterase inhibition, either of which could lead to enhanced release, or an indirect effect on noradrenergic terminals due to blockade of the tonic inhibitory input by endogenous adenosine to A_1-adenosine receptors, or an even more indirect effect

due to enhanced excitatory input to noradrenergic neurons through other neurons affected by caffeine is unknown. Depletion of brain catecholamines reduces the behavioral stimulant effects of caffeine (Finn, Iuvone, & Holtzman, 1990). Phentolamine, a general α-adrenergic agonist, blocks the caffeine cue in discrimination studies, while a selective α_1-adrenergic agonist generalizes to caffeine (Holtzman, 1986). In another study, p-chlorophenylalanine, a specific depletor of serotonin, reduced the caffeine-induced locomotor stimulation in mice (Estler, 1973). There was no effect of α- or β-adrenergic blockers.

A variety of evidence links the *in vivo* central stimulatory effects of caffeine to an activation of the function of dopaminergic systems. Caffeine does affect dopamine turnover, but results have been contradictory, with either enhanced turnover, reduced turnover, or no effect seen in different paradigms (Daly, 1993; Nehlig *et al.*, 1992). Behaviorally, caffeine generalizes to putative dopaminergic agents, such as amphetamine and cocaine, in drug-discrimination paradigms (Daly, 1993), and has effects similar to dopamine agonists on rotation in rodents with contralateral lesions to dopaminergic pathways to the striatum (Casas, Ferré, Cobos, Grau, & Jane, 1989; Fredholm, Herrara-Marschwitz, Jonzon, Lindstrom, & Ungerstedt, 1983; Garrett & Holtzman, 1995). Antagonists for either D_1- and D_2-dopamine receptors block caffeine-elicited stimulation of locomotor activity (Garrett & Holtzman, 1994b). However, 6-hydroxydopamine–induced lesions that reduce responses to the dopaminergic drugs amphetamine and caffeine do not alter the locomotor response to caffeine (Joyce & Koob, 1981). Thus, caffeine probably does not affect such dopaminergic systems to a great extent by augmenting release of dopamine. Only antagonists for D_2-dopamine receptors block the effects of caffeine on rotation in rats with contralateral lesions to dopaminergic pathways (Garrett & Holtzman, 1995). While blockade of inhibitory A_1-adenosine receptors could be involved in effects of caffeine on dopaminergic reward–arousal systems, it now appears that the blockade of striatal A_{2A}-adenosine receptors and resultant enhancement of responses of co-localized D_2-dopamine receptors to dopamine plays a greater role (Fredholm *et al.*, 1997). Activation of striatal A_{2A}-adenosine receptors decreases the affinity of dopamine for D_2-receptors (Ferré, von Euler, Johansson, Fredholm, & Fuxe, 1991). Thus, blockade by caffeine of tonic input by adenosine to such A_{2A}-receptors would increase the potency of dopamine at co-localized D_2-receptors. In addition, it has been shown that A_1-adenosine receptor agonists inhibit the binding of dopamine agonists to D_1-dopamine receptors in striatal membranes (Ferré, Popoli, Tinner-Staines, & Fuxe, 1996). Thus, interactions of caffeine with both A_{2A}- and A_1-receptors could lead to inhibition of GABAergic function, resulting in activation of dopaminergic arousal–reward pathways (Ferré, Fuxe, von Euler, Johansson, & Fredholm, 1992; Fredholm *et al.*, 1997; Fuxe *et al.*, 1993; Mukhopadhyay & Poddar, 1995; Popoli *et al.*, 1996).

There have been limited studies on effects of caffeine on cholinergic systems, but caffeine does appear to increase turnover at acetylcholine in rodents (Carter, O'Conner, Carter, & Ungerstedt, 1995; Daly, 1993; Marcuson, Myers, & Johnson, 1994; Morton & Davies, 1997). Nicotinic receptors are stimulatory to dopamine release in striatum and an enhanced release of acetylcholine caused by caffeine could thus affect dopaminergic function. The interrelated functions of adenosine-dopamine-acetylcholine-GABA systems in the basal ganglia, in particular the striatum, is currently an active area of research with respect to the behavioral pharmacology of caffeine (Fredholm *et al.*, 1997).

Interactions with Other Centrally Active Agents

Caffeine can alter behavioral responses to a variety of centrally active agents and such interactions need to be considered as relevant to mechanisms underlying the pharmacology of caffeine.

Cocaine and Amphetamines

Caffeine can potentiate the behavioral stimulant responses in rodents to cocaine, an inhibitor of dopamine uptake, and to amphetamine, an agent that releases dopamine (Daly, 1993; Kuribara, 1994; Misra, Vadlamani, & Pontani, 1984). Caffeine appears capable of priming the dopaminergic cue that is important to cocaine abuse (Horger, Wellman, Morien, Davies, & Schenk, 1991). In humans, caffeine can enhance toxic effects of cocaine and amphetamine (Derlet, Tseng, & Albertson, 1992).

Nicotine

Caffeine reverses nicotine-elicited reductions in locomotor activity in rodents and actually appears to increase locomotor activity more when administered with nicotine than when administered alone (Cohen, Welzel, & Bättig, 1991; Sansone, Battaglia, & Castellano, 1994; White, 1994). In humans, there appears a strong correlation between consumption of caffeine and nicotine (Swanson, Lee, & Hopp, 1994). Caffeine appears to ameliorate some nicotine-withdrawal symptoms (Cohen, Pickworth, Bunker, & Henningfield, 1994).

Benzodiazepines

A variety of interactions of caffeine and benzodiazepines with respect to behavior have been noted (Daly, 1993). In general, it would appear that the effects of benzodiazepines, such as diazepam, are antagonized by caffeine (White, 1994). Certainly, benzodiazepams are sedative, while caffeine is somnolytic; benzodiazepines are anxiolytic and caffeine is anxiogenic.

Alcohol

Caffeine is widely considered to be beneficial in reducing alcohol-induced sedation and functional impairment. Data supporting this are not clear; both blockade and potentiation of the effects of alcohol have been observed in humans (White, 1994) and in animals (Dar, 1988). It has been suggested that sedative effects of ethanol are mediated through increased formation of adenosine (Dar, 1990). Chronic ingestion of caffeine by mice reduces the locomotor stimulant effects of ethanol (Daly, Shi, Wong, & Nikodijević,1994).

Morphine

Caffeine has been reported to inhibit the locomotor stimulant activity of morphine without affecting the antinociceptive effect (Oliverio, Castellano, Parone, & Vetulani, 1983), but has also been reported to enhance the locomotor stimulant effect of morphine (Kuribara, 1995). Both caffeine and theophylline can in some paradigms either augment or inhibit morphine-elicited analgesia (Daly, 1993; Sawynok & Yaksh, 1993). The role of caffeine as an analgetic adjuvant and the possible mechanism involved have been reviewed in detail (Sawynok & Yaksh, 1993). Blockade of peripheral hyperalgesic responses to adenosine, perhaps produced during inflammation, may underlie some of the effects of caffeine on pain perception. Centrally, caffeine could, through enhancing norepinephrine turnover, have analgesic action, while blockade of spinal adenosine receptors, activation of which causes analgesia, should result in hyperalgesia. Antinociceptive effects of caffeine in the formalin test appear dependent on blockade of A_1-adenosine receptors (Sawynok & Reid, 1996).

Chronic Effect of Caffeine

Chronic treatment with caffeine provides a strategy to explore what systems undergo homeostatic changes in response to the pharmacological action of the caffeine. Indeed, there have been extensive studies on the behavioral and biochemical changes after chronic ingestion or administration of caffeine or theophylline. Chronic caffeine has been reported to lead to "insurmountable" tolerance in some rodent paradigms (Finn & Holtzman, 1987; Garrett & Holtzman, 1995; Holtzman, Mante, & Minneman, 1991), but this is not always the case (Chou, Khan, Forde, & Hirsh, 1985; Kaplan, Greenblatt, Kent, & Cotreau-Bibbo, 1993; Nikodijević, Jacobson, & Daly, 1993c). Such an "insurmountable" tolerance has been proposed to be explicable in terms of the biphasic effects of caffeine in which tolerance to the stimulant effects of caffeine cannot be overcome by higher doses, since such higher doses would lead to the depressant high dose effects of caffeine (Daly, 1993; Daly, Shi, Nikodijević, & Jacobson, 1994). Certainly,

complete tolerance could not occur directly at adenosine receptors, which even if up-regulated, would still be subject to blockade by a competitive antagonist, such as caffeine. In caffeine-tolerant animals, caffeine is still able to reverse the depressant effects of adenosine analogs (Holtzman et al., 1991). It should be noted that the depressant effects of adenosine analogs may be related to hypothermia, which is readily reversed by caffeine and other xanthines (Seale et al., 1988). A complete tolerance to caffeine might also be due to downstream desensitization of a neurotransmitter receptor. Interestingly, a significant behavioral depression has been reported for mice during chronic ingestion of caffeine (Kaplan et al., 1993; Nikodijević et al., 1993c).

A wide range of receptors appear to have been either up-regulated or down-regulated after chronic ingestion of caffeine (Shi, Nikodijević, Jacobson, & Daly, 1993, 1994). In some cases, alterations in behavioral responses evoked by agonists or antagonists of such receptors have been documented. *In toto,* the alterations do not provide evidence as to sites of action of caffeine but only the systems affected. Such alterations could be interpreted as resulting from blockade of the normal tonic inhibitory influence of adenosine on neurotransmitter release and a resultant change in functional activity of various neurotransmitter pathways downstream of the synapses controlled by adenosine receptors.

There can be remarkable contrast between acute and chronic effects of adenosine receptor ligands, including caffeine (Jacobson, Von Lubitz, Daly, & Fredholm, 1996). Thus, acute administration of caffeine is normally considered to improve intellectual performance (Nehlig et al., 1992; Riedel et al., 1995), but chronic administration with a resultant up-regulation in adenosine-receptor function may well prove to be detrimental to intellectual performance. Chronic treatment with a very selective A_1-adenosine receptor antagonist 8-cyclopentyl-1,3-propylxanthine does appear to slightly impair memory acquisition in a water maze paradigm, while chronic treatment with A_1-selective adenosine agonist improves acquisition and memory retention (Von Lubitz, Paul, Bartus, & Jacobson, 1993). Another contrast between acute and chronic administration of caffeine involves effects on seizures. Thus, when administered acutely, caffeine is proconvulsant, while chronic caffeine or theophylline treatment protects against drug-induced convulsions (Georgiev, Johansson, & Fredholm, 1993; Jacobson et al., 1996). Similarly, while acute administration of caffeine or theophylline exacerbates neuronal damage induced by ischemia, chronic treatment with caffeine markedly protects against ischemic damage (Rudolphi, Keil, Fastbom, & Fredholm, 1989). It would appear likely that such "effect reversals" for caffeine following chronic administration may in some cases reflect an up-regulation in adenosine receptor function.

Adenosine

Biochemically, chronic treatment with caffeine or theophylline results in a wide range of alterations in receptor densities in rodents. Not unexpectedly, an up-regulation in levels of A_1-adenosine receptors occurs (Daly, 1993). However, there have been instances where lack of up-regulation of A_1-adenosine receptors has been reported after chronic caffeine (Holtzman et al., 1991; Kaplan et al., 1993). The mRNA for A_1-adenosine receptors can be unchanged even when receptor levels are increased (Johansson et al., 1993). Levels of A_1-adenosine receptors appeared to return to control levels from 4 to 15 days after cessation of caffeine (Boulenger & Marangos, 1989; Shi et al., 1993, 1994). Levels of the A_{2A}-adenosine receptor in striatum appear unchanged in some studies, but have been reported to be up-regulated in other studies (Traversa, Rosati, Florio, & Vertua, 1994). Behavioral alterations related to up-regulation of adenosine receptors include an enhancement of the behavioral depressant effects of adenosine analogs (Nikodijević et al., 1993b, 1993c; Shi et al., 1994). Behavioral responses to adenosine analogs appear enhanced after chronic caffeine in mice, but often not in rats (Daly, 1993). The analgetic potency of an adenosine analog is increased in mice after chronic caffeine (Ahlijanian & Takemori,

1986a). Chronic caffeine treatment in rats results in an enhancement of the inhibitory effects of an adenosine on activity of central neurons (Y. Lin & Phillis, 1990a). A_1-adenosine receptor levels in adipocytes are increased after chronic caffeine in rats, but the effects of adenosine analog on adenylate cyclase and lipolysis appear unaffected (Zhang & Wells, 1990). Activity of an adenosine analog as an inhibitor of platelet aggregation, mediated through an A_{2A}-adenosine receptor, is increased after chronic caffeine in rats, but so is the inhibitory effect of a prostaglandin (Zhang & Wells, 1990). A similar increase in sensitivity of platelets to an adenosine analog has been reported in humans (Biaggioni, Paul, Puckett, & Arzubiaga, 1991). In humans, chronic caffeine increases the hypotensive effects of adenosine (Von Borstel, Wurtman, & Conlay, 1983). Adenosine deaminase activity was reported to be increased in spleen and thymus after caffeine treatment in rats (Bandyopadhyay & Poddar, 1994).

Norepinephrine

Levels of β-adrenergic receptors in cortex and cerebellum are significantly down-regulated after chronic caffeine in rats and mice (Fredholm, Jonzon, & Lindgren, 1984; Goldberg, Curatolo, & Robertson, 1982; Shi et al., 1993) clearly indicating an enhanced functional activity of noradrenergic neurons. Levels of α_1- and α_2-adrenergic receptors are unaltered. Behavioral correlates of such down-regulation of β-adrenergic receptors after chronic caffeine does not appear to have been explored. There is a reduction in the stimulation of cyclic AMP production by a β-adrenergic agonist during withdrawal from chronic caffeine in humans (MacKenzie, Popkin, Dziubinski, & Sheppard, 1981).

Dopamine

Remarkably, since a variety of evidence indicates that caffeine affects dopaminergic functions (Daly, 1993; Fredholm et al., 1997), the levels of dopamine receptors in striatum appear unaffected after chronic ingestion of caffeine by mice (Shi et al., 1993, 1994).

There are also no apparent effects on striatal dopamine uptake sites or on stimulation of striatal adenylate cyclase by dopamine. Behaviorally, the stimulant effects of cocaine and amphetamine, two drugs that act via dopaminergic systems, are virtually unaltered after chronic caffeine ingestion by mice, although the threshold for behavioral stimulation for both drugs seems lowered (Nikodijević et al., 1993b, 1993c). Selective D_1- and D_2-dopamine receptor agonists were studied after chronic caffeine ingestion by rats (Garrett & Holtzman, 1994a). Tolerance to the locomotor stimulant effects of either a D_1-dopamine receptor agonist or D_2-dopamine receptor agonists was complete after chronic caffeine, but the rats were not tolerant to the synergistic stimulation of locomotor activity elicited by a combination of D_1- and D_2-receptor agonists.

Acetylcholine

Cerebral cortical levels of muscarinic receptors are significantly increased after chronic caffeine ingestion in mice (Shi et al., 1993, 1994), suggesting a reduced functional activity of the cholinergic neurons associated with such receptors. From a behavioral standpoint, the potency of the muscarinic antagonist scopolamine in stimulating locomotor activity in the mice is decreased, consonant with up-regulation of muscarinic receptors and function. The locomotor depressant effects of the muscarinic agonist oxotremorine are not significantly altered after chronic caffeine in mice (Shi et al., 1994). However, chronic caffeine in rats results in a reduction in the excitatory effects of acetylcholine, elicited via muscarinic receptors, on cerebral cortical neurons (Y. Lin & Phillis, 1990b). Nicotinic receptors and function appear to be desensitized after chronic caffeine ingestion in mice (Shi et al., 1993, 1994). Thus, levels of high-affinity (desensitized) $\alpha_4\beta_2$-nicotinic receptors are increased in cortex (but not in striatum) and the behavioral depression normally elicited by nicotine in these mice is virtually eliminated (Shi et al., 1994). A similar increase in high-affinity (desensitized) nicotinic receptors and tolerance to nicotine occurs after chronic

nicotine (Marks, Grady, & Collins, 1993). Mecamylamine, a nicotinic antagonist, causes a somewhat greater depression of locomotor activity after chronic caffeine (Shi et al., 1994).

Serotonin

Cerebral cortical levels of both 5-HT_1-serotonin and 5-HT_2-serotonin receptors are increased after chronic caffeine ingestion in mice (Shi et al., 1993, 1994). Behavioral correlates were not investigated. In another study, the effects of the serotonin precursor 5-hydroxytryptophan, the serotonin depletor p-chlorophenylalanine, and the serotonin antagonist methylsergide on caffeine-induced stimulation of locomotor activity led to the suggestion that tolerance to caffeine was related to an enhanced sensitivity of serotonin receptors (Ray & Poddar, 1990).

GABA

Cerebral cortical levels of diazepam-binding sites associated with GABA receptor-channels are increased after chronic caffeine ingestion in rats and mice (Shi et al., 1993, 1994; Wu & Coffin, 1984; Wu & Phillis, 1988). Relevant to such changes are the decreases in convulsant activity of agents that affect GABA systems that are seen after chronic caffeine (Daly, 1993). Chronic exposure of neurons from chick embryos with either caffeine or a benzodiazepine caused apparent "uncoupling" of GABA and benzodiazepine sites (Roca, Schiller, & Farb, 1988).

Glutamate

Cerebral cortical levels of dizocilpine (MK 801) binding sites associated with the NMDA glutamate receptors are unaltered after chronic caffeine ingestion in mice (Shi et al., 1993). It should be noted that dizocilpine does antagonize caffeine-induced convulsions (Toray & Kulkarni, 1991).

Opioids

Cerebral cortical levels of μ-opioid and κ-opioid receptors are unaltered, while δ-opioid receptors are increased after chronic ingestion of caffeine in mice (Shi *et al.*, 1994). Chronic treatment of mice with caffeine results in an increase in the potency of morphine as an analgetic (Ahlijanian & Takemori, 1986b).

Other Systems

There was no effect on so-called *sigma* receptors in cerebral cortex after caffeine ingestion in mice (Shi *et al.*, 1994). There is, however, a significant increase in nifedipine-binding sites associated with L-type calcium channels in mouse cerebral cortex (Shi *et al.*, 1994). Behavioral correlates of the apparent change in levels of L-type calcium channels apparently have not been reported. Central levels of the binding sites for forskolin that are associated with adenylate cyclase were reported to be increased in rats after chronic caffeine (Daval, Deckert, Weiss, Post, & Marangos, 1989).

Summary

It should be clear that in spite of an incredible amount of research directed toward defining the molecular mechanisms underlying the pharmacology of caffeine, completely satisfactory answers have not yet been obtained. The stimulatory behavioral effects of caffeine appear to reflect blockade of tonic input of endogenous adenosine to A_1- and A_{2A}-adenosine receptors associated with dopaminergic arousal–reward systems. However, the apparent effects of caffeine on striatal adenosine, dopamine, acetylcholine, and GABA systems are complex and difficult to define probably because of multiple sites of adenosine receptor blockade. At present, the blockade of striatal A_{2A}-adenosine receptors appears to be one major mechanism involved in the behavioral stimulation elicited by caffeine. The interactions of caffeine with adenosine analogs can be quite different from those expected from caffeine administered alone. Chronic caffeine and other xanthines through up-regulation or down-regulation of receptor function can have effects opposite to those seen on acute administration. It should be stressed that caffeine is not a particularly selective drug and levels

that would block adenosine receptors will also have some effects on calcium mobilization, phosphodiesterase activity, and GABA receptors. Such sites may be relevant to the negative behavioral effects of high doses of caffeine. There remains the possibility that there is some other unsuspected site at which caffeine, theophylline, and other xanthines act to exert pharmacological effects. Until such a site is discovered, blockade of adenosine receptors remains the most viable explanation for the pharmacological effects of caffeine at doses commonly attained in humans.

Acknowledgment

The past support of the International Life Science Institute for our research on "Mechanisms of Action of Caffeine and Theophylline" is gratefully acknowledged.

References

Ahlijanian, M. K., & Takemori, A. E. (1986a). Cross-tolerance studies between caffeine and (–)-N$_6$-(phenylisopropyl)adenosine (PIA) in mice. *Life Sciences, 88,* 577–588.

Ahlijanian, M. K., & Takemori, A. E. (1986b). The effect of chronic administration of caffeine on morphine-induced analgesia, tolerance and dependence in mice. *European Journal of Pharmacology, 120,* 25–32.

Anderson, R., Sheehan, M. J., & Strong, P. (1994). Characterization of the adenosine receptors mediating hypothermia in the conscious mouse. *British Journal of Pharmacology, 113,* 1386–1390.

Axelsson, J., & Thesleff, S. (1958). Activation of the contractile mechanism in striated muscle. *Acta Physiologica Scandinavica, 44,* 55–66.

Baldwin, H. A., & File, S. E. (1989). Caffeine-induced anxiogenesis: The role of the adenosine, benzodiazepine and noradrenergic receptors. *Pharmacology, Biochemistry and Behavior, 32,* 181–186.

Bandyopadhyay, B. C., & Poddar, M. K. (1994). Caffeine-induced increase in adenosine deaminase activity in mammalian lymphoid organs. *Methods and Findings in Experimental and Clinical Pharmacology, 16,* 731–733.

Barraco, R. A., Coffin, V. L., Altman, H. J., & Phillis, J. W. (1983). Central effects of adenosine analogs on locomotor activity in mice and antagonism of caffeine. *Brain Research, 272,* 392–395.

Berkowitz, B. A., Tarver, J. H., & Spector, S. (1970). Release of norepinephrine in the central nervous system by theophylline and caffeine. *European Journal of Pharmacology, 10,* 64–71.

Biaggioni, I., Paul, S., Puckett, A., & Arzubiaga, C. (1991). Caffeine and theophylline as adenosine receptor antagonists in humans. *Journal of Pharmacology and Experimental Therapeutics, 258,* 588–593.

Bianchi, C. P. (1961). Effects of caffeine on radiocalcium movement in the frog sartorius. *Journal of General Physiology, 44,* 845–858.

Boulenger, J.-P., & Marangos, P. J. (1989). Caffeine withdrawal affects central adenosine receptors but not benzodiazepine receptors. *Journal of Neural Transmission, 78,* 9–19.

Brackett, L. E., Shamim, M. T., & Daly, J. W. (1990). Activities of caffeine, theophylline, and enprofylline analogs as tracheal relaxants. *Biochemical Pharmacology, 39,* 1897–1904.

Carter, A. J., O'Conner, W. T., Carter, M. J., & Ungerstedt. U. (1995). Caffeine enhances acetylcholine release in the hippocampus in vivo by a selective interaction with adenosine A$_1$ receptors. *Journal Pharmacology and Experimental Therapeutics, 273,* 637–642.

Casas, M., Ferré, S., Cobos, A., Grau, J. A., & Jane, F. (1989). Relationship between rotational behavior induced by apomorphine and caffeine in rats with unilateral lesion of the nigrostriatal pathway. *Neuropharmacology, 28,* 407–409.

Choi, O. H., Shamim, M. T., Padgett, W. L., & Daly, J. W. (1988). Caffeine and theophylline analogues: Correlation of behavioral effects with activity as adenosine receptor antagonists and as phosphodiesterase inhibitors. *Life Sciences, 43,* 387–398.

Chou, D. T., Khan, S., Forde, J., & Hirsh, K. R. (1985). Caffeine tolerance: Behavioral, electrophysiological and neurochemical evidence. *Life Sciences, 36,* 2347–2358.

Coffin, V. L., Taylor, J. A., Phillis, J. W., Altman, H. J., & Barraco, R. A. (1984). Behavioral interaction of adenosine and methylxanthines on central purinergic systems. *Neuroscience Letters, 47,* 91–98.

Cohen, C., Welzel, H., & Bättig, K. (1991). Effects of nicotine, caffeine, and their combination on locomotor activity in rats. *Pharmacology, Biochemistry and Behavior, 40,* 121–123.

Cohen, C., Pickworth, W. B., Bunker, E. B., & Henningfield, J. E. (1994). Caffeine antagonizes EEG effects of tobacco withdrawal. *Pharmacology, Biochemistry and Behavior, 47,* 919–926.

Conlay, L. A., Conant, J. A., deBros, F., & Wurtman, R. (1997). Caffeine alters plasma adenosine levels. *Nature, 389,* 136.

Daly, J. W. (1993). Mechanism of action of caffeine. In S. Garrattini (Ed.), *Caffeine, coffee and health* (pp 97–150). New York: Raven.

Daly, J. W., & Jacobson, K. A. (1995). Adenosine Receptors: Selective agonists and antagonists. In L. Belardinelli & A. Pelleg (Eds.), *Adenosine and adenine nucleotides: Molecular biology to integrative physiology* (pp. 157–166). Boston: Kluwer Academic.

Daly, J. W., Padgett, W., Shamim, M. T., Butts-Lamb, P., & Waters, J. (1985). 1,3-Dialkyl-8-(p-sulfophenyl)-xanthines: Potent water soluble antagonists for A$_1$- and A$_2$-adenosine receptors. *Journal of Medicinal Chemistry, 28,* 487–492.

Daly, J. W., Shi, D., Nikodijević, O., & Jacobson, K. A. (1994). The role of adenosine receptors in the central action of caffeine. *Pharmacopsychoecologia, 7,* 201–213.

Daly, J. W., Shi, D., Wong, V., & Nikodijević, O. (1994). Chronic effects of ethanol on central adenosine function of mice. *Brain Research, 650,* 153–156.

Dar, M. S. (1988). The biphasic effects of centrally and peripherally administered caffeine on ethanol-induced motor incoordination in mice. *Journal of Pharmacy and Pharmacology, 40,* 482–487.

Dar, M. S. (1990). Central adenosinergic system involvement in ethanol-induced motor incoordination in mice. *Journal of Pharmacology and Experimental Therapeutics, 255,* 1202–1209.

Daval, J. I., Deckert, J., Weiss, S. R. B., Post, R. M., & Marangos, P. J. (1989). Up-regulation of adenosine A$_1$ receptors and forskolin binding sites following chronic treatment with caffeine or carbamazepine: A quantitative autoradiographic study. *Epilepsia, 30,* 26–33.

Derlet, R. W., Tseng, J. C., & Albertson, T. E. (1992). Potentiation of cocaine and d-amphetamine toxicity with caffeine. *American Journal of Emergency Medicine, 10,* 211–216.

Dixon, A. K., Widdowson, L., & Richardson, P. J. (1997). Desensitization of the adenosine A$_1$ receptor by the A$_{2A}$ receptor in the rat striatum. *Journal of Neurochemistry, 69,* 315–3321.

Durcan, M., & Morgan, P. F. (1989). Evidence for A$_2$ receptor involvement in the hypomotility effects of adenosine analogs in mice. *European Journal of Pharmacology, 168,* 285–290.

Durcan, M. J., & Morgan, P. F. (1991). Hypothermic effects of alkylxanthines: Evidence for a calcium-independent phosphodiesterase action. *European Journal of Pharmacology, 204,* 15–20.

Ehrlich, B. E., Kaftan, E., Bezprozvannayan, S., & Bezprozvanny, I. (1994). The pharmacology of intracellular Ca^{2+}-release channels. *Trends in Pharmacological Sciences, 15,* 145–148.

Estler, C. J. (1973). Effect of α- and β-adrenergic blocking agents and parachlorophenylalanine on morphine- and caffeine-stimulated locomotor activity of mice. *Psychopharmacologia, 28,* 261–268.

Ferré, S., von Euler, G., Johansson, B., Fredholm, B. B., & Fuxe, K. (1991). Stimulation of high affinity A$_2$ receptors decreases the affinity of dopamine D$_2$ receptors in rat striatal membranes. *Proceedings of the National Academy of Sciences USA, 88,* 7237–7241.

Ferré, S., Fuxe, K., von Euler, G., Johansson, B., & Fredholm, B. B. (1992). Adenosine–dopamine interactions in the brain. *Neuroscience, 51,* 501–512.

Ferré, S., O'Conner, W. T., Svenningsson, P., Bjorklund, L., Lindberg, J., Tinner, B., Stromberg, I., Goldstein, M., Ogren, S. O., Ungerstedt, U., Fredholm, B. B., & Fuxe, K. (1996). Dopamine D_1 receptor-mediated facilitation of GABAergic neurotransmission in the rat strioentopenduncular pathway and its modulation by adenosine A_1 receptor-mediated mechanisms. *European Journal of Neuroscience, 8,* 1545–1553.

Ferré, S., Popoli, P., Tinner-Staines, B., & Fuxe, K. (1996). Adenosine A_1 receptor-dopamine interaction in the rat limbic system: Modulation of dopamine D_1 receptor antagonist binding sites. *Neuroscience Letters, 208,* 109–112.

Finn, I. B., & Holtzman, S. G. (1987). Pharmacologic specificity of tolerance to caffeine-induced stimulation of locomotor activity. *Psychopharmacology, 93,* 428–434.

Finn, I. B., Iuvone, P. M., & Holtzman, S. G. (1990). Depletion of catecholamines in the brain of rats differentially affects stimulation of locomotor activity by caffeine, D-amphetamine, and methylphenidate. *Neuropharmacology, 29,* 625–631.

Francis, A., & Fochtmann, L. (1994). Caffeine augmentation of electroconvulsive seizures. *Psychopharmacology, 110,* 320–323.

Frank, G. B. (1960). Effect of changes in extracellular calcium concentration on the potassium-induced contracture of frog's skeletal muscle. *Journal of Physiology, 151,* 518–538.

Fredholm, B. B., & Lindgren, E. (1983). Inhibition of soluble 5'-nucleotidase from rat brain by different xanthine derivatives. *Biochemical Pharmacology, 32,* 2832–2834.

Fredholm, B. B., Herrara-Marschwitz, M., Jonzon, B., Lindstrom, K., & Ungerstedt, U. (1983). On the mechanism by which methylxanthines enhance apomorphine-induced rotation in the rat. *Pharmacology, Biochemistry and Behavior, 19,* 535–54.

Fredholm, B. B., Jonzon, B., & Lindgren, E. (1984). Changes in noradrenaline release and in beta receptor number in rat hippocampus following long-term treatment with theophylline or L-phenylisopropyladenosine. *Acta Physiologica Scandinavica, 122,* 55–59.

Fredholm, B. B., Arslan, G., Johansson, B., Kull, B., & Svenningsson, P. (1997). Adenosine A_{2A} receptors and the actions of caffeine. In Y. Okada (Ed.), *The role of adenosine in the nervous system* (pp. 51–74). Amsterdam: Elsevier Science.

Fuxe, K., Ferré, S., Snaprud, P., von Euler, G., Johansson, B., & Fredholm, B. B. (1993). Antagonistic A_{2a}/D_2 receptor interactions in the striatum as a basis for adenosine/dopamine interactions in the central nervous system. *Drug Development Research, 28,* 374–380.

Garrett, B. E., & Holtzman, S. G. (1994a). Caffeine cross-tolerance to selective dopamine D_1 and D_2 receptor agonists but not to their synergistic interaction. *European Journal of Pharmacology, 262,* 65–75.

Garrett, B. E., & Holtzman, S. G. (1994b). D_1 and D_2 dopamine receptor antagonists block caffeine-induced stimulation of locomotor activity in rats. *Pharmacology, Biochemistry and Behavior, 47,* 89–94.

Garrett, B. E., & Holtzman, S. G. (1995). Does adenosine receptor blockade mediate caffeine-induced rotational behavior? *Journal of Pharmacology and Experimental Therapeutics, 274,* 207–214.

Georgiev, V., Johansson, B., & Fredholm, B. B. (1993). Long-term caffeine treatment leads to a decreased susceptibility to NMDA-induced clonic seizures in mice without a change in adenosine A_1 receptor number. *Brain Research, 612,* 271–277.

Goldberg, M. R., Curatolo, P. W., & Robertson, D. (1982). Caffeine down regulates β-adrenoceptors in rat forebrain. *Neuroscience Letters, 31,* 47–51.

Griffiths, R. R., & Mumford, G. K. (1996). Caffeine reinforcement, discrimination, tolerance and physical dependence in laboratory animals and humans. In C. R. Schuster & M. J. Kuhar (Eds.), *Handbook of experimental pharmacology* (pp. 315–341). Heidelberg, Germany: Springer-Verlag.

Holloway, F. A., Modrow, H. E., & Michaelis, R. C. (1985). Methylxanthine discrimination in the rat: Possible benzodiazepine and adenosine mechanisms. *Pharmacology, Biochemistry and Behavior, 22,* 815–824.

Holtzman, S. G. (1986). Discriminative stimulus properties of caffeine in the rat: Noradrenergic mediation. *Journal of Pharmacology and Experimental Therapeutics, 239,* 706–714.

Holtzman, S. G., Mante, S., & Minneman, K. P. (1991). Role of adenosine receptors in caffeine tolerance. *Journal of Pharmacology and Experimental Therapeutics, 256,* 62–68.

Horger, B. A., Wellman, P. J., Morien, A., Davies, B. T., & Schenk, S. (1991). Caffeine exposure sensitizes rats to the reinforcing effects of cocaine. *Neuroreport, 2,* 53–56.

Imaizumi, M., Miyazaki, S., & Onodera, K. (1994). Effects of xanthine derivatives in a light/dark test in mice and contribution of adenosine receptors. *Methods and Findings in Experimental and Clinical Pharmacology, 16,* 639–644.

Jacobson, K. A., Von Lubitz, D. K. J. E., Daly, J. W., & Fredholm, B. B. (1996). Adenosine receptor ligands: Differences with acute versus chronic treatment. *Trends in Pharmacological Sciences, 17,* 108–113.

Jain, N., Kemp, N., Adeyemo, O., Buchanan, P., & Stone, T. W. (1995). Anxiolytic activity of adenosine receptor activation in mice. *British Journal of Pharmacology, 116,* 2127–2133.

Johansson, B., Ahlberg, S., van der Ploeg, I., Brene, S., Lindefors, N., Persson, H., & Fredholm, B. B. (1993). Effect on long term caffeine treatment on A_1 and A_2 adenosine receptor binding and on mRNA levels in rat brain. *Naunyn-Schmideberg's Archives of Pharmacology, 347,* 407–414.

Joyce, E. M., & Koob, G. F. (1981). Amphetamine-, scopolamine- and caffeine-induced locomotor activity following 6-hydroxydopamine lesions in the mesolimbic dopamine system. *Psychopharmacology, 73*, 311–313.

Kaplan, G. B., Greenblatt, D. J., Kent, M. A., Cotreau, M. M., Arcelin, G., & Shader, R. I. (1992). Caffeine-induced behavioral stimulation is dose-dependent and associated with A_1 adenosine receptor occupancy. *Neuropsychopharmacology, 6*, 145–153.

Kaplan, G. B., Greenblatt, D. J., Kent, M. A., & Cotreau-Bibbo, M. M. (1993). Caffeine treatment and withdrawal in mice: Relationships between dosage, concentrations, locomotor activity and A_1 adenosine receptor binding. *Journal of Pharmacology and Experimental Therapeutics, 266*, 1563–1572.

Kaplan, G. B., Greenblatt, D. J., Leduc, B. W., Thompson, M. L., & Shader, R. I. (1989). Relationship of plasma and brain concentrations of caffeine and metabolites to benzodiazepine receptor binding and locomotor activity. *Journal of Pharmacology and Experimental Therapeutics, 248*, 1078–1083.

Katims, J. J., Annau, Z., & Snyder, S. H. (1983). Interactions in the behavioral effects of methylxanthines and adenosine derivatives. *Journal of Pharmacology and Experimental Therapeutics, 227*, 167–173.

Kuribara, H. (1994). Caffeine enhances the stimulant effects of methamphetamine, but may not affect induction of methamphetamine sensitization of ambulation in mice. *Psychopharmacology, 116*, 125–129.

Kuribara, H. (1995). Caffeine enhances acute stimulant effect of morphine but inhibits morphine sensitization when assessed by ambulation of mice. *Progress Neuropsychopharmacology, 19*, 313–321.

Kuribara, H., & Tadokoro, S. (1992). Behavioral effects of cocoa and its main active compound theobromine: Evaluation by ambulatory activity and discrete avoidance in mice. *Japanese Journal of Alcohol and Drug Dependence, 27*, 168–179.

LeBlanc, J., Richard, D., & Racotta, I. S. (1995). Metabolic and hormone-related responses to caffeine in rats. *Pharmacological Research, 32*, 129–134.

Lin, M. T., Chandra, A., & Lui, G. G. (1980). The effects of theophylline and caffeine on thermoregulatory functions of rats at different ambient temperatures. *Journal of Pharmacy and Pharmacology, 32*, 204–208.

Lin, Y., & Phillis, J. W. (1990a). Chronic caffeine exposure enhances adenosinergic inhibition of cerebral cortical neurons. *Brain Research, 520*, 322–323.

Lin, Y., & Phillis, J. W. (1990b). Chronic caffeine exposure reduces the excitant action of acetylcholine on cerebral cortical neurons. *Brain Research, 524*, 316–318.

Lopez, F., Miller, L. G., Greenblatt, D. J., Kaplan, G. B., & Shader, R. I. (1989). Interaction of caffeine with the $GABA_A$ receptor complex: Alterations in receptor function but not ligand binding. *European Journal of Pharmacology, 172*, 453–459.

MacKenzie, T. B., Popkin, M. K., Dziubinski, J., & Sheppard, J. R. (1981). Effects of caffeine withdrawal on isoproterenol-stimulated cyclic adenosine monophosphate. *Clinical Pharmacology and Therapeutics, 30*, 436–438.

Marangos, P. J., Paul, S. M., Parma, A. M., Goodwin, F. K., Syapin, P., & Skolnick, P. (1979). Purinergic inhibition of diazepam binding to rat brain (*in vitro*). *Life Sciences, 24*, 851–858.

Marangos, P. J., Martino, A. M., Paul, S. M., & Skolnick, P. (1981). The benzodiazepines and inosine antagonize caffeine induced seizures. *Psychopharmacology, 72*, 269–273.

Marcuson, D. E., Myers, J. P., & Johnson, D. A. (1994). The role of caffeine in the modulation of neurotransmission in the brain. *Pharmacopsychoecologia, 7*, 109–117.

Marks, M. J., Grady, S. R., & Collins, A. C. (1993). Down regulation of nicotinic receptor function after chronic nicotine infusion. *Journal of Pharmacology and Experimental Therapeutics, 266*, 1268–1276.

Mehta, A. K., & Kulkarni, S. K. (1983). Effect of purinergic substances on rectal temperature in mice: Involvement of P1-purinoceptors. *Archives Internationales de Pharmacodynamie et de Therapie, 264*, 180–186.

Misra, A. L., Vadlamani, N. L., & Pontani, R. B. (1984). Effect of caffeine on cocaine locomotor stimulant activity in rats. *Pharmacology, Biochemistry and Behavior, 24*, 761–764.

Miyamoto, K., Kurita, M., Ohmae, S., Sakai, R., Sanae, F., & Takagi, K. (1994). Selective tracheal relaxation and phosphodiesterase-IV inhibition by xanthine derivatives. *European Journal of Pharmacology, 267*, 317–322.

Moraidis, I., & Bingmann, D. (1994). Epileptogenic actions of xanthines in relation to their affinities for adenosine A_1 receptors in CA3 neurons of hippocampal slices (guinea pigs). *Brain Research, 640*, 140–145.

Morton, R. A., & Davies, C. H. (1997). Regulation of muscarinic acetylcholine receptor-mediated synaptic responses by adenosine in the rat hippocampus. *Journal of Physiology* (London), *502*, 75–90.

Mueller, K., Saboda, S., Palmour, R., & Nyhan, W. L. (1982). Self-injurious behavior produced in rats by daily caffeine and continuous amphetamine. *Pharmacology, Biochemistry and Behavior, 17*, 613–617.

Mukhopadhyay, S., & Poddar, J. K. (1995). Caffeine-induced locomotor activity: Possible involvement of GABAergic-dopaminergic-adenosine interaction. *Neurochemical Research, 20*, 39–44.

Müller, C. E., & Daly, J. W. (1993). Stimulation of calcium release by caffeine analogs in pheochromocytoma cells. *Biochemical Pharmacology, 46*, 1825–1829.

Nehlig, A. (1994). Caffeine, brain energy metabolism and blood flow: A basis for understanding the behavioral effects of the methylxanthines. *Pharmacopsychoecologia, 7*, 97–107.

Nehlig, A., Daval, J.-L., Boyet, S., & Vert, P. (1986). Comparative effects of acute and chronic administration of caffeine on local cerebral glucose utilization in the conscious rat. *European Journal of Pharmacology, 129*, 93–103.

Nehlig, A., Daval, J.-L., & Debry, G. (1992). Caffeine and the central nervous system: Mechanisms of action, biochemical, metabolic and psychostimulant effects. *Brain Research Reviews, 17*, 139–170.

Nikodijević, O., Sarges, R., Daly, J. W., & Jacobson, K. A. (1991). Behavioral effects of A_1- and A_2-selective adenosine agonists and antagonists: Evidence for synergism and antagonism. *Journal of Pharmacology and Experimental Therapeutics, 259*, 286–294.

Nikodijević, O., Jacobson, K. A., & Daly, J. W. (1993a). Acute treatment of mice with high doses of caffeine: An animal model for choreiform movement. *Drug Development Research, 30*, 121–128.

Nikodijević, O., Jacobson, K. A., & Daly, J. W. (1993b). Effects of combinations of methylxanthines and adenosine analogs on locomotor activity in control and chronic caffeine-treated mice. *Drug Development Research, 30*, 104–110.

Nikodijević, O., Jacobson, K. A., & Daly, J. W. (1993c). Locomotor activity in mice during chronic treatment with caffeine and withdrawal. *Pharmacology, Biochemistry and Behavior, 44*, 199–216.

Oliverio, A., Castellano, C., Parone, F., & Vetulani, J. (1983). Caffeine interferes with morphine-induced hyperactivity but not analgesia. *Polish Journal of Pharmacology and Pharmacy, 35*, 336–346.

Poisner, A. M. (1973). Caffeine-induced catecholamine secretion: Similarity to caffeine-induced muscle contraction. *Proceedings of the Society for Experimental Biology and Medicine, 142*, 102–105.

Popoli, P., Giménez-Llort, L., Pezzola, A., Reggio, R., Martínez, E., Fuxe, K., & Ferré, S. (1996). Adenosine A_1 receptor blockade selectivity potentiates the motor effects induced by dopamine D_1 receptor stimulation in rodents. *Neuroscience Letters, 218*, 209–213.

Rall, T. W., & Sutherland, E. W. (1958). Fractionation and characterization of a cyclic adenine ribonucleotide formed by tissue particles. *Journal of Biological Chemistry, 232*, 1077–1091.

Ray, S. K., & Poddar, M. K. (1990). Role of central serotonin in caffeine-induced stimulation of locomotor activity in rat. *Biogenic Amines, 7*, 153–164.

Riedel, W., Hogervorst., E., Leboux, R., Verhey, F., van Praag, L., & Jollos, J. (1995). Caffeine alters scopolamine-induced memory impairment in humans. *Psychopharmacology, 122*, 158–168.

Roca, D. J., Schiller, G. D., & Farb, D. H. (1988). Chronic caffeine or theophylline exposure reduces γ-aminobutyric acid/benzodiazepine receptor site interactions. *Molecular Pharmacology, 33*, 481–485.

Rudolphi, K. A., Keil, M., Fastbom, J., & Fredholm, B. B. (1989). Ischaemic damage in gerbil hippocampus is reduced following up-regulation of adenosine (A_1)

receptors by caffeine treatment. *Neuroscience Letters, 103*, 275–280.

Sansone, M., Battaglia, M., & Castellano, C. (1994). Effect of caffeine and nicotine on avoidance learning in mice: Lack of interaction. *Journal of Pharmacy and Pharmacology, 46*, 765–767.

Sattin, A., & Rall, T. W. (1970). The effect of adenosine and adenine nucleotides on the cyclic adenosine $3',5'$-phosphate content of guinea pig cerebral cortex slices. *Molecular Pharmacology, 6*, 13–23.

Sawynok, J., & Reid, A. (1996). Caffeine antinociception: Role of formalin concentration and A_1 and A_2 receptors. *European Journal of Pharmacology 298*, 105–111.

Sawynok, J., & Yaksh, T. L. (1993). Caffeine as an analgesic adjuvant: A review of pharmacology and mechanisms of action. *Pharmacological Reviews, 45*, 43–85.

Seale, T. W., Abla, K. A., Shamim, M. T., Carney, J. M., & Daly, J. W. (1988). 3,7-Dimethyl-1-propargylxanthine: A potent and selective in vivo antagonist of adenosine analogs. *Life Sciences, 43*, 1671–1684.

Shi, D., Nikodijević, O., Jacobson, K. A., & Daly, J. W. (1993). Chronic caffeine alters the density of A_1-adenosine, β-adrenergic, serotonin, cholinergic, and GABA$_A$ receptors and calcium channels in mouse brain. *Cellular and Molecular Neurobiology, 13*, 247–261.

Shi, D., Nikodijević, O., Jacobson, K. A., & Daly, J. W. (1994). Effects of chronic caffeine on adenosine, dopamine and acetylcholine systems in mice. *Archives Internationales de Pharmacodynamie et de Therapie, 328*, 261–287.

Snyder, S. H., Katims, J. J., Annau, Z., Bruns, R. F., & Daly, J. W. (1981). Adenosine receptors and behavioral actions of methylxanthines. *Proceedings of the National Academy of Sciences USA, 78*, 3260–3264.

Svenningsson, P., Strom, A., Johansson, B., & Fredholm, B. B. (1995). Increased expression of C-*jun, jun* B, AP-1 and preproenkephalin mRNA in rat striatum following a single injection of caffeine. *Journal of Neuroscience, 15*, 3583–3593.

Svenningsson, P., LeMoine, C., Kull, B., Sunahara, R., Bloch, B., & Fredholm, B. B. (1997). Antagonism of adenosine A_{2A} receptors underlies the behavioral activating effect of caffeine and is associated with reduced expression of messenger RNA for NGFI-A and NGFI-B in caudate-putamen and nucleus accumbens. *Neuroscience, 79*, 753–764.

Swanson, J. A., Lee, J. W., & Hopp, J. W. (1994). Caffeine and nicotine. A review of their joint use and possible interactive effects in tobacco withdrawal. *Addictive Behavior, 19*, 229–256.

Toray, S. N., & Kulkarni, S. K. (1991). Antagonism of caffeine-induced convulsions by ethanol and dizocilpine (MK-801) in mice. *Methods and Findings in Experimental and Clinical Pharmacology, 13*, 413–417.

Traversa, U., Rosati, A. M., Florio, C., & Vertua, R. (1994). Effects of chronic administration of adenosine antagonists on adenosine A_1 and A_{2A} receptors in mouse brain. *In Vivo, 8,* 1073–1078.

Ukena, D., Schudt, C., & Sybrecht, G. W. (1993). Adenosine receptor-blocking xanthines as inhibitors of phosphodiesterase isozymes. *Biochemical Pharmacology, 45,* 847–851.

Virus, R. M., Ticho, S., Pildtich, M., & Radulovacki, M. (1990). A comparison of the effects of caffeine, cyclopentyltheophylline, and alloxazine on sleep in rats: Possible roles of central nervous system adenosine receptors. *Neuropsychopharmacology, 3,* 243–249.

Von Borstel, R. W., Wurtman, R. J., & Conlay, L. A. (1983). Chronic caffeine consumption potentiates the hypotensive action of circulating adenosine. *Life Sciences, 32,* 1151–1158.

Von Lubitz, D. K. J. E., Paul, I. A., Bartus, R. T., & Jacobson, K. A. (1993). Effects of chronic administration of adenosine A_1 receptor agonist and antagonist on spatial learning and memory. *European Journal of Pharmacology, 249,* 271–280.

White, J. M. (1994). Behavioral effects of caffeine coadministered with nicotine, benzodiazepines and alcohol. *Pharmacopsychoecologia, 7,* 119–126.

Wu, P. H., & Coffin, V. L. (1984). Up-regulation of brain [^{3}H]diazepam binding sites in chronic caffeine-treated rats. *Brain Research, 294,* 186–189.

Wu, P. H., & Phillis, J. W. (1988). Up-regulation of brain [^{3}H]diazepam binding sites in chronic caffeine treated rats. *General Pharmacology, 17,* 501–503.

Zhang, Y., & Wells, J. M. (1990). Effects of chronic administration on peripheral adenosine receptors. *Journal of Pharmacology and Experimental Therapeutics, 254,* 270–276.

5

Behavioral Pharmacology of Caffeine

SUZETTE M. EVANS

Introduction

Caffeine, a central nervous system (CNS) stimulant, is the most widely used psychotropic drug in the world (Gilbert, 1984). In the United States, more than 85% of adults consume caffeine daily (Gilbert, 1976; Graham, 1978) and the average daily consumption is estimated to be 200 mg (Barone & Roberts, 1984). Caffeine is found in a wide variety of beverages (e.g., coffee, tea, colas), prescription drugs and over-the-counter stimulants, analgesics and cold preparations, and food items such as chocolate. Caffeine has been considered to be a model drug for studying and understanding drugs of abuse (Holtzman, 1990; Rush, Sullivan, & Griffiths, 1995), in part due to caffeine's widespread use, and because caffeine produces a range of behavioral effects that are common to classic drugs of abuse.

This chapter will focus specifically on those behavioral effects shared with drugs of abuse: subjective (and discriminative) effects, reinforcing effects, development of tolerance, and physical dependence. This chapter is not intended to be a comprehensive review of the entire range of caffeine's behavioral effects; it is

designed to provide an overview of the numerous advances made in this area and emphasize the important role caffeine plays in the lives of many individuals. Specific aspects of caffeine are intentionally ignored in this chapter. For instance, neither caffeine's mechanism of action nor its effects on cognition and performance are reviewed. Further, the interaction of caffeine with other drugs is not reviewed here; that topic warrants a separate discussion. Readers are referred to several excellent review papers regarding the various behavioral aspects of caffeine (Bättig & Welzl, 1993; Griffiths & Mumford, 1995, 1996; Griffiths & Woodson, 1988a, 1988c; Nehlig, Daval, & Debry, 1992).

Subjective and Discriminative Stimulus Effects of Caffeine

Discriminative Stimulus Effects of Caffeine in Animals

Over the past 35 years, drug discrimination procedures have been developed to examine the discriminative stimulus (DS) effects, or interoceptive cues, of psychoactive drugs in animals. The traditional drug discrimination procedure involves training animals to respond differentially under two different drug conditions. For example, animals are reinforced (usually with food) for responding on one lever following administration of a stimulant

SUZETTE M. EVANS • The New York State Psychiatric Institute, New York, New York 10032.

Handbook of Substance Abuse: Neurobehavioral Pharmacology, edited by Tarter *et al.* Plenum Press, New York, 1998.

and on another lever following administration of the drug vehicle (usually saline). A wide range of species can be trained to discriminate between psychotropic drugs and a striking concordance has been found between drug classes formed on the basis of similarities in the subjective effects produced in humans and those formed on the basis of similarities as DS in animals (Kamien, Bickel, Hughes, Higgins, & Smith, 1993; Schuster & Johanson, 1988; Schuster, Fischman, & Johanson, 1981).

Several early studies were either unsuccessful at training caffeine as a DS (Overton, 1973) or could establish the discrimination at only high caffeine doses of 125 mg/kg using a shock-escape procedure (Overton & Batta, 1977). Winter (1981) was one of the first to establish a reliable caffeine versus saline discrimination in rats using a training dose of 60 mg/kg. Rats acquired the discrimination within 11–32 training sessions (average of 22 sessions). In the same year, another group showed that rats could learn to discriminate 32 mg/kg caffeine from saline (Modrow, Holloway, & Carney, 1981; Modrow, Holloway, Christensen, & Carney, 1981). Further, Modrow, Holloway, and Carney (1981) showed that caffeine-appropriate responding corresponded to increasing caffeine plasma levels, but caffeine-appropriate responding dropped off rapidly even though caffeine plasma levels were still elevated. Subsequently, numerous studies have been able to establish caffeine as a DS at similar and lower doses and all of the studies to date have used rats (e.g., Holtzman, 1986; Modrow & Holloway, 1985; Mumford & Holtzman, 1991).

A range of xanthines related to caffeine have been tested in animals trained to discriminate caffeine from saline. In rats trained to discriminate a relatively high dose of caffeine (60 mg/kg), the xanthine aminophylline completely substituted for caffeine (Winter, 1981). Several studies have demonstrated that theophylline also substitutes for caffeine in rats trained to discriminate 32 mg/kg caffeine from saline (Carney, Holloway, & Modrow, 1985; Modrow & Holloway, 1985; Modrow, Holloway, & Carney, 1981) and, similarly, caffeine cross-substitutes for theophylline (Carney

et al., 1985). Other methylxanthines shared DS effects with caffeine, although theobromine did not (Carney *et al.,* 1985). Interestingly, in rats trained to discriminate either 10 or 30 mg/kg caffeine, a range of methylxanthine drugs did not share DS effects with caffeine (Holtzman, 1986). In that same study, theophylline substituted only partially for caffeine and this was most evident in the group trained to discriminate 30 mg/kg caffeine. Somewhat different results were obtained in another study by the same laboratory (Mumford & Holtzman, 1991). This study trained rats to discriminate either 10 or 56 mg/kg caffeine from saline and several xanthines completely substituted (including theophylline) for the lower training dose of caffeine. In contrast, the only xanthine to share DS effects with the higher training dose of caffeine was theophylline, and these findings did not appear to be a result of tolerance development in rats trained to discriminate 56 mg/kg. Of note, animals trained to the lower dose in the study by Mumford and Holtzman (1991) took twice as long to acquire the discrimination compared with animals trained to the higher dose, although the sessions to criteria for the 10 mg/kg dose was substantially longer than in a previous study that used the same training dose (Holtzman, 1986). Taken together, the ability of other xanthines to share DS effects with caffeine may depend on the training dose of caffeine.

Psychomotor stimulants have been shown to share some DS effects with caffeine, although the results across studies have been inconsistent. Several studies have demonstrated that *d*-amphetamine (Modrow & Holloway, 1985; Modrow, Holloway, & Carney, 1981), methylphenidate, and nicotine (Modrow, Holloway, & Carney, 1981) do not share DS effects with caffeine in rats trained to discriminate 32 mg/kg caffeine from saline. Other studies have shown that *d*-amphetamine (Winter, 1981) or cocaine (Mariathasan & Stolerman, 1992) partially substitutes for caffeine. In another study, the ability of psychomotor stimulants, including *d*-amphetamine, methylphenidate, and cocaine, to substitute for caffeine depended on the training dose (Mumford & Holtzman, 1991).

These stimulants shared DS effects with the low training dose (10 mg/kg), but not the high training dose (56 mg/kg) of caffeine, suggesting that the discrimination is based on behavioral stimulation. However, in a previous study (Holtzman, 1986), both methylphenidate and cocaine substituted completely for either 10 mg/kg or 30 mg/kg caffeine, whereas other psychomotor stimulants (d-amphetamine and ephedrine), produced more, but not complete, caffeine-appropriate responding in the rats trained to discriminate the lower dose of caffeine. However, in animals trained to discriminate 20 mg/kg caffeine from saline, d-amphetamine produced 86% caffeine-appropriate responding (Mariathasan & Stolerman, 1992).

Caffeine has also produced mixed results when tested in animals trained to discriminate other xanthines or psychomotor stimulants. At high doses, caffeine partially substituted for theophylline in one study (Carney et al., 1985); another study by the same group showed complete cross-substitution between caffeine and theophylline (Modrow & Holloway, 1985). Caffeine has shown only partial substitution in animals trained to discriminate d-amphetamine (Evans & Johanson, 1987; Holloway, Michaelis, & Huerta, 1985; Kuhn, Appel, & Greenberg, 1974; Rosen, Young, Beuthin, & Louis-Ferdinant, 1986) or cocaine (Gauvin, Harland, Michaelis, & Holloway, 1989; Harland et al., 1989). There was no cross-substitution between caffeine and phenylpropanolamine; that is, neither drug completely substituted in rats trained to discriminate the other training drug (Mariathasan & Stolerman, 1992). Interestingly, caffeine has been shown to substitute for the atypical antidepressant, bupropion (Jones, Howard, & Bennett, 1980). Although caffeine and other psychomotor stimulants do not consistently cross-substitute for one another, several studies have shown that when caffeine and psychomotor stimulants are combined, the DS effects of stimulants are enhanced (e.g., Gauvin et al., 1989; Harland et al., 1989; Holloway, Michaelis, & Huerta, 1985; Schechter, 1977, 1989).

By and large, drugs from other pharmacological classes have failed to share DS effects with caffeine (e.g., Mumford & Holtzman, 1991) and caffeine has failed to share DS effects with other drugs (e.g., Gauvin, Peirce, & Holloway, 1994), suggesting that the caffeine versus saline discrimination is relatively pharmacologically specific. The mechanism(s) underlying the DS effects of caffeine have been investigated and several studies have provided evidence for the involvement of adenosine, in that caffeine and other adenosine receptor antagonists block the DS effects of adenosine agonists (Coffin & Carney, 1983; Spencer & Lal, 1983). However, the results from some studies suggest that the caffeine discrimination is not mediated via adenosine receptor mechanisms, but by an interaction with the benzodiazepine/GABA receptor complex and/or c-AMP (Holloway, Modrow, & Michaelis, 1985) or alpha adrenergic mechanisms (Holtzman, 1986). Another study showed that the DS effects of 60 mg/kg caffeine were not antagonized by either a serotonin or dopamine antagonist (Winter, 1981).

Subjective and Discriminative Stimulus Effects of Caffeine in Humans

Subjective Effects of Caffeine

The subjective effects, or mood altering effects, of caffeine have varied considerably across studies and the range of these subjective effects seems to depend primarily on dose, the habitual use of the same subjects and whether or not there was a period of caffeine deprivation (see Griffiths & Mumford, 1995). In a questionnaire distributed to a group of housewives, coffee drinkers indicated that they drank coffee for the enjoyable and pleasant effects, although some differences were observed between light and heavy coffee drinkers (A. Goldstein & Kaizer, 1969). For instance, heavy users reported positive effects of coffee more frequently than light users and they reported other positive symptoms including increased well-being and fewer adverse effects such as nervousness and wakefulness. In a subsequent study in some of these same women (A. Goldstein, Kaizer, &

Whitby, 1969), administration of 150 and 300 mg caffeine to caffeine abstainers resulted in predominantly adverse effects (e.g., jitteriness and nervousness) while these doses of caffeine made the heavy coffee drinkers feel alert and content. In an earlier study (A. Goldstein, Kaizer, & Warren, 1965) medical students reported feeling more physically active, mentally alert, and nervous following a single dose of 300 mg caffeine, whereas 150 mg did not produce significant increases in mood relative to placebo.

Across a number of studies, when acute doses of caffeine greater than 300 mg were administered to subjects, adverse effects such as jitteriness, tension, and anxiety were generally reported (Chait & Griffiths, 1983; Charney, Heninger, & Jatlow, 1985; Cole, Pope, Labrie, & Ionescu-Pioggia, 1978; Evans & Griffiths, 1992; Griffiths & Woodson, 1988b; Loke, 1988). Not all studies have shown such negative effects following higher caffeine doses. For instance, doses of caffeine of approximately 210–420 mg increased ratings of wakefulness and activated but did not significantly increase anxiety (Hasenfratz & Bättig, 1994). Some studies have failed to demonstrate changes in mood following doses of caffeine even up to 750 mg (e.g. File, Bond, & Lister, 1982; Froberg, Karlsson, Levi, Linde, & Seeman, 1969).

At low to intermediate doses (less than 300 mg), caffeine has been shown to produce a range of positive subjective effects (Bättig, 1985; Gilbert, 1976; Griffiths et al., 1990a; Leathwood & Pollet, 1983; Lieberman, Wurtman, Emde, Roberts, & Coviella, 1987). One of the earliest studies to show significant positive effects from a low dose of caffeine (64 mg) was conducted by Lieberman, Wurtman, Emde, Roberts, and Coviella (1987). Interestingly, in another study by the same group (Lieberman, Wurtman, Emde, & Coviella, 1987), low doses of caffeine (32, 64, 128 and 256 mg) enhanced performance on auditory vigilance and reaction time tasks, but there was no corresponding change in subjective effects even at the highest dose of 256 mg. In fact, the studies that have shown the clearest

and most reliable positive effects of caffeine are those that have either trained subjects to discriminate low doses of caffeine from placebo or have maintained subjects on low doses of caffeine (e.g., Griffiths et al., 1990a, 1990b; Silverman & Griffiths, 1992). Among subjects trained to discriminate 100 mg caffeine from placebo (Griffiths et al., 1990a), caffeine produced increases in well-being, social disposition, motivation for work, and euphoria (as measured by the Addiction Research Center Inventory; Haertzen, 1974), and virtually no adverse effects. In another study, positive subjective effects were demonstrated following doses as low as 18 mg in subjects trained to discriminate progressively lower doses of caffeine from placebo (Silverman & Griffiths, 1992). However, even at doses of 100 mg or less, caffeine increased ratings of trembling, shakiness, and jitteriness. The ability of these more recent studies to show such robust subjective effects at low doses may be directly related to the fact that subjects had extensive discrimination training and were monetarily reinforced in the study by Silverman and Griffiths (1992).

While the adverse effects of caffeine, particularly increases in anxiety symptoms, can vary widely across individuals, several studies have documented a relationship between caffeine intake and anxiety (see Nelig et al., 1992). Individuals who are highly anxious, particularly those who suffer from an anxiety or panic disorder, are more likely to experience anxiety symptoms following caffeine intake; they often reduce or eliminate caffeine consumption to avoid these adverse effects (e.g., Boulenger & Uhde, 1982; Boulenger, Uhde, Wolff, & Post, 1984; Charney et al., 1985; Lee, Cameron, & Greden, 1985). However, excessive caffeine consumption can produce a Caffeine-Induced Anxiety Disorder (American Psychiatric Association, 1994) which can resemble either a panic disorder or generalized anxiety disorder (Uhde, 1990; Uhde, Boulenger, Jimerson, & Post, 1984). Results in normal volunteers have also shown a relationship between anxiety and caffeine consumption in that those subjects who scored higher on trait anxiety were less likely to choose caffeine over placebo (Evans & Griffiths, 1992; Griffiths & Woodson, 1988b).

Discriminative Stimulus Effects of Caffeine in Humans

One approach to providing information related to subjective effects is to use a drug discrimination paradigm in which subjects are trained to make one response if a certain drug dose is administered and to make a different response if a different drug condition, or no drug, is administered. In contrast to the large number of drug discrimination studies conducted in nonhumans, relatively few have been conducted in humans (Kamien et al., 1993). Typically, humans are instructed to respond differentially to two different drug conditions, usually identified by letter code as Drug "A" and Drug "B" and correct responses are reinforced with money. Simultaneously, subjects usually complete various subjective effects questionnaires.

To date, eight studies have trained humans to discriminate caffeine capsules from placebo capsules under double-blind conditions (Evans & Griffiths, 1991a; Griffiths et al., 1990a; Heishman, Taylor, Goodman, Evans, & Henningfield, 1993; Mumford et al., 1994; Oliveto, Bickel, et al., 1992; Oliveto et al., 1993; Silverman & Griffiths, 1992; Silverman, Mumford, & Griffiths, 1994b). The first study to train human subjects to discriminate caffeine from placebo used a fading procedure in which subjects continued to attempt to discriminate lower doses of caffeine (178 to 10 mg) from placebo (Griffiths et al., 1990a). At each session, subjects ingested two capsules sequentially, one of which contained caffeine and the other placebo. All seven subjects acquired the discrimination between 178 mg caffeine and placebo and as the dose decreased, the number of subjects who could reliably make the discrimination decreased. The threshold of discrimination was 56 mg caffeine for 3 subjects, 18 mg for 3 subjects, and 10 mg for 1 subject. These results indicated that caffeine has behavioral effects at lower doses than previously recognized. However, all of these subjects were scientists in the area of behavioral

pharmacology, knew that they were being trained to discriminate caffeine from placebo, and abstained from all other sources of caffeine throughout the entire study, which spanned several months. Similar thresholds of detectability for caffeine were observed in a subsequent study conducted in some of the same subjects, which also used a fading procedure (Mumford et al., 1994). More importantly, a similar fading procedure was conducted in normal volunteers from the community (Silverman & Griffiths, 1992). Seventy-three percent of subjects acquired the caffeine (178 mg) versus placebo discrimination and the threshold of discrimination across subjects ranged from 178 mg to 18 mg, which was similar to the previous study by Griffiths and colleagues (Griffiths et al., 1990a).

Most drug discrimination studies conducted in normal volunteers (rather than scientists) have used higher training doses of caffeine and subjects who have not been explicitly told that they were being trained to discriminate caffeine. For instance, Evans and Griffiths (1991a) trained 5 volunteers to discriminate either 200 or 300 mg caffeine from placebo and a full caffeine dose-response function (50 to 400 or 600 mg) was determined repeatedly under test conditions in each subject. All subjects acquired the discrimination within 6–14 sessions and the discrimination remained stable over the 5–9 months of the study. Caffeine produced orderly dose-related increases in caffeine identification, although doses of 50 and 100 mg were infrequently identified as caffeine. Similarly, two other studies trained subjects to discriminate 320 mg per 70 kg caffeine from placebo (Oliveto, Bickel, et al., 1992; Oliveto et al., 1993) and 78% of subjects acquired the discrimination within 4–16 sessions. In those subjects tested with other caffeine doses, caffeine was correctly identified in a dose-related manner, although doses lower than 180 mg were primarily identified as placebo. Interestingly, in subjects who were not given explicit instructions and sampling sessions, the caffeine versus placebo discrimination took 20–40 sessions to acquire (Silverman & Griffiths, 1992). Finally, one study trained subjects to discriminate between *d*-amphetamine (30 mg), caffeine (400 mg) and placebo (Heishman *et al.,* 1993). When various doses of caffeine were tested, there was a dose-related increase in caffeine-appropriate responding and lower doses produced primarily placebo responding.

Across the various caffeine–drug discrimination studies, the degree of caffeine abstinence has varied considerably. For instance, in the studies using behavioral pharmacologists (Griffiths *et al.,* 1990a; Mumford *et al.,* 1994), subjects were completely abstinent from all other dietary sources of caffeine. In the study by Silverman and Griffiths (1992), subjects were also completely abstinent from all other dietary sources of caffeine and saliva samples were analyzed to monitor compliance. However, to maintain subjects on the same daily dose of caffeine during each phase of the study, subjects were given a second capsule after the discrimination session (which varied in caffeine content based on the first capsule) and capsules for weekends and holidays. Three other studies, which used higher training doses, required only overnight caffeine abstinence (Evans & Griffiths, 1991a; Oliveto, Bickel, *et al.,* 1992; Oliveto *et al.,* 1993), which was verified in one study (Evans & Griffiths, 1991a).

Only three studies have evaluated the DS effects of other drugs in humans trained to discriminate caffeine from placebo (Heishman *et al.,* 1993; Oliveto, Bickel, *et al.,* 1992; Oliveto *et al.,* 1993). In one study, a range of triazolam doses was tested in 3 individuals; triazolam produced predominantly placebo responding (Oliveto, Bickel, *et al.,* 1992). In a subsequent study (Oliveto *et al.,* 1993), theophylline, methylphenidate, and buspirone were also tested in subjects trained to discriminate caffeine from placebo. Theophylline produced caffeine-appropriate responding in all 4 subjects (although not at the same doses), whereas methylphenidate produced caffeine-appropriate responding in 3 of 4 subjects. In contrast, buspirone produced primarily placebo-appropriate responding. In humans trained to discriminate *d*-amphetamine versus caffeine versus placebo (Heishman *et al.,* 1993), doses of *d*-amphetamine lower than the training dose produced approximately 40% caffeine-appropriate responding and mazindol produced a mixture of caffeine and *d*-amphetamine–appropriate responding.

Caffeine has been substituted for another training drug in two studies (Chait & Johanson, 1988; Heishman *et al.,* 1993). In normal volunteers trained to discriminate 10 mg *d*-amphetamine from placebo, caffeine produced 40% to 60% *d*-amphetamine identification at 100 and 300 mg caffeine and the 300 mg dose produced some subjective effects similar to *d*-amphetamine, including increased anxiety, vigor, arousal, and positive mood (Chait & Johanson, 1988). The lower dose (100 mg) altered only two subjective measures; this may be related to the fact that subjects were not instructed to abstain from caffeine before the session. In contrast, within a three-drug discrimination design (Heishman *et al.,* 1993), caffeine produced relatively little *d*-amphetamine responding. The difference between these two studies may be related to the training doses of caffeine and *d*-amphetamine or the use of a two- versus three-drug discrimination. Overall, these limited results in humans are consistent with other drug discrimination studies in animals indicating the relative pharmacological specificity of the caffeine discrimination.

The subjective effects reported within the context of caffeine–drug discrimination studies has varied as a function of the subject population and, more importantly, the training dose. However, most studies have shown that at doses that produce significant subjective effects, reliable discrimination has been observed (Evans & Griffiths, 1991a; Griffiths *et al.,* 1990a; Oliveto, Bickel, *et al.,* 1992; Oliveto *et al.,* 1993; Silverman & Griffiths, 1992). Subjective effects (Griffiths *et al.,* 1990a) among subjects trained to discriminate 100 mg caffeine from placebo were predominantly positive; that is, caffeine increased ratings of well-being, social disposition, motivation for work, and euphoria. These primarily positive effects of caffeine may be related to the low dose used and the fact that subjects were otherwise completely caffeine abstinent.

However, Silverman and Griffiths (1992) found that doses of 18–100 mg produced dysphoric subjective effects in some subjects. Similarly, large individual differences have been observed in the subjective effects and self-reported cues in subjects trained to discriminate 200–300 mg caffeine from placebo (Evans & Griffiths, 1991a), although increased jitteriness, nervousness, shakiness, tension, anxiety, vigor, and alertness were common at these doses. Some of these differences may be related to the caffeine history of the subjects, in that 2 individuals were complete caffeine abstainers. For instance, the 2 subjects who had the highest levels of caffeine consumption reported adverse effects (e.g., headache, tiredness) on days they received the placebo condition, suggesting that caffeine withdrawal might have been a salient stimulus for the caffeine versus placebo discrimination. Among subjects trained to discriminate 320 mg per 70 kg caffeine from placebo, the most common subjective effects reported following caffeine have included increases in lysergic acid diethylamide (LSD) scores, stimulant–bad effects and decreases on measures related to sedation (Oliveto, Bickel, et al., 1992; Oliveto et al., 1993). Further, Oliveto, Bickel, and colleagues (1992) showed that the subjective effects of the training dose of caffeine and placebo were related to whether subjects made a correct discrimination.

Reinforcing Effects of Caffeine

Reinforcing Effects of Caffeine in Animals

Numerous studies and reviews demonstrate that drugs function as reinforcers in both animals and humans (e.g., Griffiths, Bigelow, & Henningfield, 1980; Johanson, 1978). The reinforcing efficacy of a drug, like any other positive reinforcer, is the ability to initiate and maintain responding that leads to its delivery. The intravenous drug self-administration model has proven to be a valid model for assessing the reinforcing effects of psychoactive drugs in animals (Bozarth, 1987), although

other routes of administration have been used, including oral, smoked, and inhalation (Balster, 1987; Meisch, 1977; Wood, 1990). For intravenous self-administration, an animal is surgically implanted with an intravenous catheter and when the animal responds (usually by pressing a lever) to stimuli associated with drug delivery, the drug is delivered. The efficacy of the drug in functioning as a positive reinforcer is typically compared with responding for a vehicle.

In a recent review, Griffiths and Mumford (1995) summarized all intravenous caffeine self-administration studies conducted in animals. Of the six administration studies conducted in nonhuman primates, three showed that caffeine was self-administered by all animals at one or more doses, although the pattern of self-administration was intermittent across animals (Deneau, Yanagita, & Seevers, 1969; Griffiths, Brady, & Bradford, 1979; Griffiths, Sannerud, & Kaminski, cited in Table 1 in Griffiths & Mumford, 1995). Further, these studies involved extended access to caffeine (as long as 18 weeks) and they all involved a small number of animals. In another study, caffeine self-administration was demonstrated in only 1 of 4 monkeys (Schuster, Woods, & Seevers, 1969). Reliable self-administration was not maintained in animals in two other studies (Hoffmeister & Wuttke, 1973; Yanagita, 1970). However, in both of those studies caffeine was available for only a brief period of time and it was being substituted for a drug that was self-administered.

Of the three intravenous caffeine self-administration studies conducted in rats, only one reported caffeine self-administration by all animals (Dworkin, Vrana, Broadbent, & Robinson, 1993), although no vehicle data were presented. In the two other studies, caffeine self-administration was demonstrated in only a subset of animals (Atkinson & Enslen, 1976; Collins, Weeks, Cooper, Good, & Russell, 1984).

Oral caffeine self-administration has been demonstrated to some extent in rats, but only under certain conditions. For instance, the level of caffeine consumption was increased by food deprivation (Heppner, Kemble, & Cox, 1986) or chronic nicotine exposure (Schulte-Daxboek & Opitz, 1981). In another study, oral caffeine was self-administered only after a period of forced caffeine exposure (Vitiello & Woods, 1975). In fact, naive rats injected with caffeine avoided a novel flavor associated with caffeine whereas rats who had received caffeine injections for 12 consecutive days actually avoided the flavor associated with the absence of caffeine (Vitiello & Woods, 1977).

The studies that have demonstrated the most reliable caffeine self-administration allowed animals to self-administer caffeine intravenously for extended periods of time (Deneau et al., 1969; Dworkin et al., 1993; Griffiths et al., 1979; Griffiths, Sannerud, & Kaminski, cited in Table 1 in Griffiths & Mumford, 1995). Even though the majority of these studies used a fixed ratio 1 schedule of reinforcement, most still did not obtain reliable caffeine self-administration in a substantial number of animals. These findings contrast with studies involving the intravenous self-administration of other psychoactive stimulants such as cocaine and d-amphetamine, in which self-administration is established rapidly and the drugs are self-administered at consistently high rates (Griffiths et al., 1979). These results indicate that caffeine is not as robust a reinforcer as other classic drugs of abuse (e.g., cocaine, morphine), although caffeine is self-administered at higher rates than other behaviorally active drugs (Johanson, 1978). Finally, there is some evidence that chronic caffeine exposure, or caffeine withdrawal, may potentiate the reinforcing effects of caffeine in rats (Vitiello & Woods, 1975, 1977).

Reinforcing Effects of Caffeine in Humans

Experimental procedures of self-administration or choice have been developed to assess the reinforcing effects of drugs in humans (Johanson, 1978). Despite the high prevalence of caffeine consumption, relatively few laboratory studies have investigated the reinforcing effects of caffeine and, surprisingly, this has been difficult to demonstrate reliably in the

laboratory (Griffiths & Mumford, 1995). Several early studies (A. Goldstein et al., 1969; Kozlowski, 1976; Podboy & Malloy, 1977) provided suggestive evidence that caffeine played a role in coffee consumption. A series of studies by Griffiths and colleagues (Griffiths, Bigelow, & Liebson, 1986; Griffiths, Bigelow, Liebson, O'Keefe, et al., 1986; Griffiths, Bigelow, & Liebson, 1989) provided the first unequivocal demonstration of the reinforcing effects of caffeine in heavy coffee drinkers who resided on a residential research ward and had histories of other substance abuse. When coffee was freely available, subjects tended to consume it in a regular pattern and when the dose of caffeine was manipulated, the total number of cups consumed was a U-shaped function of dose (Griffiths, Bigelow, Liebson, O'Keefe, et al., 1986). In a subsequent study (Griffiths, Bigelow, & Liebson, 1986), a choice procedure was used in which caffeinated and decaffeinated coffee was available under two different background conditions. When subjects were maintained on caffeinated coffee (i.e., tolerant) they chose caffeinated coffee on 92% of the occasions whereas when subjects were maintained on decaffeinated coffee (i.e., not tolerant), caffeinated coffee was chosen on only 50% of the occasions. Finally, when similar subjects had 13 opportunities each day to administer either a caffeine capsule (100 mg) or a placebo capsule, all subjects developed a clear preference for caffeine even when capsule color codes were changed. The results of these last two studies provide clear evidence for the reinforcing effects of caffeine, both in coffee and capsules, using choice procedures.

In contrast to inpatient studies with heavy coffee drinkers who had histories of alcohol and/or other drug abuse, most other double-blind studies, using various outpatient choice and/or self-administration procedures, have failed to detect reliable caffeine reinforcement in the majority of moderate caffeine users without histories of drug abuse. That is, reliable caffeine self-administration has generally been shown to occur in only small subsets of subjects tested. The percentage of subjects showing significant caffeine choice across studies using caffeine versus placebo choice procedures has ranged from a low of 10% (Oliveto, Hughes, et al., 1992) to a high of 50% (Hughes, Hunt, et al., 1992; Oliveto, Hughes, Pepper, Bickel, & Higgins, 1991), with other studies producing intermediate values (Griffiths & Woodson, 1988b; Hale, Hughes, Oliveto, & Higgins, 1995; Hughes et al., 1991; Hughes, Oliveto, Bickel, Higgins, & Valliere, 1992; Hughes, Oliveto, Bickel, Higgins, & Badger, 1995). Nonetheless, there are two recent studies which have demonstrated caffeine reinforcement in the majority of subjects. In one study, caffeine choice was shown to be a function of different behavioral requirements (Silverman, Mumford, & Griffiths, 1994a). All subjects chose caffeine over placebo when they were scheduled to perform a vigilance task, but chose placebo over caffeine when they were scheduled to engage in relaxation. The generalizability of these results is unclear because caffeine choice was demonstrated only in a specific and highly controlled laboratory context (i.e., a vigilance task). The generalizability is also questionable because all subjects had experimental histories of discriminating caffeine from placebo, and it is unclear whether discrimination training contributed to the caffeine choice observed. A study by Evans, Critchfield, and Griffiths (1994) provides the clearest demonstration to date of caffeine reinforcement in a majority of normal subjects who were allowed to engage in their normal daily routines. The study used a mutually exclusive choice procedure in which subjects ingested capsules containing either caffeine (50 or 100 mg/capsule) or placebo throughout the day. Overall, caffeine was chosen over placebo on 80% of choice occasions. Further, this choice was demonstrated in 82% of subjects and caffeine choice was replicable despite changes in capsule colors across 8-week blocks.

One of the difficulties inherent to the inconsistent reinforcing effects observed with caffeine, particularly the outpatient studies mentioned above, is that no standardized experimental procedures exist for assessing caffeine reinforcement in humans. Two general types of choice procedures have been employed to assess reinforcing effects of caffeine in humans; both employ forced exposure sessions in which caffeine and placebo are administered according to an experimenter-determined schedule. The two procedures differ on choice sessions. In concurrent access choice procedures, subjects can choose to ingest doses of caffeine, placebo, or both in the same choice session. Hughes and colleagues have used a concurrent access choice procedure in studies in which subjects ingest multiple daily doses of caffeinated or decaffeinated coffee or soda (e.g., Hughes et al., 1991; Hughes, Oliveto, Bickel, et al., 1992). Although this procedure appears to most closely simulate the natural environment in that the vehicle (coffee or soda) is similar to what subjects would consume outside the laboratory, reliable caffeine self-administration has been demonstrated in only about 25% to 45% of subjects under this procedure (Hughes, Oliveto, Bickel, Higgins, & Badger, 1993; Ligori & Hughes, 1997; Ligori, Hughes, & Oliveto, 1997). In contrast, with mutually exclusive choice procedures, subjects must make a single drug choice that remains in effect for the duration of the choice session. However, a mutually exclusive choice procedure alone is not sufficient to guarantee high rates of caffeine choice and several studies using this procedure have not shown high levels of caffeine choice (Evans & Griffiths, 1992; Griffiths & Woodson, 1988b; Stern, Chait, & Johanson, 1989). It is possible, however, that the type of choice procedure interacts with other procedural variables in determining caffeine choice.

Caffeine reinforcement is dose-related and has a U-shaped function. Several studies have shown that doses as low as 25 mg can function as a reinforcer under conditions in which subjects could self-administer multiple cups or capsules each day (Evans et al., 1994; Hale et al., 1995; Hughes, Hunt, et al., 1992; Hughes et al., 1995; Kozlowski, 1976; Oliveto, Hughes, et al., 1992; Oliveto et al., 1991). Previous studies have shown that increasing doses above 50 to 100 mg tends to decrease choice of caffeine or rates of caffeine self-administration (Griffiths & Woodson, 1988b; Griffiths, Bigelow, Liebson, O'Keefe, et al., 1986; Hughes, Hunt, et al., 1992; Stern et al., 1989). Relatively high acute doses of caffeine (e.g., 400 or 600 mg as a single dose) have been shown to produce significant caffeine avoidance (Griffiths & Woodson, 1988b).

A factor related to caffeine dose is the extent to which subjects have control over dosing. It would seem reasonable to speculate that caffeine choice procedures may be more sensitive to the reinforcing effects of caffeine if subjects have the ability to control the number of doses and the interval between doses over the session. There is some suggestive evidence to support this from a choice study conducted by Evans and colleagues (1994). Six of 9 subjects who showed significant caffeine choice actually self-administered less caffeine on choice days than they had been required to ingest on sampling days and 1 subject consistently chose caffeine, thereby demonstrating caffeine reinforcement, but ingested only the one required capsule (100 mg caffeine).

Although the vehicle in which caffeine is self-administered would seem to be a potentially important variable, the available experimental data have not shown that vehicle affects caffeine reinforcement. For example, among heavy coffee drinkers, there was no statistical difference in self-administration when caffeine was administered in capsules or coffee (Griffiths et al., 1989). Further, studies in normal subjects using caffeine administered in capsules (e.g., Griffiths & Woodson, 1988b) have found similar rates of caffeine choice as studies in which caffeine was administered in coffee (e.g., Hughes, Oliveto, Bickel, et al., 1993) or soda (Hughes, Oliveto, Bickel, et al., 1992). In fact, the two studies which have shown the highest rates of caffeine reinforcement administered capsules (Evans et al., 1994; Silverman et al., 1994a). Overall, these results provide no support for the idea that caffeine reinforcement might be more readily demonstrated in a familiar vehicle such as coffee or soda.

Several other variables may interact with caffeine reinforcement. Most studies thus far have focused on the role of caffeine physical dependence and withdrawal as a predictor of caffeine reinforcement (see "Caffeine Physical Dependence and Withdrawal," later in this chapter, for details). Behavioral context has also been shown to influence caffeine choice (Silverman et al., 1994a). When subjects were required to perform a vigilance task, caffeine was always chosen, whereas when subjects engaged in relaxation, caffeine was not chosen by the majority of subjects. A prolonged history of exposure to experimental conditions before reinforcement testing may facilitate the demonstration of caffeine reinforcement (Evans et al., 1994; Silverman et al., 1994a). Another, often overlooked variable is the restriction and verification of nonexperimental caffeine consumption. In two studies by Griffiths and colleagues (Griffiths, Bigelow, & Liebson, 1986; Griffiths et al., 1989), in which reliable caffeine choice was demonstrated, caffeine consumption was limited to experimentally administered caffeine; other sources of caffeine were easy to restrict and monitor since the subjects lived on a residential research ward. In contrast, caffeine choice studies using normal volunteers in outpatient settings have not consistently restricted dietary caffeine intake or monitored compliance. For example, some studies made no attempt to restrict nonexperimental dietary sources of caffeine (e.g., Stern et al., 1989) and others asked subjects to refrain from caffeine-containing products, but compliance was not monitored (e.g., Hughes et al., 1991). In a study by Griffiths and Woodson (1988b), overnight caffeine abstinence was verified via analysis of saliva samples, but subjects were allowed to consume dietary caffeine between the end of the experimental session and bedtime. In each case, nonexperimental caffeine use could have contaminated the results, perhaps helping to explain intersubject variability in caffeine reinforcement. Recently, researchers are requiring total abstinence from dietary caffeine for extended periods of time (i.e., ≥ 24 hr) and are verifying compliance by analyzing saliva samples (Evans & Griffiths, 1992; Oliveto, Hughes, et al., 1992; Silverman, Evans, Strain, & Griffiths, 1992).

For the majority of studies, there is a strong correspondence between caffeine choice–reinforcement and the self-reported subjective effects of caffeine. For instance, when subjects were categorized into caffeine choosers and nonchoosers in a choice study (Evans & Griffiths, 1992), caffeine choosers tended to report positive subjective effects of caffeine (e.g., increased liking, alertness, friendliness) and negative subjective effects of placebo (e.g., increased headache, fatigue). In contrast, nonchoosers tended to report negative subjective effects of caffeine (increased tension, anxiety, and jitteriness). In another study, in which subjects were not caffeine abstinent (Stern *et al.,* 1989), caffeine produced positive subjective effects in choosers and negative effects in nonchoosers, but there was little evidence that placebo produced negative subjective effects in choosers. Two earlier studies (A. Goldstein & Kaizer, 1969; A. Goldstein *et al.,* 1969), reported that after overnight abstinence, heavy coffee drinkers (≥ 5 cups a day) felt positive effects after their morning coffee and dysphoric effects if they did not have their morning coffee, or if decaffeinated coffee was substituted. In contrast, abstainers felt normal following placebo and dysphoric following caffeine (A. Goldstein *et al.,* 1969). The results of several other studies are consistent with these findings (Griffiths & Woodson, 1988b; Griffiths, Bigelow, & Liebson, 1986; Griffiths, Bigelow, Liebson, O'Keefe, *et al.,* 1986; Griffiths *et al.,* 1989; Hughes, Oliveto, Bickel, *et al.,* 1993). Nonetheless, Hughes, Oliveto, Bickel, and colleagues (1993) have also reported that this relationship does not necessarily hold for all subjects.

Tolerance to Caffeine

Tolerance to Caffeine in Animals

Tolerance is defined as a reduction in responsiveness to an effect of a drug as a result of repeated or chronic exposure to the drug such that increased doses are necessary to produce the same magnitude of effect. The most relevant behavioral dimension of caffeine tolerance is the tolerance that develops to the CNS effects of caffeine. Caffeine tolerance has been demonstrated for three behavioral effects in animals: locomotor activity, operant conditioning, and DS effects.

Tolerance to caffeine-induced stimulation of locomotor activity has been demonstrated in a number of studies in which rats or mice were chronically maintained on caffeine ranging from doses of 5 to 220 mg/kg (Ahlijanian & Takemori, 1986; Chou, Khan, Forde, & Hirsh, 1985; File, Baldwin, Johnston, & Wilks, 1988; Finn & Holtzman, 1986, 1987; Holtzman, 1983; Kaplan, Greenblatt, Kent, & Cotreau-Bibbo, 1993). One of the first studies to demonstrate tolerance development to the increased locomotor activity produced by caffeine was conducted by Holtzman (1983). Compared with a control group that drank caffeine-free water, rats chronically maintained on caffeine (approximately 160 mg/kg daily doses in drinking water), did not show any increases in locomotor activity following a wide range of caffeine doses. In a more recent study (Lau & Falk, 1994), differences in the rate of tolerance development to caffeine-induced locomotor stimulation were reported as a function of route and schedule of chronic caffeine administration. When rats were chronically administered caffeine via the intraperitoneal (i.p.) route (20 mg/kg/day), tolerance developed to the locomotor stimulant effect of caffeine within 4 days, but this tolerance was still not complete after 21 days of administration. In contrast, following schedule-induced oral caffeine self-administration (36.5 mg/kg/day), tolerance developed over 13 days and remained incomplete at day 17.

Caffeine-induced tolerance to locomotor activity is not always surmountable (Ahlijanian & Takemori, 1986; Finn & Holtzman, 1986; Lau & Falk, 1995). For instance, in a study by Finn and Holtzman (1986), a wide range of caffeine doses tested in caffeine-tolerant rats failed to increase locomotor activity; that is, the caffeine dose-response function was shifted downward rather than to the right as has been observed in other studies (Carney, 1982; Chou *et al.,* 1985; Holtzman & Finn,

1988; Wayner, Jolicoeur, Rondeu, & Barone, 1976).

Tolerance to increased locomotor activity produced by caffeine appears to be pharmacologically specific in that cross-tolerance to the locomotor activity has been demonstrated with other xanthines including theophylline (Finn & Holtzman, 1988; Holtzman, 1991), as well as other drugs that act via the same mechanism; that is, block adenosine receptors (Holtzman, 1991). This cross-tolerance is not observed with other stimulants such as *d*-amphetamine (Finn & Holtzman, 1987, 1988; Holtzman, 1983), methamphetamine (Ahlijanian & Takemori, 1986), methylphenidate, and cocaine (Finn & Holtzman, 1987).

Several studies have demonstrated that tolerance develops to rate-altering effects of caffeine using operant schedules of food reinforcement or shock avoidance. Wayner and colleagues (1976) used a fixed interval schedule of food reinforcement and showed substantial tolerance to the effects of 100 mg/kg caffeine. Similarly, Carney (1982) reported that stable tolerance developed to the rate-decreasing effects of caffeine in rats injected with caffeine (32 mg/kg, i.p.) for 7 days. Specifically, a sixfold shift to the right in the caffeine dose-response curve for food responding was observed. Holtzman and Finn (1988) also demonstrated tolerance to the rate-decreasing effects of caffeine on schedule-controlled responding in rats. In squirrel monkeys (Katz & Goldberg, 1987), tolerance to the response rate increases for both food-reinforcement and shock-avoidance developed in monkeys maintained on 15 mg/kg caffeine daily. Rapid tolerance development (1 day) has also been demonstrated to the increased reinforcement threshold for electrical self-stimulation in rats (Mumford, Neill, & Holtzman, 1988). Insurmountable caffeine tolerance has also been demonstrated to responding under a fixed-interval schedule of stimulus termination in rhesus monkeys (Howell & Landrum, 1997).

Tolerance development to the DS effects of caffeine has also been demonstrated (Holtzman, 1987; Modrow & Holloway, 1985;

Modrow, Holloway, & Carney, 1981). The first suggestion of tolerance development to this behavioral effect of caffeine was reported by Modrow and colleagues (Modrow & Holloway, 1985; Modrow, Holloway, & Carney, 1981). In rats trained to discriminate 32 mg/kg caffeine from saline, responding for caffeine was higher on days following saline than on days following caffeine, suggesting some level of short-term tolerance development to the DS effects of caffeine. Tolerance was more clearly demonstrated in a study by Holtzman (1987). Rats trained to discriminate either 10 or 30 mg/kg caffeine from saline were then injected with 30 mg/kg caffeine twice each day for a period of 3.5 days during which discrimination training was suspended. When retested with caffeine, the dose-response functions for the DS effects of caffeine were shifted to the right following chronic caffeine exposure, but not following a similar duration of saline exposure. This tolerance development was greater for the group trained to discriminate the lower dose of caffeine. Further, cross-tolerance was demonstrated between caffeine and methylphenidate.

The development of behavioral tolerance in animals appears to depend on the frequency of dosing, the route of dosing, the duration of dosing, and the behavior being measured. As described earlier, the majority of caffeine tolerance studies in rodents have measured tolerance to locomotor activity. Tolerance to the increased locomotor effects of caffeine developed within 2 weeks of exposure to doses as low as 5–10 mg/kg/day in the drinking water of rats (Chou *et al.*, 1985). In a study by Finn and Holtzman (1986), tolerance development to caffeine-induced increases in locomotor activity was rapid; that is within 1–3 days of chronic caffeine administration (40–65 mg/kg caffeine daily in drinking water). This tolerance was almost completely lost within 3–4 days on the discontinuation of chronic caffeine. However, in more recent studies (Lau & Falk, 1994, 1995), tolerance to locomotor activity in rats depended on the route, dose, and schedule of chronic caffeine administration. Further, tolerance to this effect was not complete after 2–3 weeks of chronic caffeine (Lau & Falk, 1994).

Overall, tolerance development to the stimulation of locomotor activity appears to be rapid, insurmountable (complete with dose-response functions shifted to the right) and pharmacologically specific. In contrast, tolerance to the rate-decreasing effects on operant responding or the DS effects develops more gradually and the tolerance is surmountable (incomplete). Further, there appears to be less pharmacological specificity to these behaviors, as opposed to locomotor activity, in that cross-tolerance occurs with other non-xanthine stimulants.

Tolerance to Caffeine in Humans

The phenomenon of caffeine tolerance has been only incompletely characterized in human research. The majority of studies have investigated tolerance development to the physiological effects of caffeine, whereas relatively few studies have evaluated tolerance to the CNS effects of caffeine, such as sleep disruption and subjective effects. At this time, there are no published studies which have assessed tolerance development to other behavioral effects of caffeine in humans including the DS effects and the reinforcing effects. Further, no studies have evaluated the parameters involved in caffeine tolerance, including dosing, dosing interval, and length of abstinence needed to reinstate a caffeine effect.

Tolerance has been demonstrated to a range of physiological effects increased by caffeine including diuretic (Eddy & Downs, 1928), parotid gland secretory (Winsor & Strongin, 1933), and cardiovascular and catecholamine (Ammon, Bieck, Mandalaz, & Verspohl, 1983; Denaro, Brown, Jacob, & Benowitz, 1991; Robertson, Wade, Workman, & Woosley, 1981) effects. Several studies have shown that complete tolerance to the cardiovascular effects (increased blood pressure and decreased heart rate) of caffeine develops within a few days of repeated caffeine administration (Ammon et al., 1983; Denaro et al., 1991; Robertson et al., 1981; Shi, Benowitz, Denaro, & Sheiner, 1993). However, other studies have found that caffeine can still increase blood pressure in regular caffeine users (I. B. Goldstein,

Shapiro, Hui, & Yu, 1990; Lane & Manus, 1989). Similarly, even after 5 days of caffeine (12 mg/kg given in 6 divided doses), subjects still showed an increase in plasma norepinephrine and free fatty acids (Denaro et al., 1991). The duration of caffeine abstinence needed for caffeine to reinstate blood pressure increases has varied from overnight abstinence (Lane & Williams, 1987) to 1–3 days (Haigh et al., 1993; Robertson et al., 1981; Shi et al., 1993); these differences are most likely related to the total amount and pattern of caffeine consumption and the elimination rate.

Several studies have either indirectly or directly evaluated tolerance to the disruptive effects of caffeine on sleep. In one study (Colton, Gosselin, & Smith, 1968), in which medical students were given 150 mg of caffeinated or decaffeinated coffee shortly before bedtime, light coffee drinkers reported more sleep-disturbing effects, particularly delayed sleep onset, following caffeine ingestion than regular coffee drinkers. Consistent results on the sleep-disturbing effects of caffeine were not found in other studies using similar subject populations (A. Goldstein, 1964; A. Goldstein, Warren, & Kaizer, 1965), and, in fact, the authors concluded that tolerance did not occur to these effects (A. Goldstein, Warren, & Kaizer, 1965). A more direct demonstration of tolerance development to a CNS effect of caffeine was provided by a study which assessed the effects of caffeine (250 mg b.i.d.) or placebo on daytime alertness using the Multiple Sleep Latency Test (Zwyghuizen-Doorenbose, Roehrs, Lipschutz, Timms, & Roth, 1990). Sleep latency was shown to be significantly longer on the first day of caffeine administration than on the second day, although caffeine continued to produce a longer sleep latency relative to placebo on the second day, suggesting incomplete tolerance development. A more recent study demonstrated complete tolerance to a number of sleep measures after repeated caffeine administration (400 mg t.i.d.) for 7 days (Bonnet & Arand, 1992).

To date, only one study has clearly documented tolerance development to the subjective effects of caffeine (Evans & Griffiths,

1992). Subjects received either chronic caffeine (300 mg t.i.d.) or chronic placebo (t.i.d.) for 18 consecutive days. After this period of chronic dosing, administration of caffeine produced significant subjective effects (including increases in tension, anxiety, jitteriness, nervousness, shakiness) in the placebo group, but not in the caffeine group. In fact, in the caffeine group, the effects of caffeine were not different from the effects of placebo, suggesting complete tolerance to the subjective effects of caffeine. Further, during the last 2 weeks of chronic dosing, the placebo group and the caffeine group did not differ meaningfully on ratings of mood and subjective effects.

Caffeine Physical Dependence and Withdrawal

Caffeine Physical Dependence and Withdrawal in Animals

Physical dependence on a drug is defined as the expression of withdrawal symptoms following cessation of chronic or repeated drug administration. The withdrawal symptoms are often in the direction opposite from the acute drug effects and are time limited. Further, readministration of the drug can reverse or relieve the withdrawal symptoms. Interestingly, despite animal models for evaluating drug dependence and withdrawal for various drugs (e.g., Carroll, 1987; Holtzman & Villarreal, 1973), relatively few animal laboratory studies have investigated caffeine physical dependence and withdrawal. This is in sharp contrast to the numerous reports and studies of caffeine withdrawal in humans that is reviewed in the following section.

The most robust behavioral effect of caffeine withdrawal in animal studies is a decrease in spontaneous locomotor activity. The termination of 190 mg/kg/day caffeine, administered intragastrically to rats, reduced spontaneous locomotor activity by 50% and lasted 1 week (Boyd, Dolman, Knight, & Sheppard, 1965). Similarly, when caffeine was removed from the drinking water of rats chronically

maintained on caffeine (65–160 mg/kg/day), spontaneous locomotor activity decreased 50%–80%. This reduction in locomotor activity was maximal the first 2 days of withdrawal and did not return to control levels for 2–5 days (Finn & Holtzman, 1986; Holtzman, 1983). However, rats maintained on lower doses of caffeine did not show a reduction in locomotor activity on the removal of caffeine (Finn & Holtzman, 1986). Studies conducted in mice have demonstrated a similar suppression of locomotor activity on the termination of chronic caffeine (Kaplan et al., 1993; Nikodijevic, Jacobson, & Daly, 1993).

Some, but not all, studies have demonstrated a disruption in schedule-controlled behavior following the termination of caffeine. For example, when saline was substituted for the caffeine maintenance dose (32 mg/kg) in rats, there was a substantial reduction (50%) in response rate (Carney, 1982). Similarly, in rats responding for intracranial self-stimulation, removal of caffeine (72 mg/kg/day) from the drinking water led to decreases in both reinforcement threshold and operant responding which were maximal 24–48 hr after withdrawal and did not return to baseline levels for 3–4 days (Mumford et al., 1988). A disruption in food-maintained responding was also observed in rhesus monkeys when noncaffeinated food pellets were substituted for caffeinated food pellets for a period of several days, although the severity and time course following caffeine removal was less than that following phencyclidine (Carroll, Hagen, Asencio, & Hartman Brauer, 1989). However, not all studies have been able to show that caffeine withdrawal produces a disruption in operant responding (Holtzman & Finn, 1988) at doses that disrupted locomotor activity.

Only one other preclinical study has provided evidence for a caffeine withdrawal phenomenon. Using a taste-aversion paradigm, naive rats injected with caffeine avoided a novel flavor associated with caffeine, whereas rats that had received caffeine injections for 12 consecutive days actually avoided the flavor associated with the absence of caffeine (Vitiello & Woods, 1977).

Caffeine Physical Dependence and Withdrawal in Humans

Evidence of caffeine physical dependence and withdrawal in humans has been documented in numerous case reports and clinical observations from as early as 1833 (see review by Griffiths & Woodson, 1988a). Subsequently, many surveys and experimental studies have more thoroughly characterized caffeine withdrawal in various populations, including students, housewives, hospital and psychiatric patients, drug and alcohol abusers, and normal volunteers (see reviews by Griffiths & Mumford, 1995; Griffiths & Woodson, 1988a). Recent studies have demonstrated that the incidence of caffeine physical dependence is higher, the daily dose level at which withdrawal occurs is lower, and the range of symptoms experienced is broader than previously recognized. This section will briefly summarize our current knowledge of caffeine withdrawal including the signs and symptoms, severity, incidence, time course, minimum dosing parameters, and clinical significance.

Headache is the most commonly reported, as well as the most reliable and sensitive, caffeine withdrawal symptom (e.g., Dreisbach & Pfeiffer, 1943; A. Goldstein et al., 1969; Griffiths, Bigelow, & Liebson, 1986; Griffiths et al., 1990a; Hughes, Oliveto, Bickel, et al., 1993). Dreisbach and Pfeiffer (1943) conducted one of the first studies to characterize caffeine withdrawal headaches following placebo substitution for chronic caffeine (600–750 mg/day in capsules). Headache occurred in 82% of subjects and for some it was the most severe headache they had ever experienced; readministration of caffeine was the most effective treatment. Despite the fact that headache is considered the prominent symptom of caffeine withdrawal, not all individuals, including heavy caffeine users, reliably experience headache when caffeine is removed. Further, the incidence and severity of headache is not consistent across subjects or within an individual with repeated exposures to caffeine withdrawal. In subjects who were maintained on 100 mg/day caffeine, placebo was substituted for caffeine on six different occasions (Griffiths et al., 1990b). The magnitude of peak headache varied across each of these occasions in all 7 subjects, but it did not vary in an orderly fashion and did not appear to be related to the duration of caffeine exposure prior to placebo substitution.

In addition to headache, symptoms of fatigue (e.g., tiredness, sleepiness, decreased energy and alertness, lethargy) are routinely reported during caffeine withdrawal (Griffiths & Mumford, 1995; Griffiths & Woodson, 1988a; Hughes, Oliveto, Bickel, et al., 1993). Other less frequently reported caffeine withdrawal symptoms include difficulty concentrating, decreased motivation for work, decreased contentment, decreased sociability and friendliness, irritability, flu-like feelings, nausea and vomiting, anxiety, and even depression (e.g., Griffiths et al., 1990b; Silverman et al., 1992). Of interest, the symptoms of caffeine withdrawal vary in severity across repeated exposure to caffeine withdrawal and do not necessarily covary with one another (Griffiths & Woodson, 1988a; Griffiths et al., 1990b). For instance, on one occasion of caffeine termination, the typical constellation of withdrawal symptoms may occur, but on another occasion, only isolated symptoms, such as extreme sleepiness, may occur without a headache or other symptoms.

The range of caffeine withdrawal symptoms, and the reports from some individuals that caffeine withdrawal significantly interferes with their normal activities (Griffiths et al., 1990b; Silverman et al., 1992), would suggest that performance would be severely compromised if caffeine was terminated. However, relatively few laboratory studies have been able to document clear impairments in psychomotor performance during caffeine withdrawal. When decaffeinated coffee was substituted for caffeinated coffee among heavy coffee consumers, performance on a circular lights task decreased during the first 2 days of caffeine withdrawal; however, this decrease was not statistically significant (Griffiths, Bigelow, & Liebson, 1986). Another study showed that reaction time decreased over two sessions in nonusers of caffeine, whereas individuals who abstained from caffeine for 2 days did not show any change (Rizzo, Stamps, & Fehr, 1988), although this difference could be attributed to a practice effect. When placebo capsules were substituted for caffeinated capsules for a 2-day period in low to moderate caffeine consumers, performance on a range of psychomotor performance tasks was assessed (Silverman et al., 1992). Of the five tasks measured, performance on only a tapping task was significantly impaired following placebo compared to either baseline or caffeine. Tapping was also significantly different in individuals abstinent from caffeine for 24 hr (Bruce, Scott, Shine, & Lader, 1991). The general lack of performance impairment in the study by Silverman and colleagues (1992) may be due to the fact that subjects were only required to perform the tasks on a single occasion during the withdrawal period (presumably at peak withdrawal). These findings suggest that psychomotor performance effects may be observed only when periods of sustained performance and attention are required during caffeine abstinence. However, in a recent study (Comer, Haney, Fottin, & Fischman, 1977), the substitution of placebo for 2 consecutive days in individuals maintained on 300 mg caffeine did not alter performance on a range of tasks that were measured multiple times each day. While another study also failed to show that caffeine deprivation altered psychomotor performance (Richardson, Rogers, Elliman, & O'Dell, 1995), this study did not verify caffeine abstinence, making the results uninterpretable.

The incidence of caffeine withdrawal has varied considerably across studies and depends on the specific withdrawal symptom (cf. Griffiths & Woodson, 1988a). Among prospective studies, the incidence of headache has ranged from 17% to 100% and drowsiness or fatigue has ranged from 8% to 100% (Hughes, Oliveto, Bickel, et al., 1993). There is also evidence that the incidence is related to caffeine dose (Evans & Griffiths, 1991b; Fennelly, Galletly, & Purdie, 1991; A. Goldstein & Kaizer, 1969; Weber, Ereth, & Danielson, 1993). With

respect to the incidence of caffeine withdrawal in the general population, A. Goldstein and Kaizer (1969) conducted one of the first surveys in a group of housewives and found a dose-related increase, based on level of coffee consumption, in the number of effects reported if morning caffeine was omitted. Overall, 38% reported that not having their morning coffee made them feel half awake while only 6% reported getting a headache. The low rate of headache is not totally surprising given that the onset of headache usually requires a substantially longer period of caffeine deprivation. Among several other survey questionnaires, 11%–24% of respondents have reported withdrawal headache (Greden, Fontaine, Lubetsky, & Chamberlain, 1978; Greden, Victor, Fontaine, & Lubetsky, 1980; Victor, Lubetsky, & Greden, 1981). More recently, a random digit–dial telephone survey was conducted in Vermont, and among regular caffeine consumers who indicated that they had at some point abstained for at least 24 hr, 42% reported symptoms of caffeine withdrawal (Hughes, Oliveto, Helzer, Bickel, & Higgins, 1993).

In general, the results of experimental studies suggest that the incidence of caffeine withdrawal may be higher than the results obtained in surveys or questionnaires. In an early study by Dreisbach and Pfeiffer (1943), headache occurred in 82% of subjects. In a retrospective analysis of four studies (Hughes, Oliveto, Bickel, et al., 1993), the incidence of caffeine withdrawal ranged from 35% to 49%, depending on the criteria used. Two controlled laboratory studies, which required and verified caffeine abstinence, demonstrated caffeine withdrawal symptoms in 100% of subjects (Griffiths, Bigelow, & Liebson, 1986; Griffiths et al., 1990b). However, it should be noted that both studies used select subject populations; one study used heavy coffee drinkers who also had histories of alcohol or drug abuse (Griffiths, Bigelow, & Liebson, 1986) and the other study used scientists in the field (Griffiths et al., 1990b). Nevertheless, Griffiths and colleagues (1990b) established that moderate to severe caffeine withdrawal occurred reliably following chronic consumption of low caffeine doses (100 mg/day), which was subsequently replicated among a group of community volunteers (Evans & Griffiths, 1991b). Moderate to severe headache following a 2-day placebo substitution for caffeine was reported in 52% of low to moderate caffeine consumers recruited from the general community and several withdrawal symptoms (e.g., headache, drowsiness, sleepiness) were correlated with the dose of caffeine that subjects consumed (Silverman *et al.,* 1992). The incidence of withdrawal symptoms is also related to the duration of caffeine abstinence. For example, when subjects had to abstain from caffeine only after lunch or overnight, the frequency of headache was only 8% to 25% among heavy coffee drinkers when decaffeinated coffee was given (A. Goldstein, 1964; A. Goldstein *et al.,* 1969).

The time-course of caffeine withdrawal is orderly (Griffiths & Woodson, 1988a). The onset of withdrawal symptoms typically occurs 12–24 hr after termination of caffeine (e.g., Dreisbach & Pfeiffer, 1943; Goldstein *et al.,* 1969; Griffiths, Bigelow, & Liebson, 1986; Griffiths *et al.,* 1990b), although for some individuals the onset can be delayed for as long as 36 hr (Griffiths *et al.,* 1990b). The results of some studies suggest that the onset of symptoms such as fatigue and sleepiness occur prior to the onset of headache (Dreisbach & Pfeiffer, 1943; Evans & Griffiths, 1992; A. Goldstein *et al.,* 1969). Maximal withdrawal symptoms occur within the first 24–48 hr of caffeine deprivation and the symptoms usually persist for 2 days, to as long as 1 week or more; however, few studies have rigorously evaluated caffeine withdrawal beyond 48 hr (Dreisbach & Pfeiffer, 1943; Evans & Griffiths, 1992; Griffiths, Bigelow, & Liebson, 1986; Griffiths *et al.,* 1990b).

Although the incidence of caffeine withdrawal is relatively high, particularly in experimental studies, not all caffeine consumers experience caffeine withdrawal on discontinuation of caffeine. The reasons for this are unclear. As just described, there are a wide range of caffeine withdrawal symptoms that individuals endorse. While the symptoms experienced

after the termination of caffeine seem to vary as a function of caffeine dose, the magnitude and scope of symptoms varies both within and across individuals. This variability may be a true representation of caffeine withdrawal, but another set of factors that may contribute to this variable caffeine withdrawal syndrome is the variation across studies. Studies have differed in the doses of caffeine administered, the vehicle (e.g., coffee vs. capsules), the dosing interval, the duration of caffeine administration, and the duration of caffeine abstinence. For instance, if caffeine intake is terminated for 24 hr or less, a full caffeine withdrawal syndrome may not be manifested. Also, some studies have measured only one or two withdrawal symptoms as opposed to multiple symptoms, and nonexperimental studies have relied on retrospective reports rather than prospective reports. Last, but not least, many studies have not confirmed abstinence (i.e., measuring caffeine in biological samples), and this may have reduced the prevalence and magnitude of withdrawal symptoms (e.g., A. Goldstein *et al.,* 1969; Hughes, Oliveto, Bickel, *et al.,* 1993). If subjects are surreptitiously consuming caffeinated products during a presumed period of abstinence, withdrawal symptoms may be obscured.

The minimum dosing conditions needed to demonstrate caffeine withdrawal have not been adequately addressed until recently. Several studies have shown that consumption of high doses of caffeine for as little as 6–15 days can result in caffeine withdrawal upon abrupt cessation of caffeine (Dreisbach & Pfeiffer, 1943; Griffiths, Bigelow, & Liebson, 1986). In a subsequent study, with individuals maintained on a low dose of caffeine (100 mg/day) for a relatively long time (125–278 consecutive days), caffeine withdrawal symptoms were observed when placebo was substituted (Griffiths *et al.,* 1990b). In that same study, when a single day of placebo was intermittently substituted for caffeine every 5–17 days, caffeine withdrawal was still observed. However, as mentioned before, this study used a select, highly motivated and compliant subject population. A series of studies have been conducted to determine the specific parameters and conditions that determine dependence on caffeine, and the subsequent withdrawal symptoms on cessation of caffeine in low to moderate caffeine consumers (Evans & Griffiths, submitted). One experiment investigated the role of caffeine maintenance dose on the magnitude of withdrawal symptoms. Using a double-blind crossover design, subjects were maintained on either 100, 300 or 600 mg/day caffeine in capsules given b.i.d. Placebo was intermittently substituted for periods of 2 consecutive days after 5–9 days on a given caffeine maintenance dose. This study showed that the severity and range of withdrawal symptoms is a function of caffeine maintenance dose. Significant withdrawal symptoms were observed when subjects were maintained on as little as 100 mg caffeine each day (Evans & Griffiths, 1991b). In another study, using a similar design, the frequency of caffeine dosing on caffeine withdrawal was assessed by maintaining subjects on 300 mg caffeine each day either as a single dose in the morning or as 100 mg t.i.d. (Evans & Griffiths, submitted). When placebo was substituted for 300 mg/day caffeine, reliable caffeine withdrawal symptoms were observed and caffeine withdrawal was independent of the dosing interval, that is, whether caffeine was ingested as a single dose in the morning or in 3 doses divided throughout the day. Two other parametric studies have determined that doses as low as 100 mg caffeine can suppress caffeine withdrawal symptoms in subjects normally maintained on 300 mg caffeine each day, and caffeine physical dependence and withdrawal symptoms can develop following the relatively short duration of caffeine exposure of 3–7 days (Evans & Griffiths, submitted).

The results of several studies suggest that there is a relationship between caffeine physical dependence, or avoidance of caffeine withdrawal, and caffeine reinforcement (Evans et al., 1994; Griffiths, Bigelow, & Liebson, 1986; Griffiths & Woodson, 1988c; Hughes, Oliveto, Bickel, et al., 1993; Richardson & Rogers, 1993; Schluh & Griffiths, 1997; Garrett & Griffiths, in press). One of the first studies to experimentally test this hypothesis was conducted by Griffiths, Bigelow, and Liebson (1986). When subjects were maintained on caffeinated coffee for at least 1 week (presumably caffeine tolerant/dependent), after sampling both caffeinated and decaffeinated coffee, they chose caffeinated coffee almost exclusively. In contrast, when subjects were maintained on decaffeinated coffee for at least 1 week (presumably no longer tolerant or dependent), there was no preference for caffeinated coffee. When Hughes, Oliveto, Bickel, and colleagues (1993) combined data across four different studies in which subjects were exposed to caffeinated coffee (100 mg/cup) and decaffeinated coffee, the subjects who reported headaches and drowsiness on days they received decaffeinated coffee (i.e., experienced caffeine withdrawal) were 2.6 times more likely to choose caffeinated coffee. In another study, which maximized the likelihood that subjects were physically dependent on caffeine, comments made on an open-ended questionnaire and the choices of caffeine or placebo suggested that some subjects experienced caffeine withdrawal symptoms on placebo sampling days and subsequently chose caffeine to avoid these adverse effects (Evans et al., 1994). Two recent studies (Garrett & Griffiths, in press; Schuh & Griffiths, 1997) provide the strongest evidence to date that caffeine physical dependence increases the reinforcing effects of caffeine and that continued caffeine self-administration may have more to do with relieving or avoiding caffeine withdrawal than with the reinforcing effects of caffeine.

However, caffeine withdrawal is not a necessary condition for demonstrating caffeine choice. In most studies, there are some subjects who show reliable caffeine self-administration but do not report any caffeine withdrawal symptoms on placebo days (e.g., Hughes, Oliveto, Bickel, et al., 1993). Also, caffeine choice can be demonstrated in individuals who are not tolerant to caffeine and/or do not have a history of substantial caffeine intake (Griffiths & Woodson, 1988b; Griffiths, Bigelow, & Liebson, 1986a; Silverman et al., 1994a). For example, in the study by Silverman and colleagues (1994a), subjects were abstinent from nonexperimentally administered caffeine and caffeine administration was specifically scheduled to prevent the development of physical dependence, yet all subjects reliably chose caffeine over placebo when they had to engage in a vigilance task. Finally, a recent study directly assessed caffeine self-administration following various levels of caffeine deprivation (Mitchell, de Wit, & Zacny, 1995). Although complete caffeine deprivation produced reliable caffeine withdrawal symptoms, there was no subsequent increase in coffee self-administration. This however, does not mean that the self-administered coffee did not relieve the caffeine withdrawal. There are no data to suggest that individuals need to consume more caffeine that usual following a period of caffeine deprivation. In fact, as described above, as little as one-third the dose is sufficient to suppress caffeine withdrawal symptoms (Evans & Griffiths, submitted). A more direct assessment of this would have been to offer subjects a choice between caffeinated and decaffeinated coffee after different periods of caffeine deprivation.

Predisposing Factors

Relatively little is known regarding predisposing factors to the various behavioral effects of caffeine in humans, although this topic has been reviewed recently (Strain & Griffiths, 1997). There is some evidence suggesting that there may be a genetic predisposition for caffeine consumption (Gurling, Grant, & Dangl, 1985; Pedersen, 1981). Further, as described in "Reinforcing Effects of Caffeine," earlier in this chapter, there appears to be an inverse relationship between caffeine intake and anxiety (Nelig *et al.*, 1992). It also appears that certain subgroups of individuals, such as smokers, prisoners, psychiatric patients, and abusers of alcohol and/or other substances, are more likely to consume more caffeine than the normal population (see Strain & Griffiths, 1997), although the reasons for these differences are not understood. With respect to predisposition to caffeine withdrawal symptoms during caffeine abstinence, individuals prone to headache are more likely to experience caffeine withdrawal headaches (Weber *et al.*, 1993). The level of daily caffeine consumption is a relatively good predictor of caffeine withdrawal symptoms (e.g., Dreisbach & Pfeiffer, 1943; Evans & Griffiths, submitted).

Caffeine Abuse and Dependence

Historically, caffeine has been identified as having characteristics of a drug of abuse (e.g., Gilbert, 1976; Greden, 1981). In addition, while caffeine has been viewed as an excellent model for studying the behavioral effects of abused drugs (e.g., Holtzman, 1990; Rush *et al.*, 1995) and many studies reviewed in this chapter have shown that caffeine meets some of the clinical criteria for substance abuse (e.g., tolerance development, reinforcing effects, physical dependence; see review by Griffiths & Mumford, 1995), there remains insufficient data to conclude that caffeine should be considered a drug of abuse using *DSM-IV* criteria (Heishman & Henningfield, 1992; Hughes, 1992; Hughes, Oliveto, Helzer, Higgins, & Bickel, 1992; Strain & Griffiths, 1997). The primary substance dependence criteria that have been difficult to demonstrate with caffeine have included criterion 4 (unsuccessful attempts to cut down or control use) and criterion 7 (continued use despite knowledge of having a physical or psychological problem that may be related or due to use of the substance). At this time caffeine is the one drug class to which a clinical diagnosis of Substance Dependence cannot be given (American Psychiatric Association, 1994). Further, several of the criteria for Substance Dependence do not seem to apply to caffeine, which is widely available and culturally acceptable. Recently, two studies have provided some preliminary clinical data to suggest that some caffeine users could meet criteria for a caffeine dependence syndrome (Hughes, Oliveto, Helzer, *et al.*, 1993; Strain, Mumford, Silverman, & Griffiths, 1994). Using a random telephone survey in Vermont, individuals were interviewed and *DSM-III-R* (American Psychiatric Association, 1987) criteria (meeting 3 out of 9 criteria) for drug dependence were applied (Hughes, Oliveto, Helzer, *et al.*, 1993). Out of 166 caffeine users, 44% met the criteria for drug dependence to caffeine in the past year. A more controlled study conducted structured diagnostic interviews using the general *DSM-IV* criteria for substance dependence with individuals who reported that they were psychologically or physically dependent on caffeine (Strain *et al.*, 1994). In this study, to meet the criteria of caffeine dependence, subjects had to fulfill 3 of 4 criteria (tolerance, withdrawal, persistent attempts to reduce or control use, continued use despite a medical or psychological problem that may have caused or exacerbated the problem) rather than the traditional 3 of 7 criteria. Out of 27 individuals who were interviewed, 59% met the criteria for caffeine dependence; 6 of these subjects had been instructed by their physicians to reduce or eliminate caffeine. Further, when a double-blind withdrawal study was conducted in 11 of these individuals, 82% experienced caffeine withdrawal symptoms when they received placebo. At this time, the actual prevalence of caffeine dependence syndrome is not known and further clinical research is needed to determine whether enough individuals meet the criteria to consider it a clinical disorder.

Therapeutic Effects of Caffeine

Caffeine is primarily consumed in beverages for its mild behavioral stimulant effects. However, caffeine does have some therapeutic benefits for a variety of conditions including headaches, sleepiness, respiratory depression in neonates, hypotension in the elderly, obesity, and postoperative pain (Sawynok, 1995). Primarily, caffeine is used in combination with ergotamine to treat migraine headaches (see Sawynok, 1995), but is also an effective treatment for headaches following lumbar puncture (e.g., Sechzer, 1979). One of the most obvious therapeutic uses of caffeine is for headaches induced by habitual caffeine consumers abstaining from caffeine prior to a surgical procedure or fasting (Fennelly *et al.*, 1991; Galletly, Fennelly, & Whitman, 1989; Shorof-

sky & Lamm, 1977). The incidence of perioperative headache appears to be related to the level of caffeine intake and can be reduced by ingesting caffeine (Fennelly *et al.*, 1991; Weber *et al.*, 1993, 1997).

Caffeine is commonly used as an adjuvant to numerous analgesic medications, primarily aspirin-like drugs. There is a reasonable amount of preclinical data to suggest that caffeine is an adequate analgesic, both alone and in combination with other analgesics (Sawynok & Yaksh, 1993). While the evidence is less clear in humans, studies evaluating postoperative pain have shown that caffeine, in combination with other analgesics, is more potent than analgesics without caffeine (Forbes *et al.*, 1991; Laska *et al.*, 1984), whereas caffeine alone appears to be relatively ineffective (Forbes *et al.*, 1991).

Other therapeutic uses of caffeine include respiratory stimulation in premature infants (e.g., Bairam, Boutroy, Badonnel, & Vert, 1987), the blockade of postprandial and postural hypotension in the elderly (Ahmad & Watson, 1990; Heseltine, Dakkak, Woodhouse, Macdonald, & Potter, 1991) and enhancement of seizure duration for electroconvulsive therapy (e.g., Coffey, Figiel, & Weiner, 1990).

The doses of caffeine that have been used therapeutically range from approximately 65 mg in analgesic combinations to as high as 1,000 mg for electroconvulsive therapy. The range of therapeutic effects of caffeine also appears to involve several mechanisms. For instance, for the treatment of migraine headaches, caffeine is thought to enhance ergotamine's effects on vasoconstriction and reduction of cerebral blood flow. With respect to the analgesic effects, caffeine may be blocking either the central or peripheral actions of adenosine receptors, which are nociceptive (see Sawynok, 1995).

References

Ahlijanian, M. K., & Takemori, A. E. (1986). Cross-tolerance studies between caffeine and (–)-N^6-(phenyl isopropyl)-adenosine (PIA) in mice. *Life Sciences, 38,* 577–588.

Ahmad, R. A., & Watson, R. D. (1990). Treatment of postural hypotension. A review. *Drugs, 39*, 74–85.

American Psychiatric Association. (1987). *Diagnostic and statistical manual of mental disorders* (3rd ed., rev.). Washington, DC: Author.

American Psychiatric Association. (1994). *Diagnostic and statistical manual of mental disorders* (4th ed.). Washington, DC: Author.

Ammon, H. P. T., Bieck, P. R., Mandalaz, D., & Verspohl, E. J. (1983). Adaptation of blood pressure to continuous heavy coffee drinking in young volunteers. A double-blind crossover study. *British Journal of Clinical Pharmacology, 15*, 701–706.

Atkinson, J., & Enslen, M. (1976). Self-administration of caffeine by the rat. *Arzneimittel-Forschung, 26*, 2059–2061.

Bairam, A., Boutroy, M. J., Badonnel, Y., & Vert, P. (1987). Theophylline versus caffeine: Comparative effects in treatment of idiopathic apnea in the preterm infant. *Journal of Pediatrics, 110*, 636–639.

Balster, R. L. (1987). Abuse potential evaluation of inhalants. *Drug and Alcohol Dependence, 19*, 7–15.

Barone, J. J., & Roberts, H. (1984). Human consumption of caffeine. In P. B. Dews (Ed.), *Caffeine: Perspectives from recent research* (pp. 59–73). Berlin: Springer-Verlag.

Bättig, K. (1985). The physiological effects of coffee consumption. In M. N. Clifford & C. K. Wilson (Eds.), *Coffee: Botany, biochemistry and production of beans and beverages* (pp. 394–439). London: Croom Helm.

Bättig, K., & Welzl, H. (1993). Psychopharmacological profile of caffeine. In S. Garattini (Ed.), *Caffeine, coffee, and health* (pp. 213–253). New York: Raven.

Bonnet, M. H., & Arand, D. L. (1992). Caffeine use as a model of acute and chronic insomnia. *Sleep, 15*, 526–536.

Boulenger, J. P., & Uhde, T. W. (1982). Biochemical aspects of anxiety. *Semaine des Hopitaux, 58*, 2573–2579.

Boulenger, J. P., Uhde, T. W., Wolff, E. A., III, & Post, R. M. (1984). Increased sensitivity to caffeine in patients with panic disorders. Preliminary evidence. *Archives of General Psychiatry, 41*, 1067–1071.

Boyd, E. M., Dolman, M., Knight, L. M., & Sheppard, E. P. (1965). The chronic oral toxicity of caffeine. *Canadian Journal of Physiology and Pharmacology, 43*, 995–1007.

Bozarth, M. A. (1987). An overview of assessing drug reinforcement. In M. A. Bozarth (Ed.), *Methods of assessing the reinforcing properties of abused drugs* (pp. 635–658). New York: Springer-Verlag.

Bruce, M., Scott, N., Shine, P., & Lader, M. (1991). Caffeine withdrawal: A contrast of withdrawal symptoms in normal subjects who have abstained from caffeine for 24 hours and for 7 days. *Journal of Psychopharmacology, 5*, 129–134.

Carney, J. M. (1982). Effects of caffeine, theophylline and theobromine on scheduled controlled responding in rats. *British Journal of Clinical Pharmacology, 75*, 451–454.

Carney, J. M., Holloway, F. A., & Modrow, H. E. (1985). Discriminative stimulus properties of methylxanthines and their metabolites in rats. *Life Sciences, 36*, 913–920.

Carroll, M. E. (1987). A quantitative assessment of phencyclidine dependence produced by oral self-administration in rhesus monkeys. *Journal of Pharmacology and Experimental Therapeutics, 242*, 405–412.

Carroll, M. E., Hagen, E. W., Asencio, M., & Hartman Brauer, L. (1989). Behavioral dependence on caffeine and phencyclidine in rhesus monkeys: Interactive effects. *Pharmacology, Biochemistry and Behavior, 31*, 927–932.

Chait, L. D., & Griffiths, R. R. (1983). Effects of caffeine on cigarette smoking and subjective response. *Clinical Pharmacology and Therapeutics, 34*, 612–622.

Chait, L. D., & Johanson, C. E. (1988). Discriminative stimulus effects of caffeine and benzphetamine in amphetamine-trained volunteers. *Psychopharmacology, 96*, 302–308.

Charney, D. S., Heninger, G. R., & Jatlow, P. I. (1985). Increased anxiogenic effects of caffeine in panic disorder. *Archives of General Psychiatry, 42*, 233–243.

Chou, D. T., Khan, S., Forde, J., & Hirsh, K. R. (1985). Caffeine tolerance: Behavioral, electrophysiological and neurochemical evidence. *Life Sciences, 36*, 2347–2358.

Coffey, C. E., Figiel, S., & Weiner, R. D. (1990). Caffeine augmentation of ECT. *American Journal of Psychiatry, 147*, 579–85.

Coffin, V. L., & Carney, J. M. (1983). Behavioral pharmacology of adenosine analogs. In J. W. Daly, Y. Kuroda, J. W. Phillis, H. Shimizu, & M. Ui (Eds.), *Physiology and pharmacology of adenosine derivatives* (pp. 267–274). New York: Raven.

Cole, J. O., Pope, H. G., Jr., Labrie, R., & Ionescu-Pioggia, M. (1978). Assessing the subjective effects of stimulants in casual users. A methodology and preliminary results. *Clinical Pharmacology and Therapeutics, 24*, 243–252.

Collins, R. J., Weeks, J. R., Cooper, M. M., Good, P. I., & Russell, R. R. (1984). Prediction of abuse liability of drugs using IV self-administration by rats. *Psychopharmacology* (Berlin), *82*, 6–13.

Colton, T., Gosselin, R. E., & Smith, R. P. (1968). The tolerance of coffee drinkers to caffeine. *Clinical Pharmacology and Therapeutics, 9*, 31–39.

Comer, S. D., Haney, M., Foltin, R. W., & Fischman, M. W. (1997). Effects of caffeine withdrawal on humans living in a residential laboratory. *Experimental and Clinical Psychopharmacology, 5*, 399–403.

Denaro, C. P., Brown, C. R., Jacob, P., III, & Benowitz, N. L. (1991). Effects of caffeine with repeated dosing. *European Journal of Clinical Pharmacology, 40*, 273–278.

Deneau, G., Yanagita, T., & Seevers, M. H. (1969). Self-administration of psychoactive substances by the monkey. *Psychopharmacologia, 16,* 30–48.

Dreisbach, R. H., & Pfeiffer, C. (1943). Caffeine-withdrawal headache. *Journal of Laboratory and Clinical Medicine, 28,* 1212–1219.

Dworkin, S. I., Vrana, S. L., Broadbent, J., & Robinson, J. H. (1993). Comparing the effects of nicotine, caffeine, methylphenidate and cocaine. *Medicinal Chemistry Research, 2,* 593–602.

Eddy, N. B., & Downs, A. W. (1928). Tolerance and cross-tolerance in the human subject to the diuretic effect of caffeine, theobromine and theophylline. *Journal of Pharmacology and Experimental Therapeutics, 33,* 167–174.

Evans, S. M., & Griffiths, R. R. (1991a). Dose-related caffeine discrimination in normal volunteers: Individual differences in subjective effects and self-reported cues. *Behavioral Pharmacology, 2,* 345–356.

Evans, S. M., & Griffiths, R. R. (1991b). Low-dose caffeine physical dependence in normal subjects: Dose-related effects. In L. S. Harris (Ed.), *Problems of drug dependence, 1990* (NIDA Research Monograph No. 105, pp. 446–447). Washington, DC: U.S. Government Printing Office.

Evans, S. M., & Griffiths, R. R. (1992). Caffeine tolerance and choice in humans. *Psychopharmacology, 108,* 51–59.

Evans, S. M., & Griffiths, R. R. Caffeine withdrawal: A parametric analysis of caffeine dosing conditions. Manuscript submitted for publication.

Evans, S. M., & Johanson, C. E. (1987). Amphetamine-like effects of anorectics and related compounds in pigeons. *Journal of Pharmacology and Experimental Therapeutics, 241,* 817–825.

Evans, S. M., Critchfield, T. S., & Griffiths, R. R. (1994). Caffeine reinforcement demonstrated in a majority of moderate caffeine users. *Behavioral Pharmacology, 5,* 231–238.

Fennelly, M., Galletly, D. C., & Purdie, G. I. (1991). Is caffeine withdrawal the mechanism for postoperative headache? *Anesthesia and Analgesia, 72,* 449–53.

File, S. E., Bond, A. J., & Lister, R. G. (1982). Interaction between effects of caffeine and lorazepam in performance tests and self-ratings. *Journal of Clinical Psychopharmacology, 2,* 102–106.

File, S. E., Baldwin, H. A., Johnston, A. L., & Wilks, L. J. (1988). Behavioral effects of acute and chronic administration of caffeine in the rat. *Pharmacology, Biochemistry and Behavior, 30,* 809–815.

Finn, I. B., & Holtzman, S. G. (1986). Tolerance to caffeine-induced stimulation of locomotor activity in rats. *Journal of Pharmacology and Experimental Therapeutics, 238,* 542–546.

Finn, I. B., & Holtzman, S. G. (1987). Pharmacologic specificity of tolerance to caffeine-induced stimulation of locomotor activity. *Psychopharmacology, 93,* 428–434.

Finn, I. B., & Holtzman, S. G. (1988). Tolerance and cross-tolerance to theophylline-induced stimulation of locomotor activity in rats. *Life Sciences, 42,* 2475–2482.

Forbes, J. A., Beaver, W. T., Jones, K. F., Kehm, C. J., Smith, W. K., Gongloff, C. M., Zeleznock, J. R., & Smith, J. W. (1991). Effect of caffeine on ibuprofen analgesia in postoperative oral surgery pain. *Clinical Pharmacology and Therapeutics, 49,* 674–684.

Froberg, J., Karlsson, C. G., Levi, L., Linde, L., & Seeman, K. (1969). Test performance and subjective feelings as modified by caffeine-containing and caffeine-free coffee. In F. Heim, H. P. T. Ammon, & F. K. Schattauer (Eds.), *Koffein und andere methylxanthine* (pp. 15–20). Stuttgart, Germany: Springer.

Galletly, D. C., Fennelly, M., & Whitman, J. G. (1989). Does caffeine withdrawal contribute to postanaesthetic morbidity? *Lancet, 1,* 1335.

Garrett, B. E., & Griffiths, R. R. (in press). Physical dependence increases the relative reinforcing effects of caffeine versus placebo. *Psychopharmacology.*

Gauvin, D. V., Harland, R. D., Michaelis, R. C., & Holloway, F. A. (1989). Caffeine-phenylethylamine combinations mimic the cocaine discriminative cue. *Life Sciences, 44,* 67–73.

Gauvin, D. V., Peirce, J. M., & Holloway, F. A. (1994). Perceptual masking of the chlordiazepoxide discriminative cue by both caffeine and buspirone. *Pharmacology, Biochemistry and Behavior, 47,* 153–159.

Gilbert, R. M. (1976). Caffeine as a drug of abuse. In R. J. Gibbins, Y. Israel, H. Kalant, R. E. Popham, W. I. Schmidt, & R. G. Smart (Eds.), *Research advances in alcohol and drug problems* (pp. 49–176). New York: Wiley.

Gilbert, R. M. (1984). Caffeine consumption. In G. A. Spiller (Ed.), *The methylxanthine beverages and foods: Chemistry, consumption, and health effects* (pp. 185–213). New York: Liss.

Goldstein, A. (1964). Wakefulness caused by caffeine. *Naunyn Schmiedeberg's Archiv fur Experimentelle Pathologie und Pharmakologie, 248,* 269–278.

Goldstein, A., & Kaizer, S. (1969). Psychotropic effects of caffeine in man: 3. A questionnaire survey of coffee drinking and its effects in a group of housewives. *Clinical Pharmacology and Therapeutics, 10,* 477–488.

Goldstein, A., Kaizer, S., & Warren, R. (1965). Psychotropic effects of caffeine in man: II. Alertness, psychomotor coordination, and mood. *Journal of Pharmacology and Experimental Therapeutics, 150,* 146–151.

Goldstein, A., Warren, R., & Kaizer, S. (1965). Psychotropic effects of caffeine in man. I. Individual differences in sensitivity to caffeine-induced wakefulness. *Journal of Pharmacology and Experimental Therapeutics, 149,* 156–159.

Goldstein, A., Kaizer, S., & Whitby, O. (1969). Psychotropic effects of caffeine in man: IV. Quantitative and qualitative differences associated with habituation to coffee. *Clinical Pharmacology and Therapeutics, 10,* 489–497.

Goldstein, I. B., Shapiro, D., Hui, K. K., & Yu, J. L. (1990). Blood pressure response to the "second cup of coffee." *Psychosomatic Medicine, 52,* 337–345.

Graham, D. M. (1978). Caffeine—Its identity, dietary sources, intake and biological effects. *Nutritional Reviews, 36,* 97–102.

Greden, J. F. (1981). Caffeinism and caffeine withdrawal. In J. H. Lowinson & P. Reiz (Eds.), *Substance abuse: Clinical problems and perspectives* (pp. 274–286). Baltimore: Williams and Wilkins.

Greden, J. F., Fontaine, P., Lubetsky, M., & Chamberlin, K. (1978). Anxiety and depression associated with caffeinism among psychiatric inpatients. *American Journal of Psychiatry, 135,* 963–966.

Greden, J. F., Victor, B. S., Fontaine, P., & Lubetsky, M. (1980). Caffeine-withdrawal headache: A clinical profile. *Psychosomatics, 21,* 411–418.

Griffiths, R. R., & Mumford, G. K. (1995). Caffeine—A drug of abuse? In F. E. Bloom & D. J. Kupfer (Eds.), *Psychopharmacology: The fourth generation of progress* (pp. 1699–1713). New York: Raven.

Griffiths, R. R., & Mumford, G. K. (1996). Caffeine reinforcement, discrimination, tolerance and physical dependence in laboratory animals and humans. In C. R. Schuster & M. J. Kuhar (Eds.), *Handbook of experimental pharmacology* (Vol. 118, pp. 315–341). Heidelberg, Germany: Springer-Verlag.

Griffiths, R. R., & Woodson, P. P. (1988a). Caffeine physical dependence: A review of human and laboratory animal studies. *Psychopharmacology, 94,* 437–451.

Griffiths, R. R., & Woodson, P. P. (1988b). Reinforcing effects of caffeine in humans. *Journal of Pharmacology and Experimental Therapeutics, 246,* 21–29.

Griffiths, R. R., & Woodson, P. P. (1988c). Reinforcing properties of caffeine: Studies in humans and laboratory animals. *Pharmacology, Biochemistry and Behavior, 29,* 419–427.

Griffiths, R. R., Brady, J. V., & Bradford, L. D. (1979). Progressive ratio and fixed ratio schedules of cocaine-maintained responding in baboons. *Psychopharmacology, 65,* 125–136.

Griffiths, R. R., Bigelow, G. E., & Henningfield, J. E. (1980). Similarities in animal and human drug-taking behavior. In N. K. Mello (Ed.), *Advances in substance abuse* (Vol. 1, pp. 1–90). Greenwich, CT: JAI.

Griffiths, R. R., Bigelow, G. E., & Liebson, I. A. (1986). Human coffee drinking: Reinforcing and physical dependence producing effects of caffeine. *Journal of Pharmacology and Experimental Therapeutics, 239,* 416–425.

Griffiths, R. R., Bigelow, G. E., Liebson, I. A., O'Keefe, M., O'Leary, D., & Russ, N. (1986). Human coffee drinking: Manipulation of concentration and caffeine dose. *Journal of the Experimental Analysis of Behavior, 45,* 133–148.

Griffiths, R. R., Bigelow, G. E., & Liebson, I. A. (1989). Reinforcing effects of caffeine in coffee and capsules. *Journal of the Experimental Analysis of Behavior, 52,* 127–140.

Griffiths, R. R., Evans, S. M., Heishman, S. J., Preston, K. L., Sannerud, C. A., Wolf, B., & Woodson, P. P. (1990a). Low-dose caffeine discrimination in humans. *Journal of Pharmacology and Experimental Therapeutics, 252,* 970–978.

Griffiths, R. R., Evans, S. M., Heishman, S. J., Preston, K. L., Sannerud, C. A., Wolf, B., & Woodson, P. P. (1990b). Low-dose caffeine physical dependence in humans. *Journal of Pharmacology and Experimental Therapeutics, 255,* 1123–1132.

Gurling, H. M., Grant, S., & Dangl, J. (1985). The genetic and cultural transmission of alcohol use, alcoholism, cigarette smoking and coffee drinking: A review and an example using a log linear cultural transmission model. *British Journal of Addiction, 80,* 269–279.

Haertzen, C. A. (1974). *An overview of Addiction Research Center Inventory Scales (ARCI): An appendix and Manual of Scales* (U.S. Department of Health and Human Services Publication No. (ADM) 74-92). Rockville, MD.

Haigh, R. A., Harper, G. D., Fotherby, M., Hurd, J., Macdonald, I. A., & Potter, J. F. (1993). Duration of caffeine abstention influences the acute blood pressure responses to caffeine in elderly normotensives. *European Journal of Clinical Pharmacology, 44,* 549–553.

Hale, K. L., Hughes, J. R., Oliveto, A. H., & Higgins, S. T. (1995). Caffeine self-administration and subjective effects in adolescents. *Experimental and Clinical Psychopharmacology, 3,* 364–370.

Harland, R. D., Gauvin, D. V., Michaelis, R. C., Carney, J. M., Seale, T. W., & Holloway, F. A. (1989). Behavioral interaction between cocaine and caffeine: A drug discrimination analysis in rats. *Pharmacology, Biochemistry and Behavior, 32,* 1017–1023.

Hasenfratz, M., & Bättig, K. (1994). Acute dose-effect relationships of caffeine and mental performance, EEG, cardiovascular and subjective parameters. *Psychopharmacology, 114,* 281–287.

Heishman, S. J., & Henningfield, J. E. (1992). Stimulus functions of caffeine in humans: Relation to dependence potential. *Neuroscience and Biobehavioral Reviews, 16,* 273–287.

Heishman, S. J., Taylor, R. C., Goodman, M. L., Evans, S. M., & Henningfield, J. E. (1993). Discriminative stimulus effects of d-amphetamine, caffeine, and mazindol in humans. *Pharmacology, Biochemistry and Behavior, 46,* 502–503.

Heppner, C. C., Kemble, E. D., & Cox, W. M. (1986). Effects of food deprivation on caffeine consumption in male and female rats. *Pharmacology, Biochemistry and Behavior, 24,* 1555–1559.

Heseltine, D., Dakkak, M., Woodhouse, K., Macdonald, I. A., & Potter, J. F. (1991). The effect of caffeine on postprandial hypotension in the elderly. *Journal of the American Geriatric Society, 39,* 160–164.

Hoffmeister, F., & Wuttke, W. (1973). Negative reinforcing properties of morphine-antagonists in naive rhesus monkeys. *Psychopharmacologia, 33,* 247–258.

Holloway, F. A., Michaelis, R. C., & Huerta, P. L. (1985). Caffeine-phenylethylamine combinations mimic the amphetamine discriminative cue. *Life Sciences, 36,* 723–730.

Holloway, F. A., Modrow, H. E., & Michaelis, R. C. (1985). Methylxanthine discrimination in the rat: Possible benzodiazepine and adenosine mechanisms. *Pharmacology, Biochemistry and Behavior, 22,* 815–824.

Holtzman, S. G. (1983). Complete, reversible, drug-specific tolerance to stimulation of locomotor activity by caffeine. *Life Sciences, 33,* 779–787.

Holtzman, S. G. (1986). Discriminative stimulus properties of caffeine in the rat: Noradrenergic mediation. *Journal of Pharmacology and Experimental Therapeutics, 239,* 706–714.

Holtzman, S. G. (1987). Discriminative stimulus effects of caffeine: Tolerance and cross-tolerance with methylphenidate. *Life Sciences, 40,* 381–389.

Holtzman, S. G. (1990). Caffeine as a model drug of abuse. *Trends in Pharmacologic Science, 11,* 355–356.

Holtzman, S. G. (1991). CGS 15943, a nonxanthine adenosine receptor antagonist: Effects on locomotor activity of nontolerant and caffeine-tolerant rats. *Life Sciences, 49,* 1563–1570.

Holtzman, S. G., & Finn, I. B. (1988). Tolerance to behavioral effects of caffeine in rats. *Pharmacology, Biochemistry and Behavior, 29,* 411–418.

Holtzman, S. G., & Villarreal, J. (1973). Operant behavior in the morphine-dependent rhesus monkey. *Journal of Pharmacology and Experimental Therapeutics, 184,* 528–541.

Howell, L. L., & Landrum, A. M. (1997). Effects of chronic caffeine administration on respiration and schedule-controlled behavior in rhesus monkeys. *Journal of Pharmacology and Experimental Therapeutics, 283,* 190–199.

Hughes, J. R. (1992). Clinical importance of caffeine withdrawal. *New England Journal of Medicine, 327,* 1160–1161.

Hughes, J. R., Higgins, S. T., Bickel, W. K., Hunt, W. K., Fenwick, J. W., Gulliver, S. B., & Mireault, G. C. (1991). Caffeine self-administration, withdrawal, and adverse effects among coffee drinkers. *Archives of General Psychiatry, 48,* 611–617.

Hughes, J. R., Hunt, W. K., Higgins, S. T., Bickel, W. K., Fenwick, J. W., & Pepper, S. L. (1992). Effect of dose on the ability of caffeine to serve as a reinforcer in humans. *Behavioural Pharmacology, 3,* 211–218.

Hughes, J. R., Oliveto, A. H., Bickel, W. K., Higgins, S. T., & Valliere, W. (1992). Caffeine self-administration and withdrawal in soda drinkers. *Journal of Addictive Diseases, 4,* 178.

Hughes, J. R., Oliveto, A. H., Helzer, J. E., Higgins, S. T., & Bickel, W. K. (1992). Should caffeine abuse, dependence or withdrawal be added to DSM-IV or ICD-10? *American Journal of Psychiatry, 149,* 33–40.

Hughes, J. R., Oliveto, A. H., Bickel, W. K., Higgins, S. T., & Badger, G. J. (1993). Caffeine self-administration and withdrawal: Incidence, individual differences and interrelationships. *Drug and Alcohol Dependence, 32,* 239–246.

Hughes, J. R., Oliveto, A. H., Helzer, J. E., Bickel, W. K., & Higgins, S. T. (1993). Indications of caffeine dependence in a population-based sample. In L. S. Harris (Ed.), *Problems of drug dependence, 1992* (p. 194). Washington, DC: U.S. Government Printing Office.

Hughes, J. R., Oliveto, A. H., Bickel, W. K., Higgins, S. T., & Badger, G. J. (1995). The ability of low doses of caffeine to serve as reinforcers in humans: A replication. *Experimental and Clinical Psychopharmacology, 3,* 358–363.

Johanson, C. E. (1978). Drugs as reinforcers. In D. E. Blackman & D. J. Sanger (Eds.), *Contemporary research in behavioral pharmacology* (pp. 325–390). New York: Plenum.

Jones, C. N., Howard, J. L., & Bennett, S. T. (1980). Stimulus properties of antidepressants in the rat. *Psychopharmacology* (Berlin), *67,* 111–118.

Kamien, J. B., Bickel, W. K., Hughes, J. R., Higgins, S. T., & Smith, B. J. (1993). Drug discrimination by humans compared to nonhumans: Current status and future directions. *Psychopharmacology, 111,* 259–270.

Kaplan, G. B., Greenblatt, D. J., Kent, M. A., & Cotreau-Bibbo, M. M. (1993). Caffeine treatment and withdrawal in mice: Relationships between dosage, concentrations, locomotor activity and A_1 adenosine receptor binding. *Journal of Pharmacology and Experimental Therapeutics, 266,* 1563–1572.

Katz, J. L., & Goldberg, S. R. (1987). Psychomotor stimulant effects of caffeine alone and in combination with an adenosine analog in the squirrel monkey. *Journal of Pharmacology and Experimental Therapeutics, 242,* 179–187.

Kozlowski, L. T. (1976). Effect of caffeine on coffee drinking. *Nature, 264,* 354–355.

Kuhn, D. M., Appel, J. B., & Greenberg, I. (1974). An analysis of some discriminative properties of d-amphetamine. *Psychopharmacologia, 39,* 57–66.

Lane, J. D., & Manus, D. C. (1989). Caffeine may potentiate adrenocortical stress responses in hypertension-prone men. *Hypertension, 14,* 170–176.

Lane, J. D., & Williams, R. B. (1987). Cardiovascular effects of caffeine and stress in regular coffee drinkers. *Psychophysiology, 24,* 157–64.

Laska, E. M., Sunshine, A., Mueller, F., Elvers, W. B., Siegel, C., & Rubin, A. (1984). Caffeine as an analgesic adjuvant. *Journal of the American Medical Association, 251,* 1711–1718.

Lau, C. E., & Falk, J. L. (1994). Tolerance to oral and IP caffeine: Locomotor activity and pharmacokinetics. *Pharmacology, Biochemistry and Behavior, 48*, 337–344.

Lau, C. E., & Falk, J. L. (1995). Dose-dependent surmountability of locomotor activity in caffeine tolerance. *Pharmacology, Biochemistry and Behavior, 52*, 139–143.

Leathwood, P. D., & Pollet, P. (1983). Diet-induced mood changes in normal populations. *Journal of Psychiatric Research, 17*, 147–154.

Lee, M. A., Cameron, O. G., & Greden, J. F. (1985). Anxiety and caffeine consumption in people with anxiety disorders. *Psychiatry Research, 15*, 211–217.

Lieberman, H. R., Wurtman, R. J., Emde, G. G., & Coviella, I. L. (1987). The effects of caffeine and aspirin on mood and performance. *Journal of Clinical Psychopharmacology, 7*, 315–320.

Lieberman, H. R., Wurtman, R. J., Emde, G. G., Roberts, C., & Coviella, I. L. (1987). The effects of low doses of caffeine on human performance and mood. *Psychopharmacology, 92*, 308–312.

Ligori, A., & Hughes, J. R. (1997). Caffeine self-administration in humans: 2. A within-subjects comparison of coffee and cola vehicles. *Experimental and Clinical Psychopharmacology, 5*, 195–303.

Ligori, A., Hughes, J. R., & Oliveto, A. H. (1997). Caffeine self-administration in humans: 1. Efficacy of cola vehicle. *Experimental and Clinical Psychopharmacology, 5*, 286–294.

Loke, W. H. (1988). Effects of caffeine on mood and memory. *Physiology and Behavior, 44*, 367–372.

Mariathasan, E. A., & Stolerman, I. P. (1992). Drug discrimination studies in rats with caffeine and phenylpropanolamine administered separately and as mixtures. *Psychopharmacology* (Berlin), *109*, 99–106.

Meisch, R. A. (1977). Ethanol self-administration: Infrahuman studies. In T. Thompson & P. B. Dews (Eds.), *Advances in behavioral pharmacology* (Vol. 1, pp. 35–84). New York: Academic Press.

Mitchell, S. H., de Wit, H., & Zacny, J. P. (1995). Caffeine withdrawal symptoms and self-administration following caffeine deprivation. *Pharmacology, Biochemistry and Behavior, 51*, 941–945.

Modrow, H. E., & Holloway, F. A. (1985). Drug discrimination and cross generalization between two methylxanthines. *Pharmacology, Biochemistry and Behavior, 23*, 425–429.

Modrow, H. E., Holloway, F. A., & Carney, M. (1981). Caffeine discrimination in the rat. *Pharmacology, Biochemistry and Behavior, 14*, 683–688.

Modrow, H. E., Holloway, F. A., Christensen, H. D., & Carney, M. (1981). Relationship between caffeine discrimination and caffeine plasma levels. *Pharmacology, Biochemistry and Behavior, 15*, 323–325.

Mumford, G. K., & Holtzman, S. G. (1991). Qualitative differences in the discriminative stimulus effects of low and high doses of caffeine in the rat. *Journal of Pharmacology and Experimental Therapeutics, 258*, 857–865.

Mumford, G. K., Neill, D. B., & Holtzman, S. G. (1988). Caffeine elevates reinforcement threshold for electrical brain stimulation: Tolerance and withdrawal changes. *Brain Research, 459*, 163–167.

Mumford, G. K., Evans, S. M., Kaminski, B. J., Preston, K. L., Sannerud, C. A., Silverman, K., & Griffiths, R. R. (1994). Discriminative stimulus and subjective effects of theobromine and caffeine in humans. *Psychopharmacology, 115*, 1–8.

Nehlig, A., Daval J., & Debry G. (1992). Caffeine and the central nervous system: Mechanisms of action, biochemical, metabolic and psychostimulant effects. *Brain Research Reviews, 17*, 139–170.

Nikodijevic, O., Jacobson, K. A., & Daly, J. W. (1993). Locomotor activity in mice during chronic treatment with caffeine and withdrawal. *Pharmacology, Biochemistry and Behavior, 44*, 199–216.

Oliveto, A. H., Hughes, J. R., Pepper, S. L., Bickel, W. K., & Higgins, S. T. (1991). Low doses of caffeine can serve as reinforcers in humans. In L. S. Harris (Ed.), *Problems of drug dependence, 1990* (NIDA Research Monograph No. 105, p. 442). Washington, DC: U.S. Government Printing Office.

Oliveto, A. H., Bickel, W. K., Hughes, J. R., Shea, P. J., Higgins, S. T., & Fenwick, J. W. (1992). Caffeine drug discrimination in humans: Acquisition, specificity and correlation with self-reports. *Journal of Pharmacology and Experimental Therapeutics, 261*, 885–894.

Oliveto, A. H., Hughes, J. R., Higgins, S. T., Bickel, W. K., Pepper, S. L., & Shea, P. J. (1992). Forced-choice versus free-choice procedures: Caffeine self-administration in humans. *Psychopharmacology, 109*, 85–91.

Oliveto, A. H., Bickel, W. K., Hughes, J. R., Terry, S. Y., Higgins, S. T., & Badger, G. J. (1993). Pharmacological specificity of the caffeine discriminative stimulus in humans: Effects of theophylline, methylphenidate and buspirone. *Behavioural Pharmacology, 4*, 237–246.

Overton, D. A. (1973). State dependent learning produced by addicting drugs. *Psychopharmacology Bulletin, 9*, 29–31.

Overton, D. A., & Batta, S. K. (1977). Relationship between abuse liability of drugs and their degree of discriminability in the rat. In T. Thompson & K. Unna (Eds.), *Predicting dependence liability of stimulant and depressant drugs* (pp. 125–135). Baltimore: University Park Press.

Pedersen, N. (1981). Twin similarity for usage of common drugs. *Progress in Clinical and Biological Research, 69*, 53–59.

Podboy, J. W., & Malloy, W. A. (1977). Caffeine reduction and behavior change in the severely retarded. *Mental Retardation, 15*, 40.

Richardson, N. J., & Rogers, P. J. (1993). Caffeine, caffeine withdrawal, and preference for caffeine-containing beverages. *Appetite, 21,* 201.

Richardson, N. J., Rogers, P. J., Elliman, N. A., & O'Dell, R. J. (1995). Mood and performance effects of caffeine in relation to acute and chronic caffeine deprivation. *Pharmacology, Biochemistry and Behavior, 52,* 313–320.

Rizzo, A. A., Stamps, L. E., & Fehr, L. A. (1988). Effects of caffeine withdrawal on motor performance and heart rate changes. *International Journal of Psychophysiology, 6,* 9–14.

Robertson, D., Wade, D., Workman, R., & Woosley, R. L. (1981). Tolerance to the humoral and hemodynamic effects of caffeine in man. *Journal of Clinical Investigation, 67,* 1111–1117.

Rosen, J. B., Young, A. M., Beuthin, F. C., & Louis-Ferdinant, R. T. (1986). Discriminative stimulus properties of amphetamine and other stimulants in lead-exposed and normal rats. *Pharmacology, Biochemistry and Behavior, 24,* 211–215.

Rush, C. R., Sullivan, J. T., & Griffiths, R. R. (1995). Intravenous caffeine in stimulant drug abusers: Subjective reports and physiological effects. *Journal of Pharmacology and Experimental Therapeutics, 273,* 351–358.

Sawynok, J. (1995). Pharmacological rationale for the clinical use of caffeine. *Drugs, 49,* 37–50.

Sawynok, J., & Yaksh, T. L. (1993). Caffeine as an analgesic adjuvant: A review of pharmacology and mechanisms of action. *Pharmacological Reviews, 45,* 43–85.

Schechter, M. D. (1977). Caffeine potentiation of amphetamine: Implications for hyperkinesis therapy. *Pharmacology, Biochemistry and Behavior, 6,* 359–361.

Schechter, M. D. (1989). Potentiation of cathinone by caffeine and nikethamide. *Pharmacology, Biochemistry and Behavior, 33,* 299–301.

Schuh, K. J., & Griffiths, R. R. (1997). Caffeine reinforcement: The role of withdrawal. *Psychopharmacology, 130,* 320–326.

Schulte-Daxboek, G., & Opitz, K. (1981). Increased caffeine consumption following chronic nicotine treatment in rats. *IRCS Journal of Medical Science, 9,* 1062.

Schuster, C. R., & Johanson, C. E. (1988). Relationship between the discriminative stimulus properties and subjective effects of drugs. *Psychopharmacology Series, 4,* 161–175.

Schuster, C. R., Woods, J. H., & Seevers, M. H. (1969). Self-administration of central stimulants by the monkey. In F. Sjoqvist & M. Tottie (Eds.), *Abuse of central stimulants* (pp. 339–347). New York: Raven.

Schuster, C. R., Fischman, M. W., & Johanson, C. E. (1981). Internal stimulus control and subjective effects of drugs. In C. E. Johanson & T. Thompson (Eds.), *Behavioral pharmacology of human drug dependence* (NIDA Research Monograph No. 37, pp. 116–129). Washington, DC: U.S. Government Printing Office.

Sechzer, P. H. (1979). Post spinal anesthesia headache treated with caffeine: Part II. Intracranial vascular distension, a key factor. *Current Therapeutic Research, 26,* 440–448.

Shi, J., Benowitz, N. L., Denaro, C. P., & Sheiner, L. B. (1993). Pharmacokinetics and drug disposition. Pharmacokinetic-pharmacodynamic modeling of caffeine: Tolerance to pressor effects. *Clinical Pharmacology and Therapeutics, 53,* 6–14.

Shorofsky, M. A., & Lamm, R. N. (1977). Caffeine-withdrawal headache and fasting. *New York State Journal of Medicine, 77,* 217–218.

Silverman, K., & Griffiths, R. R. (1992). Low-dose caffeine discrimination and self-reported mood effects in normal volunteers. *Journal of the Experimental Analysis of Behavior, 57,* 91–107.

Silverman, K., Evans, S. M., Strain, E. C., & Griffiths, R. R. (1992). Withdrawal syndrome after the double-blind cessation of caffeine consumption. *New England Journal of Medicine, 327,* 1109–1114.

Silverman, K., Mumford, G. K., & Griffiths, R. R. (1994a). Enhancing caffeine reinforcement by behavioral requirements following drug ingestion. *Psychopharmacology, 114,* 424–432.

Silverman, K., Mumford, G. K., & Griffiths, R. R. (1994b). A procedure for studying the within-session onset of human drug discrimination. *Journal of the Experimental Analysis of Behavior, 61,* 181–189.

Spencer, D. G., & Lal, H. (1983). Discriminative stimulus properties of L-phenylisopropyladenosine: Blockade by caffeine and generalization to 2-chloradenosine. *Life Science, 32,* 2329–2333.

Stern, K. N., Chait, L. D., & Johanson, C. E. (1989). Reinforcing and subjective effects of caffeine in normal human volunteers. *Psychopharmacology, 98,* 81–88.

Strain, E. C., & Griffiths, R. R. (1997). Caffeine. In A. Tasman, J. Kay, & J. A. Lieberman (Eds.), *Psychiatry* (Vol. 1, pp. 779–794). Philadelphia: Saunders.

Strain, E. C., Mumford, G. K., Silverman, K., & Griffiths, R. R. (1994). Caffeine dependence syndrome: Evidence from case histories and experimental evaluations. *Journal of the American Medical Association, 272,* 1043–1048.

Uhde, T. W. (1990). Caffeine provocation of panic: A focus on biological mechanisms. In J. C. Ballenger (Ed.), *Neurobiology of panic disorder* (pp. 219–242). New York: Liss.

Uhde, T. W., Boulenger, J. P., Jimerson, D. C., & Post, R. M. (1984). Caffeine: Relationship to human anxiety, plasma MHPG and cortisol. *Psychopharmacology Bulletin, 20,* 426–430.

Victor, B. S., Lubetsky, M., & Greden, J. F. (1981). Somatic manifestations of caffeinism. *Journal of Clinical Psychiatry, 42,* 185–188.

Vitiello, M. V., & Woods, S. C. (1975). Caffeine: Preferential consumption by rats. *Pharmacology, Biochemistry and Behavior, 3,* 147–149.

Vitiello, M. V., & Woods, S. C. (1977). Evidence for withdrawal from caffeine by rats. *Pharmacology, Biochemistry and Behavior, 6,* 553–555.

Wayner, M. L., Jolicoeur, F. B., Rondeu, D. B., & Barone, F. C. (1976). Effects of acute and chronic administration of caffeine on schedule dependent and schedule induced behavior. *Pharmacology, Biochemistry and Behavior, 5,* 343–348.

Weber, J. G., Ereth, M. H., & Danielson, D. R. (1993). Perioperative ingestion of caffeine and postoperative headache. *Mayo Clinic Proceedings, 68,* 843–845.

Weber, J. G., Klindworth, J. T., Arnold, J. J., Danielson, D. R., & Ereth, M. H. (1997). Prophylactic intravenous administration of caffeine and recovery after ambulatory surgical procedures. *Mayo Clinic Proceedings, 72,* 621–626.

Winsor, A. L., & Strongin, E. I. (1933). A study of the development of tolerance for caffeinated beverages. *Journal of Experimental Psychology, 16,* 725–744.

Winter, J. C. (1981). Caffeine-induced stimulus control. *Pharmacology, Biochemistry and Behavior, 15,* 157–159.

Wood, R. W. (1990). Animal models of drug self-administration by smoking. In C. N. Chiang & R. L. Hawks (Eds.), *Research findings on smoking of abused substances* (NIDA Research Monograph No. 99, pp. 159–171). Washington, DC: U.S. Government Printing Office.

Yanagita, T. (1970). Self-administration studies on various dependence-producing agents in monkeys. *University of Michigan Medical Center Journal, 36,* 216–224.

Zwyghuizen-Doorenbose, A., Roehrs, T. A., Lipschutz, L., Timms, V., & Roth, T. (1990). Effects of caffeine on alertness. *Psychopharmacology, 100,* 36–39.

6

Psychological and Psychiatric Consequences of Caffeine

MARILYN E. CARROLL

The widespread and long-term use of caffeine in adults as well as children raises the question of whether there are psychological and psychiatric consequences of caffeine use in normal individuals. A related question regards the effects of caffeine on various psychological states such as stress, or in those diagnosed with specific psychiatric disorders. This chapter reviews some of the main psychological and psychiatric conditions in which caffeine has been shown to have effects. The medical consequences of caffeine use, and the therapeutic uses of caffeine, are also briefly discussed, because with serious acute or chronic medical conditions, or long-term therapeutic use of a drug, there are often associated psychological and psychiatric consequences. A discussion of caffeine use in children is also included, because caffeine is the only psychoactive drug legally available to children, and methylxanthines, including caffeine, have been used therapeutically in disorders that are common to children such as asthma and Attention-Deficit/Hyperactivity Disorder.

MARILYN E. CARROLL • Department of Psychiatry, University of Minnesota, Minneapolis, Minnesota 55455.

Handbook of Substance Abuse: Neurobehavioral Pharmacology, edited by Tarter *et al.* Plenum Press, New York, 1998.

Medical Consequences of Caffeine Use

Caffeine use has been implicated in more illnesses than any other psychoactive agent. There is often comorbidity between psychological and psychiatric disorders and chronic illness. Major studies have investigated the role of caffeine in myocardial infarction, arrhythmias, hypertension, hyperlipidemia, gout, fibrocystic breast disease, various forms of cancer, osteoporosis, and birth defects. Although isolated reports may suggest that caffeine use is related to these illnesses, the majority of studies, including the larger multisite investigations, show no strong relationship (Heyden, 1993). Animal studies of the association between caffeine and cholesterol have been conducted over the past 30 years, and they concur with findings from human research that caffeine has little influence on cardiovascular disease (Heyden, 1993).

Therapeutic Uses of Caffeine

Caffeine has useful effects on respiratory function. It can be used as a bronchodilator for patients with asthma, although most other asthma drugs are more effective. Dietary use of caffeine may be helpful when specific agents for treating asthma are unavailable.

One of the major uses of caffeine is to stabilize breathing in neonatal apnea (Benowitz, 1990). Caffeine has also been used to treat migraine headaches when combined with ergotamine and nonsteroidal anti-inflammatory agents (Sawynok, 1995). Caffeine may also provide direct adjuvant analgesic effects. Caffeine has been useful for enhancing seizure duration in electroconvulsive therapy. Caffeine's therapeutic effects are attributed to its actions as an adenosine receptor antagonist. Other actions such as mobilization of intracellular calcium and inhibition of phosphodiesterases occur only at very high doses. Caffeine increases metabolism throughout the brain but decreases cerebral blood flow. It also activates noradrenaline neurons, affects local dopamine release, and may have an effect on serotonin neurons.

Mood

Caffeine produces significant changes in mood that are dose-dependent and may differ in regular caffeine users versus nonusers (Lieberman, Wurtman, Emde, & Coviella, 1987; Lieberman, Wurtman, Emde, Roberts, & Coviella, 1987). Doses ranging from 64 to 300 mg are associated with positive mood, especially in regular caffeine users (Griffiths, Bigelow, & Liebson, 1989; Lieberman, Wurtman, Emde, Roberts, & Coviello, 1987; Stern, Chait, & Johanson, 1989). Improved mood is often expressed in terms of increased contentedness, friendliness, and talkativeness (Griffiths et al., 1989). It is also a common belief that performance may be improved, for example, in clearer flow of thought, association of ideas, and reduced reaction time (Loke, 1988). Higher doses (e.g., 420–800 mg) result in negative mood and dysphoric reactions such as increased tension and feeling jittery or nervous (Chait & Griffiths, 1983; Loke, Hinrichs, & Ghonheim, 1985; Roache & Griffiths, 1987). Caffeine improves mood under conditions that are associated with lower mood, such as boredom (Lieberman, Wurtman, Emde, Roberts, & Coviello, 1987; van der Stelt & Snel, 1993), age (Jarvis, 1993;

Swift & Tiplady, 1988), midafternoon slump (Smith, Rusted, Eaton-Williams, Savory, & Leathwood, 1990), menstruation (M. E. Arnold, Petros, Beckwith, Coons, & Gorman, 1987), or sleep deprivation (Penetar et al., 1993). In most of these studies, caffeine restores mood to near-normal levels.

In contrast to the beneficial mood-altering effects of moderate caffeine doses, there are negative effects on mood produced by caffeine deprivation. Mood effects were compared in young adults who were moderate caffeine consumers after 90 min, overnight, or 7 days of caffeine deprivation, and similar dysphoric effects were reported in the overnight and 7-day deprivation groups (Richardson, Rogers, Elliman, & O'Dell, 1995). Overnight-deprived subjects had higher self-ratings of being tired, angry, drowsy, and dejected, while both the overnight and 7-day groups reported increased headache and decreased levels of clear-headedness. Other studies have reported that some of these withdrawal effects may last up to 7-10 days (Griffiths, Bigelow, & Liebson, 1986; James, 1991). In another study, when heavy and habitual coffee users were deprived of coffee for 4 hr they reported a more negative overall mood after receiving decaffeinated coffee than did those receiving caffeinated coffee (Ratliff-Crain, O'Keeffe, & Baum, 1989). Subjects receiving herbal tea showed less arousal than either the caffeinated or decaffeinated coffee groups, and those given herbal tea desired coffee more than the two coffee groups. Thus, some of the stimulus effects of decaffeinated coffee slightly alleviated some of the discomfort produced by caffeinated coffee deprivation.

Psychomotor Performance

The general belief that caffeine improves clarity of thought, mood, social competence, and reaction time has led to the common assumption that caffeine can improve physical or mental performance or both. There has been great interest in these positive aspects of caffeine, and a large body of literature exists on caffeine and performance on psychomotor tasks. In general, caffeine aids rapid responding, especially when performance has been depressed (Carpenter, 1959), and vigilance is improved after a level of fatigue has been reached (Battig & Buzzi, 1986). Caffeine has been reported to decrease reaction time (Clubley, Bye, Henson, Peck, & Riddington, 1979; Kerr, Sherwood, & Hindemarch, 1991; Lieberman, Wurtman, Emde, Roberts, & Coviello, 1987), to improve vigilance (Zwyghuizen-Doorenbos, Roehrs, Liipschutz, Timms, & Roth, 1990), and to enhance workshift performance (Walsh et al., 1990). The interpretation of the results of these studies is complicated by the question of whether caffeine improves performance above normal levels, or, as in the case of regular caffeine users, restores deficits that occur during acute or chronic withdrawal back to normal levels (Rogers, Richardson, & Dernoncourt, 1995). Thus, it is important to compare performance in high and low users as well as in nonusers. Another consideration for this type of study is to control for practice effects when within-subject comparisons are made on tasks given repeatedly.

Caffeine deprivation has little or no effect on psychomotor performance. Even when an abrupt change from caffeinated to decaffeinated coffee consumption in heavy coffee drinkers produced subjective withdrawal effects, performance on a short-term psychomotor test was unaffected (Griffiths, Bigelow, Liebson, O'Keeffe, et al., 1986). There is some evidence of disruption in a study by Bruce, Scott, Shine, and Lader (1991), which showed that 24-hr caffeine-deprived subjects tired more quickly on a tapping test. In another study, low and high caffeine users were given a simple reaction-time test after overnight caffeine deprivation, with either placebo or a caffeine capsule equivalent to 1 cup of coffee (Rogers et al., 1995). Performance was not impaired in either group by caffeine withdrawal, but it significantly improved in the heavy users after a caffeine dose.

Cognitive Performance

Studies of caffeine's effect on motor tasks have shown that individuals are less tired and able to move faster after caffeine use. However, tasks requiring cognitive processes, or tasks varying in duration, may differ in their sensitivity to caffeine administration. Consensus is lacking on the effects of caffeine on cognitive functioning (James, 1991; Sawyer, Julia, & Turin, 1982; Truitt, 1971), and little or no data exist to suggest that caffeine withdrawal alters cognitive performance (Richardson et al., 1995; Rogers et al., 1995). The lack of consistent results regarding caffeine and cognitive performance may be due to the wide variety of cognitive tasks that have been used. It has been argued that only tasks demanding rapid processing (Foreman, Barraclough, Moore, Mehta, & Madon, 1989) or that high demands on the short-term memory load (Humphreys & Revelle, 1984) may be sensitive to caffeine-induced deficits. Foreman and coworkers (1989) reported a clear disruption in Stroop test (rapid processing of ambiguous or confusing stimuli) performance in men after consuming 250 mg caffeine; however, they did not show a deficit in a test involving free recall of word lists. In contrast, Terry and Phifer (1986) tested college students in a word list recall after 100 mg of caffeine, and they found deficits due to caffeine, particularly in recall of the middle to end portions of the list. Erickson and colleagues (1985) used a similar word list task presented to subjects at either a slow or fast rate. Caffeine-related deficits were found for the slow rate condition in females but not for the fast rate task, nor on either task in males. These findings suggest that there are some areas such as working memory that may be sensitive to the effects of caffeine, but the results are neither robust nor consistent across studies.

In a recent study, Jarvis (1993) examined performance in more than 7,000 adults on four simple tests of cognitive function: simple reaction time, choice reaction time, incidental verbal memory, and visuospatial memory. Subjects provided self-reports of coffee and tea intake and performance was related to amount consumed. Increased levels of coffee and tea consumption were associated with better performance on the four tasks. The effects were more pronounced for coffee than for tea. The enhancement of performance was proportionally similar for all tests, suggesting that caffeine affects a basic process that is common to all tests. It was suggested that level of arousal or vigilance is a likely candidate, since consistent results have been obtained on this type of test in many studies (e.g., Frewer & Lader, 1991; Zwyghuizen-Doorenbos et al., 1990). This study also reported that older adults were more sensitive to caffeine's performance-enhancing effects than younger adults (Jarvis, 1993). Others have reported sex differences in caffeine-induced deficits in cognitive performance (Erikson et al., 1985). Caffeine inhibited recall rate for word lists in females but not males. In another study by this group (M. E. Arnold et al., 1987), caffeine facilitated recall in females after practice with a task, but it impaired recall in males at the medium dose.

A few studies indicate that caffeine has beneficial effects on performance that has deteriorated due to fatigue or other factors (James, 1991). The laboratory model for testing this hypothesis has been the administration of drugs, usually benzodiazepines, that interfere with cognitive and psychomotor tasks. For example, lorazepam impaired performance on several tasks, and caffeine restored performance to baseline levels (File, Bond, & Lister, 1982). However, caffeine did not elevate performance above lorazepam placebo levels. Similarly, the antiemetic drug cyclizine impaired performance on an arithmetic task; the impairment was reversed by 100 mg of caffeine (Clubley et al., 1979).

Stress

Caffeine use may be initiated by nonusers or increased among users during times of stress (Mosqueda-Garcia, Robertson, & Robertson, 1993). Occupational stress is particularly related to elevated caffeine consumption. Chronic, excessive caffeine use and stress may have additive physiological consequences such as gastric ulceration or kidney disease (Gilbert, 1986). Caffeine and stress are associated with elevated levels of adrenaline in the blood. High but not low doses of caffeine can also increase serum cortisol levels 2 hr after ingestion (Spindel & Wurtman, 1984). Caffeine and emotional stress may cause delirium in some individuals (Gilbert, 1986). The cardiovascular effects resulting from combined stress and caffeine consumption have recently been investigated. Stress resulting from behavioral tasks such as numerical problems can be measured by increased blood pressure, which adds to the pressor effect of caffeine to reach hypertensive levels (e.g., France & Ditto, 1988; Pincomb, Lorallo, Passey, & Wilson, 1988).

Aggression

There are few studies of the effects of any psychoactive drugs on aggressive behavior in humans. A methodology developed by Cherek (1981), Cherek, Steinberg, and Brauchi (1983, 1984), is well suited for answering this question experimentally by their investigation of the effects of caffeine tablets and coffee. In this paradigm, subjects respond on two buttons and a switch on a response console. Pressing button A under a fixed-ratio 100 schedule yields 1 point ($.10). Pressing button B subtracts a point from a fictitious "other subject," and responding on switch C gives the "other subject" a blast of noise. The latter two responses were used as measures of aggression. In the first study (Cherek et al., 1983) orally administered caffeine was compared to placebo in male volunteers (ages 18–35), and results indicated that caffeine compared to placebo decreased aggression while increasing nonaggressive responding. The second study was similar in design, except that caffeinated and decaffeinated coffee were used (Cherek et al., 1984). Similar results were obtained. The increased responding for points indicated that the decreased aggressive responding was not due to some nonspecific depressant action.

Caffeine in Children

Caffeine is the psychoactive drug most commonly used by children. Unlike any other psychoactive drug, it is legal and readily available to children in the form of carbonated soft drinks. At least 77% of children ingest caffeine in their diet, and the amounts per capita are steadily increasing (Arbeit et al., 1988; Baer, 1987). The short- and long-term psychological consequences of this early and continuous use of caffeine have not been studied. One review indicates that children are not more sensitive to caffeine than adults (Nehlig, Daval, & Debry, 1992), but controlled comparisons are lacking. One study of 19 prepubertal boys and 20 college-age men showed greater sensitivity in the children. They had higher scores on motor activity, increased speech rate, decreased reaction time, and improved attention on a continuous performance task (Reichard & Elder, 1977).

Results of recent studies on prepubertal children indicate enhanced performance over controls on a motor task and test of attention (Bernstein et al., 1994). Studies of caffeine in children reveal dose-dependent increases in nervous and jittery feelings (Rapoport et al., 1981; Rapoport, Berg, Ismond, Zahn, & Neims, 1984), restlessness (Elkins et al., 1981), and other anxiety symptoms (Rumsey & Rapoport, 1983). In a recent study children reported feeling "less sluggish" and "more anxious" after caffeine use (Bernstein et al., 1994). It has been suggested that caffeine may be a pharmacological model for anxiety in children (Rapoport et al., 1981). Caffeine withdrawal may cause significant changes in mood and performance in children as in adults (Damrau & Damrau, 1963; Greden, Victor, Fontaine, & Lubetsky, 1980; Silverman, Evans, Strain, & Griffiths, 1992; Strain & Griffiths, 1995; Strain, Mumford, Silverman, & Griffiths, 1994;); however, studies designed to prospectively examine caffeine dependence in children are still in progress (Bernstein et al., personal communication). A recent meta-analysis of caffeine's behavioral effects in children revealed no significant deleterious effects, and there was a small positive effect on parental report of externalizing behavior (Stein, Krasowski, Leventhal, Phillips, & Bender, 1996).

Psychiatric Disorders Associated with Caffeine Use

Intoxication

The only psychiatric disorder recognized by the American Psychiatric Association (1994) manual is Caffeine Intoxication. Intoxication can occur after recent caffeine use as low as 250 mg, but for most patients it has been much higher (1 g). The diagnostic criteria for the disorder are (1) recent consumption of at least 250 mg of caffeine and (2) at least five of the following signs: restlessness, nervousness, excitement, insomnia, flushed face, diuresis, gastrointestinal disturbance, muscle twitching, rambling flow of speech and thought, tachycardia or cardiac arrhythmia, periods of inexhaustibility or psychomotor agitation, and (3) other physical or mental disorders such as anxiety disorders must first be ruled out.

Other caffeine-related disturbances, such as ringing in the ears and flashes of light, have been reported at high doses. Extremely high doses (e.g., 10 g) may result in grand mal seizures, respiratory failure, and death. Chronic use of caffeine has been associated with peptic ulcer, cardiac arrhythmia, hypotension, and circulatory failure. Caffeine intoxication can mimic manic episodes, panic disorder, and a generalized anxiety disorder. These factors are easy to rule out by monitoring the temporal relationship between caffeine use and psychiatric symptoms.

Caffeinism is an older term that described a group of symptoms related to chronic excessive caffeine use (Greden, 1974). Caffeinism is characterized by many of the same signs as described for caffeine intoxication; the difference is that caffeinism is a chronic condition. It is believed that caffeinism is a chronic problem because patients who are anxious enter into a cycle whereby they drink a lot of coffee, become tolerant, and then continue to drink large amounts to avoid withdrawal symptoms that tend to make them even more anxious.

Dependence

While the condition of caffeine dependence is not recognized in the *DSM-IV* (American Psychiatric Association, 1994) as a psychiatric disorder, there is evidence that caffeine is a psychoactive drug that produces dependence (Strain *et al.,* 1994). Strain and coworkers (1994) interviewed 99 subjects and diagnosed 16 with caffeine dependence. The diagnoses were based on subjects satisfying four of seven *DSM-IV* criteria for psychoactive substance use disorders. The four criteria were tolerance, withdrawal, persistent desire or unsuccessful efforts to cut down or control use, and continued use despite knowledge of a persistent or recurrent physical or psychological problem that is likely to have been caused or exacerbated by caffeine use. Seventy-five to 94 percent of the 16 subjects met each of these criteria. In addition, 11 of the subjects were tested in a double-blind caffeine withdrawal study, and 9 of 11 showed objective evidence of caffeine withdrawal such as headache and elevated ratings of fatigue and depression. Eight of the subjects reported functional impairment in daily activities during caffeine withdrawal.

Anxiety Disorders

In some cases, caffeine use seems to aggravate psychiatric disease. For example, caffeine induces panic attacks or anxiety symptoms in patients with panic disorders, generalized anxiety disorders, or agoraphobia, but does not generate these conditions in normal controls unless used to excess (Boulenger, Wade, Wolff, & Post, 1984; Charney, Heninger, & Jatlow, 1985; Gilbert, 1986). High doses of caffeine (500 mg) have been reported to induce panic attacks in normal individuals (Uhde, Boulenger, Jimerson, & Post, 1984), and caffeine intoxication can mimic anxiety disorders. Patients diagnosed with panic disorder appear to be even more sensitive than normal controls to the anxiogenic effects of caffeine. Klein, Zohar, Geraci, Murphy, and Uhde (1991) reported that

caffeine (480 mg) produced greater anxiogenic and panic-inducing effects than placebo in panic disorder patients. There were also significant increases in plasma cortisol concentrations. Other studies have reported abnormal sensitivity to caffeine in panic disorder patients (Boulenger *et al.,* 1984; Charney *et al.,* 1985; Lee, Flegel, Greden, & Cameron, 1988; Uhde *et al.,* 1984). Charney and coworkers (1985) presented caffeine challenges to panic disorder patients and showed increased diastolic blood pressure and self-reports of nervousness, anxiousness, fearfulness, restlessness, palpitations, nausea, and tremor as well as some reports of being mellow or happy. When compared with normal control subjects, caffeine increased anxiety more often in the patients with panic disorder than in normals (Newman, Stein, Trettau, Coppola, & Uhde, 1992). In another study, 12 patients with panic disorder, 12 normals, and 12 generalized anxiety disorder patients were compared on electroencephalographic (EEG) and self-report measures (Bruce, Scott, Shine, & Lader, 1992). Patients with generalized anxiety disorder showed different EEG activity, greater systolic and diastolic blood pressure, and higher self-ratings of anxiety and sweating than normals. Patients with panic disorder showed different EEG activity and physical tiredness, compared with normals, but they were less reactive than generalized anxiety disorder patients on some measures, such as systolic blood pressure and subjective sweating. In addition to these clinical findings, there are animal models of anxiety, such as the social interaction test and the conflict situation test in mice, indicating that caffeine has anxiogenic effects (Lapin, 1993). These findings are consistent with previous reports of enhanced sensitivity to caffeine in patients diagnosed with anxiety and panic disorders, and they also suggest that this population may benefit by limiting caffeine intake.

Schizophrenia

One study conducted on 98 psychiatric patients included 41 patients with diagnosis of schizophrenia or other psychoses, while other diagnoses included major depression, mood disorders, adjustment disorders, anxiety disorders, and organic mental disorders (Rihs, Müller, & Baumann, 1996). Of all categories, the psychotic patients had the highest caffeine intake. Psychotic patients with greater disability (longer illness, greater number of hospitalizations, more lost jobs) seemed to be at higher risk for caffeine consumption. Another study of schizophrenic patients revealed no correlation between caffeine consumption and levels of anxiety or depression and no changes in these measures when the wards changed to decaffeinated products (Mayo, Falkowski, & Jones, 1993). These results are in contrast to an earlier study that found that caffeine aggravated psychotic episodes (Mikkelson, 1978). The mixed findings and limited literature concerning caffeine's effects on psychotic patients suggest that there is not yet evidence to limit caffeine consumption in this group of patients.

Depression/Suicide

Long-term use of high doses of caffeine is associated with depressive symptoms in humans (Uhde *et al.*, 1984). A deficiency of 5 HT is related to depression, and preliminary findings imply that depression resulting from caffeine withdrawal may be 5-HT mediated (Haleem, Yasmeen, Haleem, & Zafar, 1995). Several reports suggest that depressed psychiatric patients have higher than normal caffeine intake (Greden, Fontaine, Lubetsky, & Chamberlin, 1978; James & Crosbie, 1987; Neill, Himmelhock, Mallinger, Mallinger, & Hamin, 1978). Clinical studies with depressed patients have shown that coffee drinking improves mood (Furlong, 1975) and decreases irritability (Stephanson, 1977). However, population-based studies of caffeine intake and depression are not available. In a cross-sectional study of Japanese medical students, it was found that high intake of caffeine was associated with fewer depressive symptoms among female students but not among male college students (Mino, Yasuda, Fujimura, & Ohara, 1990).

An interesting relationship exists between suicide, for which there is a high incidence among depressed patients, and caffeine use. In one study, 56 cases of suicide in women were examined, and a strong inverse relationship was found for caffeine intake and risk of suicide (Kawachi, Willett, Colditz, Stampfer, & Speizer, 1996). Caffeine may have improved mood or prevented depression. The results of this study were not expected, since heavy coffee drinking is associated with smoking (Hemenway, Solnick, & Colditz, 1993; Kawachi *et al.*, 1993), higher alcohol intake, and stress (Shaffer, 1993), all factors that are correlated with increased risk of suicide. In general, depression seems to be the psychiatric disorder that has the most positive response to caffeine.

ADHD in Children

Attention-Deficit/Hyperactivity Disorder (ADHD) is a common disorder, occurring in 10%–13% of all children. Earlier studies reported that caffeine may be useful to treat ADHD in children (L. E. Arnold, Christopher, Huestis, & Smeltzer, 1978; Garfinkel, Webster, & Sloman, 1981; Schnackenberg, 1973). However, other studies found no therapeutic effect (Conners, 1975; Firestone, Davey, Goodman, & Peters, 1978; Garfinkel, Webster, & Sloman, 1975; Huestis, Arnold, & Smeltzer, 1975). Others have shown that the combination of the standard medication for ADHD, methylphenidate (Ritalin), and caffeine yielded a more efficacious treatment than either drug alone (Garfinkel *et al.*, 1981).

Other Psychiatric Disorders

There is only limited information available on the effect of caffeine on other psychiatric disorders. In contrast to depression, social phobics reported a lower intent to drink caffeinated coffee in meetings than did a normal community control group (Holle, Heimberg, Sweet, & Holt, 1995). However, actual intake from a weekly log was the same as controls. These findings suggest that social phobics intend to control caffeine intake, possibly to reduce anxiety symptoms and negative evaluations from others.

Premenstrual Syndrome (PMS)

Premenstrual syndrome has been associated with caffeine use to the extent that some over-the-counter medications contain caffeine. However, a study of 102 women with PMS and an equal number without PMS indicated that there was no significant difference in caffeine intake during either the premenstrual or postmenstrual period (Caan *et al.,* 1993). These data suggest that women with PMS are not self-medicating with caffeinated beverages.

Comorbidity of Caffeine Use and Substance Abuse Disorders

Caffeine's ability to increase mental activity, aid wakefulness, and elevate mood, combined with its low cost and easy access, have resulted in its widespread use, including concurrent use with other legal and illegal psychoactive drugs. Nicotine is the drug that is most commonly used with caffeine. A mutually synergistic effect seems to exist (Istvan & Matarazzo, 1984). More cigarette smokers consume coffee (86.4%) than do nonsmokers (77.2%) (Swanson, Lee, & Hopp, 1994), and more cigarettes are consumed during coffee drinking than other equal time periods (Emurian, Nellis, Brady, & Ray, 1982; Nellis, Emurian, Brady, & Ray, 1982). The nature of this interaction is unclear; factors that may account for it include increased caffeine metabolism in smokers, the same stimuli (e.g., stress, social pressures) may trigger the ingestion of both drugs, or the drug combination produces a different pharmacological effect than either caffeine or nicotine alone.

The correlations between caffeine and nicotine use in epidemiological studies (e.g., Istvan & Matarazzo, 1984) are not supported by the results of laboratory studies or experimental studies in the natural environment. Conflicting reports indicate no effect of a fivefold caffeine dose range on smoking behavior (Lane & Rose, 1995) and a trend for greater cigarette consumption in smokers consuming a moderate caffeine dose compared to decaffeinated coffee (Brown & Benowitz, 1989). Others found that more nicotine was taken in by smokers on decaffeinated versus caffeinated coffee (Kozlowski, 1976), or that caffeine tended to suppress smoking behavior

(Chait & Griffiths, 1983; Nil, Buzzi, & Bättig, 1984).

Pritchard, Robinson, de Bethizy, Davis, and Stiles (1995) examined the effects of caffeine (2.5 mg/kg) and smoking on cognitive performance, subjective measures, heart rate, and EEG. Smoking and caffeine did not interact on any measure, suggesting that the epidemiological link between nicotine and caffeine may not be a true drug interaction. In an earlier study by Rose and Behm (1991), mood and physiological measures were studied in 12 subjects exposed to caffeinated or decaffeinated coffee and nicotine or nicotine-free cigarettes, and measures of mood (Profile of Mood States [POMS]) such as "awake," "lively," and "not tired," and physiological measures such as skin temperature, expired air carbon monoxide, blood pressure, and heart rate were compared. The only measures that showed interactive effects of caffeine and nicotine were arousal and diastolic blood pressure. Nicotine smoke reduced arousal in the caffeinated coffee condition but not in the decaffeinated condition. Caffeine potentiated the nicotine-induced increases in diastolic blood pressure. A recent study of the effects of caffeine and nicotine consumption on mood and somatic variables was conducted in 144 penitentiary inmates (Hughes & Boland, 1992). An interaction was found between level of smoking and caffeine use. Nonsmokers who consumed high levels of caffeine experienced poorer mood than any other group. There was also greater dissatisfaction with somatic factors such as appetite, concentration, and sleep as smoking level increased.

Another important aspect of the concurrent use of caffeine and nicotine is the effect of nicotine (tobacco) withdrawal syndrome on caffeine metabolism. Caffeine use usually persists during attempts at smoking cessation, and increased caffeine blood levels may account for the anxiety, anorexia, restlessness, and insomnia that are attributed to tobacco withdrawal (Benowitz, Hall, & Modin, 1989; Oliveto *et al.,* 1991; Sachs & Benowitz, 1988). Caffeine consumption may actually decrease during tobacco withdrawal, and for an extended period after, but caffeine concentrations in blood increase up to 250% due to a return to normal metabolic rates from a higher rate that existed during smoking (Benowitz *et al.*, 1989). A recent study showed that when relatively low doses of caffeine (50, 100 mg) were given during a 4-day tobacco withdrawal period, caffeine blood levels did not increase. There were typical tobacco withdrawal symptoms, but they were not affected by caffeine, except for decreased severity of withdrawal-induced hunger (Oliveto *et al.*, 1991).

Cocaine is another drug, like caffeine, from the class of psychomotor stimulants that raises concern because it is widely abused in those who also consume caffeine, and since drug actions are similar (increased intercellular dopamine), effects may be additive. Caffeine has been shown to enhance the locomotor (Misra, Vadlamani, & Pontani, 1986) or motor activating (Schenk, Horger, & Snow, 1989) effects of cocaine in rats. In a study of operant, schedule-controlled behavior in rats, a caffeine–cocaine combination did not produce results that were different from caffeine alone. Local rates of responding increased across the fixed interval. Cocaine had little effect on local response rates. However, in recent studies of the reinforcing effects of cocaine, caffeine did seem to have a consistent role in enhancing the reinforcing effects of cocaine. Horger, Wellman, Morien, Davies, and Schenk (1991) found that prior exposure to caffeine reduced the latency for the acquisition of intravenous cocaine self-administration. These findings were replicated in rats that had access to dietary caffeine during cocaine acquisition (Carroll & Lac, 1998) and in rhesus monkeys smoking cocaine base (Comer & Carroll, 1996). In tests of ongoing steady-state cocaine self-administration, Schenk, Valadez, Horger, Snow, and Wellman (1994) reported that caffeine increased cocaine-reinforced responding when low, sub-threshold doses of cocaine were available for self-administration. Caffeine has also been shown to dose-dependently reinstate responding that was previously reinforced by cocaine when given in a single intraperitoneal priming injection (Schenk, Worley, McNamara, &

Valadez, 1996). These findings strongly suggest that caffeine enhances the acquisition of cocaine abuse in new users and may stimulate relapse in experienced abstinent cocaine users.

There are few reports of caffeine interactions with other drugs of abuse. An earlier study by Jones (1981) investigated the effect of caffeine pretreatment on naloxone-precipitated morphine withdrawal signs and symptoms. He reported that caffeine pretreatment resulted in a more intense and longer lasting morphine withdrawal syndrome 5 and 24 hr following morphine. Caffeine and other xanthine derivatives have also been shown to alter the rate and magnitude of opiate tolerance and dependence in animals (Butt, Collier, Cuthberg, Francis, & Saeed, 1979). The benzodiazepines constitute another class of potentially abused substances that have been studied in combination with caffeine. Benzodiazepines, which are sedatives and muscle relaxants, generally impair psychomotor performance in humans and animals (Lau & Falk, 1991; Woods, Katz, & Winger, 1987). This impairment can be enhanced by administration of alcohol (Mattila, 1984; Taylor & Tinklenburg, 1987), but caffeine attenuates the psychomotor impairment (Taylor & Tinklenburg, 1987). In contrast, a recent study (Lau & Falk, 1991) examined the effect of chronic caffeine on a fine-motor-control deficit produced by the benzodiazepine midazolam in rats. Rats were trained to hold a force transducer (lever) within fixed band width to obtain food pellets. Similar forceband discrimination tasks have been shown to be sensitive to caffeine effects in humans (Miller, Lombardo, & Fowler, 1995). This synergistic effect of caffeine and midazolam may be particularly relevant for panic disorder patients whose anxiety may be treated with a benzodiazepine. These results contraindicate the use of caffeine in a benzodiazepine-treated panic disorder population. Panic disorder patients consume less caffeine than normals or a clinically depressed group (Boulenger *et al.*, 1984; Lee, Flegel, Greden, & Cameron, 1988); however, the concern would be that caffeine would be used to offset the sedative effects of the benzodiazepines.

Finally, there has been a recent increase in over-the-counter stimulant "lookalikes" such as caffeine, ephedrine, and phenylpropanolamine. Since caffeine and ephedrine occur naturally in plant material, they can be purchased as health food products with names such as "Herbal Ecstasy" without strict regulation by the Food and Drug Administration. Several overdose deaths have been reported from excessive use of these products. There is laboratory evidence to suggest that rats trained to discriminate between cocaine and saline recognize a caffeine, ephedrine, and phenylpropanolamine combination as a cocaine cue. A high dose of caffeine (56 mg/kg) and the other drugs alone only partially generalized to the cocaine cue.

ACKNOWLEDGMENTS

The assistance of Ms. Sylvie Lac and Dr. Joshua Rodefer with the literature review is greatly appreciated. This work was supported by NIDA Grants R 01 DA02486 (M. E. Carroll, P. I.) and P 01 DA08131 (Horace Loh, P. I.).

References

American Psychiatric Association. (1994). *Diagnostic and statistical manual of mental disorders* (4th ed.). Washington, DC: Author.

Arbeit, M. L., Nicklas, T. A., Frank, G. C., Webber, L. S., Miner, M. H., & Berenson, G. S. (1988). Caffeine intakes of children from a biracial population: The Bogalusa Heart Study. *Journal of the American Dietetic Association, 88,* 466–471.

Arnold, L. E., Christopher, J., Huestis, R., & Smeltzer, D. J. (1978). Methylphenidate vs dextroamphetamine vs caffeine in minimal brain dysfunction. *Archives of General Psychiatry, 35,* 463–473.

Arnold, M. E., Petros, T. V., Beckwith, B. E., Coons, G., & Gorman, N. (1987). The effects of caffeine, impulsivity, and sex on memory for word lists. *Physiology and Behavior, 41,* 25–30.

Baer, R. A. (1987). Effects of caffeine on classroom behavior, sustained attention, and a memory task in preschool children. *Journal of Applied Behavior Analysis, 20,* 225–234.

Battig, J., & Buzzi, R. (1986). The effect of coffee on the speed of subject-paced information processing. *Neuropsychobiology, 16,* 126–130.

Benowitz, N. L. (1990). Clinical pharmacology of caffeine. *Annual Review of Medicine, 41,* 277–288.

Benowitz, N. L., Hall, S. M., & Modin, G. (1989). Persistent increase in caffeine concentrations in people who stop smoking. *British Medical Journal, 298,* 1075–1076.

Bernstein, G. A., Carroll, M. E., Crosby, R. D., Perwein, A. R., Go, F. S., & Benowitz, N. L. (1994). Caffeine effects on learning, performance and anxiety in normal school-age children. *Journal of the American Academy of Child and Adolescent Psychiatry, 33,* 407–415.

Boulenger, J. P., Wade, T. W., Wolff, E. A., III, & Post, R. M. (1984). Increased sensitivity to caffeine in patients with panic disorders: Preliminary evidence. *Archives of General Psychiatry, 41,* 1067–1071.

Brown, C. R., & Benowitz, N. L. (1989). Caffeine and cigarette smoking: Behavioral, cardiovascular, and metabolic interactions. *Pharmacology, Biochemistry and Behavior, 34,* 565–570.

Bruce, M., Scott, N., Shine, P., & Lader, M. (1991). Caffeine withdrawal: A contrast of withdrawal symptoms in normal subjects who have abstained from caffeine for 24 hours and 7 days. *Journal of Psychopharmacology, 5,* 129–134.

Bruce, M., Scott, N., Shine, P., & Lader, M. (1992). Anxiogenic effects of caffeine in patients with anxiety disorders. *Archives of General Psychiatry, 49,* 867–869.

Butt, N. M., Collier, H. O. J., Cuthberg, N. J., Francis, D. L., & Saeed, S. A. (1979). Mechanism of quasi-morphine withdrawal behaviour induced by methylxanthines. *European Journal of Pharmacology, 53,* 375–378.

Caan, B., Duncan, D., Hiatt, R., Lewis, J., Chapman, J., & Armstrong, M. A. (1993). Association between alcoholic and caffeinated beverages and premenstrual syndrome. *Journal of Reproductive Medicine, 38,* 630–636.

Carpenter, J. A. (1959). The effect of alcohol and caffeine on simple visual reaction time. *Journal of Comparative and Physiological Psychology, 52,* 491–496.

Carroll, M. E., & Lac, S. T. (1998). Dietary additives and the acquisition of cocaine self-administration in rats. *Psychopharmacology, 137,* 81–89.

Chait, L. D., & Griffiths, R. R. (1983). Effects of caffeine on cigarette smoking and subjective response. *Clinical Pharmacological Therapy, 34,* 612–622.

Charney, D. S., Heninger, G. R., & Jatlow, P. I. (1985). Increased anxiogenic effects of caffeine in panic disorders. *Archives of General Psychiatry, 42,* 233–243.

Cherek, D. R. (1981). Effects of smoking different doses of nicotine on human aggressive behavior. *Psychopharmacology, 75,* 339.

Cherek, D. R., Steinberg, J. L., & Brauchi, J. T. (1983). Effects of caffeine on human aggressive behavior. *Psychiatry Research, 8,* 137.

Cherek, D. R., Steinberg, J. L., & Brauchi, J. T. (1984). Regular or decaffeinated coffee and subsequent human aggressive behavior. *Psychiatry Research, 11,* 251–258.

Clubley, M., Bye, C. E., Henson, T. A., Peck, A. W., & Riddington, C. J. (1979). Effects of caffeine and cyclizine alone and in combination on human performance, subjective effects and EEG activity. *British Journal of Clinical Pharmacology, 7,* 157–163.

Comer, S. D., & Carroll, M. E. (1996). Oral caffeine pretreatment produced modest increase in cocaine administration in rhesus monkeys. *Psychopharmacology, 126,* 281–285.

Conners, C. K. (1975). A placebo-crossover study of caffeine treatment of hyperkinetic children. *International Journal of Mental Health, 4,* 132–143.

Damrau, F., & Damrau, A. M. (1963). Use of soft drinks by children and adolescents. *Rocky Mountain Medical Journal 60,* 37–39.

Elkins, R. N., Rapoport, J. L., Zahn, T. P., Buchsbaum, M. S., Weingartner, H., Kopin, I. J., Langer, D., & Johnson, C. (1981) Acute effects of caffeine in normal prepubertal boys. *American Journal of Psychiatry, 138,* 178–183.

Emurian, H. H., Nellis, M. J., Brady, J. V., & Ray, R. L. (1982). Event time-series relationship between cigarette smoking and coffee drinking. *Addictive Behaviors, 7,* 441–444.

Erikson, G. C., Hager, L. B., Houseworth, C., Dungan, J., Petros, T., & Beckwith, B. E. (1985). The effects of caffeine on memory for word lists. *Physiology and Behavior, 35,* 47–51.

File, S. E., Bond, A. J., & Lister, R. G. (1982). Interaction between effects of caffeine and lorazepam in performance tests and self-ratings. *Journal of Clinical Psychopharmacology, 2,* 102–106.

Firestone, P., Davey, J., Goodman, J. T., & Peters, S. (1978). The effects of caffeine and methylphenidate on hyperactive children. *Journal of the American Academy of Child Psychiatry, 17,* 445–456.

Foreman, N., Barraclough, S., Moore, C., Mehta, A., & Madon, M. (1989). High doses of caffeine impair performance on a numerical version of the Stroop test in men. *Pharmacology, Biochemistry and Behavior, 32,* 349–403.

France, C., & Ditto, B. (1988). Caffeine effects on several indices of cardiovascular activity at rest and during stress. *Journal of Behavioral Medicine, 11,* 473–482.

Frewer, L. J., & Lader, M. (1991). The effects of caffeine on two computerised tests of attention and vigilance. *Human Psychopharmacology, 6,* 119–128.

Furlong, F. W. (1975). Possible psychiatric significance of excessive coffee consumption. *Canadian Journal of Psychiatry, 20,* 577–583.

Garfinkel, B. D., Webster, C. D., & Sloman, L. (1975). Methylphenidate and caffeine in the treatment of children with minimal brain dysfunction. *American Journal of Psychiatry, 132,* 723–728.

Garfinkel, B. D., Webster, C. D., & Sloman, L. (1981). Responses to methylphenidate and varied doses of caffeine in children with attention deficit disorder. *Canadian Journal of Psychiatry, 26,* 395–401.

Gilbert, R. M. (1986). *Caffeine, the most popular stimulant.* New York: Chelsea House.

Greden, J. F. (1974). Anxiety or caffeinism: A diagnostic dilemma. *American Journal of Psychiatry, 131,* 1089–1092.

Greden, J. F., Fontaine, P., Lubetsky, M., & Chamberlin, K. (1978). Anxiety and depression associated with caffeinism among psychiatric patients. *American Journal of Psychiatry, 135,* 963–966.

Greden, J. F., Victor, B. S., Fontaine, P., & Lubetsky, M. (1980). Caffeine-withdrawal headache: A clinical profile. *Psychosomatics, 21,* 411–418.

Griffiths, R. R., Bigelow, G. E., & Liebson, I. A. (1986). Human coffee drinking: Reinforcing and physical dependence producing effects. *Journal of Pharmacology and Experimental Therapeutics, 239,* 416–425.

Griffiths, R. R., Bigelow, G. E., Liebson, I. A., O'Keeffe, M., O'Leary, D., & Russ, N. (1986). Human coffee drinking: Manipulation of concentration and caffeine dose. *Journal of Experimental Analysis of Behavior, 45,* 133–148.

Griffiths, R. R., Bigelow, G. E., & Liebson, I. A. (1989). Reinforcing effect of caffeine in coffee and capsules. *Journal of Experimental Analysis of Behavior, 52,* 127–140.

Haleem, D., Yasmeen, A., Haleem, M. A., & Zafar, A. (1995). 24-h withdrawal following repeated administration of caffeine attenuates brain serotonin but not tryptophan in rat brain: Implications for caffeine-induced depression. *Life Sciences 57,* PL285–292.

Hemenway, D., Solnick, S. J., & Colditz, G. A. (1993). Smoking and suicide among nurses. *American Journal of Public Health, 83,* 249–251.

Heyden, S. (1993) Coffee and cardiovascular diseases: A personal view after 30 years of research. In S. Garattini (Ed.), *Coffee, caffeine, and health* (pp. 177–193). New York: Raven.

Holle, C., Heimberg, R. G., Sweet, R. A., & Holt, C. S. (1995). Alcohol and caffeine use by social phobics: An initial inquiry into drinking patterns and behavior. *Behavior Research and Therapy, 33,* 561–566.

Horger, B. A., Wellman, P. J., Morien, A., Davies, B. T., & Schenk, S. (1991). Caffeine exposure sensitizes rats to the reinforcing effects of cocaine. *NeuroReport, 2,* 53–56.

Huestis, R. D., Arnold, L. E., & Smeltzer, D. J. (1975). Caffeine versus methylphenidate and d-amphetamine in minimal brain dysfunction: A double-blind comparison. *American Journal of Psychiatry, 132,* 868–870.

Hughes, G. V., & Boland, F. J. (1992). The effects of caffeine and nicotine consumption on mood and somatic variables in a penitentiary inmate population. *Addictive Behaviors, 17,* 447–457.

Humphreys, M. S., & Revelle, W. (1984). Personality, motivation and performance: A theory of the relationship between individual differences and information processing. *Psychological Review, 91,* 153–184.

Istvan, J., & Matarazzo, J. D. (1984). Tobacco, alcohol, and caffeine use: A review of their interactions. *Psychological Bulletin, 95,* 301–326.

James, J. E. (1991). *Caffeine and health.* London: Academic Press.

James, J. E., & Crosbie, J. (1987). Somatic and psychological health implications of heavy caffeine use. *British Journal of Addiction, 82,* 503–509.

Jarvis, M. J. (1993). Does caffeine intake enhance absolute levels of cognitive performance? *Psychopharmacology, 110,* 45–52.

Jones, R. T. (1981). Caffeine enhances morphine dependence in humans. In *Advances in endogenous and exogenous opioids* (pp. 472–474). *Proceedings of the International Narcotic Research Conference, Kyoto, Japan.* Tokyo: Kodansha.

Kawachi, I., Colditz, G. A., Stampfer, M. J., Willett, W. C., Manson, J. E., Rosner, B., Hunter, D. T., Hennekens, C. H., & Speizer, F. E. (1993). Smoking cessation in relation to total mortality rates in women: A prospective cohort study. *Annals of Internal Medicine, 119,* 992–1000.

Kawachi, I., Willett, W. C., Colditz, G. A., Stampfer, M. J., & Speizer, F. E. (1996). A prospective study of coffee drinking and suicide in women. *Archives of Internal Medicine, 156,* 521–525.

Kerr, J. S., Sherwood, N., & Hindemarch, I. (1991). Separate and combined effects of the social drugs on psychomotor performance. *Psychopharmacology, 104,* 113–119.

Klein, E., Zohar, J., Geraci, M. F., Murphy, D. L., & Uhde, T. W. (1991). Anxiogenic effects of m-CPP in patients with panic disorder: Comparison to caffeine's anxiogenic effects. *Biological Psychiatry, 30,* 973–984.

Kozlowski, L. T. (1976). Effects of caffeine consumption on nicotine consumption. *Psychopharmacology, 47,* 165–168.

Lane, J. D., & Rose, J. E. (1995). Effects of daily caffeine intake on smoking behavior in the natural environment. *Experimental and Clinical Psychopharmacology, 3,* 49–55.

Lapin, I. P. (1993). Anxiogenic effect of phenethylamine and amphetamine in the elevated plus-maze in mice and its attenuation by ethanol. *Pharmacology, Biochemistry and Behavior, 44,* 241–243.

Lau, C. E., & Falk, J. L. (1991). Sustained synergism by chronic caffeine of the motor control deficit produced by midazolam. *Pharmacology, Biochemistry and Behavior, 40,* 723–31.

Lee, M. A., Flegel, P., Greden, J. F., & Cameron, O. G. (1988). Anxiogenic effects of caffeine on panic and depressed patients. *American Journal of Psychiatry, 145,* 632–635.

Lieberman, H. R., Wurtman, R. J., Emde, G. G., & Coviella, I. G. L. (1987). The effects of caffeine and aspirin on mood and performance. *Journal of Clinical Psychopharmacology, 7,* 315–320.

Lieberman, H. R., Wurtman, R. J., Emde, G. G., Roberts, C., & Coviella, I. G. L. (1987). The effects of low doses of caffeine on human performance and mood. *Psychopharmacology, 92,* 308–312.

Loke, W. H. (1988). Effects of caffeine on mood and memory. *Physiology and Behavior, 44,* 367–372.

Loke, W. H., Hinrichs, J. V., & Ghonheim, M. M. (1985). Caffeine and diazepam: Separate and combined effects on mood, memory, psychomotor performance. *Psychopharmacology, 87,* 344–350.

Mattila, M. J. (1984). Interactions of benzodiazepines on psychomotor skills. *British Journal of Clinical Pharmacology, 18,* 21S–26S.

Mayo, K. M., Falkowski, W., & Jones, C. A. (1993). Caffeine: Use and effects in long-stay psychiatric patients. *British Journal of Psychiatry, 162,* 543–545.

Mikkelsen, E. J. (1978). Caffeine and schizophrenia. *Journal of Clinical Psychiatry, 39,* 732–736.

Miller, L. S., Lombardo, T. W., & Fowler, S. C. (1995). Caffeine and time of day effects on a force discrimination task in humans. *Physiology and Behavior, 57,* 1117–1125.

Mino, Y., Yasuda, N., Fujimura, T., & Ohara, H. (1990). Caffeine consumption and anxiety and depressive symptomatology among medical students. *Japanese Journal of Alcohol Studies and Drug Dependence, 25,* 486–496.

Misra, A. L., Vadlamani, N. L., & Pontani, R. B. (1986). Effect of caffeine on cocaine locomotor stimulant activity in rats. *Pharmacology, Biochemistry and Behavior, 24,* 761–764.

Mosqueda-Garcia, R., Robertson, D., & Robertson, R. M. (1993). The cardiovascular effects of caffeine. In S. Garattini (Ed.), *Caffeine, coffee, and health* (pp. 157–176). New York: Raven.

Nehlig, A., Daval, J. L., & Debry, G. (1992). Caffeine and the central nervous system: Mechanisms of action, biochemical, metabolic, and psychostimulant effects. *Brain Research—Brain Research Reviews, 17,* 139–170.

Neill, J. F., Himmelhock, J. M., Mallinger, A. G., Mallinger, J., & Hamin, I. (1978). Caffeinism complicating hypersomnic depressive episodes. *Comprehensive Psychiatry, 19,* 377–385.

Nellis, M. J., Emurian, H. H., Brady, J. V., & Ray, R. L. (1982). Behavior analysis of cigarette smoking. *Pavlovian Journal of Biological Sciences, 17,* 140–149.

Newman, F., Stein, M. B., Trettau, J. R., Coppola, R., & Uhde, T. W. (1992). Quantitative electroencephalographic effects of caffeine in panic disorder. *Psychiatry Research, 45,* 105–113.

Nil, R., Buzzi, R., & Bättig, K. (1984). Effects of single doses of alcohol and caffeine on cigarette smoke puffing behavior. *Pharmacology, Biochemistry and Behavior, 20,* 583–590.

Oliveto, A. H., Hughes, J. R., Terry, S. Y., Bickel, W. K., Higgins, S. T., Pepper, S. L., & Fenwick, J. W. (1991). Effects of caffeine on tobacco withdrawal. *Clinical Pharmacological Therapy, 50,* 157–164.

Penetar, D., McCann, U., Thorne, D., Kamimori, G., Galinski, C., Sing, H., Thomas, M., & Belenky, G.

(1993). Caffeine reversal of sleep deprivation effects on alertness and mood. *Psychopharmacology, 112,* 359–365.

Pincomb, G. A., Lorallo, W. R., Passey, R. B., & Wilson, M. F. (1988). Effects of behavior state on caffeine's ability to alter blood pressure. *American Journal of Cardiology, 61,* 798–802.

Pritchard, W. S., Robinson, J. H., de Bethizy, J. D., Davis, R. A., & Stiles, M. F. (1995). Caffeine and smoking: Subjective, performance, and physiological effects. *Psychophysiology, 32,* 19–27.

Rapoport, J. L., Jensvold, M., Elkins, R., Buchsbaum, M. S., Weingartner, H., Ludlow, C., Zahn, T. P., Berg, C. J., & Neims, A. H. (1981). Behavioral and cognitive effects of caffeine in boys and adult males. *Journal of Nervous and Mental Disease, 169,* 726–732.

Rapoport, J. L., Berg, C. J., Ismond, D. R., Zahn, T. P., & Neims, A. (1984). Behavioral effects of caffeine in children. *Archives of General Psychiatry, 41,* 1073–1079.

Ratliff-Crain, J., O'Keeffe, M. K., & Baum, A. (1989). Cardiovascular reactivity, mood and task performance in deprived and nondeprived coffee drinkers. *Health Psychology, 8,* 427–447.

Reichard, C., & Elder, S. T. (1977). Effects of caffeine on reaction time in hyperkinetic and normal children. *American Journal of Psychiatry, 134,* 144–148.

Richardson, N. J., Rogers, P. J., Elliman, N. A., & O'Dell, R. J. (1995). Mood and performance effects of caffeine in relation to acute and chronic caffeine deprivation. *Pharmacology, Biochemistry and Behavior, 52,* 313–320.

Rihs, C., Müller, C., & Baumann (1996). Caffeine consumption in hospitalized psychiatric patients. *European Archives of Psychiatry and Clinical Neuroscience, 246,* 83–92.

Roache, J. D., & Griffiths, R. R. (1987). Interactions of diazepam and caffeine: Behavioral and subjective dose effects in humans. *Pharmacology, Biochemistry and Behavior, 26,* 801–812.

Rogers, P. J., Richardson, N. J., & Dernoncourt, C. (1995). Caffeine use: Is there a net benefit for mood and psychomotor performance? *Neuropsychobiology, 31,* 195–199.

Rose, J. E., & Behm, F. M. (1991). Psychophysiological interactions between caffeine and nicotine. *Pharmacology, Biochemistry and Behavior, 38,* 333–337.

Rumsey, J., & Rapoport, J. (1983). Behavioral effects of diet in children. In R. J. Wurtman & J. J. Wurtman (Eds.), *Nutrition and the brain* (Vol. 6, pp. 101–161). New York: Raven.

Sachs, D., & Benowitz, N. (1988). The nicotine withdrawal syndrome: Nicotine absence or caffeine excess? In *Proceedings of the Committee on Problems of Drug Dependence, 1988* (National Institute on Drug Abuse Research Monograph No. 90, p. 38). Washington, DC: U.S. Government Printing Office.

Sawyer, D. A., Julia, H. L., & Turin, A. C. (1982). Caffeine and human behavior: Arousal, anxiety, and performance effects. *Journal of Behavioral Medicine, 5,* 415–439.

Sawynok, J. (1995). Pharmacological rationale for the clinical use of caffeine. *Drugs, 39,* 37–50.

Schenk, S., Horger, B. A., & Snow, S. (1989). Caffeine preexposure sensitizes rats to the motor activating effects of cocaine. *Behavioural Pharmacology, 1,* 447–451.

Schenk, S., Valadez, A., Horger, B. A., Snow, S., & Wellman, P. J. (1994). Interactions between caffeine and cocaine in tests of self-administration. *Behavioural Pharmacology, 5,* 153–158.

Schenk, S., Worley, C. M., McNamara, C., & Valadez, A. (1996). Acute and repeated exposure to caffeine: Effects on reinstatement of extinguished cocaine-taking behavior in rats. *Psychopharmacology, 126,* 17–23.

Schnackenberg, R. C. (1973). Caffeine as a substitute for schedule II stimulants in hyperkinetic children. *American Journal of Psychiatry, 130,* 796–798.

Shaffer, D. (1993). Suicide: Risk factors and the public health. *American Journal of Public Health, 83,* 171–172.

Silverman, K., Evans, S. M., Strain, E. C., & Griffiths, R. R. (1992). Withdrawal syndrome after the double-blind cessation of caffeine consumption. *New England Journal of Medicine, 327,* 1109–1114.

Smith, A. P., Rusted, J. M., Eaton-Williams, P., Savory, M., & Leathwood, P. (1990). Effects of caffeine given before and after lunch on sustained attention. *Neuropsychobiology, 23,* 160–163.

Spindel, E. R., & Wurtman, R. J. (1984). Neuroendocrine effects of caffeine in rat and man. In P. B. Dews (Ed.), *Caffeine* (pp. 129–141). Berlin: Springer-Verlag.

Stein, M. A., Krasowski, M., Leventhal, B. L., Phillips, W., & Bender, B. G. (1996). Behavioral and cognitive effects of methylxanthines: A meta-analysis of theophylline and caffeine. *Archives of Pediatrics and Adolescent Medicine, 150,* 284–288.

Stephenson, P. E. (1977). Physiologic and psychotropic effects of caffeine on man. *Journal of the American Dietetic Association, 71,* 240–247.

Stern, K. N., Chait, L. D., & Johanson, C. E. (1989). Reinforcing and subjective effects of caffeine in normal volunteers. *Psychopharmacology, 98,* 81–88.

Strain, E. C., & Griffiths, R. R. (1995). Caffeine dependence: Fact or fiction? *Journal of the Royal Society of Medicine, 88,* 437–440.

Strain, E. C., Mumford, G. H., Silverman, K., & Griffiths, R. R. (1994). Caffeine dependence syndrome: Effects from case histories and experimental evaluations. *Journal of the American Medical Association, 272,* 1043–1048.

Swanson, J. A., Lee, J. W., & Hopp, J. W. (1994). Caffeine and nicotine: A review of their joint use and possible interactive effects in tobacco withdrawal. *Addictive Behaviors, 19,* 229–256.

Swift, C. G., & Tiplady, B. (1988). The effects of age on the response to caffeine. *Psychopharmacology, 94,* 29–21.

Taylor, J. L., & Tinklenburg, J. R. (1987). Cognitive impairment and benzodiazepines. In H. Y. Meltzer (Ed.), *Psychopharmacology: The third generation of progress* (pp. 1449–1454). New York: Raven.

Terry, W. S., & Phifer, B. (1986). Caffeine and memory performance on the AVLT. *Journal of Clinical Psychology, 42,* 860–863.

Truitt, E. B., Jr. (1971). The xanthines. In J. R. DiPalma (Ed.), *Drill's pharmacology in medicine* (pp. 83–99). New York: McGraw-Hill.

Uhde, T. W., Boulenger, J. P., Jimerson, D. C., & Post, R. M. (1984). Caffeine: Relationship to human anxiety, plasma MHPG, and cortisol. *Psychopharmacology. Bulletin, 20,* 426–430.

van der Stelt, O., & Snel, J. (1993). Effects of caffeine on human information processing. In S. Garattini (Ed.), *Caffeine, coffee, and health* (pp. 291–316). New York: Raven.

Walsh, J. K., Muehlbach, M. J., Humm, T. M., Dickins Q. S., Sugerman, J. L., & Schweitzer, P. K. (1990). Effect of caffeine on physiological sleep tendency and ability to sustain wakefulness at night. *Psychopharmacology, 101,* 271–273.

Woods, J. H., Katz, J. L., Winger, G. (1987). Abuse liability of benzodiazepines. *Pharmacological Reviews, 39,* 251–419.

Zwyghuizen-Doorenbos, A., Roehrs, T. A., Lipschutz, L., Timms, V., & Roth, T. (1990). Effects of caffeine on alertness. *Psychopharmacology, 100,* 36–39.

III

Cannabis

7

Pharmacology of Cannabis

ALLYN C. HOWLETT

Introduction

The biological actions of cannabinoid compounds in humans have received the attention of several excellent reviews within the last 20 years (Abood & Martin, 1992; Bhargava, 1978; Dewey, 1986; Hollister, 1986; Lemberger, 1980; Paton, 1975). It is now believed that many of the effects of cannabimimetic compounds can be attributed to their actions via two receptors, the CB_1 and the CB_2 cannabinoid receptors. The central nervous system (CNS) responses to cannabinoid compounds are believed to be mediated by the CB_1 subtype. The CB_1 subtype also exists as a splice variant isoform, $CB_{1(b)}$, which is truncated at an extracellular site and whose mRNA is found in much lower abundance (Rinaldi-Carmona et al., 1996; Shire et al., 1995). The $CB_{1(a)}$ and $CB_{1(b)}$ isoforms exhibit relatively similar pharmacological properties when expressed in Chinese hamster ovary (CHO) cells (Rinaldi-Carmona et al., 1996). The CB_1 receptor is a G protein coupled receptor that inhibits adenylate cyclase activity and regulates ion channels. Several recent reviews have described the pharmacology, biochemistry, and CNS distribution of this receptor subtype (Abood & Martin, 1992; Howlett, Bidaut-Russell, et al., 1990; Howlett, Evans, & Houston, 1992; R. Pertwee, 1993). The CB_2 receptor is

found in immune tissue, and is also a G protein coupled receptor that mediates inhibition of cyclic AMP synthesis. As discussed in reviews by Howlett (1995a), Martin (1986), and Pertwee (1988), certain in vitro effects of cannabinoid drugs have been reported that may not be mediated by a receptor mechanism.

Both CB_1 and CB_2 receptor subtypes respond to CNS-active constituents of Cannabis sativa as well as synthetic bicyclic and tricyclic cannabinoid analogs, aminoalkylindole and eicosanoid cannabimimetic compounds. The structural features of many of these compounds have been recently reviewed (Howlett, 1995b; Howlett, Berglund, & Melvin, 1995; Johnson & Melvin, 1986; Razdan, 1986). An antagonist for the CB_1 receptor has recently been described (Rinaldi-Carmona et al., 1994; Rinaldi-Carmona et al., 1995). This chapter describes the prototype compounds from these classes of agonists and antagonists that act upon CB_1 and CB_2 cannabinoid receptors, discusses the localization of these receptors and their relevance to biological actions, and describes the mechanism of action of these compounds at the cellular level.

Pharmacological Classes of Cannabimimetic Compounds

Cannabinoid Pharmacology

A large number of compounds having a "cannabinoid" tricyclic structure have been isolated from Cannabis sativa. These com-

ALLYN C. HOWLETT • Saint Louis University School of Medicine, St. Louis, Missouri 63104.

Handbook of Substance Abuse: Neurobehavioral Pharmacology, edited by Tarter et al. Plenum Press, New York, 1998.

pounds have been tested for biological activity in animal models, for example, drug discrimination and behaviors in monkeys, ataxia in dogs, and drug discrimination and biological actions (hypoactivity, hypothermia, antinociception, and immobility) in rodents (see Razdan, 1986). Of these, Δ^9-THC and Δ^8-THC are those that produce biological responses that we refer to as cannabimimetic. Cannabinol, cannabidiol, and cannabichromene are also found in organic extracts of *Cannabis*, but their cannabimimetic activity is poor. The pharmacokinetics and metabolism of these compounds have been reviewed (Agurell *et al.*, 1986). Δ^9-THC is hydroxylated at many positions on the molecule, and several of these positions can be further oxidized to carboxylic acid. These modifications generally lead to less active metabolites. However, the 11-hydroxy metabolites of Δ^9-THC and Δ^8-THC were more potent than the parent compounds in producing analgesia (Wilson & May, 1975) and signal transduction within neurons (Howlett, 1987). A structural analog of this metabolite, 9-nor,9-β-hydroxy-hexahydrocannabinol (HHC) is a prototype cannabinoid analgesic (Bloom, Dewey, Harris, & Brosius, 1977; Wilson, May, Martin, & Dewey, 1976) on which more potent compounds are based. One of the most potent tricyclic cannabinoid agonists used in research today is HU210 (11-hydroxy-Δ^8-THC-dimethylheptyl) (Howlett, Champion, *et al.*, 1990; Little, Compton, Mechoulam, & Martin, 1989). Radiolabeled compounds that bind to cannabinoid receptors have been synthesized based on dimethylheptyl analogs of these structures (Devane *et al.*, 1992; Thomas, Wei, & Martin, 1992).

Researchers at Pfizer, Inc. extensively examined the structure–activity relationships for analgesia based on HHC. They developed the analgesic and antiemetic drug levonantradol in addition to a series of bicyclic and tricyclic cannabinoid structures (see reviews by Howlett, 1995b, Howlett *et al.*, 1996, and Johnson & Melvin, 1986, for original references). Levonantradol produced analgesia in various models of antinociception in rodents and was taken through clinical trials for acute postoperative pain relief (Jain, Ryan, McMahon, & Smith, 1981). Levonantradol and its first pass metabolite, desacetyllevonantradol, were potent cannabimimetic agonists in tests of spontaneous activity, hypothermia, and immobility, and for regulation of adenylate cyclase in vitro. Pfizer, Inc. also developed a series of nonclassical bicyclic and tricyclic structures having a defined pharmacophore for analgesic activity, changes in spontaneous activity, hypothermia, and immobility in rodents, and signal transduction in neuronal cells. The prototype bicyclic compound, CP-47,497, is a simple bicyclic structure based on HHC but missing the pyran ring and modified with a dimethylheptyl side chain. Adding a hydroxypropyl group produced the potent bicyclic cannabinoid, CP-55,940. CP-55,940 was the first radiolabeled cannabinoid compound available for use in ligand binding determinations of the cannabinoid receptors (Devane, Dysarz, Johnson, Melvin, & Howlett, 1988).

Aminoalkylindole Pharmacology

Sterling Research Institute developed a series of structural analogs based on the nonsteroidal anti-inflammatory agent, pravadoline (reviewed in Howlett, 1995b; Howlett *et al.*, 1996). As the structure was modified, a potent analgesic was developed (WIN-55212-2), which no longer had the properties of a nonsteroidal anti-inflammatory agent to inhibit prostaglandin synthesis. WIN-55212-2 has been shown to bind to the cannabinoid receptor in brain and to evoke the same responses in animal models as the cannabinoid agonists. WIN-55212-2 has been radiolabeled for use in radioligand binding assays (Kuster, Stevenson, Ward, D'Ambra, & Haycock, 1993). Low-affinity cannabinoid receptor antagonist derivatives have also come out of the pravadoline series of compounds.

Eicosanoid Pharmacology

Arachidonylethanolamide (anandamide) is an eicosanoid metabolite that produces cannabimimetic responses in animal models via its association with cannabinoid receptors (see DiMarzo & Fontana, 1995; Howlett *et al.*,

1995b; Mechoulam, Manus, & Martin, 1994, for review and references). Analogs that behave as cannabimimetic agonists also have been found in biological preparations. One modification is the ethanolamide of alternative long-chain unsaturated fatty acids (Hanus, Gopher, Almog, & Mechoulam, 1993; Priller *et al.*, 1995). A second modification is a glycerol ester rather than an ethanolamine amide of arachidonic acid (Mechoulam *et al.*, 1995; Sugiura *et al.*, 1995). 2-Arachidonylglycerol does not exhibit as high an affinity for the CB_1 receptor as does arachidonylethanolamide. However, 2-arachidonylglycerol is found in much greater abundance in the brain than arachidonylethanolamide, leading to speculation that the former may have greater potential to influence cannabinoceptive cells in the brain (Sugiura *et al.*, 1995; Kempe, Hsu, Bohrer, & Turk, 1996). Mechanisms for the synthesis and the metabolism of 2-arachidonylglycerol have been proposed (Sugiura *et al.*, 1995).

A mechanism exists for arachidonyl-ethanolamide to be taken up into cells and metabolized to free arachidonic acid and ethanolamine (Deutsch & Chin, 1993; DiMarzo *et al.*, 1994; Hillard, Wilkison, Edgemond, & Campbell, 1995; Koutek *et al.*, 1994; Ueda, Kurahashi, Yamamoto, & Tokunaga, 1995). The characterization and partial purification of the activity has identified an N-acylethanolamine amidohydrolase found in membrane fractions from brain (Desarnaud, Cadas, & Piomelli, 1995; Hillard *et al.*, 1995; Ueda *et al.*, 1995). An alternative metabolic pathway, catalyzed in the presence of NADPH by microsomal cytochrome P450 isozymes in brain and liver, has been shown to produce multiple oxidative metabolites (Bornheim, Kim, Chen, & Correia, 1993, 1995). These epoxides or hydroxylated eicosanoids, although produced in small quantities, might exhibit as yet undetermined biological activity.

A controversy exists regarding the biologically relevant mechanism of synthesis of arachidonylethanolamide in cells. One method might be the condensation of arachidonic acid with ethanolamine (Deutsch & Chin, 1993; Devane & Axelrod, 1994; Kruszka & Gross,

1994; Ueda *et al.*, 1995). Evidence suggests that the condensation enzyme is the hydrolase operating in the reverse direction (Hillard *et al.*, 1995; Ueda *et al.*, 1995). A concern regarding the condensation synthesis mechanism is the high concentrations of substrates required (K_m for ethanolamine = 25–130 mM, and for arachidonic acid = 7–100 µM (Devane & Axelrod, 1994; Kruszka & Gross, 1994; Ueda *et al.*, 1995) in the absence of an apparent allosteric mechanism to regulate the K_m values for the substrates. An alternative method of synthesis is the hydrolysis by phospholipase D of arachidonylethanolamide from a precursor N-acylphosphatidylethanolamine (DiMarzo *et al.*, 1994; Schmid, Schmid, & Natarajan, 1990). This mechanism has been demonstrated in cultured neurons and can be stimulated as a manifestation of neurotoxic events following glutamate stimulation of the cells (DiMarzo *et al.*, 1994; Hansen, Lauritzen, Strond, Moesgaard, & Frandsen, 1995).

SR-141716A Antagonist

Sanofi Recherche characterized an antagonist selective for the CB_1 receptor subtype, SR-141716A (Rinaldi-Carmona *et al.*, 1994, 1995). This compound is able to produce competitive inhibition of the biological responses to CP-55,940, WIN-55212-2, and anandamide in animal models and in signal transduction in cells (Compton, Aceto, Lowe, & Martin, 1996; Felder *et al.*, 1995; Rinaldi-Carmona *et al.*, 1994, 1995, 1996). SR-141716A exhibited autonomous biological effects (increased locomotor activity) at high concentrations, by an unknown mechanism (Compton *et al.*, 1996). Drug discrimination studies in rats and monkeys demonstrated that SR141716A could antagonize the discriminative stimulus response to CP-55,940 or Δ^9-THC (Wiley, Barrett, Lowe, Balster, & Martin, 1995; Wiley, Lowe, Balster, & Martin, 1995). SR-141716A precipitated withdrawal in rats chronically exposed to Δ^9-THC (Aceto, Scates, Lowe, & Martin, 1995; Tsou, Patrick, & Walker, 1995). The abstinence signs included "head shakes, facial tremors, tongue rolling, biting, wet-dog shakes, eyelid ptosis, paw treading, retropulsion, immobility, ear twitch, chewing, licking, stretching and arched back" (Aceto *et al.*, 1995), "hyperactivity and disorganization, rapidly alternating sequences of behavior, increased time grooming" (Tsou *et al.*, 1995).

Comparison of CB_1 and CB_2 Receptor Pharmacology

Compared with the extensive structure–activity relationship studies that have been performed for the CB_1 receptor, a paucity of data exist describing the pharmacology of the CB_2 receptor. The existing data suggest no remarkable difference in the way the two receptor subtypes recognize agonist molecules. In membranes of COS cells (CV-1 transformed monkey kidney fibroblast cells) expressing the CB_2 receptor, [^{3}H]CP-55,940 and [^{3}H]WIN-55212-2 both bound with K_d values similar to those reported for the CB_1 receptor (Munro, Thomas, & Abu-Shaar, 1993). The order of potency in heterologous displacement studies was 11-OH-Δ^9-THC > Δ^9-THC = cannabinol >> cannabidiol. This pattern generally resembled that for binding to the CB_1 receptor with the exception that cannabinol was equipotent with Δ^9-THC in affinity for the CB_2 receptor. Bouaboula and coworkers (1993) reported binding of [^{3}H]CP-55,940 to myelomonocytic U937 membranes (the ratio of CB_1:CB_2 mRNA was about 1:5), which could be displaced in the nM range by Δ^9-THC, CP-55,940 and WIN-55225. This displacement pattern differed from that expected for the CB_1 receptor in that Δ^9-THC and CP-55,940 were equipotent. Felder and colleagues (1995) expressed cloned CB_1 and CB_2 receptors in AtT-20 and L cells, respectively, for comparisons of heterologous displacement of [^{3}H]CP-55,940 by agonists. The K_i values for agonists selected from the three structural classes were similar for both receptor subtypes. The major exceptions were that HU210 exhibited 10-fold greater affinity for the CB_1 receptor, and WIN-55212-2 exhibited 20-fold greater affinity for the CB_2 receptor. The major pharmacological difference between the CB_1 and the CB_2 receptor pharmacology is that SR-141716A has a 100-fold selectivity as an antagonist for the

CB_1 receptor (Rinaldi-Carmona *et al.*, 1994, 1995; Felder *et al.*, 1995).

Localization and Biological Actions of CB_1 Receptors

CB_1 receptors, quantitated by [^{3}H]CP-55,940 binding to rat brain membranes, are found in greatest abundance in the rat cortex, cerebellum, hippocampus, and striatum, with smaller but significant binding also found in the hypothalamus, brainstem, and spinal cord (Bidaut-Russell, Devane, & Howlett, 1990). Herkenham and colleagues employed quantitative autoradiography of [^{3}H]CP-55,940 binding to cannabinoid receptors in brain slices from rat and higher species including humans to define the regional localization (Herkenham *et al.*, 1990; Herkenham, Lynn, Johnson, *et al.*, 1991). These studies were confirmed by Mailleux and colleagues (Mailleux & Vanderhaeghen, 1992a; Mailleux, Verslijpe, & Vanderhaegen, 1992) and also confirmed with alternative radioligands [^{3}H]WIN-55212-2 (Jansen, Haycock, Ward, & Seybold, 1992) and [^{3}H]11-OH-Δ^9-THC-dimethylheptyl (Thomas *et al.*, 1992), with comparable results. Localization of CB_1 mRNA was reported by Matsuda and colleagues (Matsuda, Lolait, Brownstein, Young, & Bonner, 1990; Matsuda, Bonner, & Lolait, 1993) using *in situ* hybridization, and these results were confirmed by Vanderhaeghen and colleagues (Mailleux & Vanderhaeghen, 1992a; Mailleux, Parmentier, & Vanderhaeghen, 1992). Generalizations to be made from these investigations are summarized below, with specific references listed for unique observations only.

Moderately dense receptor binding is found throughout the rat cortex, particularly in layers I and VI. Although a majority of cells in layers II, V and VI appear to express low levels of mRNA for the CB_1 receptor, there exist sporadic isolated cells that express very high levels of mRNA. Specific binding has also been noted in the anterior commissure using either [^{3}H]CP-55,940 or [^{3}H]WIN-55212-2, and in the corpus callosum using the latter ligand (Jansen *et al.*, 1992), suggesting that cannabinoid receptors may be present on axons of passage within these fiber bundles. Cannabinoid receptors are of low to moderate density within the amygdalar nuclei and the stria terminalis, mammillary bodies, and lateral hypothalamus. Moderate levels of mRNA are found in the nucleus of the diagonal band and medial septum in the majority of cells, with sporadic highly positive cells. Cannabinoid receptors in these regions of the brain could be important for the reported effects of euphoria, muddled thinking, dreamy states, altered perception of visual or auditory stimuli, and distortions in duration of time (Hollister & Gillespie, 1973).

Areas of the hippocampal formation exhibiting the densest CB_1 receptor binding are the CA3 field of Ammon's horn and the molecular layer of the dentate gyrus; however, the remaining areas also exhibit fairly high binding (Herkenham, Lynn, Johnson, et al., 1991). Using [^{3}H]WIN-55212-2, cannabinoid receptor binding appeared greater in the CA1 and CA2 regions than in the CA3 (Jansen et al., 1992); however, the authors could not exclude the possibility that methodological differences may have resulted in this deviation from the observations of Herkenham, Lynn, Johnson, and colleagues (1991) using [^{3}H]CP-55,940. CB_1 mRNA has been found in abundance in granule cells in the dentate gyrus as well as in cells in the pyramidal and molecular layers of Ammon's horn and in the entorhinal cortex. Small amounts of mRNA exist in the majority of the pyramidal cells, but greater levels are present in a moderate number of interneurons. In controlled studies, humans exposed acutely to cannabimimetic compounds exhibit attention deficits and failure to consolidate short-term memory (Chait & Pierri, 1992; Ferraro, 1980; Miller, 1984). Cannabimimetic agonists administered to rats increased the number of errors committed and retarded the completion time in a radial-maze model of memory impairment (A. R. Lichtman, Dimen, & Martin, 1995). The impaired maze performance could be reproduced by microinjections of CP-55,940 bilaterally into the dorsal hippocampus in the region of fields CA1, CA2, or CA3 of Ammon's horn or in the dentate gyrus (A. R.

Lichtman et al., 1995). Rats administered Δ^9-THC exhibited an impaired tone discrimination behavior concurrent with a diminished response of the dentate granule cells to incoming information via the perforant path from the entorhinal cortex (Campbell, Foster, Hampson, & Deadwyler, 1986a, 1986b). It was shown that Δ^9-THC disrupted temporally specific information as it was processed by the hippocampus (Hampson, Foster, & Deadwyler, 1989). The impairment caused by Δ^9-THC was associated with a specific decrease in hippocampal cell discharge during the learning phase (Heyser, Hampson, & Deadwyler, 1993).

CB_1 cannabinoid receptor density is fairly low in hypothalamic nuclei, and particularly sparse in the median eminence. However, some mRNA could be found in cells intrinsic to the hypothalamus, particularly in the ventromedial hypothalamic nucleus. Cannabinoid compounds have been shown to impair thyrotropin, prolactin, and gonadotropin release from the pituitary, and these effects probably involve hypothalamic regulatory mechanisms (Hillard, Farber, Hagen, & Bloom, 1984; Murphy, Steger, & Bartke, 1990; Wenger, Croix, Tramu, & Leonardelli, 1992). Δ^9-THC stimulates corticotropin release, probably as the result of a response to stress (Dewey, Peng, & Harris, 1970; Eldridge, Murphy, & Landfield, 1991; Kokka & Garcia, 1974).

Regions of the basal ganglia that exhibited very high receptor binding included the lateral striatum (caudate-putamen), a region that receives input from the cortical regions involved in sensorimotor functions (Herkenham et al., 1990; Herkenham, Lynn, deCosta, & Richfield, 1991; Mailleux & Vanderhaeghen, 1992b). The greatest cannabinoid receptor density in the basal ganglia coincides with those regions that process motor behaviors (Herkenham et al., 1990; Herkenham, Lynn, deCosta, & Richfield, 1991; Herkenham, Lynn, Johnson, et al., 1991). CB_1 mRNA was expressed moderately in the majority of medium-size neurons in the ventrolateral putamen and in cells in the medial putamen and caudate. It was not possible to discern a clear matrix-striosome localization of receptors or mRNA. Neither receptor binding nor mRNA were detected in the substantia nigra pars compacta, which contains neurons that project to the striatum. Cannabinoid receptors are on the terminals of those striatal cells that project to the globus pallidus, entopeduncular nucleus, and substantia nigra pars reticulata (Herkenham, Lynn, deCosta, & Richfield, 1991). Low levels of mRNA were found in the majority of cells in the subthalamic nucleus. Within the olfactory tubercle, cannabinoid receptors were most dense in the ependymal and subependymal layers, and were moderately dense in the internal granular and plexiform layers. CB_1 mRNA was localized to neurons of the anterior olfactory nucleus. Cannabinoid-induced catalepsy in mice (Gough & Olley, 1978) and the synergistic effects of cannabinoids on immobility in rats that had been administered reserpine (Moss, McMaster, & Rogers, 1981) may be regulated in part at the level of the basal ganglia as evidenced by stereotaxic implantation of Δ^9-THC or levonantradol. Neurons possessing cannabinoid receptors also possess dopaminergic D1 and D2 receptors and opioid receptors (Bidaut-Russell & Howlett, 1991; Herkenham, Lynn, deCosta, & Richfield, 1991). A synergistic hypokinesia in rats resulted from subeffective doses of Δ^9-THC in combination with either reserpinization or treatment with dopaminergic antagonists (Moss et al., 1981; Moss, Manderscheid, Kobayashi, & Montgomery, 1988). This effect could be blocked by nicotinic antagonists and mimicked by nicotinic agonists. Immobility in mice in response to Δ^9-THC was synergistic with cholinergic stimulation, and this response was attenuated by muscarinic antagonists (R. G. Pertwee & Ross, 1991). Pretreatment of mice with benzodiazepines was shown to enhance the cataleptic response to Δ^9-THC, suggesting an interaction with GABAergic systems (R. G. Pertwee & Greentree, 1988; R. G. Pertwee, Greentree, & Swift, 1988).

Within the cerebellum, cannabinoid receptors were predominantly within the molecular layer and were extremely sparse in the deep nuclei (Herkenham et al., 1990; Herkenham, Groen, Lynn, De Costa, & Richfield, 1991;

Herkenham, Lynn, Johnson, et al., 1991). Autoradiographic evidence localized these receptors to the axons of granule cells (Herkenham, Groen, et al., 1991; Herkenham, Lynn, Johnson, et al., 1991). This was confirmed by examination of mutant mice strains (Herkenham, Groen, et al., 1991; Pacheco, Ward, & Childers, 1993). Homozygous strains deficient in granule cells (Weaver and Reeler) exhibited considerably reduced [^{3}H]CP-55,940 binding compared with heterozygous controls and homozygous strains deficient in Purkinje cells (Purkinje-degeneration and Nervous) (Herkenham, Groen, et al., 1991). Inhibition of adenylate cyclase by CP-55,940 or WIN-55212-2 in cerebellar membranes prepared from homozygous Weaver and Staggerer mutants was attenuated (Pacheco et al., 1993). Inhibition of rat cerebellar or granule cell adenylate cyclase by the $GABA_B$ agonist baclofen was not additive with that produced by maximally effective concentrations of the cannabimimetic agonists, suggesting that these two receptor types share a common signal transduction pathway (Pacheco et al., 1993). The static ataxia described as a measure of cannabimimetic activity in larger animals such as the dog (B. R. Martin, Balster, Razdan, Harris, & Dewey, 1981; B. R. Martin et al., 1991) may be the result of cannabinoid interactions with the receptors present in the cerebellum.

The brain stem notably lacked cannabinoid receptors. Cannabinoid compounds decrease body temperature (R. G. Pertwee, 1985), and the structure–activity relationships for this response parallel that for other CB_1 receptor-mediated effects (Compton et al., 1993). Cannabinoid compounds also produce changes in heart rate in man and animals (Hosko, Schmeling, & Hardman, 1984; Jones, 1985), suppress nausea and vomiting (Vincent, McQuiston, Einhorn, Nagy, & Brames, 1983), and decrease intraocular pressure (Adler & Geller, 1986). Although these functions are regulated at the level of the brain stem, it could be that the effects of the cannabinoid compounds may be at a higher level. On the other hand, microinjection of CP-55,940 into the posterior ventrolateral periaqueductal gray in the vicinity of the dorsal raphe of rats resulted in antinociception, immobility, and hypothermia, and these responses could be precluded by coinjection of pertussis toxin (A. H. Lichtman, Cook, & Martin, 1996).

Some cannabinoid receptor binding and the presence of mRNA were found in the substantia gelatinosa and the dorsal horn of the spinal cord, regions expected to be important to antinociceptive mechanisms. (The thalamus was virtually devoid of cannabinoid receptors or mRNA.) Cannabinoid antinociception is probably due to both spinal and supraspinal mechanisms (A. H. Lichtman & Martin, 1991b). Intrathecally administered cannabinoid agonists were able to induce analgesia determined by the tail-flick or hot plate tests in rats or mice (A. H. Lichtman & Martin, 1991b; Welch & Stevens, 1992; Yaksh, 1981) but could not be blocked by the μ opioid antagonist naloxone (Welch & Stevens, 1992; Yaksh, 1981). However, cannabinoid analgesia could be attenuated by intrathecal norbinaltorphimine, a κ opioid antagonist (Welch, 1993). Cross-tolerance could be demonstrated for Δ^9-THC and κ opioid agonists (Smith, Welch, & Martin, 1994), suggesting that a neuronal pathway involving κ opioid receptors may be distal to or converging with a pathway involving cannabinoid receptors in spinal analgesia. The central actions of cannabimimetic analgesics have been demonstrated by tail-flick analgesia in rats after intraventricular injection of either CP-55,940 or WIN-55212-2 (W. J. Martin, Lai, Patrick, Tsou, & Walker, 1993). Intrathecal administration of the α_2-adrenergic antagonist yohimbine attenuated antinociception by Δ^9-THC, suggesting the involvement of supraspinal noradrenergic descending projections to the spinal cord (A. H. Lichtman & Martin, 1991a).

Cannabimimetic compounds inhibit neuronally mediated smooth muscle contraction in model preparations including the mouse vas deferens and guinea pig ileum (Pacheco, Childers, Arnold, Casiano, & Ward, 1991; R. G. Pertwee, Stevenson, Elrick, Mechoulam, & Corbett, 1992; Rosell, Agurell, & Martin, 1976; Roth, 1978). This response may be due to presynaptic cannabinoid receptors (perhaps CB_1?) that regulate release of neurotransmitters.

Localization and Biological Actions of CB_2 Cannabinoid Receptors

The CB_2 receptor was originally cloned from a human promyelocytic leukemia cell, HL60 (Munro et al., 1993). The content of CB_2 mRNA was of greater abundance in HL60 cells that had been differentiated into granulocytes or macrophages. CB_2 mRNA was also found in splenic macrophages and monocytes but not in splenic T cells, mature blood neutrophils, thymus, liver, brain, lung, or kidney, indicating that the distribution is distinctly different from that of the CB_1 receptor. [³H]CP-55,940 binding has also been found in membranes from the myeloid cell line U937 (Bouaboula et al., 1993), consistent with the myeloid localization of CB_1 proposed by Munro and colleagues (1993).

Lynn and Herkenham (1994) localized [³H]CP-55,940 binding within the marginal zone of the spleen, cortex of the lymph nodes, and nodular corona of Peyer's patches, in support of the B lymphocytic origin of the binding sites. CB_2 mRNA was expressed in high quantities in human spleen and tonsils (and in lesser amounts in bone marrow, thymus, and pancreas), suggesting that the CB_2 subtype was responsible for the [³H]CP-55,940 binding (Galiegue et al., 1995). CB_2 mRNA was found to the greatest extent in B-cells and natural killer cells, to a moderate extent in monocytes, and only minimally in polymorphonuclear leukocytes, T4- and T8-cells (Galiegue et al., 1995).

Cannabinoid Actions at the Cellular Level

Cellular Membranes and Cannabinoid Compounds

Cellular and biochemical studies of cannabinoid compounds prior to the mid 1980s centered on the hydrophobic nature of this class of compounds and the concomitant effects of these compounds on cellular membranes. Lawrence and Gill (1975) used the electron spin resonance of a nitroxide-labeled dipalmitoyl lecithin in lecithin/cholesterol liposomes to study the effects of Δ^9-THC. This molecular probe would detect membrane order within the bilayer approximately 8 carbons away from the phospholipid headgroups. The "order parameter" is decreased by the active (–) isomer of Δ^9-THC, and somewhat less by the poorly active (+) isomer, the 11-OH metabolite of Δ^9-THC, and the dimethylheptyl analog, which has a longer hydrophobic alkyl side chain. In contrast, cannabinol and cannabidiol increased the order of the model membranes. No further membrane disorder resulted from increasing the Δ^9-THC concentration beyond a Δ^9-THC: lecithin ratio of 1:30. This may represent the limits of solubility of Δ^9 THC in the phospholipids. The maximum membrane disorder achieved by Δ^9-THC is small compared with that expected for general anesthetics, and thus, Δ^9-THC has been called a "partial anesthetic" (Lawrence & Gill, 1975; Seeman, Chau-Wong, & Moyyen, 1972). Subsequent studies by Hillard and Bloom (Hillard, Harris, & Bloom, 1985; Hillard, Pounds, Boyer, & Bloom, 1990) demonstrated that the phospholipid headgroups in the lipid vesicles and the initial bilayer rigidity were factors in determining the influence of cannabinoid compounds on membrane fluidity. The properties of the cannabinoid structure on the bilayer perturbation have been examined by X-ray diffraction (Mavromoustakos, Yang, Charalambous, Herbette, & Makriyannis, 1990; Mavromoustakos, Yang, Broderick, Fournier, & Makriyannis, 1991) and solid state ^{2}H-nuclear magnetic resonance (Yang, Banijamali, Charalambous, Marciniak, & Makriyannis, 1991) in Makriyannis's laboratory. Those studies determined that the phenolic hydroxyl of Δ^9-THC interacts with phospholipid headgroups at the membrane surface, probably via hydrogen bonding. This interaction orients the tricyclic cannabinoid ring system to be parallel to the plane of the membrane, and the alkyl side chain to be parallel to the phospholipid aliphatic chains. Membrane perturbation results from the intercalation of the cannabinoid structure between neighboring phospholipid headgroups, thereby forcing their separation at the membrane surface and allowing greater flexibility at the long aliphatic chains within the core. Modifications of the Δ^9-THC molecule that preclude the hydrogen bonding allow the hydrophobic ring structure to insert parallel to the aliphatic chains, and the membrane disruption is minimized.

The scientific literature is replete with studies that document cellular effects that can be attributed to membrane fluidity changes in response to the cannabinoid class of compounds (reviewed by Howlett, 1995a, B. R. Martin, 1986, and R. Pertwee, 1993). Because these responses are not mediated by a specific cannabinoid receptor, many of these effects occur at high concentrations of drug, and are not pharmacologically correlated with potency values reported for biological responses in humans and animal models. Membrane effects would not be expected to be antagonized by specific cannabinoid receptor antagonists. Of particular interest to signal transduction, membrane fluidity changes have been reported to increase activity of adenylate cyclase (Houslay & Gordon, 1983). This effect has clearly been demonstrated for the cannabinoid class of membrane fluidizing agents (Hillard et al., 1990). Additional effects of membrane perturbation by cannabinoid compounds have been manifest as alterations in the ligand binding parameters in *in vitro* assays for several receptor systems including dopamine, adrenergic, and opioid receptors (see Howlett, 1995a, for review and references).

Cannabinoid-Evoked Arachidonic Acid Accumulation

Another cellular effect of cannabinoid compounds is the accumulation of free arachidonic acid (see Howlett, 1995a, and Howlett et al., 1992, for reviews and references). Evidence has attributed this to activation of phospholipases or inhibition of arachidonic acid esterification or both. Subsequent production of arachidonic acid metabolites would be dependent upon the particular cell type involved. Indirect effects of cannabinoid compounds may result from the production of prostaglandins or other eicosanoids *in vitro*. An example is the demonstration of cannabinoid-stimulated cyclic AMP accumulation in brain preparations that can be blocked by the cyclooxygenase inhibitor indomethacin (Hillard & Bloom, 1983).

Cannabinoid Compounds and Estrogen Receptors

Environmental estrogens have been a source of concern in recent years, and *Cannabis sativa* has been included on lists of environmental estrogens with the implication that cannabinoid components exhibit estrogenic properties. Biologically active cannabinoid compounds were reported to displace specific binding of [^{3}H]estrogen to rat uterine estrogen receptors, and [^{14}C]Δ^9-THC cosedimented with estrogen receptors on sucrose density gradients (Rawitch, Schultz, Ebner, & Vardaris, 1977). Similar results were reported by Sauer, Rifka, Hawks, Cutler, and Lariaux (1983) using crude extracts of *Cannabis* or cannabidiol (which is not an active cannabimimetic). In contrast, Okey and Bondy (1977) failed to detect Δ^9-THC binding to estrogen receptors in rodent uterine cytosol. Ruh, Taylor, Howlett, and Welshons (1997) investigated whether cannabinoid compounds exert estrogenic effects on the proliferation of MCF-7 cells or on the ability to interact with a reporter gene for the estrogen receptor that had been transiently transfected into MCF-7 cells. Under conditions in which estradiol evoked an increase in MCF-7 cell proliferation and activated the reporter gene, no response was observed with biologically relevant concentrations of Δ^9-THC, desacetyllevonantradol, or with cannabidiol. The cannabinoid compounds also failed to block either response to estradiol under conditions in which the estrogen antagonist raloxifene was effective. It can be concluded that psychoactive or inactive compounds of the cannabinoid class fail to behave as estrogen receptor agonists or antagonists in appropriate assays of estrogen receptor responses *in vitro*. The endocrine effects of cannabimimetic compounds are likely to be primarily attributed to CNS mechanisms that govern pituitary functions (Murphy *et al.*, 1990; Wenger *et al.*, 1992).

Cannabinoid Receptors as G Protein-Coupled Receptors

CB_1 cannabinoid receptors in the brain are coupled to the G_i/G_o family of G protein heterotrimers (α, β, γ subunits) (see Howlett, 1995a, and Howlett *et al.*, 1992, for review). The G_i proteins transduce the signals between the receptor and adenylate cyclase to cause an inhibition of its activity, and Ca^{2+} channels to cause an inhibition of current flow into the cell. The G_o proteins are believed to transduce the signals to K^+ channels. When a cannabimimetic agonist binds to the CB_1 receptor, a conformational change in the receptor facilitates a change in the α subunit of the G protein to allow the release of a GDP molecule. Subsequently, a GTP molecule binds to that site and facilitates the dissociation of the α and $\beta\gamma$ proteins. These proteins are then free to interact with effector molecules such as adenylate cyclase or ion channels. The G proteins remain active until the GTP on the α subunit is hydrolyzed to GDP and the α and $\beta\gamma$ subunits reassociate.

One way that the CB_1 receptor interaction with G proteins in the brain has been detected is by determining the rate of [^{32}P]-GTP hydrolysis in response to agonists (Childers & Deadwyler, 1996; Pacheco, Ward, & Childers, 1994). A second method measures GDP displacement by substituting radiolabeled [^{35}S] GTPγS for GTP (Childers & Deadwyler, 1996; Selley, Stark, & Childers, 1996; Sim, Selley, & Childers, 1995). Because GTPγS cannot be readily hydrolyzed to GDP, it remains on the α subunit and accumulates in response to agonist-stimulation of the receptor. This has been demonstrated for cannabinoid, aminoakylindole, and eicosanoid CB_1 receptor agonists in rat brain membrane preparations and brain slices, and the response could be blocked by the CB_1 receptor antagonist SR141716A (Selley *et al.*, 1996; Sim *et al.*, 1995). This method detected cannabimimetic G protein activation in the substantia nigra, globus pallidus, striatum, hippocampus, amygdala, cortex, and cerebellum, areas previously recognized to possess CB_1 receptors. However, quantitative differences between CB_1 receptor autoradiography and $[^{35}S]GTP\gamma S$ autoradiography suggest that the efficiency of receptor-G protein coupling may exhibit regional differences (Childers & Deadwyler, 1996; Sim et al., 1995).

Biochemical evidence also suggests regional differences in CB_1 receptor-G protein interactions. Sodium ion is a modulator of the coupling of some receptors to G proteins. For the CB_1 cannabinoid receptors in the striatal and hippocampal membranes, 50 mM NaCl enhanced CP-55,940- or WIN55212-1-stimulated $[^{32}P]GTP$ hydrolysis (Pacheco et al., 1994). However, NaCl attenuated the response in cerebellar membranes. This diversity of responses may be the result of coupling to different G proteins rather than to diversity in the cannabinoid receptors.

Cannabinoid Receptors Negatively Coupled to Adenylate Cyclase

Cannabinoid receptors in various brain regions are coupled via G_i proteins to adenylate cyclases. Adenylate cyclases comprise a family of isoforms that are regulated by various mechanisms (reviewed by Mons & Cooper, 1995; Sunahara, Dessauer, & Gilman, 1996). Several isoforms are potentially subject to inhibition via G_i and therefore via cannabinoid receptors. Cannabinoid receptors in the cerebellum, cortex, and hippocampus are probably coupled to type I adenylate cyclase. Type I adenylate cyclase is predominantly stimulated by Ca^{2+} via a calmodulin mechanism in response to agents such as glutamate that increase intracellular Ca^{2+}. Type I adenylate cyclase is only slightly stimulated by G_s and the neuromodulator receptors that are coupled to G_s. Hippocampal CA1 and CA3 pyramidal cells and dentate gyrus neurons possess a related Ca^{2+}-calmodulin-stimulated type VIII isoform. Cerebellar granule cells express type VII adenylate cyclase, an isoform that can be stimulated both by neuromodulators via G_s and by agents that stimulate protein kinase C. The granule cell adenylate cyclase enzymes are transported to the molecular layer, as are the cannabinoid receptors.

Cannabinoid receptors in the basal ganglia are found on GABAergic cells which express type V adenylate cyclase mRNA. Adenylate cyclase enzymes are synthesized in the striatum and are transported to presynaptic locations in the globus pallidus and substantia nigra pars reticulata as are the cannabinoid receptors. Type V adenylate cyclase is stimulated via G_s by neuromodulator receptors such as D_1 dopaminergic receptors.

Cannabinoid Receptors Coupled to Ion Channels

Inhibition of a Ca^{2+} channel via CB_1 receptors in response to Δ^9-THC, CP-55,940, and WIN-55212-2 was demonstrated in differentiated NG108-15 cells (Caulfield & Brown, 1992; Mackie & Hille, 1992). This response was not related to cAMP because inhibition of the Ca^{2+} current was not reversed by cAMP analogs or a phosphodiesterase inhibitor. The Ca^{2+} channel was sensitive to ω-conotoxin, implicating the N-type Ca^{2+} channel. Rat CB_1 receptors transiently expressed in rat superior cervical ganglion neurons also inhibited N-type Ca^{2+} channels in response to WIN-55212-2 and CP-55,940 (Pan, Ikeda, & Lewis, 1996). WIN-55212-2 or arachidonylethanolamide also inhibited Q-type Ca^{2+} currents in AtT-20 cells expressing a cloned rat or human CB_1 receptor (Felder et al., 1995; Mackie, Lai, Westenbroek, & Mitchell, 1995).

Cannabinoid agonists WIN-55212-2 and arachidonylethanolamide activate an inwardly rectifying K^+ current in two model systems. This was demonstrated in AtT-20 cells expressing the rat CB_1 receptor (Mackie et al., 1995), and this effect was blocked by pertussis toxin to confirm its mediation by Gi/o. A similar demonstration was made in Xenopus oocytes that had been cotransfected with both the rat CB_1 receptor and the G protein coupled inwardly rectifying K^+ channel (Henry & Chavkin, 1995).

Using whole-cell patch clamp recording from primary cultures of hippocampal cells,

Deadwyler and coworkers (1993) demonstrated that a voltage-sensitive K^+ current, I_A, was modified by cannabinoid compounds. CP-55,940, levonantradol and WIN-55212-2 decreased the inactivation of I_A by producing a positive shift in the voltage dependence; these drugs also increased the residual I_A current. In contrast to the cannabinoid effects on the Ca^{2+} current, the cannabinoid regulation of the I_A current is dependent on cannabinoid regulation of cAMP production (Childers & Deadwyler, 1996). A negative voltage-dependence shift resulted from application of the cyclic AMP analog, 8-bromo-cyclic AMP, or the adenylate cyclase activator, forskolin (Hampson et al., 1995). The response to forskolin was reversed by WIN-55212-2. Furthermore, protein kinase A inhibitors prevented the cannabinoid actions. These data support a model in which the I_A current is regulated by phosphorylation in response to an increase in intracellular cAMP, and this process is attenuated when cannabinoid agonists diminish cAMP production (Childers & Deadwyler, 1996).

Signal Transduction for the CB_2 Receptor

The CB_2 receptor utilizes the G_i signal transduction pathway to inhibit adenylate cyclase. Δ^9-THC at high micromolar concentrations was able to inhibit both forskolin-stimulated cyclic AMP production in spleen cells (Schatz, Kessler, & Kaminski, 1992) and NaF-stimulated adenylate cyclase activity in membranes from ML2 human leukemia cells (Rowley & Rowley, 1990). Cannabimimetic agonists were able to inhibit cAMP accumulation in CHO cells expressing the human CB_2 receptor with a pharmacology that approximated that for the CB_2 receptor expressed in CHO cells (Felder et al., 1995). In those same CB_2-CHO cells, neither WIN-55212-2 nor arachidonylethanolamine were able to stimulate phospholipase C or phospholipase D signal transduction pathways, mobilize intracellular Ca^{2+} stores, or stimulate arachidonic acid release in a receptor-dependent manner (Felder et al., 1995). CB_2 receptors expressed in AtT-20 cells were not able to inhibit

voltage-gated Ca^{2+} currents or to activate inwardly rectifying K^+ currents (Felder et al., 1995).

Conclusions

Our understanding of cannabinoid receptor pharmacology has advanced in the past 10 years largely due to the development of high-potency agonists of both cannabinoid and aminoalkylindole structural classes. These high-potency agonists have been utilized to define the two cannabinoid receptor subtypes, CB_1 and CB_2, to describe their biochemical and signal transduction properties and their distribution in the brain and the immune system, and to correlate these findings with the biological functions that are altered by these drugs in humans and intact animal models. The advent of an antagonist to the CB_1 receptor subtype has provided researchers with a powerful tool to describe the pharmacology of numerous biological functions that may not have been readily approached given the limitations of agonist ligands. It can be predicted that new antagonists will become available, including those selective for the CB_2 receptor. The scientific community will continue to utilize these tools to expand our understanding of how cannabinoid receptors influence behaviors and biological functions in the body.

ACKNOWLEDGMENT

The majority of the studies referenced in this chapter were supported by the National Institute on Drug Abuse.

References

Abood, M. E., & Martin, B. R. (1992). Neurobiology of marijuana abuse. Trends in Pharmacological Sciences, 13, 201–206.

Aceto, M. D., Scates, S. M., Lowe, J. A., & Martin, B. R. (1995). Cannabinoid precipitated withdrawal by the selective cannabinoid receptor antagonist, SR 141716A. European Journal of Pharmacology, 282, R1–R2.

Adler, M. W., & Geller, E. B. (1986). Ocular effects of cannabinoids. In R. Mechoulam (Ed.), Cannabinoids as therapeutic agents (pp. 51–70). Boca Raton, FL: CRC.

Agurell, S., Halldin, M., Lindgren, J. E., Ohlsson, A., Widman, M., Gillespie, H., & Hollister, L. (1986). Pharmacokinetics and metabolism of delta 1-tetrahydrocannabinol and other cannabinoids with emphasis on man. *Pharmacological Reviews, 38,* 21–43.

Bhargava, H. N. (1978). Potential therapeutic applications of naturally occurring and synthetic cannabinoids. *General Pharmacology, 9,* 195–213.

Bidaut-Russell, M., & Howlett, A. C. (1991). Cannabinoid receptor-regulated cyclic AMP accumulation in the rat striatum. *Journal of Neurochemistry, 57,* 1769–1773.

Bidaut-Russell, M., Devane, W. A., & Howlett, A. C. (1990). Cannabinoid receptors and modulation of cyclic AMP accumulation in the rat brain. *Journal of Neurochemistry, 55,* 21–26.

Bloom, A. S., Dewey, W. L., Harris, L. S., & Brosius, K. K. (1977). 9-nor-9β-Hydroxyhexahydrocannabinol, a cannabinoid with potent antinociceptive activity: Comparisons with morphine. *Journal of Pharmacology and Experimental Therapeutics, 200,* 263–270.

Bornheim, L. M., Kim, K. Y., Chen, B., & Correia, M. A. (1993). The effect of cannabidiol on mouse hepatic microsomal cytochrome P450-dependent anandamide metabolism. *Biochemical and Biophysical Research Communications, 197,* 740–746.

Bornheim, L. M., Kim, K. Y., Chen, B., & Correia, M. A. (1995). Microsomal cytochrome P450-mediated liver and brain anandamide metabolism. *Biochemical Pharmacology, 50,* 677–686.

Bouaboula, M., Rinaldi, M., Carayon, P., Carillon, C., Delpech, B., Shire, D., Le Fur, G., & Casellas, P. (1993). Cannabinoid-receptor expression in human leukocytes. *European Journal of Biochemistry, 214,* 173–180.

Campbell, K. A., Foster, T. C., Hampson, R. E., & Deadwyler, S. (1986a). Δ⁹-Tetrahydrocannabinol differentially affects sensory-evoked potentials in the rat dentate gyrus. *Journal of Pharmacology and Experimental Therapeutics, 239,* 936–940.

Campbell, K. A., Foster, T. C., Hampson, R. E., & Deadwyler, S. A. (1986b). Effects of Δ⁹-tetrahydrocannabinol on sensory-evoked discharges of granule cells in the dentate gyrus of behaving rats. *Journal of Pharmacology and Experimental Therapeutics, 239,* 941–945.

Caulfield, M. P., & Brown, D. A. (1992). Cannabinoid receptor agonists inhibit Ca current in NG108-15 neuroblastoma cells via a pertussis toxin-sensitive mechanism. *British Journal of Pharmacology, 106,* 231–232.

Chait, L. D., & Pierri, J. (1992). Effects of smoked marijuana on human performance: A critical review. In L. Murphy & A. Bartke (Eds.), *Marijuana/cannabinoids neurobiology and neurophysiology* (pp. 387–424). Boca Raton, FL: CRC.

Childers, S. R., & Deadwyler, S. A. (1996). Role of cyclic AMP in the actions of cannabinoid receptors. *Biochemical Pharmacology, 52,* 819–827.

Compton, D. R., Rice, K. C., De Costa, B. R., Razdan, R. K., Melvin, L. S., Johnson, M. R., & Martin, B. R. (1993). Cannabinoid structure–activity relationships: Correlation of receptor binding and in vivo activities. *Journal of Pharmacology and Experimental Therapeutics, 265,* 218–226.

Compton, D. R., Aceto, M. D., Lowe, J., & Martin, B. R. (1996). In vivo characterization of a specific cannabinoid receptor antagonist (SR141716A): Inhibition of Δ⁹-tetrahydrocannabinol-induced responses and apparent agonist activity. *Journal of Pharmacology and Experimental Therapeutics, 277,* 586–594.

Deadwyler, S. A., Hampson, R. E., Bennett, B. A., Edwards, T. A., Mu, J., Pacheco, M. A., Ward, S. J., & Childers, S. R. (1993). Cannabinoids modulate potassium current in cultured hippocampal neurons. *Receptors and Channels, 1,* 121–134.

Desarnaud, F., Cadas, H., & Piomelli, D. (1995). Anandamide amidohydrolase activity in rat brain microsomes: Identification and partial characterization. *Journal of Biological Chemistry, 270,* 6030–6035.

Deutsch, D. G., & Chin, S. A. (1993). Enzymatic synthesis and degradation of anandamide, a cannabinoid receptor agonist. *Biochemical Pharmacology, 46,* 791–796.

Devane, W. A., & Axelrod, J. (1994). Enzymatic synthesis of anandamide, an endogenous ligand for the cannabinoid receptor, by brain membranes. *Proceedings of the National Academy of Sciences of the United States of America, 91,* 6698–6701.

Devane, W. A., Dysarz, F. A., Johnson, M. R., Melvin, L. S., & Howlett, A. C. (1988). Determination and characterization of a cannabinoid receptor in rat brain. *Molecular Pharmacology, 34,* 605–613.

Devane, W. A., Breuer, A., Sheskin, T., Jarbe, T. U. C., Eisen, M. S., & Mechoulam, R. (1992). A novel probe for the cannabinoid receptor. *Journal of Medicinal Chemistry, 35,* 2065–2069.

Dewey, W. L. (1986). Cannabinoid pharmacology. *Pharmacological Reviews, 38,* 151–178.

Dewey, W. L., Peng, T. C., & Harris, L. S. (1970). The effect of 1-trans-Δ⁹-tetrahydrocannabinol on the hypothalamo-hypophyseal-adrenal axis of rats. *European Journal of Pharmacology, 12,* 382–384.

DiMarzo, V., & Fontana, A. (1995). Anandamide, an endogenous cannabinomimetic eicosanoid: "Killing two birds with one stone." *Prostaglandins Leukotrienes and Essential Fatty Acids, 53,* 1–11.

DiMarzo, V., Fontana, A., Cadas, H., Schinelli, S., Cimino, G., Schwartz, J.-C., & Piomelli, D. (1994). Formation and inactivation of endogenous cannabinoid anandamide in central neurons. *Nature, 372,* 686–691.

Eldridge, J. C., Murphy, L. L., & Landfield, P. W. (1991). Cannabinoids and the hippocampal glucocorticoid receptor: Recent findings and possible significance. *Steroids, 56,* 226–231.

Felder, C. C., Joyce, K. E., Briley, E. M., Mansouri, J., Mackie, K., Blond, O., Lai, Y., Ma, A. L., & Mitchell,

R. L. (1995). Comparison of the pharmacology and signal transduction of the human cannabinoid CB1 and CB2 receptors. *Molecular Pharmacology, 48,* 443–450.

Ferraro, D. P. (1980). Acute effects of marijuana on human memory and cognition. In R. C. Peterson (Ed.), *Marijuana research findings: 1980* (NIDA Research Monograph Series No. 31, pp. 98–119). Bethesda, MD: National Institute on Drug Abuse.

Galiegue, S., Sophie, M., Marchand, J., Dussossoy, D., Carriere, D., Carayon, P., Bouaboula, M., Shire, D., LeFur, G., & Casellas, P. (1995). Expression of central and peripheral cannabinoid receptors in human immune tissues and leukocyte subpopulations. *European Journal of Biochemistry, 232,* 54–61.

Gough, A. L., & Olley, J. E. (1978). Catalepsy induced by intrastriatal injections of delta9-THC and 11-OH-delta9-THC in the rat. *Neuropharmacology, 17,* 137–144.

Hampson, R. E., Foster, T. C., & Deadwyler, S. A. (1989). Effects of Δ^9-tetrahydrocannabinol on sensory evoked hippocampal activity in the rat: Principal components analysis and sequential dependency. *Journal of Pharmacology and Experimental Therapeutics, 251,* 870–877.

Hampson, R. E., Evans, G. J. O., Mu, J., Zhuang, S., King, V. C., Childers, S. R., & Deadwyler, S. A. (1995). Role of cyclic AMP dependent protein kinase in cannabinoid receptor modulation of potassium "A-current" in cultured rat hippocampal neurons. *Life Sciences, 56,* 2081–2088.

Hansen, H. S., Lauritzen, L., Strand, A. M., Moesgaard, B., & Frandsen, A. (1995). Glutamate stimulates the formation of N-acylphosphatidylethanolamine and N-acylethanolamine in cortical neurons in culture. *Biochimica Et Biophysica Acta, 1258,* 303–308.

Hanus, L., Gopher, A., Almog, S., & Mechoulam, R. (1993). Two new unsaturated fatty acid ethanolamides in brain that bind to the cannabinoid receptor. *Journal of Medicinal Chemistry, 36,* 3032–3034.

Henry, D. J., & Chavkin, C. (1995). Activation of inwardly rectifying potassium channels (GIRK1) by co-expressed rat brain cannabinoid receptors in Xenopus oocytes. *Neuroscience Letters, 186,* 91–94.

Herkenham, M., Lynn, A. B., Little, M. D., Johnson, M. R., Melvin, L. S., de Costa, B. R., & Rice, K. C. (1990). Cannabinoid receptor localization in brain. *Proceedings of the National Academy of Sciences of the United States of America, 87,* 1932–1936.

Herkenham, M., Groen, B. G., Lynn, A. B., De Costa, B. R., & Richfield, E. K. (1991). Neuronal localization of cannabinoid receptors and second messengers in mutant mouse cerebellum. *Brain Research, 552,* 301–310.

Herkenham, M., Lynn, A. B., De Costa, B. R., & Richfield, E. K. (1991). Neuronal localization of cannabinoid receptors in the basal ganglia of the rat. *Brain Research, 547,* 267–274.

Herkenham, M., Lynn, A. B., Johnson, M. R., Melvin, L. S., de Costa, B. R., & Rice, K. C. (1991). Characterization and localization of cannabinoid receptors in rat brain: A quantitative in vitro autoradiographic study. *Journal of Neuroscience, 11,* 563–583.

Heyser, C. J., Hampson, R. E., & Deadwyler, S. A. (1993). Effects of Δ^9-tetrahydrocannabinol on delayed match to sample performance in rats: Alterations in short-term memory associated with changes in task specific firing of hippocampal cells. *Journal of Pharmacology and Experimental Therapeutics, 264,* 294–307.

Hillard, C. J., & Bloom, A. S. (1983). Possible role of prostaglandins in the effects of the cannabinoids on adenylate cyclase activity. *European Journal of Pharmacology, 91,* 21–27.

Hillard, C. J., Farber, N. E., Hagen, T. C., & Bloom, A. S. (1984). The effects of Δ^9-tetrahydrocannabinol on serum thyrotropin levels in the rat. *Pharmacology, Biochemistry and Behavior, 20,* 547–550.

Hillard, C. J., Harris, R. A., & Bloom, A. S. (1985). Effects of the cannabinoids on physical properties of brain membranes and phospholipid vesicles: Fluorescence studies. *Journal of Pharmacology and Experimental Therapeutics, 232,* 579–588.

Hillard, C. J., Pounds, J. J., Boyer, D. R., & Bloom, A. S. (1990). Studies of the role of membrane lipid order in the effects of delta 9-tetrahydrocannabinol on adenylate cyclase activation in heart. *Journal of Pharmacology and Experimental Therapeutics, 252,* 1075–1082.

Hillard, C. J., Wilkison, D. M., Edgemond, W. S., & Campbell, W. B. (1995). Characterization of the kinetics and distribution of N-arachidonylethanolamine (anandamide) hydrolysis by rat brain. *Biochimica Et Biophysica Acta, 1257,* 249–256.

Hollister, L. E. (1986). Health aspects of cannabis. *Pharmacological Reviews, 38,* 1–20.

Hollister, L. E., & Gillespie, H. K. (1973). Delta-8- and delta-9-tetrahydrocannabinol comparison in man by oral and intravenous administration. *Clinical Pharmacology and Therapeutics, 14,* 353–357.

Hosko, M. J., Schmeling, W. T., & Hardman, H. F. (1984). Δ^9-tetrahydrocannabinol: Site of action for autonomic effects. In S. Agurell, W. L. Dewey, & R. E. Willette (Eds.), *The cannabinoids: Chemical, pharmacologic and therapeutic aspects* (pp. 635–648). New York: Academic Press.

Houslay, M. D., & Gordon, L. M. (1983). The activity of adenylate cyclase is regulated by the nature of its lipid environment. *Current Topics Membranes and Transport, 18,* 179–231.

Howlett, A. C. (1987). Cannabinoid inhibition of adenylate cyclase: Relative activity of constituents and metabolites of marihuana. *Neuropharmacology, 26,* 507–512.

Howlett, A. C. (1995a). Cannabinoid compounds and signal transduction mechanisms. In R. G. Pertwee (Ed.),

Cannabinoid receptors: Molecular biology and pharmacology (pp. 167–204). London: Academic Press.

Howlett, A. C. (1995b). Pharmacology of cannabinoid receptors. *Annual Review of Pharmacology and Toxicology, 35,* 607–634.

Howlett, A. C., Bidaut-Russell, M., Devane, W. A., Melvin, L. S., Johnson, M. R., & Herkenham, M. (1990). The cannabinoid receptor: Biochemical, anatomical and behavioral characterization. *Trends in Neurosciences, 13,* 420–423.

Howlett, A. C., Champion, T. M., Wilken, G. H., & Mechoulam, R. (1990). Stereochemical effects of 11-OH-delta 8-tetrahydrocannabinol-dimethylheptyl to inhibit adenylate cyclase and bind to the cannabinoid receptor. *Neuropharmacology, 29,* 161–165.

Howlett, A. C., Evans, D. M., & Houston, D. B. (1992). The cannabinoid receptor. In L. Murphy & A. Bartke (Eds.), *Marijuana/cannabinoids: Neurobiology and neurophysiology* (pp. 35–72). Boca Raton, FL: CRC.

Howlett, A. C., Berglund, B. A., & Melvin, L. S. (1995). Cannabinoid receptor agonists and antagonists. *Current Pharmaceutical Design, 1,* 343–354.

Jain, A. K., Ryan, J. R., McMahon, F. G., & Smith, G. (1981). Evaluation of intramuscular levonantradol and placebo in acute postoperative pain. *Journal of Clinical Pharmacology, 21,* 320S–326S.

Jansen, E. M., Haycock, D. A., Ward, S. J., & Seybold, V. S. (1992). Distribution of cannabinoid receptors in rat brain determined with aminoalkylindoles. *Brain Research, 575,* 93–102.

Johnson, M. R., & Melvin, L. S. (1986). The discovery of nonclassical cannabinoid analgetics. In R. Mechoulam (Ed.), *Cannabinoids as therapeutic agents* (pp. 121–145). Boca Raton, FL: CRC.

Jones, R. T. (1985). Cardiovascular effects of cannabinoids. In D. J. Harvey (Ed.), *Marihuana '84* (pp. 325–334). Oxford, England: IRL.

Kempe, K., Hsu, F. F., Bohrer, A., & Turk, J. (1996). Isotope dilution mass spectrometric measurements indicate that arachidonylethanolamide, the proposed endogenous ligand of the cannabinoid receptor, accumulates in rat brain tissue post mortem but is contained at low levels in or is absent from fresh tissue. *Journal of Biological Chemistry, 271,* 17287–17295.

Kokka, N., & Garcia, Y. F. (1974). Effects of Δ^9-tetrahydrocannabinol on growth hormone and adrenocorticotrophic hormone secretions in rats. *Life Sciences, 15,* 329–338.

Koutek, B., Prestwich, G. D., Howlett, A. C., Chin, S. A., Salehani, D., Akhavan, N., & Deutsch, D. G. (1994). Inhibitors of arachidonoyl ethanolamide hydrolysis. *Journal of Biological Chemistry, 269,* 22937–22940.

Kruszka, K. K., & Gross, R. W. (1994). The ATP- and CoA-independent synthesis of arachidonoylethanolamide. *Journal of Biological Chemistry, 269,* 14345–14348.

Kuster, J. E., Stevenson, J. I., Ward, S. J., D'Ambra, T. E., & Haycock, D. A. (1993). Aminoalkylindole binding

in rat cerebellum: Selective displacement by natural and synthetic cannabinoids. *Journal of Pharmacology and Experimental Therapeutics, 264,* 1352–1363.

Lawrence, D. K., & Gill, E. W. (1975). The effects of delta1-tetrahydrocannabinol and other cannabinoids on spin-labeled liposomes and their relationship to mechanisms of general anesthesia. *Molecular Pharmacology, 11,* 595–602.

Lemberger, L. (1980). Potential therapeutic usefulness of marijuana. *Annual Review of Pharmacology and Toxicology, 20,* 151–172.

Lichtman, A. H., & Martin, B. R. (1991a). Cannabinoid-induced antinociception is mediated by a spinal alpha 2-noradrenergic mechanism. *Brain Research, 559,* 309–314.

Lichtman, A. H., & Martin, B. R. (1991b). Spinal and supraspinal components of cannabinoid-induced antinociception. *Journal of Pharmacology and Experimental Therapeutics, 258,* 517–523.

Lichtman, A. H., Cook, S. A., & Martin, B. R. (1996). Investigation of brain sites mediating cannabinoid-induced antinociception in rats: Evidence supporting periaqueductal gray involvement. *Journal of Pharmacology and Experimental Therapeutics, 276,* 585–593.

Lichtman, A. R., Dimen, K. R., & Martin, B. R. (1995). Systemic or intrahippocampal cannabinoid administration impairs spatial memory in rats. *Psychopharmacology, 119,* 282–290.

Little, P. J., Compton, D. R., Mechoulam, R., & Martin, B. R. (1989). Stereochemical Effects of 11-OH-Δ^8-THC-dimethylheptyl in mice and dogs. *Pharmacology, Biochemistry and Behavior, 32,* 661–666.

Lynn, A. B., & Herkenham, M. (1994). Localization of cannabinoid receptors and nonsaturable high-density cannabinoid binding sites in peripheral tissues of the rat: Implications for receptor-mediated immune modulation by cannabinoids. *Journal of Pharmacology and Experimental Therapeutics, 268,* 1612–1623.

Mackie, K., & Hille, B. (1992). Cannabinoids inhibit N-type calcium channels in neuroblastoma-glioma cells. *Proceedings of the National Academy of Sciences of the United States of America, 89,* 3825–3829.

Mackie, K., Lai, Y., Westenbroek, R., & Mitchell, R. (1995). Cannabinoids activate an inwardly rectifying potassium conductance and inhibit Q-type calcium currents in AtT20 cells transfected with rat brain cannabinoid receptor. *Journal of Neuroscience, 15,* 6552–6561.

Mailleux, P., & Vanderhaeghen, J.-J. (1992a). Distribution of neuronal cannabinoid receptor in the adult rat brain: A comparative receptor binding radioautography and in situ hybridization histochemistry. *Neuroscience, 48,* 655–668.

Mailleux, P., & Vanderhaeghen, J. J. (1992b). Localization of cannabinoid receptor in the human developing and adult basal ganglia. Higher levels in the striatonigral neurons. *Neuroscience Letters, 148,* 173–176.

Mailleux, P., Parmentier, M., & Vanderhaeghen, J. J. (1992). Distribution of cannabinoid receptor messenger RNA in the human brain: An in situ hybridization histochemistry with oligonucleotides. *Neuroscience Letters, 143,* 200–204.

Mailleux, P., Verslijpe, M., & Vanderhaeghen, J.-J. (1992). Initial observations on the distribution of cannabinoid receptor binding sites in the human adult basal ganglia using autoradiography. *Neuroscience Letters, 139,* 7–9.

Martin, B. R. (1986). Cellular effects of cannabinoids. *Pharmacological Reviews, 38,* 45–74.

Martin, B. R., Balster, R. L., Razdan, R. K., Harris, L. S., & Dewey, W. L. (1981). Behavioral comparisons of the stereoisomers of tetrahydrocannabinols. *Life Sciences, 29,* 565–574.

Martin, B. R., Compton, D. R., Thomas, B. F., Prescott, W. R., Little, P. J., Razdan, R. K., Johnson, M. R., Melvin, L. S., Mechoulam, R., & Ward, S. J. (1991). Behavioral, biochemical, and molecular modeling evaluations of cannabinoid analogs. *Pharmacology, Biochemistry and Behavior, 40,* 471–478.

Martin, W. J., Lai, N. K., Patrick, S. L., Tsou, P. K., & Walker, J. M. (1993). Antinociceptive actions of cannabinoids following intraventricular administration in rats. *Brain Research, 629,* 300–304.

Matsuda, L. A., Lolait, S. J., Brownstein, M. J., Young, A. C., & Bonner, T. I. (1990). Structure of a cannabinoid receptor and functional expression of the cloned cDNA. *Nature, 346,* 561–564.

Matsuda, L. A., Bonner, T. I., & Lolait, S. J. (1993). Localization of cannabinoid receptor mRNA in rat brain. *Journal of Comparative Neurology, 327,* 535–550.

Mavromoustakos, T., Yang, D. P., Charalambous, A., Herbette, L. G., & Makriyannis, A. (1990). Study of the topography of cannabinoids in model membranes using X-ray diffraction. *Biochimica Et Biophysica Acta, 1024,* 336–344.

Mavromoustakos, T., Yang, D. P., Broderick, W., Fournier, D., & Makriyannis, A. (1991). Small angle x-ray diffraction studies on the topography of cannabinoids in synaptic plasma membranes. *Pharmacology, Biochemistry and Behavior, 40,* 547–552.

Mechoulam, R., Hanus, L., & Martin, B. R. (1994). Search for endogenous ligands of the cannabinoid receptor. *Biochemical Pharmacology, 48,* 1537–1544.

Mechoulam, R., Ben-Shabat, S., Hanus, L., Ligumsky, M., Kaminski, N. E., Schatz, A. R., Gopher, A., Almog, S., Martin, B. R., Compton, D. R., Pertwee, R. G., Griffin, G., Bayewitch, M., Barg, J., & Vogel, Z. (1995). Identification of an endogenous 2-monoglyceride, present in canine gut, that binds to cannabinoid receptors. *Biochemical Pharmacology, 50,* 83–90.

Miller, L. L. (1984). Marijuana: Acute effects on human memory. In S. Agurell, W. L. Dewey, & R. E. Willette (Eds.), *The cannabinoids: Chemical, pharmacological, and therapeutic aspects* (pp. 21–46). Orlando, FL: Academic Press.

Mons, N., & Cooper, D. M. F. (1995). Adenylate cyclases: Critical foci in neuronal signaling. *Trends in Neurosciences, 18,* 536–542.

Moss, D. E., McMaster, S. B., & Rogers, J. (1981). Tetrahydrocannabinol potentiates reserpine-induced hypokinesia. *Pharmacology, Biochemistry and Behavior, 15,* 779–783.

Moss, D. E., Manderscheid, P. Z., Kobayashi, H., & Montgomery, S. P. (1988). Evidence for the nicotinic cholinergic hypothesis of cannabinoid action within the central nervous system: Extrapyramidal motor behaviors. In G. Chesher, P. Consroe, & R. Musty (Eds.), *Marijuana: An international research report* (pp. 359–364). Canberra, Australia: Australian Government Publishing Service.

Munro, S., Thomas, K. L., & Abu-Shaar, M. (1993). Molecular characterization of a peripheral receptor for cannabinoids. *Nature, 365,* 61–65.

Murphy, L. L., Steger, R. W., & Bartke, A. (1990). Psychoactive and nonpsychoactive cannabinoids and their effects on reproductive neuroendocrine parameters. In R. R. Watson (Ed.), *Biochemistry and physiology of substance abuse* (Vol. 2, pp. 73–93). Boca Raton, FL: CRC.

Okey, A. B., & Bondy, G. P. (1977). Is delta-9-tetrahydrocannabinol estrogenic? [Letter]. *Science, 195,* 904–906.

Pacheco, M., Childers, S. R., Arnold, R., Casiano, F., & Ward, S. J. (1991). Aminoalkylindoles: Actions on specific G-protein–linked receptors. *Journal of Pharmacology and Experimental Therapeutics, 257,* 170–183.

Pacheco, M. A., Ward, S. J., & Childers, S. R. (1993). Identification of cannabinoid receptors in cultures of rat cerebellar granule cells. *Brain Research, 603,* 102–110.

Pacheco, M. A., Ward, S. J., & Childers, S. R. (1994). Differential requirements of sodium for coupling of cannabinoid receptors to adenylyl cyclase in rat brain membranes. *Journal of Neurochemistry, 62,* 1773–1782.

Pan, X., Ikeda, S. R., & Lewis, D. L. (1996). Rat brain cannabinoid receptor modulates N-type Ca^{2+} channels in a neuronal expression system. *Molecular Pharmacology, 49,* 707–714.

Paton, W. D. (1975). Pharmacology of marijuana. *Annual Review of Pharmacology, 15,* 191–220.

Pertwee, R. (1993). The evidence for the existence of cannabinoid receptors. *General Pharmacology, 24,* 811–824.

Pertwee, R. G. (1985). Effects of cannabinoids on thermoregulation: A brief review. In D. J. Harvey (Ed.), *Marihuana '84* (pp. 263–277). Oxford, England: IRL.

Pertwee, R. G. (1988). The central neuropharmacology of psychotropic cannabinoids. *Pharmacology & Therapeutics, 36,* 189–261.

Pertwee, R. G., & Greentree, S. G. (1988). Δ^9-tetrahydrocannabinol-induced catalepsy in mice is enhanced by pretreatment with flurazepam or chlordiazepoxide. *Neuropharmacology, 27,* 485–491.

Pertwee, R. G., & Ross, T. M. (1991). Drugs which stimulate or facilitate central cholinergic transmission interact synergistically with delta-9-tetrahydrocannabinol to produce marked catalepsy in mice. *Neuropharmacology, 30,* 67–71.

Pertwee, R. G., Greentree, S. G., & Swift, P. A. (1988). Drugs which stimulate or facilitate central GABAergic transmission interact synergistically with Δ^9-tetrahydrocannabinol to produce marked catalepsy in mice. *Neuropharmacology, 27,* 1265–1270.

Pertwee, R. G., Stevenson, L. A., Elrick, D. B., Mechoulam, R., & Corbett, A. D. (1992). Inhibitory effects of certain enantiomeric cannabinoids in the mouse vas deferens and the myenteric plexus preparation of guinea-pig small intestine. *British Journal of Pharmacology, 105,* 980–984.

Priller, J., Briley, E. M., Mansouri, J., Devane, W. A., Mackie, K., & Felder, C. C. (1995). Mead ethanolamide, a novel eicosanoid, is an agonist for the central (CB1) and peripheral (CB2) cannabinoid receptors. *Molecular Pharmacology, 48,* 288–292.

Rawitch, A. B., Schultz, G. S., Ebner, K. E., & Vardaris, R. M. (1977). Competition of delta 9-tetrahydrocannabinol with estrogen in rat uterine estrogen receptor binding. *Science, 197,* 1189–1191.

Razdan, R. K. (1986). Structure–activity relationships in cannabinoids. *Pharmacological Reviews, 38,* 75–149.

Rinaldi-Carmona, M., Barth, F., Heaulme, M., Shire, D., Calandra, B., Congy, C., Martinez, S., Maruani, J., Neliat, G., Caput, D., Ferrara, P., Soubrie, P., Breliere, J. C., & LeFur, G. (1994). SR141716A, a potent and selective antagonist of the brain cannabinoid receptor. *FEBS Letters, 350,* 240–244.

Rinaldi-Carmona, M., Barth, F., Heaulme, M., Alonso, R., Shire, D., Congy, C., Soubrie, P., Breliere, J.-C., & LeFur, G. (1995). Biochemical and pharmacological characterization of SR141716A, the first potent and selective brain cannabinoid receptor antagonist. *Life Sciences, 56,* 1941–1947.

Rinaldi-Carmona, M., Calandra, B., Shire, D., Bouaboula, M., Oustric, D., Barth, F., Casellas, P., Ferrara, P., & LeFur, G. (1996). Characterization of two cloned human CB1 cannabinoid receptor isoforms. *Journal of Pharmacology and Experimental Therapeutics, 278,* 871–878.

Rosell, S., Agurell, S., & Martin, B. (1976). Effects of cannabinoids on isolated smooth muscle preparations. In G. G. Nahas (Ed.), *Marihuana: Chemistry, biochemistry and cellular effects* (pp. 397–406). New York: Springer-Verlag.

Roth, S. H. (1978). Stereospecific presynaptic inhibitory effect of Δ^9-tetrahydrocannabinol on cholinergic transmission in the myenteric plexus of the guinea pig. *Canadian Journal of Physiology and Pharmacology, 56,* 968–975.

Rowley, J. T., & Rowley, P. T. (1990). Tetrahydrocannabinol inhibits adenyl cyclase in human leukemia cells. *Life Sciences, 46,* 217–222.

Ruh, M. F., Taylor, J. A., Howlett, A. C., & Welshons, W. V. (1997). Cannabinoid compounds fail to stimulate estrogen receptors. *Biochemical Pharmacology, 53,* 35–41.

Sauer, M. A., Rifka, S. M., Hawks, R. L., Cutler, G. B., Jr., & Loriaux, D. L. (1983). Marijuana: Interaction with the estrogen receptor. *Journal of Pharmacology and Experimental Therapeutics, 224,* 404–407.

Schatz, A. R., Kessler, F. K., & Kaminski, N. E. (1992). Inhibition of adenylate cyclase by Δ^9-tetrahydrocannabinol in mouse spleen cells: A potential mechanism for cannabinoid-mediated immunosuppression. *Life Sciences, 51,* PL25–PL30.

Schmid, H. H. O., Schmid, P. C., & Natarajan, V. (1990). N-Acylated glycerophospholipids and their derivatives. *Progress in Lipid Research, 29,* 1–43.

Seeman, P., Chau-Wong, M., & Moyyen, S. (1972). The membrane binding of morphine, diphenylhydantoin, and tetrahydrocannabinol. *Canadian Journal of Physiology and Pharmacology, 50,* 1193–1200.

Selley, D. E., Stark, S., & Childers, S. R. (1996). Cannabinoid receptor stimulation of [^{35}S]GTPγS binding in rat brain membranes. *Life Sciences, 59,* 659–668.

Shire, D., Carillon, C., Kaghad, M., Calandra, B., Rinaldi-Carmona, M., LeFur, G., Caput, D., & Ferrara, P. (1995). An amino-terminal variant of the central cannabinoid receptor resulting from alternative splicing. *Journal of Biological Chemistry, 270,* 3726–3731.

Sim, L. J., Selley, D. E., & Childers, S. R. (1995). In vitro autoradiography of receptor-activated G proteins in rat brain by agonist-stimulated guanylyl 5'-[γ[^{35}S]thio]-triphosphate binding. *Proceedings of the National Academy of Sciences of the United States of America, 92,* 7242–7246.

Smith, P. B., Welch, S. P., & Martin, B. R. (1994). Interactions between Δ^9-tetrahydrocannabinol and kappa opioids in mice. *Journal of Pharmacology and Experimental Therapeutics, 268,* 1381–1387.

Sugiura, T., Kondo, S., Sukagawa, A., Nakane, S., Shinoda, A., Itoh, K., Yamashita, A., & Waku, K. (1995). 2-arachidonoylglycerol: A possible endogenous cannabinoid receptor ligand in brain. *Biochemical and Biophysical Research Communications, 215,* 89–97.

Sunahara, R. K., Dessauer, C. W., & Gilman, A. G. (1996). Complexity and diversity of mammalian adenylate cyclases. *Annual Review of Pharmacology and Toxicology, 36,* 461–480.

Thomas, B. F., Wei, X., & Martin, B. R. (1992). Characterization and autoradiographic localization of the cannabinoid binding site in rat brain using [^{3}H]11-OH-Δ^9-THC-DMH. *Journal of Pharmacology and Experimental Therapeutics, 263,* 1383–1390.

Tsou, K., Patrick, S. L., & Walker, J. M. (1995). Physical withdrawal in rats tolerant to Δ⁹-tetrahydrocannabinol precipitated by a cannabinoid receptor antagonist. *European Journal of Pharmacology, 280,* R13–R15.

Ueda, N., Kurahashi, Y., Yamamoto, S., & Tokunaga, T. (1995). Partial purification and characterization of the porcine brain enzyme hydrolyzing and synthesizing anandamide. *Journal of Biological Chemistry, 270,* 23823–23827.

Vincent, B. J., McQuiston, D. J., Einhorn, L. H., Nagy, C. M., & Brames, M. J. (1983). Review of cannabinoids and their antiemetic effectiveness. *Drugs, 25,* 52–62.

Welch, S. P. (1993). Blockade of cannabinoid-induced antinociception by norbinaltorphimine, but not N,N-di-allyl-tyrosine-aib-phenylalanine-leucine, ICI 174,864 or naloxone in mice. *Journal of Pharmacology and Experimental Therapeutics, 265,* 633–640.

Welch, S. P., & Stevens, D. L. (1992). Antinociceptive activity of intrathecally administered cannabinoids alone, and in combination with morphine, in mice. *Journal of Pharmacology and Experimental Therapeutics, 262,* 10–18.

Wenger, T., Croix, D., Tramu, G., & Leonardelli, J. (1992). Effects of Δ⁹-tetrahydrocannabinol on pregnancy, puberty, and the neuroendocrine system. In L. Murphy & A. Bartke (Eds.), *Marijuana /cannabinoids. Neurobiology and neurophysiology* (pp. 539–560). Boca Raton, FL: CRC.

Wiley, J. L., Barrett, R. L., Lowe, J., Balster, R. L., & Martin, B. R. (1995). Discriminative stimulus effects of CP 55,940 and structurally dissimilar cannabinoids in rats. *Neuropharmacology, 34,* 669–676.

Wiley, J. L., Lowe, J. A., Balster, R. L., & Martin, B. R. (1995). Antagonism of the discriminative stimulus effects of Δ⁹-tetrahydrocannabinol in rats and rhesus monkeys. *Journal of Pharmacology and Experimental Therapeutics, 275,* 1–6.

Wilson, R. S., & May, E. L. (1975). Analgesic properties of the tetrahydrocannabinols, their metabolites, and analogs. *Journal of Medicinal Chemistry, 18,* 700–703.

Wilson, R. S., May, E. L., Martin, B. R., & Dewey, W. L. (1976). 9-Nor-9-hydroxyhexahydrocannabinols: Synthesis, some behavioral and analgesic properties, and comparison with the tetrahydrocannabinols. *Journal of Medicinal Chemistry, 19,* 1165–1167.

Yaksh, T. L. (1981). The antinociceptive effects of intrathecally administered levonantradol and desacetyl-levonantradol in the rat. *Journal of Clinical Pharmacology, 21,* 334S–340S.

Yang, D. P., Banijamali, A., Charalambous, A., Marciniak, G., & Makriyannis, A. (1991). Solid state 2H-NMR as a method for determining the orientation of cannabinoid analogs in membranes. *Pharmacology, Biochemistry and Behavior, 40,* 553–557.

8

Behavioral Pharmacology of Cannabinoids

HARRIET DE WIT, JEFFREY M. KIRK, AND ANGELA JUSTICE

Introduction

Many cannabinoids, including both naturally occurring constituents of the plant *Cannabis sativa* and their synthetic analogs, are psychoactive and produce a distinctive profile of behavioral effects. These effects have been most completely documented for Δ^9-tetrahydrocannabinol (Δ^9-THC), the major psychoactive constituent of the marijuana plant, and to a lesser extent for other cannabinoids. The other cannabinoids, which vary in their potencies and efficacies on various measures of central effects according to their chemical structures (Compton, Johnson, Melvin, & Martin, 1992; Pertwee, Greentree, & Swift, 1988), provide a useful means for investigating central sites of action. This review focuses primarily on the acute behavioral effects of Δ^9-THC, and other cannabinoids are mentioned when pertinent. The reader is referred to Martin (1986), Pertwee (1990), Chait and Pierri (1992), Grinspoon and Bakalar (1995), Howlett (1995), and Compton, Harris, Lichtman, and Martin (1996) for more extensive reviews of cannabinoid pharmacology.

Recently, there has been a surge of interest in central cannabinoid pharmacology because of several major discoveries in cannabinoid receptor pharmacology. These discoveries have the potential to significantly advance our understanding of brain and behavior. First, in 1988, a specific cannabinoid receptor was discovered (Devane et al., 1988), and shortly thereafter the receptor was cloned (Gerard, Mollereau, Vassart, & Parmentier, 1991; Matsuda, Lolait, Brownstein, Young, & Bonner, 1990). Then, in 1992, Devane and colleagues identified an endogenous ligand that binds to the receptor, strongly suggesting the existence of a cannabinoid-like neurotransmitter system. The endogenous ligand is known as anandamide, and it has been found to share many, but not all, of the behavioral effects of Δ^9-THC. Even more recently, researchers have developed specific receptor antagonists (e.g., Rinaldi-Carmona et al., 1994), which will allow them to characterize the function of the endogenous system. These discoveries provide exciting opportunities to advance our understanding of the mechanisms underlying the behavioral effects of this interesting class of psychoactive drugs. Already, new highly specific receptor ligands have been developed and significant progress has been made in identifying brain structures mediating cannabinoid effects on memory and analgesia.

HARRIET DE WIT, JEFFREY M. KIRK, AND ANGELA JUSTICE • Department of Psychiatry, University of Chicago, Chicago, Illinois 60637.

Handbook of Substance Abuse: Neurobehavioral Pharmacology, edited by Tarter *et al.* Plenum Press, New York, 1998.

Memory and Cognition

Laboratory Animals

One of the most reliable and distinctive effects of Δ^9-THC is its ability to impair memory. In laboratory animals, Δ^9-THC and related compounds consistently impair memory and behaviors involving temporal differentiation, while leaving many other aspects of cognitive performance relatively unaffected. Heyser, Hampson, and Deadwyler (1993) recently assessed the effects of Δ^9-THC on a delayed-matching-to-sample (DMTS) task in rats. On this prototypic test of memory, Δ^9-THC specifically impaired performance in a dose-dependent (0.75–2.0 mg/kg) and a delay-dependent (1–30 sec) manner. The fact that the impairment was delay dependent provides strong support for the specificity of the deficit to memory-related processes. The impairment in the Heyser and colleagues (1993) study was completely reversible after 24 hr, and was not evident after administration of the nonpsychoactive cannabinoid, cannabidiol. In another test of memory, Lichtman, Dimen, and Martin (1995) showed that Δ^9-THC and related compounds impaired performance on the radial arm maze in rats. These investigators found that systemic administration of Δ^9-THC and two other cannabinoids, WIN-55-212-2 and CP-55,940, increased the number of errors and the time taken to complete the task, in a manner that suggested specific memory effects rather than locomotor or motivational effects. Neither the putative endogenous ligand anandamide nor cannabidiol affected memory on this task. Schulze and colleagues (1988) examined the acute effects of Δ^9-THC on performance of a series of complex operant tasks in rhesus monkeys. They concluded that the effects of Δ^9-THC on performance were consistent with an impairment in temporal differentiation, a phenomenon similar to that reported in studies with humans (see the following discussion). Notably, they reported that these effects in monkeys occurred at concentrations of Δ^9-THC comparable to the concentrations reached by humans who smoke marijuana.

In contrast, Δ^9-THC does not impair performance on many tasks that do not rely strongly on memory or timing. For example, Δ^9-THC did not impair acquisition of behavioral chains in either squirrel monkeys (Evans & Wenger, 1992) or pigeons (McMillan, 1988), at least until doses were reached that produced general response suppression. Aigner (1988) found that visual discrimination performance was unaffected by Δ^9-THC in rhesus monkeys, even after repeated daily administration. Taken together, these findings suggest that the main cognitive impairments produced by Δ^9-THC in laboratory animals are related to the drug's specific effects on memory and timing.

Important advances have been made recently in the neural mechanisms by which Δ^9-THC produces impairments in memory, attention, and information processing. In an elegant series of studies, Deadwyler and colleagues (e.g., Campbell, Foster, Hampson, & Deadwyler, 1986; Hampson, Foster, & Deadwyler, 1989; Heyser *et al.,* 1993) have investigated the neural processes underlying cannabinoid-induced impairments in memory processes by studying sensory evoked potentials in the rat. Their results implicate the hippocampus as a brain site strongly involved in the memory-impairing effects of cannabinoids. For example, Heyser and colleagues (1993) found that the impaired memory performance observed after administration of Δ^9-THC on the DMTS task coincided specifically with a suppression of firing in hippocampal cells during the sampling phase of the DMTS. Lichtman and colleagues (1995) found that the potent cannabinoid analog CP-55,940 specifically impaired memory on the radial arm maze when it was administered directly into the hippocampus. This impairment of memory was observed at a dose that did not produce other cannabinoid effects such as antinociception, hypothermia, or catalepsy.

Humans

The effects of cannabinoids on memory and cognition have been studied extensively in humans, most often using the whole plant form of marijuana by the smoked route. Less is known about the effects of other cannabinoids, or cannabinoids administered by other routes. The results of many of these studies were recently reviewed by Chait and Pierri (1992). Unfortunately, many of the tasks typically used in studies with humans involve multiple cognitive and attentional processes, making it difficult to specify the exact nature of the impairment. Nevertheless, the findings can be summarized in several general categories, including impairments in short-term memory and learning, time perception, psychomotor ability, attention, and complex cognitive skills.

The two most consistent effects of marijuana are on memory and on time perception. The impairment of memory appears to be predominantly related to acquisition of new information, as measured by free-recall tasks. Retrieval of material learned before drug administration is unaffected. For example, Wetzel, Janowsky, and Clopton (1982) demonstrated that after having smoked marijuana, subjects were able to remember details of 14-year-old television shows, but their ability to learn word lists was impaired. More recently, Kamien, Bickel, Higgins, and Hughes (1994) also reported that oral Δ^9-THC produced a moderate impairment on a repeated acquisition task, a measure of learning that has some memory components. Marijuana also produces a distinctive distortion in time perception, such that perceived time appears to pass more slowly than real time (Chait & Pierri, 1992). After smoking marijuana, subjects tend to overestimate the duration of a discrete time interval, and when they are asked to produce an interval of a specified time, they produce intervals of significantly shorter duration than control subjects. This effect has not, to our knowledge, been reported with any other class of psychoactive drugs.

Marijuana also has been shown to impair performance on other, more complex cognitive tasks. Block, Farinpour, and Braverman (1992) tested the effects of smoked marijuana (2.57%) or placebo in experienced users on a range of complex cognitive tasks, some of which were designed to test educational development and ability and others to test learning, associative processes, abstraction, and psychomotor performance. Marijuana significantly impaired learning of a word list and of associations between words, verbal expression,

and ability to do quantitative thinking. In contrast, it had little effect on tests of abstraction, concept formation, long-term memory, or vocabulary. The authors noted that one of the noteworthy aspects of the drug's effects was its tendency to increase uncommon associations. These authors also point out that there are some commonalities between the impairments observed after acute administration and those observed after chronic use.

Chait and Pierri (1992) conclude from their review of the literature that smoked marijuana has inconsistent effects on psychomotor ability, as measured by reaction time and hand–eye coordination. Several more recent studies have shown that smoked marijuana (Kelly, Foltin, & Fischman, 1993; Wilson, Ellinwood, Matthew, & Johnson, 1994) and oral Δ^9-THC 10 or 20 mg (Kamien *et al.,* 1994) impairs Digit–Symbol Substitution Task (DSST) performance, another general measure of both cognition and psychomotor ability. Marijuana has inconsistent effects on attention, as measured by either divided attention tasks or vigilance (sustained attention) tasks (Chait & Pierri, 1992). Although marijuana appears to impair psychomotor and attentional functions, as measured either by simple laboratory tests or by more complex simulated driving and flying tests, in some individuals and in some studies, it does not do so consistently. Some of the variability may be due to individual differences in subjects' habitual use of cannabis (i.e., tolerance), and some may be due to the subjects' ability to overcome mild deficits in laboratory settings. The lack of consistent effect across studies indicates that the effects of marijuana on psychomotor performance are modest. Nevertheless, it should be noted that any drug taken in high enough doses is likely to impair functioning, and that even at lower doses in some individuals cannabis use may be hazardous under certain circumstances.

Although the focus of this chapter is on the acute effects of cannabinoids, it is noteworthy that several recent findings have suggested that the effects of smoked marijuana on memory and cognition may be relatively long-lasting. Block and Ghoneim (1993) examined the long-term effects of chronic marijuana use using a unique database which permitted them to control for the subjects' intellectual status before the chronic drug use. These authors obtained fourth-grade intellectual performance scores for a large sample of individuals who as adults reported either no use of marijuana or light, moderate, or heavy use. The fourth-grade scores provided a measure of pre-drug functioning, and the researchers assessed the cognitive performance of these individuals after years of marijuana use. Heavy marijuana use (7 or more times per week) was associated with impairment in mathematical skills and verbal expression, and with selective impairments in memory retrieval. Intermediate use of marijuana was associated with superior performance on one aspect of concept formation. In another study of lasting impairments after marijuana use, Pope and Yurgelun-Todd (1996) found that performance on a memory task and on the Wisconsin Card Sort task (Heaton, 1981), a measure of abstraction ability, after 24 hr of supervised abstinence from smoking was poorer in heavy marijuana smokers than in light marijuana smokers. It was not clear from this study whether the impairments were lasting changes associated with chronic marijuana use, "drug residue" effects that would disappear after days or weeks of abstinence, or withdrawal-related impairments. Nevertheless, these studies are consistent with the possibility that chronic marijuana use may have lasting adverse effects on certain measures of memory and cognition.

Stimulus Effects

Laboratory Animals: Drug Discrimination

Drug discrimination studies in laboratory animals provide a measure of the interoceptive stimulus effects of drugs. The drug discrimination procedure can be used to assess sensitivity to different doses of a drug, and it can be used to assess similarities in stimulus effects across drugs. The discriminative stimulus effects of drugs in animals are thought to correspond to subjective drug effects in humans, and the pro-

cedure with animals may be used to model pharmacological processes underlying the subjective drug effects, including, for example, pharmacological specificity, brain mechanisms underlying the drugs' effects, and changes in stimulus effects related to tolerance. Balster and Prescott (1992) extensively reviewed the literature on the discriminative stimulus effects of Δ^9-THC in rats, and the authors recently extended their review with additional empirical data (Barrett, Wiley, Balster, & Martin, 1995). They conclude that full generalization to Δ^9-THC has been reported only with cannabinoid analogs, and at best, partial generalization (usually less than 40%) is observed with drugs from other pharmacological classes. In the 1992 review they cite examples of 23 cannabinoids with full Δ^9-THC-like discriminative effects, and 11 other cannabinoids that show partial substitution. In contrast, none of the drugs from other pharmacological classes showed complete generalization to Δ^9-THC. Some other drugs, particularly those with sedative-like effects such as benzodiazepines, barbiturates, and, in one study, the muscle relaxant muscimol, show partial generalization, suggesting that Δ^9-THC and sedative drugs share some discriminative stimulus effects (e.g., Jarbe & Hiltunen, 1988). Notably, however, generalization did not occur with stimulants such as amphetamine, hallucinogens such as LSD, or opioids such as morphine, suggesting that Δ^9-THC does not produce effects similar to these drugs in rats. Interestingly, the authors report a good correspondence between the cannabinoids that produce generalization to Δ^9-THC in rats and monkeys, and those that produce cannabis-like intoxication in humans. This latter correspondence lends support to the use of the drug discrimination model in animals as a model for the subjective effects of Δ^9-THC in humans.

In an extensive series of recent studies, Wiley, Barrett, Balster, and Martin (1993) have further explored various aspects of cannabinoid pharmacology using the drug discrimination procedure in rats and rhesus monkeys. For example, Wiley, Barrett, Balster, and Martin (1993) and Wiley, Barrett, Britt, Balster, and

Martin (1993) examined the development of tolerance to the stimulus effects of Δ^9-THC after repeated administration of the drug. They found that tolerance did develop to the effects of Δ^9-THC (i.e., the threshold for detecting the drug increased), in animals that received the Δ^9-THC repeatedly without further drug discrimination training or testing. Previously, researchers had failed to observe tolerance to the discriminative stimulus effects of Δ^9-THC after repeated administration (e.g., Hirschlorn & Rosecrans, 1974), but this may have been because in those studies training was not suspended during repeated administration, resulting in continuous retraining (i.e., to a changing drug stimulus cue) as the animals became tolerant. Wiley, Barrett, Britt, and colleagues (1993) characterized the effects of Δ^{9-11} tetrahydrocannabinol, and showed that it generalized to Δ^9-THC but was less potent, and that it did not antagonize the effects of Δ^9-THC as some had previously reported. Wiley, Barrett, Lowe, Balster, and Martin (1995), Wiley, Huffman, Balster, and Martin (1995), Wiley, Lowe, Balster, and Martin (1995), and others (Mansbach, Rovetti, Winston, & Lowe, 1996; Perio *et al.*, 1996) have also shown that the newly developed cannabinoid antagonist SR141716A blocks the discriminative stimulus effects of Δ^9-THC, WIN55,212-2, and CP 55,940 in rats and monkeys. Further, Wiley, Balster, and Martin (1995) showed that the putative endogenous cannabinoid ligand, anandamide, produced surprisingly poor generalization to Δ^9-THC: Anandamide generalized to Δ^9-THC and CP 55,940 at only one dose, and at this dose response rates were also substantially decreased. In summary, the discriminative stimulus effects of Δ^9-THC and its analogs have been well characterized and have provided useful information about the nature of the stimulus in laboratory animals, about tolerance, potential antagonists, and potential endogenous ligands.

Humans: Subjective Effects

The subjective effects of cannabinoids in humans have been assessed using standardized self-report questionnaires, mainly in studies with smoked marijuana. Notably, most of these studies have been conducted with subjects who have prior histories of marijuana use, and relatively few systematic data exist concerning the subjective effects of cannabinoids in nonusers. Whether the subjective effects of cannabis are similar in users and nonusers is not certain. In addition, there are few studies of the effects in humans of cannabinoids other than Δ^9-THC. As more centrally acting cannabinoids are discovered and as our knowledge about the receptor mechanisms underlying their effects increases, the number of studies examining other cannabinoids in humans is likely to increase.

Most of the studies measuring the subjective effects of cannabinoids in humans have assessed two major aspects of the drugs' effects: (a) the quality, or nature of the effects produced by the drugs, and (b) the subjects' affective valuations, or liking, of these effects.

One of the most common measures of subjective effects is the visual analog scale, which consists of a line on which subjects indicate the magnitude of effect they are experiencing, from "not at all" to "very much." On these scales, marijuana typically increases ratings on descriptors such as "high," "stoned," and "intoxicated" (e.g., Chait & Zacny, 1992; Heishman, Stitzer, & Bigelow, 1988; Heishman, Stitzer, & Yingling, 1989; Kelly *et al.*, 1993; Lukas, Mendelson, & Benedikt, 1995). Subjects report increased ratings of "sedated," and sometimes also "stimulated" (Chait, 1989; Chait & Burke, 1994; Chait & Perry, 1994; Chait *et al.*, 1988). Subjects also typically report feeling more "impaired" and "confused," and less "clearheaded" after smoking marijuana (Azorlosa, Heishman, Stitzer, & Mahaffey, 1992).

Another measure commonly used to measure the psychoactive effects of cannabinoids and other abused drugs is the Addiction Research Center Inventory (ARCI; Haertzen, 1974), a true–false questionnaire sensitive to several classes of drugs' effects. The ARCI has a scale specifically designed to detect the effects of marijuana (the M scale), which includes questions such as "My thoughts seem to come and go," "I have difficulty in remembering," and "My mouth seems very dry." The M scale is sensitive to dose and time-course of the subjective effects of marijuana. In one study (Chait & Zacny, 1992) the effects of smoked marijuana were compared to the effects of oral Δ^9-THC. The two drugs produced a highly similar profile of effects despite the different constituents and different routes of administration, but they differed in their timecourse. Both drugs produced similar peak ratings of "high," "like," and "overall effect," but the peak effects of the smoked marijuana occurred sooner after administration than the effects of oral Δ^9-THC. Smoked marijuana also typically increases scores on the LSD scale of the ARCI, a subscale that measures dysphoria, somatic effects, and confusion (Chait, 1989; Chait & Burke, 1994; Chait & Perry, 1994; Chait & Zacny, 1992; Chait et al., 1988). There are occasional reports that marijuana increases scores on the sedation scale (PCAG) (Chait et al., 1988; Huestis, Sampson, Holickey, Henningfield, & Cone, 1992), but this effect has been inconsistent across studies. Interestingly, increases in both sedation (PCAG) and visual analog scale ratings of "stimulated" have been reported to occur at the same time (Chait et al., 1988). This finding is interesting because sedation and stimulation are usually thought to be opposites on a single dimension. The finding that they can occur simultaneously may indicate that the dimensions are more complex and may be comprised of different, independently functioning subdimensions. In summary, marijuana produces complex subjective effects that may be either sedative-like or a mixture of sedative- and stimulant-like effects. These mixed stimulant and sedative effects of Δ^9-THC appear to be distinctive to cannabinoids and are consistent with studies using laboratory animals.

One way to study the relationship between subjective drug effects and drug discrimination performance is to conduct drug discrimination studies in human volunteers and obtain self-report data concurrently. Chait and colleagues (1988) trained normal volunteers to discriminate marijuana-containing cigarettes (2.7% Δ^9-THC) from placebo cigarettes, and then tested them with cigarettes containing lower doses of Δ^9-THC. Subjects were able to dis-

criminate cigarettes containing 1.7% Δ^9-THC from placebo but they were not able to discriminate a lower dose (0.9% Δ^9-THC) from placebo. Future studies of this type that include generalization tests with other drugs will be informative for interpreting the data from laboratory animals.

The self-reported subjective effects of smoked marijuana and oral Δ^9-THC are dose- and time-related. Higher doses are generally associated with greater ratings of "high" and "like" (e.g., Azorlosa et al., 1992; Chait, 1989; Chait et al., 1988; Chesher, Bird, Jackson, Perrignon, & Starmer, 1990; Kelly et al., 1993; Perez-Reyes, Di Guiseppi, Davis, Schindler, & Cook, 1982), and "stimulated" (Chait, 1989; Chait & Burke, 1994; Chait & Perry, 1994). One study reports that higher doses of marijuana produced greater and more delayed sedative effects (Huestis et al., 1992). The onset and duration of the drugs' subjective effects are related to the route of administration. After marijuana is smoked or after Δ^9-THC is administered intravenously, plasma Δ^9-THC levels peak within 10 min (Hollister et al., 1981; Huestis et al., 1992), and self-reported subjective effects peak within 30 min. In contrast, when marijuana or Δ^9-THC is ingested orally, peak levels of Δ^9-THC do not appear until 1–2 hr after ingestion, and peak ratings do not appear until approximately 2–3 hr after ingestion (Chesher et al., 1990; Hollister et al., 1981). In one study (Cone, Johnson, Paul, Mell, & Mitchell, 1988), subjects ate marijuana-laced brownies. They reported peak ratings of "like" and "high" 2–3 hr after ingestion and some drug effects endured for up to 12 hr.

Rewarding Effects

Laboratory Animals

In marked contrast to most other drugs that are abused by humans, cannabinoids are not readily self-administered by laboratory animals (Carney, Uwaydah, & Balster, 1977; Harris, Waters, & McLendon, 1974; Takahashi & Singer, 1979). Whereas most drugs that are used recreationally or abused by humans serve as positive reinforcers in laboratory animal models (i.e., self-administration or place preference tests; Johanson and Balster, 1978), cannabinoids have consistently failed in these tests, by either the oral or the intravenous route. These findings are surprising in view of the widespread recreational use of this class of drugs in humans (Richards, 1981). Mansbach, Nicholson, Martin, and Balster (1994) recently addressed the possibility that the difficulty in demonstrating Δ^9-THC self-administration was due to its relatively slow onset and long duration of effect. They provided rhesus monkeys with opportunities to self-administer intravenous Δ^9-THC and CP 55,940 three times each day, at intervals that were spaced widely enough for the drug's effects to be perceptible. In addition, they paired each infusion with a distinctive visual stimulus. Even under these conditions, Δ^9-THC was a poor reinforcer. Conflicting results have been reported using the place preference procedure. Lepore, Stanislav, Lowinson, and Gardner (1995) showed that Δ^9-THC (1.0–4.0 mg/kg, ip) produced a significant place preference in rats, comparable to that produced by cocaine, morphine, and food. However, Parker and Gillies (1995) found that Δ^9-THC (0.2–1.5 mg/kg ip) produced only place avoidance, as well as taste avoidance and aversive taste reactivity in two strains of rats. In another putative model of rewarding drug effects, it has been shown that Δ^9-THC, like other abused drugs, decreases thresholds in brain stimulation reward (Gardner et al., 1988). Unfortunately, not only are the brain stimulation findings inconsistent with most other studies of rewarding effects of Δ^9-THC in animals, but the model also lacks the face validity of the other animal models of drug reinforcement, making the results somewhat difficult to interpret. In summary, despite repeated attempts using a range of experimental conditions, it has been extremely difficult to demonstrate any positive reinforcing effects of Δ^9-THC in laboratory animals.

Humans

In humans, rewarding, or pleasurable, effects of drugs have been assessed both with self-report measures of ratings of hedonic value, or "liking," and with objective measures of actual drug taking (e.g., drug-vs.-placebo choice, rate of self-administration, latency to consume, or amount consumed). Although laboratory studies that have used both of these measures indicate that the subjective reports of drug liking are generally well correlated with the objective measures of their reinforcing effects (i.e., drug taking), the fact that the two measures are occasionally dissociated (e.g., Lamb et al., 1991) indicates that they may be independent and that both measures should be obtained. Generally, however, drugs that increase ratings of liking and high are also self-administered. For example, Mendelson and Mello (1984) provided subjects with the opportunity to smoke marijuana (1.83% Δ^9-THC) and ingest a dose of oral Δ^9-THC (17.5 mg). Subjects reported greater ratings of "high" for smoked marijuana than for oral Δ^9-THC, at the doses tested, and when subjects were allowed to choose between the smoked marijuana and oral substances, they preferred the smoked form. Chait and Zacny (1992) examined the effects of oral Δ^9-THC (10 or 15 mg, depending on subjects' sensitivity to a low sampling dose) and smoked marijuana (2.3% or 3.6% Δ^9-THC, depending on subjects' sensitivity to a low sampling dose) in experienced marijuana smokers. Relative to placebo, both the marijuana and the Δ^9-THC increased subjects' ratings of "like," "high," and "overall effect," and in both cases the subjects chose to administer the active drugs over placebo. Chait and Burke (1994) examined the effects of two doses of marijuana (0.63% and 1.95% Δ^9-THC) in regular marijuana users. The subjective effects were greater at the higher dose, and when subjects were given a choice to smoke one of the two doses they consistently chose the higher dose. Although these studies demonstrate the dose dependence of the effects of marijuana, dose-dependent effects have not been reliably demonstrated for all measures. For example, several researchers have reported that subjects failed to titrate their smoke intake with increases in drug potency (Chait, 1989; Perez-Reyes et al., 1982; Wu, Tashkin, Rose,

& Djahed, 1988). Thus, in the marijuana-using populations who have served as subjects in these studies, cannabinoids appear to be rewarding insofar as subjects rate their effects as being pleasurable and liked, and the subjects ingest the drugs repeatedly when given the opportunity, even under double-blind conditions.

Locomotor Activity

Cannabinoids decrease spontaneous locomotor activity in laboratory animals and produce several other distinctive behavioral effects in activity tests. In particular, they produce a distinctive stimulatory effect at low doses or even, paradoxically, during the depressant phase of the drugs' effects (Abood & Martin, 1992; Compton et al., 1996; Dewey, 1986; Fride & Mechoulam, 1993). These stimulatory effects appear to take the form of hyperreflexia, which is characterized by a hyperreactivity to environmental stimuli. This hyperreflexia distinguishes psychoactive cannabinoids from other, purely depressant, drugs. For example, whereas the prototypic psychoactive cannabinoid Δ^9-THC reliably produces this effect, nonpsychoactive cannabinoids such as cannabidiol do not (Dewey, 1986). Cannabinoids also produce static ataxia in dogs, impair rotorod performance in mice, and produce catalepsy and hypomotility at high doses in several species (see Consroe & Mechoulam, 1987; Little, Compton, Johnson, Melvin, & Martin, 1988).

Locomotor activity or other measures of gross bodily movement are rarely assessed in humans. Cannabinoids have been reported to increase both self-reported feelings of sedation and stimulation, sometimes only producing stimulation (Chait, 1989), sometimes only sedation (Azorlosa et al., 1992), and sometimes producing both (Chait et al., 1988). To whatever extent self-reported feelings of sedation and stimulation are related to overt behavioral manifestations of those feelings, these findings suggest that there are commonalities in effects between humans and nonhumans. However, the exact nature of the paradoxical stimulant-sedative effects, or the phenomenon of hyper-

reflexia in response to environmental stimuli, to our knowledge, have not been examined in detail in humans.

Analgesia

The analgesic effects of cannabinoids in laboratory animals are well documented, and have been demonstrated in standardized tests of analgesia including the tail-flick, hot plate, acetic acid writhing and pinch tests (Howlett, 1995; Martin, 1986; Pertwee, 1990). Indeed, the antinociceptive effects of cannabinoids have served as one of identifying features used to classify novel compounds as cannabimimetic. The cloning of the cannabinoid receptor (Gerard et al., 1991; Matsuda et al., 1990) and the discovery of an endogenous ligand for this receptor (Devane et al., 1992) have stimulated considerable research on the receptor mechanisms underlying cannabinoid-induced analgesia. Although it was initially believed that cannabinoids might exert their analgesic effects through interactions with the opioid system, it is now believed that both opioid and cannabinoid systems can mediate analgesic effects independently of one another (Compton et al., 1996). The analgesic effects of cannabinoids have been shown to be mediated both through spinal mechanisms (Lichtman & Martin, 1991) and through direct actions on the brain (Martin et al., 1993). The products of this active area of research are likely to further our understanding of cannabinoid pharmacology and the function of this newly discovered neurotransmitter system.

Few studies have examined the antinociceptive effects of cannabinoids in humans. Noyes, Brunk, Avery, and Canter (1975) and Noyes, Brunk, Baram, and Canter (1975) reported that Δ^9-THC (20 mg) was as effective as codeine in decreasing pain in patients suffering from neoplastic disease. Notably, these patients were not experienced marijuana users, and they found the psychoactive effects unpleasant. Milstein, MacCannell, Karr, and Clark (1975) conducted a laboratory study to examine the analgesic effects of marijuana in normal volunteers, half of whom had previous experience with marijuana and half of whom did not. Both groups exhibited higher pain tolerance, and the analgesic effects were greater in the experienced users than in the naive subjects. Although the unpleasant psychoactive effects experienced by non-drug-experienced individuals may limit the clinical usefulness of cannabinoids as analgesics, further studies with healthy volunteers who are experienced marijuana users may be useful to elucidate the basic processes underlying cannabinoid-induced analgesia.

Antiemetic Effects

Oral Δ^9-THC and its analogs have been shown to be effective at preventing emesis and vomiting in cancer patients undergoing chemotherapy (e.g., Levitt, 1986; Ungerleider *et al.,* 1982; Vincent, McQuiston, Einhorn, Nagy, & Brames, 1983). A dosage of 5–10mg/m^2 is generally administered 1–2 hr before chemotherapy and repeated every 4–6 hr after, up to 24 hr. These drugs have been shown to be as effective or more effective at reducing nausea when compared with phenothiazines, drugs traditionally used as antiemetics in this context (e.g., Orr, McKerman, & Bloone, 1980; Sallan, Cronin, Zelen, & Zinberg, 1980; Ungerleider *et al.,* 1982). The antiemetic effects may indirectly affect appetite and food intake (see the following discussion). For example, oral Δ^9-THC has also been shown to increase appetite and decrease weight loss in AIDS patients being treated with antiviral chemotherapy (Plasse *et al.,* 1991). Despite the efficacy of Δ^9-THC as an antiemetic drug, its clinical usefulness may be limited because of unpleasant psychoactive side effects, including dizziness, confusion, and dysphoria (e.g., Plasse *et al.,* 1991; Sweet, Miller, Weddington, Senay, & Sushelsky, 1981; Ungerleider *et al.,* 1982). However, there is limited evidence to suggest that, when Δ^9-THC is used in combination with phenothiazines, these side effects are somewhat attenuated and its antiemetic efficacy increases (Chang *et al.,* 1979; Plasse *et al.,* 1991).

Because the administration of Δ^9-THC by the oral route results in lower and more variable bioavailability as compared with smoking or iv administration, and because oral drug administration may be difficult in subjects who repeatedly vomit, several studies have recently explored the antiemetic effectiveness of Δ^9-THC administered by other routes. For example, Vinciguerra, Moore, and Brennan (1988) found that smoked marijuana was effective at reducing emesis in 78% of cancer chemotherapy patients. However, it is unclear how practical this method would be for patients for whom smoking is unpleasant or medically contraindicated (e.g., those with respiratory conditions). Mattes, Shaw, Edling-Owens, Engelman, and Elsohly (1993) recently explored the kinetics of Δ^9-THC administered in the form of a suppository, comparing plasma Δ^9-THC levels after the suppository (11.8 mg) to an oral dose (9 mg) in healthy volunteers. Plasma levels of Δ^9-THC were significantly higher and endured for a longer period of time after using the suppository than by the oral route. However, the relationship between concentrations of Δ^9-THC (or its metabolites) and the drug's antiemetic efficacy or psychotropic side effect profile has not been fully investigated.

Abrahamov, Abrahamov, and Mechoulam (1995) recently examined Δ^8-THC, a less psychoactive cannabinoid than Δ^9-THC, as a potential antiemetic in children being treated with cancer chemotherapy. In doses higher than doses of Δ^9-THC usually given to adults (18 mg/m^2), Δ^8-THC completely blocked emesis and prevented vomiting in all subjects and, in contrast to Δ^9-THC, few psychotropic side effects were reported. Thus, this agent may have potential as a clinically useful antiemetic drug.

Appetite and Food Intake

Laboratory Animals

In laboratory animals, a primary effect of Δ^9-THC has been to decrease food intake, but there have also been reports of increases in food intake at low doses. The most commonly reported effect, from both acute and chronic administration of Δ^9-THC, is a decrease in appetite and food consumption. This effect has been shown in rats (Abel & Schiff, 1969; Drewnowski & Grinker, 1978a; Johansson, Jarbe, & Henriksson, 1975; Miczek & Dixit, 1980; Sofia & Barry, 1974; Sofia & Knobloch, 1976; Stark & Dews, 1980), mice (Weinberg, Dimon, Simon, Harris, & Borzelleca, 1977), beagles (Huy & Roy, 1976), and chickens (Abel, Cooper & Harris, 1974). In rats, this depression of appetite has been demonstrated to be dose dependent (Drewnowski & Grinker, 1978a; Johansson *et al.,* 1975; Sofia & Barry, 1974; Stark & Dews, 1980), and to recover after chronic administration has ceased (Drewnowski & Grinker, 1978b; Johansson *et al.,* 1975; Miczek & Dixit, 1980). In contrast, increases in food intake have been reported at low doses of Δ^9-THC. For example, Glick and Milloy (1972) reported that an acute dose of 1.0 mg/kg Δ^9-THC increased food intake in rats, whereas a higher dose (2.0 mg/kg) decreased intake. Gluck and Ferraro (1974) reported that 1.0 mg/kg Δ^9-THC continued to increase food intake even when it was administered daily over a 12-day period. McLaughlin, Baile, and Bender (1979) demonstrated that low doses (i.e., 10 µg/kg iv) of l-Δ^9-THC increased food intake in sheep, whereas d-Δ^9-THC did not. The l-isomer of THC has also been found to increase food intake in sated rats when administered intragastrically and when microinjected into the ventralmedial hypothalamus (VMH) (Anderson-Baker, McLaughlin, & Baile, 1979). In the Anderson-Baker and colleagues (1979) study, the d-isomer did not increase feeding when administered into the VMH, but did increase feeding when administered into the lateral hypothalamus.

Differences in testing conditions, fed and fasted states, fluid intake, and route of administration across studies make it difficult to identify factors that might account for the disparate effects of Δ^9-THC on food intake. There is some evidence to indicate a biphasic dose response, with low doses increasing, and higher doses decreasing food intake. The findings with laboratory animals are difficult to compare with those involving humans because the doses used in most of the animal studies are substantially higher than those that produce a "high" in humans, 1000 µg/kg vs. 19 µg/kg (Perez-Reyes, Timmons, Davis, & Wall, 1973). At these very high doses, behavioral measures of food intake may be confounded by nonspecific factors such as increases in sedation.

Humans

In humans, anecdotal evidence indicates that marijuana may increase both food intake and taste sensitivity (Foltin, Fischman, & Byrne, 1988; Halikas, Goodwin, & Guze, 1971; Hollister, 1971). Laboratory studies involving acute marijuana administration by both oral (Hollister, 1971) and smoked routes (Abel, 1971) have supported these anecdotal accounts, although the results have been variable and sensitive to methodological conditions. For example, Hollister (1971) found that an acute oral dose of marijuana prepared as an extract and calibrated for Δ^9-THC (0.5 mg/kg; mean dose 32 mg) increased consumption of a single test beverage (chocolate milkshake) in fed, but not fasted subjects. However the effect was observed in only 7 of 12 of the subjects, and 4 of the fasted subjects reported a decrease in appetite.

Chronic marijuana administration has been reported to increase caloric intake, which may result in weight gain (Foltin, Brady, & Fischman, 1986; Greenberg, Kuehnle, Mendelson, & Bernstein, 1976). However, the results of these chronic dosing studies have also been variable and dependent on dose, test conditions, and test environment. For example, Foltin and colleagues (1986) reported that subjects who smoked in a social setting reported a greater increase in food intake than subjects who smoked alone. Subjects who smoked two or three marijuana cigarettes (1.84% Δ^9-THC) daily for 25 days in a social context, increased their food consumption by 20%, whereas subjects who smoked one cigarette per day alone in their individual rooms did not increase their food intake. In a later study this group reported that when subjects smoked four regularly spaced marijuana cigarettes (2%–3%

Δ^9-THC) every day in either private or social settings, food consumption was increased by 40% in both settings.

There is some evidence to suggest that this appetite stimulation effect may be susceptible to tolerance following chronic smoking. Greenberg and colleagues (1976) studied both heavy and casual marijuana users before, during, and after 21 days of marijuana smoking in a research ward. They found that both groups of smokers significantly increased their caloric intake and gained weight (heavy users, 3.7 lbs; casual users, 2.8 lbs) during the marijuana smoking period. In contrast, control subjects who did not smoke marijuana displayed only a slight increase in weight (0.2 lbs) during the same time period. The researchers also noted that the number of marijuana cigarettes smoked per day increased progressively during the 21-day period.

There is some evidence that marijuana- or Δ^9-THC-induced hunger appears to be specific to certain types of foods, particularly sweet-solid snacks such as candy bars (Foltin et al., 1986; Foltin et al., 1988). However, a recent study (Mattes, Shaw, & Engelman, 1994) reported contradictory findings. Light marijuana users received an acute oral dose of Δ^9-THC (15 mg for males, 10 mg for females) or placebo, a marijuana cigarette (2.57 ± 0.06% Δ^9-THC), sublingual Δ^9-THC (15 mg for males, 10 mg for females), or a chronic (3-day) dose of Δ^9-THC given orally or via a rectal suppository. Subjects were presented with salty, sweet, sour, and bitter solutions and asked to rate, on Likert-type scales, the intensity of the taste and how much they liked or disliked the taste. Subjects were also asked what kinds of foods they would prefer to eat, and their food intake was recorded. Following marijuana or Δ^9-THC administration, no significant increases were observed, compared to placebo, in taste intensity, hedonics, or caloric intake during any dosing condition. The authors suggested that previously reported shifts in taste responses may have been due to alterations of memory and cognition, rather than gustatory function.

The effects of marijuana on appetite in humans may be influenced by social factors and environmental familiarity. Foltin and colleagues (1986) observed that marijuana increased food intake only in subjects who were allowed to socialize after smoking. Others have observed that increased food intake is highly correlated with experience of a "high" (Sallan et al., 1980), and such a sensation is strongly related to social cues (Jones, 1971). Other researchers failed to detect a correlation between reported "high" and food intake; they noted that approximately 20% of subjects informed researchers that, upon returning home after the study, they experienced a resurgence of a "high" and ate voraciously (Mattes, Engelman, Shaw, & Elsohly, 1994). It is possible that the drug's effects on appetite were suppressed in the laboratory setting but emerged in the naturalistic setting of the home. The influence of social setting on marijuana's potential effects on appetite stimulation may account for the low incidence of appetite stimulation in controlled studies (about 50%) relative to descriptive accounts (about 90%) in which the drugs were used in more naturalistic, usually social, settings (Mattes et al., 1994).

Amotivational Syndrome

There are anecdotal reports that chronic marijuana use results in an "amotivational syndrome," characterized by lethargy and loss of goal-oriented activity (McGlothin & West, 1968; Smith, 1968). Although there has been a great deal of interest in this purported phenomenon, it has been difficult to document empirically. Among the difficulties in studying this effect in the laboratory are defining "heavy" smoking, determining which individual characteristics predated the drug use and which resulted from the drug use, separating other lifestyle factors from pharmacological effects, and finding valid behavioral measures of motivation (Mendelson, Kuehnle, Greenberg, & Mello, 1976).

Recent experiments with humans and laboratory animals have yielded mixed results. Foltin and his colleagues (1989, 1990) performed two experiments in which subjects resided in a research laboratory for up to 2 weeks. In these experiments, subjects were required to work at low-probability activities (i.e., activities in which subjects would be unlikely to participate if given a choice, such as performing cognitive tasks on a computer) in order to earn time to participate in high-probability activities (e.g., socializing) under the effects of marijuana and placebo. In one of these studies (Foltin *et al.*, 1989), marijuana decreased the amount of time subjects worked on the low-probability activity. This observation was interpreted as a decrease in "motivation" to work. However, a subsequent experiment by this group (Foltin *et al.*, 1990) yielded the opposite result. Paule and colleagues (1992) reported that chronic exposure to marijuana smoke in monkeys decreased responding on a progressive ratio schedule for food reinforcement. Although the authors interpreted this decrease in progressive ratio break point as a decrease in motivation, further studies are needed to rule out alternative interpretations.

Conclusion

Marijuana and other cannabinoids have a distinctive profile of behavioral and subjective effects. Many of these effects have been well documented in laboratory animals and human subjects, using standardized measures in carefully controlled laboratory settings. There have been significant advances in our understanding of the effects of cannabinoids on memory, cognition, and analgesia, and modest advances in our knowledge of the drugs' antiemetic effects and effects on appetite. Much remains to be learned about the long-term effects of marijuana and other cannabinoids on each of these measures. Research is needed to elucidate the basis for individual differences in subjective and behavioral responses to this class of drugs, including individual differences that are related to expectancies and histories of prior drug use. The pharmacologic effects of cannabinoids other than Δ^9-THC may shed light on the role of the endogenous cannabinoid system in normal function and in patho-

logical conditions. The subjective and behavioral effects of these compounds, after both acute and chronic administration, and administered alone or in combination with other drugs, are important for identifying the therapeutic uses and limitations of this class of drugs.

ACKNOWLEDGMENTS

This work was supported by the National Institute on Drug Abuse (DA02812, DA03517 and T32 07255). The authors thank Robert Block and Jenny Wiley for their helpful comments on an earlier draft.

References

Abel, E. L. (1971). Effects of marijuana on the solution of anagrams, memory and appetite. *Nature, 231,* 260–261.

Abel, E. L., & Schiff, B. B. (1969). Effects of the marijuana homologue, parahexyl, on food and water intake and curiosity in the rat. *Psychopharmacology, 35,* 335–339.

Abel, E. L., Cooper, C. W., & Harris, L. S. (1974). Effects of Δ^9-tetrahydrocannabinol on body weight and brain electrolytes in the chicken. *Behavioral Biology, 15,* 1–27.

Abood, M. E., & Martin, B. R. (1992). Neurobiology of marijuana abuse. *Trends in Pharmacological Sciences, 13,* 201–206.

Abrahamov, A., Abrahamov, A., & Mechoulam, R. (1995). An efficient new cannabinoid antiemetic in pediatric oncology. *Life Sciences, 56,* 2097–2102.

Aigner, T. G. (1988). Delta-9 tetrahydrocannabinol impairs visual recognition memory but not discrimination learning in rhesus monkeys. *Psychopharmacology, 95,* 507–511.

Anderson-Baker, W. C., McLaughlin, C. L., & Baile, C. A. (1979). Oral and hypothalamic injections of barbiturates, benzodiazepines and cannabinoids and food intake in rats. *Pharmacology, Biochemistry and Behavior, 11,* 487–491.

Azorlosa, J. L., Heishman, S. J., Stitzer, M. L., & Mahaffey, J. M. (1992). Marijuana smoking: Effect of varying Δ^9-tetrahydrocannabinol content and number of puffs. *Journal of Pharmacology and Experimental Therapeutics, 261,* 114–122.

Balster, R. L., & Prescott, W. R. (1992). Δ^9-tetrahydrocannabinol discrimination in rats as a model of cannabis intoxication. *Neuroscience and Biobehavioral Reviews, 16,* 55–62.

Barrett, R. L., Wiley, J. L., Balster, R. L., & Martin, B. R. (1995). Pharmacological specificity of Δ^9-tetrahydrocannabinol discrimination in rats. *Psychopharmacology, 118,* 419–424.

Block, R. I., & Ghoneim, M. M. (1993). Effects of chronic marijuana use on human cognition. *Psychopharmacology, 110,* 219–228.

Block, R. I., Farinpour, R., & Braverman, K. (1992). Acute effects of marijuana on cognition: Relationships to chronic effects and smoking techniques. *Pharmacology, Biochemistry and Behavior, 43,* 907–917.

Campbell, K. A., Foster, T. C., Hampson, R. E., & Deadwyler, S. A. (1986). Delta-9 tetrahydrocannabinol differentially affects sensory-evoked potentials in the rat dentate gyrus. *Journal of Pharmacology and Experimental Therapeutics, 239,* 936–940.

Carney, J. M., Uwaydah, I. M., & Balster, R. L. (1977). Evaluation of a suspension system for intravenous self-administration studies of water-insoluble compounds in the rhesus monkey. *Pharmacology, Biochemistry and Behavior, 7,* 357–364

Chait, L. D. (1989). Δ^9-tetrahydrocannabinol content and human marijuana self-administration. *Psychopharmacology, 98,* 51–55.

Chait, L. D., & Burke, K. A. (1994). Preference for high- versus low-potency marijuana. *Pharmacology, Biochemistry and Behavior, 49,* 643–647.

Chait, L. D., & Perry, J. L. (1994). Acute and residual effects of alcohol and marijuana, alone and in combination, on mood and performance. *Psychopharmacology, 115,* 340–349.

Chait, L. D., & Pierri, J. (1992). Effects of smoked marijuana on human performance: A critical review. In L. Murphy & A. Bartke (Eds.), *Marijuana/cannabinoids: Neurobiology and neurophysiology* (pp. 387–423). Ann Arbor, MI: CRC.

Chait, L. D., & Zacny, J. P. (1992). Reinforcing and subjective effects of oral Δ^9-THC and smoked marijuana in humans. *Psychopharmacology, 107,* 255–262.

Chait, L. D., Evans, S. M., Grant, K. A., Kamien, J. B., Johansen, C. E., & Schuster, C. R. (1988). Discriminative stimulus effects of smoked marijuana in humans. *Psychopharmacology, 94,* 206–212.

Chang, A. E., Shiling, D. J., Stillman, R. C., Goldberg, N. H., Seipp, C. A., Barofsky, I., Simon, R. M., & Rosenberg, S. A. (1979). ^{9}-tetrahydrocannabinol as an antiemetic in cancer patients receiving high-dose methotrexate. *Annals of Internal Medicine, 91,* 819–824.

Chesher, G. B., Bird, K. D., Jackson, D. M., Perrignon, A., & Starmer, G. A. (1990). The effects of orally administered Δ^9-tetrahydrocannabinol in man on mood and performance measure: A dose-response study. *Pharmacology, Biochemistry and Behavior, 35,* 861–864.

Compton, D. R., Johnson, M. R., Melvin, L. S., & Martin, B. R. (1992). Pharmacological profile of a series of bicyclic cannabinoid analogs: Classification as cannabimimetic agents. *Journal of Pharmacology and Experimental Therapeutics, 260,* 275–280.

Compton, D. R., Harris, L. S., Lichtman, A. H., & Martin, B. R. (1996). Marihuana. In C. R. Schuster & M. J. Kuhar (Eds.), *Pharmacological aspects of drug dependence: Toward an integrated neurobehavioral approach* (pp. 83–158). Berlin: Springer-Verlag.

Cone, E. J., Johnson, R. E., Paul, B. D., Mell, L. D., & Mitchell, J. (1988). Marijuana-laced brownies: Behavioral effects, physiologic effects, and urinalysis in humans following ingestion. *Journal of Analytical Toxicology, 12,* 169–175.

Consroe, P., & Mechoulam, R. (1987). Anticonvulsant and neurotoxic effects of tetrahydrocannabinol stereoisomers. In R. S. Rapaka & A. Markiyannis (Eds.), *Structure–activity relationships of the cannabinoids* (pp. 59–66). Washington, DC: U.S. Government Printing Office.

Devane, W. A., Dysarz, F. A., III, Johnson, M. R., Melvin, L. S., Howlett, A. C., & Mechoulam, R. (1988). Isolation and structure of a brain constituent that binds to the cannabinoid receptor. *Science, 258,* 1946–1949.

Devane, W. A., Hanus, L., Breuer, A., Pertwee, R. G., Stevenson, L. A., Griffin, G., Gibson, D., Mandelbaum, A., Etinger, A., & Mechoulam, R. (1992). Isolation and structure of a brain constituent that binds to the cannabinoid receptor. *Science, 258,* 1946–1949.

Dewey, W. L. (1986). Cannabinoid pharmacology. *Pharmacological Reviews, 38,* 151–178.

Drewnowski, A., & Grinker, J. A. (1978a). Food and water intake, meal patterns and activity of obese and lean zucker rats following chronic and acute treatment with Δ^9-tetrahydrocannabinol. *Pharmacology, Biochemistry and Behavior, 9,* 619–630.

Drewnowski, A., & Grinker, J. A. (1978b). Temporal effects of Δ^9-tetrahydrocannabinol on feeding patterns and activity of obese and lean zucker rats. *Behavioral Biology, 23,* 112–117.

Evans, E. B., & Wenger, G. R. (1992). Effects of drugs of abuse on acquisition of behavioral chains in squirrel monkeys. *Psychopharmacology, 107,* 55–60.

Foltin, R. W., Brady, J. V., & Fischman, M. W. (1986). Behavioral analysis of marijuana effects on food intake in humans. *Pharmacology, Biochemistry and Behavior, 25,* 577–582.

Foltin, R. W., Fischman, M. W., & Byrne, M. F. (1988). Effects of smoked marijuana on food intake and body weight of humans living in a residential laboratory. *Appetite, 11,* 1–14.

Foltin, R. W., Fischman, M. W., Brady, J. V., Kelly, T. H., Bernstein, D. J., & Nellis, M. J. (1989). Motivational effects of smoked marijuana: Behavioral contingencies and high-probability recreational activities. *Pharmacology, Biochemistry and Behavior, 34,* 871–877.

Foltin, R. W., Fischman, M. W., Brady, J. V., Bernstein, D. J., Capriotti, R. M., Nellis, M. J., & Kelly, T. H. (1990). Motivational effects of smoked marijuana: Behavioral contingencies and low-probability activities. *Journal of the Experimental Analysis of Behavior, 53,* 5–19.

Fride, E., & Mechoulam, R. (1993). Pharmacological activity of the cannabinoid receptor agonist, anandamide, a brain constituent. *European Journal of Pharmacology, 231,* 313–314.

Gardner, E. L., Paredes, W., Smith, D., Donner, A., Milling, C., Cohen, D., & Morrison, D. (1988). Facilitation of brain stimulation reward by Δ^9-tetrahydrocannabinol. *Psychopharmacology, 96,* 142–144.

Gerard, C. M., Mollereau, C., Vassart, G., & Parmentier, M. (1991). Molecular cloning of a human cannabinoid receptor which is also expressed in testis. *Biochememistry Journal, 279,* 129–134.

Glick, S. D., & Milloy, S. (1972). Increased and decreased eating following THC administration. *Psychonomic Science, 29,* 6.

Gluck, J. P., & Ferraro, D. P. (1974). Effects of Δ^9-THC on food and water intake of deprivation experienced rats. *Behavioral Biology, 11,* 395–398.

Greenberg, I., Kuehnle, J., Mendelson, J., & Bernstein, J. (1976). Effects of marihuana use on body weight and caloric intake in humans. *Psychopharmacology, 49,* 79–84.

Grinspoon, L., & Bakalar, J. B. (1995). Marihuana as medicine: A plea for reconsideration. *Journal of the American Medical Association, 273,* 1875–1876.

Haertzen, C. A. (1974). *An overview of Addiction Research Center Inventory Scales (ARCI): An appendix and manual of scales.* Washington, DC: U.S. Government Printing Office.

Halikas, J. A., Goodwin, D. W., & Guze, S. B. (1971). Marijuana effects—A survey of regular users. *Journal of the American Medical Association, 217,* 692–694.

Hampson, R. E., Foster, T. C., & Deadwyler, S.A. (1989). Effects of Δ^9-tetrahydrocannabinol on sensory evoked hippocampal activity in the rat: Principal components analysis and sequential dependency. *Journal of Pharmacology and Experimental Therapeutics, 251,* 870–879.

Harris, R. T., Waters, W., & McLendon, D. (1974). Evaluation of reinforcing capability of delta-9 tetrahydrocannabinol in rhesus monkeys. *Psychopharmacologia, 37,* 23–29.

Heaton, R. K. (1981). *Wisconsin Card Sorting Test Manual.* Odessa, FL: Psychological Assessment Resources.

Heishman, S. J., Stitzer, M. L., & Bigelow, G. E. (1988). Alcohol and marijuana: Comparative dose effect profiles in humans. *Pharmacology, Biochemistry and Behavior, 31,* 649–655.

Heishman, S. J., Stitzer, M. L., & Yingling, J. E. (1989). Effects of tetrahydrocannabinol content on marijuana smoking behavior, subjective reports, and performance, *Pharmacology, Biochemistry and Behavior, 34,* 173–179.

Heyser, C. J., Hampson, R. E., & Deadwyler, S. A. (1993). Effects of Δ^9-tetrahydrocannabinol on delayed match to sample performance in rats: Alterations in short-term memory associated with changes in task specific

firing of hippocampal cells. *Journal of Pharmacology and Experimental Therapeutics, 264,* 294–307.

Hirschlorn, I. D., & Rosecrans, J. A. (1974). Morphine and Δ^9-tetrahydrocannabinol: Tolerance to the stimulus effects. *Psychopharmacologia, 36,* 243–253.

Hollister, L. E. (1971). Hunger and appetite after single doses of marihuana, alcohol, and dextroamphetamine. *Clinical Pharmacology & Therapeutics, 12,* 44–49.

Hollister, L. E., Gillespie, H. K., Ohlsson, A., Lindgren, J.-E., Wahlen, A., & Agurell, S. (1981). Do plasma concentrations of Δ^9-tetrahydrocannabinol reflect the degree of intoxication? *Journal of Clinical Pharmacology, 21,* 171S–177S.

Howlett, A. C. (1995). Pharmacology of cannabinoid receptors. *Annual Review of Pharmacology & Toxicology, 35,* 607–634.

Huestis, M. A., Sampson, A. H., Holickey, B. J., Henningfield, J. E., & Cone, E. J. (1992). Characterization of the absorption phase of marijuana smoking. *Clinical Pharmacology & Therapeutics, 52,* 31–41.

Huy, N. D., & Roy, P. E. (1976). Inhalation of tobacco and marijuana in dog over a period of 30 months: Effect on body weight, food intake and organ weight. *Research Communications in Chemical Pathology & Pharmacology, 13,* 465–472.

Jarbe, T. U. C., & Hiltunen, A. J. (1988) Limited stimulus generalization between Δ^9-tetrahydrocannabinol and diazepam in pigeons and gerbils. *Psychopharmacology, 94,* 328–331.

Johanson, C. E., & Balster, R. L. (1978). A summary of the results of a drug self-administration study using substitution procedures in rhesus monkeys. *Bulletin on Narcotics, 30,* 43–54.

Johansson, J. O., Jarbe, T. U., & Henriksson, B. G. (1975). Acute and subchronic influences of tetrahydrocannabinols on water and food intake, body weight, and temperature in rats. *T.I.T. Journal of Life Sciences, 5,* 17–27.

Jones, R. T. (1971). Tetrahydrocannabinol and the marijuana-induced social "high" or the effects on the mind of marijuana. *Annals of the New York Academy of Sciences, 191,* 155–165.

Kamien, J. B., Bickel, W. K., Higgins, S. T., & Hughes, J. R. (1994). The effects of Δ^9-tetrahydrocannabinol on repeated acquisition and performance of response sequences and on self-reports in humans. *Behavioural Pharmacology, 5,* 71–78.

Kelly, T. H., Foltin, R. W., & Fischman, M. W. (1993). Effects of smoked marijuana on heart rate, drug ratings and task performance by humans. *Behavioural Pharmacology, 4,* 167–178.

Lamb, R. J., Preston, K. L., Schindler, C. W., Meisch, R. A., Davis, F., Katz, J. L., Henningfield, J. E., & Goldberg, S. R. (1991). The reinforcing and subjective effects of morphine in post-addicts: A dose-response study. *Journal of Pharmacology and Experimental Therapeutics, 259,* 1165–1173.

Lepore, M., Stanislav, V. R., Lowinson, J., & Gardner, E. L. (1995). Conditioned place preference induced by Δ⁹-tetrahydrocannabinol: Comparison with cocaine, morphine, and food reward. *Life Sciences, 56,* 2073–2080.

Levitt, M. (1986). Cannabinoids as antiemetics in cancer chemotherapy. In R. Mechoulam (Ed.), *Cannabinoids as therapeutic agents* (pp. 71–83). Boca Raton, FL: CRC.

Lichtman, A. H., & Martin, B. R. (1991). Cannabinoid induced antinociception is mediated by a spinal α_2 noradrenergic mechanism. *Brain Research, 559,* 309–314.

Lichtman, A. H., Dimen, K. R., & Martin, B. R. (1995). Systemic or intrahippocampal cannabinoid administration impairs spatial memory in rats. *Psychopharmacology, 119,* 282–290.

Little, P. J., Compton, D. R., Johnson, M. R., Melvin, L. S., & Martin, B. R. (1988). Pharmacology and stereoselectivity of structurally novel cannabinoids in mice. *Journal of Pharmacology and Experimental Therapeutics, 247,* 1046–1051.

Lukas, S. E., Mendelson, J. H., & Benedikt, R. (1995). Electroencephalographic correlates of marihuana-induced euphoria. *Drug and Alcohol Dependence, 37,* 131–140.

Mansbach, R. S., Nicholson, K. L., Martin, B. R., & Balster, R. L. (1994). Failure of Δ⁹-tetrahydrocannabinol and CP 55,940 to maintain intravenous self-administration under a fixed-interval schedule in rhesus monkeys. *Behavioral Pharmacology, 5,* 219–225.

Mansbach, R. S., Rovetti, C. C., Winston, E. N., & Lowe, J. A. (1996) Effects of the cannabinoid CB1 receptor antagonist SR141716A on the behavior of pigeons and rats. *Psychopharmacology, 124,* 315–322.

Martin, B. R. (1986). Cellular effects of cannabinoids. *Psychological Review, 38,* 45–74.

Martin, B. R., Compton, D. R., Thomas, B. F., Prescott, W. R., Little, P. J., Razdan, R. K., Johnson, M. R., Melvin, L. S., Mechoulam, R., & Ward, S. J. (1993). Behavioral, biochemical, and molecular modeling evaluations of cannabinoid analogs. *Pharmacology, Biochemistry and Behavior, 40,* 471–478.

Matsuda, L. A., Lolait, S. J., Brownstein, M. J., Young, A. C., & Bonner, T. I. (1990). Structure of cannabinoid receptor: Functional expression of the cloned cDNA. *Nature, 346,* 561–563.

Mattes, R. D., Shaw, L. M., Edling-Owens, J., Engelman, K., & Elsohly, M. A. (1993). Bypassing the first-pass effect for the therapeutic use of cannabinoids. *Pharmacology, Biochemistry and Behavior, 44,* 745–747.

Mattes, R. D., Engelman, K., Shaw, L. M., & Elsohly, M. A. (1994). Cannabinoids and appetite stimulation. *Pharmacology, Biochemistry and Behavior, 49,* 187–195.

Mattes, R. D., Shaw, L. M., & Engelman, K. (1994). Effects of cannabinoids (marijuana) on taste intensity and hedonic ratings and salivary flow of adults. *Chemical Senses, 19,* 125–140.

McGlothin, W. H., & West, L. J. (1968). The marijuana problem: An overview. *American Journal of Psychiatry, 125,* 370–378.

McLaughlin, C. L., Baile, C. A., & Bender, P. E., (1979). Cannabinols and feeding in sheep. *Psychopharmacology, 64,* 321–323.

McMillan, D. E. (1988). Failure of acute and chronic administration of Δ⁹-tetrahydrocannabinol to affect the repeated acquisition of serial position responses in pigeons. *Pavlovian Journal of Biological Science, 23,* 57–66.

Mendelson, J. H., & Mello, N. K. (1984). Reinforcing properties of oral Δ⁹-tetrahydrocannabinol, smoked marijuana, and nabilone: Influence of previous marijuana use. *Psychopharmacology, 83,* 351–356.

Mendelson, J. H., Kuehnle, J. C., Greenberg, I., & Mello, N. K. (1976). Operant acquisition of marihuana in man. *Journal of Pharmacology and Experimental Therapeutics, 198,* 482–486.

Miczek, K. A., & Dixit, B. N. (1980). Behavioral and biochemical effects of chronic Δ⁹-tetrahydrocannabinol in rats. *Psychopharmacology, 67,* 195–202.

Milstein, S. L., MacCannell, K., Karr, G., & Clark, S. (1975). Marijuana-produced changes in pain tolerance: Experienced and nonexperienced subjects. *International Pharmacopsychiatry, 10,* 177–182.

Noyes, R., Brunk, S., Avery, D., & Canter, A. (1975). The analgesic properties of delta-9-tetrahydrocannabinol and codeine. *Clinical Pharmacology & Therapuetics, 18,* 84–89.

Noyes, R., Brunk, S., Baram, D., & Canter, A. (1975). Analgesic effect of delta-9-tetrahydrocannabinol. *Journal of Clinical Pharmacology, 15,* 139–143.

Orr, L. E., McKerman, J. F., & Bloone, B. (1980). Antiemetic effect of tetrahydrocannabinol. *Archives of Internal Medicine, 140,* 1431–1433.

Parker, L. A., & Gillies, T. (1995). THC-induced place and taste aversions in Lewis and Sprague–Dawley rats. *Behavioral Neuroscience, 109,* 71–78.

Paule, M. G., Allen, R. R., Bailey, J. R., Scallet, A. C., Ali, S. F., Brown, R. M., & Slikker, W., Jr. (1992). Chronic marijuana smoke exposure in the rhesus monkey: II. Effects of responding on progressive ration and conditioned position responding. *Journal of Pharmacology and Experimental Therapeutics, 260,* 210–222.

Perez-Reyes, M., Timmons, M. C., Davis, K. H., & Wall, E. M. (1973). A comparison of the pharmacological activity in man of intravenously administered Δ⁹-tetrahydrocannabinol, cannabinol, and cannabidiol. *Experientia, 29,* 1368–1369.

Perez-Reyes, M., Di Guiseppi, S., Davis, K. H., Schindler, V. H., & Cook, E. (1982). Comparison of effects of marihuana cigarettes of three different potencies. *Clinical Pharmacology & Therapeutics, 31,* 617–624.

Perio, A., Rinaldi-Carmona, M., Maruani, J., Barth, F., LeFur, G., & Soubrie, P. (1996). Central mediation of the cannabinoid cue: Activity of a selective CB1 antagonist, SR 141716A. *Behavioural Pharmacology, 7*, 65–71.

Pertwee, R. G. (1990). The central neuropharmacology of psychotropic cannabinoids. *International Encyclopedia of Pharmacology and Therapeutics, 130*, 355–419.

Pertwee, R. G., Greentree, S. G., & Swift, P. A. (1988). Drugs which stimulate or facilitate central GABAergic transmission interact synergistically with Δ^9-tetrahydrocannabinol to produce marked catalepsy in mice. *Neuropharmacology, 27*, 1256–1270.

Plasse, T. F., Gorter, R. W., Krasnow, S. H., Lane, M., Shepard, K. V., & Wadleigh, R. G. (1991). Recent clinical experience with dronabinol. *Pharmacology, Biochemistry and Behavior, 40*, 695–700.

Pope, H. G., Jr., & Yurgelun-Todd, D. (1996). The residual cognitive effects of heavy marijuana use in college students. *Journal of the American Medical Association, 275*, 521–561.

Richards, L. G. (1981). *Demographic trends and drug abuse, 1980–1985* (NIDA Research Monograph Series 35). Rockville, MD: National Institute on Drug Abuse.

Rinaldi-Carmona, M., Barth, F., Heaulme, M., Shire, D., Calandra, B., Congy, C., Martinez, S., Maruani, J., Neliat, G., Caput, D., Ferrara, P., Soubrie, P., Breliere, J. C., & Le Fur, G. (1994). SR141716A, a potent and selective antagonist of the brain cannabinoid receptor. *FEBS Letters, 350*, 240–244.

Sallan, S. E., Cronin, C., Zelen, M., & Zinberg, N. E. (1980). Antiemetics in patients receiving chemotherapy for cancer. *New England Journal of Medicine, 302*, 135–138.

Schulze, G. E., McMillan, D. E., Bailey, J. R., Scallett, A., Ali, S. F., Slikker, W., Jr., & Paule, M. G. (1988). Acute effects of ^{9}-tetrahydrocannabinol in rhesus monkeys as measured by performance in a battery of complex operant tests. *Journal of Pharmacology and Experimental Therapeutics, 245*, 178–186.

Smith, D. E. (1968). Acute and chronic toxicity of marijuana. *Journal of Psychedelic Drugs, 2*, 37–47.

Sofia, R. D., & Barry, H. (1974). Acute and chronic effects of Δ^9-tetrahydrocannabinol on food intake by rats. *Psychopharmacologia, 39*, 213–222.

Sofia, R. D., & Knobloch, L. C. (1976). Comparative effects of various naturally occurring cannabinoids on food, sucrose and water consumption by rats. *Pharmacology, Biochemistry and Behavior, 4*, 591–599.

Stark, P., & Dews, P. (1980). Cannabinoids: I. Behavioral effects. *Journal of Pharmacology and Experimental Therapeutics, 214*, 124–130.

Sweet, D. L., Miller, N. J., Weddington, W., Senay, E., & Sushelsky, L. (1981). Δ^9-Tetrahydrocannabinol as an antiemetic for patients receiving cancer chemotherapy. A pilot study. *Journal of Clinical Pharmacology, 21*, 70S–75S.

Takahashi, R. N., & Singer, G. (1979). Self-administration of Δ^9-tetrahydrocannabinol by rats. *Pharmacology, Biochemistry and Behavior, 11*, 737–740.

Ungerleider, J. T., Andrysiak, T., Fairbanks, L., Goodnight, J., Sarna, G., & Jamison, K. (1982). Cannabis and cancer chemotherapy: A comparison of oral Δ^9-THC and prochlorperazine. *Cancer, 50*, 636–645.

Vincent, B. J., McQuiston, D. J., Einhorn, L. H., Nagy, C. M., & Brames, M. J. (1983). Review of cannabinoids and their antiemetic effectiveness. *Drugs, 25*, 52–62.

Vinciguerra, V., Moore, T., & Brennan, E. (1988). Inhalation marijuana as an antiemetic for cancer chemotherapy. *New York State Journal of Medicine, 88*, 525–527.

Weinberg, A. D., Dimon, E. M., Simon, G. S., Harris, L. S., & Borzelleca, J. F. (1977). Measurements of weight and activity in male mice following inhalation of cannabis smoke in a controlled smoke exposure chamber. *Toxicology & Applied Pharmacology, 42*, 301–307.

Wetzel, C. D., Janowsky, D. S., & Clopton, P. L. (1982). Remote memory during marijuana intoxication. *Psychopharmacology, 76*, 278–281.

Wiley, J. L., Barrett, R. L., Balster, R. L., & Martin, B. R. (1993). Tolerance to the discriminative stimulus effects of Δ^9-tetrahydrocannabinol. *Behavioral Pharmacology, 4*, 581–585.

Wiley, J. L., Barrett, R. L., Britt, D. T., Balster, R. L., & Martin, B. R. (1993). Discriminative stimulus effects of Δ^9-tetrahydrocannabinol and Δ^{9-11} tetrahydrocannabinol in rats and rhesus monkeys. *Neuropharmacology, 32*, 359.

Wiley, J. L., Balster, R. L., & Martin, B. R. (1995). Discriminative stimulus effects of anandamide in rats. *European Journal of Pharmacology, 276*, 49–54.

Wiley, J. L., Barrett, R. L., Lowe, J., Balster, R. L., & Martin, B. R. (1995). Discriminative stimulus effects of CP 55,940 and structurally dissimilar cannabinoids in rats. *Neuropharmacology, 34*, 669–676.

Wiley, J. L., Huffman, J. W., Balster, R. L., & Martin, B. R. (1995). Pharmacological specificity of the discriminative stimulus effects of Δ^9-tetrahydrocannabinol in rhesus monkeys. *Drug and Alcohol Dependence, 40*, 81–86.

Wiley, J. L., Lowe, J. A., Balster, R. L., & Martin, B. R. (1995). Antagonism of the discriminative stimulus effects of Δ^9-tetrahydrocannabinol in rats and rhesus monkeys. *Journal of Pharmacology and Experimental Therapeutics, 275*, 1–6.

Wilson, W. H., Ellinwood, E. H., Matthew, R. J., & Johnson, K. (1994). Effects of marijuana on performance of a computerized cognitive–neuromotor test battery. *Psychiatry Research, 51*, 115–125.

Wu, T-C, Tashkin, D. P., Rose, J. E., & Djahed, B. (1988). Influence of marijuana potency and amount of cigarette consumed on marijuana smoking pattern. *Journal of Psychoactive Drugs, 20*, 43–46.

9

Psychological and Psychiatric Consequences of Cannabis

BRUCE PHARISS, ROBERT B. MILLMAN, AND

ANN BORDWINE BEEDER

Introduction

Cannabis, particularly as smoked as marijuana cigarettes ("joint," "reefer," "herb"), is the most frequently abused illicit substance in the United States. Not surprisingly, psychologists and other mental professionals are asked to evaluate large numbers of often youthful people with psychiatric and behavioral problems who also use cannabis. In some individuals, the cannabis use clearly leads to the psychological and psychiatric consequences observed by the clinician. In others, the psychopathology noted antedates the cannabis use or dependence and is a determinate of drug use. Both the drug use and the psychopathology may also occur concurrently and be relatively independent of each other. Further complicating the picture, other illicit drugs and alcohol are often used in association with cannabis. The intermittent or occasional use of cannabis may not be associated with any psychological or psychiatric consequences.

BRUCE PHARISS, ROBERT B. MILLMAN, AND ANN BORDWINE BEEDER • Cornell University Medical College, New York, New York 10036.

Handbook of Substance Abuse: Neurobehavioral Pharmacology, edited by Tarter *et al.* Plenum Press, New York, 1998.

Epidemiology

It is clear that marijuana use is increasing in all population groups. The National Institute of Mental Health Epidemiological Catchment Area (ECA) Survey found about 4.4% of the household population met criteria for cannabis dependence or abuse. In a longitudinal sample of young men and women in New York State, Kandel and Davies (1992) estimated that almost one half of young male marijuana users had started near-daily marijuana use by ages 28–29, and about 37% of the young female marijuana users had also done so. The Preliminary Estimates From the 1995 National Household Survey on Drug Use, published by the U.S. Department of Health and Human Services (Substance Abuse and Mental Health Services Administration, 1995), notes that marijuana use increased from 6.0% to 8.2% from 1994 to 1995 (based on past month use) among the civilian noninstitutionalized population age 12 years and older.

Increases in marijuana use for adolescents are more striking in the National Institute on Drug Abuse, the Monitoring the Future Study (MTF), 1995. According to this study, marijuana use has increased steadily among 8th, 10th, and 12th graders. The upswing in marijuana use rates from 1994 to 1995 represents an increase for the 3rd consecutive year among

10th and 12th graders, and an increase for the 4th consecutive year among 8th graders. For 8th graders, the increase is from slightly more than 6% to more than 12% for the period 1992 to 1995; for the same period, the increased use of marijuana rose from 22% to 35%. The MTF survey reveals a decrease in the percentage of 8th-, 10th-, and 12th-grade students who say that trying marijuana or smoking it occasionally is a "great risk." As perceived risk decreases, use increases.

Controversy persists as to whether marijuana use leads to the use of stronger drugs, the so-called stepping stone hypothesis (O'Donnell & Clayton, 1979). It has been well demonstrated that there is a hierarchy to drug use and that marijuana is generally used before depressants, hallucinogens, cocaine, or heroin (Jessor, 1975). Moreover, the frequency of use of cannabis correlates with the use of stronger drugs (Kandel, Kessler, & Margulies, 1978). One nationwide study (O'Donnell, Voss, Clayton, Slatin, & Room, 1976) showed that of those young men who had never used marijuana, less than 1% subsequently used heroin or cocaine. Of those who had used marijuana 1,000 times or more, 73% used cocaine and 33% used heroin. In a study (Clayton & Voss, 1981) of young men in Manhattan, no non-marijuana-using subjects had used psychedelics, whereas 37% of marijuana-using subjects had used psychedelics. Similarly, whereas only 1%–5% of non-marijuana-using subjects had used prescription stimulants, sedatives, or opioids, 34%–36% of the marijuana-using subjects had used these drugs. A national survey confirmed this association (O'Malley, Johnston, & Bachman, 1985). Of the survey subjects who had ever tried cocaine, 98% had used marijuana and 93% used marijuana first. Of those survey subjects who have used cannabis at least 100 times, 75% had used cocaine. Of high school students who used cocaine in 1985, 84% also used marijuana (O'Malley *et al.,* 1985). Marijuana use usually precedes other illicit drug use and individuals who smoke cannabis more frequently are more likely to use other illicit drugs.

As with other substance abuse disorders, appropriate referral and treatment depends on determining the nature of the relationship of the drug use to the behaviors and psychopathology noted in each individual. Though it may be useful to determine whether the psychopathology preceded or followed the drug use or dependence, these behaviors are often inextricably intertwined.

Intoxicating Effects

The acute psychoactive effects of cannabis are remarkably varied and are profoundly dependent on the psychological set of the user and the social setting in which the drug is used (Zinberg, 1984). Relaxation, mild euphoria, a sense of well-being, and altered time perception (such that time seems to pass more slowly) are typical effects of intoxication. Enhanced somatosensory perceptions (or altered concentration) are commonly reported. While under the influence of the drug, users report enhanced perception of details that might not otherwise be so vividly noted. For example, some users report that colors seem brighter and richer and that aspects of music or art that previously had little or no meaning to the viewer are now appreciated in greater depth. Many jazz and rock musicians have said that they are more creative or may perform better under the influence of marijuana. Although it is difficult to study these effects objectively, the beliefs are widely held. In addition, ideas may seem to change in importance and relevance.

Marijuana intoxication is frequently associated with labile affects and impaired short-term memory. The onset of effects from smoked marijuana occurs in minutes and the effects may persist for 2–4 hr; the onset of effects from ingestion are delayed for one half to 1 hr and may persist for 5–12 hr. The memory effects may be a function of altered attention or executive functions. There is often a splitting of consciousness, so that the smoker experiences the high while he or she objectively observes his or her own intoxication. This ability to retain a degree of objectivity may explain how some experienced users of marijuana manage to behave in a sober fashion in public even when they are highly intoxicated. Enhanced sociability may occur, but so may social withdrawal and extreme self-consciousness. Information processing is altered, such that boring and repetitive tasks may be performed with enhanced interest and concentration, while the ability to carry out complex goal-oriented tasks may be impaired. Neuropsychological effects are addressed in detail in the following sections.

Adverse Psychological Effects

Anxiety/Panic Reactions

The most frequently reported adverse reactions to cannabis include anxiety reactions and panic attacks. These generally occur during the period of intoxication and abate within minutes to hours, rarely persisting for more than 24 hr (Knight, 1976). These reactions are more likely to occur in naive users who are unfamiliar with the drug's effects and who take it in an unfamiliar or threatening setting (Hall, Solowij, & Lemon, 1994; Khantzian & McKenna, 1979). They are quite variable in intensity and characteristics and range from mild discomfort to frank hysteria, sometimes associated with the sensation of being unable to move or breathe or of an impending heart attack. Restlessness, paranoia, derealization, depersonalization, frank panic, a sense of loss of control, and the idea that one will never regain sanity are also often associated with these anxiety reactions (Millman & Sbriglio, 1986). It is likely that psychologically predisposed individuals are more susceptible to these reactions and may be vulnerable to the persistence of symptoms, the development of a cannabis-induced psychotic disorder, or even the development of a persistent psychotic reaction (Millman & Sbriglio, 1986).

Most people experiencing anxiety or panic do not seek medical attention and these reactions resolve spontaneously in minutes or hours. Calm and gentle reassurance by trusted friends or experienced users in a warm and supportive atmosphere is often the only treat-

ment required. It is useful to remind the patient gently, firmly, and continuously that the symptoms are related to the drug, are quite common, and will wane rapidly. When necessary, an anxiolytic may be administered, preferably one with a rapid onset of effects and long duration of action (diazepam 10 to 30 mg). Neuroleptics may precipitate anticholinergic effects or other adverse reactions and should be avoided in acute episodes.

Cannabis-Induced Psychotic Disorder

It is generally agreed by most experienced observers that ingestion of cannabis can precipitate an acute psychotic disorder. According to the *Diagnostic and Statistical Manual of Mental Disorders,* 4th edition (American Psychiatric Association, 1994) and other sources, the disorder may develop shortly after cannabis use and usually involves persecutory and other delusions, ideas of reference, and angry, fearful, or jealous feelings. This disorder is apparently rare and is most likely to occur with the ingestion of larger amounts of cannabis by inexperienced or predisposed users in unusual or threatening circumstances. These doses may be far in excess of those required for a euphoric effect (Kiplinger & Manno, 1971), though in some people the precipitating dose may be quite small. When this disorder does occur it usually remits within hours or a day, although in some cases it has lasted a few days. Anxiety, emotional lability, depersonalization, derealization, and, rarely, subsequent amnesia relative to the episode are associated with this disorder (Ames, 1958; Chopra & Smith, 1974). Frank hallucinations are rare except when very high doses are ingested or individuals have premorbid psychopathology such as in schizophrenia or borderline personality disorder. Acute psychotic reactions occurring in a setting of clear consciousness may also occur. This may resemble manic or schizophrenic psychosis.

It has been suggested that a higher incidence of psychosis associated with cannabis use may occur in Asian cultures, where preparations of the drug are more commonly taken orally, compared with Western cultures, where it is usually smoked (Chaudry, Moss, Bashir,

& Suliman, 1991). Chaudry and colleagues proposed the hypothesis that oral administration of cannabis, which results in a different profile of metabolites compared with smoking, may produce an unidentified psychotogenic metabolite that accounts for these observed differences.

Treatment includes close observation in a warm and supportive environment with gentle and continual reassurance, again reminding the patient that the thoughts and feelings are due to the drug and will abate. When necessary, an anxiolytic should be administered (diazepam 10–30 mg). In patients with persistent and severe symptoms, it may be necessary to administer neuroleptic medication (haloperidol 2–4 mg). The typical neuroleptics may be particularly useful in this population because adverse psychological effects are decreased. Clozapine is probably the most effective, though risperidol or olanzapine do not lead to agranulocytosis. Adverse effects are often treated by self-medication with other drugs such as alcohol, sedatives, or opiates. (Breier, *et al.,* 1994; Marder & Meibach, 1994).

Acute Toxic Psychosis

An acute toxic psychosis or delirium may occur from the smoking or more often the oral ingestion of large amounts of cannabis (Brill & Nahas, 1984; Estroff & Gold, 1986; Ghodse, 1986; Johnson, 1990; Negrete, 1988; Thornicroft, 1990; Tien & Anthony, 1990; Tunving, 1985). It is marked by clouding of consciousness, confusion, depersonalization, impaired and sluggish thinking, and motor imbalance. There may be memory impairment, visual and auditory hallucinations, paranoia, and violent or bizarre behavior. Speech is disconnected; nystagmus is often present. Four cases of mutism in addition to symptoms of delirium have been reported (Marlotte, 1972). The syndrome lasts from a few hours to a few days and is indistinguishable from other acute reactions that have been described variously as acute toxic psychoses, ganja psychoses, or acute organic brain syndrome (Keup, 1970). The episodes are generally short-lived and self-limiting, but may occur upon subsequent exposure to the drug. It may be difficult to distinguish an acute toxic psychosis from an acute psychotic disorder precipitated by cannabis. Treatment may involve the use of both anxiolytics and neuroleptics to treat the symptoms.

Flashback Syndrome

A flashback is the transitory recurrence of feelings and perceptions originally experienced while under the influence of a psychedelic drug in the absence of intoxication. They may be precipitated by cannabis use. Flashbacks with cannabis use alone are rare. (Edwards, 1983; Johnson, 1990; Solomons & Neppe, 1989). Marijuana smoking some time after the use of a psychedelic drug is the most common cause of flashbacks. Flashbacks may also occur in the context of emotional stress, fatigue, or altered ego functioning. Flashbacks are quite variable in character, intensity, and duration, may last from seconds to hours, and may be pleasant or horrifying. Most flashbacks are episodes of visual distortion, reexperienced intense emotion, depersonalization, or physical symptoms. They generally decrease in number and intensity over time. However, in rare cases they have become more frequent repetitions of frightening images or thoughts (Grinspoon & Bakalar 1986).

Frequent cannabis or psychedelic drug use may increase the incidence of flashbacks. They generally follow acute and profound reactions to the original drug experience ("bad trips"). Although the etiology is unclear, flashback experiences have been variously explained as similar to traumatic neuroses, as based on persisting neurochemical change, and as a type of visual seizure (Chopra & Smith, 1974). A pharmacological explanation could be that psychoactive components are released from body fat where they are stored during periods of drug use. Individual differences in tissue retention capacities and factors that may accelerate release of cannabinoids into the bloodstream have not yet been explored (Negrete, 1988).

The treatment for flashbacks consists of reassurance. Occasionally, anxiolytic medication is useful if the flashback is severe. Individuals should be cautioned against the continued use of marijuana or psychedelic drugs. Psychotherapy might be indicated to relieve the anxiety or to resolve the conflicts that may precipitate the episodes, although there is little evidence to confirm this point. Rarely, chronic neuroleptic medication might be indicated in a severe case with frequent recurrences.

Neuropsychological Consequences

Evidence supporting or refuting neuropsychological deficits secondary to cannabis use must first be separated from evidence regarding the acute intoxicating effects of the drug, the psychiatric and social attributes of heavy cannabis users, and actual psychiatric disorders caused or exacerbated by cannabis. There is no question that cannabis produces a syndrome of acute intoxication, with characteristic cognitive and perceptual changes, lasting for some hours after the drug is ingested. Individuals who consume the drug several times a day will display this effect almost continuously. It must then be determined if the data supports either a drug residue effect lasting 12–24 hr after acute intoxication ("drug residue effect") or a more lasting toxic effect on the central nervous system (CNS) and cognitive functioning that persists even after all drug residue has left the system ("CNS alteration effect").

Drug residue effects 12–24 hr after intoxication must be differentiated from simple attributes of heavy cannabis users as compared to nonusing controls. Some studies have found that heavy users of cannabis differ from nonusers on various psychological or neuropsychological measures (Kouri, Pope, Yurgelun-Todd, & Gruber, 1995; Mendhiratta *et al.,* 1988). Although part of this difference might be attributable to the drug residue effect of cannabis, much of the difference might be due to acute effects, which may become virtually continuous in heavy users; premorbid differences between users and nonusers in intellectual, cognitive, or psychological functions; other risk factors which covary with cannabis use, such as use of other drugs; or

different values with respect to academic or occupational achievement. With these many confounding factors, it is difficult to draw conclusions about the drug residue effect of cannabis from a simple comparison of the attributes of users versus nonusers. This diminishes the usefulness of many research studies examining this effect.

A recent study by Pope and Yurgelun-Todd (1996) compared frequent users to infrequent users to control for some of these variables and found that heavy marijuana use was associated with residue effects even after a day of supervised abstinence from the drug. The controlled study examined residual cognitive effects of heavy marijuana use in college students using a single-blind comparison of regular users versus infrequent users of marijuana. The study found that regular users displayed significantly greater impairment than light users on attention-executive functions, as evidenced particularly by greater perseverations on card sorting and reduced learning of words lists. These differences remained after controlling for potential confounding variables, such as estimated levels or premorbid cognitive functioning, and for use of alcohol and other substances in the two groups.

In examining studies of neuropsychological consequences, one must also bear in mind the complex pharmacokinetics of cannabinoids. The principal active component of cannabis, delta-9-tetrahydrocannabinol (9-THC) displays a plasma half-life of 2–60 hr (Johannson, Agurell, Hollister, & Halldin, 1988; Seth & Sinha, 1991; Wall & Perez-Reyes, 1981), but much of this decline reflects redistribution of drug from the plasma compartment into tissues. Thus, 9-THC may persist at CNS receptor sites far longer than in plasma, and serial plasma levels will not reflect the time-course of CNS activity. In chronic users, both 9-THC and other metabolites accumulate in fat stores, from which they are slowly released back into the circulation (Seth & Sinha, 1991). Thus, chronic users may display cannabinoid metabolites in the urine after weeks or even months of abstinence (Ellis, Mann, Judson, Schramm, & Taschian, 1985). Chronic users also differ from infrequent users in their rates of metabolism of cannabinoids (Seth & Sinha, 1991), and may display effects of both tolerance and withdrawal (Hunt & Jones, 1980; Jones & Benowitz, 1976; Jones, Benowitz, & Bachman, 1976). Thus, when single doses of cannabis are administered to relatively drug-naive volunteers, a simple decay in residual effects may be observed as 9-THC is quickly redistributed into various tissue compartments. But in naturalistic studies of chronic users, the duration of impairment due to the drug residue effect may be much longer and more difficult to estimate.

Also complicating interpretation, several studies have suggested that abrupt discontinuation of heavy cannabis use may precipitate a withdrawal syndrome characterized by insomnia, restlessness, and irritability (Jones, Benowitz, & Herning, 1981; Mendelson, Mello, Lex, & Bavli, 1984; Rohr, Showlund, & Martin, 1989). Such a syndrome might also influence the findings of neuropsychological functioning. Only a study with a much longer abstinence period could fully resolve this issue.

Most studies examine the CNS alteration effect by looking at heavy users a short time after their last cannabis ingestion. This complicates assessment because observed impairment could be attributable to a protracted drug residue effect from a large accumulated CNS burden of cannabis rather than a frank CNS alteration effect above and beyond the drug residue effect. Examining heavy cannabis users weeks after their last exposure to the drug, when cannabis components would reasonably be expected to have disappeared from the CNS, would avoid this confounding factor (Pope, Gruber, & Yugelun-Todd, 1995).

Mendhiratta and colleagues (1988) examined a subsample of patients previously tested 10 years earlier. Subjects were abstinent for a supervised 12-hr period. Users performed more poorly than nonusers on virtually all tests in the study. On response time and the Bender visuomotor gestalt test, users had deteriorated more from their performance 10 years earlier than had the nonusers. However, the study did not control for many of the confounding factors detailed earlier.

In a small study by Schwartz, Gruenwald, Klitzner, and Fedio (1989), cannabis-dependent adolescents performed significantly worse than control groups on the Benton visual retention test and the Wechsler memory scale prose passages, both after 2 days and again after 6 weeks of abstinence. Finding differences even at 6 weeks, despite the fact that users were matched with nonusers on age, socioeconomic status, home environment, parents' education, and IQ, favors the existence of the CNS alteration effect due to cannabis. The small study size may render the study vulnerable to the effects of one or two outliers in a given group (Pope *et al.*, 1995).

Presently, only very limited conclusions about the residual effects of cannabis can be drawn. There is reasonable evidence for a brief drug residue effect of 12–24 hr after even a single episode of smoking. Given laboratory evidence that frequent daily smoking may accumulate a large CNS burden of 9-THC and other psychoactive substances, one might reasonably expect this drug residue effect to persist longer in chronic heavy users, but evidence is as yet inadequate to support or refute this speculation. Similarly, the evidence is inadequate to answer the CNS alteration effect question. Given that many studies have found modest or absent differences between even heavy users and controls, one might be tempted to assume that any CNS alteration effect with cannabis is slight or nonexistent. But findings such as those of Pope and Yurgelun-Todd (1996), and the deterioration noted by Mendhiratta and colleagues (1988) on a 10-year follow-up of an earlier sample of users, as well as the impairment found by Schwartz and colleagues (1989) even after 6 weeks of abstinence, indicate that the case is not closed on the issue of lasting CNS toxicity.

In studies where residual effects have been reported, the most consistent findings are subtle drug-induced deficits in the attention-executive system, with recall memory functions per se remaining relatively unaffected. The data suggest that multiple brain systems may be affected by marijuana, but the most pronounced effects may be in sustained attention, mediated by brain stem structures, and in the capacity to shift attention, associated with prefrontal cortical regions. However, comparisons between individual studies are difficult because most studies have examined only a subset of cognitive measures. Given that the ability to learn new information, or memory, is dependent on a number of cognitive components—including the ability to attend, organize, encode, store, and retrieve new information—conclusions must be reserved until specific subprocesses that are compromised by the residual effects of the drug are studied. Nevertheless, subtle changes may cause important difficulties in adapting to intellectual and interpersonal tasks (Pope & Yurgelun-Todd, 1996). These changes may in turn relate to the chronic cannabis syndrome that has received much attention and has become a source of much concern on the part of parents, educators, and mental health professionals.

Chronic Cannabis Syndrome

Effects on Personality

Smith (1968) used the term "amotivational syndrome" to describe the apathy, diminished goal-directed activity, and the inability to master new problems in individuals who chronically use high doses of marijuana. The syndrome is sometimes called chronic cannabis syndrome. The term "aberrant motivational syndrome" has been suggested as a more precise description of the phenomenon (Millman & Sbriglio, 1986). The syndrome describes individuals whose personal habits have deteriorated; that is, they are withdrawn, passive, and easily distracted, with poor judgment and impaired communication skills (Stefanis, Boulougouris, & Liakos, 1976). The syndrome has been invoked to explain poor school performance and personality deterioration particularly in adolescents. In other young individuals, chronic heavy cannabis use has been associated with profound changes in perspective, dress, and behavior, although they have demonstrated

considerable energy and ambition in the pursuit of their particular goals, such as intense involvement with popular music and the pursuit of musical groups such as the Grateful Dead or identification with drug-using cults such as Rastafarians. These reports are compromised by the absence of control subjects and the inability to distinguish the pharmacologic effects of the drug from antecedent psychological and social conditions.

The pharmacologic effect of cannabis, interacting with psychological and social factors, may be responsible for the clinical picture seen. In other highly motivated, productive people, the drug is reported to facilitate performance and productivity, perhaps due to the reduction of incapacitating anxiety and enhanced relaxation in experienced users. The dose and frequency of the drug used is generally lower than used by most compulsive users.

Other studies have found that comorbid depression may be the contributing factor in the amotivational syndrome (Musty & Kaback, 1995). Depression and learned helplessness are common problems that interfere with motivation to achieve. Zablocki, Aidala, Hansell, and White (1991) found that marijuana use was significantly associated with psychological distress (depression, anxiety, or both) for highly introspective individuals. It is possible that heavy users with depressive symptoms may be highly introspective and may be more sensitive to contingencies and challenges in their environments, which may in turn interact with heavy marijuana use (either consciously or unconsciously) to contribute to lower motivation.

The amotivational syndrome occurs more frequently in individuals who are required to master complex and often intimidating tasks or information, for example, students or skilled workers required to do complex thinking. The drug may facilitate performance in groups in which repetitive or boring tasks are required (Rubin & Comitas, 1976; Stefanis et al., 1976).

The chronic cannabis syndrome may also be considered to be a variant of the cannabis dependence disorder that has been described. Cessation of cannabis use in the absence of severe psychopathology and committed involvement to a treatment program frequently results in a marked and rapid improvement in mental clarity and energy levels. In addition to being a result of the waning of drug effects, the often remarkable behavioral changes seen may be a function of decreased feelings of isolation and demoralization that many previously chemically dependent individuals experience on rejoining the ranks of consensual society, however intensely it was previously shunned. (Millman & Beeder, 1994).

Other reports of chronic users have not supported the idea of cannabis use leading to personality deterioration (Beaubrun & Knight, 1973; Carter, 1980; Rubin & Comitas, 1975). These reports are also flawed in that they focused on low-level workers doing relatively menial tasks. Some studies of personality and concomitant drug use make it difficult to establish that any decrease in motivation is due to cannabis use per se (Alcoholism and Drug Addiction Research Foundation/World Health Organization, 1981; Nicholi, 1983). The syndrome has not been demonstrated in controlled laboratory studies (Brady, Foltin, Fischman, & Capriotti, 1986).

Mood Disturbance

Brief, self-limiting, depressive reactions are well-recognized consequences of cannabis use. There is some anecdotal evidence that more serious or prolonged mood disturbances can occur, but this has not been supported by controlled studies.

Depressive symptoms may follow euphoria (Ames, 1958) or come after a psychotic episode (Palsson, Thulin, & Tunving, 1982). Heavy marijuana users have been reported to consistently have higher negative moods and lower positive moods than light marijuana users (Lex, Griffin, Mello, & Mendelson, 1989). In addition, marijuana use may precipitate relapse in patients with preexisting depressive disorders.

Psychosocial Correlates

Chronic psychopathology noted in chronic marijuana users, as with all other drug abusers, is determined by the interaction of the psychobiology of the user with the pharmacology and psychoactive effects of the drug. It remains difficult in individual patients to differentiate what came before the drug use from what is seen after, to distinguish the correlates of abuse and dependence from the consequences. Chronic marijuana use may reflect impaired premorbid social or occupational functioning and psychopathology and also may be a cause of psychiatric symptomatology and behavioral disability (Beeder & Millman, 1992).

Surveys in the 1970s and the early 1980s revealed that the psychosocial correlates of marijuana use include less value placed on academic achievement, higher value of independence relative to achievement values, greater social criticism and tolerance of deviant behavior, and less religiosity (Jessor & Jessor, 1977; Kandel, 1978). Social measures that relate to marijuana use include psychosocial unconventionality, less perceived control from friends, lower compatibility between the expectations of friends and of parents, greater influence of friends relative to parents, and greater involvement in other problem behaviors such as excessive drinking, delinquency, and precocious sexual behavior (Kandel et al., 1978). These findings demonstrate that marijuana use and other drug use are associated with a larger network of personal, social, and behavioral attributes (Jessor, Donovan, & Costa, 1986).

Drug use in many young people may represent purposeful, goal-directed behavior: They may feel older, more mature, or more in control when using drugs. The drug is used to cope with dysphoric feelings of boredom, anxiety, frustration, and inadequacy in relation to the demands or expectations of peers, parents, and school authorities. Marijuana may serve to alter perceptions sufficiently such that these feelings are less intense and the situations attendant to these feelings may be perceived as less important (Jessor, Chase, & Donovan, 1980). Compulsive marijuana use may facilitate a regressive avoidance of stress. Persistence and cessation of cannabis use has been related to the ability to assume an adult role, for example, maintaining a long-term relationship, having children, and maintaining employment (Hammer, 1990).

Cannabis as Self-Medication

Cannabis abuse and dependency is often associated with significant premorbid psychopathology ranging from personality and affective disorders to psychotic disorders. In some of these disorders, the drug is used as self-medication. It is necessary to define the meaning of the drug use for each patient (Beeder & Millman, 1992). The anxiolytic and sedative properties of the drug may serve to reduce painful affects of depression, rage, shame, and loneliness in people who are postulated to have major defects in affect defense (McLellan, Woody, & O'Brien, 1979; Millman & Sbriglio, 1986). The drug may alleviate the symptomatology associated with these personality disorders.

A variety of workers have reported on patients with schizophrenic and manic or hypomanic disorders who self-medicated their psychotic symptoms with marijuana, with a consequent deterioration of the clinical picture (Andreasson, Allenbeck, & Rydberg, 1989; O'Connell, 1990). A study (Mathers, Ghodse, Cann, & Scott, 1991) of 908 psychiatric inpatients in the United Kingdom found a significant correlation between urines positive for cannabis and an initial diagnosis of psychosis. Because cannabis weakens perceptual cues and is itself psychotomimetic, it has been difficult to understand why cannabis would be used as self-medication by psychotic individuals. Certainly alcohol, depressants, and particularly the opioids would be more effective as self-medication for these disorders. Schizophrenic patients often report that the antipsychotic medications they may take produce feelings of emptiness, being uninspired, passive, and subdued. With cannabis, patients reported a two-phased experience, with initial feelings of relaxation, increased energy, and improved mood followed by a deterioration marked by increased severity of auditory hallucinations and disorganization. This suggests that schizophrenic patients might be willing to

accept predictably worsening symptomatology to be able to experience fleeting moments of escape and euphoria. It has also been postulated that the anticholinergic effect of cannabis may diminish the therapeutic efficacy of neuroleptic agents (Bernhardson & Gunne, 1972; Knudsen & Vilmar, 1984). The manic and hypomanic patients described may have been attempting to control their symptomatology and experienced a worsening of symptoms leading to a transient marijuana-induced schizophreniform phase of manic illness (Harding & Knight, 1973; Knight, 1976). Some of these patients seem to have been trying to distance themselves from threatening symptomatology in any way possible. It has been shown that a major determinant of schizophrenic patients' returning to psychiatric hospitals is cannabis use and failure to take neuroleptic medication. For these patients, the issue often seems to be whether they should take the prescribed medication and feel empty and sad, although their function improves, or take illicit drugs that offer them moments of joy and pleasure, although the symptoms are likely to worsen (Millman & Beeder, 1994).

A related phenomenon may be the attempt by some individuals, particularly adolescents, to rationalize their psychopathology, abnormal or bizarre behavior, and inability to relate to their peers (Millman & Sbriglio, 1986). They would prefer to attribute their strange thoughts and feelings to the drug and not to their own psychopathology. The deviant subculture of "potheads" and "druggies" is certainly more tolerant of the strange ways of psychologically impaired people than conventional society. Some of these people become expert in acquiring, selling, and using drugs such that they have honored roles in their group, albeit an antisocial role in a bizarre society.

The type of treatment for patients with premorbid psychopathology depends on the characterization of their disorder when they have ceased marijuana use. It is often necessary to institute treatment presumptively based on the clinical picture. Psychotic symptoms associated with cannabis use should be treated in the same manner as functional psychotic symptoms. Patients should be carefully educated with respect to issues such as their attempt at self-medication and at rationalization of their psychopathology. Patients on neuroleptics must be specifically cautioned against the use of cannabis and may require group support in this effort.

Afterword

It should be appreciated, however, that experimental or intermittent use of marijuana is very different from compulsive use and dependence on marijuana or other drugs. Dependence is determined by psychosocial factors in addition to pharmacological ones. Though at times not dangerous in itself, cannabis use often leads to experimentation with other drugs, and these drugs may be much more difficult to control.

References

Alcoholism and Drug Addiction Research Foundation/World Health Organization. (1981). *Report of an ARF/WHO Scientific Meeting on Adverse Health and Behavioral Consequences of Cannabis Use.* Toronto, Ontario, Canada: Author.

American Psychiatric Association. (1994). *Diagnostic and statistical manual of mental disorders* (4th ed.). Washington, DC: Author.

Ames, F. (1958). A clinical and metabolic study of acute intoxication with Cannabis sativa and its role in the model psychoses. *Journal of Mental Science, 104,* 972–999.

Andreasson, S., Allenbeck, P., & Rydberg, U. (1989). Schizophrenia in users and non-users of cannabis: A longitudinal study in Stockholm county. *Acta Psychiatrica Scandinavica, 79,* 505–510.

Beaubrun, M., & Knight, F. (1973). Psychiatric assessment of 30 chronic users of cannabis and 30 matched controls. *American Journal of Psychiatry, 130,* 309–311.

Beeder, A. B., & Millman, R. B. (1992). Treatment of patients with psychopathology and substance abuse. In J. H. Lowinson, P. Ruiz, R. B. Millman, & John Langrod (Eds.), *Substance abuse: A comprehensive textbook* (2nd ed., pp. 675–690). Baltimore: Williams & Wilkins.

Bernhardson, G., & Gunne, L. M. (1972). Forty-six cases of psychosis in cannabis abusers. *International Journal of the Addictions, 7,* 9–16.

Brady, J. V., Foltin, R. W., Fischman, M. W., & Capriotti, R. M. (1986). Behavioral interactions and the effects of marijuana. *Alcohol, Drugs, and Driving, 2,* 93–103.

Breier, A., Buchanan, R. W., Kirkpatrick, B., Davis, O. R., Irish, D., Summerfelt, A., & Carpenter, W. T. (1994). Effects of Clozapine on positive and negative symptoms in outpatients with schizophrenia. *American Journal of Psychiatry, 151,* 20–26.

Brill, H., & Nahas, G. G. (1984). Cannabis intoxication and mental illness. In G. G. Nahas (Ed.), *Marijuana in science and medicine* (pp. 263–305). New York: Raven.

Carter, W. E. (1980). *Cannabis in Costa Rica: A study of chronic marijuana use.* Philadelphia: Institute for the Study of Human Issues.

Chaudry, H. R., Moss, H. B., Bashir, A., & Suliman, T. (1991). Cannabis psychosis following bhang ingestion. *British Journal of Addiction, 86,* 1075–1081.

Chopra, G., & Smith, J. (1974). Psychotic reactions following cannabis use in East Indians. *Archives of General Psychiatry, 30,* 24–27.

Clayton, R. R., & Voss, H. L. (1981). *Young men and drugs in Manhattan: A casual analysis* (NIDA Research Monograph No. 39). Washington, DC: U.S. Government Printing Office.

Edwards, G. (1983). Psychopathology of a drug experience. *British Journal of Psychiatry, 143,* 509–512.

Ellis, G. M., Mann, M. A., Judson, B. A., Schramm, N. T., & Taschian, A. (1985). Excretion patterns of cannabinoid metabolites after last use in a group of chronic users. *Clinical Pharmacology & Therapeutics, 38,* 572–578.

Estroff, T. W., & Gold, M. S. (1986). Psychiatric presentations of marijuana abuse. *Psychiatric Annals, 16,* 221–224.

Ghodse, H. (1986). Cannabis psychosis. *British Journal of Addiction, 81,* 473–478.

Grinspoon, L., & Bakalar, J. B. (1986). Psychedelics and arylcyclohexylamines. In A. J. Frances & R. E. Hales (Eds.), *Psychiatry update: American Psychiatric Association annual review* (Vol. 5, pp. 212–225). Washington, DC: American Psychiatric Press.

Hall, W., Solowij, N., & Lemon, J. (1994). *The health and psychological effects of cannabis* (National Drug Strategy Monograph No. 25). Canberra, Australia: Australian Government Publishing Service.

Hammer, T. (1990). Per Vaglum: Initiation, continuation, or discontinuation of cannabis use in the general population. *British Journal of Addiction, 85,* 899–909.

Harding, T., & Knight, F. (1973). Marijuana-modified mania. *Archives of General Psychiatry, 29,* 635–637.

Hunt, C. A., & Jones, R. T. (1980). Tolerance and disposition of tetrahydrocannabinol in man. *Journal of Pharmacology and Experimental Therapeutics, 215,* 35–44.

Jessor, R. (1975). Predicting time of marijuana use: A developmental study of high school youths. In D. J. Lettieri (Ed.), *Predicting adolescent drug abuse: A review of issues, methods, and correlates: Research issues, II.* Rockville, MD: National Institute on Drug Abuse.

Jessor, R., & Jessor, S. L. (1977). *Problem behavior and psychosocial development: A longitudinal study of youth.* New York: Academic Press.

Jessor, R., Chase, J. A., & Donovan, J. E. (1980). Psychosocial correlates of marijuana use and problem drinking in a national sample of adolescents. *American Journal of Public Health, 70*, 604–613.

Jessor, R., Donovan, J., & Costa, F. (1986). Psychoactive correlates of marijuana in adolescent and young adulthood: The past as prologue, in marijuana, cocaine, and traffic society. In H. Moskowitz (Ed.), *Alcohol, drugs and driving* (Vol. 2, pp. 31–49). Santa Monica, CA.

Johansson, E., Agurell, S., Hollister, L. E., & Halldin, M. M. (1988). Prolonged apparent half-life of delta-1-tetrahydrocannabinol in plasma of chronic marijuana users. *Journal of Pharmacy and Pharmacology, 40*, 374–375.

Johnson, B. A. (1990). Psychopharmacological effects of cannabis. *British Journal of Hospital Medicine, 43*, 114–122.

Jones, R. T., & Benowitz, N. (1976). The 30-day trip—Clinical studies of cannabis tolerance and dependence. In M. C. Braude & S. Szara (Eds.), *The pharmacology of marijuana* (pp. 627–642). New York: Raven.

Jones, R. T., Benowitz, N., & Bachman, J. (1976). Clinical studies of cannabis tolerance and dependence. *Annals of the New York Academy of Sciences, 282*, 221–239.

Jones, R. T., Benowitz, N. L., & Herning, R. I. (1981). Clinical relevance of cannabis tolerance and dependence. *Journal of Clinical Pharmacology, 21* (Suppl.), 143S–152S.

Kandel, D. B. (Ed.). (1978). *Longitudinal research on drug use: Empirical findings and methodological issues.* Washington, DC: Hemisphere.

Kandel, D. B., & Davies, M. (1992). Progression to regular marijuana involvement: Phenomenology and risk factors for near-daily use. In M. Glantz & R. Pickens (Eds.), *Vulnerability to drug abuse* (pp. 211–254). Washington, DC: American Psychological Association.

Kandel, D. B., Kessler, R., & Margulies, R. (1978). Antecedents of adolescent initiation into stages of drug use: A developmental analysis. In D. B. Kandel (Ed.), *Longitudinal research on drug use: Empirical findings and methodological issues* (pp. 73–99). Washington, DC: Hemisphere.

Keup, W. (1970). Psychotic symptoms due to cannabis abuse. *Diseases of the Nervous System, 31*, 119–126.

Khantzian, E. J., & McKenna, G. J. (1979). Acute toxic and withdrawal reactions associated with drug use and abuse. *Annals of Internal Medicine, 90*, 361–373.

Kiplinger, G. G., & Manno, J. E. (1971). Dose response relationships to cannabis in human subjects. *Pharmacological Review, 23*, 339–347.

Knight, F. (1976). Role of cannabis in psychiatric disturbance. *Annals of the New York Academy of Sciences, 282*, 64–71.

Knudsen, P., & Vilmar, T. (1984). Cannabis and neuroleptic agents in schizophrenia. *Acta Psychiatrica Scandinavica, 69*, 162–174.

Kouri, E., Pope, H. G., Yurgelun-Todd, D., & Gruber, S. (1995). Attributes of heavy vs. occasional marijuana smokers in a college population. *Biological Psychiatry. 38*, 475–481.

Lex, B. W., Griffin, M. L., Mello, N. K., & Mendelson, J. (1989). Alcohol, marijuana and mood states in young women. *International Journal of the Addictions, 24*, 405–424.

Marder, S. R., & Meibach, R. C. (1994). Risperidone in the treatment of schizophrenia. *American Journal of Psychiatry, 151*, 825–835.

Marlotte, D. B. (1972). Marijuana and mutism. *American Journal of Psychiatry, 129*, 475–477.

Mathers, D. C., Ghodse, A. H. , Cann, A. W. , & Scott, S. A. (1991). Cannabis use in a large sample of acute psychiatric admissions. *British Journal of Addiction, 86*, 779–784.

McLellan, A. T., Woody, G. E., & O'Brien, C. P. (1979). Development of psychiatric illness in drug abusers: Possible role of drug preference. *New England Journal of Medicine, 301*, 1310–1314.

Mendelson, J. H., Mello, N. K., Lex, B. W., & Bavli, S. (1984). Marijuana withdrawal syndrome in a woman. *American Journal of Psychiatry, 141*, 1289–1290.

Mendhiratta, S. S., Varma, V. K., Dang, R., Malhotra, A. K., Das, K., & Nehra, R. (1988). Cannabis and cognitive functions: A re-evaluation study. *British Journal of Addictions, 20*, 57–65.

Millman, R. B., & Beeder, A. B. (1994). Treatment of patients for specific drugs of abuse: Cannabis. In M. Galanter & H. D. Kleber (Eds.), *The American Psychiatric Press textbook of substance abuse treatment* (pp. 91–109). Washington, DC: American Psychiatric Press.

Millman, R. B., & Sbriglio, R. (1986). Patterns of use and psychopathology in chronic marijuana users. *Psychiatric Clinics of North America, 9*, 533–545.

Musty, R. E., & Kaback, L. (1995). Relationships between motivation and depression in chronic marijuana users. *Life Sciences, 56*, 2151–2158.

National Institute on Drug Abuse. (1995). *The monitoring the future study, Institute for Social Research.* Ann Arbor: University of Michigan Press.

Negrete, J. C. (1988). What's happened to the cannabis debate? *British Journal of Addiction, 83*, 359–372.

Nicholi, A. A. (1983). The non-therapeutic use of psychoactive drugs: A modern epidemic. *New England Journal of Medicine, 308*, 925–933.

O'Connell, D. F. (1990). Managing the dually diagnosed patient. In D. F. O'Connell (Ed.), *Current issues and clinical approaches.* New York: Haworth.

O'Donnell, J. A., & Clayton, R. R. (1979). The stepping stone hypothesis: A reappraisal. In G. M. Beschner & A. S. Friedman (Eds.), *Youth drug abuse: Problems, issues and treatment.* Lexington, MA: Lexington Books.

O'Donnell, J. A., Voss, H. L., Clayton, R. R., Slatin, G. T., & Room, R. G. (1976). *Young men and drugs: A na-*

tionwide survey (NIDA Research Monograph No. 5; DHEW Publication No. ADM-76-311). Washington, DC: U.S. Government Printing Office.

O'Malley, P. M., Johnston, L. D., & Bachman, J. G. (1985). Cocaine use among American adolescents and young adults. In N. J. Kozel & E. H. Adams (Eds.), *Cocaine use in America: Epidemiologic and clinical perspectives* (NIDA Research Monograph No. 61, pp. 50–75). Washington, DC: National Institute on Drug Abuse.

Palsson, A., Thulin, S. O., & Tunving, K. (1982). Cannabis psychosis in South Sweden. *Acta Psychiatrica Scandinavica, 66,* 311–321.

Pope, H. G., & Yurgelun-Todd, D. (1996). The residual cognitive effects of heavy marijuana use in college students. *Journal of the American Medical Association, 7,* 521–527.

Pope, H. G., Gruber, A. J., & Yurgelun-Todd, D. (1995). The residual neuropsychological effects of cannabis: The current status of research. *Drug and Alcohol Dependence, 38,* 25–34.

Rohr, J. M., Showlund, S. W., & Martin, T. E. (1989). Withdrawal sequelae to cannabis use. *International Journal of the Addictions, 24,* 627–631.

Rubin V., & Comitas, L. (1975). Psychological assessment. In V. Rubin & L. Comitas (Eds.), *Ganja in Jamaica: A medical-anthropological study of chronic marijuana use* (pp. 111–119). The Hague, Netherlands: Mouton.

Rubin, V., & Comitas, L. (1976). *Ganja in Jamaica: The effects of marijuana.* New York: Anchor/Doubleday.

Schwartz, R. H., Gruenwald, P. J., Klitzner, M., & Fedio, P. (1989). Short-term memory impairment in cannabis-dependent adolescents. *American Journal of Diseases of Children, 143,* 1214–1219.

Seth, R., & Sinha, S. (1991). Chemistry and pharmacology of cannabis. *Progress in Drug Research, 36,* 71–115.

Smith, D. E. (1968). Acute and chronic toxicity of marijuana. *Journal of Psychedelic Drugs, 2,* 37–47.

Solomons, K., & Neppe, V. M. (1989). Cannabis—Its clinical effects. *South African Medical Journal, 76,* 102–104.

Stefanis, C., Boulougouris. I., & Liakos, A. (1976). Clinical and psychophysiological effects of cannabis in long-term users. In M. C. Brause & S. Szara (Eds.), *Pharmacology of marijuana.* New York: Raven.

Substance Abuse and Mental Health Services Administration. (1995). *Preliminary estimates from the 1994 National Household Survey on Drug Abuse,* Advance Report No. 10. Washington, DC: U.S. Government Printing Office.

Thornicroft, G. (1990). Cannabis and psychosis—Is there epidemiological evidence for an association? *British Journal of Psychiatry, 157,* 25–33.

Tien, A. Y., & Anthony, J. C. (1990). Epidemiological analysis of alcohol and drug use as risk factors for psychotic experiences. *Journal of Nervous and Mental Disease, 178,* 473–480.

Tunving, K. (1985). Psychiatric effects of cannabis use. *Acta Psychiatrica Scandinavica, 72,* 209–217.

Wall, M. E., & Perez-Reyes, M. (1981). The metabolism of delta-9-tetrahydrocannabinol and related cannabinoids in man. *Journal of Clinical Pharmacology, 21,* 1785–1795.

Zablocki, B., Aidala, A., Hansell, S., & White, H. R. (1991). Marijuana use, introspectiveness, and mental health. *Journal of Health and Social Behavior, 32,* 65–79.

Zinberg, N. (1984). *Drug, set and setting.* New Haven, CT: Yale University Press.

IV

Cocaine

10

Pharmacology of Cocaine

S. JOHN GATLEY, ANDREW N. GIFFORD,

NORA D. VOLKOW, AND JOANNA S. FOWLER

Introduction

Cocaine is a naturally occurring alkaloid extracted from the leaves of the South American shrub *Erythroxylon coca*. Early European explorers reported the habit of chewing of coca leaves by native populations, and systematic investigations of the effects of cocaine were conducted in the late nineteenth century by Sigmund Freud and others. For a review of the older literature on cocaine, the reader is referred to VanDyke and Byck (1974). Cocaine possesses short-acting local anesthetic and vasoconstrictor properties, which make it clinically useful for topical application. Its actions as a local anesthetic are due to inhibition of neuronal sodium channels which results in blockage of the initiation and conduction of nerve impulses. This area is not discussed in detail in this chapter. Cocaine is a Schedule II drug in the United States. Its abuse is associated with enormous costs to both addicted individuals and to society as a whole. Valuable perspectives on the abuse of cocaine and other stimulants were provided by Gawin and Ellinwood (1988).

Chemically, cocaine can be described as 2β-carbomethoxy-3β-benzoyloxytropane, or the benzoic acid ester of ecgonine methylester. Only one of the several possible optical isomers, the one found in nature, possesses significant pharmacological activity. Figure 1 indicates the stereochemistry at each of the chiral carbon atoms of cocaine, and summarizes many of cocaine's properties. Cocaine is a weak base and is readily soluble in common organic solvents. Salts including the hydrochloride are easily soluble in water. Cocaine hydrochloride tends to decompose before becoming volatile on heating, but the free base forms a vapor readily at temperatures above about 100°. This is the basis for the recent epidemic of smoked free base ("crack") cocaine.

The enormous amount of literature on cocaine precludes a comprehensive review in this chapter. A detailed review was presented by Johanson and Fischman (1989), and some recent advances were discussed by Johanson and Schuster (1995). The purpose of this chapter is to describe some of the important features of the pharmacokinetics and metabolism of cocaine, and some aspects of the mechanisms involved in cocaine's reinforcing effects. We emphasize the results of recent studies using positron emission tomography (PET) and carbon-11 labeled cocaine, which have allowed

S. JOHN GATLEY, ANDREW N. GIFFORD, AND NORA D. VOLKOW • Medical Department, Brookhaven National Laboratory, Upton, New York 11973. JOANNA S. FOWLER • Chemistry Department, Brookhaven National Laboratory, Upton, New York 11973.

Handbook of Substance Abuse: Neurobehavioral Pharmacology, edited by Tarter *et al.* Plenum Press, New York, 1998.

structure	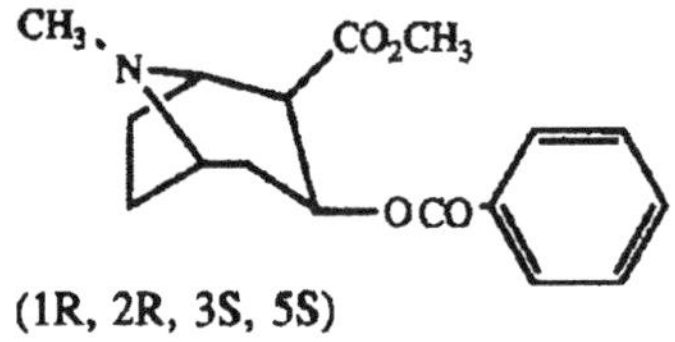 (1R, 2R, 3S, 5S)
chemical name	(-)-2β-carbomethoxy-3β-benzoyloxytropane [1R-(exo, exo)]-3-(Benzoyloxy)-8-methyl-8-azabicyclo[3.2.1]octane-2-carboxylic acid methyl ester
molecular weight	303 (free base); 340 (hydrochloride
source	*Erythroxylon coca* leaves
pharmacological classifications	psychomotor stimulant, anesthetic-vasoconstrictor (mucosal-local)
legal classification	schedule II
legitimate medical use	local anesthesia (topical)
pK	8.4
log P	1.1
plasma free fraction	10%
volume of distribution	100-200 L
plasma clearance half-time	40-90 min
peak brain uptake (i/v)	11% of injected dose
time to peak brain uptake (i/v)	4-6 min
brain clearance half-time (i/v)	20 min
major excretion pathway	urinary metabolites
major metabolites	benzoylecgonine (40%) ecgonine methylester (20%)
pharmacological target for abuse	dopamine transporter
affinity for dopamine transporter (rat)	120 nM
LD_{50} (rat)	17.5 mg/kg
typical single dose for abuser (i/v)	40 mg
consumption in typical "binge"	1 g
major medical complications	cardiovascular
most common co-abused drug	alcohol

FIGURE 1. Cocaine and some of its properties. The chemical structure of cocaine is shown, together with its major characteristics.

direct measurements of cocaine kinetics in individual tissues in human subjects. Developments in medicinal chemistry, which have resulted in new analogs of cocaine and other dopamine reuptake blockers, are also emphasized because of their potential importance in the search for pharmacotherapies of cocaine abuse (Kleber, 1995). Molecular biological studies of reinforcement and addiction have been reviewed elsewhere (Self & Nestler, 1995).

Route of Administration and Plasma Pharmacokinetics

As expected for a molecule with its physicochemical properties, cocaine is readily absorbed through all mucous membranes.

However, the major routes of self-administration are nasal insufflation, smoking, and intravenous injection. Although the oral administration route is reinforcing in animal models (Seidman, Lau, Chen, & Falk, 1992) and has been reported to induce a more intense "high" in humans than intranasal administration (VanDyke, Jatlow, Ungerer, Barash, & Byck, 1978), this is not a common form of cocaine abuse. Studies in animals have shown that the reinforcing efficacy of cocaine depends on the rate of delivery of cocaine to the brain (Balster & Schuster, 1973), presumably because brain reward mechanisms (Gardner, 1992) are sensitive to increases in the degree of occupancy of cocaine receptors. This is consistent with the prevalence of the intravenous route of cocaine abuse, which avoids time delays involved in absorption of drug at peripheral sites. The recent increase in popularity of "crack" smoking in drug abuse populations also supports this notion, because cocaine vapor deposited in the lungs is expected to be very rapidly absorbed through the large area of the alveolar membranes. The cocaine can then be transported to the brain in a shorter time than after intravenous administration (Cone, 1995). Foltin and Fischman (1992) reported that addicts preferred 25 mg of smoked cocaine to 32 mg of intravenous cocaine, despite the fact that some of the smoked cocaine is lost to decomposition and condensation in the smoking apparatus (Cook, Jeffcoat, & Perez-Reyes, 1985). By contrast with intravenous or smoked cocaine, the slower absorption of cocaine after intranasal administration results in a more gradual delivery to the brain, and cocaine abuse by this route appears to be associated with fewer medical and societal problems. Several authors have conducted traditional pharmacokinetic analyses of human plasma concentrations of cocaine after its administration by various routes (Barnet, Hawks, & Resnick, 1981; Chow et al., 1985; Cone, 1995; Cone, Kumor, Thompson, & Sherer, 1988; Cook et al., 1985; Javaid, Musa, Fischman, Schuster, & Davis, 1983; Jeffcoat, Perez-Reyes, Hill, Sadler, & Cook, 1989; Wilkinson, VanDyke, Jatlow, Barash, & Byck, 1980).

These studies have provided average elimination half-lives of 40–90 min and volumes of distribution of 100–200 L. The half-life for absorption of cocaine from the nasal mucosa is about 10 min. Cone (1995) recently reported the results of pharmacokinetic, physiological, and neuropsychological testing after administration of cocaine by the intravenous, intranasal, and smoked routes to each of 6 subjects. While venous plasma concentrations of intravenous and smoked cocaine peaked within 5 min, peak concentrations after intranasal cocaine occurred at about 30 min and were about 0.25–0.5 those seen for the intravenous or smoked routes. Although no significant pharmacokinetic differences between intravenous and smoked cocaine were measured for doses of equivalent bioavailability, the smoked route gave higher scores for self-reported "high" (Cone, 1995; Foltin & Fischman, 1992). These recent studies confirm that the euphoric effects of a given dose of cocaine do not depend on its concentration in the venous plasma so much as on the speed with which the bolus of cocaine is delivered to the brain in the arterial plasma (Evans, Cone, Marco, & Henningfield, 1992). Cocaine appears to be similar to other drugs of abuse, including nicotine (Henningfield & Keenan, 1993; Wakasa, Takada, & Yanagita, 1995) and heroin (Jaffe, 1990), in this respect. Traditional pharmacokinetic analyses based on measurements of drug concentrations in venous plasma are probably not particularly useful in predicting or interpreting the subjective effects of these abused drugs.

PET Studies of the Distribution of Cocaine

Until recently, drug pharmacokinetics required the investigation of samples of tissues and fluids taken at particular times after drug administration, which precluded the collection of a complete set of data in a given individual. With the availability of PET and appropriate labeled compounds it is now feasible to assess the pharmacokinetics of drugs directly in the brain while monitoring physiological and behavioral effects as well as plasma pharmacokinetics in a single subject. Furthermore, because experiments are nonterminal, the same subject can be used to investigate the effects of a drug at more than one concentration or on more than one neurochemical system.

Initial PET experiments with [^{11}C]cocaine demonstrated its selective binding in the basal ganglia of human and baboon brains (Fowler et al., 1989). The time-course of this binding (peak uptake of 0.008% injected activity per cc at 5 min, and a clearance half-time of 20 min) was very similar to that of the "high" previously reported by cocaine abusers (Cook et al., 1985). Furthermore, blockade of dopamine transporters by pretreatment with the dopamine reuptake inhibitor nomifensine reduced [^{11}C]cocaine binding in the striatum but not in the cerebellum, which lacks dopamine transporters. These observations were a further indication that cocaine binding to the dopamine transporter may be the initial event in reinforcement. The PET experiments indicate that the peak concentration of cocaine in basal ganglia after administration of a euphorigenic dose of cocaine (40 mg) would be about 10 μM, more than 10-fold higher than peak concentrations in venous plasma (e.g., Cone, 1995).

Subsequent PET studies with [^{11}C]cocaine examined its distribution in other parts of the human body following intravenous injection (Volkow, Fowler, et al., 1992). The results are summarized in Table 1. An hour after injection, whole-body PET images showed a diffuse background level of radioactivity with higher levels only in the liver, urinary bladder, and gastrointestinal tract. Although the extent to which radioactivity represents free cocaine, cocaine bound to specific target sites, and labeled metabolites at later times is uncertain, the early high concentrations of cocaine in human heart, kidneys, adrenals, and liver (Table 1) could contribute to its toxicity.

Cardiac toxicity is the most frequent complication of cocaine abuse, which can induce myocardial infarction and lethal arrythmias (Gradman, 1988; Huester, 1987; Isner, Estes, & Thompson, 1986; Kloner, Hale, Alker, & Rezkalla, 1992). The pharmacokinetics of [^{11}C]cocaine in the human heart were faster than in the brain (Table 1), and may represent binding to the norepinephrine transporter. Furthermore, in baboon PET studies the myocardial uptake of 6-[^{18}F]norepinephrine was profoundly decreased by pretreatment with cocaine (Fowler et al., 1994). These observations support the idea that noradrenergic stimulation contributes to the cardiotoxicity of cocaine. However, local anesthetic action of cocaine may also directly damage the myocardium, (Przywara & Dambach, 1989). The high uptake of [^{11}C]cocaine in the adrenals also presumably results from binding to catecholamine transporters. It may be related to the large increases in plasma catecholamines after acute cocaine administration, which increases are expected to further enhance cocaine's cardiotoxicity (Chiueh & Kopin, 1978).

In contrast to experiments with tracer amounts of [^{11}C]cocaine (< 5 μg/kg), when

TABLE 1. Tissue Distribution and Kinetics of [^{11}C]Cocaine in Human Subjects

Organ	Peak uptake (% injected C-11)	Time to peak (min)	Peak concentration (μM)[a]	Clearance half-time (min)
Brain	11.0%	4–6	11	20
Heart	2.2%	2–3	9	10
Kidney	4.1%	2–3	19	10
Liver	24.0%	10–15	19	[c]
Adrenals	0.5%	10	45	22
Lungs	[b]	2–3	[b]	5

[a]Peak concentrations were calculated assuming injection of 40 mg of cocaine free base, homogeneous distributions in organs, and no metabolism. Organ weights and specific gravities were taken from Snyder et al. (1975).
[b]C-11 in lungs paralleled that in plasma.
[c]C-11 in liver remained approximately constant after 15 minutes.

doses of cocaine known to induce euphoria in humans (0.5 mg/kg) were given simultaneously with [^{11}C]cocaine there was no preferential uptake of C-11 in the basal ganglia (Volkow, Fowler, *et al.*, 1995). This demonstrates near saturation of the dopamine transporters at this dose of cocaine. The peak uptake in striatum, expressed as a fraction of injected activity, occurred earlier (3 min versus 5 min) but was slightly higher than for [^{11}C]cocaine of high specific activity, perhaps because of saturation of binding sites in the blood which modulate the distribution of cocaine (Tella & Goldberg, 1993).

PET Studies in Cocaine Abusers

In addition to studies in control human and baboon subjects, PET studies with several radiotracers have been conducted to evaluate acute and chronic effects of cocaine on various physiological and neurochemical parameters.

Brain Uptake of Cocaine

A group of 12 detoxified cocaine abusers was studied (Volkow *et al.*, 1996). They showed globally decreased uptake of cocaine in the brain, relative to nonabusers, but no changes in dopamine transporter availability as assessed by tracer kinetic modeling (Logan *et al.*, 1990).

Cerebral Blood Flow

In early PET studies of cocaine abusers, widespread brain perfusion abnormalities were detected using the blood flow tracer [^{15}O]water (Volkow, Mullani, Gould, Adler, & Krajewski, 1988). Fourteen of 20 abusers exhibited perfusion defects which were widely distributed through the brain but predominantly in the frontal cortex and left hemisphere. Cerebellar abnormalities were rare. These findings have been replicated in single photon emission computed tomography (SPECT) studies among moderate and heavy cocaine abusers (Strickland *et al.*, 1993; Tumeh, Nagel, & English, 1990). They corroborate the clinical documentation of a high incidence of cerebral strokes and hemorrhages associated with cocaine abuse (Levin &

Welch, 1988; Lichtenfeld, Rubin, & Feldman, 1984). The perfusion defects could arise from vascular damage and ischemia secondary to prolonged cocaine-induced vasoconstriction. They are distinct from the transient effects of cocaine administration on cerebral blood flow (Stein & Fuller, 1993).

Acute Cocaine Challenge and Glucose Metabolism

In PET studies in cocaine abusers with 2-[^{18}F]fluorodeoxyglucose (FDG), intravenous administration of 40 mg of cocaine decreased glucose metabolic rates in both cortical and subcortical structures (London *et al.*, 1990). Decreases were correlated with the subjective sense of intoxication. The authors postulated that the cocaine's mechanism of reinforcement may involve a reduction in brain metabolic activity. In interpreting PET/FDG studies it must be remembered that the time required for measurements (> 30 min) is long compared to cocaine's pharmacokinetics. The average metabolic rates may therefore mask increases or decreases in brain function that occur on a shorter time-scale (Stein & Fuller, 1993). Decreased glucose utilization has been reported in PET/FDG studies after acute administration of alcohol, diazepam, amphetamine, or morphine (deWit, Metz, Wagner, & Cooper, 1990; deWit, Metz, & Cooper, 1994; London *et al.*, 1990; Volkow *et al.*, 1990; Volkow, Wang, *et al.*, 1995; Wolkin *et al.*, 1987). The finding is not general to all drugs of abuse, however, since tetrahydrocannabinol (THC; the active principle of marijuana) did not reduce global FDG uptake (Volkow, Gillespie, *et al.*, 1991).

Chronic Cocaine Abuse and Glucose Metabolism

Glucose metabolic rates appear to be sensitive to the period of abstinence from cocaine, as subjects tested within 1 week of last cocaine use had significantly higher metabolic rates in the orbitofrontal cortex and basal ganglia than either normal controls or abusers tested 1 month after detoxification (Volkow, Fowler, *et al.*, 1991). These increases were negatively correlated with the duration of abstinence and with the intensity of cocaine craving. Another study was conducted in inpatient cocaine abusers who were tested 8–60 days after last use of cocaine and again after a 3–4-month drug-free period (Volkow, Hitzemann, *et al.,* 1992). These subjects showed significant reductions in frontal metabolic activity compared with normal controls. The decreases were larger for the left frontal cortex than for the right, and they persisted when the subjects were retested 3–4 months after detoxification. Relative changes in metabolic activity in the frontal cortex were correlated with the intensity of depressive symptoms. These two studies together suggest different metabolic changes in the early and late phases of detoxification. In the early phase there is increased metabolic activity in basal ganglia and orbitofrontal cortex, whereas in the late phase there is decreased metabolic activity in the frontal cortex which persists for at least several months.

Chronic Cocaine Abuse and Neurotransmitter Receptors

Dopamine D2 receptor availability measured using $[^{18}F]N$-methylspiroperidol 1–4 weeks after detoxification was decreased in a group of 10 cocaine abusers compared with normal controls (Volkow *et al.,* 1993; Volkow *et al.,* 1996). These decreases may represent adaptation to dopaminergic overstimulation by chronic exposure to cocaine. A second study of 20 cocaine abusers demonstrated that the decrease in D2 receptor availability was positively correlated with the decreases in glucose metabolism in the frontal cortex (Volkow *et al.,* 1993). No changes were noted between cocaine abusers and control subjects in terms of availability of 5HT2 receptors (Wang *et al.,* 1995).

Distribution of Cocaine in the Primate Brain

Madras has recently reported the results of autoradiographic measurements of cocaine concentrations in the brains of squirrel monkeys 15 min after intravenous administration of $[^{3}H]$cocaine (Madras & Kaufman, 1994).

The autoradiographic measurements were supplemented by thin-layer chromatographic analysis of radioactivity extracted from different brain regions. Although complex and requiring sacrifice of the animals, these studies permitted the distribution of cocaine to be mapped in much greater anatomical detail than is possible in PET studies.

In addition to its high level of localization in caudate nucleus, putamen, and nucleus accumbens/olfactory tubercle, $[^{3}H]$cocaine also localized to a moderate extent in the stria terminalis, medial septum, and substantia nigra/ventral tegmental area. Uptake in these regions was expected on the basis of previous studies of the distribution of cocaine binding sites in primate brains (Biegon *et al.,* 1992; Kaufman, Spealman, & Madras, 1991). In addition, however, moderate $[^{3}H]$cocaine concentrations were found in the locus coeruleus, hippocampus, and amygdala, where norepinephrine is an important neurotransmitter. The cerebellum, which is almost devoid of dopamine transporters, contained the lowest concentration of cocaine, and cortex contained a low-to-moderate concentration. The regional distribution of $[^{3}H]$cocaine administered at a dose which is behaviorally active in squirrel monkeys (0.3 mg/kg) was well correlated with the regional distribution of tracer $[^{3}H]$cocaine (0.001 mg/kg). This observation confirms the relevance of PET studies with high specific activity $[^{11}C]$cocaine to the effects of behaviorally active doses of cocaine (Fowler *et al.,* 1989). In addition the finding that radioactivity in caudate-putamen, cortex, and hippocampus appeared to be about 90% unchanged cocaine was further confirmation that labeled metabolites do not significantly affect PET scans with $[^{11}C]$cocaine in primates (Gatley *et al.,* 1994). However, labeled metabolites did account for approximately 20% and 30% of the tritium in hypothalamus and substantia nigra, respectively. Another important finding was that the regional distribution of $[^{11}C]$cocaine administered *in vivo* to squirrel monkeys was well correlated with the distribution of the cocaine analog $[^{3}H]$WIN 35,428 obtained in *in vitro* autoradiographic experiments in the same species (Kaufman *et al.,* 1991). This supports the use of labeled high-affinity cocaine congeners for *in vitro* studies, when the congeners are experimentally more convenient to use than cocaine.

The main conclusion drawn by Madras and Kaufman (1994) from their study is that cocaine may exert some of its actions through binding to sites in locus coeruleus, amygdala, and hippocampus, as well to brain areas with predominantly dopaminergic innervation. They also pointed out that a good correlation was obtained when the uptake of cocaine in several brain regions was plotted against the cocaine-induced increases in glucose utilization previously found in the same regions of rat brain (Porrino, 1993), which suggests a direct relationship between occupancy of cocaine binding sites and an increase in terminal synaptic activity.

Metabolism

General

Cocaine metabolism proceeds by three major initial transformations: cleavage of the benzoyl ester to give ecgonine methylester, cleavage of the methyl ester to give benzoylecgonine, and N-demethylation to give norcocaine (Inaba, 1989; Stewart, Inaba, Lucassen, & Kalow, 1979). Formation of benzoylecgonine occurs spontaneously at body temperature and blood pH with a half-life of several hr (Garrett & Seyda, 1983). Enzymatically catalyzed cleavage also occurs, in liver and possibly other tissues (Dean, Christian, Sample, & Bosron, 1991). Ecgonine methylester is formed from cocaine by the action of butyrylcholinesterase, which is found in plasma and other tissues (Gatley, 1991; Stewart, Inaba, Tang, & Kalow, 1977). This reaction is probably also catalyzed by other enzymes. Benzoylecgonine is the principal metabolite of cocaine in humans; it accounts for 30%–40% of its urinary excretion, while ecgonine methyl ester accounts for about 20% (Ambre, 1985). Norcocaine is produced in the liver as a result of microsomal mixed-function oxidases. Cocaine induced hepatotoxicity has been linked to the N-oxidative metabolism of cocaine (Roth, Harbison, James, Tobin, & Roberts, 1992). In addition to benzoylecgonine, ecgo-

nine methylester and norcocaine, benzoyl norecgonine, methyl ecgonidine, ecgonine and norecgonine, and other trace metabolites have been identified in urine of cocaine abusers (Peterson, Logan, & Christian, 1995).

Of the three initial cocaine catabolites, ecgonine methylester and benzoylecgonine are not expected to cross the blood brain barrier because of their low lipophilicity, and are also inactive at the dopamine transporter (Ritz, Cone, & Kuhar, 1990). They are thus not expected to contribute to the actions of cocaine on the central nervous system if formed peripherally (Mule, Casella, & Misra, 1976). However, norcocaine does bind to the dopamine transporter (Ritz *et al.*, 1990) and is lipophilic (octanol/water partition coefficient 19 versus 12 for cocaine (Mule *et al.*, 1976); therefore, it is not surprising that it is behaviorally active in a manner similar to cocaine (Hawks, Kopin, Colburn, & Thoa, 1975; Spealman *et al.*, 1979). Thus, norcocaine formed extracerebrally from cocaine could in principle enter the brain and contribute to cocaine's pharmacological actions (Hawks *et al.*, 1975; Spealman *et al.*, 1979).

It has been confirmed using carbon-11 labeled compounds and PET scanning that norcocaine but not ecgonine methyl ester or benzoyl ecgonine can readily enter the primate brain following intravenous injection (Gatley *et al.*, 1990; Gatley *et al.*, 1994). The potential contributions of labeled metabolites to PET images were further addressed by labeling the cocaine molecule in three different positions so that different patterns of labeled metabolites would be produced. The nearly identical brain kinetics for the labeled forms of cocaine indicated that labeled metabolites do not significantly affect PET images of the brain (Gatley *et al.*, 1994). This result also strongly suggests that benzoylecgonine, ecgonine methylester, and norcocaine do not contribute to the subjective effects experienced immediately after intravenous administration of pharmacologically active doses of cocaine.

It is possible, however, that cocaine metabolites contribute to delayed effects of cocaine including toxicity (Erzouki, Allen, Newman, Goldberg, & Schindler, 1995; Madden & Powers, 1990). Benzoylecgonine was found to be a potent contractile agent when tested in an isolated cat cerebral artery model; it caused a 50% reduction in cross-sectional area at a concentration of 10 µM. This was a 10-fold greater effect than found with cocaine. The other major metabolite, ecgonine methylester, had weak relaxing properties.

An issue related to that of pharmacologically active metabolites is the possibility that pyrolysis products formed during crack cocaine smoking might have subjective or toxic properties (Erzouki et al., 1995; Sisti, Fowler, & Fowler, 1989). This is potentially relevant not only to the high potency of smoked cocaine, but also to pulmonary problems such as the fatal bronchoconstriction reported in crack smokers (Rao, Polos, & Walther, 1990). The major pyrolysis products are benzoic acid and methyl ecgonidine (also known as anhydroecgonine methyl ester). In studies with isolated guinea pig tracheal rings, methyl ecgonidine has been demonstrated to antagonize acetylcholine-induced contraction at concentrations as low as 10 nM (El-Fawal & Wood, 1995).

Cocaine and Alcohol

Cocaine abusers frequently consume alcohol during binges. Co-abuse of cocaine and ethanol is associated with detection of significant amounts of the O-ethyl homolog of cocaine, cocaethylene, in urine and post mortem tissue samples (Hearn et al., 1991). Rodent studies have confirmed this finding (Dean, Bosron, Zachman, Zhang, & Brzezinski, 1996). Cocaethylene is formed by a transesterification reaction between cocaine and ethanol; a human liver enzyme which catalyzes this reaction, and also the formation of benzoylecgonine when ethanol is absent, has been purified and characterized (Brzezinski, Abraham, Stone, Dean, & Bosron, 1994). Cocaine and cocaethylene bind with similar affinities to the dopamine transporter, and equimolar doses of the two drugs raise extracellular dopamine in the caudate nucleus to the same extent (Iyer, Nobiletti, Jatlow, & Bradberry, 1995). However, cocaethylene is more lethal in animal models (Hearn et al., 1991; Meehan & Schechter, 1995). The recog-

nition of cocaethylene as a contingent metabolite of cocaine prompted a number of further studies, because it may be relevant to the greater toxicity of cocaine when it is coabused with alcohol (Farre et al., 1993). The effects of cocaine may be increased because in the presence of alcohol some of the inactive metabolite benzoylecgonine is replaced by the active metabolite cocaethylene. A further hypothesis is that cocaethylene, although pharmacologically similar to cocaine, might have a longer tissue residence time, and thus more time to damage organs. This possibility was addressed by preparing [^{11}C]cocaethylene and comparing its distribution in baboon brain to that of [^{11}C]cocaine after intravenous injection (Fowler, Volkow, MacGregor, et al., 1992). Distribution volumes (Logan et al., 1990) for the two radioactive drugs were identical in striatum but significantly greater for cocaethylene in thalamus, cerebellum, and whole brain. In addition, the rate of debenzoylation of cocaethylene in baboon plasma was found to be about one third that of cocaine (Fowler, Volkow, MacGregor, et al., 1992). The slower clearance of cocaethylene could thus lead to accentuated physiological effects relative to cocaine. However, the maximum differences between the two drugs in terms of brain clearance were only about 50%. Another conjecture, that alcohol might increase the exposure of tissues to cocaine by slowing its clearance, was also examined using PET. However, alcohol intoxication (1 g/kg) did not alter the pharmacokinetics of [^{11}C]cocaine in human brain or heart (Fowler, Volkow, Logan, et al., 1992). Furthermore, labeled cocaethylene was not detected in the subjects' blood at 10 min after administration of [^{11}C]cocaine, which is consistent with other studies (Perez-Reyes & Jeffcoat, 1992). It is possible that cocaethylene is formed more readily from pharmacological doses of cocaine than tracer doses, or that the enzyme responsible for transesterification of cocaine is inducible and therefore present in greater activities after chronic abuse.

The results of these PET studies suggested that the enhanced behavioral and toxic properties of cocaine and alcohol when they are coadministered largely result from direct actions of the two drugs, rather than from a pharmacokinetic interaction or via formation of cocaethylene. This direct action might be mediated by the dopamine system, because both cocaine and alcohol increase brain extracellular dopamine (Di Chiara & Imperato, 1988). Similarly, alcohol has an acute stimulatory effect on the sympathetic nervous system (Rall, 1993), which could act synergistically with that caused by cocaine's blockade of the norepinephrine transporter (Ritz et al., 1990). Other observations, such as the increased toxicity of amphetamine and alcohol after co-administration (Rech, Vomachka, Rickert, & Braude, 1976) and the enhanced lethality of cocaethylene itself when alcohol is co-administered (Meehan & Schechter, 1995), argue against a large role for cocaethylene in mediating the effects of alcohol on the toxicity of cocaine.

Mechanism of Action

Inhibition of the Dopamine Transporter

Cocaine blocks reuptake of the monoamine neurotransmitters, dopamine, norepinephrine, and serotonin (Table 2). Cocaine also affects other processes involved in nervous transmission, including sodium channels, muscarinic and glutamate receptors, and butyrylcholinesterase (Gatley, 1991; Ritchie & Greene, 1985; Sharkey, Glen, Wolfe, & Kuhar, 1988; Sharkey, Ritz, Schenden, Hanson, &

Kuhar, 1988; Turkanis, Partlow, & Karler, 1989), although these occur at higher concentrations than the inhibition of serotonin or dopamine uptake. The reinforcing efficacies of psychostimulant drugs have been shown to be better correlated with their abilities to block the dopamine transporter than with their actions at norepinephrine and serotonin transporter (Calligaro & Eldefrawi, 1988; Ritz, Lamb, Goldbeg, & Kuhar, 1987). During the last decade it has become increasingly accepted that cocaine's subjective and behavioral effects are largely caused by inhibition of the dopamine transporter (Galloway, 1988; Johanson & Fischman, 1989; Kennedy & Hanbauer, 1983). In vivo microdialysis experiments (e.g., Table 3) have shown that psychostimulant drugs elevate extracellular dopamine in terminal dopaminergic fields including the nucleus accumbens (Butcher, Liptrot, & Aburthnot, 1991; Hurd & Ungerstedt, 1989), where iontophoretic application of dopamine (Guerin, Goeders, Dworkin, & Smith, 1984) or reuptake blockers (Carlezon, Devine, & Wise, 1995) also activates reward circuits. Furthermore, the concentration of cocaine in striatum has been shown to parallel that of elevated extracellular dopamine (Hurd & Ungerstedt, 1989; Pettit, Pan, Parsons, & Justice, 1990). The recent demonstration that dopamine transporter "knock out" mice exhibit hyperlocomotion and are insensitive to cocaine has provided important new support for the view that the transporter is the critical target (Giros, Jaber, Jones, Wightman, & Caron, 1996). On a

TABLE 2. Inhibition Constants (Ki Values, μM) of Cocaine at Dopamine, Norepinephrine, and 5-Hydroxytryptamine Transporter

Drug	Study	Ki value (μM) at reuptake site		
		DA	NE	5HT
Cocaine	1[a]	0.64	1.6	0.14
	2[b]	0.12	1.5	0.13

[a]Ritz et al. (1987).
[b]Gatley, Pan, et al. (1996).
Values obtained in other studies can be found in Seeman (1993).
 Cocaine is more potent at the 5HT and dopamine reuptake sites
 than the norepinephrine site.

TABLE 3. Kinetics of the Rise in Extracellular Dopamine Measured by Microdialysis for Different Routes of Administration of Cocaine

Route	Time to peak (min)	Clearance half-time (min)
Intravenous[a]	<10	30–45
Intraperitoneal[b]	20–30	60
Subcutaneous[c]	40–60	60–90

[a]Di Chiara & Imperato (1988).
[b]Nicolaysen et al. (1988).
[c]Lienau & Kuschinsky (1997).

neuroanatomical level the reinforcing properties of cocaine are believed to be mediated by
dopamine transporters on mesolimbic, rather
than mesostriatal, nerve terminals.

Amphetamine and related compounds share
many of cocaine's actions, but act by releasing
dopamine via the transporter, rather than by
blocking its reuptake (Braestrup, 1977). The
behavioral and dopamine-enhancing effects of
cocaine, unlike those of amphetamine, are sensitive to reserpine and inhibition of calcium influx, suggesting that increases in extracellular
dopamine caused by cocaine are vesicular
rather than cytoplasmic in origin.

Neurophysiology

The effects of cocaine on neuronal activity
have been examined in several regions of the
brain. In the case of the dopamine terminal regions these studies have involved applying cocaine directly onto cells in the nucleus
accumbens and corpus striatum in anesthetized
rats (Qiao, Dougherty, Wiggins, & Dafney,
1990; F. J. White, Hu, & Henry, 1993). These
investigations have revealed that cocaine has
an inhibitory influence on neurotransmission
that appears to result from a local potentiation
of dopamine levels (F. J. White *et al.*, 1993).
As expected for a dopamine uptake inhibitor,
cocaine will also enhance the inhibitory effects
of exogenously applied dopamine (Uchimura
& North, 1990). However, the previously men-

tioned studies indicating an inhibitory action
of cocaine in dopamine terminal regions contrast with those obtained in the nucleus accumbens of awake rats self-administering
intravenous cocaine, where no direct inhibitory
pharmacological effects resulting from the actions of cocaine were observed (Carelli, King,
Hampson, & Deadwyler, 1993).

The effects of cocaine on the activity of
monoaminergic neurons in the ventral tegmental area, locus coeruleus, and dorsal raphe
nucleus have been better established. In the
ventral tegmental area, intravenously applied
cocaine produces an inhibition of the activity
of dopamine neurons (Einhorn, Johansen, &
White, 1988). This appears to be a result of
activation of negative feedback mechanisms
resulting from elevation of extracellular dopamine levels. In the norepinephrine neurons in
the locus coeruleus and serotonin neurons in
the dorsal raphe nucleus, systemically administered cocaine also has an inhibitory effect on
activity, although in these cases the inhibition
is mediated by its elevation of extracellular
norepinephrine and serotonin levels, respectively (Lakoski & Cunningham, 1988; Pitts &
Marwah, 1987).]

Structure–Activity Relationships

The molecular structures of several dopamine
transport inhibitors are shown in Figure 2.

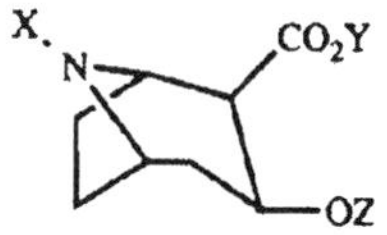

Compound	Group		
	X	Y	Z
cocaine	CH_3	CH_3	benzoyl
norcocaine	H	CH_3	benzoyl
benzoylecgonine	CH_3	H	benzoyl
ecgonine methylester	CH_3	CH_3	H
cocaethylene	CH_3	C_2H_5	benzoyl

FIGURE 2. Cocaine metabolites.

Cocaine Analogs

Many compounds that are structural analogs of cocaine have been investigated. Cocaethylene and norcocaine possess reinforcing properties similar to cocaine and have similar affinity for the dopamine transporter (Hawks et al., 1975; Hearn et al., 1991; Ritz et al., 1990; Spealman et al., 1979). However, cocaethylene has a lower affinity than cocaine for the serotonin transporter, whereas norcocaine has a higher affinity for the serotonin transporter. Benzoylecgonine does not inhibit dopamine transport (Ritz et al., 1990). Substitution of a fluorine or iodine atom on the para position of the aromatic ring has little effect on affinity for the dopamine transporter, while substitution of iodine at the meta or ortho positions decreased affinity (Gatley et al., 1994; Yu et al., 1992). Cocaine analogs with a methoxy group substituted on the 6 or 7 position of the tropane ring are weaker inhibitors of synaptosomal dopamine transport than of the binding of [^{3}H]mazindol (Simoni et al., 1993); it has been suggested that they might be weak "cocaine antagonists."

A cocaine analog having a direct linkage between the tropane and phenyl rings in place of the benzoyl ester linkage (WIN 35, 065) was reported in 1973, together with several related compounds bearing substituents on the phenyl group (Clarke et al., 1973). WIN 35,428, the para-fluorophenyl compound of this series, appears to have been the most heavily investigated of the phenyltropanes, both as an experimental drug (Spealman, Kelleher, & Goldberg, 1983) and as a radiotracer in the tritiated and carbon-11 labeled forms (Frost et al., 1993; Madras, 1994; Madras, Fahey, Bergman, Canfield, & Spealman, 1989). It is about 10-fold more potent than cocaine in in vitro assays of the dopamine transporter (Ki ≅ 10 nM and 100 nM, respectively) (Gatley, Pan, Chen, Charurvedi, & Ding, 1996; Ritz et al., 1990). Since the original report of the WIN compounds, additional members of the series have been prepared. The most potent so far described is the 3,4-dichlorophenyl compound (Carroll, Lewin, Boja, & Kuhar, 1992), but the para-iodophenyl congener (termed RTI-55 or β-CIT) is also very potent (Ki = 1–2 nM), and in radioiodinated forms has been extensively used as a radioligand for both dopamine and serotonin transporters (Boja et al., 1990; Boja et al., 1991; Laruelle et al., 1993).

The direct phenyltropane linkage in the WIN compounds reduces their susceptibility to metabolic degradation, since the benzoyl ester functionality in cocaine is readily hydrolyzed by plasma and liver enzymes. More recently, cocaine analogs have been described with high affinities for the dopamine and/or the serotonin transporter which are WIN compounds further modified to bear an alkyl ketone group on the 2β position. They thus lack the methyl ester as well as the benzoyl ester, and are presumably even more metabolically stable (Davies, Saikali, Sexton, & Childers, 1993). Other recent studies have shown that the dopamine transporter has a relatively high tolerance for substituents on both the 2β position and the nitrogen atom (Kosikowski, Salah, Johnson, & Bergmann, 1995).

Other Dopamine Transporter Inhibitors

Benztropine, a muscarinic antagonist drug, is also a potent dopamine reuptake blocker. Benztropine has a diphenylmethyl ether substituent in the 3α position of the tropane ring, in place of cocaine's 3β benzoyloxy substituent, but a hydrogen in place of the 2β carbomethoxy substituent on carbon atom 2 (Figure 3). Recently, the effect of adding the 2β carbomethoxy group was investigated (Meltzer, Liang, Brownell, Elmaleh, & Madras, 1993; Meltzer, Liang, & Madras, 1994). Remarkably, the most active compound (difluoropine) was stereochemically related to the inactive (+)-cocaine, rather than to the naturally occurring (−)-cocaine.

Besides cocaine and other compounds containing the tropane ring substructure, many other structurally distinct compounds bind to the dopamine transporter and block dopamine reuptake. They include bupropion, pyrovalerone, pemoline, methylphenidate, nomifensine, mazindol, BTCP, LR5182 (Wong &

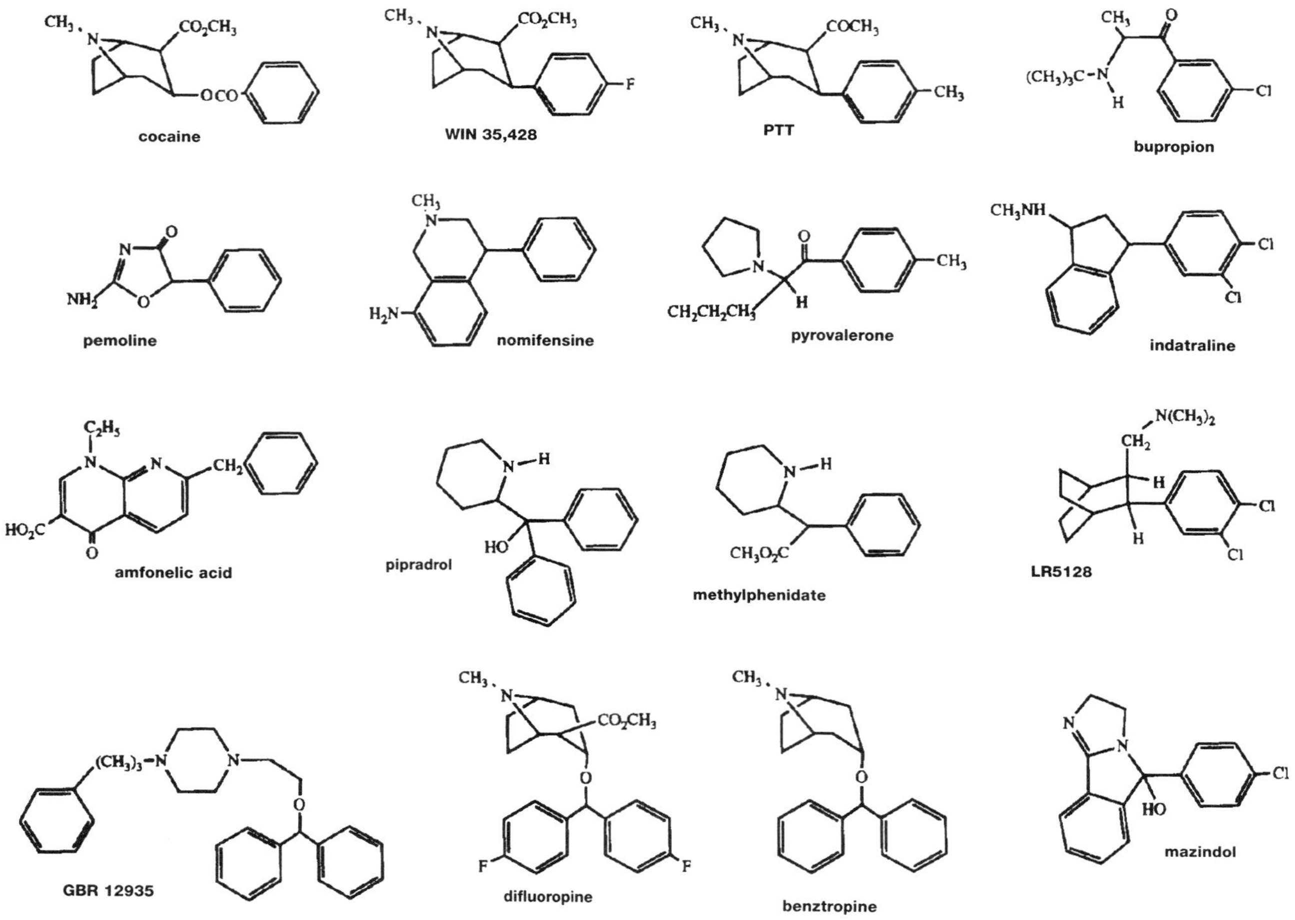

FIGURE 3. Structures of cocaine and some other dopamine transport inhibitors.

Bymaster, 1978), amfonelic acid, and GBR 12909. In recent years, medicinal chemists have synthesized derivatives of most of these parent structures as part of the search for effective pharmacotherapies of cocaine abuse. Currently, known dopamine transport inhibitors with high (submicromolar) affinity probably number in the several hundreds.

Search for a Cocaine "Antagonist" or "Partial Agonist"

Some dopamine reuptake blockers are commonly prescribed therapeutic drugs. They include mazindol, which has anorectic properties, and methylphenidate which is given to millions of American children for attention-deficit/hyperactivity disorder. Mazindol does not appear to have rewarding properties in humans (Chait, Uhlenhuth, & Johanson, 1987), but methylphenidate is sometimes abused by the intravenous route (Parran & Jasinski, 1991). Cocaine abusers given intravenous methylphenidate under experimental conditions report that the "high" from the two drugs is almost identical (Volkow, Ding, et al., 1995; Wang et al., 1996). The various classes of dopamine (DA) reuptake blockers differ in terms of pharmacokinetic profiles, pharmacological specificities, and affinity for the dopamine transporter. These differences may account for their diverse apparent abuse potentials in humans. However, it has also been suggested that the abuse potentials of these drugs may depend on their detailed interactions with the transporter. Rothman proposed that DA reuptake inhibitors could be classified into two groups (Rothman, 1990). Type 1 inhibitors (including cocaine and methylphenidate) produce euphoria and addiction in humans. Type 2 inhibitors (including benztropine, mazindol, nomifensine, and bupropion) do not. This categorization implies that drug binding sites on the transporter can differ from each other and from the dopamine binding site. The type 2 inhibitors might be "partial agonists" which would induce a smaller rise in synaptic dopamine at a particular degree of occupancy of the transporter than the type 1 inhibitors. In that case the type 2 inhibitors might be thera-

peutically useful, since by displacing cocaine from its binding site they would be able to mitigate the elevation in dopamine caused by cocaine. Several observations have supported the possibility that the dopamine and cocaine binding sites are distinct, including:

1. GBR 12909 given ip attenuated the rise in rat striatal extracellular dopamine concentration after administration of cocaine by means of the microdialysis probe (Rothman et al., 1991).
2. The Ki value for [^{3}H]cocaine displacement by dopamine depended on the dopamine concentration, leading to the suggestion that cocaine and dopamine binding sites are distinct and that dopamine can be considered an allosteric modulator which stabilizes the transporter in a low-affinity state for cocaine (Calligaro & Eldefrawi, 1988).
3. Binding requirements of [^{125}I]RTI-55 binding to the dopamine transporter (DAT) differed from those of dopamine, in that it was inhibited by low pH and insensitive to chloride ion concentration (Wall, Innis, & Rudnick, 1993).
4. Inhibition of the specific binding of [^{3}H]mazindol (Johnson, Bergmann, & Kozikowski, 1992) to the dopamine transporter was completely protected by 10 μM cocaine, but unaffected by 300 μM dopamine or amphetamine (Johnson et al., 1992).
5. Mazindol, GBR 12935, bupropion, nomifensine, and benztropine inhibited the spontaneous efflux of dopamine from cells transfected with the dopamine transporter, whereas phencyclidine, cocaine, methylphenidate, and WIN 35438 had no effect on efflux (Eshleman, Henningsen, Neve, & Janowsky, 1994).
6. Molecular biological studies of the dopamine transporter have established that an aspartate residue in hydrophobic domain 1 and two serine residues in hydrophobic domain 7 are critical to transporter function. Whereas mutations in the domain 1 aspartate greatly decreased both [^{3}H]dopamine

and [^{3}H]WIN 35428 binding, mutations in the domain 7 serines had a large effect on uptake but only a weak effect on binding (Kitayama *et al.*, 1992).

7. Most binding studies with [^{3}H]cocaine and cocaine analogs indicate the existence of 2 binding sites in striatal tissue (Calligaro & Eldefrawi, 1988; Madras, Fahey, *et al.*, 1989; Madras, Spealman, *et al.*, 1989). The same protein is believed to be responsible for the two binding sites detected with cocaine and other tropane compounds, since a single cDNA causes expression of both sites in transfected human cells (Boja *et al.*, 1992; Pristupa, Nelson, Hoffman, Kish, & Niznik, 1994). In contrast to cocaine and its congeners, [^{3}H]mazindol appears to bind only to a single site (Johnson *et al.*, 1992).

8. Studies of the cloned and native human DAT have indicated that [^{3}H]WIN 35428 and [^{3}H]GBR 12935 do not bind to the same functional form or state of the DAT, since the rank order of Ki values for various other dopamine transport inhibitors varied, and also inhibitors varied in whether binding curves indicated the presence of 1 or 2 binding sites (Pristupa *et al.*, 1994).

9. *In vitro* kinetic studies of dopamine uptake by striatal synaptosomal suspensions using rotating disk voltammetry have suggested that cocaine does not bind to the dopamine site on the transporter, but to a sodium ion site (McElvain & Schenk, 1992).

These studies, which suggest differences among reuptake inhibitors and substrates in terms of binding sites on the dopamine transporter, have encouraged the search for compounds that might be able to prevent the binding of cocaine without blocking reuptake of dopamine. Many compounds have been screened for such "cocaine antagonist" activity using assays of synaptosomal [^{3}H]dopamine uptake and *in vitro* radioligand binding. These studies have so far failed to identify compounds that exhibit large discrepancies between Ki values for binding and uptake, although modest "discrimination ratios" (Deutsch & Schweri, 1994) of up to about sixfold have been reported. Compounds with Ki values for inhibition of DA uptake larger than expected from the Ki values for radioligand binding include, with radioligand(s) shown in parenthesis, two cocaine derivatives substituted with methoxy groups on the tropane-ring ([^{3}H]mazindol)(Simoni *et al.*, 1993); the N,N-dibutyl derivative of 1-(2-benzo[b]thienyl)-cyclohexylamine ([^{3}H]cocaine and [^{3}H]BTCP) (He, Raymon, Mattson, Eldefrawi, & DeCosta, 1993); the isopropyl ester analog of RTI-55 ([^{3}H]WIN 35,428) (Carroll *et al.*, 1995); and p-methoxymethylphenidate ([^{3}H]WIN 35,428) (Gatley, Pan, *et al.*, 1996). However, the results for p-methoxymethylphenidate were not confirmed by other workers using different assay conditions (Deutsch, Shi, Gruszecka-Kowalik, & Schweri, 1996). Discrepant binding and uptake data should not be accepted as indicating cocaine antagonist properties unless other possible explanations can be excluded. For example, since the uptake and binding assays are usually done under different conditions (Rothman *et al.*, 1993), a drug could bind to low-affinity but high-capacity "non-specific" sites in the uptake assay system to a greater extent than in the binding assay system. This could decrease the free concentration available to bind to the transporter in the uptake assay system, and thus increase the observed IC$_{50}$. Another possibility is that compounds could interact with other binding sites in synaptosomes that modulate the reuptake rate or otherwise alter the net uptake of dopamine.

The dopamine transporter is a complex molecule that transports in a concerted manner two sodium ions, a chloride ion, and a dopamine molecule across the neuronal membranes (McElvain & Schenk, 1992). It is easy to see that even small perturbations in its tertiary structure caused by interactions of other molecules at any of its binding sites could interfere with transport. Thus, despite the fact that dopamine and cocaine do not bind to precisely the same site on the transporter, it is not obvious that binding of cocaine and transport of dopamine are dissociable to a significant degree. In fact, binding and uptake are well correlated for dopamine transporter ligands of all known structural classes of such compounds, including cocaine, WIN compounds, GBR compounds, benztropine, nomifensine, mazindol and methylphenidate (Deutsch et al., 1996; Gatley, Pan, et al., 1996; Ritz et al., 1987). Furthermore, competition studies have indicated that DA, cocaine, WIN 35428, mazindol, BTCP, and GBR 12935 share a common binding region in mouse striatum (Reith, DeCosta, Rice, & Jacobson, 1992). It is too soon to totally discount the possibility of the discovery of a drug which is able to inhibit cocaine binding much more than dopamine reuptake. However, given the number and diversity of compounds already investigated, it appears less likely than it did in 1990 (Rothman, 1990) that a compound with cocaine antagonist properties will be developed from currently known structural types. At present, therefore, it seems more likely that the differences between type 1 and type 2 inhibitors result from pharmacokinetic factors, effects on other neurotransmitter systems, or both.

In Vivo Studies with Dopamine Transporter Inhibitors

Some in vivo studies also suggest that type 2 inhibitors have partial agonist properties. For example, intraperitoneally administered GBR 12909 was found to attenuate the increase in rat striatal extracellular dopamine caused by locally applied cocaine (Rothman et al., 1991). However, the partial agonist explanation for these results has been challenged. Gifford, Bergmann, and Johnson (1993) found that GBR 12909 did not antagonize the effects of cocaine on efflux of dopamine from superfused rat striatal slices, and also that GBR 12909 inhibited uptake of DA by striatal synaptosomes in a competitive manner. Two alternative explanations were proposed for the 1991 results of Rothman and colleagues (Gifford et al., 1993). First, the dopamine compartment(s) labeled by [³H]dopamine in synaptosomes and tissue slices might be different from the compartment(s) probed by mi-

crodialysis. Second, GBR 12909 administered systemically might attenuate the nigrostriatal neuronal firing rate, for example by raising extracellular dopamine in the substantia nigra and activating impulse-regulating autoreceptors. This would have the consequence of decreasing the elevation of extracellular dopamine by topically administered cocaine, since to increase dopamine levels by cocaine, firing of the dopaminergic neurons must be maintained. Another possible explanation for the results of Rothman and colleagues (1991) has been advanced by Reith, Coffey, Xu, and Chen (1994), who found that GBR 12909 and GBR 12935 are potent (10-fold weaker than synaptosomal) inhibitors of dopamine uptake into brain synaptic vesicles. In contrast, cocaine is a thousand-fold weaker inhibitor of synaptic uptake than of nerve terminal uptake. Inhibition of vesicular uptake could in part account for the attenuation of cocaine's elevation of extracellular DA by GBR 12909, because exocytotic release may be occurring from partially depleted vesicles (Reith et al., 1994). These studies (Gifford et al., 1993; Reith et al., 1994; Rothman et al., 1991) show that apparent partial agonism of cocaine might be caused by a variety of mechanisms. Developing a better understanding of the behavior of high-affinity dopamine reuptake blockers in vivo might lead to drugs with useful therapeutic properties based on interactions at other neurochemical sites.

In another in vivo study interpreted to support partial agonism, cocaine, WIN 35,428, or nomifensine were reported to maximally stimulate rat locomotor activity with transporter occupancies of 60%, whereas, for GBR 12783, total occupancy was required for maximum locomotor activity (Rothman et al., 1992). The experimental design involved injection of animals with the test drug 15 min before injection of [³H]BTCP, and sacrifice after a further 15 min. The degree of occupancy was calculated by comparing the specific binding of [³H]BTCP in the striatum with that of control animals. However, in experiments of this kind, the degree of displacement of radioligand binding by the test drug depends on several factors including the pharmacokinetics and the binding kinetics of the radioligand and the test drug, and the time of sacrifice. GBR 12909 may indicate a higher occupancy than cocaine because of its much higher affinity for the transporter, relative to the radioligand. Similar considerations presumably explain recent results of mouse experiments in our laboratory in which nonradioactive cocaine and RTI-55 were used as test drugs (Gatley, Volkow, *et al.*, 1996). When [^{123}I]RTI-55 was used as the radioligand, both cocaine and RTI-55 failed to produce a significant displacement of [^{123}I]RTI-55, but when [^{3}H]cocaine was used as radioligand, displacements of 40% and 70%, respectively, were measured. Thus the results of occupancy experiments clearly depend on relative affinities of test drug and radioligand, as well as other factors.

To date, attempts to treat cocaine abusers with other dopamine transporter blockers have not met with success. The type 1 inhibitor methylphenidate was found to lack therapeutic efficacy for treating cocaine abuse, and in fact led to increased craving and cocaine consumption (Gawin, Riordan, & Kleber, 1985). The type 2 inhibitor mazindol did not differ in efficacy from placebo in a recent 6-week-long double-blind study (Stine, Krystal, Kosten, & Charney, 1995). Furthermore, pretreatment with 2 mg mazindol did not decrease the subjective effects of cocaine (Preston, Sullivan, Berger, & Bigelow, 1993). The results of these studies suggest that treatment of cocaine abusers with drugs that partially block the dopamine transporters does not remove the incentive to self-administer cocaine. However, it is possible that maintenance of partial occupancy of the transporter with an appropriate drug might have a therapeutically beneficial effect via other mechanisms, such as reducing craving.

Behavioral Sensitization to Cocaine

Unlike the situation with opioid receptor agonists, psychostimulants are less generally associated with the phenomenon of tolerance, in which abusers escalate drug doses. In rodents repeated daily injections of cocaine results in a progressive enhancement of its locomotor- and stereotypy-inducing effects (Post & Rose, 1976). This process is called behavioral sensitization or reverse tolerance. A similar phenomenon occurs with repeated injection in rodents of other direct and indirect dopamine agonists such as apomorphine and amphetamine, and of opioid receptor agonists (Vezina & Stewart, 1989). Behavioral sensitization to cocaine and other stimulant drugs has been intensively studied with the idea that its underlying changes may be the same as those accounting for the drug-induced paranoid schizophrenia-like psychotic episodes that often develop in humans with the repeated use of cocaine or amphetamine (Connell, 1958; Post, 1975).

Studies of behavioral sensitization to cocaine have examined the nature of the neurochemical changes resulting in sensitization and the mechanism and locus for these changes. The progressive enhancement in the behavioral response to repeated injections of cocaine does not appear to be a result of a decreased rate of metabolism of this drug in sensitized animals (Nayak, Misra, & Mule, 1976; Reith, Benuck, & Lajtha, 1987), although see Cass and Zahniser (1993). It is thus thought that the enhanced behavioral response to cocaine is a result of an upregulation in the functioning of the dopamine system itself, resulting either from a presynaptic increase in dopamine release or a postsynaptic supersensitivity to dopamine. On the postsynaptic side, some evidence has been obtained that neurons in the nucleus accumbens and corpus striatum are supersensitive to dopamine in sensitized animals (Henry & White, 1991; S. R. White, Harris, Imel, & Wheaton, 1995). However, the literature on whether cocaine-sensitized animals show an increased behavioral response to apomorphine and amphetamine, which would be expected if there was a postsynaptic supersensitivity to dopamine, is controversial (Hoffman & Wise, 1993; Shuster, Yu, & Bates, 1977; Ujike, Akiyama, & Otsuki, 1990). There is more evidence for an increase in the cocaine-induced elevation of extracellular dopamine levels in the accumbens and striatum as the mechanism for sensitization (Akimoto, Hamamura, & Otsuki, 1989; Pettit *et al.,* 1990). A number of investigations have been carried out to determine whether this enhancement is a result of a decreased functioning of the negative feedback mechanisms that serve to regulate the levels of extracellular dopamine in the accumbens and striatum. These studies have indicated that terminal release-regulating DA autoreceptors are probably not subsensitive in cocaine-sensitized animals (Fitzgerald & Reid, 1991; Gifford & Johnson, 1992). There is, however, some evidence for a subsensitivity of impulse-regulating DA autoreceptors in sensitized animals (Henry, Greene, & White, 1989), although the duration of the impulse-regulating autoreceptor subsensitivity after cocaine sensitization and that observed after amphetamine sensitization appear to be short relative to that of the sensitization phenomenon (Ackerman & White, 1990; Wolf & Jeziorski, 1993; Wolf, White, Nassar, Brooderson, & Khansa, 1993); the latter can still be observed many months after daily cocaine or amphetamine treatments have ended (Shuster *et al.,* 1977).

Studies designed to elucidate the molecular targets responsible for translating the repeated injections of cocaine into an eventual upregulated behavioral and neurochemical response to this drug have implicated N-methyl-D-aspartate (NMDA) receptors as essential, since injection of NMDA antagonists immediately prior to the daily cocaine injections effectively blocks the development of behavioral sensitization (Karler, Calder, Chaudhry, & Turkanis, 1989; Wolf & Jeziorski, 1993). In addition to NMDA antagonists, some studies have reported that dopamine receptor antagonists also block the development of sensitization to amphetamine and cocaine (Karler, Calder, & Bedingfield, 1994; Vezina & Stewart, 1989), although this was not confirmed by another study (Mattingly, Hart, Lim, & Perkins, 1994). As for the locus of action of cocaine in inducing behavioral sensitization, accumulating evidence implicates the ventral tegmental area (VTA) as the primary area. Thus, injections of NMDA antagonists or protein synthesis inhibitors directly into this region immediately prior to the daily cocaine injections attenuate or block the development of sensitization (Kalivas & Alesdatter, 1993; Sorg & Ulibarri, 1995). Conversely, daily amphetamine injections directly into the VTA have been found to produce a sensitized response when the animals were subsequently given systemically administered cocaine (Kalivas & Weber, 1988).

Withdrawal and Dysphoria

It has been suggested that the dysphoric state (the "crash") induced by withdrawal of dependent individuals from chronic exposure to cocaine results from decreased synaptic dopamine (Dackis & Gold, 1985). Such a decrease could involve a persistence of an elevation in the concentration of dopamine transporters, or of kinetic upregulation of the transporters caused by chronic cocaine. The available data are confusing on this issue. Some investigators have documented decreased radioligand binding to the rat accumbens dopamine transporter in withdrawal (Sharpe, Pilotte, Mitchell, & DeSouza, 1991), and in postmortem striatum from cocaine abusers (Hurd & Herkenham, 1993). In contrast, increased high-affinity binding of the cocaine congener RTI-55 has been reported in postmortem brains of cocaine abusers (Staley, Hearn, Ruttenber, Wetli, & Mash, 1994). Studies of dopamine uptake in synaptosomes prepared from cocaine-treated rats have also given conflicting results (Izenwasser & Cox, 1990; Masserano, Venable, & Wyatt, 1994). Furthermore, although microdialysis experiments have indicated no change in extracellular dopamine in the rat nucleus accumbens 1 day after withdrawal from chronic cocaine treatment (Parsons & Justice, 1994), the data did indicate a reduced resistance to diffusion of extracellular dopamine, and after 10 days, extracellular dopamine was reduced to about half the concentration in control rats (Parsons & Justice, 1994). These observations suggest that other factors besides the concentration of dopamine transporters can affect extracellular dopamine during withdrawal.

The recent finding that the dopamine D2 receptor antagonist haloperidol decreased cocaine craving and anxiety provoked by cocaine-related cues suggests that craving is associated with increased, rather than decreased, dopamine (Berger *et al.*, 1996).

ACKNOWLEDGMENTS

This work was carried out at Brookhaven National Laboratory under contract DE-AC02-76CH00016 with the U.S. Department of Energy and supported by its Office of Health and Environmental Research. The research was also supported by the National Institute on Drug Abuse (DA 06278 and DA 09490).

References

Ackerman, J. M., & White, F. J. (1990). A10 somatodendritic dopamine autoreceptor sensitivity following withdrawal from repeated cocaine treatment. *Neuroscience Letters, 117*, 181–187.

Akimoto, K., Hamamura, T., & Otsuki, S. (1989). Subchronic cocaine treatment enhances cocaine induced dopamine efflux, studied by in vivo intracerebral dialysis. *Brain Research, 490*, 339–344.

Ambre, J. (1985). The urinary excretion of cocaine and metabolites in humans: A kinetic analysis of published data. *Journal of Analytic Toxicology, 9*, 241–245.

Balster, R. L., & Schuster, C. R. (1973). Fixed-interval schedule of cocaine reinforcement: Effect of dose and infusion duration. *Journal of Experimental and Analytic Behavior, 20*, 119–129.

Barnet, G., Hawks, R., & Resnick, R. (1981). Cocaine pharmacokinetics in humans. *Journal of Ethnopharmacology, 3*, 353–366.

Berger, S. P., Hall, S., Mickalian, J. D., Reid, M. S., Crawford, C. A., Delucchi, K., Carr, K., & Hall, S. (1996). Haloperidol antagonism of cue-elicited cocaine craving. *Lancet, 347*, 504–508.

Biegon, A., Dillon, K., Volkow, N. D., Hitzemann, R. J., Fowler, J. S., & Wolf, A. P. (1992). Quantitative autoradiography of cocaine binding sites in human brain postmortem. *Synapse, 10*, 126–130.

Boja, J. W., Carroll, F. I., Rahman, M. A., Philip, A., Lewin, A. H., & Kuhar, M. J. (1990). New, potent cocaine analogs: Ligand binding and transport studies in rat striatum. *European Journal of Pharmacology, 184*, 329–332.

Boja, J. W., Patel, A., Carroll, F. I., Rahman, M. A., Philip, A., Lewin, A., Kopajtic, T. A., & Kuhar, M. J. (1991). [^{125}I]RTI-55: A potent ligand for dopamine transporters. *European Journal of Pharmacology, 194*, 133–134.

Boja, J. W., Markham, L., Patel, A., Uhl, G., & Kuhar, M. J. (1992). Expression of a single dopamine transporter cDNA can confer two cocaine binding sites. *Neuroreport, 3*, 247–248.

Braestrup, C. (1977). Biochemical differentiation of amphetamine vs methylphenidate and nomifensine in rats. *Journal of Pharmacy and Pharmacology, 26*, 463–470.

Brzezinski, M. R., Abraham, T. R., Stone, C. L., Dean, R. A., & Bosron, W. F. (1994). Purification and characterization of a human liver cocaine carboxylesterase that catalyzes the production of benzoylecgonine and the formation of cocaethylene from alcohol and cocaine. *Biochemical Pharmacology, 48*, 1747–1755.

Butcher, S., Liptrot, J., & Aburthnot, G. (1991). Characterization of methylphenidate and nomifensine induced dopamine release in rat striatum using in vivo brain microdialysis. *Neuroscience Letters, 122*, 245–248.

Calligaro, D. O., & Eldefrawi, M. E. (1988). High affinity stereospecific binding of [^{3}H]cocaine in striatum and its relationship to the dopamine transporter. *Membrane Biochemistry, 7*, 87–106.

Carelli, R. M., King, V. C., Hampson, R. E., & Deadwyler, S. A. (1993). Firing patterns of nucleus accumbens neurons during cocaine self-administration in rats. *Brain Research, 626*, 14–22.

Carlezon, W. A., Devine, D. P., & Wise, R. A. (1995). Habit-forming actions of nomifensine in nucleus accumbens. *Psychopharmacology, 122*, 194–197.

Carroll, F. I., Lewin, A. H., Boja, J. W., & Kuhar, M. J. (1992). Cocaine receptor: Biochemical characterization and structure–activity relationships of cocaine analogues at the dopamine transporter. *Journal of Medicinal Chemistry, 35*, 969–981.

Carroll, F. I., Kotian, P., Dehghani, A., Gray, J. L., Kuzemko, M. A., Parham, K. A., Abraham, P., Lewin, A. H., Boja, J. W., & Kuhar, M. J. (1995). Cocaine and 3b-(4′-substituted phenyl)tropane-2b-carboxylic acid ester and amide analogues: New high-affinity and selective compounds for the dopamine transporter. *Journal of Medicinal Chemistry, 38*, 379–388.

Cass, W. A., & Zahniser, N. R. (1993). Cocaine levels in striatum and nucleus accumbens: Augmentation following challenge injection in rats withdrawn from repeated cocaine administration. *Neuroscience Letters, 152*, 177–180.

Chait, L. D., Uhlenhuth, E. H., & Johanson, C. E. (1987). Reinforcing and subjective effects of several anorectics in normal human volunteers. *Journal of Pharmacology and Experimental Therapeutics, 242*, 777–783.

Chiueh, C. C., & Kopin, I. J. (1978). Endogenous epinephrine and norepinephrine from the synpathoadrenal medullary system of unanesthetized rats. *Journal of Pharmacology and Experimental Therapeutics, 205*, 14–154.

Chow, M. J., Ambre, J. J., Ruo, T. I., Atkinson, A. J., Bowsher, D. J., & Fischman, M. W. (1985). Kinetics of cocaine distribution, elimination and chronotropic effects. *Clinical Pharmacology Therapy, 38*, 318–324.

Clarke, R. L., Daum, S. J., Gambino, A. J., Aceto, M. D., Pearl, J., Levitt, M., Cumisky, W. R., & Bogado, E. F. (1973). Compounds affecting the central nervous system 4 3-b-phenyltropane-2-carboxylic esters and analogs. *Journal of Medicinal Chemistry, 16,* 1260–1267.

Cone, E. J. (1995). Pharmacokinetics and pharmacodynamics of cocaine. *Journal of Analytic Toxicology, 19,* 459–478.

Cone, E. J., Kumor, K., Thompson, L. K., & Sherer, M. (1988). Correlation of saliva cocaine levels with plasma levels and with pharmacological effects after intravenous cocaine administration in human subjects. *Journal of Analytic Toxicology, 12,* 200–206.

Connell, P. H. (1958) *Amphetamine psychosis.* London: Chapman and Hill.

Cook, C. E., Jeffcoat, A. R., & Perez-Reyes, M. (1985) Pharmacokinetic studies of cocaine and phencyclidine in man. In G. Barnett & N. C. Chang (Eds.), *Pharmacokinetics and pharmacodynamics of psychoactive drugs* (pp. 48–74). Foster City, CA: Biomedical Publications.

Dackis, C. A., & Gold, M. S. (1985). New concepts in cocaine addiction: The dopamine depletion hypothesis. *Neuroscience and Behavior Review, 9,* 469–477.

Davies, H. M. L., Saikali, E., Sexton, T., & Childers, S. R. (1993). Novel 2-substituted cocaine analogs–binding-properties at dopamine transport sites in rat striatum. *European Journal of Pharmacology, 244,* 93–97.

Dean, R. A., Christian, C. D., Sample, R. H. B., & Bosron, W. F. (1991). Human liver cocaine esterases: Ethanol mediated formation of ethylcocaine. *Federation of the American Societies for Experimental Biology Journal, 5,* 2735–2739.

Dean, R. A., Bosron, W. F., Zachman, F. M., Zhang, J., & Brzezinski, M. R. (1997). Effects of ethanol on cocaine metabolism and disposition in the rat. NIDA Research Monograph No. 173, pp. 35–47). Washington, DC: U.S. Government Printing Office.

Deutsch, H. M., & Schweri, M. M. (1994). Can stimulant binding and dopamine transport be differentiated— studies with GBR-12783 derivatives. *Life Science, 55,* 1115–1120.

Deutsch, H. M., Shi, Q., Gruszecka-Kowalik, E., & Schweri, M. M. (1996). Synthesis and pharmacology of potential cocaine antagonists: 2. Structure–activity relationship studies of aromatic ring substituted methylphenidate analogs. *Journal of Medicinal Chemistry, 39,* 1201–1209.

deWit, H., Metz, J. T., Wagner, N., & Cooper, M. D. (1990). Behavioral and subjective effects of alcohol: Relationship to cerebral metabolism using PET. *Alcoholism: Clinical and Experimental Research, 14,* 482–489.

deWit, H., Metz, J. T., & Cooper, M. D. (1994) The effects of drugs of abuse on regional cerebral metabolism and mood. In B. N. Dhawan, R. C. Srimal, R. Raghubir, & R. S. Rapaka (Eds.), *Recent advances in the study of neurotransmitter receptors* (pp. 482–489). Lucknow, India: Central Drug Research Institute.

Di Chiara, G., & Imperato, A. (1988). Drugs abused by humans preferentially increase synaptic dopamine concentrations in the mesolimbic system of freely moving rats. *Proceedings of the National Academy of Science, 85,* 5274–5278.

Einhorn, L. C., Johansen, P. A., & White, F. J. (1988). Electrophysiological effects of cocaine in the mesoaccumbens dopamine system: Studies in the ventral tegmental area. *Journal of Neuroscience, 8,* 100–112.

El-Fawal, H. A. N., & Wood, R. W. (1995). airway smooth muscle relaxant effects of the cocaine pyrolysis product, methylecgonidine. *Journal of Pharmacology and Experimental Therapeutics, 272,* 991–996.

Erzouki, H. K., Allen, A. C., Newman, A. H., Goldberg, S. R., & Schindler, C. W. (1995). Effects of cocaine, cocaine metabolites and cocaine pyrolysis products on the hindbrain cardiorespiratory centers of the rabbit. *Life Science, 57,* 1861–1868.

Eshleman, E. J., Henningsen, R. A., Neve, K. A., & Janowsky, A. (1994). Release of dopamine via the human transporter. *Molecular Pharmacology, 45,* 312–316.

Evans, S. M., Cone, E. J., Marco, A. P., & Henningfield, J. E. (1992) A comparison of the kinetics of smoked and intravenous cocaine. In L. Harris (Ed.), *Problems of drug dependence* (p. 343). Rockville, MD: U.S. Department of Health and Human Services.

Farre, M., Torre, R. D. L., Llorente, M., Lamas, X., Ugena, B., Segura, J., & Cami, J. (1993). Alcohol and cocaine interactions in humans. *Journal of Pharmacology and Experimental Therapeutics, 266,* 1364–1373.

Fitzgerald, J. L., & Reid, J. J. (1991). Chronic cocaine treatment does not alter rat striatal D2 autoreceptor sensitivity to pergolide. *Brain Research, 541,* 327–333.

Foltin, R. W., & Fischman, M. W. (1992). Self-administration of cocaine by humans: Choice between smoked and intravenous cocaine,. *Journal of Pharmacology and Experimental Therapeutics, 261,* 841–849.

Fowler, J. S., Volkow, N. D., Wolf, A. P., Dewey, S. L., Schlyer, D. J., & MacGregor, R. R. (1989). Mapping cocaine binding sites in human and baboon brain in vivo. *Synapse, 4,* 371–377.

Fowler, J. S., Volkow, N. D., Logan, J., MacGregor, R. R., Wang, G. J., & Wolf, A. P. (1992). Alcohol intoxication does not change [11C] cocaine pharmacokinetics in human brain and heart. *Synapse, 12,* 228–135.

Fowler, J. S., Volkow, N. D., MacGregor, R. R., Logan, J., Dewey, S. L., Gatley, S. J., & Wolf, A. P. (1992). Comparative PET studies of the kinetics and distribution of cocaine and cocaethylene baboon brain. *Synapse, 12,* 220–227.

Fowler, J. S., Ding, Y.-S., Volkow, N. D., Martin, T., MacGregor, R. R., Dewey, S., King, P., Pappas, N., Alexoff, D., Shea, C., Gatley, S. J., Schlyer, D. J., & Wolf, A. P.

(1994). PET studies of cocaine inhibition of the my-ocardial norepinephrine uptake. *Synapse, 16,* 312–317.

Frost, J. J., Rosier, A. J., Reich, S. G., Smith, J. S., Ehlers, M. D., Snyder, S. H., Ravert, H. T., & Dannals, R. F. (1993). Positron emission tomographic imaging of the dopamine transporter with ^{11}C-WIN 35,428 reveals marked declines in mild Parkinson's disease. *Annals of Neurology, 34,* 423–431.

Galloway, M. P. (1988). Neurochemical interactions of cocaine with the dopaminergic system. *Trends in Pharmacological Science, 9,* 451–454.

Gardner, E. L. (1992). Brain reward mechanisms. In J. H. Lowinson, P. Ruiz, J. G. Millman, & J. G. Langrod (Eds.), *Substance abuse: A comprehensive textbook* (pp. 70–99). Baltimore, MD: Williams and Wilkins.

Garrett, E. R., & Seyda, K. (1983). Prediction of stability in pharmaceutical preparations XX: Stability, evaluation and bioanalysis of cocaine and benzoylecgonine by high performance liquid chromatography. *Journal of Pharmacy and Science, 72,* 258–271.

Gatley, S. J. (1991). The activities of the enantiomers of cocaine, and some related compounds as substrates and inhibitors of plasma butyrylcholinesterase. *Biochemical Pharmacology, 41,* 1249–1254.

Gatley, S. J., MacGregor, R. R., Fowler, J. S., Wolf, A. P., Dewey, S. L., & Schlyer, D. J. (1990). Rapid stereoselective hydrolysis of (+) cocaine in baboon plasma prevents its uptake in the brain: Implications for behavioral studies. *Journal of Neurochemistry, 54,* 720–723.

Gatley, S. J., Yu, D.-W., Fowler, J. S., MacGregor, R. R., Schlyer, D. J., Dewey, S. L., Wolf, A. P., Shea, C. E., Martin, T. P., & Volkow, N. D. (1994). Studies with differentially labeled C-11 cocaine, C-11 norcocaine, C-11 benzoylecgonine, and C-11 and F-18 4′-fluorococaine, to probe the extent to which C-11 cocaine metabolites contribute to PET images of the baboon brain. *Journal of Neurochemistry, 62,* 1154–1162.

Gatley, S. J., Pan, D., Chen, R., Chatrurvedi, G., & Ding, Y.-S. (1996). Affinities of methylphenidate derivatives for dopamine, norepinephrine and serotonin transporters. *Life Science, 58,* PL231–PL239.

Gatley, S. J., Volkow, N. D., Chen, R., Fowler, J. S., Carroll, F. I., & Kuhar, M. J. (1996). Displacement of rti-55 from the dopamine transporter by cocaine: implications for pharmacotherapy of stimulant abuse and in vivo imaging studies. *European Journal of Pharmacology, 296,* 145–151.

Gawin, F. H., & Ellinwood, E. H. (1988). Cocaine and other stimulants. *New England Journal of Medicine, 318,* 1173–1182.

Gawin, F. H., Riordan, C., & Kleber, H. D. (1985). Methylphenidate use in non-ADD cocaine abusers: A negative study. *American Journal of Drug and Alcohol Abuse, 11,* 193–197.

Gifford, A. N., & Johnson, K. M. (1992). Comparison of the role of local anaesthetic properties with dopamine

uptake blockade in the inhibition of striatal and nucleus accumbens [^{3}H]acetylcholine release by cocaine. *Journal of Pharmacology and Experimental Therapeutics, 263,* 757–761.

Gifford, A. N., Bergmann, J. S., & Johnson, K. M. (1993). GBR 12909 fails to antagonize cocaine induced elevation of dopamine in striatal slices. *Drug and Alcohol Dependence, 93,* 65–71.

Giros, B., Jaber, M., Jones, S. R., Wightman, R. M., & Caron, M. G. (1996). Hyperlocomotion and indifference to cocaine and amphetamine in mice lacking the dopamine transporter. *Nature 379 Issue,* 606–612.

Gradman, A. H. (1988). Cardiac effects of cocaine: A review. *Yale Journal of Biological Medicine, 61,* 137–141.

Guerin, G. F., Goeders, N. E., Dworkin, S. I., & Smith, J. E. (1984). Intracranial self-administration of dopamine into the nucleus accumbens. *Society of Neuroscience Abstracts, 10,* 1072.

Hawks, R. L., Kopin, I. J., Colburn, R. W., & Thoa, N. B. (1975). Norcocaine: A pharmacologically active metabolite of cocaine found in brain. *Life Science, 15,* 2189–2195.

He, X. S., Raymon, L. P., Mattson, M. V., Eldefrawi, M. E., & DeCosta, B. R. (1993). Further studies of the structure–activity relationships of 1-[1-(2-benzo[b]thienyl)cyclohexyl]piperidine. synthesis and evaluation of 1-(2-benzo[b]thienyl)-N,N-dialkylcyclohexylamines at dopamine uptake and phencyclidine binding sites. *Journal of Medicinal Chemistry, 36,* 4075–4081.

Hearn, W. L., Flynn, D. D., Hime, G. W., Rose, S., Confino, J. C., ManteroAtienza, E., Wetli, C. W., & Mash, D. C. (1991). Cocaethylene: A unique cocaine metabolite displays high-affinity for the dopamine transporter. *Journal of Neurochemistry, 56,* 698–701.

Henningfield, J. E., & Keenan, R. M. (1993). Nicotine delivery kinetics and abuse liability. *Journal of Consulting and Clinical Psychiatry, 61,* 743–750.

Henry, D. J., & White, F. J. (1991). Repeated cocaine administration caused persistent enhancement of D1 dopamine receptor sensitivity within the rat nucleus accumbens. *Journal of Pharmacology and Experimental Therapeutics, 258,* 882–890.

Henry, D. J., Greene, M. A., & White, F. J. (1989). Electrophysiological effects of cocaine in the mesoaccumbens dopamine system: Repeated administration. *Journal of Experimental Therapeutics, 251,* 833–839.

Hoffman, D. C., & Wise, R. A. (1993). Lack of cross-sensitization between the locomotor-activating effects of bromocriptine and those of cocaine or heroin. *Psychopharmacology, 110,* 402–408.

Huester, D. C. (1987). Cardiovascular effects of cocaine. *Journal of the American Medical Association, 257,* 979–980.

Hurd, Y. L., & Herkenham, M. (1993). Molecular alterations in the neostriatum of human cocaine addicts. *Synapse, 13,* 357–369.

Hurd, Y. L., & Ungerstedt, U. (1989). Cocaine: An in vivo microdialysis evaluation of its acute action on dopamine transmission in rat striatum. *Synapse, 3,* 48–54.

Inaba, T. (1989). Cocaine: Pharmacokinetics and biotransformation in man. *Canadian Journal of Physiology and Pharmacology, 67,* 1154–1157.

Isner, J., Estes, M., & Thompson, P. D. (1986). Acute cardiac events temporally related to cocaine abuse. *New England Journal of Medicine, 15,* 1438–1443.

Iyer, R. N., Nobiletti, J. B., Jatlow, P. I., & Bradberry, C. W. (1995). cocaine and cocaethylene: Effects on extracellular dopamine in the primate. *Psychopharmacology, 120,* 150–155.

Izenwasser, S., & Cox, B. M. (1990). Daily cocaine treatment produces a persistent reduction in [3H]dopamine uptake in vitro in rat nucleus accumbens but not in striatum. *Brain Research, 531,* 338–341.

Jaffe, J. H. (1990). Trivializing dependence. *British Journal of Addiction, 85,* 1425–1427.

Javaid, J. I., Musa, M. N., Fischman, M., Schuster, C. R., & Davis, J. M. (1983). Kinetics of cocaine in humans after intravenous and intranasal administration. *Biopharmacology of Drug Disposition, 4,* 9–18.

Jeffcoat, A. R., Perez-Reyes, M., Hill, J. M., Sadler, B. M., & Cook, C. E. (1989). Cocaine disposition in humans after intravenous injection, nasal insufflation (snorting), or smoking. *Drug Metabolism and Disposition, 17,* 153–159.

Johanson, C.-E., & Fischman, M. W. (1989). The pharmacology of cocaine related to its abuse. *Pharmacological Review, 41,* 3–52.

Johanson, C.-E., & Schuster, C. R. (1995) Cocaine. In F. E. Bloom & D. J. Kupfer (Eds.), *Psychopharmacology: The fourth generation of progress* (pp. 1685–1697). New York: Raven.

Johnson, K. M., Bergmann, J. S., & Kozikowski, A. P. (1992). Cocaine and dopamine differentially protect [3H]mazindol binding sites from alkylation by N-ethylmaleimide. *European Journal of Pharmacology, 227,* 411–427.

Kalivas, P. W., & Alesdatter, J. E. (1993). Involvement of NMDA receptor stimulation in the VTA and amygdala in behavioral sensitization to cocaine. *Journal of Pharmacology and Experimental Therapeutics, 267,* 486–495.

Kalivas, P. W., & Weber, B. (1988). Amphetamine injection into the ventral mesencephalon sensitizes rats to peripheral amphetamine and cocaine. *Journal of Pharmacology and Experimental Therapeutics, 245,* 1095–1101.

Karler, R., Calder, L. D., Chaudhry, I. A., & Turkanis, S. A. (1989). Blockade of "reverse tolerance" to cocaine and amphetamine by MK-801. *Life Science, 45,* 599–606.

Karler, R., Calder, L. D., & Bedingfield, J. B. (1994). Cocaine behavioral sensitization and the excitatory amino acids. *Psychopharmacology, 115,* 305–310.

Kaufman, M. J., Spealman, R. D., & Madras, B. K. (1991). Distribution of cocaine recognition sites in monkey brain. In vitro autoradiography with [3H]CFT. *Synapse, 9,* 177–187.

Kennedy, L. T., & Hanbauer, I. (1983). Sodium sensitive cocaine binding to rat striatal membrane: Possible relationship to dopamine uptake. *Journal of Neurochemistry, 41,* 172–178.

Kitayama, S., Shimada, S., Xu, H., Markham, L., Donovan, D. M., & Uhl, G. R. (1992). Dopamine transporter site-directed mutations differentially alter substrate transport and cocaine binding. *Proceedings of the National Academy of Science, 89,* 7782–7785.

Kleber, H. D. (1995). Pharmacotherapy, current and potential, for the treatment of cocaine dependence. *Clinical Neuropharmacology, 18* (Suppl. 1), S96–S109.

Kloner, R. A., Hale, S., Alker, K., & Rezkalla, S. (1992). The effects of acute and chronic cocaine use on the heart. *Circulation, 85,* 407–419.

Kosikowski, A. P., Salah, M. K. E., Johnson, K. M., & Bergmann, J. M. (1995). Chemistry and biology of the 2β-alkyl-3β-phenyl analogues of cocaine: Subnanomolar affinity ligands that suggest a new pharmacophore at the C-2 position. *Journal of Medicinal Chemistry, 38,* 3086–3093.

Lakoski, J. M., & Cunningham, K. A. (1988). Cocaine interaction with central monoaminergic systems: Electrophysiological approaches. *Trends in Pharmacological Science, 9,* 177–180.

Laruelle, M., Baldwin, R. M., Malison, R. T., Zea-Ponce, Y., Zoghbi, S. S., Al-Tikriti, M., Sybirska, E. H., Zimmermann, R. C., Wisniewski, G., Neumeyer, J. L., Milius, R. A., Wang, R. A., Smith, E. O., Roth, R. H., Charney, D., Hoffer, P. B., & Innis, R. B. (1993). SPECT imaging of dopamine and serotonin transporters with [I-123] beta-CIT: Pharmacological characterization of brain uptake in non-human primates. *Synapse, 13,* 295–309.

Levin, S. R., & Welch, K. M. A. (1988). Cocaine and stroke: Current concepts of cerebrovascular disease. *Stroke, 19,* 779–7883.

Lichtenfeld, P. J., Rubin, D. B., & Feldman, R. S. (1984). Subarachnoid hemorrhage precipitated by cocaine snorting. *Archives of Neurology, 41,* 223–224.

Lienau, A. K., & Kuschinsky, K. (1997). Sensitization phenomena after repeated administration of cocaine or D-amphetamine in rats: Associative and nonassociative mechanisms and the role of dopamine in the striatum. *Naunyn Schmiedebergs Archives of Pharmacology, 355,* 531–537.

Logan, J., Fowler, J. S., Volkow, N. D., Wolf, A. P., Dewey, S. L., Schlyer, D. J., MacGregor, R. R., Hitzemann, R., Bendirem, B., Gatley, S. J., & Christman, D. R. (1990). Graphical analysis of reversible radiolig and binding from time activity measurements applied to [N-^{11}C-methyl]-(–)cocaine PET studies in human subjects. *Journal of Cerebral Blood Flow and Metabolism, 10,* 740–747.

London, E. D., Cascella, N. G., Wong, D. F., Phillips, R. L., Dannals, R. F., Links, J. M., Herning, R., Grayson, R., Jaffe, J. H., & Wagner, H. N. J. (1990). Cocaine-induced reduction of glucose utilization in human brain: A study using positron emission tomography and [Fluorine 18]-Fluorodeoxyglucose. *Archives of General Psychiatry, 47,* 567–574.

Madden, J. A., & Powers, R. H. (1990). Effect of cocaine and cocaine metabolites on cerebral arteries in vitro. *Life Sciences, 47,* 1109–1114.

Madras, B. K. (1994). ^{11}C-WIN 35,428 for detecting dopamine depletion in mild Parkinson's disease. *Annals of Neurology, 35,* 376–377.

Madras, B. K., & Kaufman, M. J. (1994). Cocaine accumulates in dopamine rich regions of primate brain after I.V. administration: Comparison with mazindol distribution. *Synapse, 18,* 261–275.

Madras, B. K., Fahey, M. A., Bergman, J., Canfield, D. R., & Spealman, R. D. (1989). Effects of cocaine and related drugs in non-human primates. I [^{3}H]Cocaine binding sites in caudate-putamen. *Journal of Pharmacology and Experimental Therapeutics, 251,* 131–141.

Madras, B. K., Spealman, R. D., Fahey, M. A., Neumeyer, J. L., Saha, J. K., & Milius, R. A. (1989). Cocaine receptors labeled by [^{3}H]2b-carbomethoxy-3b-(4-fluorophenyl)tropane. *Molecular Pharmacology, 36,* 518–524.

Masserano, J. M., Venable, D., & Wyatt, R. J. (1994). Effect of chronic cocaine administration on [3H]dopamine uptake in the nucleus accumbens, striatum and frontal cortex of rats. *Journal of Pharmacology and Experimental Therapeutics, 270,* 133–141.

Mattingly, B. A., Hart, T. C., Lim, K., & Perkins, C. (1994). Selective antagonism of dopamine D1 and D2 receptors does not block the development of behavioral sensitization to cocaine. *Psychopharmacology, 114,* 239–242.

McElvain, J. S., & Schenk, J. O. (1992). A multisubstrate mechanism of striatal dopamine uptake and its inhibition by cocaine. *Biochemical Pharmacology, 43,* 2189–2199.

Meehan, S. M., & Schechter, M. D. (1995). Cocaethylene-induced lethality in mice is potentiated by alcohol. *Alcohol, 12,* 383–385.

Meltzer, P. C., Liang, A. Y., Brownell, A. L., Elmaleh, D. R., & Madras, B. K. (1993). Substituted 3-phenyltropane analogs of cocaine: Synthesis and inhibition of binding at cocaine recognition sites, and positron emission tomography imaging. *Journal of Medicinal Chemistry, 36,* 855–862.

Meltzer, P. C., Liang, A. Y., & Madras, B. K. (1994). The discovery of an unusually selective and novel cocaine analog: Difluoropine (O-620). synthesis and inhibition of binding at cocaine recognition sites. *Journal of Medicinal Chemistry, 37,* 2001–2010.

Mule, S. J., Casella, G. A., & Misra, A. L. (1976). Intracellular disposition of [^{3}H]cocaine, [^{3}H]norcocaine, [^{3}H]benzoylecgonine and [^{3}H]benzoylnorecgonine in the brain of rats. *Life Sciences, 19,* 1585–1596.

Nayak, P. K., Misra, A. L., & Mulé, S. J. (1976). Physiological disposition and biotransformation of [^{3}H]cocaine in acutely and chronically treated rats. *Journal of Pharmacology and Experimental Therapeutics, 196,* 556–569.

Nicolaysen, L. C., Pan, H. T., & Justice, J. B., Jr. (1988). Extracellular cocaine and dopamine concentrations are linearly related in rat striatum. *Brain Research, 456,* 317–323.

Parran, T. V., & Jasinski, D. R. (1991). Intravenous methylphenidate abuse: Prototype for prescription drug abuse. *Archives of Internal Medicine, 151,* 781–783.

Parsons, L. H., & Justice, J. B. (1994). Quantitative approaches to in vivo brain microdialysis. *Critical Review of Neurobiology, 8,* 189–220.

Perez-Reyes, M., & Jeffcoat, A. R. (1992). Ethanol/cocaine interaction: Cocaine and cocaethylene plasma concentrations and their relationship to subjective and cardiovascular effects. *Life Sciences, 51,* 553–563.

Peterson, K. I., Logan, B. K., & Christian, G. D. (1995). Detection of cocaine and its polar transformation products and metabolites in human urine. *Forensic Science International, 73,* 183–196.

Pettit, H. O., & Justice, J. B., Jr. (1989). Dopamine in the nucleus accumbens during cocaine self-administration as studied by in vivo microdialysis. *Pharmacology, Biochemistry and Behavior, 34,* 899–904.

Pettit, H. O., Pan, H.-T., Parsons, L. H., & Justice, J. B. (1990). Extracellular concentrations of cocaine and dopamine are enhanced during chronic cocaine administration. *Journal of Neurochemistry, 55,* 798–804.

Pitts, D. K., & Marwah, J. (1987). Electrophysiological actions of cocaine on noradrenergic neurons in rat locus ceruleus. *Journal of Pharmacology and Experimental Therapeutics, 240,* 345–351.

Porrino, L. J. (1993). Functional consequences of acute cocaine treatment depend on route of administration. *Psychopharmacology, 112,* 343–351.

Post, R. M. (1975). Cocaine psychoses: A continuum model. *American Journal of Psychiatry, 132,* 225–231.

Post, R. M., & Rose, H. (1976). Increasing effects of repetitive cocaine administration in the rat. *Nature, 260,* 731–732.

Preston, K. L., Sullivan, J. T., Berger, P., & Bigelow, G. E. (1993). Effects of cocaine alone and in combination with mazindol in human cocaine abusers. *Journal of Pharmacology and Experimental Therapeutics, 258,* 296–307.

Pristupa, Z. B., Wilson, J. M., Hoffman, B. J., Kish, S. J., & Niznik, H. B. (1994). Pharmacological heterogeneity of the cloned and native human dopamine transporter: Disassociation of the [^{3}H]WIN 35,428 and [3H]GBR 12,935 binding. *Molecular Pharmacology, 45,* 125–135.

Przywara, D. A., & Dambach, G. E. (1989). Direct actions of cocaine on cardiac cellular activity. *Circulation Research, 65,* 185–192.

Qiao, J.-T., Dougherty, P. M., Wiggins, R. C., & Dafny, N. (1990). Effects of microiontophoretic application of cocaine, alone and with receptor antagonists, upon the neurons of the medial prefrontal cortex, nucleus accumbens and caudate nucleus of rats. *Neuropharmacology, 29,* 379–385.

Rall, T. W. (1993) Hypnotics and sedatives: Ethanol. In A. Goodman-Gilman, L. S. Goodman, T. W. Rall, & F. Murad (Eds.), *Goodman and Gilman's the pharmacological basis of therapeutics* (pp. 345–382). New York: Macmillan.

Rao, A. N., Polos, P. G., & Walther, F. A. (1990). Crack abuse and asthma: A fatal combination. *New York State Journal of Medicine, 90,* 511–512.

Rech, R. H., Vomachka, M. K., Rickert, D., & Braude, M. C. (1976). Interactions between amphetamine and alcohol, and their effects on rodent behavior. *Annals of the New York Academy of Science, 281,* 426–440.

Reith, M. E. A., Benuck, M., & Lajtha, A. (1987). Cocaine disposition in the brain after continuous or intermittent treatment and locomotor stimulation in mice. *Journal of Pharmacology and Experimental Therapeutics, 243,* 281–287.

Reith, M. E. A., DeCosta, B., Rice, K. C., & Jacobson, A. E. (1992). Evidence for mutually exclusive binding of cocaine, BTCP, GBR 12935 and dopamine to the dopamine transporter. *European Journal of Pharmacology, 227,* 417–425.

Reith, M. E. A., Coffey, L. L., Xu, C., & Chen, N. H. (1994). GBR 12909 and GBR 12935 block dopamine uptake into brain synaptic vesicles as well as nerve endings. *European Journal of Pharmacology, 253,* 175–178.

Ritchie, J. M., & Greene, N. M. (1993). Local anesthetics. In A. Goodman-Gilman, T. N. Rall, A. S. Nies, & P. Taylor (Eds.), *Goodman and Gilman's the pharmacological basis of therapeutics* (8th ed., pp. 311–331). New York: Macmillan.

Ritz, M. C., Lamb, R. J., Goldberg, S. R., & Kuhar, M. J. (1987). Cocaine receptors on dopamine transporters are related to self administration of cocaine. *Science, 237,* 1219–1223.

Ritz, M. C., Cone, E. J., & Kuhar, M. J. (1990). Cocaine inhibition of ligand binding at dopamine norepinephrine and serotonin transporters: A structure–activity study. *Life Sciences, 46,* 635–645.

Roth, L., Harbison, R. B., James, R. C., Tobin, T., & Roberts, S. M. (1992). Cocaine hepatotoxicity: Influence of hepatic enzyme inducing and inhibiting agents on the site of necrosis. *Hepatology, 15,* 934–940.

Rothman, R. B. (1990). High affinity dopamine reuptake inhibitors as potential cocaine antagonists: A strategy for drug development. *Life Sciences, 46,* PL17–PL21.

Rothman, R. B., Mele, A., Reid, A. A., Hyacinth, C. A., Greg, N., Thurkauf, A., DeCosta, B. R., Rice, K. C.,

& Pert, A. (1991). GBR 12909 antagonizes the ability of cocaine to elevate extracellular levels of dopamine. *Pharmacology, Biochemistry and Behavior, 40,* 387–397.

Rothman, R. B., Grieg, N., Kim, A., De Costa, B. R., Rice, K. C., Carroll, F., & Pert, A. (1992). Cocaine and GBR 12909 produce equivalent motoric responses at different occupancy of the dopamine transporter. *Pharmacology, Biochemistry and Behavior, 43,* 1135–42.

Rothman, R. B., Becketts, K. M., Radesca, L. R., DeCosta, B. R., Rice, K. C., Carroll, F. I., & Dersch, C. M. (1993). Studies of the biogenic amine transporters: II. A brief study on the use of [^{3}H]DA-uptake-inhibition to transporter-binding-inhibition ratios for the in vitro evaluation of putative cocaine antagonists. *Life Sciences, 53,* PL267–PL272.

Seeman, P. (1993). *Receptor tables. Volume 2: Drug dissociation constants for neuroreceptors and transporters.* Toronto, Ontario, Canada: SZ Resarch.

Seidman, M. H., Lau, C. E., Chen, R., & Falk, J. L. (1992). Orally self-administered cocaine: Reinforcing efficacy by the place preference method. *Pharmacology, Biochemistry and Behavior, 43,* 235–241.

Self, D. W., & Nestler, E. J. (1995). Molecular mechanisms of drug reinforcement and addiction. *Annual Review of Neuroscience, 43,* 463–495.

Sharkey, J., Glen, K. A., Wolfe, S., & Kuhar, M. J. (1988). Cocaine binding at sigma receptors. *European Journal of Pharmacology, 149,* 171–174.

Sharkey, J., Ritz, M. C., Schenden, J. A., Hanson, R. C., & Kuhar, M. J. (1988). Cocaine inhibits muscarinic cholinergic receptors in heart and brain. *Journal of Pharmacology and Experimental Therapeutics, 246,* 1048–1052.

Sharpe, L. G., Pilotte, N. S., Mitchell, W. M., & DeSouza, E. B. (1991). Withdrawal of repeated cocaine decreases autoradiographic [^{3}H]mazindol labelling of dopamine transporter in rat nucleus accumbens. *European Journal of Pharmacology, 203,* 141–144.

Shuster, L., Yu, G., & Bates, A. (1977). Sensitization to cocaine stimulation in mice. *Psychopharmacology, 52,* 185–190.

Simoni, D., Stoelwinder, J., Kozikowski, A. P., Johnson, K. M., Bergmann, J. S., & Ball, R. G. (1993). Methoxylation of cocaine reduces binding affinity and produces compounds of differential binding and dopamine uptake inhibitory activity: Discovery of a weak cocaine "antagonist." *Journal of Medicinal Chemistry, 36,* 3975–3977.

Sisti, N. J., Fowler, F. W., & Fowler, J. S. (1989). The flash vacuum thermolysis of (–)-cocaine. *Tetrahydron Letters, 30,* 5977–5980.

Snyder, W. S., Cook, M. J., Nasset, E. S., Karhausen, L. R., Parry-Howells, G., & Tipton, I. H. (1975). *Report on the task group on Reference Man* (ICRP Publication 23). Oxford, England: Pergamon.

Sorg, B. A., & Ulibarri, C. (1995). Application of a protein synthesis inhibitor into the ventral tegmental area, but not the nucleus accumbens, prevents behavioral sensitization to cocaine. *Synapse, 20,* 217–224.

Spealman, R. D., Goldberg, S. R., Kelleher, R. T., Morse, W. H., Goldberg, D. M., Hakansson, C. G., Nieforth, K. A., & Lazer, E. S. (1979). Effects of norcocaine and some norcocaine derivatives on schedule-controlled behavior of pigeons and squirrel monkeys. *Journal of Pharmacology and Experimental Therapeutics, 210,* 196–205.

Spealman, R. D., Kelleher, R. T., & Goldberg, S. R. (1983). Stereoselective effects of cocaine and a phenyltropane analog. *Journal of Pharmacology and Experimental Therapeutics, 225,* 509–514.

Staley, J. K., Hearn, W. L., Ruttenber, A. J., Wetli, C. V., & Mash, D. C. (1994). High affinity cocaine recognition sites on the dopamine transporter are elevated in fatal cocaine overdose victims. *Journal of Pharmacology and Experimental Therapeutics, 271,* 1678–1685.

Stein, E. A., & Fuller, S. A. (1993). Cocaine time action profile on regional cerebral blood flow in the rat. *Brain Research, 626,* 117–126.

Stewart, D. J., Inaba, T., Tang, B. K., & Kalow, W. (1977). Hydrolysis of cocaine in human plasma by cholinesterase. *Life Sciences, 20,* 1557–1564.

Stewart, D. J., Inaba, T., Lucassen, M., & Kalow, W. (1979). Cocaine metabolism: Cocaine and norcocaine hydrolysis by liver and serum esterases. *Clinical Pharmacology and Therapeutics, 25,* 464–468.

Stine, S. M., Krystal, J. H., Kosten, T. R., & Charney, D. S. (1995). Mazindol treatment for cocaine dependence. *Drug and Alcohol Dependence, 39,* 245–253.

Strickland, T. L., Mena, I., Villanueva-Meyer, J., Miller, B. L., Cummings, J., Mehringer, C. M., Satz, P., & Myers, H. (1993). Cerebral perfusion and neuropsychological consequences of chronic cocaine use. *Journal of Neuropsychiatry, 5,* 1–9.

Tella, S. R., & Goldberg, S. R. (1993). Monoamine uptake inhibitors alter cocaine pharmacokinetics. *Psychopharmacology, 112,* 497–502.

Tumeh, S., Nagel, J. S., & English, R. J. (1990). Cerebral abnormalities in cocaine abusers: Demonstration by SPECT perfusion brain scintigraphy. *Radiology, 176,* 821–24.

Turkanis, S. A., Partlow, L. M., & Karler, R. (1989). Effects of cocaine on neuromuscular transmission in the lobster. *Neuropharmacology, 28,* 971–975.

Uchimura, N., & North, R. A. (1990). Actions of cocaine on rat nucleus accumbens neurones *in vitro. British Journal of Pharmacology, 99,* 736–740.

Ujike, H., Akiyama, K., & Otsuki, S. (1990). D-2 but not D-1 dopamine agonists produce augmented behavioral response in rats after subchronic treatment with methamphetamine or cocaine. *Psychopharmacology, 102,* 459–464.

Van Dyke, C., & Byck, R. (1974) Cocaine: 1884–1974. In E. H. Elinwood (Ed.), *Advances in behavioral biology* (pp. 1–30). New York: Plenum.

Van Dyke, C., Jatlow, P., Ungerer, J., Barash, P. G., & Byck, R. (1978). Oral cocaine: Plasma concentrations and central effects. *Science, 200,* 211–213.

Vezina, P., & Stewart, J. (1989). The effect of dopamine receptor blockade on the development of sensitization to the locomotor activating effects of amphetamine and morphine. *Brain Research, 499,* 108–120.

Volkow, N. D., Mullani, N., Gould, K. L., Adler, S., & Krajewski, K. (1988). Cerebral blood flow in chronic cocaine users: A study with positron emission tomography. *British Journal of Psychiatry, 152,* 641–648.

Volkow, N. D., Hitzemann, R., Wolf, A. P., Logan, J., Fowler, J., Christman, D., Dewey, S., Schlyer, D., Burr, G., Vitkun, S., & Hirschowitz, J. (1990). Acute effects of ethanol on regional brain glucose metabolism and transport. *Psychiatry Research, 35,* 39–48.

Volkow, N. D., Fowler, J. S., Wolf, A. P., Hitzemann, R., Dewey, S. L., Bendriem, B., Alpert, R., & Hoff, A. (1991). Changes in brain glucose metabolism in cocaine dependence and withdrawal. *American Journal of Psychiatry, 148,* 621–626.

Volkow, N. D., Gillespie, H., Mullani, N., Tancredi, L., Grant, C., Ivanovic, M., & Hollister, L. (1991). Cerebellar metabolic activation by delta-9-tetrahydrocannabinol in human brains: A study with positron emission tomography and ^{18}F-2-deoxy-2-fluoro-D-glucose. *Psychiatric Research, 40,* 69–80.

Volkow, N. D., Fowler, J. S., Wolf, A. P., Wang, G.-J., Logan, J., MacGregor, R. R., Dewey, S. L., Schlyer, D. J., & Hitzemann, R. (1992). Distribution and kinetics of carbon-11-cocaine in the human body measured with PET. *Journal of Nuclear Medicine, 33,* 521–525.

Volkow, N. D., Hitzemann, R., Wang, G.-J., Fowler, J. S., Wolf, A. P., Dewey, S. L., Burr, G., Piscani, K., Handlesman, L., & Hoff, A. (1992). Long term frontal brain metabolic changes in cocaine abusers. *Synapse, 11,* 184–190.

Volkow, N. D., Fowler, J. S., Wang, G.-J., Hitzemann, R., Wolf, A. P., Logan, J., Schlyer, D., MacGregor, R. R., Angrist, B., Liebermann, J., Burr, G., & Pappas, N. (1993). PET studies of the function of the dopamine transporter in cocaine abusers. *Journal of Nuclear Medicine, 34,* 67.

Volkow, N. D., Ding, Y.-S., Fowler, J. S., Wang, G.-J., Logan, J., Gatley, S. J., Dewey, S., Ashby, C., Liebermann, J., Hitzemann, R., & Wolf, A. P. (1995). Is methylphenidate like cocaine? Studies on their pharmacokinetics and distribution in human brain. *Archives of General Psychiatry, 52,* 456–463.

Volkow, N. D., Fowler, J. S., Logan, J., Gatley, S. J., Dewey, S. L., MacGregor, R. R., Schlyer, D. J., Pappas, N., King, P., & Wolf, A. P. (1995). Comparison of [11C]cocaine binding at sub-pharmacological and pharmacological doses in baboon brain. *Journal of Nuclear Medicine, 36,* 1289–1297.

Volkow, N. D., Wang, G.-J., Hitzemann, R., Fowler, J. S., Burr, G., & Wolf, A. P. (1995). Recovery of brain glucose metabolism in detoxified alcoholics. *American Journal of Psychiatry, 151,* 178–183.

Volkow, N. D., Wang, G. J., Fowler, J. S., Logan, J., Hitzemann, R., Gatley, S. J., Macgregor, R. R., & Wolf, A. P. (1996). Cocaine uptake is decreased in the brain of detoxified cocaine abusers. *Neuropsychopharmacology, 14,* 159–168.

Wakasa, Y., Takada, K., & Yanagita, T. (1995). Reinforcing effect as a function of infusion speed in intravenous self-administration of nicotine in rhesus monkeys. *Japanese Journal of Psychopharmacology, 15,* 53–59.

Wall, S. C., Innis, R. B., & Rudnick, G. (1993). Binding of the cocaine analog 2b-carbomethoxy-3b-(4-[^{125}I]iodophenyl)tropane to serotonin and dopamine transporters: Different ionic requirements for substrate and 2β-carbomethoxy-3β-(4-[^{125}I]iodophenyl)tropane binding. *Molecular Pharmacology, 43,* 264–270.

Wang, G. J., Volkow, N. D., Logan, J., Fowler, J. S., Schlyer, D. J., MacGregor, R. R., Hitzemann, R. J., Gjedde, A., & Wolf, A. P. (1995). Serotonin 5-HT2 receptor availability in chronic cocaine abusers. *Life Sciences, 56,* PL299–PL303.

Wang, G. J., Volkow, N. D., Hitzemann, R. J., Wong, C., Angrist, B., Burr, G., Pascani, K., Pappas, N., Lu, A., Cooper, T., & Lieberman, J. A. (1997). Behavioral and cardiovascular effects of intravenous methylphenidate in normal subjects and cocaine abusers. *European Addiction Research, 3,* 49–54.

White, F. J., Hu, X.-T., & Henry, D. J. (1993). Electrophysiological effects of cocaine in the rat nucleus accumbens: Microiontophoretic studies. *Journal of Pharmacology and Experimental Therapeutics, 266,* 1075–1084.

White, S. R., Harris, G. C., Imel, K. M., & Wheaton, M. J. (1995). Inhibitory effects of dopamine and methylenedioxymethamphetamine (MDMA) on glutamate-evoked firing of nucleus accumbens and caudate/putamen cells are enhanced following cocaine self-administration. *Brain Research, 681,* 167–176.

Wilkinson, P., VanDyke, C., Jatlow, P., Barash, P., & Byck, R. (1980). Intranasal and oral cocaine kinetics. *Clinical Pharmacologic Therapeutics, 27,* 386–394.

Wolf, M. E., & Jeziorski, M. (1993). Coadministration of MK-801 with amphetamine, cocaine or morphine prevents rather than transiently masks the development of behavioral sensitization. *Brain Research, 613,* 291–294.

Wolf, M. E., White, F. J., Nassar, R., Brooderson, R. J., & Khansa, M. R. (1993). Differential development of autoreceptor subsensitivity and enhanced dopamine release during amphetamine sensitization. *Journal of Pharmacology and Experimental Therapeutics, 264,* 249–255.

Wolkin, A., Angrist, B., Wolf, A., Brodie, J., Wolkin, B., Jaeger, J., Cancro, R., & Rotrosen, J. (1987). Effects of amphetamine on local cerebral metabolism in normal and schizophrenic subjects as determined by positron emission tomography. *Psychopharmacology, 92,* 241–252.

Wong, D. T., & Bymaster, F. P. (1978). An inhibitor of dopamine reuptake, LR5182, cis-3-(3,4-dichlorophenyl)-2-N,N-dimethylaminomethyl-bicyclo [2,2,2]octane, hydrochloride. *Life Sciences, 23,* 1041–1047.

Yu, D. W., Gatley, S. J., Wolf, A. P., MacGregor, R. R., Dewey, S. L., Fowler, J. S., & Schlyer, D. (1992). Synthesis of carbon-11 labeled iodinated cocaine derivatives and their distribution in baboon brain measured using positron emission tomography. *Journal of Medicinal Chemistry, 35,* 2178–2183.

11

Behavioral Pharmacology of Cocaine

SHARON L. WALSH

Introduction

The behavioral pharmacological characteristics of cocaine have been investigated in nonhumans and humans for several decades. Various experimental approaches have been utilized to explore the physiological, subjective, behavioral, and psychological effects of cocaine. This chapter reviews findings regarding the behavioral pharmacology of cocaine use encompassing data from both animal and human laboratory studies. The first two sections provide an overview of the pharmacological actions of cocaine and the patterns of cocaine abuse. The next three sections review select studies characterizing (1) the subjective effects of cocaine in humans, (2) the discriminative stimulus properties of cocaine, and (3) the reinforcing properties of cocaine assessed using the drug self-administration paradigm. Preclinical drug-discrimination and self-administration studies of cocaine are abundant and a complete review of these studies is beyond the scope of this chapter. Thus, preclinical data will be synthesized to illustrate principal findings and more

detailed analysis of the results from studies with humans, when available, will be provided.

Cocaine Pharmacology

Cocaine is a natural substance found in the leaves of the coca shrub grown primarily in the highlands of the Andes mountains. For thousands of years, the indigenous peoples of this region have chewed coca leaves during religious rituals and to enhance physical performance and vigor (Goddard, deGoddard, & Whitehead, 1969; Grinspoon & Bakalar, 1981). The cocaine alkaloid was isolated in the mid-1800s and, thereafter, cocaine became a widely used additive in a variety of commercial products. The therapeutic benefits of cocaine for the treatment of various ailments, including morphine addiction, alcoholism, hayfever, and general malaise, were widely extolled, and cocaine could be in found a wide range of medicinal tonics, wines, and soft drinks (Musto, 1992; Van Dyke & Byck, 1983). Over a period of decades, concern grew about the potential medical risks and addictive properties of cocaine. The uncontrolled use of cocaine was banned in the United States by the Harrison Narcotics Act of 1914.

Cocaine exerts many actions in the peripheral and central nervous system (CNS); however, it has two prominent actions that are most relevant to its therapeutic effects and abuse liability, respectively. The therapeutic benefits of cocaine

SHARON L. WALSH • Behavioral Pharmacology Research Unit, Department of Psychiatry and Behavioral Sciences, Johns Hopkins University School of Medicine, Baltimore, Maryland 21224.

Handbook of Substance Abuse: Neurobehavioral Pharmacology, edited by Tarter *et al.* Plenum Press, New York, 1998.

are derived from its potent action as a local anesthetic. Cocaine inhibits sodium ion movement within the cell membrane, thus blocking the initiation or conduction of nerve impulses. Cocaine is legally available only as a topical solution in the United States and is currently classified as a Schedule II drug under the Controlled Substances Act of 1970. This preparation is used primarily to induce local anesthesia for surgery of the eyes, mouth, nose, and throat; however, the availability of structural analogs of cocaine without prominent CNS effects, such as lidocaine, has significantly diminished the medical use of cocaine (see Brain & Coward, 1989; Middleton & Kirkpatrick, 1993).

Cocaine is also a potent psychomotor stimulant, and it is this pharmacological property that is believed to account for its high abuse potential. Cocaine binds to the monoamine transporters for dopamine, norepinephrine, and serotonin, and inhibits neurotransmitter reuptake from the synapse (Harris & Baldessarini, 1973; Koe, 1976). Reuptake inhibition leads to increased synaptic concentrations of monoamines and results in prolonged receptor stimulation. Cocaine also binds to peripheral and central receptors including muscarinic and serotonergic receptors (Kilpatrick, Jones, & Tyers, 1989; Sharkey, Ritz, Schenden, Hanson, & Kuhar, 1988). Although cocaine has multiple pharmacologic actions, the ability of cocaine to inhibit dopamine transport is commonly believed to underlie its reinforcing and psychomotor stimulant properties (de Wit & Wise, 1977; Heikkila, Cabbat, Manzino, & Duvoisin, 1979; Ritz, Lamb, Goldberg, & Kuhar, 1987; Scheel-Kruger, Braestrup, Nielson, Golembiowska, & Modilnicka, 1976). For more information on selected topics, one may refer to thorough reviews on the pharmacology (Johanson & Fischman, 1989, and elsewhere in this volume), neuropharmacology (Fibiger, Phillips, & Brown, 1992; Koob, 1992a, 1992b), and therapeutic safety of cocaine (Warner, 1993).

Patterns of Abuse

The patterns of cocaine use and abuse vary across different geographic regions. In the South American regions where the coca plant is grown, there are several million people who use cocaine regularly, with the highest prevalence of use in Bolivia, Colombia, and Peru (Negrete, 1992). In South America, cocaine is primarily consumed orally either by chewing on coca leaves to extract the active alkaloid (Goddard et al, 1969) or by drinking tea made from the leaves of the coca plant. When cocaine is administered by the oral route, the onset of effects is fairly slow, with plasma concentrations peaking at approximately 1 hr after ingestion. The bioavailability of oral cocaine is estimated to be only about 20% (Mayersohn & Perrier, 1978), and thus the total amount of cocaine consumed by leaf chewing or tea drinking is fairly low. In contrast to South America, the history of cocaine use in the United States is relatively recent. Cocaine was introduced to Europe and the United States only in the latter part of the 19th century. The contemporary patterns of use in the United States and other western countries (e.g., Gossop, Griffiths, Powis, & Strang, 1994) also differ greatly from that seen in South America. Cocaine is rarely consumed by the oral route and the coca plant product is not available. The cocaine alkaloid is extracted from the coca plant in the countries of origin and transported to the United States as a relatively pure substance.

After the United States government illegalized the possession and sale of cocaine earlier in the 1900s, cocaine use declined precipitously until the recent epidemic that began in the 1970s. During the rise of cocaine use through the 1980s, the drug was most commonly administered by the intranasal route. However, for the past decade, the intravenous administration of cocaine and smoking of the base form of cocaine, known as crack, have risen dramatically (for review, see Hatsukami & Fischman, 1996). Both of these routes of administration deliver the drug rapidly to the CNS and produce an intense euphorigenic effect as well as an increased risk of adverse medical consequences. It is typical for cocaine abusers to readminister the drug repeatedly in quick succession; the interval of repeated dosing may vary from as little as a few minutes as occurs with smoking to as long as 30 min or more with intranasal use. This repeated use pattern has become known as a binge. Binges may last for a few hours or up to a few days, and typically end because of physical exhaustion or the exhaustion of economic resources, drug supply, or both. Although this is a common pattern of abuse, there is wide individual variation and some cocaine users consume limited quantities on a more regular basis. Recent epidemiological studies suggest that the prevalence of cocaine use has reached a plateau over the past few years in the United States. However, the most recent National Household Survey on Drug Abuse (1995) estimates that approximately 1.4 million people used cocaine and another 520,000 used crack in the month preceding the survey. These estimates indicate that cocaine use continues to pose a major public health problem in this country.

Subjective Effects of Cocaine in Humans

The mood-altering properties of drugs are believed to contribute largely to their abuse liability and reinforcing efficacy. Because changes in mood or internal subjective states are not observable to others, determining the qualitative and quantitative features of these subjective experiences can be difficult. The most commonly used procedure for evaluating the characteristics of the subjective response to drugs in humans is to collect verbal or written reports. Structured self-report questionnaires can assess the presence or absence of an interoceptive drug effect, or descriptive information can be collected to characterize the qualitative nature and magnitude of the subjective drug experience.

In the majority of studies evaluating the effects of cocaine in human subjects, participants are enrolled who report using cocaine illicitly, and these reports are objectively verified prior to study initiation. In a typical study, cocaine is administered under close medical supervision in a controlled inpatient or outpatient laboratory setting. The subject is asked to

respond to a number of questionnaires before and at multiple points after drug administration to characterize the complete time-course of the drug effect. Various subjective instruments have been used to assess the effects of cocaine in humans. The characteristics of the specific questionnaires vary widely (e.g., analog, ordinal, and binomial scales). Tests of validity and reliability are available for some instruments, but for many of the most widely used questionnaires (e.g., visual analog measures) investigators rely on the face validity of the instruments. These questionnaires may be designed or selected to detect the euphorigenic, stimulant, or anxiogenic properties of cocaine, or a combination of these properties.

The profile of subjective effects produced by cocaine has been characterized for several routes of administration including the oral (Oliveto, Rosen, Woods, & Kosten, 1995; Rowbotham, Jones, Benowitz, & Jacob, 1984; Van Dyke, Jatlow, Ungerer, Barash, & Byck, 1978), intravenous (Foltin & Fischman, 1991; Javaid, Fischman, Schuster, Dekirmenjian, & Davis, 1978; Resnick, Kestenbaum, & Schwartz, 1977), intranasal (Javaid et al., 1978; Resnick et al., 1977), and smoking routes (Foltin & Fischman, 1991; Hatsukami, Thompson, Pentel, Flygare, & Carroll, 1994; Perez-Reyes, DiGuiseppi, Ondrusek, Jeffcoat, & Cook, 1982). Cocaine produces subjective effects that are consistent with both its euphorigenic and stimulant actions. Subjects describe feeling "high," "rush," "good effects," "pleasantness," and "liking for the drug" after cocaine administration. Dose response studies find that ratings on these variables are positively related to both dose and plasma concentrations of cocaine regardless of route of administration (e.g., Perez-Reyes et al., 1982; Resnick et al., 1977; Van Dyke & Byck, 1983; Walsh, Preston, Sullivan, Fromme, & Bigelow, 1994). These global drug effect indices are very sensitive and are commonly used in abuse liability test procedures (Bigelow, 1991; Jasinski, Johnson, & Henningfield, 1984). While they are useful for assessing global euphorigenic properties, more specific questionnaires may be needed to qualitatively distinguish cocaine from other drugs with euphorigenic properties, such as opioids (Walsh, Sullivan, Preston, Garner, & Bigelow, 1996).

Adjective rating scales are designed to assess specific subjective and somatic symptoms. These instruments are typically composed of a list of single adjectives or phrases that are scored on an ordinal scale. Following cocaine administration, scores on items descriptive or symptomatic of psychomotor stimulation are elevated including "stimulated," "excited," "tremor," "fidgety," "energetic and nervous"; measures of sedation, such as "drowsy," "sleepy," and "fatigued," are typically decreased (Foltin, Fischman, Pedroso, & Pearlson, 1988; Preston, Sullivan, Strain, & Bigelow, 1992; Sherer, 1988). Items describing somatic sensations that are commonly altered by cocaine include increased ratings of "dizziness," "lightheadedness," "tingling sensations," "numbness," "dry mouth," "sweating," and decreased ratings of "hunger" (Foltin *et al.,* 1988; Preston *et al.,* 1992; Resnick *et al.,* 1977).

The Addiction Research Center Inventory (ARCI) is an empirically derived structured questionnaire that is widely used in drug abuse research. In its original form the questionnaire consisted of 550 items (Haertzen, 1974; Hill, Haertzen, Wolbach, & Miner, 1963), but a shortened version is most frequently used (Martin, Sloan, Sapira, & Jasinksi, 1971). The short form of the ARCI consists of 49 true–false questions and contains five major subscales: the Morphine-Benzedrine Group (MBG; an index of euphoria); the Pentobarbital-Chlorpromazine-Alcohol Group (PCAG; an index of sedation); the Lysergic Diethylamide scale (LSD; an index of somatic and dysphoric changes) and the Benzedrine (BG) and Amphetamine (A or AMPH) scales (empirically derived stimulant-sensitive scales). Many studies have employed the ARCI to evaluate the subjective effects of cocaine in humans and the results of these are summarized across studies (Fischman *et al.,* 1976; Haberny *et al.,* 1995; Kumor, Sherer, & Jaffe., 1989; Oliveto *et al.,* 1995; Perez-Reyes *et al.,* 1982; Preston *et al.,* 1992, Preston, Sullivan,

Berger, & Bigelow, 1993; Sherer, 1988). As would be expected, cocaine typically increases ratings on the two scales empirically derived for sensitivity to psychomotor stimulants, the BG and A scales. Conversely, scores on the PCAG scale, a measure of sedation, are frequently decreased by cocaine. Cocaine administration usually results in increased scores on the MBG scale consistent with its euphorigenic and stimulant effects. Finally, scores on the LSD scale are reliably increased by acute doses of cocaine. Although this scale has been previously described as a general index of dysphoria, it actually detects some somatic symptoms that may not necessarily be considered unpleasant (e.g., "I have a weird feeling" or "I feel drowsy" [this item is weighted negatively in the scale]). Moreover, several items on the LSD scale may detect the stimulant anxiogenic-like effects of cocaine (e.g., "I notice my hand shakes when I try to write" or "I feel anxious and upset"). The effects of cocaine on these ARCI scales are usually dose related regardless of route of administration.

The Profile of Mood States (POMS) is a structured questionnaire that was originally developed to assess mood effects in psychiatric populations (McNair, Lorr, & Droppleman, 1971); however, it is commonly used in drug abuse research. This questionnaire consists of several adjective items that are rated on a 5-point scale from "not at all" (0) to "extremely" (4). The items are weighted and grouped by factor analysis into eight subscales as follows: tension-anxiety, depression-dejection, anger-hostility, vigor, fatigue, confusion-bewilderment, friendliness, and elation. Cocaine typically produces increased scores on vigor, friendliness, and elation and decreased scores on fatigue; these effects are typically dose dependent and occur across routes of administration (Fischman *et al.,* 1976; Foltin & Fischman, 1992; Foltin, Fischman, Pippen, & Kelly, 1993; Perez-Reyes *et al.,* 1982)

Numerous studies have reported that the onset and peak subjective effects of cocaine closely correspond to the concentration of cocaine in plasma and parallel the expected distribution of the drug by these different routes of administration (Javaid *et al.,* 1978; Perez-Reyes *et al.,* 1982; Resnick *et al.,* 1977; Van Dyke *et al.,* 1978). A more recent study reported that arterial, rather than venous, concentrations of cocaine correspond more closely to the pharmacodynamic time-course of cocaine (Evans, Cone, & Henningfield, 1996). Thus, when cocaine is smoked or administered intravenously, the onset of subjective effects is almost immediate, occurring within 1–2 min of drug administration, and the peak response occurs shortly thereafter. A recent study reported that even modest variations in the speed of intravenous infusion (2 s versus 60 s) can significantly alter the magnitude of the subjective response to cocaine, with a faster infusion speed producing subjective responses of greater magnitude compared with a slower infusion speed (Abreu, Walsh, Bonson, Ginn, & Bigelow, 1997). The time to onset of the effects of intranasal cocaine is slower than intravenous and smoked cocaine; subjective ratings of drug effects increase within 5 min and peak between 20–30 min after insufflation, although there may be substantial intersubject variability. The euphorigenic effects of cocaine dissipate fairly quickly following administration by all three of these routes of administration. The onset of effects is slowest after administration of oral cocaine, appearing at about 30 min and reaching peak effect by approximately 1 hr after ingestion; thus the oral route actually produces a more sustained drug effect compared to the more rapid delivery methods.

Discriminative Stimulus Effects of Cocaine

The drug discrimination procedure has been developed as a means of studying interoceptive drug stimuli in animals. These discriminative stimulus effects are often considered analogous to subjective drug effects in humans (Preston & Bigelow, 1991; Schuster & Johanson, 1988). Although this procedure has been used primarily in laboratory animals, this paradigm has more recently been applied to stud-

ies of drug action in humans (see Preston, Walsh, & Sannerud, 1997, for review). The typical drug discrimination paradigm employs the use of differential reinforcement in order to train a discrimination between two or even three experimental conditions (e.g., drug vs. placebo [2-choice] or placebo vs. Drug A vs. Drug B [3-choice]). During training sessions, reinforcer delivery is dependent on the subject performing a specific response that is associated with either the presence or the absence of the drug stimulus. For example, the training drug may be administered prior to the experimental session and subsequent responses on one of two manipulanda will result in reinforcer delivery (e.g., food in a food-deprived subject). Following administration of placebo or a different training drug, responses on an alternate manipulanda will be reinforced. It is in this manner that over repeated training sessions stimulus control by the training drug(s) is eventually achieved. Subsequent testing can be conducted to determine (1) whether a novel drug will "substitute" for the training drug (engender drug-appropriate responding rather than placebo-appropriate) or (2) whether a novel compound administered before or in combination with the training drug modifies its discriminative stimulus properties. While drug discrimination procedures can be very sensitive, drug discrimination performance can be modulated by a number of experimental manipulations such as training dose or number of training conditions, and changes in these independent variables can significantly alter the study outcome (for reviews on this topic, see Overton, 1987; Stolerman, 1991; A. M. Young, 1991).

The drug discrimination procedure has been widely used to study the interoceptive stimuli of cocaine in nonhumans and more recently in humans.* Some of the most common applications of drug discrimination research with cocaine have focused on characterizing the behavioral profile of cocaine in comparison

*A complete updated bibliography of drug discrimination studies has been created by Dr. Ian Stolerman and can be accessed on the Internet at: http://www.arf.org/dd.

with other psychomotor stimulants and other classes of drugs, investigating the role of specific neurotransmitter systems in mediating the dynamic effects of cocaine, and evaluating potential pharmacotherapeutic agents for their ability to modulate the stimulus effects of cocaine. Cocaine can support discrimination performance in a variety of species, including rats (e.g., Colpaert, Niemegeers, & Janssen, 1976; Wood & Emmett-Oglesby, 1988), pigeons (Jarbe, 1981; Johanson & Barrett, 1993), nonhuman primates (e.g., Ando & Yanagita, 1978; de la Garza & Johanson, 1983; Woolverton & Trost, 1978), and, more recently, humans (Oliveto *et al.*, 1995). Numerous studies have also indicated that cocaine can be discriminated from placebo when administered by various routes of administration in laboratory animals including intraperitoneal (e.g., Cunningham & Callahan, 1991; Wood & Emmett-Oglesby, 1988 [most common in studies with rats]), intramuscular (e.g., de la Garza & Johanson, 1986; Lamas, Negus, Hall, & Mello, 1995 [most common in studies with nonhuman primates]), intravenous and intragastric (de la Garza & Johanson, 1986), and oral and intranasal routes in humans (Oliveto *et al.*, 1995).

Review of the cocaine drug discrimination literature reveals three common factors that influence or regulate cocaine discrimination behavior across species and routes. These include the training dose of cocaine, concentration of drug at the site of action, and specificity of stimulus effects for the pharmacological class. The influence of the training dose on subsequent discrimination performance has been evaluated for cocaine as well as other drugs (Colpaert & Janssen, 1982; Shannon & Holtzman, 1979; Stolerman & D'Mello, 1981). When cocaine doses other than the training dose are evaluated during substitution testing, cocaine-appropriate responses are emitted, and the frequency of the cocaine-appropriate responding is positively related to dose. Moreover, the cocaine dose–effect curve shifts leftward when animals are trained to discriminate progressively lower cocaine doses (Colpaert & Janssen, 1982; Terry, Witkin, & Katz, 1994). The degree of discriminative control exerted by the cocaine stimulus has been shown to be positively related to the concentration of cocaine in plasma in drug discrimination studies with concurrent pharmacokinetic analyses (Lamas *et al.*, 1995).

Preclinical studies report that the discriminative stimulus effects of cocaine are similar to other psychomotor stimulants, thus demonstrating specificity within the drug class. Animals trained to discriminate cocaine from saline will emit cocaine-appropriate responses when other stimulant compounds are administered; the array of stimulants that can substitute for cocaine under specified training conditions include, but are not limited to, *d*-amphetamine, methamphetamine, methylphenidate, phentermine, diethylproprion, methcathinone, and GBR 12909 (Johanson & Barrett, 1993; R. Young & Glennon, 1993; Witkin, Nichols, Terry, & Katz, 1991; Wood & Emmett-Oglesby, 1988). In contrast, substitution with drugs from other pharmacological classes (e.g., benzodiazepines, barbiturates, neuroleptics, morphine, or LSD) produce primarily placebo or nondrug responding in both nonhuman (e.g., de la Garza & Johanson, 1983; Jarbe, 1981; Witkin *et al.*, 1991) and human subjects (Oliveto *et al.*, 1995).

Drug discrimination studies with cocaine reveal information germane to the pharmacological mechanisms underlying the subjective and reinforcing effects of cocaine. While cocaine produces both central and peripheral pharmacologic effects, discrimination studies have revealed that the discriminative stimulus effects of cocaine are primarily related to its CNS actions. In one study, rats acquired a cocaine versus placebo discrimination in which cocaine was administered by the intraperitoneal route; subsequent substitution testing with cocaine administered through indwelling cannulae in the cerebral ventricles revealed that the centrally administered cocaine substituted for the intraperitoneal training dose of cocaine (Wood, Retz, & Emmett-Oglesby, 1987). Another method employed to assess the central versus peripheral mediation of the discriminative stimulus effects of cocaine is to conduct substitution tests with cocaine methiodide in cocaine-trained animals. Two studies used cocaine methiodide, a quaternary form of cocaine that mimics its peripheral actions but does not cross the blood-brain barrier, to evaluate whether the discriminative effects of cocaine were centrally mediated. Both studies reported that cocaine methiodide did not substitute for cocaine in rats trained to discriminate cocaine from placebo (McKenna & Ho, 1980; Witkin et al., 1991). In summary, these studies provide corroborative evidence that the central effects of cocaine are primarily responsible for mediating its discriminative stimulus properties. Moreover, although cocaine exerts pharmacological effects at a number of central receptor and transporter sites, the majority of studies support a role for dopamine over other neurotransmitters in mediating the discriminative stimulus effects of cocaine. Compounds that enhance dopamine transmission, such as reuptake inhibitors or some receptor agonists, can substitute for cocaine, while dopamine receptor antagonists attenuate the discriminative stimulus effects of cocaine (Callahan, Appel, & Cunningham, 1991; Kleven, Anthony, & Woolverton, 1990; Spealman, Bergman, Madras, & Melia, 1991; Witkin et al., 1991). In contrast, drugs such as desipramine and fluoxetine that share cocaine's ability to inhibit the reuptake of norepinephrine and serotonin, respectively, do not substitute for cocaine in the drug discrimination procedure (Cunningham & Callahan, 1991; Johanson & Fischman, 1989).

While most drug discrimination studies have been conducted with laboratory animals, human drug discrimination studies are becoming increasingly more common. The methodology applied in human studies is a modification of that used in animal studies. Subjects initially receive each training drug during separate sessions and are instructed to learn to recognize differences between the training drugs. During early training, the drugs are identified to the subject prior to administration by using either randomly assigned labels such as a letter code (A versus B) or by using identifiers that provide information about the training conditions, such as "drug" or "placebo" (Chait, Uhlenhuth, & Johanson, 1985; Grif-

fiths et al., 1990). Acquisition of the discrimination is determined by assessing whether the subject can identify the correct drug label after drug administration in subsequent trials. Another notable difference is that the reinforcer used in human studies is typically money in contrast to the traditional appetitive reinforcers (i.e., food or water) commonly used in animal studies. To date, only one study has been published evaluating the discriminative stimulus effects of cocaine in humans (Oliveto et al., 1995). In this study, human subjects with cocaine abuse histories were trained to discriminate oral cocaine (80 mg/70 kg) from placebo. Following acquisition, substitution tests revealed that a range of cocaine doses given both orally and intranasally substituted for the cocaine training dose, while the benzodiazepine drug, triazolam, produced predominately placebo responding. One of the unique features of drug discrimination research with humans is that subjective reports can be collected concurrently with discrimination measures. In this study, the range of cocaine doses that produced cocaine-appropriate responding also produced significant elevations on subjective report measures of prototypic cocaine effects. Thus, the limited data from human subjects suggest that a cocaine discrimination can be trained in humans, that it has specificity for the drug class, and that discriminative and subjective effects occur in concert.

Cocaine Reinforcement: Laboratory Studies

Self-Administration Studies with Nonhuman Subjects

A review of the cocaine self-administration literature reveals that there are more than 400 published studies on this topic. Numerous variables are known to influence the outcome of cocaine self-administration studies including the operant schedule (e.g., fixed ratio, second-order), the chosen self-administration paradigm (e.g., choice procedure, progressive ratio), cocaine dose, availability of alternative reinforcers, and several other factors. Indeed, there are a substantial number of published studies that have systematically investigated the influence of parametric manipulations of one or more of these variables. A detailed discussion of these determinants and their influence on cocaine self-administration is beyond the scope of this chapter and can be found elsewhere (Bickel, DeGrandpre, & Higgins, 1995; Johanson & Fischman, 1989; Mello & Negus, 1996; Woolverton, 1992). Thus, preclinical studies are summarized briefly to illustrate some of the general characteristics of cocaine self-administration in the laboratory; a detailed discussion of human self-administration studies follows.

It was first discovered nearly three decades ago that animals would self-administer cocaine. In these earliest studies, it was demonstrated that cocaine was a potent reinforcer, the delivery of which maintained high rates of operant behavior in laboratory animals (Pickens & Thompson, 1968; Woods & Schuster, 1968). In studies providing 24-hr unrestricted access to cocaine, self-administration occurred in irregular episodes; periods of high rates of responding would be followed by periods of varying duration during which no responding occurred. With unrestricted access to cocaine, both rats and monkeys would self-administer cocaine to the exclusion of engaging in other behaviors, such as feeding and grooming; lethal overdose was a common outcome (Deneau, Yanagita, & Seevers, 1969; Johanson, Balster, & Bonese, 1976). In contrast, when conditions are arranged so that access is restricted to a fixed period of time (e.g., one 4-hr session a day), the temporal pattern of responding for cocaine becomes very regular within sessions and total intake of cocaine may be stable for several months (Wilson, Hitomi, & Schuster, 1971). Consistent with the finding that total cocaine intake can remain stable over time, it has been demonstrated that modifying the available unit dose of cocaine (i.e., cocaine dose per injection) does not necessarily alter the total intake of cocaine. Thus, self-administration of cocaine increases when the unit dose of cocaine is decreased, and, conversely, self-administration of cocaine decreases when the unit dose of cocaine is increased (Wilson et al., 1971; Woods & Schuster, 1968). This inverse relationship between the unit dose of cocaine and the frequency of self-administration leads to an inverted U-shaped dose response function for response rate while the actual intake of daily cocaine under restricted access conditions remains fairly constant.

Studies conducted in nonhumans have shown that cocaine is self-administered under a wide range of experimental conditions and by various routes of administration. The majority of cocaine self-administration studies have employed the intravenous route. Indeed, intravenous cocaine is such a powerful reinforcer that it is commonly used to initiate or train self-administration behavior in studies designed to assess the effects of novel compounds with unknown abuse liability (e.g., Griffiths, Llamb, Sannerud, Ator, & Brady, 1991; Sannerud, Kaminsky, & Griffiths, 1996). Cocaine also acts as a reinforcer when it is administered by the intramuscular (Goldberg, Morse, & Goldberg, 1976) or intragastric route (Woolverton & Schuster, 1983), although these routes are not commonly used. Oral cocaine can also act as a reinforcer in spite of its slow onset of pharmacodynamic effects; however, it may require greater experimental effort to engender this behavior. Self-administration of oral cocaine has been demonstrated in several species including rhesus monkeys (Meisch & Stewart, 1995; Meisch, George, & Lemaire, 1990), rats (Lau, Falk, & King, 1992; Tang & Falk, 1987), and mice (George, Elmer, Meisch, & Goldberg, 1991).

Similar to the findings for the discriminative stimulus effects of cocaine, evidence from neuropharmacological studies suggests that the reinforcing effects of cocaine are largely mediated through its actions on central dopamine systems. Preclinical studies have shown that pharmacological blockade of dopamine receptors by pretreatment with neuroleptic agents decreases or completely extinguishes responding for cocaine (Bergman, Kamien, & Spealman, 1990; de Wit & Wise, 1977; Wilson & Schuster, 1972). Destruction of dopamine nerve terminals within these mesolimbic regions results in extinction of cocaine-reinforced responding, suggesting that the integrity of this pathway is critical to the reinforcing actions of cocaine (Goeders & Smith, 1986; Petit, Ettenbeg, Bloom, & Koob, 1984; Roberts, Koob, Klonoff, & Fibiger, 1980). Specifically, it is the ability of cocaine to bind to the dopamine transporter in these regions that appears to underlie its reinforcing properties. Studies in rodents and nonhuman primates indicate that the potency for inhibiting dopamine reuptake closely corresponds to the reinforcing efficacy of compounds that are structurally related to cocaine (Bergman, Madras, Johson, & Spealman, 1989; Ritz et al., 1987). Moreover, reuptake inhibitors of norepinephrine and serotonin are not typically reinforcing (see Woolverton, 1992). Thorough reviews of studies evaluating the role of dopamine in the reinforcing effects of cocaine can be found elsewhere (Fibiger et al., 1992; Koob, 1992a, 1992b; Woolverton, 1992; but see also Gratton, 1996).

Self-Administration Studies with Humans

Human self-administration studies draw on experimental methodology that has been developed with laboratory animals. However, the safety and ethical concerns regarding the use of human subjects in these studies limits the range of experimental factors that can be explored and influences the experimental design. For example, both the range of cocaine doses and the frequency of within-session dosing are limited to ensure that cocaine administration is safely tolerated by all volunteers. Moreover, session duration and frequency can be limited by such practical considerations as the availability of medical staff to administer the drug and to monitor the safety of the volunteers. The majority of human cocaine self-administration studies have employed the choice procedure, first developed in rhesus monkeys (Johanson & Schuster, 1975), because this procedure eliminates some of the logistic difficulties associated with employing standard operant procedures and the progressive ratio paradigm in the human laboratory. Some stud-

ies have incorporated an operant work requirement that produces a conditioned reinforcer (e.g., a token) exchangeable for cocaine or alternative reinforcers (Dudish, Pentel, & Hatsukami, 1996; Foltin & Fischman, 1994). As in human drug discrimination studies, human self-administration studies can also incorporate concurrent subjective effect measures, thus directly evaluating the relationship between the subjective response to cocaine and drug-taking behavior (Fischman & Schuster, 1982; Fischman, Foltin, Nestadt, & Pearlson, 1990; Hatsukami et al., 1994; Higgins, Bickel, & Hughes, 1994).

Evidence from laboratory studies demonstrates that cocaine functions as a positive reinforcer under controlled experimental conditions in humans as well as in nonhumans. Human subjects with cocaine abuse histories reliably choose to self-administer cocaine over placebo. This has been demonstrated for cocaine administered by the intravenous (Fischman & Schuster, 1982) and intranasal (Higgins et al., 1994) routes and with smoking freebase cocaine (Foltin & Fischman, 1992; Hatsukami et al., 1994). In studies using a choice procedure in which subjects may choose between two active doses of cocaine, higher doses are reliably chosen over lower doses, and this occurs independent of route of administration (Dudish et al., 1996; Foltin & Fischman, 1992; Hatsukami et al., 1994). Similar to findings with nonhumans, studies with human subjects report that cocaine intake is fairly stable over repeated trials (Hatsukami et al., 1994) and, in most cases, subjects choose the maximum number of available cocaine doses within a session when alternative reinforcers are not available.

The concurrent availability of nondrug reinforcers and their effect on cocaine self-administration has also been evaluated in humans. In one recent study, volunteers were given the option to choose either a dose of intranasal cocaine or placebo (Higgins et al., 1994). In subsequent sessions subjects could choose either cocaine or money, and the amount of money was varied over several trials. Cocaine was reliably chosen over placebo, and the number of cocaine choices systematically increased as the amount of available money decreased, demonstrating the influence of alternative reinforcers on cocaine self-administration. This relationship between money as an alternative reinforcer and cocaine choice has also been investigated with smoked cocaine (Hatsukami *et al.*, 1994). The findings were quite similar to those obtained with intranasal cocaine; that is, as the dollar value of available token increased, cocaine self-administration decreased, although this relationship was more orderly for low doses of cocaine compared with high doses of cocaine.

Several studies with humans have suggested that there may be a dissociation between the subjective effects of cocaine and its reinforcing properties as assessed in these laboratory procedures. In one study aimed at evaluating the potential therapeutic efficacy of desipramine for cocaine abuse, it was reported that desipramine pretreatment did not alter cocaine self-administration despite declines on the subject-rated measure of "want" for cocaine (Fischman *et al.*, 1990). Repeated dosing studies have shown that acute tolerance to the subjective effects of cocaine occurs following the initial dose; however, subjects continue to self-administer cocaine over repeated trials despite the decrease in its capacity to produce positive mood effects (Fischman *et al.*, 1990; Foltin *et al.*, 1988). Finally, a recent study utilized a choice procedure to assess preference for route of administration (intravenous versus smoking) in volunteers who predominately reported intravenous administration as their preferred route for illicit use. More frequent choices for smoking free-base cocaine were made compared with choices for intravenous injections of cocaine, despite the fact that cocaine doses for both routes produced equivalent effects on subjective and cardiovascular indices (Foltin & Fischman, 1992). These data suggest that there is not a perfect correspondence between subjective reports and self-administration of cocaine in the laboratory setting. Collectively, these self-administration studies indicate that cocaine functions as a reinforcer in humans and that self-administration

behavior may be influenced by factors similar to those shown to modulate drug intake in studies with nonhuman subjects, including dose of cocaine and the availability of alternative reinforcers.

Conclusions

Cocaine abuse continues to pose a significant health problem in the United States and, for this reason, cocaine remains the focus of numerous preclinical and clinical studies aimed at identifying its behavioral pharmacologic actions and variables that may modulate its abuse liability. Subjective effect studies indicate that cocaine produces euphorigenic, stimulant, and anxiogenic effects in humans, and these effects are positively related to dose regardless of the route of administration. The onset and peak subjective effects closely parallel the concentration of cocaine in plasma in single-dose studies; however, acute tolerance occurs after the first dose in repeated dose procedures decreasing the subjective and physiological response to subsequent doses. Preclinical data indicate that the discriminative stimulus effects of cocaine are related to dose and are qualitatively similar for other stimulant compounds. These effects are centrally, not peripherally, mediated, and, as with the reinforcing effects of cocaine, it appears that mesolimbic dopamine plays a principal role in the discriminative stimulus properties of cocaine. Limited data from human subjects indicates that the discriminative stimulus effects of cocaine closely correspond to its subjective effects, while self-administration studies have reported some dissociations between subjective responses and cocaine-taking in the laboratory. Finally, self-administration of cocaine in humans can be modified by variables known to influence self-administration in nonhumans, including the dose of cocaine and the availability of alternative reinforcers.

ACKNOWLEDGMENT

Preparation of this chapter was supported by grants from the National Institute on Drug Abuse (DA 05196, DA 10029 and DA 10753).

References

Abreu, M. E., Walsh, S. L., Bonson, K. R., Ginn, D., & Bigelow, G. E. (1997). Effects of intravenous injection speed on responses to cocaine or hydromorphone in humans. In *Problems of Drug Dependence 1996, Proceedings of the 58th Annual Scientific Meeting,* The College on Problems of Drug Dependence, Inc. (NIDA Research Monographs, NIDA Research Monograph No. 174, p. 139). Rockville, MD: U.S. Government Printing Office.

Ando, K., & Yanagita, T. (1978). The discriminative stimulus properties of intravenously administered cocaine in rhesus monkeys. In G. C. Colpaert & J. A. Rosecrans (Eds.), *Stimulus properties of drugs: Ten years of progress* (pp. 125–136). Amsterdam: Elsevier/North.

Bergman, J., Madras, B. K., Johson, S. E., & Spealman, R. D. (1989). Effects of cocaine and related drugs in nonhuman primates. III. Self-administration by squirrel monkeys. *Journal of Pharmacology and Experimental Therapeutics, 251,* 150–155.

Bergman, J., Kamien, J. B., & Spealman, R. D. (1990). Antagonism of cocaine self-administration by selective D_1 and D_2 antagonists. *Behavioural Pharmacology, 1,* 355–363.

Bickel, W. K., DeGrandpre, R. J., & Higgins, S. T. (1995). The behavioral economics of concurrent drug reinforcers: A review and reanalysis of drug self-administration research. *Psychopharmacology, 118,* 250–259.

Bigelow, G. E. (1991). Human drug abuse liability assessment: Opioids and analgesics. *British Journal of Addiction, 86,* 1615–1628.

Brain, P. F., & Coward, G. A. (1989). A review of the history, actions and legitimate uses of cocaine. *Journal of Substance Abuse, 11,* 431–451.

Callahan, P. M., Appel, J. B., & Cunningham, K. A. (1991). Dopamine D_1 and D_2 mediation of the discriminative stimulus properties of *d*-amphetamine and cocaine. *Psychopharmacology, 103,* 50–55.

Chait, L. D., Uhlenhuth, E. H., & Johanson, C-E. (1985). The discriminative stimulus and subjective effects of d-amphetamine in humans. *Psychopharmacology, 86,* 307–312.

Colpaert, F. C., & Janssen, P. A. J. (1982). Factors regulating drug cue sensitivity: Limits of discriminability and the role of a progressively decreasing training dose in cocaine-saline discrimination. *Neuropharmacology, 21,* 1187–1194.

Colpaert, F. C., Niemegeers, C. J. E., & Janssen, P. A. J. (1976). Cocaine cue in rats as it relates to subjective drug effects: A preliminary report. *European Journal of Pharmacology, 10,* 195–199.

Cunningham, K. A., & Callahan, P. M. (1991). Monoamine reuptake inhibitors enhance the discriminative state induced by cocaine in the rat. *Psychopharmacology, 104,* 177–180.

de la Garza, R., & Johanson, C-E. (1983). The discriminative stimulus properties of cocaine in the rhesus monkey. *Pharmacology, Biochemistry and Behavior, 19,* 145–148.

de la Garza, R., & Johanson, C-E. (1986). The discriminative stimulus properties of cocaine and *d*-amphetamine: The effects of three routes of administration. *Pharmacology, Biochemistry and Behavior, 24,* 765–768.

Deneau, F., Yanagita, T., & Seevers, M. H. (1969). Self-administration of psychoactive substances by the monkey: A measure of psychological dependence. *Psychopharmacologia, 16,* 30–48.

de Wit, H., & Wise, R. A. (1977). Blockade of cocaine reinforcement in rats with the dopamine receptor blocker pimozide, but not with the noradrenergic blockers phentolamine or phenoxybenzamine. *Canadian Journal of Psychology, 31,* 195–203.

Dudish, S. A., Pentel, P. R., & Hatsukami, D. K. (1996). Smoked cocaine self-administration in females. *Psychopharmacology, 123,* 79–87.

Evans, S. M., Cone, E. J., & Henningfield, J. E. (1996). Arterial and venous cocaine plasma concentrations in humans: Relationship to route of administration, cardiovascular effects and subjective effects. *Journal of Pharmacology and Experimental Therapeutics, 279,* 135–1356.

Fibiger, H. C., Phillips, A. G., & Brown, E. E. (1992). The neurobiology of cocaine-induced reinforcement. In R. Bock & J. Whelan (Eds.), *Cocaine: Scientific and social dimensions* (Ciba Foundation Symposium, Vol. 166, pp. 96–111). New York: Wiley.

Fischman, M. W., & Schuster, C. R. (1982). Cocaine self-administration in humans. *Federation Proceedings, 41,* 241–246.

Fischman, M. W., Schuster, C. R., Resnekov, L., Schick, J. F. E., Krasnegor, N. A., Fennell, W., & Freedman, D. X. (1976). Cardiovascular and subjective effects of intravenous cocaine administration in humans. *Archives of General Psychiatry, 33,* 983–989.

Fischman, M. W., Foltin, R. W., Nestadt, G., & Pearlson, G. D. (1990). Effects of desipramine maintenance on cocaine self-administration by humans. *Journal of Pharmacology and Experimental Therapeutics, 253,* 760–770.

Foltin, R. W., & Fischman, M. W. (1991). Smoked and intravenous cocaine in humans: Acute tolerance, cardiovascular and subjective effects. *Journal of Pharmacology and Experimental Therapeutics, 257,* 247–261.

Foltin, R. W., & Fischman, M. W. (1992). Self-administration of cocaine by humans: Choice between smoked and intravenous cocaine. *Journal of Pharmacology and Experimental Therapeutics, 261,* 841–849.

Foltin, R. W., & Fischman, M. W. (1994). Effects of buprenorphine on the self-administration of cocaine by humans. *Behavioural Pharmacology, 5,* 79–89.

Foltin, R. W., Fischman, M. W., Pedroso, J. J., & Pearlson, G. D. (1988). Repeated intranasal cocaine administration: Lack of tolerance to pressor effects. *Drug and Alcohol Dependence, 22,* 169–177.

Foltin, R. W., Fischman, M. W., Pippen, P. A., & Kelly, T. H. (1993). Behavioral effects of cocaine alone and in combination with ethanol or marijuana in humans. *Drug and Alcohol Dependence, 32,* 93–106.

George, F. R., Elmer, G. I., Meisch, R. A., & Goldberg, S. R. (1991). Orally delivered cocaine functions as a positive reinforcer in C57BL/6J mice. *Pharmacology, Biochemistry and Behavior, 38,* 897–903.

Goddard, D., de Goddard, S. N., & Whitehead, P. C. (1969). Social factors associated with coca use in the Andean region. *International Journal of the Addictions, 4,* 577–590.

Goeders, N. E., & Smith, J. E. (1986). Reinforcing properties of cocaine in the medial prefrontal cortex: Primary action on presynaptic dopaminergic terminals. *Pharmacology, Biochemistry and Behavior, 25,* 191–196.

Goldberg, S. R., Morse, W. H., & Goldberg, D. M. (1976). Behavior maintained under a second-order schedule by intramuscular injection of morphine or cocaine in rhesus monkeys. *Journal of Pharmacology and Experimental Therapeutics, 199,* 278–286.

Gossop, M., Griffiths, P., Powis, B., & Strang, J. (1994). Cocaine: Patterns of use, route of administration and severity of dependence. *British Journal of Psychiatry, 164,* 660–664.

Gratton, A. (1996). In vivo analysis of the role of dopamine in stimulant and opiate self-administration. *Journal of Psychiatry and Neuroscience, 21,* 264–279.

Griffiths, R. R., Evans, S. M., Heishman, S. J., Preston, K. L., Sannerud, C. A., Wolf, B., & Woodson, P. O. (1990). Low-dose caffeine discrimination in humans. *Journal of Pharmacology and Experimental Therapeutics, 252,* 970–978.

Griffiths, R. R., Lamb, R. J., Sannerud, C. A., Ator, N. A., & Brady, J. V. (1991). Self-injection of barbiturates, benzodiazepines and other sedative-anxiolytics in baboons. *Psychopharmacology, 103,* 154–161.

Grinspoon, L., & Bakalar, J. B. (1981). Coca and cocaine as medicines: A historical review. *Journal of Ethnopharmacology, 3,* 149–159.

Haberny, K. A., Walsh, S. L., Ginn, D. H., Wilkins, J. N., Garner, J. E., Setoda, D., & Bigelow, G. E. (1995). Absence of acute cocaine interactions with the MAO-B inhibitor selegiline. *Drug and Alcohol Dependence, 39,* 55–62.

Haertzen, C. A. (1974). An overview of the Addiction Research Center Inventory (ARCI): An appendix and manual of scales (DHEW Publication No. 79). Washington, DC: U.S. Department of Health, Education and Welfare.

Harris, J. E., & Baldessarini, R. J. (1973). Uptake of [³H]-catecholamines by homogenates of rat corpus striatum and cerebral cortex: Effects of amphetamine analogues. *Neuropharmacology, 12,* 659–679.

Hatsukami, D. K., & Fischman, M. W. (1996). Crack cocaine and cocaine hydrochloride. Are the differences myth or reality? *Journal of the American Medical Association, 276,* 1580–1588.

Hatsukami, D. K., Thompson, T. N., Pentel, P. R., Flygare, B. K., & Carroll, M. E. (1994). Self-administration of smoked cocaine. *Experimental and Clinical Psychopharmacology, 2,* 115–125.

Heikkila, R. E., Cabbat, F. S., Manzino, R. C., & Duvoisin, R. C. (1979). Rotational behavior induced by cocaine analogs in rats with unilateral 6-hydroxydopamine lesions of the substantia nigra: Dependence upon dopamine uptake inhibition. *Journal of Pharmacology and Experimental Therapeutics, 211,* 189–194

Higgins, S. T., Bickel, W. K., & Hughes, J. R. (1994). Influence of an alternative reinforcer on human cocaine self-administration. *Life Sciences, 55,* 179–187.

Hill, H. E., Haertzen, C. A., Wolbach, A. B., & Miner, E. J. (1963). The Addiction Research Inventory: Standardization of scales which evaluate subjective effects of morphine, amphetamine, pentobarbital, alcohol, LSD-25, pyrahexyl and chlorpromazine. *Psychopharmacologia, 4,* 167–183.

Jarbe, T. U. C. (1981). Cocaine cue in pigeons: Time course studies and generalization to structurally related compounds (norcocaine, WIN 35,428 and 35,065-2) and (+)-amphetamine. *British Journal of Pharmacology, 73,* 843–852.

Jasinski, D. R., Johnson, R. E., & Henningfield, J. E. (1984). Abuse liability assessment in human subjects. *Trends in Pharmacological Sciences, 5,* 196–200.

Javaid, J. I., Fischman, M. W., Schuster, C. R., Dekirmenjian, H., & Davis, J. M. (1978). Cocaine plasma concentration: Relation to physiological and subjective effects in humans. *Science, 202,* 227–228.

Johanson, C-E., & Barrett, J. E. (1993). The discriminative stimulus effects of cocaine in pigeons. *Journal of Pharmacology and Experimental Therapeutics, 267,* 1–8.

Johanson, C-E., & Fischman M. W. (1989). The pharmacology of cocaine related to its abuse. *Pharmacological Reviews, 41,* 3–52.

Johanson, C-E., & Schuster, C. R. (1975). A choice procedure for drug reinforcers: Cocaine and methylphenidate in the rhesus monkey. *Journal of Pharmacology and Experimental Therapeutics, 193,* 676–688.

Johanson, C-E., Balster, R. L., & Bonese, K. (1976). Self-administration of psychomotor stimulant drugs: The effects of unlimited access. *Pharmacology, Biochemistry and Behavior, 4,* 45–51.

Kilpatrick, G. J., Jones, B. J., & Tyers, M. B. (1989). Binding of the 5-HT₃ ligand GR65630, to rat area postrema vagus nerve and the brain of several species. *European Journal of Pharmacology, 159,* 157–164.

Kleven, M. S., Anthony, E. W., & Woolverton, W. L. (1990). Pharmacological characterization of the discriminative stimulus effects of cocaine in rhesus monkeys. *Journal of Pharmacology and Experimental Therapeutics, 254,* 312–317.

Koe, B. K. (1976). Molecular geometry of inhibitors of the uptake of catecholamines and serotonin in synaptosomal preparations of rat brain. *Journal of Pharmacology and Experimental Therapeutics, 199,* 649–661.

Koob, G. F. (1992a). Drugs of abuse: Anatomy, pharmacology and function of reward pathways. *Trends in Pharmacological Sciences, 13,* 177–184.

Koob, G. F. (1992b). Neural mechanisms of drug reinforcement. *Annals of the New York Academy of Sciences, 654,* 171–191.

Kumor, K, Sherer, M., & Jaffe, J. (1989). Effects of bromocriptine pretreatment on subjective and physiological responses to IV cocaine. *Pharmacology, Biochemistry and Behavior, 33,* 829–837.

Lamas, X., Negus, S. S., Hall, E., & Mello, N. K. (1995). Relationship between the discriminative stimulus effects and plasma concentrations of intramuscular cocaine in rhesus monkeys. *Psychopharmacology, 121,* 331–338.

Lau, C. E., Falk, J. L., & King, G. R. (1992). Oral cocaine self-administration: relation of locomotor activity to pharmacokinetics. *Pharmacology, Biochemistry and Behavior, 43,* 45–51.

Martin, W. R., Sloan, B. S., Sapira, J. D., & Jasinksi, D. R. (1971). Physiologic, subjective and behavioral effects of amphetamine, methamphetamine, ephedrine, phenmetrazine and methylphenidate in man. *Clinical Pharmacology & Therapeutics, 12,* 245–258.

Mayersohn, M., & Perrier, D. (1978). Kinetics of pharmacologic response to cocaine. *Research Communications in Chemistry, Pathology and Pharmacology, 22,* 465–474.

McKenna, M. L., & Ho, B. T. (1980). The role of dopamine in the discriminative stimulus properties of cocaine. *Neuropharmacology, 19,* 297–303.

McNair, D. M., Lorr, M., & Droppleman, L. F. (1971). *EITS manual for the profile of mood states.* San Diego, CA: Educational and Industrial Testing Service.

Meisch, R. A., & Stewart, R. B. (1995). Relative reinforcing effects of different doses of orally delivered cocaine. *Drug and Alcohol Dependence, 37,* 141–147.

Meisch, R. A., George, F. R., & Lemaire, G. A. (1990). Orally delivered cocaine as a reinforcer for Rhesus monkeys. *Pharmacology, Biochemistry and Behavior, 35,* 245–249.

Mello, N. K., & Negus, S. S. (1996). Preclinical evaluation of pharmacotherapies for treatment of cocaine and opioid abuse using drug self-administration procedures. *Neuropsychopharmacology, 14,* 375–424.

Middleton, R. M., & Kirkpatrick, M. B. (1993). Clinical use of cocaine: A review of the risks and benefits. *Drug Safety, 9,* 212–217.

Musto, D. F. (1992). Cocaine's history, especially the American experience. In R. Bock & J. Whelan (Eds.), *Cocaine: Scientific and social dimensions* (Ciba Foundation Symposium, Vol. 166, pp. 7–14). New York: Wiley.

National Household Survey on Drug Abuse. (1995). *Population estimates 1994* (U.S. Department of Health and Human Services, Substance Abuse Mental Health Service Administration [SAMHSA], DHHS 95-3063). Washington, DC: U.S. Government Printing Office.

Negrete, J. C. (1992). Cocaine problems in the coca-growing countries of South America. In R. Bock & J. Whelan (Eds.), *Cocaine: Scientific and social dimensions* (Ciba Foundation Symposium, Vol. 166, pp. 40–50). New York: Wiley.

Oliveto, A., Rosen, M. I., Woods, S. W., & Kosten, T. R. (1995). Discriminative stimulus, self-reported and cardiovascular effects of orally administered cocaine in humans. *Journal of Pharmacology and Experimental Therapeutics, 272,* 231–241.

Overton, D. A. (1987). Applications and limitations of the drug discrimination method for the study of drug abuse. In M. A. Bozarth (Ed.), *Methods for assessing the reinforcing properties of abused drugs* (pp. 91–340). New York: Springer-Verlag.

Perez-Reyes, M., Di Guiseppi, S., Ondrusek, G., Jeffcoat, A. R., & Cook, C. E. (1982). Free-base cocaine smoking. *Clinical Pharmacology & Therapeutics, 32,* 459–465.

Petit, H. O., Ettenberg, A., Bloom, F. E., & Koob, G. F. (1984). Destruction of dopamine in the nucleus accumbens selectively attenuates cocaine but not heroin self-administration in rats. *Psychopharmacology, 84,* 167–173.

Pickens, R., & Thompson, T. (1968). Cocaine-reinforced behavior in rats: Effects of reinforcement magnitude and fixed-ratio size. *Journal of Pharmacology and Experimental Therapeutics, 161,* 122–129.

Preston, K. L., & Bigelow, G. E. (1991). Subjective and discriminative effects of drugs. *Behavioural Pharmacology, 2,* 293–313.

Preston, K. L., Sullivan, J. T., Strain, E. C., & Bigelow, G. E. (1992). Effects of cocaine alone and in combination with bromocriptine in human cocaine abusers. *Journal of Pharmacology and Experimental Therapeutics, 262,* 279–291.

Preston, K. L., Sullivan, J. T., Berger, P. B., & Bigelow, G. E. (1993). Effects of cocaine alone and in combination with mazindol in human cocaine abusers. *Journal of Pharmacology and Experimental Therapeutics, 267,* 296–307.

Preston, K. L., Walsh, S. L., & Sannerud, C. A. (1997). Measures of interoceptive stimulus effects: Relationship to drug reinforcement. In J. D. Roache & B. A. Johnson (Eds.), *Drug addiction and its treatment: Nexus of neuroscience and behavior* (pp. 91–114). Philadelphia: Lippincott-Raven.

Resnick, R. B., Kestenbaum, R. S., & Schwartz, L. K. (1977). Acute systemic effects of cocaine in man: A controlled study by intranasal and intravenous routes. *Science, 195,* 696–699.

Ritz, M. C., Lamb, R. J., Goldberg, S. R., & Kuhar, M. J. (1987). Cocaine receptors on dopamine transporters are related to self-administration of cocaine. *Science, 237,* 1219–1223.

Roberts, D. C. S., Koob, G. F., Klonoff, P., & Fibiger, H. C. (1980). Extinction and recovery of cocaine self-administration following 6-hydroxydopamine lesions of the nucleus accumbens. *Pharmacology, Biochemistry and Behavior, 12*, 781–787.

Rowbotham, M. C., Jones, R. T., Benowitz, N. L., & Jacob, P. (1984). Trazodone–oral cocaine interactions. *Archives of General Psychiatry, 41*, 895–899.

Sannerud, C. A., Kaminski, B. J., & Griffiths, R. R. (1996). Intravenous self-injection of four novel phenethylamines in baboons. *Behavioural Pharmacology, 7*, 315–323.

Scheel-Kruger, J., Braestrup, C., Nielson, M., Golembiowska, K., & Modilnicka, E. (1976). Cocaine: Discussion on the role of dopamine in the biochemical mechanism of action. In E. H. Ellinwood & M. M. Kilbey (Eds.), *Cocaine and other stimulants* (pp. 373–407). New York: Plenum.

Schuster, C. R., & Johanson, C-E. (1988). Relationship between the discriminative stimulus properties and subjective effects of drugs. In F. C. Colpaert & R. L. Balster (Eds.), *Transduction mechanisms of drug stimuli* (pp. 161–175). Berlin: Springer-Verlag.

Shannon, H. E., & Holtzman, S. G. (1979). Morphine training dose: A determinant of stimulus generalization to narcotic antagonists in the rat. *Psychopharmacology, 61*, 239–244.

Sharkey, J., Ritz, M. C., Schenden, J. A., Hanson, R. C., & Kuhar, M. J. (1988). Cocaine inhibits muscarinic cholinergic receptors in heart and brain. *Journal of Pharmacology and Experimental Therapeutics, 246*, 1048–1052.

Sherer, M. A. (1988). Intravenous cocaine: Psychiatric effects, biological mechanisms. *Biological Psychiatry, 24*, 865–885.

Spealman, R. D., Bergman, J., Madras, B. K., & Melia, K. F. (1991). Discriminative stimulus effects of cocaine in squirrel monkeys: Involvement of dopamine receptor subtypes. *Journal of Pharmacology and Experimental Therapeutics, 258*, 945–953.

Stolerman, I. P. (1991). Measures of stimulus generalization in drug discrimination experiments. *Behavioural Pharmacology, 2*, 265–282.

Stolerman, I. P., & D'Mello, G. D. (1981). Role of training conditions in discrimination of central nervous system stimulants by rats. *Psychopharmacology, 73*, 295–303.

Tang, M., & Falk, J. L. (1987). Oral self-administration of cocaine: Chronic excessive intake by schedule induction. *Pharmacology, Biochemistry and Behavior, 28*, 517–519.

Terry, P., Witkin, J. M., & Katz, J. L. (1994). Pharmacological characterization of the novel discriminative stimulus effects of a low dose of cocaine. *Journal of Pharmacology and Experimental Therapeutics, 270*, 1041–1048.

Van Dyke, C., & Byck, R. (1983). Cocaine use in man. In N. K. Mello (Ed.), *Advances in substance abuse* (Vol. 3, pp. 1–24). Greenwich, CT: JAI.

Van Dyke, C., Jatlow, P., Ungerer, J., Barash, P. G., & Byck, R. (1978). Oral cocaine: Plasma concentrations and central effects. *Science, 200*, 211–213.

Walsh, S. L., Preston, K. L., Sullivan, J. T., Fromme, R., & Bigelow, G. E. (1994). Fluoxetine alters the effects of intravenous cocaine in humans. *Journal of Clinical Psychopharmacology, 14*, 396–407.

Walsh, S. L., Sullivan, J. T., Preston, K. L., Garner, J. E., & Bigelow, G. E. (1996). The effects of naltrexone on response to intravenous cocaine, hydromorphone, and their combination in humans. *Journal of Pharmacology and Experimental Therapeutics, 279*, 524–538.

Warner, E. A. (1993). Safety and risks of cocaine use. *Annals of Internal Medicine, 119*, 226–235.

Wilson, M. C., & Schuster, C. R. (1972). The effects of chlorpromazine on psychomotor stimulant self-administration in the rhesus monkey. *Psychopharmacologia, 26*, 115–126.

Wilson, M. C., Hitomi, M., & Schuster, C. R. (1971). Psychomotor stimulant self-administration as a function of dosage per injection in the Rhesus monkey. *Psychopharmacologia, 22*, 271–281.

Witkin, J. M., Nichols, D. E., Terry, P., & Katz, J. L. (1991). Behavioral effects of selective dopaminergic compounds in rats discriminating cocaine injections. *Journal of Pharmacology and Experimental Therapeutics, 257*, 706–713.

Wood, D. M., & Emmett-Oglesby, M. W. (1988). Substitution and cross-tolerance profiles of anorectic drugs in rats trained to detect the discriminative stimulus properties of cocaine. *Psychopharmacology, 95*, 364–368.

Wood, D. M., Retz, K. C., & Emmett-Oglesby, M. W. (1987). Evidence of a central mechanism mediating tolerance to the discriminative stimulus properties of cocaine. *Pharmacology, Biochemistry and Behavior, 28*, 401–406.

Woods, J., & Schuster, C. R. (1968). Reinforcement properties of morphine, cocaine and SPA as a function of unit dose. *International Journal of the Addictions, 3*, 231–237.

Woolverton, W. L. (1992). Determinants of cocaine self-administration by laboratory animals. In R. Bock & J. Whelan (Eds.), *Cocaine: Scientific and social dimensions* (Ciba Foundation Symposium, Vol. 166, pp. 96–111). New York: Wiley.

Woolverton, W. L., & Schuster, C. R. (1983). Intragastric self-administration in rhesus monkeys under limited access conditions: Methodological studies. *Journal of Pharmacological Methods, 10*, 93–106.

Woolverton, W. L., & Trost, R. C. (1978). Cocaine as a discriminative stimulus for responding maintained by food in squirrel monkeys. *Pharmacology, Biochemistry and Behavior, 8*, 627–630.

Young, A. M. (1991). Discriminative stimulus profiles of psychoactive drugs. In N. K. Mello (Ed.), *Advances in substance abuse* (Vol. 4, pp. 139–203). London: Jessica Kingsley.

Young, R., & Glennon, R. A. (1993). Cocaine-stimulus generalization to two new designer drugs: Methcathinone and 4-methylaminorex. *Pharmacology, Biochemistry and Behavior, 45*, 229–231.

12

Psychological and Psychiatric Consequences of Cocaine

M. ELENA DENISON, ALFONSO PAREDES, SHANA BACAL, AND FRANK H. GAWIN

Introduction

Systematic observations of abuse and abstinence patterns that refine conceptualizations of street cocaine abuse and dependence are rare and, unfortunately, practical and ethical design restrictions on systematic inpatient research render clinical generalization from such studies negligible. Thus, a significant proportion of the clinical research base and clinical consensus is gleaned from experiences with heterogeneous "street" samples.

Psychological and psychiatric consequences of cocaine abuse always reflect (a) the results of recent acute use, (b) complications associated with abstinence initiation, and (c) preexisting symptoms and conditions. All must be taken into account to understand the symptoms, and their course, presented by most abusers as they seek treatment. In this chapter we discuss these three types of consequences, preceded by a brief description of the spectrum of cocaine use and abuse.

M. ELENA DENISON, ALFONSO PAREDES, SHANA BACAL, AND FRANK H. GAWIN • UCLA-VAMC Laboratory for the Study of Addictions, Los Angeles, California 90073.

Handbook of Substance Abuse: Neurobehavioral Pharmacology, edited by Tarter *et al.* Plenum Press, New York, 1998.

The Spectrum of Cocaine Use

Initial Low-Intensity Use

Cocaine use has occurred historically across a wide spectrum that ranges from casual, infrequent, intranasal use to compulsive crack use and dependence. In the mid-1980s, before the use of crack had supplanted intranasal use as the predominant route of administration of cocaine, the National Institute on Drug Abuse estimated that of the 30 million individuals who had tried cocaine in the United States, 6 million were regular users and one fourth of those were in immediate need of treatment. Most individuals who were using intranasal cocaine did so intermittently and at least a period of controlled, low-intensity use was possible (National Institute on Drug Abuse, 1986). Initially, low intranasal or oral doses enhance interactions with the environment, facilitating performance and confidence to enable productive increases in interpersonal or occupational industry and adventurousness (Connell, 1969; Ellinwood & Petrie, 1977; Gawin & Kleber, 1985a; Siegel, 1985). Such low-intensity use is devoid of significant psychiatric or psychological problems. It was typical of many users in initial phases of the cocaine epidemic, leading to erroneous early proclamations of cocaine's relative safety in the 1970s and early 1980s.

Stimulant-induced euphoria differs from opiate-, alcohol-, or other drug-induced euphoria. Acutely, cocaine produces profound, subjective well-being with alertness. Normal pleasures are magnified, anxiety is decreased, and self-confidence and self-perceptions of mastery increase. Social inhibitions are reduced and interpersonal communication is facilitated. At first, awareness level is heightened. However, once dosage increases, self-awareness decreases. Satiation of appetite occurs and emotions and sexual feelings are enhanced (Ellinwood & Petrie, 1977; Siegel, 1982; Van Dyke, Ungerer, Jatlow, Barash, & Byck, 1982). Many cocaine users experience cocaine as an aphrodisiac and, in low doses, libido is stimulated and sexual pleasure enhanced, with heightened orgasm and prolonged intercourse often described (Gawin, 1978). With negative contingencies absent or scarcely apparent, such early cocaine experiences are seductive (Ellinwood & Petrie, 1977; Kleber & Gawin, 1984). Further, state-dependent memory formation may limit later recall of adverse events.

Low-intensity use may progress to regular use with negative consequences, and abuse may rapidly escalate in degree and frequency to a dependence level, especially among crack smokers.

Transition to High-Intensity Use

Paradoxically, compulsive intranasal cocaine abusers appeared to have patterns of low-intensity use that were similar to those of the millions of noncompulsive intranasal users during their early cocaine use (Gawin & Kleber, 1985a), reporting that 2 to 4 years of relative control existed between the initial exposure to intranasal cocaine and the development of severe dependence. The advent of crack shows dependence can occur almost immediately after initiation of cocaine use with a high-intensity, very rapid administration route.

Former cocaine abusers describe the beginning of compulsive use with initiation of injection or initiation of crack smoking, or when availability and intranasal dosage increases markedly (e.g., increased resources, improved supply sources, engaging in cocaine commerce), suggesting that stimulant use may be controlled until episodes of extremely intense euphoria have occurred. Such episodes produce what become persecutory memories of intense euphoria. These memories are later contrasted to any immediate dysphoria to become the fount of cocaine craving. Intravenous administration or smoking cocaine uniformly does not produce noncompulsive use (Kleber & Gawin, 1984; Siegel, 1982, 1985); "controlled" nondependent crack use has not been described

Chronic animal studies on cocaine involve substantial boluses and usually employ intravenous administration. In effect, they start at the point in the cocaine use spectrum after the high-intensity transition, explaining the lack of animal data on the transition itself or on low-intensity use. Systematic longitudinal clinical studies to prospectively examine the transition itself were not done in the pre-crack era, but may again be possible for stimulants with the upsurge in oral amphetamine use. Both animal and clinical studies are clearly needed.

Abuse and Dependence

Animal experiments illustrate the power of the compulsion to use cocaine. Animals given free access to stimulants engage in continuous self-administration. Stimulants are chosen over food, sex, opioids, alcohol, sedatives, hallucinogens, and phencyclidine. In limited cocaine-administration paradigms, animals can be kept alive, but they adjust self-administration to attain maximum effects (Gay, 1982). Human cocaine users act similarly. That is, they report virtual exclusion of all non-cocaine–related thoughts during cocaine "binges" (i.e., episodes of repeated serial administrations usually involving substantial doses), with behavior displaying overwhelming obsession with cocaine. Sex, nourishment, sleep, safety, survival, money, morality, loved ones, and responsibilities, all become immaterial when juxtaposed with the desire to reexperience cocaine euphoria (Ellinwood & Petrie, 1977; Gawin & Kleber, 1986; Lasagna, Von Flesinger, & Beecher, 1955; Lewin, 1924;

Siegel, 1982). Abuse is limited only by the extreme cost of the drug and legal limitations on distribution.

Most abusers appearing for treatment have used cocaine in extended binges, which disrupt sleep (Gawin & Kleber, 1985a), duplicating a pattern previously observed in amphetamine-abusing subjects (Connell, 1969; Kramer, Fischman, & Littlefield, 1967). Several days of abstinence often separate binges, and some abusers report that limited daily use patterns precede binge abuse (Connell, 1969; Gawin & Kleber, 1985a). Even among subjects abusing crack daily, use generally occurs in binges that last several hours, rather than titration throughout the day as with opiates or alcohol dependence. In contrast to non-cocaine drug abuse, daily cocaine use when sleep patterns are maintained is not the maximal abuse pattern. Severe abuse can exist without incessant daily administration. Some abusers with unlimited access develop an unceasing binge lasting weeks or months with severely disrupted functioning (Siegel, 1982), but such cases are rare.

As a cocaine binge progresses, euphoria decreases and anxiety, fatigue, irritability, and depression increase. This usually leads to cocaine readministration in an attempt to relieve the discomfort of these symptoms, which may manifest within the first 30 min after a cocaine binge. However, supplies are eventually exhausted, or a state of acute tolerance occurs in which further high-dose administration produces little euphoria and instead augments anxiety or paranoia, and self-administration ends.

Acute tolerance to cocaine effects (a reduction in intensity and a shortening of the duration of effects occurring within a binge), has been clearly described clinically and in laboratory experiments. Chronic tolerance has been less well experimentally proven, and clinical consensus is that it is much less substantial.

Assessing the precise details of cocaine withdrawal remains a crucial focus of current treatment research. It is accepted that chronic high-dose cocaine use generates sustained neurophysiologic changes in brain systems that regulate psychological processes. Changes in these neurophysiologic systems produce a true physiologic dependence and withdrawal syndrome, but one with a mainly psychological clinical expression. Extensive experimental data in animals and clinical evidence support this view. Briefly, animal experiments using electrical stimulation at brain reward sites show a decrease in sensitivity, and other experiments show neurotransmitter, neurotransporter, and neuroreceptor changes in animals after chronic cocaine (Banerjee, Sharma, Kung-Cheung, Chanda, & Riggi, 1979; Borison, Hitri, Klawans, & Diamond, 1979; Colpaert, Niemegeers, & Janssen, 1979; Fitzgerald & Reid, 1991; Henry & White, 1991; Karoum, Suddath, & Wyatt, 1990; Kokkinidis, Zacharko, & Predy, 1980; Leith & Barrett, 1976; Markou & Koob, 1991; Ricaurte, Schuster, & Seiden, 1980; Robertson, Leslie, & Bennett, 1991; Simpson & Arnau, 1977; Taylor, Ho, & Fagan, 1979). Research has also shown that chronic use of cocaine produces long-term behavioral changes in animals (Utena, 1966; Yagi, 1963), and changes in positron emission tomography (PET), computerized electroencephalography, neuroendocrine system, and sleep EEG in humans (Alper, Chabot, Kim, Prichep, & John, 1990; Gawin & Kleber 1985b; Hollander *et al.*, 1990; Lee, Bowers, Nach, & Meltzer, 1990; Volkow, Mullani, Gould, Adler, & Krajewski, 1988; Watson, Hartmann, & Schidkraut, 1972; Watson, Bakos, Compton, & Gawin, 1992). Combined, these findings clearly support the presence of a neuroadaptive process. The data are complex and have been critically reviewed in more detail elsewhere (Gawin, 1991).

Psychological Complications of Acute Intoxication

Anxiety, panic attacks, paranoid psychosis, and other drug-induced disorders have all been previously described as aberrant effects of acute cocaine intoxication (Bowers, Imirowicz, Druss, & Mazure, 1995; Brody, Slovis, & Wrenn, 1990; Cowley, 1992; Rosen & Kosten, 1992). Some cocaine users, especially naive users, sometimes experience a sensation of being out of control, which is accompanied by intense feelings of impending doom, profound panic, and hopelessness.

Delusional psychoses are surprisingly frequent, occurring in as many as two thirds of chronic cocaine users (Satel, Price, et al., 1991; Satel, Southwick, & Gawin, 1991) after prolonged and intense cocaine binges (Gawin & Ellinwood, 1990). At earlier, less severe levels, the same phenomenon causes the cocaine user to become irritable, edgy, suspicious, and anxious.

Psychoses experienced by cocaine abusers are indistinguishable from those experienced by paranoid schizophrenics on acute presentation, but are easily distinguished by history and toxicology. Delusions of paranoid schizophrenics are often richer and more severe than those of the cocaine abusers, while cocaine abusers may experience more illusory visual phenomena (Mitchell & Vierkant, 1991), but enough overlap exists to render such distinctions nondiagnostic. The most classically described tactile hallucinations of cocaine abusers are "cocaine bugs," described by abusers as a sensation of insects crawling beneath the skin.

Complications Associated with Abstinence Initiation

Psychological Symptoms of Withdrawal from Cocaine Dependence

Until the 1980s, the commonly held belief was that cocaine was mainly "psychologically" addictive. Classic pharmacologic drug abuse constructs—such as withdrawal, dependence, and tolerance—did not provide models that could be applied easily to cocaine or other stimulants, as cocaine withdrawal does not seem to manifest in discrete or in universally observed physical symptoms. Thus, dependence and withdrawal reflected by gross physiologic indices verge on being imperceptible in cocaine-abusing individuals. The DSM-III (American Psychiatric Association, 1980) reflected the belief that cocaine abuse did not lead to dependence or withdrawal; consequently, there was no diagnostic category for cocaine dependence. However, its first revision moved away from this belief with its introduction of a diagnosis of "cocaine dependence" and began to define a cocaine withdrawal syndrome that included the symptoms of depression, irritability, anxiety, fatigue, insomnia or hypersomnia, and psychomotor agitation. The DSM-IV (American Psychiatric Association, 1994) added increased appetite, psychomotor retardation, and unpleasant dreams as additional cocaine withdrawal symptoms.

Still, there is significant controversy over the characteristics of cocaine withdrawal. Prior attempts at systematic investigation of cocaine withdrawal in humans have been rather unsophisticated. Most studies are problematic in many of the following dimensions: (1) Sample sizes are very small, usually less than 20 subjects; (2) formal instruments used have been developed for other disorders, or involve only partially overlapping symptom dimensions of other disorders, such that neither constructs or empirically validated instruments have been developed to measure cocaine withdrawal; (3) assessment of the subtle but principal cocaine withdrawal symptom of anhedonia has been largely ignored due to difficulties in measurement; (4) subjects are typically rated at intake, often regardless of the time since last cocaine use; (5) variations in users' intra-binge intervals, intensity of use, and other components of individual cocaine use patterns, which may have substantial impact on the time-course and intensity of symptom expression, as well as degree of counterneuroadaptation, are often ignored; (6) the symptom dimensions expressed are not each present in equivalent amounts in all abusers; (7) comparisons at single time points after admission discount substantial individual variation and assume linear trends in the resolution of withdrawal symptoms; (8) the inpatient populations used may isolate patients from conditioned cues that could play a role in eliciting the withdrawal symptoms (Satel, Price, et al., 1991; Satel,

Southwick, *et al.,* 1991; Weddington *et al.,* 1990); and (9) use of small, infrequent but prolonged dosing to approximate a "test" binge that calibrates withdrawal temporally may instead be a short-term detoxification regimen that lessens symptoms.

Gawin and Kleber (1986) proposed a time-dependent evolution of abstinence symptoms, a triphasic model in the cocaine abstinence pattern that predicts withdrawal symptoms as they fluctuate across three main phases: *Crash* (9 hr to 4 days after last cocaine use); *Withdrawal* (1 to 10 weeks after last cocaine use); and *Extinction* (indefinite) (Figure 1).

Crash: Acute Dysphoria (Phase 1)

If a cocaine-use episode involves several serial readministrations, substantial doses (a binge), or both, even in a naive, nondependent user, mood does not return to baseline when use ceases but instead rapidly descends into dysphoria. This dysphoria, called the "crash" by abusers, is usually self-limited, resolving after one or two nights of sleep. Clinically, the crash fully mimics unipolar depression with melancholia, except for its comparatively brief duration. It is a regular accompaniment of the recurrent binges that occur in cocaine dependence. The depression of the crash can be extremely intense, and may include potentially lethal, but temporary, suicidal ideation which remits completely when the crash is over. This transient suicidal ideation can occur in individuals who have no prior history of depression, suicidal ideation, or suicide attempts (Gawin & Ellinwood, 1990).

The crash is initially a descent into depressed mood with continued stimulation and anxiety. Then, a desire for rest and escape from the hyperstimulated dysphoria often cause use

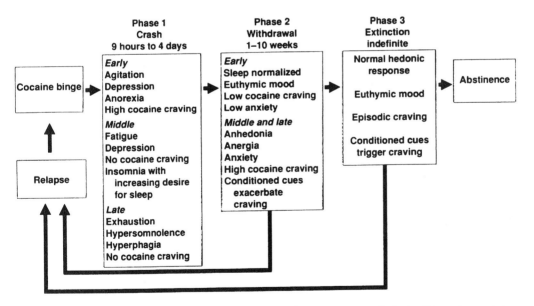

FIGURE 1. Cocaine abstinence phases. Duration and intensity of symptoms vary on the basis of binge characteristics and diagnosis. Binges range in duration from under 4 hr to 6 or more days. High cocaine craving in Phase 1 usually lasts less than 6 hr and is followed by a period of noncraving with similar duration in the next subphase (middle Phase 1). Substantial craving then returns only after a lag of 0.5–5 days, during Phase 2. *Note.* From "Cocaine Abuse: Abstinence Symptomatology and Psychiatric Diagnosis," by F. H. Gawin and H. D. Kleber, 1986, *Archives of General Psychiatry, 43,* pp. 107–113. Copyright 1986 by the American Medical Association. Adapted with permission of the authors.

of anxiolytics, sedatives, opioids, or alcohol to induce sleep.

Whether or not sleep is pharmacologically induced, a later period of hypersomnolence and hyperphagia (during brief awakenings or after the hypersomnolence) eventually occurs. The duration of these periods is related to the duration and intensity of the preceding binge (Gawin & Kleber, 1986). Ingestion of cocaine leads to a reduction in the total amount of REM sleep; yet, these changes appear to be condensed over time as opposed to those associated with amphetamines, possibly because of the shorter half-life of cocaine (Watson *et al.,* 1992). Following week-long cocaine binges, hypersomnolence may last several days (Kramer *et al.,* 1967; Siegel, 1982). The exhaustion, depression, and hypersomnolence of the crash probably result from acute neurotransmitter depletion secondary to the preceding cocaine binge. Such depletion has been demonstrated directly in animal experiments (Taylor *et al.,* 1979) and in experiments using indirect peripheral indices in humans (reviewed in Gawin & Ellinwood, 1988). Clinical recovery from the crash probably depends on sleep and time for new dopamine, serotonin, and norepinephrine synthesis.

The crash appears in first-time users if the dose and duration of cocaine administration are large. It thus appears that the crash may be similar to immediate aftereffects of high-dose alcohol use rather than to alcohol or opioid withdrawal. The crash thus appears to be a self-limiting acute state that does not itself require active treatment. It apparently does not contribute to chronic relapse and abuse, but only to prolonging cocaine binges (Gawin & Kleber, 1986).

Withdrawal: Postcocaine Mood Dysfunction (Phase 2)

After chronic, high-dose use of cocaine, abstinence is accompanied by protracted dysphoria occurring after the initial crash phase, (Connell, 1969; Gawin & Kleber, 1986). Protracted dysphoric symptoms are frequent antecedents of cocaine craving, often contributing to unceasing cycles of recurrent binges. These chronic symptoms are not quickly self-remitting and therefore have great importance to treatment. They thus have great clinical similarity to withdrawal in other abused drugs.

In most individuals who abuse stimulants at severe levels, a regular progression of symptoms follows the resolution of intoxication and crash symptoms. On awakening from hypersomnolence, an interval with normal mood and little cocaine craving occurs. In individuals who are attempting to cease use, this interval is usually associated with vivid memories of the misery of the crash and acute awareness of the psychosocial costs of continued cocaine abuse. This lasts from several hours to several days (Gawin & Kleber, 1986). It is slowly supplanted by increasing anxiety, inactivation, irritability, amotivation, and restricted pleasurable responses to the environment. These symptoms have been variously labeled anergia, depression (Connell, 1969; Kramer *et al.,* 1967), or psychasthenia (Ellinwood & Petrie, 1977) and anhedonia (Gawin & Kleber, 1984, 1986).

The dysphoric symptoms wax and wane and are often not constant or severe enough to meet restrictive psychiatric diagnostic criteria for affective disorders. Cocaine abusers display a symptom constellation that is consistent with a decreased capacity to perceive reward or pleasure. The abusers' limited hedonic reactions to existence contrasted with memories of cocaine-induced euphoria continue to make resumption of use compellingly seductive. Furthermore, the symptom intensity is responsive to environmental cues. That is, the same stimuli that trigger memories of cocaine euphoria and craving for cocaine also intensify awareness of an abuser's baseline dysphoria. During the experience of craving there is a remarkable lack of memory of the acute dysphoria of the initial crash phase or of the adverse psychosocial consequences of abuse. Such negative memories often reemerge only when an episode of craving, and possibly relapse, has passed.

The details of cocaine withdrawal symptoms, initially based on clinical observations, have been substantiated by systematic rating instruments and factor analytic studies in humans. In an ongoing analysis of a large-scale

($n = 200$) sample of treatment seeking cocaine abusers having experienced at least 1 week of cocaine abstinence, more than 90% reported one or more of 28 symptoms of withdrawal (Denison, Engelhardt, Jekel, & Gawin, in press; Gawin, Khalsa, & Anglin, 1992 [partial sample assessment]). Factor analysis revealed six factors—dysthymic mood, anhedonia, anergia, anxiety-irritability, substance craving, and somatization—using the Subjective Cocaine Abstinence Symptom Scale (SCASS) scores. The SCASS is a 17-item scale optimized from the original items using 15 SCL-90 symptoms and two craving items. Symptoms of the fatigue factor were most prevalent (> 90% reporting), followed by craving, dysthymia, somatization, anhedonia, and anxiety (70% reporting).

The crash-withdrawal sequence has been best assessed by Margolin, Avants, and Kosten (1996), who studied longitudinal cocaine abstinence in a sample of cocaine addicts on methadone maintenance ($n = 100$). Retrospective reports of 18 symptoms were obtained at 6 time points, 30 min to 2 weeks after ceasing cocaine use while on methadone. Thus, both crash and withdrawal periods were assessed, but not anchored by sleep, and intermixed at the 24-hr assessment. The authors assessed a four-factor structure, with the early crash symptoms "psychoticism" and "nervousness" dominating during the first 3 hr post-binge. This was followed by maximal sleep and hunger, "nervousness" and "depression" factors at 24 hr, decreasing by 25%–50% at 2 weeks. Psychotism declined 75% by 1 day, with 90% reduction at 1 to 2 weeks. The results clearly confirm descriptions of the initial portions of the crash, as well as the protracted endurance of depressive symptoms. The absence of sleep anchoring, however, renders assessment of the early euthymic withdrawal subphase impossible. Taken together, these two studies confirm both the details and sequence of phase 1 and 2 withdrawal symptoms.

Cocaine-abusing individuals often describe amelioration of anhedonic symptoms within days to weeks if they can sustain abstinence (Gawin, 1991; Gawin & Kleber, 1986). The severity and duration of these symptoms depend partially on the intensity of the preceding chronic abuse. In severe cases, irreversible changes may exist. In a series of PET imaging studies, Volkow has demonstrated the brain dysfunction expected to accompany withdrawal and, in subjects whose use was significantly greater than those in the clinical series engendering the triphasic abstinence model, no resolution after even 6 months of abstinence, suggesting that in some cases these changes may be irreversible.

Preexisting mood disorders may also amplify withdrawal symptoms. Conversely, in those few intermittent, controlled cocaine-using individuals without psychiatric disorders, an anhedonic-psychasthenic phase may not occur at all. High-intensity use and its coinciding neuroadaptation likely cause the psychasthenia and anhedonia to emerge and are a prerequisite for their expression. Further, drug availability and the drug-taking environment are essential for the appearance of full withdrawal symptoms because only very modest symptom expression occurs in inpatient settings (Satel, Price, et al., 1991; Satel, Southwick, & Gawin, 1991; Weddington et al., 1990), mirroring previous observations of unexpectedly low nicotine and opioid withdrawal symptom expression in inpatient studies that prohibited any chance of access to the street environment or drugs.

Extinction: Post-Withdrawal Conditioned Dysfunction (Phase 3)

Even following successful initiation of abstinence and the resolution of early anhedonia and craving, intermittent "conditioned" cocaine craving continues to be reported (Ellinwood & Petrie, 1977; Gawin & Kleber, 1986; Maier, 1926). Such craving also occurs during withdrawal, but afterwards it is not accompanied by the baseline dysphoria of the withdrawal period (Phase 2). Conditioned cravings appear in the context of such divergent factors as particular mood states, both positive and negative; specific persons, locations, events, or times of year; intoxications with other substances; interpersonal strife; or drug-related objects (e.g., money, white powder, pipes, mirrors, syringes, single-edged razor blades). These factors vary with no factor uniformly associated with craving. These are classically conditioned cues, varying according to the abuse habits of the individual abuser. All reinforcing agents produce classical and operant conditioning. Animal experiments have clearly established that cocaine is among the strongest reinforcers known; therefore, the conditioning is extreme. Such craving is intense and can reemerge months or even years after last cocaine use (Gawin & Kleber, 1986). Conditioned craving is also reported during abstinence from other drugs, although the current clinical consensus is that conditioned cravings are probably more consistently present and intense in former stimulant abusers than in those who abuse alcohol and other drugs.

Systematic studies of the reemergence of conditioned craving are being carried out but are not yet complete. Clinical impressions indicate that among ex-abusers who have been abstinent for long periods, the craving is episodic, lasting only hours, with very long periods free of craving. The magnitude and episodic nature of the craving, the variety of the cues, and their temporal contiguity to stimulant abuse episodes all support the view that this craving is conditioned.

By far the most common clinical example of a conditioned cue is alcohol. Alcohol-induced disinhibition can overcome early hesitancies toward trying cocaine based on its expense or illegality. Mild alcohol intoxication often precedes initial cocaine use or early repetitions of use. If this association occurs regularly, alcohol intoxication then becomes a conditioned cue for cocaine craving. Some abusers report little craving except immediately after alcohol intake. Relapse in such patients often follows prolonged abstinence, but occurs with regularity when social contacts are reestablished, following weeks of relative social isolation imposed to initiate abstinence, and occurs after only one or two drinks. In such cases, individuals with years of nonproblematic alcohol use and a total weekly alcohol intake of less than half a dozen drinks may require total alcohol abstinence to achieve abstinence from cocaine.

Predisposing Factors

Predictors

Findings from animal and clinical research clearly support only three clinically applicable predictors of cocaine abuse susceptibility or severity: use patterns, availability, and impairment of self-control. Reliable predictors of later heavy abuse have not been found in low-intensity cocaine users who have not yet become abusers. A cocaine "addictive" personality has not been identified. No objective, systematic assessment of the natural longitudinal course of cocaine use and abuse is yet available that could predict cocaine abuse or a subsequent symptom spectrum after dependence.

Although no personality variables predisposing individuals to cocaine abuse have been demonstrated, a spectrum of associated symptoms has been noted. In some studies, cocaine abusers are found to be more likely to be socially inhibited and self-defeating; in other studies, cocaine abusers have been described as sensation seekers and not introverted (Flynn et al., 1995). Cocaine addicts are also likely to be more distressed overall, and report or exhibit high levels of anger and rebellion, paranoid mistrust and sensitivity, confusion and alienation, agitation, and a high need for excitement (Lesswing & Dougherty, 1993). Unfortunately, the effects of recent use, the abstinence phase, and the question of whether personality distinctions preexist or are consequences of abuse all confound the interpretation and restrict clinical implications of such research.

Genetic Factors

Studies of genetic factors in drug abuse have been conducted, and their results remain controversial (Horgan, 1992). In the alcohol field, few scientists dispute that heredity affects susceptibility to alcoholism. Blum and

Noble (1990) announced the discovery of a single gene that increased the risk of alcoholism by a factor of up to nine, but those findings have been contradicted by other studies, severely disputed, and subsequent attempts to replicate Blum's findings have been largely unsuccessful (Gelernter, Goldman, & Risch, 1993; Kidd, 1993). For cocaine, genetic studies are fewer and their results even less definitive. Noble and colleagues (1993) reported on a study of white male cocaine addicts where a significantly higher proportion of addicts had the A_1 allele of the D_2 gene than did controls. Uhl, reviewing four studies with drug abusers, concludes findings in the same direction (reviewed in Holden, 1994). Most other authors report negative findings (reviewed in Holden, 1994) that are consistent with the absence of literature reporting clinical observations having any genetic implications parallel to alcohol typologies. Heuristically, it is important to remember that self-administration of alcohol occurs only in genetically selected animal subsets, but cocaine self-administration occurs almost universally, across not only all mammalian species but virtually all strains.

Family Studies

Results from cocaine familial studies are similar to those from other nonalcohol substance addictions, suggesting associations but allowing no definitive identification of predictive inferences. Several researchers (Boyd, 1993; Hagan, 1988; Handelsman *et al.,* 1993; McCaul, Turkkan, Svikis, & Bigelow, 1990; Miller, Gold, Belkin, & Klahr, 1989; Smith & Frawley, 1992) have found significant rates of alcoholism in first-degree relatives of cocaine addicts. Smith and Frawley (1992) suggested that these findings support the hypothesis that the risk for developing alcoholism may be a more general susceptibility to addiction. Yet, when dually addicted (alcohol and cocaine) individuals are distinguished from nonalcoholic cocaine addicts, there is a significant difference in the rate of familial alcoholism (Kosten, Kosten, & Rounsaville, 1991), with higher rates of familial alcoholism in alcoholic cocaine addicts than in nonalcoholic cocaine ad-

dicts. Mirin, Weiss, Griffin, and Michael (1991) found that more than 50% of their cocaine-abusing subjects also met *DSM-III* criteria for alcohol abuse/dependence. In these cocaine and alcohol addicts, the rate of familial alcoholism was, again, significantly higher than in their nonalcoholic cocaine-addicted patients. These data clearly indicate that alcoholism and cocaine abuse are not variants of the same disorder.

Regarding gender differences, Mirin and colleagues (1991) also found that male relatives of cocaine addicts had significantly higher rates of alcoholism and other substance abuse than female relatives. Smith and Frawley (1992) found that a much higher proportion of female than male nonalcoholic cocaine addicts had an alcoholic relative, but Boyd (1993) found no significant correlation between family alcohol and drug use and age at first drug use in her female cocaine-addicted patients. The absence of an as yet coherent message from such research is reflected in admonitions that variables such as gender, family history of substance abuse, antisocial disorder, and others must all be identified in any new model for cocaine dependence (e.g., Ball, 1994).

Preexisting Psychiatric Symptoms and Cocaine-Induced Psychiatric Disorders

To date, no study has established that any preexisting personality or psychological state is required for, or even contributory to, consistently predictable aspects of cocaine abuse or effects. In the context of how prevalent stimulant use has been over the last two decades, however, even paranoid psychosis during the crash, given its prevalence, presents acutely to the clinician quite infrequently. It is not certain that all reported cases of paranoia had no preexisting psychiatric disorder, but this is clearly the case in the great majority of patients reported on in the literature. Paranoia induced by cocaine has been found to be largely independent of the quantity and route of administration (Satel, Price, *et al.,* 1991; Satel, Southwick, &

Gawin, 1991), so it appears susceptibility factors do exist. Paranoia reportedly develops more rapidly and is found to be more severe as use history and severity increases (Satel, Price, *et al.,* 1991; Satel, Southwick, & Gawin, 1991) and some very heavy users nonetheless deny ever experiencing paranoia, further supporting at least a partial susceptibility dimension.

Childhood onset Attention-Deficit/Hyperactivity Disorder (ADHD) persisting into adulthood is a demonstrated risk factor for drug and alcohol dependence independent of other psychiatric comorbidity (Biederman, Wilens, Milberger, Spencer, & Faraone, 1995). Anecdotal evidence indicates that a small subgroup of severe ADHD patients, most often diagnosed and treated in childhood, are self-medicating rather than abusing illegal stimulants, and that they respond immediately to substitution therapy with methylphenidate or pemoline, ceasing illegal use (Khantzian, 1985; Weiss, 1988). High rates (30%) of ADHD in cocaine treatment samples can appear (e.g., Carroll & Rounsaville, 1993) if liberal *DSM-IV* criteria that may include some drug-induced symptomology are used, but most groups using more restrictive *DSM-IV* or Wender Utah Rating Scale criteria report 10% or less ADHD in cocaine users in treatment (Ward, Wender, & Reimherr, 1993).

Because symptoms of syndromal depression overlap with cocaine withdrawal, their discrimination is problematic. Many authors, such as Ziedonis and Kosten (1991a, 1991b), Carroll, Ball, Barbor, and Rounsaville (1995), and Nunes and colleagues (1995), have discussed depression in cocaine abuse samples. It is crucial to note that intake Beck Depression scale scores for samples of stimulant-abusing subjects average from 8, below the range for minor (dysthymic) depressive disorder, to 16, below the range for major depression. In samples of crack users in treatment, the absence of some withdrawal dysphoria is rare. Hence, most depressive symptomatology in cocaine populations is not reflecting syndromal depression, but withdrawal. Independent diagnosis of syndromal depression is clearly warranted only if such symptoms predated the onset of drug

abuse, or persist despite many weeks of confirmed abstinence. In all, more systematic long-term follow-up studies of cocaine abusers are clearly needed to examine the reversibility of the psychological and psychiatric consequences of cocaine use among posttreatment relapsers and the variability of the severity of consequences over time among chronic users. More systematic, detailed, longitudinal evaluations are in fact needed for all aspects of symptomatology associated with cocaine use.

References

Alper, K. R., Chabot, R. J., Kim, A. H., Prichep, L., & John, E. (1990). Quantitative EEG correlates of crack cocaine dependence. *Psychiatry Research, 35,* 95–105.

American Psychiatric Association. (1980). *Diagnostic and statistical manual of mental disorders* (3rd ed.). Washington, DC: Author.

American Psychiatric Association. (1994). *Diagnostic and statistical manual of mental disorders* (4th ed.). Washington, DC: Author.

Ball, J. C. (1994). Why has it proved so difficult to match drug abuse patients to appropriate treatment? *Addiction, 89,* 263–265.

Banerjee, S. P., Sharma, V. K., Kung-Cheung, L. S., Chanda, S. K., & Riggi, S. J. (1979). Cocaine and D-amphetamine induce changes in central beta-adrenoceptor sensitivity: Effects of acute and chronic drug treatment. *Brain Research, 175,* 199–239.

Biederman, J., Wilens, T., Milberger, S., Spencer, T. J., & Faraone, S. V. (1995). Psychoactive substance abuse disorders in adults with attention deficit hyperactivity disorder (ADHD): Effects of ADHD and psychiatric comorbidity. *American Journal of Psychiatry, 152,* 1652–1658.

Blum, K., & Noble, E. (1990). Allelic association of human dopamine D2 receptor gene in alcoholism. *Journal of the American Medical Association, 263,* 2055–2060.

Borison, R. L., Hitri, A., Klawans, H. L., & Diamond, B. I. (1979). A new animal model for schizophrenia: Behavioral and receptor binding studies. In E. Usdin, G. Kopin, & J. Barchas (Eds.), *Catecholamine: Basic and clinical frontiers* (pp. 719–721). New York: Pergamon.

Bowers, M. B., Imirowicz, R., Druss, B., & Mazure, C. M. (1995). Autonomous psychosis following psychotogenic substance abuse. *Biological Psychiatry, 37,* 136–137.

Boyd, C. J. (1993). The antecedents of women's crack cocaine abuse: Family substance abuse, sexual abuse, depression and illicit drug use. *Journal of Substance Abuse Treatment, 10,* 433–438.

Brody, S. L., Slovis, C. M., & Wrenn, K. D. (1990). Cocaine related medical problems: Consecutive series of

233 patients. *American Journal of Medicine, 88,* 325–331.

Carroll, K. M., & Rounsaville, B. J. (1993). History and significance of childhood attention deficit disorder in treatment-seeking cocaine abusers. *Comprehensive Psychiatry, 34,* 75–82.

Carroll, K. M., Ball, S. A., Barbor, T. F., & Rounsaville, B. J. (1995). Subtypes of cocaine abusers: Support for a type A–type B distinction. *Journal of Consulting and Clinical Psychology, 63,* 115–124.

Colpaert, F. C., Niemegeers, C. H., & Janssen, P. A. (1979). Discriminative stimulus properties of cocaine: Neuropharmacological characteristics as derived from stimulus generalization experiments. *Pharmacology, Biochemistry and Behavior, 10,* 535–546.

Connell, P. H. (1969). Some observations concerning amphetamine misuse: Its diagnosis, management, and treatment with special reference to research needs, drugs and agement, and treatment with special reference to research needs. In J. R. Wittenborn, H. Brill, J. P. Smith, & S. A. Wittenborn (Eds.), *Drugs and youth* (pp. 125–134). Springfield, IL: Thomas.

Cowley, D. S. (1992). Alcohol abuse, substance abuse, and panic disorder. *American Journal of Medicine, 92,* 41S–48S.

Denison, M. E., Engelhardt, R., Jekel, J., & Gawin, F. (in press). Cocaine withdrawal.

Ellinwood, E. H., & Petrie, W. M. (1977). Dependence on amphetamine, cocaine and other stimulants. In S. N. Pradhan (Ed.), *Drug abuse: Clinical and basic aspects* (pp. 249–262). New York: Mosby.

Fitzgerald, J. I., & Reid, J. J. (1991). Chronic cocaine treatment does not alter rat striatal D2 autoreceptor sensitivity to pergolide. *Brain Research, 541,* 327–333.

Flynn, P. M., Luckey, J. W., Brown, B. S., Hoffman, J. A., Dunteman, G. H., Thiesen, A. C., Hubbard, R. L., Needle, R., Schneider, S. J., & Koman, J. J., 3d. (1995). Relationship between drug preference and indicators of psychiatric impairment. *American Journal of Drug and Alcohol Abuse, 21,* 153–166.

Gawin, F. H. (1978). Drugs and Eros: Reflections on aphrodisiacs. *Journal of Psychoactive Drugs, 10,* 227–236.

Gawin, F. H. (1991). Cocaine addiction: Psychology and neurophysiology [published erratum appears in *Science,* Aug. 2, 253–494, 1991]. *Science, 251,* 1580–1586.

Gawin, F. H., & Ellinwood, E. H. (1988). Stimulants: Actions, abuse, and treatment. *New England Journal of Medicine, 318,* 1173–1183.

Gawin, F. H., & Ellinwood, E. H. (1990). Consequences and correlates of cocaine abuse: Clinical phenomenology. In N. D. Volkow & A. C. Swan (Eds.), *Cocaine and the brain* (pp. 155–178). New Brunswick, NJ: Rutgers University Press.

Gawin, F. H., & Kleber, H. D. (1984). Cocaine abuse treatment: An open trial with lithium and desipramine. *Archives of General Psychiatry, 41,* 903–910.

Gawin, F. H., & Kleber, H. D. (1985a). Cocaine abuse in a treatment population: Patterns and diagnostic distractions. In E. H. Adams & N. J. Kozel (Eds.), *Cocaine use in America: Epidemiologic and clinical perspectives* (NIDA Research Monograph No. 61, pp. 182–192). Rockville, MD: U.S. Department of Health and Human Services.

Gawin, F. H., & Kleber, H. D. (1985b). *Cocaine use in a treatment population: Patterns and diagnostic distinctions* (NIDA Research Monograph No. 61, pp. 182–192). Washington, DC: U.S. Department of Health and Human Services, U.S. Government Printing Office.

Gawin, F. H., & Kleber, H. D. (1986). Cocaine abuse: Abstinence symptomatoloty and psychiatric diagnosis. *Archives of General Psychiatry, 43,* 107–113.

Gawin, F. H., Khalsa, M. E., & Anglin, M. D. (1992). *Subjective symptoms of cocaine withdrawal* (NIH Publication No. 92-1888, p. 442). Washington, DC: U.S. Department of Health and Human Services.

Gay, G. R. (1982). Clinical management of acute and toxic cocaine poisoning. *Annals of Emergency Medicine, 11,* 562–572.

Gelernter, J., Goldman, D., & Risch, N. (1993). The A1 allele, at the D2 dopamine receptor gene and alcoholism: A reappraisal. *Journal of the American Medical Association, 269,* 1801–1807.

Hagan, T. (1988). *A retrospective search for the etiology of drug abuse: A background comparison of a drug-addicted population of women and a control group of non-addicted women* (NIDA Research Monograph No. 81, pp. 254–261). Washington, DC: U.S. Department of Health and Human Services, U.S. Government Printing Office.

Handelsman, L., Branchey, M. H., Buydens-Branchey, L., Gribomont, B., Holloway, K., & Silverman, J. (1993). Morbidity risks for alcoholism and drug abuse in relatives of cocaine addicts. *American Journal of Drug and Alcohol Abuse, 19,* 347–357.

Henry, D. J., & White, F. J. (1991). Repeated cocaine administration causes persistent enhancement of D1 dopamine receptor sensitivity within the rat nucleus accumbens. *Journal of Pharmacology and Experimental Therapeutics, 258,* 882–890.

Holden, C. (1994). A cautionary genetic tale: The sobering story of D2. *Science, 264,* 1696–1697.

Hollander, E., Nunes, E., Decaria, C. M., Quitkin, F., Cooper, T., Wager, S., & Klein, D. (1990). Dopaminergic sensitivity and cocaine abuse: Response to apomorphine. *Psychiatry Research, 33,* 161–169.

Horgan, J. (1992). D2 or not D2. A barroom brawl over an alcoholism gene. *Scientific American, 266,* 29–32.

Karoum, F., Suddath, R. l., & Wyatt, R. J. (1990). Chronic cocaine and rat brain catecholamines: Long term reduction in hypothalamic and frontal cortex dopamine metabolism. *European Journal of Pharmacology, 186,* 1–8.

Khantzian, E. J. (1985). The self-medication hypothesis of addictive disorders: Focus on heroine and cocaine dependence. *American Journal of Psychiatry, 142,* 1259–1264.

Kidd, K. (1993). Associations of disease with genetic markers: Deja vu all over again. *American Journal of Medical Genetics, 48,* 71.

Kleber, H. D., & Gawin, F. H. (1984). Cocaine abuse: A review of current experimental treatments. In J. Grabowski (Ed.), *Cocaine pharmacology, effects, and treatment of abuse* (NIDA Research Monograph No. 50, DHHS Publication No. 84-1326). Rockville, MD: U.S. Department of Heath and Human Services.

Kokkinidis, L., Zacharko, R. M., & Predy, P. A. (1980). Post-amphetamine depression of self-stimulation responding from substantia nigra: Reversal by tricyclic anti-depressants. *Pharmacology, Biochemistry and Behavior, 13,* 379–383.

Kosten, T. A., Kosten, T. R., & Rounsaville, B. J. (1991). *Cocaine symptoms are predicted by familial psychopathology* (NIDA Research Monograph No. 105, pp. 603–604). Washington, DC: U.S. Department of Health and Human Services, U.S. Government Printing Office.

Kramer, J. C., Fischman, V. S., & Littlefield, D. C. (1967). Amphetamine abuse patterns and effects of high doses taken intravenously. *Journal of the American Medical Association, 201,* 305–309.

Lasagna, L., Von Flesinger, J. M., & Beecher, H. K. (1955). Drug induced mood changes in man: I. Observations on healthy subjects, chronically ill patients, and post-addicts. *Journal of the American Medical Association, 157,* 1066–1020.

Lee, M. A., Bowers, M. M., Nach, J. F., & Meltzer, H. (1990). Neuroendocrine measures of dopaminergic function in chronic cocaine users. *Psychiatry Research, 33,* 151–159.

Leith, N. J., & Barrett, R. J. (1976). Amphetamine and the reward system: Evidence for tolerance and post-drug depression. *Psychopharmacology* (Berlin) *74,* 23–28.

Lesswing, N. J., & Dougherty, R. J. (1993). Psychopathology in alcohol and cocaine-dependent patients: A comparison of findings from psychological testing. *Journal of Substance Abuse Treatment, 10,* 53–57.

Lewin, L. (1924). *Phantastica.* Berlin: Verlag Von Georg Stilke.

Maier, H. W. (1926). *Der Kokainismus.* Leipzig, Germany: Georg Thieme Verlag.

Margolin, A., Avants, S. K., & Kosten, T. R. (1996). Abstinence symptomatology associated with cessation of chronic cocaine abuse among methadone-maintained patients. *American Journal of Drug and Alcohol Abuse, 22,* 377–388.

Markou, A., & Koob, G. F. (1991). Post cocaine anhedonia: An animal model of cocaine withdrawal. *Neuropsychopharmacology, 4,* 17–26.

McCaul, M. E., Turkkan, J. S., Svikis, D. S., & Bigelow, G. E. (1990). Alcohol and secobarbital effects as a function of familial alcoholism: Acute psychophysio-

logical effects. *Alcoholism, Clinical and Experimental Research, 14,* 704–712.

Miller, N. S., Gold, M. S., Belkin, B. H., & Klahr, A. L. (1989). Family history and diagnosis of alcohol dependence in cocaine dependence. *Psychiatry Research, 29,* 113–121.

Mirin, S. M., Weiss, R. D., Griffin, M. L., & Michael, J. L. (1991). Psychopathology in drug abusers and their families. *Comprehensive Psychiatry, 32,* 36–51.

Mitchell, J., & Vierkant, A. D. (1991). Delusions and hallucinations of cocaine abusers and paranoid schizophrenics: A comparative study. *Journal of Psychology, 125,* 301–310.

National Institute on Drug Abuse. (1986). *NIDA capsules: 1985 National Household Survey on Drug Abuse.* Rockville, MD: Press Office of the National Institute on Drug Abuse.

Noble, E., Blum, K., Khalsa, M. E., Ritchie, T., Montgomery, A., Wood, R., Fitch, R., Ozkaragoz, T., Sheridan, P., & Anglin, M. (1993). Allelic association of the D2 dopamine receptor gene with cocaine dependence. *Drug and Alcohol Dependence, 33,* 271–285.

Nunes, E. V., McGrath, P. J., Quitkin, F. M., Ocepek-Welikson, K., Stewart, J., Koenig, T., Wager, S., & Klein, D. (1995). Imipramine treatment of cocaine abuse: Possible boundaries of efficacy. *Drug and Alcohol Dependence, 39,* 185–195.

Ricaurte, G. A., Schuster, C. R., & Seiden, L. S. (1980). Long-term effects of repeated methylamphetamine administration on dopamine and serotonin neurons in the rat brain: A regional study. *Brain Research, 193,* 153–163.

Robertson, M. W., Leslie, C. A., & Bennett, J. P. (1991). Apparent synaptic dopamine deficiency induced by withdrawal from chronic cocaine treatment. *Brain Research, 538,* 337–339.

Rosen, M. I., & Kosten, T. (1992). Cocaine-associated panic attacks in methadone-maintained patients. *American Journal of Drug and Alcohol Abuse, 18,* 57–62.

Satel, S. L., Price, L. H., Palumbo, J. M., McDougle, C. J., Krystal, J. H., Gawin, F. H., Charney, D. S., Heninger, G. R., & Kleber, H. D. (1991). Clinical phenomenology and neurobiology of cocaine abstinence: A prospective inpatient study. *American Journal of Psychiatry, 148,* 1712–1716.

Satel, S. L., Southwick, S. M., & Gawin, F. H. (1991). Clinical features of cocaine-induced paranoia. *American Journal of Psychiatry, 148,* 495–498.

Siegel, R. K. (1982). Cocaine free base abuse: A new smoking disorder. *Journal of Psychoactive Drugs, 14,* 321–338.

Siegel, R. K. (1985). New patterns of cocaine use: Changing doses and routes. In E. H. Adams & N. J. Kozel (Eds.), *Cocaine use in America: Epidemiologic and clinical perspectives* (NIDA Research Monograph No. 61, pp. 204–220). Rockville, MD: U.S. Department of Health and Human Services.

Simpson, D. M., & Arnau, Z. (1977). Behavioral withdrawal following several psychoactive drugs. *Biochemistry and Behavior, 7,* 59–64.

Smith, J. W., & Frawley, P. J. (1992). Alcoholism in relatives of primary cocaine-dependent patients. *Journal of Substance Abuse Treatment, 9,* 153–155.

Taylor, D. L., Ho, B. T., & Fagan, J. D. (1979). Increased dopamine receptor binding in rat brain by repeated cocaine injection. *Community Psychopharmacology, 3,* 137–142.

Utena, H. (1966). Behavioral aberrations in methamphetamine intoxicated animals and chemical correlates in the brain. *Progress in Brain Research, 2,* 192–207.

Van Dyke, C., Ungerer, J., Jatlow, P., Barash, P., & Byck, R. (1982). Intranasal cocaine dose relationships of psychological effects and plasma levels. *International Journal of Psychiatry in Medicine, 12,* 1–13.

Volkow, N. D., Mullani, N., Gould, K., Adler, S., & Krajewski, K. (1988). Cerebral blood flow in chronic cocaine users: A study with positron emission tomography. *British Journal of Psychiatry, 152,* 641–648.

Ward, M. F., Wender, P. H., & Reimherr, F. W. (1993). The Wender Utah Rating Scale: An aid in the retrospective diagnosis of childhood attention deficit hyperactivity disorder. *American Journal of Psychiatry, 150,* 885–890.

Watson, R., Hartmann, E., & Schildkraut, J. J. (1972). Amphetamine withdrawal: Affective state, sleep patterns and MHPG excretion. *American Journal of Psychiatry, 129,* 263–269.

Watson, R., Bakos, L., Compton, P., & Gawin, F. (1992). Cocaine use and withdrawal: The effect on sleep and mood. *American Journal of Drug and Alcohol Abuse, 18,* 21–28.

Weddington, W., Brown, B., Haertzen, C., Cone, E., Dax, E., Herning, R., & Michaelson, B. (1990). Changes in mood, craving, and sleep during short-term abstinence reported by male cocaine addicts: A controlled, residential study. *Archives of General Psychiatry, 47,* 861–868.

Weiss, R. D. (1988). Relapse to cocaine abuse after initiating desipramine treatment. *Journal of the American Medical Association, 260,* 2545–2546.

Yagi, B. (1963). Studies in general activity: II. The effect of methamphetamine. *Annals of Animal Psychology, 13,* 37–47.

Ziedonis, D. M., & Kosten, T. R. (1991a). Depression as a prognostic factor for pharmacological treatment of cocaine dependence. *Psychopharmacology Bulletin, 27,* 337–343.

Ziedonis, D. M., & Kosten, T. R. (1991b). Pharmacotherapy improves treatment outcome in depressed cocaine addicts. *Journal of Psychoactive Drugs, 23,* 417–425.

V

Hallucinogens

13

Pharmacology of Hallucinogens

RICHARD A. GLENNON

Introduction

What constitutes a hallucinogenic agent; what is the definition of *hallucinogenic?* What effects are commonly produced by hallucinogens? How are hallucinogenic agents classified? Chemically, what are the structural requirements for hallucinogenic activity? How do hallucinogenic agents work? Interestingly, and perhaps counterintuitively, these questions are roughly listed in descending order of difficulty. Actually, there is more agreement today on how hallucinogens work than on a definition of the term hallucinogen.

Hallucinogens: A Definition

In his book *Chemical Psychoses,* Hollister (1968) stated that "one can scarcely get any agreement upon the term used to describe this class of drugs" (p. 18). According to Brimblecombe and Pinder (1975), there is "no clear definition or even agreement as to what constitutes [hallucinogenic] action" (p. 1), categorizing hallucinogens into hallucinogenic poisons or agents that produce toxic psychoses (e.g., ethanol, carbon tetrachloride), deliriants (e.g., atropine, hyoscine, benztropine), and psychotomimetics (e.g., lysergic acid diethy-

lamide or LSD). Szara (1994) has argued that the various names for hallucinogens, for example, phantastica, psychotomimetic, psychotogenic, psychedelic, hallucinogen, have largely lost their usefulness and may even be misleading. Szara proposes that these agents be termed *psychoheuristics.* In this chapter, the term *hallucinogen* is used because it is readily recognized and commonly accepted. How, then, do we define hallucinogenic? The most inclusive definition of hallucinogen was proposed by Hollister (1968). A hallucinogenic agent (Hollister actually favored the term *psychotomimetic*) meets the following criteria: (1) in proportion to other effects, changes in thought, perception, and mood should predominate; (2) intellectual or memory impairment are minimal at doses that produce the effects just mentioned; (3) stupor, narcosis, or excessive stimulation is not an integral effect; (4) autonomic nervous system side effects are neither disabling nor severely disconcerting; and (5) addictive craving is minimal. These criteria are specific and encompass a wide variety of agents. Using these criteria, Hollister (1968) narrowed the field of "psychotomimetics" to seven categories that include (1) lysergic acid derivatives, such as LSD, (2) phenylethylamines, (2) indolealkylamines, (4) other indolic derivatives (including harmala alkaloids and ibogaine), (5) piperidyl benzilate esters, (6) phenylcyclohexyl compounds (including phencyclidine or PCP), and (7) miscellaneous agents (including cannabinoids, kawain, and dimethylacetamide). Using this

RICHARD A. GLENNON • Department of Medicinal Chemistry, Virginia Commonwealth University, Richmond, Virginia 23298.

Handbook of Substance Abuse: Neurobehavioral Pharmacology, edited by Tarter *et al.* Plenum Press, New York, 1998.

definition, it has been possible to pare down psychoactive agents to a more circumscribed group. Nevertheless, this group of agents is still quite broad, and is also heterogeneous with respect to the actions of the agents. It would appear that hallucinogenic agents do not represent a behaviorally homogeneous class of agents.

Within the past decade, the term *classical hallucinogen* has evolved. No formal definition has yet been provided for this class of agents. However, the term may further aid in restricting the types and classes of agents to be considered and might, from this perspective, be useful. It is quite clear that certain agents, such as PCP, THC (Δ^9-tetrahydrocannabinol), and LSD do not produce identical effects (Hollister, 1984). In fact, PCP is thought to act via PCP receptors, tetrahydrocannabinol may act via cannabinoid receptors, and such agents are discussed separately in other chapters of this book. Using the Hollister definition as a starting point, classical hallucinogens may be considered those that also possess a basic nitrogen atom and that produce little to no cholinergic or anticholinergic effects. This extension of the original definition essentially eliminates

agents such as the piperidyl benzilates (which are potent anticholinergic agents), and the cannabinoids, kawain, and dimethylacetamide (which lack a basic nitrogen atom). Perhaps the best working definition of a classical hallucinogen is an agent that (1) binds at 5-HT_2 serotonin receptors, *and* (2) is recognized by animals trained to discriminate 1-(2,5-dimethoxy-4-methylphenyl)-2-aminopropane (DOM) from vehicle in tests of stimulus generalization (Glennon, 1996).

Hallucinogenic Agents: Classification

Classical hallucinogens can be grouped into two broad categories: indolealkylamines and phenylalkylamines. As shown in Table 1 both categories consist of several subclasses of agents; the indolealkylamines include N-substituted tryptamines, α-alkyltryptamines, ergolines, and, most likely, β-carbolines, whereas the phenylalkylamines consist of the phenylethylamines and the phenylisopropylamines. The phenylethylamines and the phenylisopropylamines differ only in the presence or absence of an α-methyl group; for example, removal of the α-methyl group of the phenylisopropylamine DOM results in the phenyl-

TABLE 1. Categories of Arylalkylamine Classical Hallucinogens

Category	Subcategory	Examples[a]
Indolealkylamines	N-Substituted Tryptamines	Dimethyltryptamine (DMT) 5-Methoxy DMT 4-Hydroxy DMT (Psilocin) N,N-Diethyltryptamine (DET)
	α-Alkyltryptamines	α-Methyltryptamine (α-MeT) 5-Methoxy-α-methyltryptamine
	Ergolines	Lysergic acid diethylamide (LSD) 1-Acetyl LSD
	β-Carbolines	Harmaline Harmine
Phenylalkylamines	Phenylethylamines	Mescaline α-Desmethyl DOM
	Phenylisopropylamines	2,4,5-TMA DOM DOB DOI

[a]For additional examples, see Nichols and Glennon (1984).

ethylamine α-desmethyl DOM. The agents now referred to as classical hallucinogens are those that Hollister (1968) classified as producing similar effects; those agents shown to produce somewhat different effects (e.g., cannabinoids, PCP, piperidyl benzilates) are excluded.

There is evidence, both from human and from animal studies, that examples of classical hallucinogens produce similar effects. Since the hallucinogenic phenomenon is not directly accessible to observers once they partake of the experience, objectivity is lost (Brimblecombe & Pinder, 1975). Nevertheless, it has been demonstrated that administration of agents such as DMT, α-MeT, mescaline, and psilocybin (the phosphate ester of psilocin) to humans results in effects that are perceived to be similar to those produced by LSD. In contrast, administration of agents such as JB 329 (Ditran®, a piperidyl benzilate) produces effects perceived to be different. Moreover, in humans, tolerance develops to repeated administration of LSD, mescaline, psilocybin, and JB 329, but cross-tolerance develops only among LSD, mescaline, and psilocybin. (For further discussion, see Brimblecombe & Pinder, 1975; Hollister, 1968). Because the effects produced by hallucinogens are primarily subjective, it would seem, given the previously mentioned caveat, that humans are the most appropriate subjects for evaluating and classifying hallucinogens. This method, however, does not readily lend itself to a rapid examination of large numbers of agents, or an examination of new agents for which toxicity data are unavailable.

Another approach is to examine agents in various tests using animals as subjects; however, it is impossible to know when, or if, animals hallucinate. Nonetheless, animal models of hallucinogenic activity have been advanced in an attempt to develop an assay system that can identify active versus inactive agents quantitatively and qualitatively (Glennon, 1992). Despite considerable effort, an animal model has not yet been developed that reliably and consistently identifies hallucinogenic agents or predicts hallucinogenic activity without producing false negatives or false positives. One reason for this finding may be that investigators may have attempted to develop global models that would identify examples of every class of hallucinogens. Is there any effective animal method of identifying or differentiating between a subset of agents such as, for example, PCP-like agents, or cannabinoids, or the classical hallucinogens? Several methods have been explored and some are quite successful. For example, classical hallucinogens routinely produce hyperthermia in rabbits. Of course, other types of agents (e.g., the stimulant amphetamine, the pyretic agent 2,4-dinitrophenol) can also produce these effects. The hyperthermia assay, therefore, represents one method for identifying classical hallucinogens, but it also results in false positives. The animal method most often employed for examining hallucinogens is the drug discrimination procedure. In this paradigm, animals are trained to recognize the stimulus effects of a given agent under standard operant conditions and then administered other agents in tests of stimulus generalization in order to answer the question, Does the novel agent (i.e., challenge drug) produce stimulus effects similar to those of the standard training drug? Results are both qualitative and quantitative. That is, stimulus generalization studies are conducted in a dose-related manner and results are not only of a "yes or no" nature, but where stimulus generalization occurs, the potency of the challenge drug relative to the training drug can be determined. This procedure detects the similarity of stimulus effects among various agents. However, if a hallucinogen is used as the training drug, it should be possible to identify other agents that produce similar effects when administered to hallucinogen-trained animals in tests of stimulus generalization. Agents such as PCP, tetrahydrocannabinol, ethanol, amphetamine, morphine, diazepam, pentobarbital, and many others have been used as training drugs (Colpaert & Slangen, 1982; Glennon, Jarbe, & Frankenheim, 1991). Classical hallucinogens that have been used as training drugs include LSD, 5-methoxy DMT, mescaline, DOM, DOI, and R(−)DOB, (Glennon, Rosecrans & Young, 1982).

Several hundred agents have now been examined in rats trained to discriminate DOM from vehicle (inactive compound). It has been found that the DOM-stimulus generalizes to the examples of classical hallucinogens shown in Table 1 (Glennon, 1994). Furthermore, stimulus generalization occurs among LSD, DOM, mescaline, and 5-methoxy DMT regardless of which agent is used as the training drug. One class of agents that has not been well investigated is the β-carbolines; however, it has recently been shown that harmaline serves as a discriminative stimulus in rats and that DOM produces harmaline-like stimulus effects (Glennon & Young, unpublished findings). These stimulus generalization studies strongly support the conclusion that classical hallucinogens produce similar stimulus effects in rats. Furthermore, consistent with research on humans, the stimulus effects are quite selective; that is, THC, LSD, PCP, and JB 329 produce distinct stimulus effects (Weissman, 1978).

It must be emphasized that hallucinogen-trained animals do not represent a model of hallucinogenic activity. Rather, stimulus generalization studies with hallucinogen-trained animals provide a means of identifying which agents produce stimulus effects similar to those of the particular hallucinogen used as training drug. There is strong evidence that the classical hallucinogens act via a specific serotonergic mechanism; that is, they act as serotonin agonists. Thus, it is not surprising that DOM-trained animals recognize the serotonin releasing agent fenfluramine. In this respect, if it had been claimed that DOM-stimulus generalization was an animal model of hallucinogenic activity, the nonhallucinogenic fenfluramine would have to be considered a false positive.

Classical Hallucinogens

The classical hallucinogens (representative chemical structures of these agents are shown in Figure 1) have now been extracted from the definition of hallucinogens (Lin & Glennon, 1994) and, from a behavioral perspective, these agents seem to constitute a reasonably homogeneous class of agents. However, even agents within the various subcategories of classical hallucinogens may not produce identical effects. Naranjo (1973) found that a dose of a given agent may produce different effects in the same individual upon different occasions of administration. Some of these differences may reflect some other action or actions common to a particular subcategory of classical hallucinogens, or may represent unique properties of a specific agent. For example, certain β-carbolines are potent inhibitors of monoamine oxidase, and LSD has significant effects on dopaminergic (and other neurotransmitter) systems, that are not commonly shared by the other classical hallucinogens. In addition, the "set and setting" of the hallucinogenic episode also seems to be a major contributing factor to its effects in humans (Shulgin & Shulgin, 1991).

Effects on Humans

Most of the studies of hallucinogenic agents in humans were conducted during the 1950s and 1960s, then essentially abandoned until recently (Strassman, 1994). The vast majority of hallucinogens (as identified by anecdotal reports or from street data) or potential hallucinogens (as identified on the basis of studies with animals) have been identified since the mid 1960s and have not been examined in carefully controlled clinical investigations. Therefore, although there is an impressive body of literature available on a small handful of classical hallucinogens (e.g., LSD, mescaline, DMT), little is known about other related agents. Most of what we know is derived from studies with LSD (Siva Sankar, 1975).

Detailed descriptions of the actions of LSD and related agents are available (Siva Sankar, 1975). In general, these agents produce alterations in perception (time, space, shape, color). Some agents produce synesthesia. Although some hallucinogens produce vivid and colorful hallucinations, this effect does not seem to be common to the class as a whole. Closed-eye imagery is more common, and auditory hallucinations, although possible, are uncommon. LSD produces effects that have

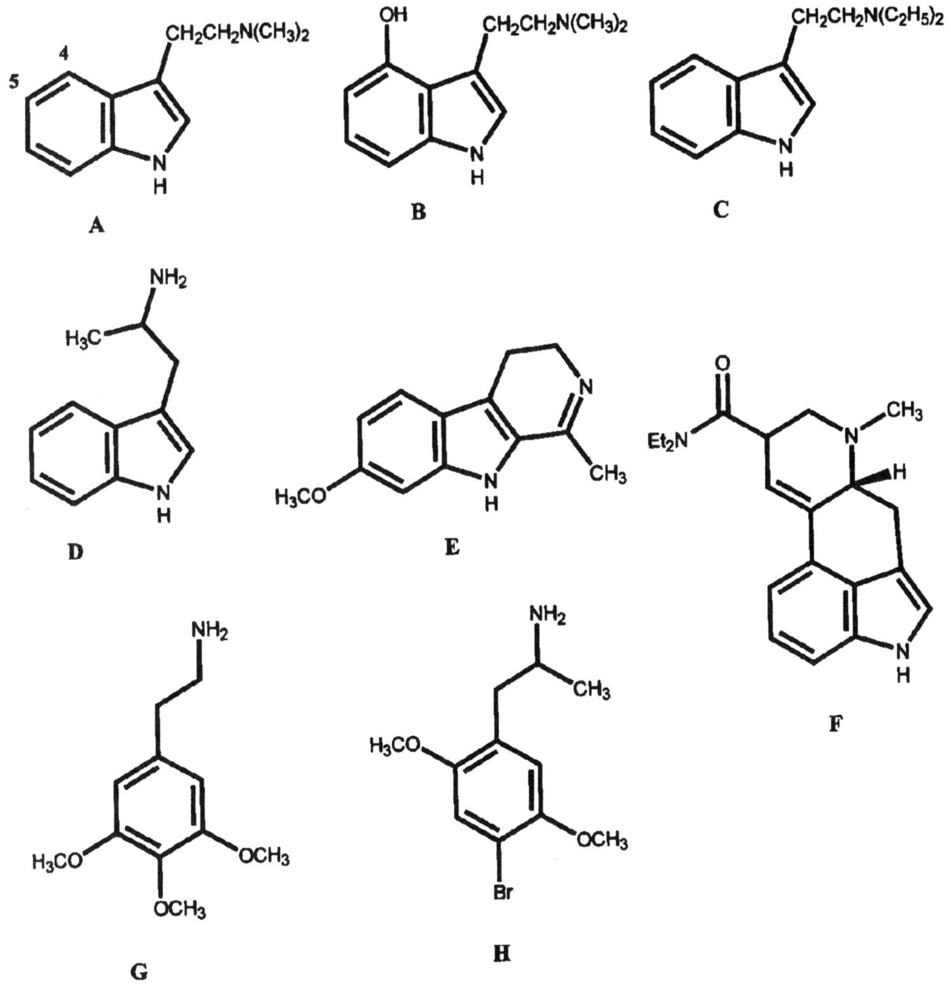

FIGURE 1. Structures of the classical hallucinogens DMT (N,N-dimethyltryptamine): (**A**), psilocin (**B**), DET (N,N-diethyltryptamine); (**C**), α-MeT (α-methyltryptamine); (**D**), harmaline (**E**), LSD (lysergic acid diethylamide); (**F**), mescaline (**G**), DOB (1-(4-bromo-2,5-dimethoxyphenyl)-2-aminopropane); (**H**).

been divided into the somatic (nausea, blurred vision, dizziness, drowsiness), perceptual (altered shapes and colors, heightened sense of hearing), and psychic (alterations in mood, depersonalization, distorted sense of time, visual hallucinations) (Hollister, 1984). In terms of principal effects and duration of action, little difference is found between LSD, psilocybin, and mescaline (Hoffer & Osmond, 1967; Hollister, 1984).

Shulgin and Shulgin (1991) have provided detailed discussions of a vast array of phenylalkylamine derivatives. On the one hand, these descriptions offer unprecedented insight into the effects produced by the agents and how effects can vary with minor molecular variation. On the other hand, the number of doses employed for an individual agent may have been limited, and the subject populations may have been small or unspecified. Nevertheless, the descriptions of effects emphasize the difficulty in defining the term *hallucinogen*. Naranjo (1973) has described the effects of certain β-carbolines in human subjects;

with these agents, both similarities and differences exist compared with other classical hallucinogens.

Mechanism of Action

It is not yet known how these agents produce their hallucinogenic effects. The neurotransmitter serotonin (5-HT) has been implicated. The most widely investigated hallucinogen is LSD. The one neurotransmitter that has been consistently implicated as being involved in the hallucinogenic action of LSD and LSD-related agents is serotonin. In fact, 5-HT was suggested to be involved in the action of these agents as far back as the mid to late 1950s (Woolley, 1962). During the 1950s through the 1980s, there was considerable controversy as to whether these hallucinogens were acting as 5-HT agonists or 5-HT antagonists. Although increasing evidence suggests an agonist mechanism of action, some reports demonstrated antagonist activity for LSD. It is likely that classical hallucinogens act as agonists or partial agonists (Glennon, 1994). In 1979, it was demonstrated that multiple populations of 5-HT receptors (5-HT$_1$ and 5-HT$_2$) exist in the brain; today, more than 15 different subpopulations of 5-HT receptors have been identified (Hoyer *et al.,* 1994). In 1984, the *5-HT$_2$ hypothesis* of hallucinogenic drug action was proposed (Glennon, Teitler, & McKenney, 1984); it was suggested that classical hallucinogens act as 5-HT$_2$ agonists. Events leading to this hypothesis were twofold. First, with the development and availability of 5-HT$_2$ antagonists, it was demonstrated in tests of stimulus antagonism that the 5-HT$_2$ antagonists ketanserin and pirenperone potently and effectively attenuate the DOM stimulus, and DOM-stimulus generalization to mescaline and LSD, in DOM-trained rats. Second, if classical hallucinogens act as direct-acting 5-HT$_2$ agonists, it should be possible to demonstrate that they bind at 5-HT$_2$ receptors. A significant correlation has also been found between 5-HT$_2$ receptor affinity and human hallucinogenic potency. A similar correlation exists between 5-HT$_2$ receptor affinity and stimulus generalization potency in DOM-

trained animals for a number of classical hallucinogens (Glennon, 1996). Finally, certain animal models of hallucinogenic activity also appear to involve a 5-HT$_2$ mechanism (Glennon, 1992). For example, 5-HT$_2$ receptors seem to be involved in thermoregulation. Specifically, 5-HT$_2$ agonists can produce hyperthermia in animals. This finding supports the use of the rabbit hyperthermia assay mentioned earlier. The hyperthermic potencies of classical hallucinogens also correlates significantly with their 5-HT$_2$ receptor affinity (Glennon, 1992).

The same year that the 5-HT$_2$ hypothesis was proposed, a new population of 5-HT receptors, 5-HT$_{1C}$ receptors, was identified. It was subsequently demonstrated that classical hallucinogens also bind at this population of receptors. Studies showed that 5-HT$_{1C}$ receptors possess greater similarity (second messenger coupling, transmembrane sequence homology) to the 5-HT$_2$ receptors than to other members of the 5-HT$_1$ family. They have since been termed 5-HT$_{2C}$ receptors, whereas the original 5-HT$_2$ receptors have been renamed 5 HT$_{2A}$ receptors (Hoyer *et al.,* 1994). A significant correlation exists between 5-HT$_{2C}$ receptor affinity and hallucinogenic potency in humans and stimulus generalization–derived ED50 values in DOM-trained rats (Glennon, 1996). These findings posed a new question: Which of the two populations of 5-HT$_2$ receptors, 5-HT$_{2A}$ or 5-HT$_{2C}$, is involved in the actions of the classical hallucinogens? Several antagonists have been developed that display selectivity for 5-HT$_{2A}$ versus 5-HT$_{2C}$ receptors. Two agents, AMI-193 and MDL 100,907, were found to effectively antagonize the effects of DOM in DOM-trained animals (Ismaiel, De Los Angeles, Teitler, Ingher, & Glennon, 1993), and the effects of DOI in DOI-trained animals (Schreiber, Brocco, & Millan, 1994). These results suggest that these agents produce their stimulus effects via 5-HT$_{2A}$, not 5-HT$_{2C}$, mechanisms. It was later demonstrated that a significant correlation exists between the potencies of a series of nonselective 5-HT antagonists to antagonize the stimulus effects of LSD, and LSD-stimulus generalization to

$(-)$DOM, in LSD-trained rats and their 5-HT_{2A} receptor affinities; the correlation with their 5-HT_{2C} receptor affinities was much less significant (Fiorella, Rabin, & Winter, 1995).

The issue of whether other populations of 5-HT receptors, other than or in addition to 5-HT_2 receptors, are involved in the actions of hallucinogens has yet to be examined. Indolealkylamines, specifically tryptamine derivatives, are fairly nonselective agents that bind at several populations of 5-HT receptors; for example, 5-methoxy DMT binds at 5-HT_{1A} receptors with high affinity. However, phenylalkylamines are much more selective and do not bind at 5-HT_{1A} receptors. Furthermore, ketanserin, which is known to block the behavioral effects of hallucinogenic indolealkylamines and phenylalkylamines, lacks affinity for 5-HT_{1A} receptors. The same holds true for other members of the 5-HT_1 family of receptors. In general ergolines, LSD-related agents, do not bind at 5-HT_3 and 5-HT_4 receptors. These receptors are thus unlikely to account for the actions of all classical hallucinogens. Certain ergolines, including LSD, bind at 5-HT_5, 5-HT_6, and 5-HT_7 receptors; thus the role of these receptors requires additional examination. The only population of receptors definitively linked to the actions of the classical hallucinogens are the 5-HT_2 receptors. This is not to say, however, that other populations may not somehow modulate the effects of hallucinogens (Glennon, 1994).

Recently, another member of the 5-HT_2 family was identified: 5-HT_{2B} receptors. Like 5-HT_{2A} and 5-HT_{2C} receptors, 17 classical hallucinogens were shown to bind at 5-HT_{2B} receptors. A significant correlation was also found between human 5-HT_{2B} receptor affinities and human hallucinogenic potencies (Nelson, Glennon, & Wainscott, 1994). It has since been demonstrated that AMI-193, an agent that antagonizes the DOM stimulus, binds with 100-fold selectivity for 5-HT_{2A} versus 5-HT_{2B} receptors (Ismaiel, Dukat, Nelson, Lucaites, & Glennon, 1996). Ketanserin, another 5-HT_2 antagonist that attenuates the stimulus effects of classical hallucinogens such as DOM and LSD, also displays low affinity at

5-HT_{2B} receptors (Nelson, 1993). These findings indicate that the stimulus effects produced by these agents involve primarily 5-HT_{2A} receptors. It is emphasized, however, that although the stimulus effects of classical hallucinogens are likely mediated via a 5-HT_{2A} mechanism, evidence for the involvement of a 5-HT_{2A} agonist mechanism in the human hallucinogenic actions of these agents is by implication only, and has yet to be conclusively demonstrated.

Structure–Activity Relationships

There is reason to conclude that classical hallucinogens act as 5-HT_2 agonists. It should thus be possible to utilize stimulus generalization techniques to formulate *in vivo* structure–activity relationships (SAR) and radioligand binding data to formulate *in vitro* structure–affinity relationships (SAFIR). Indeed, this has been done for the phenylalkylamines, and to some extent for the indolealkylamines. In general, there is good agreement between SAR and SAFIR results (except where a particular structural modification might influence bioavailability). Although SAR and SAFIR findings have been reviewed previously (Glennon, 1994; Nichols & Glennon, 1984), some of the highlights of such investigations with phenylalkylamines are shown in Table 2. For a general discussion, see Glennon (1994), Nichols and Glennon (1984), and Pfaff, Huang, Marona-Lewicka, Oberlender, and Nichols (1994). For a discussion of human structure–activity relationships, see Jacob and Shulgin (1994).

Classical Hallucinogens: Reexamination of the Definition

It was mentioned in the beginning of this chapter that classical hallucinogens are best described as agents that bind at 5-HT_2 (specifically 5-HT_{2A}) receptors and they are also agents recognized in tests of stimulus generalization in DOM-trained rats. Certain compounds meet these requirements but either seem to lack hallucinogenic activity or have not been thoroughly investigated in humans. These compounds have been termed *enigmatic*

TABLE 2. Structure–Activity Relationships for the Phenylalkylamines[a]

Substituent	Effect
Terminal amine	The primary amine (i.e., -NH$_2$) is optimal. Substitution decreases both receptor affinity and stimulus generalization potency.
Chiral center	The R(–) optical isomers are usually twice as potent as the racemates which, in turn, are two to five times more potent than the corresponding S(+) isomers.
α-Substituent	There is essentially no difference in 5-HT$_{2A}$ receptor affinity regardless of whether the α-substituent is -H or -CH$_3$. However, *in vivo*, the α-methyl derivatives are several times more potent than the unsubstituted analogs. This probably reflects bioavailability. Larger α-alkyl substituents decrease potency or abolish activity.
2-Position	A 2-position methoxy substituent appears optimal.
3-Position	Although substituents may be tolerated, an unsubstituted 3-position is optimal.
4-Position	Small polar substituents (-OH, -COOH) abolish activity and dramatically decrease affinity. Small alkyl groups are favored (-CH$_3$ = DOM; -C$_2$H$_5$ = DOET; -C$_3$H$_7$ = DOPR). Halogen, especially Br and I, are optimal (e.g., -Br = DOB; -I = DOI). Larger alkyl and arylalkyl substituents bind but may constitute 5-HT$_2$ antagonists.
5-Position	A 5-position methoxy group seems optimal.
6-Position	Not well investigated.

[a]For review, see Nichols and Glennon (1984) and Glennon (1994).

agents (Glennon, 1994). Examples include lisuride (which is not normally considered to be hallucinogenic, but for which hallucinogenic activity has been reported) (Calne, McDonald, Horowski, & Wuttke, 1983) and quipazine (whose human effects have not been extensively documented and whose hallucinogenic actions are controversial).

The issue of *designer drugs* deserves mention. During the past decade, several new agents, termed controlled substance analogs or designer drugs, have appeared on the clandestine market. Some drugs are clearly hallucinogens (e.g., NEXUS, the α-desmethyl or phenylethylamine counterpart of DOB), whereas others are amphetamine-like central stimulants (e.g., CAT or methcathinone). The actions of others are not so clearly defined. For example, MDMA (Ecstasy, XTC) is the N-methyl derivative of 1-(3,4-methylenedioxyphenyl)-2-aminopropane or MDA. MDA possesses both hallucinogenic and central stimulant properties. Interestingly, the hallucinogenic actions of MDA rest primarily with the R(–) isomer, whereas the S(+) isomer seems mostly responsible for the stimulant actions (Young & Glennon, 1996). MDA, however,

seems to possess a third type of action, namely an empathogenic effect. This effect is characterized by facilitation of communication and increased feelings of empathy. MDMA displays essentially no hallucinogenic character, some stimulant character, but enhanced empathogenic character. MDMA also saw some use as an adjunct to psychotherapy before it became a controlled substance. As shown in Figure 2, the structures of the hallucinogen DOM, the central stimulant amphetamine, MDA, and MDMA are quite similar. MBDB (Figure 2), the α-ethyl homolog of MDMA (Nichols & Oberlender, 1989), seems to lack hallucinogenic or stimulant character. It would appear that these phenylisopropylamines exist on a behavioral continuum. That is, DOM is hallucinogenic, amphetamine is a stimulant, MBDB is empathogenic, and MDA possesses remnants of all three types of action. MDMA is similar to MDA but lacks significant hallucinogenic properties. Recently, a new agent has been identified, paramethoxymethamphetamine or PMMA (Figure 2). This compound is devoid of hallucinogenic and stimulant character but possesses MDMA-like properties. Like MDMA, PMMA bears a structural similarity to DOM,

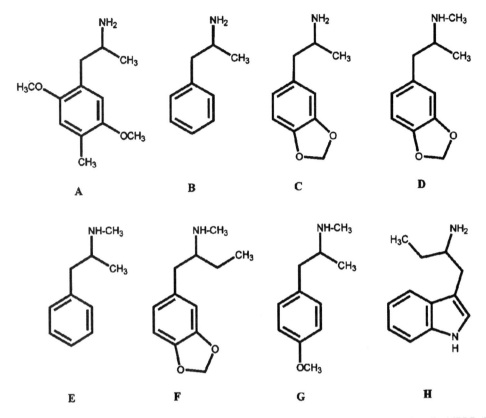

FIGURE 2. Structures of DOM (**A**), amphetamine (**B**), MDA (**C**), MDMA (**D**), methamphetamine (**E**), MBDB (**F**), PMMA (**G**), and α-EtT (**H**).

amphetamine, and methamphetamine (Figure 2). In an attempt to explain these actions, it has been proposed that the behavioral (or at least the stimulus) effects of these phenylisopropylamines may be explained by the Venn diagram shown in Figure 3 (Glennon, Young, Dukat, & Cheng, 1997). Segment H represents hallucinogenic activity, segment S represents stimulant activity, and segment O represents the "other" effect. Segments H and A are typified by agents such as DOM and amphetamine, respectively. Agents such as MBDB and PMMA typify segment O. MDA falls into the common intersect because it produces all three types of actions; the stimulant isomer of MDA, S(+)MDA, might best represent intersect 3, whereas the hallucinogenic isomer, R(−)MDA, would best represent intersect 2. MDMA, because it produces effects similar to MBDB, but also because it possesses stimulant character,

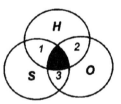

FIGURE 3. Venn diagram showing the possible relationships between agents classified as classical hallucinogens (H), amphetamine-like central stimulants (S), and other (O). Segment H is typified by DOM, segment S by (+)amphetamine, and segment O by MBDB and PMMA.

might also be represented by intersect 3. This means of classification gives us an entirely new way to view these agents.

The behavioral relationships implied in Figure 3 for phenylalkylamines may also apply to indolealkylamines. For example, α-MeT (Table 1) is considered an indolealkylamine hallucinogen (Murphree, Dippy, Jenney, & Pfeiffer, 1961). However, its homolog, α-ethyltryptamine (Figure 2), has long been recognized to possess central stimulant character (Hoffer & Osmond, 1967). α-Ethyltryptamine (α-EtT) has recently appeared on the street as the designer drug ET and has been sold as a substitute for MDMA. Consistent with this claim, α-EtT is recognized by MDMA-trained animals. Subsequently, the optical isomers of α-EtT were prepared and it has now been demonstrated that $(+)\alpha$-EtT, but not $(-)\alpha$-EtT, is recognized by DOM-trained animals, $(-)\alpha$-EtT, but not $(+)\alpha$-EtT, is recognized by $(+)$amphetamine-trained animals, and that both isomers of α-EtT are recognized by MDMA-trained animals; α-EtT also serves as an effective training drug in drug discrimination studies with rats (Young, Hong, & Glennon, 1996). Is α-EtT an indolealkylamine counterpart of the phenylisopropylamine MDA? Although additional work is obviously required to answer this question, the possibilities are quite intriguing, and may lead to a better understanding of how hallucinogens are classified. Such a behavioral relationship among the phenylalkylamines and indolealkylamines may also explain why it is occasionally so difficult to classify these agents if they are capable of producing effects that are not clearly hallucinogenic or stimulant-like. For example, α-EtT has been shown to be LSD-like in humans, but its effects could be differentiated from those produced by LSD (Murphree *et al.*, 1961).

ACKNOWLEDGMENT

Work from the author's laboratory was largely supported by PHS grant DA-01642.

References

Brimblecombe, R. W., & Pinder, R. M. (1975). *Hallucinogenic agents*. Bristol, England: Wright-Scientechnica.

Calne, D. B., McDonald, R. J., Horowski, R., & Wuttke, W. (1983). *Lisuride and other dopamine agonists*. New York: Raven.

Colpaert, F. C., & Slangen, J. L. (Eds.). (1982). *Drug discrimination: Applications in CNS pharmacology*. Amsterdam: Elsevier Biomedical Press.

Fiorella, D., Rabin, R. A., & Winter, J. C. (1995). The role of 5-HT2A and 5-HT2C receptors in the stimulus effects of hallucinogenic drugs: I. Antagonist correlation analysis. *Psychopharmacology, 121,* 347–356.

Glennon, R. A. (1992). Animal models for assessing classical hallucinogens. In A. A. Boulton, G. B. Baker, & P. H. Wu (Eds.), *Animal models for the assessment of psychoactive drugs* (pp. 345–381). Clifton, NJ: Humana.

Glennon, R. A. (1994). Classical hallucinogens: An introductory overview. In G. C. Lin & R. A. Glennon (Eds.), *Hallucinogens: An update* (pp. 4–32). Washington, DC: U.S. Department of Health and Human Services.

Glennon, R. A. (1996). Classical hallucinogens. In C. R. Schuster & M. J. Kuhar (Eds.), *Pharmacological aspects of drug dependence* (pp. 343–372). Berlin: Springer.

Glennon, R. A., Rosecrans, J. A., & Young, R. (1982). Use of the drug discrimination paradigm for studying hallucinogenic agents. In F. C. Colpaert & J. L. Slangen (Eds.), *Drug discrimination: Applications in CNS pharmacology* (pp. 69–96). Amsterdam: Elsevier Biomedical Press.

Glennon, R. A., Teitler, M., & McKenney, J. D. (1984). Evidence for involvement of 5-HT$_2$ receptors in the mechanism of action of hallucinogenic agents. *Life Sciences, 35,* 2505–2509.

Glennon, R. A., Jarbe, T. U. C., & Frankenheim, J. (Eds.). (1991). *Drug discrimination: Applications to drug abuse research*. Washington, DC: U.S. Department of Health and Human Services.

Glennon, R. A., Young, R., Dukat, M., & Cheng, Y. (1997). Initial characterization of PMMA as a discriminative stimulus. *Pharmacology, Biochemistry and Behavior, 57,* 151–158.

Hoffer, A., & Osmond, H. (1967). *The hallucinogens*. New York: Academic Press.

Hollister, L. E. (1968). *Chemical psychoses*. Springfield, IL: Thomas.

Hollister, L. E. (1984). Effects of hallucinogens in humans. In B. L. Jacobs (Ed.), *Hallucinogens: Neurochemical, behavioral, and clinical perspectives* (pp. 19–33). New York: Raven.

Hoyer, D., Clarke, D. E., Fozard, J. R., Hartig, P. R., Martin, G. R., Myelecharane, E. J., Saxena, P. R., & Humphrey, P. A. (1994). International Union of Pharmacology classification of receptors for 5-hydroxytryptamine (serotonin). *Pharmacological Reviews, 46,* 158–203.

Ismaiel, A. M., De Los Angeles, J., Teitler, M., Ingher, S., & Glennon, R. A. (1993). Antagonism of the 1-(2,5-dimethoxy-4-methylphenyl)-2-aminopropane stimulus with a newly identified 5-HT$_2$- versus 5-HT$_{1C}$-selective antagonist. *Journal of Medicinal Chemistry, 36,* 2519–2525.

Ismaiel, A. M., Dukat, M., Nelson, D. L., Lucaites, V. L., & Glennon, R. A. (1996). Binding of N2-substituted pyrido[4,3-b]indole analogs of spiperone at human 5-HT$_{2A}$, 5-HT$_{2B}$, and 5-HT$_{2C}$ serotonin receptors. *Medicinal Chemistry Research, 6*, 179–211.

Jacob, P., & Shulgin, A. T. (1994). Structure–activity relationships of the classical hallucinogens and their analogs. In G. C. Lin & R. A. Glennon (Eds.), *Hallucinogens: An update* (pp. 74–91). Washington, DC: U.S. Department of Health and Human Services.

Lin, G. C., & Glennon, R. A. (Eds.). (1994). *Hallucinogens: An update.* Washington, DC: U.S. Department of Health and Human Services.

Murphree, H. B., Dippey, R. H., Jenney, E. H., & Pfeiffer, C. C. (1961). Effects in normal man of α-methyltryptamine and α-ethyltryptamine. *Clinical Pharmacology and Therapeutics, 2*, 722–726.

Naranjo, C. (1973). *The healing journey.* New York: Pantheon.

Nelson, D. L. (1993). The serotonin$_2$ (5-HT$_2$) subfamily of receptors: Pharmacological challenges. *Medicinal Chemistry Research, 3*, 306–316.

Nelson, D. L., Glennon, R. A., & Wainscott, D. B. (1994, July–August). Comparison of the affinities of hallucinogenic phenylalkylamines at the cloned human 5-HT2A, 2B and 2C receptors. [Abstract #120, p. 116]. *Third IUPHAR Satellite Meeting on Serotonin,* Chicago.

Nichols, D. E., & Glennon, R. A. (1984). Medicinal chemistry and structure–activity relationships of hallucinogens. In B. L. Jacobs (Ed.), *Hallucinogens: Neurochemical, behavioral, and clinical perspectives* (pp. 95–142). New York: Raven.

Nichols, D. E., & Oberlender, R. (1989). Structure–activity relationships of MDMA-like substances. In K. Ashgar & E. B. De Souza (Eds.), *Pharmacology and toxicology of amphetamine and related designer drugs* (pp. 1–29). Washington, DC: U.S. Government Printing Office.

Pfaff, R. C., Huang, X., Marona-Lewicka, D., Oberlender, R., & Nichols, D. E. (1994). Lysergamides revisited.

In G. C. Lin & R. A. Glennon (Eds.), *Hallucinogens: An update* (pp. 52–73). Washington, DC: U.S. Department of Health and Human Services.

Schreiber, R., Brocco, M., & Millan, M. J. (1994). Blockade of the discriminative stimulus effects of DOI by MDL 100,907, and the atypical antipsychotics clozapine and risperidone. *European Journal of Pharmacology, 264*, 99–102.

Shulgin, A., & Shulgin, A. (1991). *Pihkal.* Berkeley, CA: Transform.

Siva Sankar, D. V. (1975). *LSD—A total study.* Westbury, NY: PJD.

Strassman, R. J. (1994). Human hallucinogenic drug research: Regulatory, clinical, and scientific issues. In G. C. Lin & R. A. Glennon (Eds.), *Hallucinogens: An update* (pp. 92–123). Washington, DC: U.S. Department of Health and Human Services.

Szara, S. (1994). Are hallucinogens psychoheuristic? In G. C. Lin & R. A. Glennon (Eds.), *Hallucinogens: An update* (pp. 33–51). Washington, DC: U.S. Department of Health and Human Services.

Weissman, A. (1978). Generalization of the discriminative stimulus properties of Δ^9-tetrahydrocannabinol to cannabinoids with therapeutic potential. In F. C. Colpaert & J. A. Rosecrans (Eds.), *Stimulus properties of drugs: Ten years of progress* (pp. 99–122). Amsterdam: Elsevier North Holland Biomedical Press.

Woolley, D. W. (1962). *The biochemical bases of psychoses.* New York: Wiley.

Young, R., & Glennon, R. A. (1996). A three-lever operant procedure differentiates the stimulus effects of R(–)MDA from S(+)MDA. *Journal of Pharmacology and Experimental Therapeutics, 276*, 594–601.

Young, R., Hong, S., & Glennon, R. A. (1996). α-ET: A tryptamine version of MDA? In L. S. Harris (Ed.), *Problems of drug dependence, 1995* (p. 357). Washington, DC: U.S. Department of Health and Human Services.

14

Behavioral Pharmacology of Hallucinogens

NANCY K. MORRISON

Introduction

All classic hallucinogens produce unique subjective effects on the basic functions of the human mind: perception, affect, cognition, volition, and interoception. Despite these usually profound effects, the individual retains contact with reality and memory during the altered state. Subtle differences are ascribed to particular compounds, although their subjective effects are more alike than different. These subjective effects account for the use of hallucinogens in established rituals of some cultures as well as the use and abuse of them in contemporary Western culture. Hallucinogens differ from other drugs of abuse in that tolerance develops rapidly and there is no physical dependence. The unique and profound effect on cognitive processes makes the hallucinogens valuable in neuroscientific research, and the discovery of LSD's psychotropic effects, as much as the contemporaneous discovery of chlorpromazine, mark the beginning of modern biological psychiatry (Strassman, 1995).

The classic hallucinogens are divided into two categories: indolylalkylamines and phenyl-alkylamines. The indolylalkylamines include DMT (n,n-dimethyltryptamine), psilocybin, psilocin, LSD (lysergic acid diethylamide), and β-carbolines. The phenylalkylamines are represented by mescaline, the psychoactive component of peyote (Glennon, 1994). Ibogaine is included because of the growing interest in this hallucinogen as a possible treatment for opiate and cocaine addiction.

Characteristics of the Hallucinogens

Hallucinogens elicit behavioral tolerance rapidly (Isbell, Belleville, Fraser, Wikler, & Logan, 1956). A diminished drug response occurs on the second consecutive day of administration and all response is essentially lost by the fourth consecutive day of administration. With the exception of DMT (Gillin, Kaplan, Stillman, & Wyatt, 1976), there is cross-tolerance between the classic hallucinogens (Milhorn, 1990). Physical dependence does not occur even with repetitive use of hallucinogens although psychological dependence has been described. Hallucinogens also do not cause an abstinence syndrome.

The rapid development of tolerance, cross-tolerance, and lack of withdrawal syndrome mean that generic dependence criteria do not apply to these drugs (*DSM-IV;* American Psychiatric Association, 1994). Those who abuse hallucinogens use them much less often than

NANCY K. MORRISON • Department of Psychiatry, The University of New Mexico, Albuquerque, New Mexico 87131.

Handbook of Substance Abuse: Neurobehavioral Pharmacology, edited by Tarter *et al.* Plenum Press, New York, 1998.

those with psychological dependence. Problems associated with their use manifest as difficulties in fulfilling obligations to school, work, or home and are due to acute intoxication rather than addiction. Individual hallucinogens are differentiated primarily on route of administration, onset, and duration of action.

Lysergic Acid Diethylamide (LSD)

LSD is traditionally considered the prototypic hallucinogen perhaps because it has been the most studied. LSD is a synthetically produced ergot derivative that is a white, odorless crystalline, water-soluble material, and is ingested orally. Average doses range between 25 and 500 micrograms (Milhorn, 1990; Strassman, 1984). LSD is reported to be 200 times as potent as psilocybin and 5000 times as potent as mescaline (O'Brien & Cohen, 1984). Preparations of LSD are often sold on blotter paper or sugar cubes. Street names for LSD include acid, blotter acid, sugar, and window panes (Milhorn, 1990). Despite the high potency of LSD, the drug is not directly toxic and deaths due to overdose have not been reported.

The initial effects of LSD are experienced after several minutes following oral ingestion. The initial experiences are the sympathomimetic physical symptoms which include dilatation of pupils, flushing, and experience of change of body temperature, dizziness, and sometimes weakness. These initial reactions may be accompanied by a subjective experience of anxiety or even panic (Strassman, 1984).

The psychological effects follow in 30–90 min. These can include visual illusions and hallucinations with occasional auditory experiences, a sense of inner tension or emotional lability, a blending of sensory modalities, and a change in the subjective experience of time. The half-life of LSD is approximately 8 hr and the peak reaction occurs between 4 and 6 hr. Most reactions subside after 8 hr (Linton & Langs, 1962).

Psilocybin and Psilocin

Psilocybin and its congener psilocin are the active hallucinogenic ingredients in the psilocybe-mexicana mushroom found in Mexico and Central America. Named the "flesh of the gods," their use dates back to at least 1500 B.C. Synthetic psilocybin is not generally available and psilocybin is taken by eating the mushrooms. The usual dose of psilocybin is 4 to 5 mg.

The initial sympathomimetic effects usually begin 10–15 min after oral ingestion and reach a maximum intensity at 1.5–2 hr. The effects subside 5–6 hr after ingestion. Tolerance and psychological dependence do develop, as well as cross-tolerance to LSD and mescaline. There is no report of physical dependence (Beck & Gordon, 1982).

Mescaline, Peyote

Mescaline is the phenylethalineamine active hallucinogen found in the peyote cactus of northern Mexico and Texas and the San Pedro cactus of Peru. Peyote has been used in religious ceremonies of the indigenous people of the southwestern United States and northern Mexico for centuries. Currently, it is used legally by members of the Native American Church in the United States. The synthetic preparations of mescaline are available for oral use, while peyote buttons have become somewhat scarce and are not as readily available. Mescaline is a low-potency hallucinogen and requires an ingestion of 300–500 mg to show effects.

DMT (N,N-Dimethyltryptamine)

DMT is the active hallucinogenic ingredient in ayahuasca (DeKorne, 1994). Ayahuasca is a preparation used in Ecuador and Peru, and yage is the name of a similar preparation used in Columbia and parts of Brazil. It is currently utilized by certain religious groups in South America. Ayahuasca requires the combination of two different plants, one containing DMT and the other containing a monoamineoxidase inhibitor. Oral DMT is deactivated in the intestine unless it is accompanied by the monoamineoxidase inhibitor. While these preparations remain an important part of certain religious practices in South America, ayahuasca and yage are not generally available in the United States. Forms of DMT utilized in the United

States are snuffed or smoked. In this form they have a rapid onset of action, usually within a few seconds, and have a short duration of action. Because of their short hallucinogenic effect they are called "the businessman's trip" (Milhorn, 1990). DMT has also been utilized in recent research. Its characteristics of rapid onset and brief duration of action made DMT an ideal hallucinogen for study in a clinical research setting (Strassman, 1994).

Ibogaine

Ibogaine and iboga are the active hallucinogenic ingredients in tabernanthe iboga, a native shrub of equatorial Africa. Ibogaine is utilized in cultural rites of the people of this region. Ibogaine is known to be an extremely potent hallucinogen and to have a long duration of action, possibly greater than 12 hr (DeKorne, 1994). Ibogaine is not generally available in the United States and is mentioned here because of research interest in ibogaine's potential use in the treatment of cocaine and heroin addiction. There have been anecdotal reports of deaths from the use of ibogaine and it has not been systematically studied in humans.

Psychological Effects

Hallucinogenic substances occur naturally in various plants on all the continents. These substances have been used in religious, spiritual, and other cultural rites throughout many cultures of the world (Dobkin de Rios, 1984) because of their psychological effects. Although a few naturally occurring hallucinogens are found in the eastern hemisphere, more than ninety species are known in the western hemisphere. Many of the indigenous people of the western hemisphere utilize hallucinogens in their cultures. In such a cultural context, hallucinogens are rarely drugs of abuse. Their use is carefully culturally prescribed and in some cultures they are entrusted to specific people and often are prohibited to children (Grinspoon & Balaker, 1979).

Western cultures did not develop significant interest in the psychological effects of hallucinogens until the 1960s, when LSD became a drug of experimentation. Of the classic hallucinogens, LSD is the only semisynthetic compound. LSD was originally synthesized by Albert Hoffman in 1938 from an ergot compound. He discovered the hallucinogenic properties of LSD through accidental ingestion at his laboratory.

Hallucinogens are perhaps the only class of abusable drugs named for their psychological effects. Despite this, there is technical argument about the correctness of this term. Hallucination is strictly defined as a "sense perception to which there is no external stimulus" (Campbell, 1989, p. 314). Actual hallucinations are reported to be rare effects of these drugs (Hollister *et al.,* 1962). While visual pattern distortions occur, the individual recognizes the cause of these distortions and only rarely are these perceived as having a real outside existence (Szara, 1994). It is suggested that these visual distortions are more appropriately termed illusions.

Psychedelic is another popular term for these drugs. Psychedelic literally means "mind manifesting" or "mind opening." Humphrey Osmond originally suggested this term in 1957 (Grof, 1980). Psychedelic suggests more of the sought-after effects of these drugs than the term hallucinogen. Individuals reporting on subjective effects more often describe the expansive affectual experiences as opposed to emphasizing the hallucinogenic experiences.

The overall experience and especially the positive or negative tone of the experience is influenced by the set and setting (Grof, 1980). Set refers to the attitude, beliefs, and expectations of the individual. The setting refers to the external circumstances: the place, security, and the attitudes and relationships with the other people present during the drug experience.

Freedman (1968) describes this aspect of the hallucinogenic experience as portentousness. By this he means "the capacity of the mind to see more than it can tell, to experience more than it can explicate, to believe in and be impressed with more than it can rationally justify, to experience boundlessness and 'boundaryless' events from the banal to the profound" (p. 331). Grof (1980) identified both a temporal and spatial expansion of consciousness. He referred to a rich and diverse phenomenon of feeling that the individual identifies as consciousness expanded beyond the usual ego boundaries and limitations of time and space.

These states of experience reflect back to the cultural use of hallucinogens that became incorporated into spiritual and religious functions. Parallels have been described between the hallucinogenic experience and the mystical experience. The "peak experience" was believed to create the potential for various kinds of psychological changes (W. A. Richards, Rhead, DiLeo, Yensen, & Kurland, 1977).

The same categories that define the peak experience are used to describe the mystical experience (R. A. Richards, 1978). The six categories of the so-called peak or mystical experience are unity, transcendence of time and space, objectivity and reality (noetic quality), deeply felt positive mood, sense of sacredness, and ineffability and paradoxicality. Unity is the experience of loss of the subject–object dichotomy of perception and a sense of merging into a unity with objects in the external world or specific ideas and images. This includes the concept of ego death and transcendence. Transcendence of time and space is the experience of feeling outside the historical drama and feeling a part of eternity or infinity. The third category, objectivity and reality, is related to a concept developed by William James called the noetic quality. This refers to insight into the depths of truth and moving beyond the discursive intellect (James, 1902). Importantly, this includes the experience of a strong intrinsic self-validation. The deeply felt positive mood includes a sense of peacefulness and a belief that there is no cause for anxiety. Fifth is the sense of sacredness with the experience of awe, majesty, and energy. Sixth is ineffability and paradoxicality, which refers to the experience of the inability to use rationality or common logic to explain the experience. It includes a strong sense of paradox such as everything remaining the same while being in a constant state of change.

These experiences are reported to be the most meaningful and sought-after by those who utilize hallucinogens. The day following the drug experience some individuals report the feeling of having acquired new meanings in life. This perception of new meaning may be separate from the direct drug effect (Linton & Langs, 1962). This change in perceived meaning raises some concerns about the long-term impact of these drugs, such as lifestyle changes.

Some early research attempted to describe more objectively the responses to the hallucinogens. Typically the initial reactions are sympathomimetic physical symptoms. These include dilatation of pupils, nausea, flushing, chilliness, increased blood pressure and heart rate, sometimes tremor, piloerection, dizziness, and weakness. These physiological reactions during the onset of drug effect are sometimes described as unpleasant by the research subjects, and may lead to anxiety and panic (Strassman, 1984).

The more psychological effects follow soon after. One of the most common experiences involves changes in thinking and flow of thought. There is difficulty with concentration and a sense that the individual's attention is captured involuntarily. Subjects have difficulty maintaining their attention on a task at hand. Many subjects report a sense of loss of control over their thoughts, body, emotions, and behavior (Linton & Langs, 1962).

Changes in the experience of the body are common and fall into two categories. First are direct physical changes that can include feeling numb, cold or hot, nauseated, weak, and having palpitations. The second category of change in bodily experience is in perceived body image. These changes include the subjective experience of changes in size, shape, proportion, skin texture, and in extreme situations the sense of loss of a body part.

Included in the perceptual changes is an experience called synethesia which refers to experiencing senses through different organs. For example, music is "seen" rather than heard, or colors are "tasted" rather than seen. These experiences occur in the context of other often compelling visual experiences.

A frequently reported change is in the experience of time. Most often is the sense of time slowing down or of time becoming nonexistent. Occasionally, individuals will report the sense of time having speeded up. The change may also be the sense of transcending the dimension of time.

Changes in affect, including lability, frequently occur. Study subjects may report the impulse to laugh without any apparent reason. The experience of euphoria is frequent but experiences of sadness, depression, and anger are also reported. Affect is often heightened and may be related to childhood memories that are retrieved during the experience. Depersonalization and derealization experiences can be disconcerting but may also be reported without affectual involvement.

Patterns of Use and Abuse

Historical and Cultural Patterns

Cultures with established rituals involving hallucinogens carefully prescribe their use, which is often associated with the sacred. Use of hallucinogens outside of these cultural rites is rare. Grob and Dobkin de Rios (1992) describe the differences in societal use of hallucinogenic plants in initiation rites of adolescents among three separate cultures. They suggest that cultures are able to create managed altered states of consciousness that can be used in rites of socialization for both religious and pedagogical purposes. Cultural rites are viewed in contrast to the use patterns found among American adolescents where cultural prescriptions are not in place.

Western culture became aware of hallucinogens and their effects from exploration of the new world, although use of hallucinogens in Western culture until the mid twentieth century was rare. Sporadic reports such as that of Aldus Huxley (1954) were cause for curiosity. It was not until the 1960s that hallucinogens became widely used. Hallucinogens were made illegal in 1966 when Congress passed the Drug Abuse Control Amendment (see Szara, 1994). Despite this, the use of hallucinogens increased slightly between 1968 (18%) and 1978 (21%) (Pope, Ionescu-Pioggia, Aizley, & Varma, 1990). During this period of time, one component of the American population believed that consciousness-altering properties of hallucinogenic drugs had positive influences. Albert Hoffman (1980), the chemist who developed LSD and first experienced its psychological effects, expressed his belief that hallucinogenic drugs offer the potential for a mystical experience and thus an alternative to materialism and other problems of the modern world. He did indicate, however, that when these substances are mistaken for pleasure drugs, wrong and inappropriate use pose a danger and possible catastrophic consequences. In these circumstances, he referred to LSD as "my problem child."

Current Patterns of Abuse

The context of hallucinogen use is reported to have changed over the past three or four decades. During the 1960s, psychedelics were used by individuals in small groups either to celebrate an event or in a quest for spiritual or cultural values (Millman & Beeder, 1994). Current use also includes these circumstances. Hallucinogens, however, are now used in a new setting called the "rave" phenomenon. Raves began in Europe in the 1980s. These events are sponsored by club owners and businessmen and are held in warehouses, basements, tenements, and other buildings that are in disrepair and disuse. Participants ingest hallucinogens and then spend the evening listening and dancing to "techno music." Alcohol, marijuana, and cocaine seem to be less desirable drugs at these events. Participants report that they usually begin to experience hallucinogenic effects after the first hour and then spend the next several hours dancing as the drug peaks. After the drug effects disappear, they may remain exhausted for several hours. While adverse psychological drug effects are reported as one problem, a greater concern is physiological effects, especially dehydration. Some raves provide handouts informing participants of the need to drink fluids, take breaks, and to leave the scene in order to control responses such as paranoia and agitation.

During the 1980s the use of hallucinogens appears to have declined. In Pope and colleagues' (1990) study conducted in 1989, 14% of college students reported having used hallucinogens at some time. These results are similar to a study done by Patterson, Myers, and Gallant (1988) comparing substance use on a college campus between 1972 and 1986, in which the reported use of LSD also declined.

Recent studies, however, suggest that hallucinogen use is rising among high school and junior high students. One study of 522,328 junior and senior high school students found that hallucinogen use rose from 4.9% to 5.3% in 1 year. Annual use of hallucinogens was 2.4% for eighth graders and 7.1% for seniors (Gold, 1994). The Pride survey data (1993) from 236,745 students in 40 states across the United States found that LSD and hallucinogen use annually increased significantly for eighth graders (2.4% to 2.7%), eleventh graders (5.6% to 6.4%), and twelfth graders (7.1% to 8.0%).

These studies also suggest changes in availability and attitudes toward the hallucinogenic drugs. Data from Gold's study (1994) indicates that disapproval of LSD experimentation fell from 91.6% in 1987 to 88% in 1992. Fifty-five percent of the high school seniors stated that they believed trying LSD a few times was not harmful. In the Pride survey (1992), more students indicated that hallucinogens were easier to obtain. Fewer students reported that none of their friends used LSD or other hallucinogens, and only 80% believed that hallucinogens were "very much harmful" to health.

A household survey of the United States population in 1990 reported 7.6% had used a hallucinogenic drug at some point in their lives (National Institute of Drug Abuse, 1991). In the population over the age of 12, 5.5% reported using LSD, 3.0%, mescaline, psilocybin, or PCP, and 1.0%, peyote (National Institute of Drug Abuse, 1989). Data on lifetime abuse or dependence suggest that hallucinogens are the fifth most common of six drugs to have been used or abused, and that 0.4% of the population would meet criteria for abuse of or dependence on hallucinogens. Of 1,330 males, 1.0% had lifetime prevalence

rates of drug abuse or dependence on hallucinogens, while only 0.1% of 1,928 females met criteria for lifetime prevalence rates of drug dependence or abuse of hallucinogens (Russell, Newman, & Bland, 1994).

Characteristics of Hallucinogen Users

Various studies have attempted to look at characteristics of individuals who are prone to the use of hallucinogens. The 1985 National Household Survey (National Institute on Drug Abuse, 1986) reports that use is consistently highest among the age group 18–34 and is consistently higher among men than women. The use of hallucinogens may be related to needs for novel or unconventional experiences as well as negative attitudes toward conventionally defined social values (Mabry & Khavari, 1986). Arousal-seeking and stimulus-screening characteristics may also be important. Individuals who preferred the experience of hallucinogens were higher in internal stimulus screening than all other drug preference groups (Kern, Kenkel, Templer, & Newell, 1986). No significant differences were found between college nonusers and users of hallucinogens on such parameters as grade-point averages, participation in athletic activities, clubs, and political organizations in a 1989 study. While in 1969 the hallucinogen user group reported a greater sense of alienation, this was not true for the users in 1989 (Pope et al., 1990).

A certain folklore exists that creative individuals are drawn to the use of hallucinogens. A study of substance abuse among 22 writers, 27 visual artists, 12 musicians, and 25 controls found no difference among the groups in the overall use of alcohol, narcotics, tranquilizers, or hallucinogens. On interview, the creative individuals held strong negative opinions about the effects of substances on creativity. Some creative individuals indicated that initially they perceived mood- and mind-altering substances as potentially useful to creativity but discovered that, eventually, they were destructive (Kerr, Shaffer, Chambers, & Hallowell, 1991).

The use of hallucinogens by psychiatric patients also has been studied. The association between a comorbid lifetime psychiatric diagnosis and the choice of drug abused among those individuals who met *DSM-IV* criteria for drug abuse or drug dependence revealed that hallucinogens accounted for only a small percentage (Russell *et al.,* 1994). In an inpatient psychiatric population, 2.6% reported the use of hallucinogens (Brady, Casto, Lydiard, & Malcolm, 1991). Hallucinogen abuse is found more frequently in association with mania than any other diagnosis and the abuse of hallucinogens is highest among individuals with a lifetime psychiatric diagnosis of affective disorder and antisocial personality disorder. Substance abuse is known to be high among individuals with borderline personality disorder. Of 137 borderline patients studied, 67% received a *DSM-III* substance use disorder diagnosis. Hallucinogen abuse was found in only 3.6% of patients and accounted for only 2.2% of the substance use diagnoses (Dulit, Fryer, Haas, Sullivan, & Francis, 1990). Among girls ages 12 to 19 in treatment for chemical dependency, many reported a history of sexual abuse. The sexual abuse victims were significantly more likely to regularly use stimulants, sedatives, tranquilizers, and hallucinogens (Harrison, Hoffman, & Edwall, 1989).

Adverse Reactions to Hallucinogenic Drugs

Adverse reactions are defined here as dysphoric, maladaptive, or dysfunctional responses, or a combination of these, to the use of these drugs which result in the need for clinical attention or that disrupt normal functioning. The perspective of investigators has sometimes made it difficult to study adverse reactions. Some define the subjective effects of hallucinogenic drugs as inherently adverse, while others view even the most extreme responses as potentially useful to an individual seeking a higher level of consciousness (Strassman, 1984). The *DSM-IV* identifies hallucinogenic intoxication as a diagnosis although it is well known that most individuals using hallucinogenics do not present for treatment.

Strassman (1984) extensively reviewed the literature on adverse effects of hallucinogens. He identified several problems in evaluating these reports. These include (1) lack of data on the pre-drug personality and history of subjects, (2) lack of control for use of other psychoactive drugs, (3) reports including street use of hallucinogens which precludes knowledge of actual substance or substances ingested and the amounts, (4) unknown frequency of exposure, and (5) unknown set and setting of ingestion experience. From this extensive review, he concluded that the incidence of adverse reactions is low in controlled studies.

Acute Reactions

The most common acute adverse reaction is the "bad trip" (Strassman, 1984). Most frequently these present with an episode of panic that lasts for the duration of the acute effects of the drug, but on occasion can last up to 24 hr. Occasionally, the dysphoric affect is depression rather than panic. Usually, the affect is congruent with the cognitions and illusions that are generated by the drug. Occasionally patients need to be protected from acting out aggressive and suicidal behaviors during this acute episode. While often reported in dramatic fashion, dangerous acting-out behaviors such as homicides, suicides, or staring into the sun are extremely rare and the circumstances often include the use of other drugs.

The diagnosis is based primarily on a careful history identifying the recent ingestion of a hallucinogenic drug (Abraham & Aldridge, 1993). It is important to obtain a description of the substance. For example, acid is often taken on blotter paper and psilocybin is most often ingested as mushrooms. Even this description cannot rule out either adulterants or that the individual has taken a completely unknown substance. PCP is one of the most important complicating adulterants in hallucinogenic drugs. Individuals who have ingested PCP are much more likely to become aggressive. Most patients respond to a psychotherapeutic intervention commonly known as "being talked down." They may also need treatment with diazepam. Neuroleptics are reported to exacerbate these symptoms.

Dependence

Physical dependence or addiction does not develop to the classic hallucinogens. Tolerance to the euphoric and psychedelic effects of hallucinogens develops rapidly and there is cross-tolerance between LSD and other hallucinogens. Consequently, even individuals who are diagnosed as being dependent limit their use to at most a few times a week. Physical withdrawal has not been demonstrated, although a psychological craving has been reported (American Psychiatric Association, 1994).

Hallucinogen Abuse

The *DSM-IV* distinguishes hallucinogen abuse from dependence based on frequency of use. Hallucinogen abuse is identified when the individual fails in one or more major role obligations such as school, work, or relationships because of frequent hallucinogen intoxication. This diagnosis also can be made when the individual participates in physically dangerous pursuits while intoxicated or develops legal difficulties related to hallucinogenic use.

Hallucinogen Persisting Perception Disorder (Flashback)

So called flashbacks may be defined as spontaneous, transient recurrences of the hallucinogen drug effect that appear after a period of normalcy (Wesson & Smith, 1976). These reexperiences include any aspect of the hallucinogen experience and are divided into three categories: perceptual, somatic, and emotional (Schick & Smith, 1970). In order to meet criteria for the disorder in D*SM-IV,* the symptoms must cause clinically significant distress or impairment in a major area of functioning. The reported incidence of flashbacks varies from 15% to 77% (Strassman, 1984).

Attempts to identify factors predisposing to flashbacks suggest some evidence that increasing numbers of drug experiences may increase the likelihood of this phenomenon. Certain situations such as decreased sensory input, fatigue, fever, relaxation, stress, and marijuana use increase the likelihood of experiencing flashbacks in predisposed individuals (Strassman, 1984). No significant psychopathological differences among those with flashbacks was found on the Minnesota Multiphasic Personality Inventory (MMPI) or attentional processes as measured by the Embedded Figures Test (Matefy & Crawl, 1974).

LSD-Psychosis

The incidence of prolonged psychotic reactions occurring after the use of hallucinogens is reported to be between 0.08% and 4.6% with a median of 2.7% (Abraham & Aldridge, 1993). The higher figures occur among patient populations, while the lower figure is derived from experimental subjects. It remains unclear whether a specific entity of "LSD-psychosis" exists or if prolonged psychotic states following hallucinogen use are actually cases of schizophrenia or other psychotic illnesses (Strassman, 1984).

Research

Hallucinogenic drugs offer unique opportunities for research into the mind–brain interface and the neurochemistry of the brain. The study of these psychoactive hallucinogens began in earnest after the demonstration of the reported effects of LSD by Albert Hoffman in the late 1940s. Much of this research was halted by the Controlled Substances Act of 1970, which defines hallucinogens as Schedule I drugs. Animal research has continued although research in humans has only recently been resumed.

Animal Model Research

As a consequence of the legal restrictions on hallucinogenic drugs, most studies since 1970 have been conducted in animal models. Animal research is hampered by the obvious limitation that only human subjects can accurately assess and describe the subjective effects of these agents (Glennon, 1994). Animal models are either investigative or interpretive. The first categorizes the effects of known hallucinogens on animals, for example, social behavior, sleep cycles, and other observable effects, and then attempts to catalogue pharmacological effects. Interpretive methods address possible mechanisms involved in the production of these hallucinogenic effects. Animal models are also used to identify novel hallucinogens.

In the drug discrimination paradigm, animals are trained to demonstrate a particular response when administered a specific dose of a known hallucinogenic agent and to give a different response when administered a placebo vehicle. Animals trained to discriminate specific hallucinogens from placebo can be utilized to test questions related to effective drug dose, time of onset, and duration of action of potential hallucinogens. This paradigm is also used to test stimulus antagonism; that is, to identify neurotransmitter agonists that block the effect of the test agents (Glennon, 1991).

Strassman (1995) suggested that the simultaneous discoveries of serotonin and LSD may have led to the description of the preeminent role of this neurotransmitter in explicating effects and mechanisms of action of hallucinogens. Other neurotransmitters including noradrenergic, dopaminergic, and cholinergic systems are also implicated but have received less attention. Currently, the mechanisms of action of classic hallucinogens are not fully understood but 5HT2A and 5HT2C receptors are thought to play a major role (Glennon, 1994).

Despite their limitations, animal models provide an important avenue for the study of the effect of hallucinogens in the neurotransmitter systems. Such research may help in developing antagonists to the behavioral effects of hallucinogens which may offer information in the treatment of schizophrenia and other psychotic states. Such strategies might also provide a treatment to reverse acute adverse reactions or to develop blockade strategies to treat chronic abuse of hallucinogens (Strassman, 1995).

Research with Human Subjects

Studies prior to 1970 on human subjects relied on careful clinical observation; while useful, these studies did not have modern research methodologies available (Strassman, 1995).

Some studies attempted to define the effects of hallucinogens on the human mind and utilized psychoanalytic or behavioral frameworks. Other studies focused on such variables as route of administration, onset of action, dose response, duration of action, development of tolerance, and physiological effects such as blood pressure and pulse.

This early research attempted to identify therapeutic uses of the hallucinogenic drugs. Savage (1952) noted that daily LSD produced strong antidepressant responses. Kast and Collins (1964) studied the effect of LSD on pain in more than 200 patients with advanced carcinomas and found the analgesic effects to be equal to and longer lasting than the effects of opiates. Hallucinogens were studied in the treatment of substance abuse (Hollister, Shelton, & Krieger, 1969) and sociopathy (Shagass & Bittle, 1967).

Hallucinogens were also utilized in an attempt to augment or shorten psychotherapeutic approaches. The psycholytic technique utilized low doses in multiple sessions over months or years (Chandler & Hartman, 1960; Hollister, Degan, & Schultz, 1962). The psychedelic approach (Pahnke, Kurland, Unger, Savage, & Grof, 1970) utilized high doses of LSD, 300 to 1500 micrograms, usually only one time after a short course of preparation. This approach encouraged the subject to undergo a peak experience, proposing a potential long-term impact on the personality. One interesting utilization of this approach was for the terminally ill. Studies suggest that terminally ill patients experienced a decrease in pain and dysphoric affect as well as increased ability to reengage with their families (Grof, Goodman, Richards, & Kurland, 1973; W. A. Richards et al., 1977).

Research studies with human subjects are restarting in the United States. DMT was administered to study its physiological and psychological effects (Strassman, 1991). A phase I study of ibogaine has been initiated at the University of Miami, MDMA is being studied at the University of California at Los Angeles, and ketamine is being studied at Yale (Strassman, 1995).

The dose response studies of DMT demonstrate that this drug can be safely administered in a controlled setting with experienced hallucinogen users (Strassman & Qualls, 1994). The biological effects including onset and duration of action, along with effects on physiological measures and blood concentrations of beta endorphins, corticotropin, cortisol, prolactin, and growth hormone, are measured. Utilizing the Hallucinogen Rating Scale (HRS), psychological effects are also determined and found to be more sensitive to dosage changes than the biological markers (Strassman, Qualls, Uhlenhuth, & Kellner, 1994).

Of current active study is the use of ibogaine in the potential treatment of substance abuse. Animal research is defining the neurotransmitter activity of ibogaine and its active metabolites. Ibogaine showed highest affinity for K-opioid receptors and its active metabolite noribogaine showed a higher affinity than ibogaine for all the opioid receptors (Pearl, Herrick-Davis, Teitler, & Glick, 1995) . Ibogaine has also been demonstrated to have acute and persistent effects on extracellular levels of dopamine and to demonstrate interactions with D-amphetamine (Glick, Rossman, Wang, Dong, & Keller, 1993). Ibogaine reduced preference for cocaine consumption in mice (Sershen, Hashim, & Lajtha, 1994) and ibogaine and other iboga-alkaloids decreased both morphine and cocaine intake in rats immediately after treatment (Cappendijk & Dzoljic, 1993), and in some the intake was reduced on the day after administration (Glick et al., 1994). Sheppard (1994) reported on 7 human subjects addicted to opioids who were administered a single dose of ibogaine. All subjects refrained from opioid use for at least 2 days and none displayed withdrawal symptoms. Subjects received doses varying from 700 to 1800 mg and duration of abstinence appeared to relate to dosage. This small study suggests that ibogaine may be of value in the treatment of substance addiction in humans.

There are many areas of future hallucinogen research that offer potential clinical relevance. One area involves hallucinogenic agonists and their relation to behavioral effects in schizophrenia and developing blockade strategies for the treatment of acute adverse reactions and chronic abuse of hallucinogens. The study of hallucinogens in psychiatric populations where presumably there are abnormalities in neurotransmitter systems is another area of potential study (Strassman, 1995). The early use of hallucinogen-assisted psychotherapy suggests many avenues of research. Utilization of these approaches in different psychopathological states such as antisocial personality and substance abuse are two areas of potential import. Early studies suggest a role of hallucinogenic drugs for those individuals with terminal illness. Flooding techniques are used to treat posttraumatic stress disorder (Grigsby, 1987) and this technique might be utilized in conjunction with hallucinogenic drugs.

References

Abraham, H. D., & Aldridge, A. M. (1993). Adverse consequences of lysergic acid diethylamide. *Addiction, 88,* 1327–1334.

American Psychiatric Association. (1994). *Diagnostic and statistical manual of mental disorders* (4th ed.). Washington, DC: Author.

Beck, J. E., & Gordon, D. V. (1982). Psilocybin mushrooms. *Pharmaceutical Chemistry Newsletter, 4,* 1–4.

Brady, K. T., Casto, S., Lydiard, R. B., & Malcolm, R. (1991). Substance abuse in an inpatient psychiatric example. *American Journal of Drug and Alcohol Abuse, 17,* 389–397.

Campbell, R. J. (1989). *Psychiatric dictionary* (6th ed.). New York: Oxford University Press.

Cappendijk, S. L., & Dzoljic, M. R. (1993). Inhibitory effects of ibogaine on cocaine self-administration in rats. *European Journal of Pharmacology, 241,* 261–265.

Chandler, A. L., & Hartman, M. A. (1960). Lysergic acid diethylamide (LSD-25) as a facilitating agent in psychotherapy. *Archives of General Psychiatry, 2,* 286–299.

Controlled Substances Act, Public L No. 91-153, 21 USC 801 *et. seq* (1970).

DeKorne, J. (1994). *Psychedelic shamanism.* Port Townsend, WA: Loompanics.

Dobkin de Rios, M. (1984). *Hallucinogens: Cross-cultural perspectives.* Albuquerque: University of New Mexico Press.

Dulit, R. A., Fryer, M. R., Haas, G. L., Sullivan, T., & Francis, A. J. (1990). Substance use in borderline personality disorder. *American Journal of Psychiatry, 147,* 1002–1007.

Freedman, D. X. (1968). On the use and abuse of LSD. *Archives of General Psychiatry, 18,* 330–347.

Gillin, J. C., Kaplan, J., Stillman, R., & Wyatt, R. J. (1976). The psychedelic model of schizophrenia: The case of n,n-dimethyltryptamine. *American Journal of Psychiatry, 133,* 203–208.

Glennon, R. A. (1991). Discriminative stimulus properties of hallucinogens and related designer drugs. In R. A. Glennon, T. Jarbe, & J. Frankenheim (Eds.), *Drug discrimination: Applications to drug research* (NIDA Research Monograph No. 116, pp. 25–44). Washington, DC: U.S. Government Printing Office.

Glennon, R. A. (1994). Classical hallucinogens: An introductory overview. In G. C. Lin & R. A. Glennon (Eds.), *Hallucinogens: An update* (NIDA Monograph Series No. 146, pp. 4–32). Washington, DC: U.S. Department of Health and Human Services.

Glick, S. D., Rossman, K., Wang, S., Dong, N., & Keller, R. W., Jr. (1993). Local effects of ibogaine on extracellular levels of dopamine and its metabolites in nucleus accumbens and striatum: Interactions with D-amphetamine. *Brain Research, 628,* 201–208.

Glick, S. D., Kuehne, M. E., Raucci, J., Wilson, T. E., Larson, D., & Keller, R. W., Jr. (1994). Effects of iboga alkaloids on morphine and cocaine self-administration in rats: Relationship to tremorigenic effects and to effects on dopamine release in nucleus accumbens and striatum. *Brain Research, 657,* 14–22.

Gold, M. S. (1994). The epidemiology, attitudes, and pharmacology of LSD use in the 1990s. *Psychiatric Annals, 24,* 124–126.

Grigsby, J. P. (1987). The use of imagery in the treatment of posttraumatic stress disorder. *Journal of Nervous and Mental Disorders, 175,* 55–59.

Grinspoon, L., & Balaker J. (1979). *Psychedelic drugs reconsidered.* New York: Basic Books.

Grob, C., & Dobkin de Rios, M. (1992). Adolescent drug use in cross-cultural perspective. *Journal of Drug Issues, 22,* 122–138.

Grof, S. (1980). *LSD Psychotherapy.* Alameda, CA: Hunter House.

Grof, S., Goodman, L. E., Richards, W. A., & Kurland, A. A. (1973). LSD-assisted psychotherapy in patients with terminal cancer. *International Pharmacopsychiatry, 8,* 129–144.

Harrison, P. A., Hoffman, N. G., & Edwall, G. E. (1989). Differential drug use patterns among sexually abused adolescent girls in treatment for chemical dependency. *International Journal of the Addictions, 24,* 499–514.

Hoffman, L. (1980). *LSD, my problem child.* New York: McGraw-Hill.

Hollister, L. E., Degan, R. O., & Schultz, S. D. (1962). An experimental approach to facilitation of psychotherapy by psychotomimetic drugs. *Journal of Mental Sciences, 108,* 99–100.

Hollister, L. E., Shelton, J., & Krieger, G. (1969). A controlled comparison of lysergic acid diethylamide (LSD) and dextroamphetamine in alcoholics. *American Journal of Psychiatry, 125,* 1352–1357.

Huxley, A. (1954). *Doors of perception.* New York: Harper & Row.

Isbell, H., Belleville, R. E., Fraser, H. F., Wikler, A., & Logan, C. R. (1956). Studies on lysergic acid diethylamide: I. Effects in former morphine addicts and development of tolerance during chronic intoxication. *Archives of General Psychiatry, 76,* 468–478.

James, W. (1902). *The varieties of religious experience.* New York: Modern Library.

Kast, E. C., & Collins, V. J. (1964). Study of lysergic acid diethylamide as an analgesic agent. *Anesthesia and Analgesia, 43,* 285–291.

Kern, M. F., Kenkel, M. B., Templer, D. I., & Newell, T. G. (1986). Drug preference as a function of arousal and stimulus screening. *International Journal of the Addictions, 21,* 255–265.

Kerr, B., Shaffer, J., Chambers, C., & Hallowell, K. (1991). Substance abuse of creatively talented adults. *Journal of Creative Behavior, 25,* 145–153.

Linton, H. B., & Langs, R. J. (1962). Subjective reactions to lysergic acid diethylamide (LSD-25). *Archives of General Psychiatry, 6,* 36–52.

Mabry, E. A., & Khavari, K. A. (1986). Attitude and personality correlates of hallucinogenic drug use. *International Journal of the Addictions, 21,* 691–699.

Matefy, R., & Krawl, R. (1974). An initial investigation of the psychedelic drug flashback phenomena. *Journal of Consulting and Clinical Psychology, 43,* 434.

Milhorn, H. T. (1990). *Chemical dependence: Diagnosis, treatment and prevention.* New York: Springer-Verlag.

Millman, R. B., & Beeder, A. B. (1994). The new psychedelic culture: LSD, ecstasy, "rave" parties and the Grateful Dead. *Psychiatric Annals, 24,* 148–150.

National Institute on Drug Abuse. (1986). *National Household Survey on Drug Abuse: Populations estimates 1985.* Rockville, MD: U.S. Department of Health and Human Services.

National Institute on Drug Abuse. (1989). *National Household Survey on Drug Abuse: Populations estimates 1988.* Rockville, MD: U.S. Department of Health and Human Services.

National Institute on Drug Abuse. (1991). *National Household Survey on Drug Abuse: Populations estimates 1990.* Rockville, MD: U.S. Department of Health and Human Services.

O'Brien, R., & Cohen, S. (1984). *The encyclopedia of drug abuse.* New York: Facts on File.

Pahnke, W. N., Kurland, A. A., Unger, S., Savage, C., & Grof, S. (1970). The experimental use of psychedelic (LSD) psychotherapy. *Journal of the American Medical Association, 212,* 1856–1863.

Patterson, E. W., Myers, G., & Gallant, D. M. (1988). Patterns of substance use on a college campus: A 14-year comparison study. *American Journal of Drug and Alcohol Abuse, 14,* 237–246.

Pearl, S. M., Herrick-Davis, K., Teitler, M., & Glick, S. D. (1995). Radioligand-binding study of noribogaine, a likely metabolite of ibogaine. *Brain Research, 675,* 342–344.

Pope, H. G., Ionescu-Pioggia, M., Aizley, H. G., & Varma, D. K. (1990). Drug use and life among college undergraduates in 1989: A comparison with 1969 and 1978. *American Journal of Psychiatry, 147,* 998–1001.

Pride Survey, 1991–92. (1992). *National summary, United States, grades 6–12.* Bowling Green KY: Pride.

Pride Survey, 1992–1993. (1993). *National summary, United States, grades 6–12.* Bowling Green, KY: Pride.

Richards, R. A. (1978). Mystical and archetypal experiences of terminal patients in DPT-assisted psychotherapy. *Journal of Religion and Health, 17,* 117–126.

Richards, W. A., Rhead, J. C., DiLeo, F. B., Yensen, R., & Kurland, A. A. (1977). The peak experience variable in DPT-assisted psychotherapy with cancer patients. *Journal of Psychedelic Drugs, 9,* 1–10.

Russell, J. M., Newman, S. C., & Bland, R. C. (1994). Drug abuse and dependence. *Acta Psychiatry Scandinavia, 376,* 54–62.

Savage, C. (1952). Lysergic acid diethylamide (LSD-25). A clinical-psychological study. *American Journal of Psychiatry, 108,* 896–900.

Schick, J., & Smith, D. (1970). Analysis of the LSD flashback. *Journal of Psychedelic Drugs, 3,* 13–19.

Sershen, H., Hashim, A., & Lajtha, A. (1994). Ibogaine-reduces preference for cocaine consumption in C57BL/6BY mice. *Pharmacology, Biochemistry and Behavior, 47,* 13–19.

Shagass, C., & Bittle, R. (1967). Therapeutic effects of LSD: A follow-up study. *Journal of Nervous and Mental Disorders, 144,* 471–478.

Sheppard, S. G. (1994). A preliminary investigation of ibogaine: Case reports and recommendations for further study. *Journal of Substance Abuse Treatment, 11,* 379–385.

Strassman, R. J. (1984). Adverse reactions to psychedelic drugs: A review of the literature. *Journal of Nervous and Mental Disease, 172,* 577–595.

Strassman, R. J. (1991). Human hallucinogenic drug research in the United States: A present-day case history and review of the process. *Journal of Psychoactive Drugs, 23,* 29–38.

Strassman, R. J. (1994). Human hallucinogenic drug research: Regulatory, clinical, and scientific issues. In G. C. Lin & R. A. Glennon (Eds.), *Hallucinogens: An update* (NIDA Monograph Series No. 146, pp. 92–123). Washington, DC: U.S. Department of Health and Human Services.

Strassman, R. J. (1995). Hallucinogenic drugs in psychiatric research and treatment: Perspectives and prospects. *Journal of Nervous and Mental Disease, 183,* 127–138.

Strassman, R. J., & Qualls, C. R. (1994). Dose-response study of n,n-dimethyltryptamine in humans: I. Neuroendocrine, autonomic, and cardiovascular effects. *Archives of General Psychiatry, 51,* 85–97.

Strassman, R. J., Qualls, C. R., Uhlenhuth, E. H., & Kellner, R. (1994). Dose-response study of n,n-dimethyltryptamine in humans: II. Subjective effects and preliminary results of a new rating scale. *Archives of General Psychiatry, 51,* 98–108.

Szara, S. (1994). Are hallucinogenics psychoheuristic? In G. C. Lin & R. A. Glennon (Eds.), *Hallucinogens: An update* (NIDA Monograph Series No. 146, pp. 33–51). Washington, DC: U.S. Department of Health and Human Services.

Wesson, D., & Smith, D. (1976). An analysis of psychedelic drug flashbacks. *American Journal of Drug and Alcohol Abuse, 3,* 425–438.

15

Psychological and Psychiatric Consequences of Hallucinogens

RICHARD B. SEYMOUR AND DAVID E. SMITH

Introduction

America is now in a second cycle of hallucinogen abuse; the first centered on lysergic acid diethylamide or LSD in the 1960s and the present one involves methylenedioxymethamphetamine or MDMA and its congeners. The long-term consequences of all hallucinogens have certain similarities, resulting from the intense effect of these drugs on the brain's cognitive centers. While all hallucinogens have some relation in action to the stimulant drugs, this relation is particularly pronounced in such drugs as MDMA and MDA that have specific stimulant components and produce a combination of hallucinogenic and stimulant effects.

In general, hallucinogens have a history of association with psychological and psychiatric consequences. When these drugs came to be studied in the laboratory, they were first called "psychotomimetic" because they were seen as mimicking the symptoms of psychoses. Studies at that time focused on what these drugs could teach scientists about the nature of mental illness. The psychotomimetic drugs were

considered capable of consistently producing short-term changes in thought, perception, and mood without causing major disturbances of the autonomic nervous system or other serious disability. Research utilizing these drugs was considered important for three reasons: (1) It could give the investigator an approximate subjective experience of mental disorder, (2) model psychoses could be studied in the same way as mental disorders, and (3) a study of the drugs' chemical natures could be expected to throw some light on the nature of the hypothetical substances believed to cause mental disorders (Seymour & Smith, 1993).

A descriptive term used for many of these substances is "hallucinogen." This means a drug that produces visual, auditory, tactile, taste, and olfactory or smell hallucinations. There has been much disagreement as to the precise definition of a hallucination. There has even been much discussion as to whether or not any of these drugs actually produce hallucinations. Some observers maintain that these drugs merely produce visual and temporal distortions. Others mention sensory crossover, such as "seeing" sounds and "hearing" colors. Some subjects and scientists postulate that what is seen or experienced via these drugs is there all the time, but that we are conditioned to be aware of only a small portion of our sensory intake. When one takes a psychedelic drug, that conditioning breaks down and one is

RICHARD B. SEYMOUR AND DAVID E. SMITH • Haight-Ashbury Free Medical Clinic, San Francisco, California 94117.

Handbook of Substance Abuse: Neurobehavioral Pharmacology, edited by Tarter *et al.* Plenum Press, New York, 1998.

aware of a whole new range of sensory material (Seymour & Smith, 1991).

During the two decades since the 1960s, LSD underwent a social and medical evolution from *psychotomimetic* to the *psychedelic* model that proposed that, under proper conditions, "the experience will be enlightening, productive and consciousness expanding" (Metzner, 1978, p. 138).

The publication of such materials as a handbook to psychedelic experience by Leary, Metzner, and Alpert (1964), as well as publications and declarations by others of like mind, added to the shaping of a drug-using subculture centered around the use of LSD and other psychedelic drugs. A variety of other psychedelic drugs became available at this time, but never enjoyed the widespread popularity or availability of LSD.

It was during this proliferation that the problem of LSD-induced negative reactions became acute. During the clinically supervised stage of LSD's sociopharmacological study, adverse reactions were rare. Cohen (1960), one of the pioneer clinical investigators of LSD, reported that the incidence of psychotic reactions lasting more than 48 hr was 0.8 per 1,000 in experimental subjects and 1.8 per 1,000 in psychiatric patients. However, by 1967, when the Haight-Ashbury Free Medical Clinic first opened its doors in San Francisco, negative LSD experiences, or "bad trips," as the acid culture called them, were frequent. In 1970, new federal legislation produced a graduated sequence of drug "schedules," based on abuse potential versus medical use. All of the known psychedelic drugs were placed in Schedule One, as highly dangerous drugs with no potential for medical use.

During the 1970s and 1980s, from a public awareness standpoint, the use of hallucinogens was eclipsed by the emergence of a massive and nationally demoralizing succession of drug epidemics involving such substances as heroin, PCP, and crack cocaine. This did not mean, however, that the street use of psychedelic drugs had ceased. It would appear that this was a period that gave rise to two distinct use phenomena. On the one hand, young people were still

using LSD, but at low doses for intoxication at rock concerts. What bad trips occurred in this population usually involved very young and inexperienced users, most often in school settings or at concerts. At the same time, ritualized use within certain psychedelic drug–using communities with a goal of changing consciousness and developing spiritual enhancement continued with members of those communities usually taking care of their own.

The contention that the drug community had learned how to handle bad trips without attracting the attention of medical or police authorities (Metzner, 1978) is echoed in data gathered by Newmeyer and Johnson (1979) at rock concerts from 1973 through 1977. Their findings indicated that while treatment incidents involving LSD accounted for only 5.9% of all drug treatment at concert sites, and alcohol accounted for 60.2%, there was a much higher proportion of LSD use without complications.

In the mid 1960s, the public use of LSD and other psychedelics was initiated at a series of gatherings called "Acid Tests." These Acid Tests were held in large auditoriums, such as San Francisco's Longshoremen's Hall, and were characterized by dancing to the electronic music of such "underground" groups as the Grateful Dead, and the presence of pulsating strobe lights and projected "light shows." According to author Tom Wolfe (1968), a punch available to one and all at these "concerts" was liberally spiked with LSD. After LSD was made illegal in 1966, "electric kool-aid" was no longer served openly at gatherings, but the use of psychedelics at many rock concerts had become a common practice.

Although drug use has been associated with rock concerts ever since, the focus diffused in the 1970s from one of inducing group altered states of consciousness to one of general intoxications by whatever means available. Psychedelic drugs were taken, if at all, in lower dosages and often in combination with alcohol, amphetamines, and other drugs. Concerts became less psychedelic rites of passage and more events at which to get high and listen to music.

In the late 1980s, a new wave of group psychedelic celebrations came into being. The first of these, appearing overseas in England and Germany, were called "Acid Houses," even though the primary drug used was methylenedioxymethampetamine, or MDMA. When these celebrations spread to the United States, they were called "raves," and rather than being based at specific venues, as most rock concerts have been, they were held at relatively impromptu sites, advertised through "rave shops" and an MDMA underground network, and attended mostly by invitation.

Rave attendees are predominantly white, middle class, over 21 and under 35 years of age, and pay a door fee of $10 to $25. Unlike the "Acid Tests," raves do not provide MDMA or any other psychedelics to attendees. LSD and MDMA, currently selling for about $25 a capsule, are usually available, however. What is served at the raves are "smart drinks." These are blender-concocted mixtures of fruit juices, vitamins, and powdered amino acids, sold at $4 to $5. These smart drinks contain no intoxicants, but the amino acids are thought to be the building blocks used by the body to manufacture such brain neurotransmitters as serotonin, a substance that can be exhausted by chronic MDMA use. The smart drinks also help to offset chronic dehydration caused by the drugs and constant dancing (Seymour & Smith, 1993).

Raves can be seen as a marriage of psychedelic and cybernetic, the twin fascinations of a new generation. At these celebrations, the music is intensely rhythmic and starkly electronic, global in its nature, the young attendees often dance all night, and some events can last for days. Often attendees will "rave" throughout weekend cycles on an ongoing basis. The stimulant qualities of MDMA probably serve to support such activity. Attendees often alternate MDMA and LSD, usually taken at low dosages in order to stay awake, a practice they call "candyflipping."

While the raves started as a grassroots movement, they seem to be taking on a more commercial, according to some attendees "hard edge," aspect that may include exploitation by outside people interested only in making money from the rave phenomenon. As the

price of admission and the cost of MDMA increase, and as endurance becomes an increasing factor, the use of less expensive but much more potent stimulant drugs such as street methamphetamine seems to be on the rise. According to Greg Hayner at the Haight-Ashbury Free Clinics, "A lot of people (at raves) seem to be changing over from Ecstasy to methamphetamine. On about $10 worth, you can keep going for a good 12 hours. If what you're looking for is a way to party, it's a much cheaper way to go" (Hallissy, 1993, p. 1). An ongoing concern is that of drug composition. There is no "illicit" food and drug administration monitoring MDMA, LSD, or any other street drug for that matter, and users are taking their chances on a commodity that is often not what it seems.

Psychological and Psychiatric Consequences of the Use of LSD, MDMA, and Other Hallucinogens

MDMA, or Methylenedioxy-Methamphetamine, Stimulant Reactions

As of 1984, anxiety and other stimulant effects were the primary presenting symptoms seen at the Haight-Ashbury Free Medical Clinic's drug abuse treatment program. In its 31 years of operation, the Haight-Ashbury Free Medical Clinic has had more than 2 million patient visits. Today, the primary drug detoxification staff alone sees an average of 460 new outpatient clients a month.

Incidents involving MDMA and methoxylated amphetamines reported in the clinical data include "mentions," in which patients may come in with a complaint related to another drug, but report use of such substances as MDMA, MDM, DOM, STP, MDA, Adam, or Ecstasy.

Often treatment centers will not know what specific drug a client may have used. It takes sophisticated drug testing equipment to tell the difference between two drugs as similar in structure as MDA and MDMA. The process is also comparatively expensive and unnecessary for symptomatic treatment of stimulant reactions, which are similar for all drugs in the category. In such cases, and if no untoward symptoms are apparent, treatment staff usually take the word of the client for what they have taken. The client, in turn, has usually taken the word of the person who sold the drug as to what is in it. With MDMA and the methoxylated amphetamines, the acute toxicity symptoms that are usually seen in treatment are similar and result from taking too much of the drug. These dose-related symptoms usually dissipate as the drug wears off, and the patient can be discharged within a few hours.

The acute toxicity symptoms for methoxylated amphetamines involve anxiety, fear reactions usually accompanied by a racing pulse and rapid heartbeat, paranoia (sometimes with delusions), and a sufficient sense of unease to prompt the individual to seek treatment. Treatment usually begins with reassuring the patient that these feelings are a result of taking too much of the drug, are not dangerous, and will wear off as the drug is metabolized. There is some variation depending on the individual. In some cases, these patients come back for a series of counseling sessions. In most cases, a talkdown similar to that used for psychedelic bad trips is sufficient.

Severe Toxic Reactions to MDMA

More severe reactions to what users believed to be MDMA have been reported, including prolonged psychotic reactions. As with any consciousness effective drug, these psychotic breaks can happen, especially if the user has underlying psychopathology. Hayner and McKinney (1986) reported two severe cases involving MDMA. These apparently involved idiosyncratic, life-threatening reactions to the drug. Although there seems to be no cross-tolerance or additive effect between MDMA and MDA or any of the methoxylated amphetamines, all stimulants do have some cumulative effect.

Psychedelic Drugs and Addictive Disease

A concern about the use of psychedelic drugs that is disputed by some researchers and clinicians but is very important to many therapists in the substance abuse treatment field involves the question of use by anyone who is vulnerable to or suffering from addictive disease.

We believe that hallucinogens have a low addiction potential with the population in general, but a high addiction potential for anyone with or vulnerable to addictive disease. Illustrative is a recent case in which a woman who reported that her husband had entered private treatment for chronic cocaine abuse and had been given MDMA. "Now," she said, "he claims that the MDMA has cured his cocaine habit. The only problem is that he takes MDMA a couple times a week and spends the rest of his time at home drinking and smoking marijuana." In this instance, the individual used the MDMA to feed his addiction denial system. This allowed him to change venues and engage in the compulsive use of alcohol and marijuana while claiming to have been cured of cocaine addiction (see Seymour & Smith, 1987).

Immediate and Chronic Problems with Hallucinogens

Smith (1967) identified the adverse effects of hallucinogens as "largely psychological in nature," and classified them as either acute toxicity, effects occurring during the use of the drug, or chronic after-effects. Although there have been some occurrences of physiological consequences, particularly with MDMA, these have been primarily of an idiosyncratic nature, while in most cases the adverse effects of these drugs still appear to be psychological in nature.

The acute toxic effects take many forms. Often individuals knowingly take a hallucinogenic drug and find themselves in a state of anxiety as the powerful hallucinogen begins to take effect. They are aware that they have taken a drug, but feel that they cannot control its effects. Some users experiencing a bad trip try to physically flee the situation, giving rise to potential physical danger. Others may become paranoid.

Not all acute toxicity is based on anxiety or loss of control. Some people taking hallucinogens display decided changes in cognition and demonstrate poor judgment. They may decide that they can fly, and jump out a window. Some users are reported to have walked into the sea, feeling that they were "at one with the universe." Such physical mishaps have been described within the acid culture as "being God, but tripping over the furniture." Susceptibility to bad trips is not necessarily dose related, but can depend on the experience, maturity, and personality of the user as well as the circumstances and the environment in which the trip takes place. Sometimes the individual will complain of unpleasant symptoms while intoxicated and later speak in glowing terms of the experience. Negative psychological set and environmental setting are the most significant contributing factors to bad hallucinogenic trips (Smith & Seymour, 1985).

We are also seeing a "new age" upper-downer cycle with MDMA and Rohypnol, a benzodiazepine, which may contribute to the growing problem of stimulant abuse. Such drug trends are ominous as a potential repetition of the shift from hallucinogens to powerful stimulants following the psychedelic "Summer of Love" in 1967–1968.

Treatment of Acute Toxicity

Techniques originally developed within the psychedelic community and adopted by free clinics and other counter-culture–oriented treatment centers, as reported by Smith and Shick (1970), are based on the findings that most psychedelic bad trips are best treated in a supportive, nonpharmacological fashion through the restoration of a positive, nonthreatening environment. Facilities in a residential setting, with little to mark them as medical, with a quiet space or calm center set aside for drug crises, and with casually dressed staff dedicated to a nonjudgmental attitude, were admirably suited for such treatment. At large rock concerts, emergency talkdown procedures are accomplished by Haight-Ashbury staff and volunteers in a quiet space set up specifically for treating acute psychedelic toxicity.

Talkdowns of most acute toxicity reactions can be accomplished without medication or hospitalization. Paraprofessionals with psychedelic drug experience have been particularly effective at such sites as large rock concerts. Amelioration of bad trips has even been accomplished by long-distance telephone calls (Alpert, 1967).

In the talkdown approach, one should maintain a relaxed, conversational tone aimed at putting the individual at ease. Quick movements should be avoided. One should make the patients comfortable, but not impede their freedom of movement. Let them walk around, stand, sit or lie down. At times, such physical movement and activity may be enough to break the anxiety reaction. Gentle suggestion should be used to divert patients from any activity that seems to be adding to their agitation. Getting the individual's mind off the frightening elements of a bad trip and onto positive elements is the key to the talkdown.

An understanding of the phases generally experienced in a hallucinogenic drug trip is most helpful in treating acute reactions. After orally ingesting an average dose of 100–250 μg of LSD, the user experiences sympathomimetic, or stimulant responses, including elevated heart rate and respiration. Adverse reactions in this phase are primarily managed by reassurances that these are normal and expected effects of psychedelic drugs. This reassurance is usually sufficient to override a potentially frightening situation.

From the first to the sixth hour, visual imagery becomes vivid and may take on frightening content. The patient may have forgotten taking the drug, and given acute time distortion, may believe this retinal circus (Michaux, 1963) will go on forever. Such fears can be dispelled by reminding the individual that these effects are drug induced, by suggesting alternative images, and by distracting the individual from those images that are frightening.

In the later stages, philosophical "insights" and ideas predominate. Adverse experiences here are most frequently due to recurring unpleasant thoughts or feelings that can become overwhelming in their impact. The therapist can be most effective by being supportive and by suggesting new trains of thought.

The therapist's attitude toward hallucinogens and their use is very important. Empathy and self-confidence are essential. Anxiety and fear in the therapist will be perceived in an amplified manner by the client. Physical contact with the individual is often reassuring, but can be misinterpreted. Ideally, the therapist should rely on intuition rather than preconceptions.

Wesson and Smith (1978) noted that medication may be necessary and should be given either after the talkdown has failed or as a supplement to the talkdown process. During the first phase of intervention, oral administration of a sedative, such as 25 mg of chlordiazepoxide or 10 mg of diazepam, can have an important pharmacological and reassuring effect.

During the second and third phases, a toxic psychosis or major break with reality may occur in which one can no longer communicate with the individual. If the individual begins acting in such a way as to be an immediate danger, antipsychotic drugs may be employed. Only if the individual refuses oral medication and is out of behavioral control should antipsychotics be administered by injection. Haloperidol (2.0–4.0 mg administered intramuscularly every hour) is the current drug of choice. Any medication, however, should be given only by qualified personnel. If antipsychotic drugs are required, hospitalization is usually indicated.

As soon as rapport and verbal contact are established, further medication is generally unnecessary. Occasionally an individual fails to respond to the regimen and must be referred to an inpatient psychiatric facility. Such a decision must be weighed carefully, however, as transfer to a hospital may of itself have an aggravating and threatening effect. Hospitalization should be used only as a last resort if all else has failed.

Treating Chronic Hallucinogenic Drug Aftereffects

Chronic hallucinogenic drug aftereffects present situations wherein a condition that may be attributable to the ingestion of a toxic substance occurs or continues long after the me-

tabolization of that substance. With the use of hallucinogens, four recognized chronic reactions have been reported (Seymour & Smith, 1987; Wesson & Smith, 1978): (1) prolonged psychotic reactions, (2) depression sufficiently severe so as to be life-threatening, (3) flashbacks, and (4) exacerbations of preexisting psychiatric illness. Since then a fifth chronic reaction has been listed in the *DSM-IV* (American Psychiatric Association, 1994), posthallucinogen perceptual disorder.

Some people who have taken many hallucinogenic drug trips, especially those who have had acute toxic reactions, show what appears to be serious long-term personality disruptions. These prolonged psychotic reactions have similarities to schizophrenic reactions and appear to occur most often in people with preexisting psychological difficulties, such as primarily prepsychotic or psychotic personalities. Hallucinogenic drug-induced personality disorganizations can be quite severe and prolonged. Appropriate treatment often requires antipsychotic medication and residential care in a mental health facility followed by outpatient counseling.

It has also been observed that some clients self-medicate their hallucinogenic-precipitated psychotic episodes with amphetamines (Seymour & Smith, 1991; Smith & Luce, 1969). Often, this self-medication results in the development of amphetamine abuse, followed by secondary heroin, barbiturate, or alcohol abuse patterns to ameliorate the side effects of the amphetamines. Thus, in certain patients, chronic psychological problems induced by LSD and other hallucinogenic drugs may lead to complicated patterns of polydrug abuse that require additional treatment approaches (Smith & Wesson, 1975).

Flashbacks

By far the most ubiquitous chronic reaction to hallucinogens is the flashback. Flashbacks are transient spontaneous occurrences of some aspect of the hallucinogenic drug effect occurring after a period of normalcy that follows the original intoxication. This period of normalcy distinguishes flashbacks from prolonged psychotic reactions. Flashbacks may occur after a single ingestion of a psychedelic drug, but more commonly occur after multiple psychedelic drug ingestions.

Flashbacks are a symptom, not a specific disease entity. They may well have multiple causes, and many cases called flashbacks may have occurred although the individual has never ingested a psychedelic drug. Some investigators have suggested that flashbacks may be due to a residue of the drug retained in the body and released into the brain at a later time. Although this is known to happen with phencyclidine (PCP) and drugs similar to it, there is no direct evidence of retention or prolonged storage of such psychedelics as LSD.

Individuals who have used psychedelic drugs several times a month have indicated that fleeting flashes of light and afterimage prolongation occurring in the periphery of vision commonly occur for days or weeks after ingestion. Active and chronic psychedelic drug users tend to accept these occurrences as part of the psychedelic experience, are unlikely to seek medical or psychiatric treatment, and frequently view them as "free trips." It is the inexperienced user and the individual who attaches a negative interpretation to these visual phenomena who are likely to be disturbed by them and seek medical or psychiatric help. While emotional reactions to the flashback are generally contained in the period of the flashback itself, prolonged anxiety states or psychotic breaks have occurred following a frightening flashback. There is no record of flashback activity specifically attributable to hallucinogenic drug use occurring more than a year after the individual's last use of a psychedelic drug (Seymour & Smith, 1987).

Long-Term Consequences of Hallucinogenic Drug Use

The long-term study of adverse hallucinogenic drug reactions has revealed the existence of low-prevalence, but quite disabling chronic consequences of LSD use (Smith & Seymour, 1985). Of particular concern is the posthallucinogen perceptual disorder (PHPD). With PHPD, individuals report a persistent perceptual disorder which they describe as being like living in a bubble under water. They also describe trails of light and images following movement of their hands, and often describe living in a purple haze. This perceptual disorder is aggravated by any psychoactive drug use, including alcohol and marijuana, and is distinguished from flashbacks, which are episodic rather than chronic phenomena. With the PHPD, the individual often experiences anxiety, even panic, and becomes phobic and depressed. With the PHPD sufferers, our experience has been that individuals do not have a disturbed psychiatric history prior to the onset of psychedelic drug use and that the PHPD can occur even after a single dose.

With the more severe, prolonged LSD reactions, such as an LSD-precipitated schizophrenic reaction or severe depressive disorder, individuals almost always have a premorbid psychiatric history and require inpatient treatment. With the prolonged psychotic reactions, antipsychotic medication is required, and with the prolonged depressive reactions, antidepressant medication is required. A major concern involves teenagers with depressive reactions to psychedelic use that may result in severe depression culminating in suicide.

With the posthallucinogen perceptual disorder, drug-free recovery with supportive counseling is often adequate treatment, although recovery may take several months and antianxiety medication may be needed to treat the secondary anxiety and panic disorder that develops when the individuals feel that they are irreversibly brain damaged and will never see normally again.

Acute MDMA Toxicity

Acute MDMA toxicity is essentially the result of taking too much MDMA in too short a period of time. This results in some physical or psychological dysfunction. The symptoms appear to be time and dose related. These symptoms range from a mild caffeine-like toxicity to potentially life-threatening stimulant overdoses.

Prolonged MDMA toxicity results from chronic or regular ingestion of MDMA. The symptoms range in severity from mild dysphoria to frank paranoid psychosis and relate to acute toxicity, chronicity of use, and secondary drug effects such as sleep and appetite suppression.

MDMA-induced anxiety syndromes are related to MDMA's ability to bring unconscious material to consciousness. We hypothesize that these anxiety syndromes are primarily caused by the lack of resolution and integration of now-conscious and often emotionally potent materials. These anxiety syndromes appear to be psychodynamic in nature and not purely toxicological. They last beyond the period of actual drug intoxication.

Low-Dose Acute Toxicity

Greer and Tolbert (1986) have described some of the low-dose, therapeutic range toxic reactions such as jitteriness, mild anxiety, mild apprehension, and jaw clenching. Because many MDMA users view the MDMA use as a relatively important event and many users even formally ritualize such use, an anticipation and apprehension of the events to come may blend with the sympathomimetic properties of MDMA to further heighten apprehension and perhaps even produce fear in predisposed people. Generally, most of the sympathomimetic reactions are dose related and are typically mild. Nonmedicinal approaches, such as support, quiet, and reassurance that the symptoms will fade over time, should be successful in reducing this apprehension. In most cases, individuals taking MDMA at the dosages used in therapy (i.e., 50–150 mg) would be aware that problems they may be experiencing are drug related.

Medium-Dose Acute Toxicity

At somewhat higher doses (i.e., 250–300 mg), MDMA dose- and setting-related psychopathology may develop. In a person with low tolerance to stimulants, there may be a medium-dose acute toxicity resulting from ingestion at this level.

Visual distortions have been reported, such as viewing an object that appears to be shim-mering, shiny, or perhaps moving in a jittery fashion, or with geometric embellishments. There is an awareness that these distortions are drug induced, and they do not appear to carry any particularly positive or negative content. Also, they do not typically interfere with the therapeutic goals of insight and empathy for most individuals. Some users have reported that they desire to be alone and some report that they become slightly concerned about others noticing their behavior and knowing that they are "high." There can be a slightly paranoid flavor or self-conscious tendency which appears to be dose related. These feelings of self-consciousness may occur only while inside a building or in crowds, and there may be a tendency to move outdoors.

For many, there may be a fairly distressing depression that may emerge rapidly, especially if there is a sudden shift in consciousness away from the particularly empathic or euphoric stage of the MDMA experience. The subjective aspect of this depression may have to do with returning to a fairly normal consciousness after having experienced often significantly beautiful or meaningful feelings.

High-Dose Acute Toxicity

The most obvious and most clinically important acute toxicological problem involves the high-dose MDMA toxic reaction. Depending on personal variables such as prior drug experience (especially with stimulants, hallucinogens, and PCP), tolerance to the effects of the drug, and setting, the toxic range for MDMA may be as low as 300 mg for some people, but 400 mg or more for others. Toxic symptomatology would be on a continuum ranging from anxiety symptoms and panic with or without tachycardia to psychotic reactions with paranoia and violence. Hypertensive crises and even cerebrovascular accidents and cardiac arrhythmias could theoretically occur as with cocaine and the amphetamines.

Some MDMA users may also use other drugs during the same time period. Others may use MDMA in combination with other drugs, such as MDA or marijuana. Other drugs that may have properties and effects similar to those of MDMA include 2-CB, or 4-bromo-2,5-dimethoxyphenethylamine, and MDE (Eve) or N-ethyl-3,4-methylenedioxymethamphetamine.

Treatment Considerations

The medical management of this problem is also on a continuum. At the lower doses, or at the least severe reactions, the appropriate medical management of clients may simply be supportive, reassuring interactions in which they are moved to a perceived safe environment with reduced stimuli. Clients should be told that the distressing symptoms will fade over time. It is best that the client is not left alone, but rather is with someone who is capable of providing psychological support.

For moderately dysfunctional anxiety symptoms that increase with severity, 5–10 mg diazepam may be given orally. For the patient who also experiences tachycardia, propanalol, 10–20 mg, can be given orally, or if given iv, administered 0.5–1 mg very slowly at a maximum of 1 mg per min up to a total of 6 mg.

If symptoms are more severe, consideration should be given to containment if (1) anxiety merges into aggressive behavior, (2) there is evidence of stimulant psychosis with violence to self or to others, or (3) there are suicidal verbalizations or behaviors. If the client has a stimulant psychosis and is markedly anxious, either (1) give haloperidol 2 mg b.i.d. and assess remaining anxiety, treating with diazepam 5–10 mg iv if necessary; or (2) give 5–10 mg diazepam orally or iv. If anxiety is still marked, give diazepam every 1–2 hr. If anxiety is effectively treated, give diazepam every 4–6 hr for a maximum of about 40 mg per 24-hr period. If stimulant psychosis remains and is an issue relative to violence or danger to self or others, give haloperidol 2 mg b.i.d. orally.

For persistent adrenergic crisis, give propanalol orally in doses of 40–60 mg at 4 to 6 hr intervals for the duration of the crisis. A pulse of 90 or less is the goal. Many stimulant psychosis patients will be resistant to haloperidol and may in fact request a sedative-hypnotic

to reduce anxiety. Some of these patients may be able to handle the stimulant psychosis if anxiolytic therapy is given. The important diagnostic criterion is, Does the psychotic break represent a clear danger to the client or to others? Note also that the amphetamines and haloperidol both lower seizure threshold, so caution should be exercised in their use. Also, some patients may be very sensitive to the sedative-hypnotics and proceed into coma with even lower doses than recommended; thus, caution is urged. The treatment of stimulant-related problems and treatment concerns is discussed in depth in Wesson and Smith (1979).

Prolonged High-Dose MDMA Toxicity

The person who uses high doses of MDMA (or any mood-altering drug) on a daily basis is likely to have a substance abuse disorder. Whereas most people who use MDMA for its psychotherapeutic benefits dislike the stimulant properties of MDMA, some people actively seek out this experience. Clearly, present cocaine problems speak to the fact that stimulant abuse is commonplace. In interviews with MDMA users, it is revealed that some cocaine dealers also sell MDMA as an adjunct to their normal trade, and many cocaine abusers and addicts are introduced to MDMA in this setting. Also, amphetamine addicts who have had access to MDMA may have used MDMA as an alternative to amphetamine or turned to MDMA as a supplement to their amphetamine use. Because drug switching is a regular part of drug abuse, a regular stimulant abuser might have a tendency to use MDMA at higher doses and for longer periods of time, and to use this drug for its stimulant rather than its empathogenic qualities. These individuals might also exhibit a cross-tolerance to MDMA and thus be able to ingest fairly large quantities of the drug.

The daily or chronic use of a central nervous system stimulant can push a person to the limit and drain their physical and psychological strengths. With the high-dose chronic user, mood swings, emotional lability, and anxiety can increase, converting to depression in times of abstinence. In time, stimulant psychosis, paranoia, and violence can emerge.

Prolonged Low-Dose MDMA Toxicity

While high-dose chronic use of MDMA suggests stimulant addiction, the lower-dose extended use may suggest a different type of drug use. The stimulant addict understands and desires the stimulant effects of amphetamines and cocaine. That is not the case with a number of people we have interviewed. Most often, these are individuals engaged in generalized drug experimentation and their chronic use is usually over a finite period of time, usually a week or two.

The effects of this prolonged MDMA use at lower doses include mild psychopathology. Interviewees describe a lack of mental clarity, being "out of sorts," having mild mental confusion and slight memory impairment. Some mention a lack of motivation, mild disorientation, and forgetfulness. There may be some sleep dysfunction and some nutritional needs may not be met if the pattern continues. These individuals did not report anxiety or hyperactivity, however, and that may be due to titrating or controlling their doses over the day. They also state that cessation of MDMA use returns them to their normal emotions and psychological state.

MDMA Treatment Considerations

It is important that the possible presence of addictive disease be assessed. The chronicity of use, as opposed to event-specific use or very rare use, may be a signal of addictive illness. Appropriate treatment for the addiction would include inpatient or outpatient chemical dependency treatment based on an abstinence model of supported recovery. Appropriate referral should be made to such 12-step programs as Alcoholics Anonymous or Narcotics Anonymous.

MDMA-Induced Anxiety Syndromes

Although it is atypical for a drug user to contact a drug treatment facility to report *positive* drug experiences, we do receive reports of unsupervised, positive psychodynamic facilitation in MDMA users who call, write, or visit the clinics for literature or questions regarding MDMA. However, the opposite is also true. For some users, MDMA will bring to the surface unconscious material that may manifest itself in a variety of negative ways.

These problems seem unrelated to volume, dose, or duration of MDMA use. We have identified it as a delayed anxiety disorder secondary to MDMA ingestion. In these cases, the MDMA user reports one or more symptoms of anxiety, typically emerging shortly after their initial MDMA experience. These symptoms range from mild anxiety or concentration difficulties to a full-blown disorder such as panic attack with hyperventilation and tachycardia, phobic disorders, paresthesias, or other anxiety states.

In some cases, the client will be particularly concerned about a certain part of the body. The client may perceive that a hand is shaking, or that the extremities are cold and clammy. Subjective reactions to these concerns can range from mild annoyance to high inhibition. The dysfunction may require psychiatric or psychological intervention.

References

Alpert, R. (1967). Psychedelic drugs and the law. *Journal of Psychedelic Drugs, 1,* 7–26.

American Psychiatric Association. (1994). *Diagnostic and statistical manual of mental disorders* (4th ed.). Washington, DC: Author.

Cohen, S. (1960). Lysergic acid diethylamide: Side effects and complications. *Journal of Nervous and Mental Disease, 130,* 30–40.

Greer, G., & Tolbert, R. (1986). Subjective reports of the effects of MDMA in a clinical setting. In R. B. Seymour, D. R. Wesson, & D. E. Smith, (Eds.), MDMA: Proceedings of the conference. *Journal of Psychoactive Drugs, 18,* 319–328.

Hallissy, E. (1993, March 24). Use of "Speed" drug rising in state. *San Francisco Chronicle,* pp. 1, 12.

Hayner, G. N., & McKinney, H. E. (1986). MDMA: The dark side of ecstasy. In R. B. Seymour, D. R. Wesson, & D. E. Smith (Eds.), MDMA: Proceedings of the Conference. *Journal of Psychoactive Drugs, 18,* 341–348.

Leary, T., Metzner, R., & Alpert, R. (1964). *The psychedelic experience: A manual based on the Tibetan Book of the Dead.* New Hyde Park, NY: University Books.

Metzner, R. (1978). Reflections on LSD—Ten years later. *Journal of Psychedelic Drugs, 10,* 137–140.

Michaux, H. (1963). *Miserable miracle* (L. Varese, Trans.). San Francisco: City Lights Books.

Newmeyer, J., & Johnson, G. (1979). Drug emergencies in crowds: An analysis of "rock medicine." *Journal of Psychedelic Drugs, 9,* 235–245.

Seymour, R. B., & Smith, D. E. (1987). *Drugfree: A unique, positive approach to staying off alcohol and other drugs.* New York: Facts on File.

Seymour, R. B., & Smith, D. E. (1991). Hallucinogens. In N. S. Miller (Ed.), *Comprehensive handbook of drug and alcohol addiction* (pp. 455–476). New York: Dekker.

Seymour, R. B., & Smith, D. E. (1993). *The psychedelic resurgence: Treatment, support, and recovery options.* Center City, MN: Hazelden.

Smith, D. E. (1967). [Editor's Note]. *Journal of Psychedelic Drugs, 1,* 1–5.

Smith, D. E., & Luce, J. (1969). *Love needs care.* Boston: Little, Brown.

Smith, D. E., & Seymour, R. B. (1985). Dream becomes nightmare: Adverse reactions to LSD. *Journal of Psychoactive Drugs, 17,* 297–303.

Smith, D. E., & Shick, J. F. E. (1970). Analysis of the LSD flashback. *Journal of Psychedelic Drugs, 3,* 13–19.

Smith, D. E., & Wesson, D. R. (1975). [Editors' Note]. *Journal of Psychoactive Drugs, 7,* 111–114.

Wesson, D. R., & Smith, D. E. (1978). Psychedelics. In A. Schecter (Ed.), *Treatment aspects of drug dependence* (pp. 148–160). West Palm Beach, FL: CRC.

Wesson, D. R., & Smith, D. E. (1979). *Amphetamine use, misuse and abuse.* New York: G. K. Hall.

Wolfe, T. (1968). *The electric kool-aid acid test.* New York: Bantam.

VI

Inhalants

16

Pharmacology of Inhalants

ERIC B. EVANS

Introduction

The recreational use of gaseous and volatile substances is not a new phenomenon. In early western civilization Greeks inhaled gases for religious purposes (Brecher, 1972). The synthesis of nitrous oxide in 1776 by Priestly could be marked as the beginning of the modern era of inhalant abuse. In fact, its abuse preceded the announcement of a legitimate medical use as an anesthetic 20 years later by Priestly and Davy (Nagle, 1968). The misuse of nitrous oxide and the other early anesthetic agents, chloroform and ether ("ether frolics"), was fashionable in the 19th century. Not surprisingly, the modern, nonflammable, inhalational anesthetic halothane has been abused by medical personnel, and there have been reports of deaths (Spencer, Raasch, & Trefny, 1976).

The rise of organic chemistry has been very rapid, and it is estimated that by 1880, approximately 12,000 compounds had been synthesized. For the first time numerous organic substances were readily available which were both volatile at room temperature and hydrophobic. This combination of properties greatly improved the performance of numerous products, for example, water resistance of shoe glues and decreased drying time of floor lacquers. As with most beneficial discoveries, no time was wasted before the dangerous properties of these substances were exploited. Methods were found to concentrate and inhale the vapors for their intoxicating effects. Contemporary inhalant abuse dates from the 1940s when adhesive abuse came to be known as "glue sniffing," with today's abusers having access to inhalants in an extensive number of ordinary products from gasoline to typewriter correction fluid. Primarily a habit of the young (12–18-year age group), this form of drug abuse is much more widespread than generally recognized, exceeded only by marijuana, ethanol, and tobacco (National Institute on Drug Abuse, 1993). In other regions of the world, such as Mexico, the magnitude of the problem is greater, with inhalant abuse exceeding that of marijuana and cocaine (Montoya, 1990).

Inhalants can be grouped many ways (e.g., by chemical family, legitimate use) but are frequently divided into four classes: volatile or organic solvents, aerosols, anesthetics, and volatile nitrites. The individual chemicals that comprise these groups of inhalants represent many chemical families and even a few therapeutic classes (Table 1). Examples include acetone-based nail polish removers, toluene-based adhesives, butane gas cigarette lighters, the anesthetic gas halothane, nitrous oxide propellant for whipping cream canisters, amyl nitrite in room deodorizers, 1,1,1-trichloroethane in typewriter correction fluid, and complex mixtures such as gasoline and kerosene. The

ERIC B. EVANS • National Starch and Chemical Company, Bridgewater, New Jersey 08807.

Handbook of Substance Abuse: Neurobehavioral Pharmacology, edited by Tarter *et al.* Plenum Press, New York, 1998.

TABLE 1. Chemical Constituents of Abused Inhalants

Inhalant	Chemical constituents
Aromatic hydrocarbons	Methylbenzene (Toluene) Dimethylbenzene (Xylene)
Cycloalkanes or cycloparaffins	Cyclohexane Methylcyclohexane
Ketones	2-Propanone (Acetone) Methyl ethyl ketone Methyl isobutyl ketone Methyl n-amyl ketone
Halogenated hydrocarbons	Dichloromethane (Methylene chloride) Trichloromethane (Chloroform) Tetrachloromethane (Carbon tetrachloride) 1,1,1-Trichloroethane (Methylchloroform) 1,1,2-Trichloroethylene (Trilene) Tetrachloroethylene (Perchloroethylene)
Esters	Methyl acetate Ethyl acetate Isopropyl acetate n-Butyl acetate Amyl acetate
Ethers	Diethyl ether (Ether)
Aliphatic hydrocarbons	n-Butane n-Propane n-Hexane n-Heptane
Alcohols	Methyl alcohol (Methanol, Wood alcohol) Ethyl alcohol (Ethanol, Grain alcohol) Isopropyl alcohol (Isopropanol, Rubbing alcohol) Butyl alcohol Amyl alcohol
Aliphatic, naphthenic, olfenic, and aromatic petroleum hydrocarbon mixtures	Gasoline Kerosene Thinners Mineral spirits Naphthas
Anesthetic agents	Nitrous oxide 2-Bromo-2-chloro-1,1,1-trifluoroethane (Halothane) 2-Chloro-1-(difluoromethoxy)-1,1,2-trifluoroethane (Enflurane) 2-Chloro-2-(difluoromethoxy)-1,1,1-trifluoroethane (Isoflurane)
Aerosol propellants and refrigerants[a]	Trichlorofluoromethane (Freon 11, Frigen 11) Dichlorodifluoromethane (Freon 12, Frigen 12, Halon) 1,2-Dichloro-1,1,2,2-tetrafluoroethane (Freon 114, Frigen 114)
Nitrites	Amyl nitrite[b,c] Isobutyl nitrite n-butyl nitrite sec-butyl nitrite tert-butyl nitrite

[a]Marketed under general names: Arcton, Freon, Frigen, Genetron.
[b]Originally used in the treatment of angina and poisoning by hydrogen sulfide or hydrogen cyanide.
[c]Primarily consists of isopentyl nitrite.

list becomes extensive by virtue of the enormous number of abused ordinary consumer products which often contain complex mixtures of volatile chemicals. The nitrites, the last group of chemicals listed in Table 1, compared with the other chemicals listed are unique in terms of pharmacological mechanism of action and thus are not discussed in this chapter (see review by Haverkos & Dougherty, 1988).

All inhalants, regardless of how they are classified, share some common physicochemical properties. Each is either a volatile liquid or gas at room temperature, and has both a low boiling point and molecular weight. All are lipophilic compounds, which in conjunction with their small molecular size facilitates their entry and distribution in the body. Once in the body these chemicals have a high affinity for lipid, and consequently readily concentrate in organs rich in fat, such as the central and peripheral nervous system, liver, and kidney.

Pharmacological Actions

Absorption, Distribution, and Metabolism

The high degree of vascularity of the lungs is the reason that a gas delivered to this site is rapidly absorbed. Therefore, whether an abuser inhales a gas or vapor evaporated from a liquid, at the lungs, the site of gas absorption, the net transfer rate from the alveoli to the blood is rapid at first. For example, the brain and blood levels of toluene and 1,1,1-trichloroethane approach final asymptotic concentrations within minutes of inhalational administration (Benignus, Muller, Barton, & Bittikofer, 1981; Dallas, Bruckner, Maedgen, & Weir, 1986). Uptake progressively slows as blood levels near a plateau at the steady state. However, considering the brief exposure typical of an inhalant abuse scenario, achievement of a steady state is unlikely. Being highly lipophilic, abused inhalants quickly distribute out of the blood into primarily lipid-rich tissues. In rats, the maximum levels of $[^{14}C]$toluene were detected throughout the brain when animals were

sacrificed immediately after a 10-min inhalation exposure (Gospe & Calaban, 1988). Many of these agents are not metabolized or excreted in any significant amount by the usual routes, but are eliminated unchanged almost entirely by the lungs (Nolan, Freshour, Rick, McCarty, & Saunders, 1984; Schumann, Fox, & Watanabe, 1982). Thus, once exposure is terminated blood and tissue concentrations quickly decrease.

Central Nervous System

The industrial worker, under normal working conditions, is exposed to a low concentration of a single, volatile chemical or a known combination of chemicals over a long period of time. In contrast, the inhalant abuser willingly inhales a high concentration of an often very complex mixture of chemicals within a very short period. It has been estimated that the concentration of toluene encountered during inhalation of a toluene-based glue from a bag exceed 10,000 ppm (Press & Done, 1967). Given the long list of substances noted in Table 1, the specific differences between inhalants are not discussed. Nevertheless, in general, it is fair to say that at the high concentrations encountered during inhalant abuse, these substances act as depressants of the central nervous system (CNS). In humans both experimental data and anecdotal accounts of industrial accidents describe a continuum of acute effects like those of classical CNS depressant drugs (Browning, 1965; Shoemaker, 1981; Stewart, Gay, Erley, Hake, & Schaffer, 1961). The onset of effects is rapid due to the inhalational route of administration, and initial stimulatory effects may be experienced that are indicative of the biphasic effects also noted with ethanol, barbiturates, and other CNS depressant drugs. However, as the concentration and/or duration of exposure increases, effects progress from numerous subjective feelings such as relaxation, giddiness, and elation, to loss of coordination, sedation, and possibly unconsciousness and death. The very rapid onset of these symptoms is evidence that the acute depressant actions are due to the parent molecule and not metabolites. Other effects associated with intoxication include alterations in mood, perceptual changes, and distortions including vivid visual and auditory hallucinations.

In laboratory animals, controlled exposures to known concentrations of a wide variety of abused inhalants have revealed a profile of depressant-like effects. For example, biphasic effects on spontaneous motor activity and other behaviors have been recorded. In rodents, low to intermediate concentrations of toluene and chlorinated hydrocarbons increased spontaneous locomotor activity, though as the exposure duration or concentration increased locomotor activity was inhibited (Kjellstrand, Holmquist, Jonsson, Romare, & Månsson, 1985; Wood & Colotla, 1990). Prolonged exposure to high levels of aromatic and halogenated hydrocarbons, ketones, alcohols, and anesthetic agents in laboratory animals consistently produce a concentration-dependent impairment of CNS activity, sensorimotor responses, righting reflex, and both motor control and activity (see review by E. B. Evans & Balster, 1991; Tegeris & Balster, 1994).

If exposure is terminated soon enough, the CNS effects are reversible or "drug-like" in nature, for recovery is most often rapid and complete (Glowa, 1985). In industries such as shipbuilding, rescue of unconscious workers from exposure to very high vapor concentrations of solvents encountered from use in confined spaces has resulted in dramatic recovery (Longley, Jones, Welsh, & Lomaev, 1967; Morley *et al.*, 1970). In fact, the reversible, drug-like depressant actions of the chlorinated hydrocarbons, particularly 1,1,1-trichloroethane and 1,1,2-trichloroethylene, were recognized and these substances were subsequently evaluated as surgical anesthetics but were abandoned due to low potency and target organ toxicity.

Tolerance and Dependence

Habitual use of inhalants may result in physical dependence. Upon cessation of use, anecdotal clinical reports have described a group of symptoms representative of CNS hyperactivity and typical of withdrawal from a depressant drug (A. C. Evans & Raistrick,

1987; Merry & Zachariadis, 1962; Westermeyer, 1987). Within 1 to 2 days of cessation of inhalant use, sleep disturbance, irritability, hallucinations, tremors, sweating, and abdominal cramps were experienced.

In mice, removal from continuous daily exposure to 2,000 ppm 1,1,1-trichloroethane evoked the appearance of handling-induced convulsions. The convulsions were suppressed by either an injection of a barbiturate or benzodiazepine or readministration of 1,1,1-trichloroethane vapor itself (E. B. Evans & Balster, 1993). Similarly, in monkeys experiencing withdrawal from barbital, inhalation of chloroform reversed the symptoms of withdrawal (Yanagita & Takahashi, 1973). Thus, controlled laboratory research has demonstrated both physical dependence to an inhalant and cross-dependence to CNS depressant drugs.

In subjects admitted to addiction treatment centers there are mentions of tolerance to toluene and butane but in experiments designed to examine tolerance results were contradictory. For commonly abused inhalants neither pharmacodynamic or dispositional tolerance has been clearly elucidated.

Adverse Effects

Inhalant abusers, unlike typical industrial workers, ignore the "warning properties" of odor, mucous membrane irritation, tearing, and nasal irritation elicited at relatively low concentrations by most inhalants and continue to subject themselves to harmful concentrations of these substances. Although the recovery from the acute depressant actions is rapid and complete, repeated prolonged abuse of inhalants may result in specific organ toxicities. Many inhalants and their metabolites are prototypic nephrotoxins, hepatotoxins, myelotoxins, and neurotoxins, although the prevalence of these toxicities among chronic abusers is unknown. Toxic neuropathies (Layzer, Fishman, & Schafer, 1978; Prockop, 1979), renal dysfunction (O'Brien, Yoeman, & Hobby, 1971; Streicher, Cabow, Moss, Kono, & Kaehny, 1981; Taher, Anderson, McCartney, Popovtzer, & Schrier, 1974), liver damage, and hepatitis (Marjot & McLeod, 1989; Press & Done, 1967) have been reported as a consequence of abuse of primarily organic solvents. The selectivity of organ damage is specific to the particular solvent involved (see review by Synder & Andrews, 1996). Impurities inherent to the preparation, synthesis, or isolation of many organic chemical constituents of inhalants may exert their own unique toxicities. For example, toluene-based adhesives and complex mixtures such as gasoline, paint, and lacquer thinners often contain small quantities of benzene or lead, rendering chronic abusers susceptible to neurologic and hematopoietic toxicities (Hansen & Sharp, 1978; Linden, 1990; Powars, 1965). In addition to the target organ toxicities already described, clinical reports have noted numerous other effects including headache, nausea, vomiting, diplopia, and tinnitus, as well as effects indicative of exposure to a primary irritant, such as rhinitis, conjunctivitis, and skin rash.

Inhalant induced damage to the peripheral nerves has been frequently described, but besides the acute intoxication, inhalant-induced toxic effects on the CNS have only recently come to light. First noted in Scandinavian countries, considerable evidence collected in workers exposed for long periods of time to solvents has brought about the identification of a new disease entity, a toxic encephalopathy often referred to as the "Painter's syndrome." Although the studies documenting the syndrome existence in workers are the subject of controversy, in these Scandinavian countries, workers who develop this syndrome receive monetary compensation (Flodin, Edling, & Axelson, 1984). The encephalopathy consists of a general cerebral and cerebellar degeneration, leading to enlargement of the fluid-filled ventricular system and basal cisterns. The principal effects that accompany the brain atrophy are an impairment of motor control and associated impairment of some intellectual and memory capacity. Clinical examination and brain imaging of chronic toluene abusers, whose exposure concentrations certainly exceed those of the average worker, revealed unequivocal brain atrophy (Fornazzari, Wilkinson, Kapur, &

Carlen, 1983; Lazar, Ho, Melen, & Daghestani, 1983; Rosenberg, Spitz, Filley, Davis, & Schaumburg, 1988; Schikler, Seitz, Rice, & Strader, 1982). In these abusers, toluene generally represents only one of many chemicals inhaled, so it cannot be identified as the causative agent in inhalant-induced CNS toxicity. Furthermore, sniffing complex mixtures such as gasoline, paint, and paint thinner has produced cerebral and cerebellar damage or dysfunction (Escobar & Aruffo, 1980; Kelly, 1975; Valpey, Sumi, Copass, & Goble, 1978). It is unknown whether the degenerative processes noted in a few clinical reports represent typical inhalant abusers and whether the atrophy is progressive or reversible. It is clear that more research and controlled studies are needed to provide a better understanding of the problem (Triebig, Bleecker, Gilioli, & Flynn, 1989).

The high level of exposure scenarios desired by abusers have resulted in many deaths but, considering the magnitude of the inhalant abuse problem, casualties are relatively rare and most often result from exacerbating circumstances (e.g., trauma) rather than from the toxic effects. Aromatic and aliphatic hydrocarbons, alcohols, ethers, esters, chlorinated hydrocarbons, and ketones all have the potential to produce unconsciousness, paralysis, convulsions, and death from respiratory or cardiovascular arrest (Browning, 1965). It is believed that the major risk of death from inhalant toxicity results from cardiac arrhythmias. Many of these deaths are attributed to inhalation of aerosol products containing chlorinated hydrocarbon propellants which can cause fatal cardiac arrhythmias, probably due to sensitization of the myocardium to endogenous epinephrine (Reinhardt, Azar, Maxfield, Smith, & Mullin, 1971). This lethal mechanism of action is also associated with the abuse of butane in cigarette lighter refills, propane, and gasoline (Adgey, Johnston, & McMechan, 1995). However, it should be noted that many aromatic and aliphatic hydrocarbons also directly depress cardiovascular function. Other factors contributing to inhalant induced death include anoxia, respiratory depression, vagal stimulation, and aspiration of vomit.

Mechanism of Action of CNS Effects

Since most inhalants are commercial, commodity chemicals, there is little direct evidence of their cellular mode of action. However, it is clear that inhalants are small, lipophilic compounds that produce CNS depression and eventually anesthesia, thus sharing physicochemical and pharmacological properties with CNS depressant drugs and anesthetics whose molecular mode of action has been extensively studied. At the turn of the century Overton and Meyer published a theory of anesthesia that accounted for depressant actions of a structurally diverse group of chemicals capable of producing anesthesia based on their physicochemical properties (Overton, 1901). Their studies and subsequent work has demonstrated that the anesthetic potency of a myriad of compounds, including volatile anesthetics, inert gases, halogenated hydrocarbons, alcohols, alkanes, and ethers, is directly proportional to their oil–water partition coefficient or solubility in fat-like solvents (for example, olive oil). The gas molecules of these highly lipophilic compounds exert their actions by partitioning into the neuronal cellular membrane, perturbing its structural integrity and subsequently altering cellular excitability. Anesthesia would be obtained, irrespective of chemical structure, when the concentration of an anesthetic reaches a critical molar concentration in the membrane (see reviews by Paton, 1984; Seeman, 1972). Although over the years minor refinements of the Overton–Meyer correlations have been made by considering such things as the space-filling volume of the anesthetic in the membrane, presently no other theory can account for the pharmacological effects of a class with such great diversity in molecular structure as found among these agents.

A discrete receptor-mediated mode of action elucidated for the CNS depressants benzodiazepines and barbiturates has been explored as a mechanism for anesthesia. These two important classes of pharmacologic agents enhance the actions of the amino acid transmitter γ-aminobutyric acid (GABA), an inhibitory transmitter prevalent in the mammalian central nervous system, by allosterically facilitating its binding to the $GABA_A$ receptor. For many years it was thought that the depressant effects of ethanol and other aliphatic alcohols, like anesthetics, were exerted by perturbation of lipid membranes. More recently, it has been demonstrated that ethanol has the capacity to augment GABA-mediated neuronal inhibition (Harris, 1990; Suzdak, Schwartz, Skolnick, & Paul, 1986; Ticku, 1990). Similarly, volatile anesthetic agents have demonstrated GABA modulatory effects in numerous assays (Cheng & Brunner, 1981; Huidobro-Toro, Bleck, Allan, & Harris, 1987; Nakahiro, Yeh, Brunner, & Narahashi, 1989).

At the molecular level, rather than exerting their effects by disturbing membrane lipids, recent studies have demonstrated that general anesthetics stereoselectively bind directly to discrete proteins (Franks & Lieb, 1991). Many investigators now agree that general anesthetics, like the barbiturates, benzodiazepines, and ethanol, do not act nonspecifically, but bind selectively at both the cellular and molecular level (see review by Franks & Lieb, 1994). Unfortunately, to date no theory of the mechanism of anesthesia yet exists and the abused inhalants which produce depressant-like pharmacological effects have not been examined for their cellular effects on these systems.

References

Adgey, A. A., Johnston, P. W., & McMechan, S. (1995). Sudden cardiac death and substance abuse. *Resuscitation, 29*, 219–221.

Benignus, V. A., Muller, K. E., Barton, C. N., & Bittikofer, J. A. (1981). Toluene levels in blood and brain of rats during and after respiratory exposure. *Toxicology and Applied Pharmacology, 61*, 326–334.

Brecher, E. M. (1972). Inhalants; solvents and glue sniffing; the historical antecedents of glue sniffing; how to launch a nationwide drug menace. In E. M. Brecher & Consumer Reports (Eds.), *Licit and illicit drugs* (pp. 309–334). Boston: Little, Brown.

Browning, E. (1965). *Toxicity and metabolism of industrial solvents.* New York: Elsevier.

Cheng, S., & Brunner, E. A. (1981). Effects of anesthetic agents on synaptosomal GABA disposal. *Anesthesiology, 55*, 34–40.

Dallas, C. E., Bruckner, J. V., Maedgen, J. L., & Weir, F. W. (1986). A method for direct measurement of systemic uptake and elimination of volatile organics in small animals. *Journal of Pharmacological Methods, 16,* 239–250.

Escobar, A., & Aruffo, C. (1980). Chronic thinner intoxication: Clinico-pathologic report of a human case. *Journal of Neurology, Neurosurgery and Psychiatry, 43,* 986–994.

Evans, A. C., & Raistrick, D. (1987). Phenomenology of intoxication with toluene-based adhesives and butane gas. *British Journal of Psychiatry, 150,* 769–773.

Evans, E. B., & Balster, R. L. (1991). CNS depressant effects of volatile organic solvents. *Neuroscience and Biobehavioral Reviews, 15,* 233–241.

Evans, E. B., & Balster, R. L. (1993). Inhaled 1,1,1-Trichloroethane-produced physical dependence in mice: Effects of drugs and vapors on withdrawal. *Journal of Pharmacology and Experimental Therapeutics, 264,* 726–733.

Flodin, U., Edling, C., & Axelson, O. (1984). Clinical studies of psychoorganic syndromes among workers with solvent exposure. *American Journal of Industrial Medicine, 5,* 287–295.

Fornazzari, L., Wilkinson, D. A., Kapur, B. M., & Carlen, P. L. (1983). Cerebellar cortical and functional impairment in toluene abusers. *Acta Neurologica Scandinavica, 67,* 319–329.

Franks, N. P., & Lieb, W. R. (1991). Stereospecific effects of inhalational general anesthetics optical isomers on nerve ion channels. *Science, 254,* 427–430.

Franks, N. P., & Lieb, W. R. (1994). Molecular and cellular mechanisms of general anesthesia. *Nature, 367,* 607–614.

Glowa, J. R. (1985). Behavioral effects of volatile organic solvents. In L. S. Seiden & R. L. Balster (Eds.), *Behavioral pharmacology: The current status* (pp. 537–552). New York: Liss.

Gospe, S. M., & Calaban, M. J. (1988). Central nervous distribution of inhaled toluene. *Fundamental and Applied Toxicology, 11,* 540–545.

Hansen, K. S., & Sharp, F. R. (1978). Gasoline sniffing, lead poisoning, and myoclonus. *Journal of the American Medical Association, 240,* 1375–1376.

Harris, R. A. (1990). Distinct actions of alcohols, barbiturates and benzodiazepines on GABA-activated chloride channels. *Alcohol, 7,* 273–275.

Haverkos, H. W., & Dougherty, J. A. (Eds.). (1988). *Health hazards of nitrite inhalants* (National Institute on Drug Abuse Research Monograph No. 83). Washington, DC: U.S. Government Printing Office.

Huidobro-Toro, J. P., Bleck, V., Allan, A. M., & Harris, R. A. (1987). Neurochemical actions of anesthetic drugs on the γ-aminobutyric acid receptor-chloride channel complex. *Journal of Pharmacology and Experimental Therapeutics, 242,* 963–969.

Kelly, T. (1975). Prolonged cerebellar dysfunction associated with paint sniffing. *Pediatrics, 56,* 605–606.

Kjellstrand, P., Holmquist, B., Jonsson, I., Romare, S., & Månsson, L. (1985). Effects of organic solvents on motor activity in mice. *Toxicology, 35,* 35–46.

Layzer, R. B., Fishman, R. A., & Schafer, J. A. (1978). Neuropathy following abuse of nitrous oxide. *Neurology, 28,* 504–505.

Lazar, R. B., Ho, S. U., Melen, O., & Daghestani, A. N. (1983). Multifocal central nervous system damage caused by toluene abuse. *Neurology, 33,* 1337–1340.

Linden, C. H. (1990). Volatile substances of abuse. *Emergency Medicine Clinics of North America, 8,* 559–578.

Longley, E. O., Jones, A. T., Welsh, R., & Lomaev, O. (1967). Two acute toluene episodes in merchant ships. *Archives of Environmental Health, 14,* 481–487.

Marjot, R., & McLeod, A. A. (1989). Chronic non-neurological toxicity from volatile solvent substance abuse. *Human Toxicology, 8,* 301–306.

Merry, J., & Zachariadis, N. (1962). Addiction to glue sniffing. *British Medical Journal, 2,* 1448.

Montoya, C. M. A. (1990). Neurotoxicology in Mexico and its relation to the general and work environment. In B. L. Johnson (Ed.), *Advances in neurobehavioral toxicology: Applications in environmental and occupational health* (pp 35–57). Chelsea, MI: Lewis.

Morley, R., Eccleston, D. W., Douglas, C. P., Greville, W. E. J., Scott, D. J., & Anderson, J. (1970). Xylene poisoning: A report on a fatal case and two cases of recovery after prolonged unconsciousness. *British Medical Journal, 3,* 442–443.

Nagle, D. R. (1968). Anesthetic addiction and drunkenness: A contemporary and historical survey. *International Journal of the Addictions, 3,* 25–39.

Nakahiro, M., Yeh, J. Z., Brunner, E., & Narahashi, T. (1989). General anesthetics modulate GABA receptor channel complex in rat dorsal root ganglia neurons. *Federation of American Societies for Experimental Biology Journal, 3,* 1850–1854.

National Institute on Drug Abuse. (1993). *National household survey on drug abuse.* Rockville, MD: U.S. Department of Health and Human Services, Division of Epidemiology and Statistical Analysis.

Nolan, R. J., Freshour, N. L., Rick, D. L., McCarty, L. P., & Saunders, J. H. (1984). Kinetics and metabolism of inhaled methyl chloroform (1,1,1-trichloroethane) in male volunteers. *Fundamental and Applied Toxicology, 4,* 654–662.

O'Brien, E. T., Yoeman, W. B., & Hobby, J. A. E. (1971). Hepatorenal damage from toluene in a "glue sniffer." *British Medical Journal, 2,* 29–30.

Overton, E. (1901). *Studien über die narkose zugleich ein beitrag zur allgemeinen pharmakologie.* Jena, Germany: Verlag von Gustav Fischer.

Paton, W. D. M. (1984). How far do we understand the mechanism of anaesthesia. *European Journal of Anesthesiology, 1,* 93–103.

Powars, D. (1965). Aplastic anemia secondary to glue sniffing. *New England Journal of Medicine, 273,* 700–702.

Press, E., & Done, A. K. (1967). Solvent sniffing: Physiologic effects and community control measures for intoxication from intentional inhalation of organic solvents. *Pediatrics, 39,* 451–461, 611–622.

Prockop, L. D. (1979). Neurotoxic volatile substances. *Neurology, 29,* 862–865.

Reinhardt, C. F., Azar, A., Maxfield, M. E., Smith, P. E., Jr., & Mullin, L. S. (1971). Cardiac arrhythmias and aerosol "sniffing." *Archives of Environmental Health, 22,* 265–279.

Rosenberg, N. L., Spitz, M. C., Filley, C. M., Davis, K. A., & Schaumburg, H. H. (1988). Central nervous system effects of chronic toluene abuse—Clinical, brainstem evoked response and magnetic resonance imaging studies. *Neurotoxicology and Teratology, 10,* 489–495.

Schikler, K. N., Seitz, K., Rice, J. F., & Strader, T. (1982). Solvent abuse associated cortical atrophy. *Journal of Adolescent Health Care, 3,* 37–39.

Schumann, A. M., Fox, T. R., & Watanabe, P. G. (1982). ^{14}C-Methyl chloroform (1,1,1-trichloroethane: Pharmacokinetics in rats and mice following inhalation exposure. *Toxicology and Applied Pharmacology, 62,* 390–401.

Seeman, P. (1972). The membrane actions of anesthetics and tranquilizers. *Pharmacological Reviews, 24,* 583–655.

Shoemaker, W. J. (1981). The neurotoxicity of alcohols. *Neurobehavioral Toxicology and Teratology, 3,* 431–436.

Spencer, J. D., Raasch, F. O., & Trefny, F. A. (1976). Halothane abuse in hospital personnel. *Journal of the American Medical Association, 236,* 139–140.

Stewart, R. D., Gay, H. H., Erley, D. S., Hake, C. L., & Schaffer, A. W. (1961). Human exposure to 1,1,1-trichloroethane vapor: Relationship of expired air and blood concentrations to exposure and toxicity. *Industrial Hygiene Journal, 22,* 252–262.

Streicher, H. Z., Cabow, P., Moss, A., Kono, D, & Kaehny, W. D. (1981). Syndromes of toluene sniffing in adults. *Annals of Internal Medicine, 94,* 758–762.

Suzdak, P. D., Schwartz, R. D., Skolnick, P., & Paul, S. M. (1986). Ethanol stimulates γ-aminobutyric acid receptor-mediated chloride transport in rat brain synaptoneursomes. *Proceedings of the National Academy of Science USA, 83,* 4071–4075.

Synder, R., & Andrews, L. S. (1996). Toxic effects of solvents and vapors. In C. D. Klaassen (Ed.) & M. O. Amdur & J. Doull (Eds. Emeriti), *Casarett and Doull's toxicology: The basic science of poisons* (pp. 737–771). New York: McGraw-Hill.

Taher, S. M., Anderson, R. J., McCartney, R., Popovtzer, M. M., & Schrier, R. W. (1974). Renal tubular acidosis associated with toluene "sniffing." *New England Journal of Medicine, 290,* 765–768.

Tegeris, J. S., & Balster, R. L. (1994). A comparison of the acute behavioral effects of alkylbenzenes using a functional observational battery in mice. *Fundamental and Applied Toxicology, 22,* 240–250.

Ticku, M. K. (1990). Alcohol and GABA-benzodiazepine receptor function. *Annals of Medicine, 22,* 241–246.

Triebig, G., Bleecker, M., Gilioli, R., & Flynn, R. R. (1989). International working group on the epidemiology of the chronic neurobehavioral effects of organic solvents. *International Archives of Occupational Environmental Health, 61,* 423–424.

Valpey, R., Sumi, S. M., Copass, M. K., & Goble, G. J. (1978). Acute and chronic progressive encephalopathy due to gasoline sniffing. *Neurology, 28,* 507–510.

Westermeyer, J. (1987). The psychiatrist and solvent-inhalant abuse: Recognition, assessment, and treatment. *American Journal of Psychiatry, 144,* 903–907.

Wood, R. W., & Colotla, V. C. (1990). Biphasic changes in mouse motor activity during exposure to toluene. *Fundamental and Applied Toxicology, 14,* 6–14.

Yanagita, T., & Takahashi, S. (1973). Dependence liability of several sedative-hypnotic agents evaluated in monkeys. *Journal of Pharmacology and Experimental Therapeutics, 185,* 307–316.

17

Behavioral Pharmacology of Inhalants

DAVID E. HARTMAN

Categories of Inhalants

Inhalants comprise a disparate group of mind-altering substances that are classified by their intake route. Despite more than 7 million users, there is a paucity of medical and neuropsychological literature. Only rarely are investigations into inhalant abuse reported in prominent substance abuse journals. This is probably due to multiple factors including (1) difficulty in studying or neglect of the population in which inhalant use is most prevalent, namely, individuals in lower socioeconomic strata; (2) the finding that use rarely occurs in isolation from other polydrug use or exposure to other inhalants; and (3) the fact that these substances are not generally classified as abused drugs because they are commonly available legal products.

Inhalants are grouped into four categories:

1. *Volatile gases and solvents* (e.g., lighter fluid, barbecue grill gas, spray paint, paint thinner, glue): The active compound is generally acetone, ethyl acetate, n-hexane, propane, n-butane, toluene, methylbutylketone.

2. *Propellant aerosols* (e.g., hair spray, deodorants, other pressurized products): The intoxicating inhalant is the propellant rather than the active ingredient. Active compounds include methylene chloride, isobutane, propane, bromochlorodifluoromethane, and various halons including trichlorofluoromethane, dichlorodifluoromethane, chlorodifluoromethane, and dichlorotetrafluorethane.

3. *Nitrites:* These compounds include butyl nitrites and amyl nitrites. The former are often known by the trade names *Rush, Locker Room, Bolt,* and *Climax.* They are intended for use as room deodorizers. The latter are packaged in capsules known as "poppers" or "snappers." They were originally administered to treat angina.

4. *Anesthetic gases:* These compounds, most notably nitrous oxide ("laughing gas"), are typically contained in small cylinders called whippets, which propel whipped cream in commercial machines. Other common compounds include halothane and enflurane.

Neurobehavioral Effects

Typically the acute effects are manifest as disinhibited behavior and euphoria. High doses are capable of precipitating an acute psychosis and seizures (Brust, 1993). Chronic

DAVID E. HARTMAN • Isaac Ray Center, Rush Presbyterian St. Luke's Hospital, Chicago, Illinois 60612.

Handbook of Substance Abuse: Neurobehavioral Pharmacology, edited by Tarter *et al.* Plenum Press, New York, 1998.

effects include tolerance and withdrawal symptoms (Evans & Raistrick, 1987; Knox & Nelson, 1966; Press & Done, 1967). Withdrawal presents as acute psychotic symptoms similar to delirium tremens (Nylander, 1962). More typically, symptoms consist of sleep disturbances, nausea, tremor, and irritability.

Overdose of inhalants is far more likely to produce lethal consequences than are noninjectable drugs. General causes of fatalities include respiratory arrest, vomiting with aspiration, or suffocation from plastic bag inhalation (Brust, 1993). The specific cause of death may depend upon the substance. For example, death from anoxia has been reported from nitrous oxide, whereas fatal cardiac arrhythmia and cerebral edema have resulted from exposure to fluoroalkane propellants, particularly trichlorofluoromethane (Freon 11), dichlorodifluoromethane (Freon 12), and solvents found in typewriter correction fluid (Aviado, 1977; King, Smialek, & Troutman, 1985). Cardiac arrhythmia may occur over a period of several hours after initial use (Brust, 1993). In one cohort of fatalities the most prevalent manner of death was suicide (28 percent), leading Garriott (1992) to suggest the possibility of an acute drug-induced disinhibitory effect on a population known to have elevated rates of clinical depression.

Alkyl Halides

Exposure to this diverse group of predominantly chlorinated and fluorinated hydrocarbons (methyl chloride, freons) typically produces nausea, vomiting, fatigue, and muscle pain. Hepatitis, acute renal tubular necrosis, or both may follow exposure in 1 to 3 days (Linden, 1990). One college-age experimenter with freon reported his reactions in an Internet discussion forum. He tried inhaling Freon after hearing that it "gave a similar buzz to nitrous (oxide)." Initially, "for about 2 seconds, I had a small buzz. Then my vision went wild. A wall about 5 feet from me seemed like it moved from two inches . . . to 100 miles . . . every second. Then my heart started beating like wild. As I collapsed to the floor, I managed to gasp out 'get an ambulance!'" The individual

was extremely frightened by the experience and concluded that he "would sooner drink gasoline than [inhale freon] again" (Dillinger, 1993). Such an individual might be considered lucky to recount his experiences, since cardiac arrhythmia and death have been known to follow exposure to fluoroalkane propellants (Aviado, 1977; Brust, 1993). Carbon monoxide poisoning is an additional complication of exposure to methylene chloride. Severe or fatal methemoglobinemia may be produced.

Amyl and Isobutyl Nitrite

Nitrite inhalants were originally used to reduce pain from angina and as an antidote to cyanide poisoning (Wood, 1988). Blood flow increase throughout the brain has been reported after administration of amyl nitrite (Mathew, Wilson, & Tant, 1989). Consequent symptoms of dizziness and headache are attributed to dilation of arteries in the brain. Test subjects administered amyl nitrite report increased feelings of anger, depression, and fatigue. Acute toxicity from anoxia-methemglobinemia is a well-known side effect, and vital organs may become starved of oxygen because of "profound peripheral vasodilation, pooling of blood in the extremities and impaired vascular return" (Wood, 1988, p. 30). Nitrite drugs are immunotoxic and render AIDS patients more susceptible to Kaposi's sarcoma.

Isobutyl nitrite, an inhalant similar to amyl nitrite, continues to be sold legally as a locker room deodorizer. Inhalation is similar to amyl nitrate. Symptoms include severe headache, blurred vision, and eye pressure (Wood, 1988). Inhalation produces a "high" lasting from a few seconds to several minutes. Intoxication is accompanied by a decrease in blood pressure followed by an increase in heart rate, flushed face and neck, dizziness, and headache. Toxicity from methemoglobin can be a cause of death (Wood, 1988).

Butane

Butane inhalation can result in burns in the case of cigarette lighter fluid abuse, or sudden death from cardiac dysrhythmia (Siegel & Wason, 1990). Tohhara, Tani, Nakajima, and

Tsuda (1989) reported the subjective experiences of two polydrug abusers who contrasted their reactions to butane and toluene. Butane gas caused visual hallucinations and a distortion of body perception.

Nitrous Oxide (N_2O)

Nitrous oxide, a slightly sweet-smelling gas with legitimate medical and dental indications, is used where sedation, anesthesia, or analgesia are required. N_2O possesses properties similar to opioids and interacts with opioid receptors to release beta-endorphin. The gas is a partial opioid agonist, that is, capable of attenuating the effects of morphine, but acting synergistically when combined with ketamine. Gillman (1992) suggests that N_2O has inherently low abuse potential from a toxicological standpoint since (1) it is a partial rather than full opioid agonist, (2) there is rapid tolerance, and (3) the euphoria experience decays within minutes after inhalation. Consequently, abuse potential is considered to be quite low. Not surprisingly, the highest percentage of abusers is found among dental professionals. In one study of 178 dentists treated for polydrug dependence, 16.3% self-administered N_2O (Willis, cited in Gillman, 1992). However, N_2O was not the preferred intoxicant.

Acute neuropsychological effects of N_2O include impairments in psychomotor speed, coordination, and auditory reaction time (Dohrn et al., 1993). Neurological symptoms include numbness, limb weakness, sensory disturbances, and disequilibrium. Polyneuropathy may occur even in the presence of adequate oxygen (Layzer, 1978). Myeloneuropathies are the most commonly reported neurological effects of chronic abuse. Lung damage and death from anoxia have also been reported (Layzer, 1985).

Nitrous oxide abuse may interact with vitamin B-12 deficiency since nitrous oxide produces irreversible oxidation to the Co^{++} and Co^{+++} forms that render vitamin B-12 inactive. Flippo and Holder (1993) report five cases where patients who had vitamin B-12 deficiency developed subacute combined degeneration of the spinal cord following nitrous oxide anesthesia. The authors concluded that patients with vitamin B-12 deficiency are extremely sensitive to neurologic deterioration following nitrous oxide exposure and that if not recognized, neurologic deterioration can become irreversible and even fatal.

One unpublished case study describes the condition of a 36-year-old electrical engineer who had inhaled 48 to 72 cartridges of nitrous oxide almost every day for 6 months. Symptoms began as paresthesia "pins and needles" in both feet. Four days later, he presented to the emergency room unable to walk. Paresthesias worsened, with complete anesthesia to touch or pain and difficulty with motor control and the sensation of electric shocks through the back and legs precipitated by neck flexion. Neurological examination showed hyperesthesia and hyperalgesia in the lower extremities up to the knees, with severe bilateral sensory dystaxia. The patient's neurological condition continued to deteriorate even following intramuscular B-12 and improvement in hematological status. Paresthesias ascended to the nipples and incontinence of urine and feces developed. The patient showed improvement over 4 weeks with regained bladder, bowel, and sexual function. The patient was able to walk "with some hesitation" (Stacey, DiRocco, & Gould, 1992).

Solvents

Solvent abuse is a problem of epidemic and international scope. In Mexico City there are an estimated 500,000 children who are addicted to these substances. Organic solvents are the drug of choice because of low cost and euphoric effects. Children as young as 4 years have been reported to have "marked addiction" to organic solvent inhalation (Montoya-Cabrera, 1990). In the United States, solvents are primarily abused by adolescents. Solvents are typically placed in a plastic bag and inhaled, soaked on a piece of cloth which is then sniffed, or inhaled directly from the container (Barnes, 1979). The addictive potential of solvents has been demonstrated in animals (Wood, 1979; Yanagita, Takahashi, Ishida, & Funamoto, 1970). Narcotic effects are common in all solvents independent of their particular chemical structure at high concentrations (Ikeda, 1992).

The effects on the nervous system are predictable from their highly lipophilic nature. Acute intoxication is caused by rapid vapor absorption into the lungs, where it is transferred within seconds to the brain and other organs. Symptom onset also occurs within seconds and peak blood level occurs 15–30 min postinhalation. Peak tissue level occurs somewhat later (Linden, 1990). Several hours after inhalation, solvent abusers are likely to be lethargic and "hung over" with a headache that may be severe (Rosenberg & Sharp, 1992).

Wyse (1973) divided acute behavioral reactions to solvent inhalation into four stages. Initial intoxication is characterized by euphoria, excitation, dizziness, and visual and auditory hallucinations. In the second stage, CNS depression occurs, with symptoms of confusion, disorientation, dullness, loss of self-control, tinnitus, blurred vision, and diplopia (Barnes, 1979). In the third stage, increasing CNS depression produces sleepiness, incoordination, ataxia, dysarthria, diminished reflexes, and nystagmus. In the fourth stage, seizures and EEG changes occur (Barnes, 1979). Paranoia and bizarre behavior may be manifest. Symptoms of carbon monoxide poisoning may emerge following methylene chloride intoxication.

Acute toxic reactions occur through anoxia because solvent vapors decrease partial pressure of oxygen. Chronic damage occurs to neuronal membranes rather than degradation of neurotransmitter function. Aliphatic and aromatic hydrocarbons, alkyl halides, and ketones are known to cause permanent neurologic damage (Linden, 1990). Importantly, solvent mixtures may complicate neurotoxicity effects because of potentiation or cancellation from their combination (Rosenberg & Sharp, 1992).

The neurotoxic properties of common solvents may be amplified if combined with other drugs, or if typical exposure conditions are changed. For example, drug abusers have experimented with smoking marijuana cigarettes that have been soaked in formaldehyde-based embalming fluid ("Wicky Sticks," "AMP"). Hawkins, Schwartz-Thompson, and Kahare (1994) reported on two individuals without prior psychiatric history who were admitted to the hospital with auditory hallucinations, disorganized thinking, and other symptoms of severe psychosis. A neuropsychological examination of the first patient, conducted 6 weeks after admission, showed complete disorientation for time and date, along with severe impairments in learning. Severe memory deficits persisted upon reexamination 7 weeks later. The second patient had no signs of psychosis but displayed disorientation and had a severe memory deficit.

Mild organic syndromes from solvent abuse are difficult to diagnose from the standard neurological examination. The clinical presentation is nonspecific and may be mistaken for demyelinating diseases, metabolic abnormalities, degenerative disease, or nutritional disorders (Rosenberg & Sharp, 1992). The sequelae of chronic solvent abuse are not completely reversible.

Most of the research conducted on solvent abuse pertains to the inhalation of toluene; however, several case reports have been published on gasoline "huffing" and inhalation of other solvents. In a cohort of 20 toluene abusers, Hormes, Filley, and Rosenberg (1986) found that 60% had cognitive deficits, 50% had pyramidal disturbances, 45% showed cerebellar abnormalities, 25% demonstrated cranial nerve or brainstem abnormalities, and 15% had tremor. Four individuals (20%) exhibited complete or partial anosmia, and two subjects (10%) had bilateral hearing loss. Another study found visual and auditory evoked potential abnormalities in 8 of 15 children with a history of inhalant abuse who did not manifest neurological abnormalities (Tenenbein & Pillay, 1993).

In the most widely studied solvent of abuse (toluene) a range of serious neurological deficits have been reported: short-term memory loss, emotional instability, cognitive impairment, slurred and "scanning" speech, wide-based ataxic gait, staggering or stumbling in trying to walk, nystagmus, ocular flutter, tremor, optic neuropathy, unilateral or bilateral hearing loss, diffuse slowing of EEG, abnormal or absent brainstem auditory evoked response, diffuse cerebral, cerebellar, and brainstem atrophy, enlarged ventricles, and widening of cortical sulci, especially in the frontal or temporal cortex (Pryor, 1992).

Uitti and colleagues (1994) reported the case of a 29-year-old woman who developed extrapyramidal symptoms following repeated inhalation of lacquer thinner. This particular solvent consists of 60% toluene with the remainder composed of methanol, ethyl acetate, and methylethylketone. The patient presented with akathisia, but was otherwise fully oriented. Short-term memory was normal but the patient's voice was monotonous and soft. Drooling was observed and upper extremities and neck were moderately to severely rigid with left side worse than right. A mild resting tremor was noted in the right hand and a prominent jaw jerk was observed. The results of a PET scan suggested decreased raclopride binding at D_2 striatal receptor sites. Treatment with sinemet, clonazepam, and trazodone was initiated and when levodopa was increased to 1,400 mg daily, a marked reduction in symptoms was observed. This case study is of particular interest because of the selective affinity of solvents and their toxicity to dopaminergic structures.

Neuropsychological studies have consistently documented a variety of cognitive deficits among individuals with chronic solvent abuse. Hormes and colleagues (1986) observed apathy, poor concentration, memory deficits, visuospatial abnormalities, and impairments in cognitive capacity. Grigsby, Rosenberg, Dreisbach, Busenbark, and Grigsby (1992) found that toluene users were impaired on a variety of cognitive measures, including verbal IQ, abstracting capacity, language comprehension, learning, and immediate memory compared with nonsolvent drug users. The authors conclude that the pattern of test scores suggested the presence of a subcortical dementia.

Gasoline sniffing is particularly neurotoxic. Prejean and Gouvier (1994) described the neuropsychological functioning of an individual who inhaled unleaded gasoline exclusively on a daily basis for over 1 year. The patient demonstrated deficits in tactile sensory perception and tactile memory, but had normal psychomotor performance. A lower verbal IQ compared to performance IQ was noted; however, it is unclear whether this difference was due to premorbid factors.

Solvent abuse may worsen neuropsychological functioning concomitant to injury of organ systems besides the brain. Pulmonary injury resulting in chronic hypoxemia, along with cardiovascular and respiratory depression, as well as renal and hepatic pathology, may contribute to impaired cognitive capacity. For example, carbon tetrachloride abuse has been shown to precipitate severe acute hepatic injury with progressive oliguria (Knox & Nelson, 1966). Pancreatitis, proteinuria, hematuria, and acute renal failure has also been reported (Durden & Chipman, 1967). Solvents that metabolize to carbon monoxide (methylene chloride and chlorobromomethane) may produce secondary toxicity related to carbon monoxide toxicokinetics.

In conclusion, there is a preponderance of evidence indicating that inhalant abuse is more damaging to brain and other organ systems than drugs that have achieved far more public attention (e.g., marijuana, heroin). The risk of fatality also is much greater from inhalant abuse. Future efforts to document the effects of inhalants must be coupled with intervention strategies that address the specific needs of this population.

References

Aviado, D. M. (1977). Preclinicial pharmacology and toxicology of halogenated solvents and propellants. In C. W. Shar & M. L. Brehm (Eds.), *Review of inhalants: Euphoria to dysfunction* (NIDA Research Monograph No. 15, pp. 164–184). Rockville, MD: National Institute on Drug Abuse.

Barnes, G. E. (1979). Solvent abuse: A review. *International Journal of the Addictions, 14,* 1–26.

Brust, J. C. M. (1993). Other agents: Phencyclidine, marijuana, hallucinogens, inhalants and anticholinergics. *Neurologic Clinics, 11,* 555–561.

Dillinger, S. (1993, May 15). Inhaling freon—Don't. *Alternate drugs.* Usenet Newsgroup.

Dohrn, C. S., Lichtor, J. L., Coalson, D. W., Uitvlugt, A., de Wit, H., & Zacny, J. P. (1993). Reinforcing effects of extended inhalation of nitrous oxide in humans. *Drug and Alcohol Dependence, 31,* 265–280.

Durden, W. D., & Chipman, D. W. (1967). Gasoline sniffing complicated by acute carbon tetrachloride poisoning. *Archives of Internal Medicine, 119,* 371.

Evans, A. C., & Raistrick, D. (1987). Phenomenology of intoxication with toluene-based adhesives and butane gas. *British Journal of Psychiatry, 150,* 769–773.

Flippo, T., & Holder, W. D. (1993). Neurologic degeneration associated with nitrous oxide anesthesia in patients with Vitamin B12 deficiency. *Archives of Surgery, 128,* 1391–1395.

Garriott J. C. (1992) Death among inhalant abusers. In C. W. Sharp, F. Beauvas, & R. Spence (Eds.), *Inhalant abuse: A volatile research agenda* (NIDA Research Monograph No. 129, pp. 181–192). Rockville, MD: National Institute on Drug Abuse.

Gillman, M. A. (1992). Nitrous oxide in perspective. *Clinical Neuropharmacology, 15,* 297–306.

Grigsby, J., Rosenberg, N. L., Dreisbach, J. N., Busenbark, D., & Grigsby, P. (1992, November). *Chronic toluene abuse produces neuropsychological deficits.* Paper presented at the annual meeting of the National Academy of Neuropsychology, Pittsburgh, PA.

Hawkins, K. A., Schwartz-Thompson, J., & Kahane, A. (1994). Abuse of formaldehyde-laced marijuana may cause dysmnesia. *Journal of Neuropsychiatry, 2,* 67.

Hormes, J. T., Filley, C. M., & Rosenberg, N. L. (1986). Neurologic sequelae of chronic solvent vapor abuse. *Neurology, 36,* 698–702.

Ikeda, M. (1992). Public health problems of organic solvents. *Toxicology Letters, 64–65,* 191–201

King, G. S., Smialek, J. E., & Troutman, W. G. (1985). Sudden death in adolescents resulting from the inhalation of typewriter correction fluid. *Journal of the American Medical Association, 253,* 1604–1606.

Knox, W. J., & Nelson, J. R. (1966). Permanent encephalopathy from toluene inhalation. *New England Journal of Medicine, 269,* 1340.

Layzer, R. B. (1978). Myeloneuropathy after prolonged exposure to nitrous oxide. *Lancet, 2,* 1227–1230.

Layzer, R. B. (1985). Nitrous oxide abuse. In E. I. Eger (Ed.), *Nitrous oxide/N₂O* (pp. 249–257). New York: Elsevier.

Linden, C. (1990). Volatile substances of abuse. *Emergency Medicine Clinics of North America, 8,* 559–578.

Mathew, R. J., Wilson, W. H., & Tant, S. R. (1989). Regional cerebral blood flow changes associated with amyl nitrite inhalation. *British Journal of Addiction, 84,* 293–299.

Montoya-Cabrera, M. A. (1990). Neurotoxicology in Mexico and its relation to the general and work environment. In B. L. Johnson (Ed.), *Advances in neurobehavioral toxicology: Applications in environmental and occupational health* (pp. 35–57). Chelsea, MI: Lewis.

Nylander, I. (1962). "Thinner" addition in children and adolescents. *Acta Paedopsychiatrica, 29,* 273–283.

Prejean, J., & Gouvier, W. D. (1994). Neuropsychological sequelae of chronic recreational gasoline inhalation. *Archives of Clinical Neuropsychology, 9,* 173–174.

Press, E., & Done, A. K. (1967). Solvent sniffing. Physiologic effects and community control measures for intoxication from the intentional inhalation of organic solvents. *Journal of Pediatrics, 39,* 451–461.

Pryor, G. T. (1992). Animal research on solvent abuse. In C. W. Sharp, F. Beauvas, & R. Spence (Eds.), *Inhalant abuse: A volatile research agenda* (NIDA Research Monograph No. 129, pp. 233–258). Rockville, MD: National Institute on Drug Abuse.

Rosenberg, N. L., & Sharp, C. W. (1992). Solvent toxicity: A neurological focus. In C. W. Sharp, F. Beauvas, & R. Spence (Eds.), *Inhalant abuse: A volatile research agenda* (NIDA Research Monograph No. 129, pp. 117–171). Rockville, MD: National Institute on Drug Abuse.

Siegel, E., & Wason, S. (1990). Sudden death caused by inhalation of butane and propane. *New England Journal of Medicine, 323,* 1638.

Stacey, C. B., DiRocco, A., & Gould, R. J. (1992). Methionine in the treatment of nitrous oxide-induced neuropathy and myeloneuropathy. *Journal of Neurology, 239,* 401–403.

Tenenbein, M., & Pillay, N. (1993). Sensory evoked potentials in inhalant (volatile solvent) abuse. *Journal of Paediatrics and Child Health, 29,* 206–208.

Tohhara, S., Tani, N, Nakajima, T., & Tsuda, E. (1989). Clinical study of butane gas abuse: In comparison with toluene-based solvent and marihuana. *Arukoru Kenkyuto Yakubutsu Ison, 6,* 504–510.

Uitti, R. J., Snow, B. J., Shinotoh, H., Vingerhoets, F. J. G., Hayward, M., Hashimoto, S., Richmond, J., Markey, S. P., Markey, C. J., & Calne, D. B. (1994). Parkinsonism induced by solvent abuse. *Annals of Neurology, 35,* 616–619.

Wood, R. W. (1979). Reinforcing properties of inhaled substances. *Neurobehavioral Toxicology, 1* (Suppl. 1), 67–72.

Wood, R. W. (1988). The acute toxicity of nitrite inhalants. In H. W. Haverkos & J. A. Dougherty (Eds.), *Health hazards of nitrite inhalants* (NIDA Research Monograph No. 83, pp. 28–38). Rockville, MD: National Institute on Drug Abuse.

Wyse, D. G. (1973). Deliberate inhalation of volatile hydrocarbons: A review. *Canadian Medical Association Journal, 108,* 71–74.

Yanagita, T. S., Takahashi, K., Ishida, K., & Funamoto, H. (1970). Voluntary inhalation of volatile anesthetics and organic solvents by monkeys. *Japanese Journal of Clinical Pharmacology, 1,* 13–16.

18

Psychological and Psychiatric Consequences of Inhalants

STEPHEN H. DINWIDDIE

Introduction

Easily available, inexpensive, simple to conceal, and legal to possess, inhalants occupy a peculiar position among substances of abuse. Even defining the group of substances to be discussed has proven difficult, and terms such as glue-sniffing, solvent use, or volatile substance use have been suggested. Classifying these substances as inhalants, though perhaps the least misleading practice, is overly broad: Many psychoactive substances are, or can be, inhaled, yet cannabis, cocaine, or heroin are not classified as inhalants. Conversely, nitrite vasodilators or anesthetic gases, though sharing with the inhalants the route of ingestion, differ markedly in pharmacologic and toxicologic properties as well as the populations at risk for use, and are generally not considered to be members of the same class of abusable substance. What is left, therefore, is a heterogeneous collection of fuel gases, industrial solvents, cleaning agents, paints, and related compounds, sharing a common route of use and some chemical and pharmacological characteristics (Beauvais & Oetting, 1987).

STEPHEN H. DINWIDDIE • Department of Psychiatry, Finch University of Health Sciences, The Chicago Medical School, North Chicago, Illinois 60064.

Handbook of Substance Abuse: Neurobehavioral Pharmacology, edited by Tarter *et al.* Plenum Press, New York, 1998.

Along with tobacco, alcohol, and cannabis, inhalants are often among the first psychoactive substances to be used by youthful experimenters; unlike those substances, however, for most lifetime users, inhalant use is often abandoned relatively rapidly. Nonetheless, even if an individual is not a current user and has sustained no medical, psychological, or psychiatric consequences of use, knowledge of his or her status as a lifetime (ever) user may be of importance in assessing risk of subsequent substance use and associated psychopathology.

Epidemiology

Worldwide, lifetime prevalence of inhalant use varies substantially. A study of Brazilian college students found a rate of 28% (Silva, Barros, & de Magalhaes, 1994). Elsewhere in Central and South America, though prevalence appears to vary significantly between countries, lifetime inhalant use is extremely common, consistently exceeded only by tobacco and alcohol, and on a par with cannabis use (Baldivieso, 1995; Carlini-Cotrim, 1995; Duque, Rodriguez, & Huertas, 1995; Medina-Mora & Berenzon, 1995). Little is known about use in Africa, though there is evidence to suggest that lifetime use may be high, with studies reporting rates of 26% among secondary students in Nigeria (Obot, 1995) and 11% in Zimbabwe (Acuda & Eide, 1994).

By contrast, lifetime use may be as low as 1.5% among Japanese junior high school students, even though inhalants, as elsewhere in the world, are among the most commonly abused substances (Wada & Fukui, 1993). Much less is known regarding prevalence of use in other Asian countries, though there is evidence to suggest that it has become more common (or at least more frequently recognized) over the past decade (Kin & Navaratnam, 1995).

In the United States, rates have been estimated to be in the range of 5%–15% (Beauvais & Oetting, 1988b). A more recent estimate of 6.8% from the National Comorbidity Survey suggests that the lower end of this range may be a more accurate reflection of the rate in the general population (Anthony, Arria, & Johnson, 1995), though it is possible that inhalant .users may have been undersampled (Frank, 1995). By contrast, estimates of rates among younger people consistently have been higher: 14%–16% of eighth graders surveyed between 1987 and 1992 for the Monitoring the Future study and nearly 10% of respondents between 18 and 25 in the 1992 National Household Survey on Drug Abuse reported some lifetime use (Edwards & Oetting, 1995).

Estimates of rates in the United Kingdom appear to be comparable, ranging from 6%–10% (Cooke, Evans, & Farrow, 1988; Diamond et al., 1988; Ramsay, 1982). Less attention, apparently, has been paid to the phenomenon in other European countries, although there is evidence to suggest that either use or recognition of use is increasing in Central and Eastern European countries (Dinwiddie, 1996; Katona, 1995).

Within the United States, while it has been suggested that rates are higher among Hispanic youth, this association appears to be mediated by lower socioeconomic status rather than ethnicity (Frank, Marel, & Schmeidler, 1988; Mata & Andrew, 1988; Padilla, Padilla, Morales, Olmedo, & Ramirez, 1979; Vega, Zimmerman, Warheit, Apospori, & Gil, 1993). Consistent with the influence of economic forces, it has been estimated that nearly a third of American Indians on reservations have used

inhalants, with substantially lower rates reported among those not residing on reservations and presumably somewhat less affected by economic disadvantage (Beauvais & Oetting, 1988a; Edwards & Oetting, 1995). Interestingly, this does not appear to be the case among African Americans, where there is considerable evidence that lifetime use is somewhat less common, with rates approximately one half to two thirds those reported by whites (Compton et al., 1994; Edwards & Oetting, 1995; Epstein & Wieland, 1978; Vega et al, 1993).

Although inhalant users tend to be young, there is some evidence to suggest that the age distribution of users has broadened. Data from the Drug Awareness Warning Network (DAWN) in 1987 indicated that only 20% of contacts involved patients ages 17 or younger, while nearly half of contacts were with patients ages 26 or older (Colliver & Gampel, 1988). On the other hand, cases ascertained in this fashion are likely to be quite atypical, and population-based studies continue to demonstrate that age at onset of use is typically quite young. In a sample of 10,198 North Carolina middle- and high-school students, Hansen and Rose (1995) found a lifetime rate of 12.8% and a past-month use rate of 4.6%, with incidence apparently increasing among younger students (grades 6–8). While this may indicate a true increase, the phenomenon of lifetime prevalence appearing to decrease among high school seniors as compared with eighth graders has been noted elsewhere (in contrast to rates for other drug use, which tend to be stable) and most probably represents differential retention in school, with those using inhalants at markedly elevated risk for dropping out (Edwards & Oetting, 1995).

As with use of other psychoactive substances, there appears to be a gender difference in lifetime inhalant use. Data from the Monitoring the Future study indicate that, among sixth graders, 10.4% of boys as compared with 7.5% of girls reported use. This gap narrowed to 16.4% of boys and 15.9% of girls by 8th grade (the age of highest reported prevalence) and increased substantially by 12th grade,

15.1% of boys versus 8.6% of girls (Johnston, O'Malley, & Bachman, 1992).

So far, the discussion has focused entirely on lifetime ("ever") use. Comparison of lifetime and current (i.e., prior month) use indicates that only a minority of users report ongoing use. Among high school seniors, while 10%–13% reported lifetime use, only 2% reported use within the prior month (Johnston et al., 1992). Similarly, data from the National Comorbidity Study indicate that the risk of addiction, given the necessary precondition of use, is low, on the order of 4%, significantly lower than for other psychoactive substances (Anthony et al., 1995). However, in the DSM-IV Field Trial for substance use disorders, it was found that, while repeated inhalant use (defined as six or more occasions of use lifetime) was uncommon even in a sample enriched for substance use disorders, 23% of those who reported such use met proposed criteria for dependence, including symptoms of tolerance and withdrawal. An additional 10% met broader dependence criteria (not requiring dependence or withdrawal), and a further 18% met criteria for abuse, but not dependence (Cottler et al., 1995). Thus, it appears that while only a small proportion of those who ever have used inhalants develop significant problems related to use, a significant percentage of those who have repeatedly used, although a small population in absolute terms, will develop abuse or dependence.

Clinical experience is consistent with these observations. In the United States there are few specialized treatment programs for inhalant abusers, and inhalant-related problems appear to be an infrequent presenting complaint for substance abuse treatment. Taken together, these observations suggest that, for the majority of lifetime inhalant users, active use will have ceased soon after initiation; only for a small minority will use continue and progress to significant medical, psychological, and social consequences stemming directly from misuse of inhalants. In most cases evaluated by clinicians, therefore, inhalant use will not be an active problem. Nonetheless, in those individuals, inhalant use, even if long

since abandoned, may still be useful as a risk marker for significant problems. This does not imply that active use should be treated casually. Any inhalant use is risky and potentially fatal. Rather, from a public health standpoint, any lifetime use may identify a group at particularly high risk for a variety of medical, psychological, and social complications.

Medical Complications of Use

Little systematic study of risk of specific toxicity conveyed by inhalant use has been done, owing to the great variety of substances available and the admixture of chemical compounds contained in many preparations. Perhaps because of the heterogeneity of compounds and, consequently, different routes of metabolism, a variety of medical complications of inhalant misuse have been identified.

It should be emphasized that any inhalant use is potentially fatal. "Sudden sniffing death" (Bass, 1970) continues to occur on a regular basis, estimated to cause an average of two to three deaths per week in the United Kingdom alone (Ramsey, Taylor, Anderson, & Flanagan, 1995). Death in such cases appears to occur very rapidly after inhalation: The user may become excited, begin to run, and collapse within seconds (Bass, 1970). It is generally believed that the cause of death is cardiac arrhythmia, since inhalants are myocardial depressants and may sensitize the myocardium to the effects of epinephrine. This effect may be further enhanced by hypoxia, vagal stimulation due to laryngeal irritation from the vapors inhaled, or both. Risk appears quite random, and it has been reported that as many as one in five inhalant-related deaths occur in first-time users, though this estimate may be inflated by ignorance or active concealment of prior use by family or other informants (Adgey, Johnston, & McMechan, 1995; Johns, 1991; Ramsey et al., 1995; Shepherd, 1989; Wodka & Jeong, 1989).

Death may also result from aspiration of vomitus, anoxia from placement of a bag over the head, or respiratory depression due to the CNS depressant qualities of the substance used. It has been estimated that as many as 20% of inhalant-related deaths may occur in this fashion; in addition, in one study, death by trauma accounted for more than 10% of inhalant-related deaths (Ashton, 1990). Cause of death, however, may differ depending on the substance used, and choice of substance may affect the choice of method of administration (e.g., "bagging," squirting directly into the mouth), further affecting risk of mortality. In the United Kingdom, as noted by Ramsey and colleagues (1995), about 40% of fatalities associated with use of adhesives resulted from trauma, versus about 20% from direct toxic effects (presumably arrhythmia). For other inhalants, trauma accounted for only about 5% of deaths, with 60% stemming from direct toxicity and the remainder from aspiration or asphyxia. By contrast, in Bexar County, Texas, of 39 inhalant-related deaths identified between 1982 and 1988, only 7 (18%) were attributable to toxicity, with the remainder attributed to suicide (28%), homicide (23%), accident (26%), or cause unknown (5%) (Garriott, 1992).

Long-term use has been associated with deleterious effects on a number of organ systems. However, it should be noted that most such reports are based on small numbers of nonsystematically ascertained subjects, and tend therefore not to control for other potential causes of pathology. Alternatively, some reports are derived from industrial exposure, and therefore may not be appropriate models for the episodic, high-concentration exposure typical of inhalant abusers. Thus, such reports are uncertain guides as to the likelihood of developing these problems.

Because of route of use, pulmonary involvement is an obvious concern, with acute use potentially resulting in either a chemical pneumonitis or aspiration pneumonia. Long-term use may also lead to emphysema.

Renal involvement, either distal renal tubular acidosis or glomerulonephritis, has been reported both among abusers and among those occupationally exposed to toluene (Daniell, Couser, & Rosenstock, 1988; Narvarte, Saba, & Ramirez, 1989; Streicher, Cabow, Moss, Kono, & Kaehny, 1981; Taher, Anderson, McCartney, Popovtzer, & Schrier, 1974), though evidence supporting a causal link has been criticized (Carlisle *et al.*, 1991).

Other potential complications of use include bone marrow suppression (Flanagan, Ruprah, Meredith, & Ramsey, 1990; Linden, 1990) and hepatic toxicity, particularly after exposure to chloroform, carbon tetrachloride, or trichloroethylene (Marjot & McLeod, 1989). There have also been reports of microcephaly and craniofacial and limb abnormalities following prenatal exposure to toluene (Hersh, 1989; Hersh, Podurch, Rogers, & Weisskopf, 1985), though teratogenicity remains to be established, particularly given the association between inhalant use on the one hand and exposure to other drugs and poverty and consequent poor prenatal care on the other.

More attention has been paid to the risk of neurologic damage from repeated inhalant use. Although there has been some interest in relating manifestations of toxicity to specific inhalants, because of small numbers, variation in substances used and duration of use, nonsystematic sampling, and confounding from potential effects of other substance use, asphyxia, and head trauma (not unlikely in this population), less can be concluded regarding the risk and specificity of neurologic damage conveyed by use of specific substances than would be desirable, even among chronic abusers (Rosenberg & Sharp, 1992).

Hormes, Filley, and Rosenberg (1986), on the basis of imaging and clinical evaluation, found evidence of CNS damage in 65% of 20 chronic inhalant users, a rate quite comparable to the 6 out of 11 reported by Rosenberg, Spitz, Filley, Davis, and Schaumburg (1988). Specific cerebellar damage has been repeatedly noted (Boor & Hurtig, 1977; Grabski, 1961; Kelly, 1975; Lolin, 1989). While this may clear with abstinence, at least one case with significant loss of Purkinje cells has been reported (Escobar & Aruffo, 1980). Widespread cerebral demyelination leading to atrophy and dementia has also been noted (Al-Alousi, 1989; King, Day, Oliver, Lush, & Watson, 1981; Knox & Nelson, 1966; Lazar,

Ho, Melen, & Daghestani, 1983), though again the role of other potential causal factors is unclear. Cranial neuropathies (most notably optic neuropathy), as well as peripheral neuropathies and muscular weakness have also been reported; some of these findings in the past may have been further exacerbated by the sniffing of leaded gas (Goldings & Stewart, 1982; Herskowitz, Ishii, & Schaumburg, 1971; Keane, 1978; Prockop, Alt, & Tison, 1974; Robinson, 1978; Rosenberg & Sharp, 1992; Streicher *et al.*, 1981).

Abnormalities on EEG and evoked potential recording have been described (Hormes *et al.*, 1986; Metrick & Brenner, 1982), as have widespread deficits on neuropsychological testing (Allison & Jerrom, 1984; Tsushima & Towne, 1977). Again, however, a causal relationship is far from established; such deficits might precede and predispose to inhalant use, rather than result from it (Chadwick & Anderson, 1989; Ron, 1986).

Relation to Other Psychoactive Substance Use

As noted above, epidemiologic data suggest that most inhalant users rapidly abandon the practice, with only a small proportion continuing to use. Oetting, Edwards, and Beauvais (1988) have proposed a three-group typology of such users: Young inhalant users who become intoxicated relatively frequently (several times a month) on alcohol, cannabis, or inhalants; inhalant-dependent adults; and polydrug-using adolescents for whom inhalants represent a small and often transient part of what is a significant involvement with psychoactive substances.

Probably most often, inhalants represent a "gateway" drug, one of the first psychoactive substances to be used by youthful experimenters. Indeed, there is recent evidence to suggest that, at least among younger cohorts, inhalant use more often than not precedes use of cannabis (Edwards & Oetting, 1995). Given the health risks noted earlier, this practice is of concern even if inhalant use is rapidly abandoned. Perhaps even more important, however,

is the question of whether inhalant use is a marker for unusual liability to substance use or abuse: Are those who use inhalants (even if they have little total exposure) likely to have more extensive substance user "careers" than those who do not?

A number of case reports documenting progression from inhalant use to dependence on opiates have appeared (Davies, Thorley, & O'Connor, 1985; Merry, 1967; Skuse & Burrell 1982), and several large retrospective studies of opiate-dependent individuals in treatment have found substantial minorities with a history of inhalant use. Langrod (1970) reported that 22% of 422 treated heroin users had used inhalants, 14% more than six times; of those, about one third had used inhalants within 2 years of admission to treatment, indicating that inhalant use in that population was more persistent.

D'Amanda, Plumb, and Taintor (1977) reported a similar rate: 26% of 133 treated heroin addicts. In that sample, inhalant users also tended to report having used a greater variety of psychoactive substances on a lifetime basis than heroin addicts without a history of inhalant use. A somewhat higher rate (44% of 50 treated heroin addicts) was reported by Kramer (1972), balanced by a lower prevalence found in a later sample by Altenkirch and Kindermann (1986), 13% of 574 heroin addicts, although they again noted that inhalant use was associated with earlier age at onset of drug use and with more criminal behavior.

Such retrospective studies would seem to indicate that lifetime inhalant use is associated with elevated risk for exposure to other substances. Such samples, derived from clinical populations, are obviously strongly biased. However, population-based studies also have found an association with polysubstance use. Whitehead (1974), in a survey of Nova Scotia secondary school students, found that individuals who endorsed inhalant use were three times as likely to have used cannabis, eight times as likely to have used barbiturates or hallucinogens, and fourteen times as likely to report opiate use.

Using data from a large family study of alcoholism and criminality, Dinwiddie, Reich, and Cloninger (1991a) found that 93% of those who reported any lifetime inhalant use had used three or more additional classes of psychoactive drugs. In fact, two thirds had used drugs from every class inquired about (cannabis, opiates, sedative-hypnotics, stimulants, and hallucinogens). In addition, those individuals tended to begin use of other substances at a younger age than those who reported using those substances but had not tried inhalants.

The association with substantial lifetime polysubstance use, and particularly opiate use, further raises a question about other high-risk drug use, particularly drug injecting. Using the same database as the earlier study, Dinwiddie, Reich, and Cloninger (1991b) found an association with later drug injecting, with odds for injecting increased by a factor of 3.2 given a lifetime history of inhalant use. Subsequent work by Schutz, Chilcoat, and Anthony (1994), using a more representative sample (the 1990 Household Survey on Drug Abuse), also found a relationship, with inhalant users 5.4 times more likely to report drug injection as compared with those reporting no inhalant use. Similarly, using a sample of 545 drug users, Compton and colleagues (1994) found that lifetime inhalant use increased the odds of reporting drug injection by a factor of 3.6. Finally, preliminary data analysis from a large-scale, multicenter family study of alcoholism indicates that (restricting analysis to relatives only, to decrease ascertainment bias) 30% of lifetime inhalant users reported drug injection, corresponding to an increase in odds of 7.5 relative to nonusers. Inhalant users in that sample also were more likely to report other behaviors associated with elevated risk for HIV exposure (Dinwiddie, 1996).

Psychiatric Comorbidity

Given such high lifetime rates of polysubstance use, it is unsurprising to find high lifetime rates of psychoactive substance abuse, dependence, or both, among lifetime inhalant users. Dinwiddie, Reich, and Cloninger (1990) found that, among relatives of alcoholic or criminal probands, 50% of those with any lifetime inhalant use met diagnostic criteria for alcoholism, compared with 22% of those without a history of inhalant use. Preliminary analyses of data derived from a large, multicenter family study of alcoholism (the COGA project) are consistent with this observation, with 82% of users (versus 30% of nonusers) meeting *DSM-III-R* (American Psychiatric Association, 1987) criteria for Alcohol Dependence on a lifetime basis. Any history of inhalant use also conveyed elevated odds for dependence on cannabis, cocaine, other CNS stimulants, sedative-hypnotics, and opiates (Dinwiddie, 1996).

Regarding major psychiatric disorders, it is notable that few reports have linked inhalant use to chronic psychotic conditions. However, little systematic study of inhalant use among such individuals has appeared, and given the high rates of substance use in general among populations of schizophrenics, a high rate of lifetime inhalant use would not be surprising.

Mood disorders, although more commonly reported, also do not appear to be specifically associated with inhalant use. Primary depression appears to be uncommon, and while secondary depression is not infrequent, it appears more strongly associated with alcoholism, other substance dependence, and Antisocial Personality Disorder (ASPD), rather than inhalant use per se (Dinwiddie *et al.,* 1990).

Over the past three decades, delinquency has frequently been noted to be strongly associated with inhalant use (e.g. Barker & Adams, 1963; Jacobs & Ghodse, 1988; Lockhart & Lennox, 1983; Oetting & Webb, 1992; Press & Done, 1967). Such an association is unsurprising, given that early studies focused primarily on youths ascertained through contact with the legal system. Nonetheless, the finding that youths with significant behavioral difficulties or who had been remanded to residential treatment had markedly elevated rates of inhalant use was suggestive, again, that inhalant use might be an indicator of multiple difficulties, extending beyond involvement in substance use. Indeed, there is evidence that even compared with other delinquents, inhalant users tend to develop behavioral problems earlier and commit a wider variety of crimes than delinquents without a history of inhalant use (Reed & May, 1984).

Diagnostically, this finding (particularly given the association with polysubstance use) suggests elevated risk for ASPD. Crites and Schuckit (1979), evaluating 757 youths referred to an alcohol counseling program, found that 23% of those with a history of inhalant use met criteria for this diagnosis. Similarly, Dinwiddie and colleagues (1990) found a rate of 63% among inhalant users derived from the alcoholism family study noted earlier. Preliminary analysis using data from the COGA project also indicates a very powerful association, with 44% of men and 16% of women with a history of inhalant use meeting diagnostic criteria for ASPD.

It should be noted that these figures are likely to be overestimates, given what is known of the population base rates of lifetime inhalant use and ASPD. Nonetheless, they strongly suggest that individuals at high risk for ASPD and polysubstance use are differentially likely to have experimented with inhalants. Furthermore, given that inhalant use typically begins at an early age, these data further suggest that identification of current inhalant users might define a population at markedly elevated risk for a myriad of behavioral difficulties and progression of substance use.

Precursors to Inhalant Use and Prevention Efforts

As mentioned, inhalant use appears to be associated with delinquent behavior, family disruption, early onset of experimentation with other substances, and premature termination of education (Oetting & Webb, 1992)—factors which, rather than representing a clear causal chain, are perhaps better conceived as being powerfully interrelated and interacting to result in an outcome which often is poor. In most cases, therefore, inhalant use might best be conceived of as a marker of risk for such problems rather than necessarily being an etiologic

factor in later development of addiction, other significant psychopathology, or both.

These observations may in turn shape prevention efforts. Efforts at primary prevention, by decreasing exposure, are likely to be of some benefit; there is evidence that measures designed to reduce access to inhalants can be successful. In theory at least, such measures are likely to be most effective among those individuals with least liability to use (and presumably with less liability to other substance use, as well). Nonetheless, prevention of exposure should at least decrease risk of inhalant-related fatalities: Given that most users use inhalants only a few times, the population "at risk" for sudden death will be composed primarily of casual users, even though a small number of long-term users will have higher exposure and, hence, higher risk.

However, because of the ubiquitous nature of inhalants, comprehensive restriction is impossible, and one result of restriction may be a shift to use of more dangerous and toxic compounds (Anderson, 1990; Ramsey, Anderson, Bloor, & Flanagan, 1989). Thus, further prevention and treatment efforts might be focused on that group identified through inhalant use and differentially made up of individuals with multiple risk factors, at elevated risk for substance dependence and antisocial personality disorder, who might respond to more structured and focused interventions.

There appears to be little information on specialized treatment of those individuals dependent primarily on inhalants. Such individuals, obviously, are at elevated risk for end-organ diseases related to inhalant use, as well to as the deleterious effects of other psychoactive substances. What little information is available about treatment indicates that response is disappointing. The finding of substantial overlap with other substance abuse and dependence and substantial psychiatric comorbidity suggests that such individuals are, as a group, likely to have unusually numerous problems and few resources. There appears to be little role for pharmacotherapy (at least trials are lacking), and little empirical work evaluating the role of psychosocial treatments has appeared (Dinwiddie, Zorumski, & Rubin, 1987; Jumper-Thurman & Beauvais, 1992; McSherry, 1988; Skuse & Burrell, 1982).

Conclusion

Easily available and potentially lethal, inhalants represent one of the first psychoactive substances to be used by young substance experimenters. Use may also be instituted secondarily, by those with substantial drug abuse histories, when unable to obtain their drug of choice. Even though for most, inhalant use represents a relatively brief period of experimentation, any history of use may be an indicator of significant exposure to illicit psychoactive substances, or of substantially elevated risk for such exposure in the near future, as well as being a clinical indicator of risk for family disruption, premature termination of education, and involvement in delinquent activities.

References

Acuda, S. W., & Eide, A. H. (1994). Epidemiological study of drug use in urban and rural secondary schools in Zimbabwe. *Central African Journal of Medicine, 40,* 207–212.

Adgey, A. A., Johnston, P. W., & McMechan, S. (1995). Sudden cardiac death and substance abuse. *Resuscitation, 29,* 219–221.

Al-Alousi, L. M. (1989). Pathology of volatile substance abuse: A case report and a literature review. *Medicine Science and the Law, 29,* 189–202.

Allison, W. M., & Jerrom, D. W. (1984). Glue sniffing: A pilot study of the cognitive effects of long-term use. *International Journal of the Addictions, 19,* 453–458.

Altenkirch, H., & Kindermann, W. (1986). Inhalant abuse and heroin addiction: A comparative study on 574 opiate addicts with and without a history of sniffing. *Addictive Behaviors, 11,* 93–104.

American Psychiatric Association. (1987). *Diagnostic and statistical manual of mental disorders* (3rd ed., rev.). Washington, DC: Author.

Anderson, H. R. (1990). Increase in deaths from deliberate inhalation of fuel gases and pressurized aerosols. *British Medical Journal, 301,* 41.

Anthony, J. C., Arria, A. M., & Johnson, E. O. (1995). Epidemiological and public health issues for tobacco, alcohol, and other drugs. In J. M. Oldham & M. B. Riba (Eds.), *Annual review of psychiatry* (Vol. 14, pp. 15–49). Washington, DC: American Psychiatric Press.

Ashton, C. H. (1990). Solvent abuse. *British Medical Journal, 300,* 135–136.

Baldivieso, L. E. (1995). Inhalant use in Bolivia. In N. Kozel, Z. Sloboda, & M. De La Rosa (Eds.), *Epidemiology of inhalant abuse: An international perspective* (NIDA Research Monograph No. 148, pp. 50–63). Rockville, MD: National Institute on Drug Abuse.

Barker, G. H., & Adams, W. T. (1963). Glue sniffers. *Sociology and Social Research, 47,* 298–310.

Bass, M. (1970). Sudden sniffing death. *Journal of the American Medical Association, 212,* 2075–2079.

Beauvais, F., & Oetting, E. R. (1987). Toward a clear definition of inhalant abuse. *International Journal of the Addictions, 22,* 779–784.

Beauvais, F., & Oetting, E. R. (1988a). Indian youth and inhalants: An update. In R. A. Crider & B. A. Rouse (Eds.), *Epidemiology of inhalant abuse: An update* (NIDA Research Monograph No. 85, pp. 34–48). Rockville, MD: National Institute on Drug Abuse.

Beauvais, F., & Oetting, E. R. (1988b). Inhalant abuse by young children. In R. A. Crider & B. A. Rouse (Eds.), *Epidemiology of inhalant abuse: An update* (NIDA Research Monograph No. 85, pp. 30–33). Rockville, MD: National Institute on Drug Abuse.

Boor, J. W., & Hurtig, H. I. (1977). Persistent cerebellar ataxia after exposure to toluene. *Annals of Neurology, 2,* 440–442.

Carlini-Cotrim, B. (1995). Inhalant use among Brazilian youths. In N. Kozel, Z. Sloboda, & M. De La Rosa (Eds.), *Epidemiology of inhalant abuse: An international perspective* (NIDA Research Monograph No. 148, pp. 64–78). Rockville, MD: National Institute on Drug Abuse.

Carlisle, E. J., Donnelley, S. M., Vasuvattakul, S., Kamel, K. S., Tobe, S., & Halperin, S. L. (1991). Glue-sniffing and distal renal tubular acidosis: Sticking to the facts. *Journal of the American Society of Nephrology, 1,* 1019–1027.

Chadwick, O. F., & Anderson, H. R. (1989). Neuropsychological consequences of volatile substance abuse: A review. *Human Toxicology, 8,* 307–312.

Colliver, J. D., & Gampel, J. C. (1988). *Inhalant data in DAWN* (Paper prepared for the Division of Epidemiology and Statistical Analysis, NIDA, pp. 1–28). Rockville, MD: National Institute on Drug Abuse.

Compton, W. M., Cottler, L. B., Dinwiddie, S. H., Spitznagel, E., Mager, D. E., & Asmus, G. (1994). Inhalant use: Characteristics and predictors. *American Journal on Addictions, 3,* 263–274.

Cooke, B. R., Evans, D. A., & Farrow, S. C. (1988). Solvent misuse in secondary schoolchildren: A prevalence study. *Community Medicine, 10,* 8–13.

Cottler, L. B., Schuckit, M. A., Helzer, J. E., Crowley, T., Woody, G., & Nathan, P. (1995). The *DSM-IV* Field Trial for Substance Use Disorders: Major results. *Drug and Alcohol Dependence, 38,* 59–69.

Crites, J., & Schuckit, M. A. (1979). Solvent misuse in adolescents at a community alcohol center. *Journal of Clinical Psychiatry, 40,* 39–43.

D'Amanda, C., Plumb, M. M., & Taintor, Z. (1977). Heroin addicts with a history of glue sniffing: A deviant group within a deviant group. *International Journal of the Addictions, 12,* 255–270.

Daniell, W. E., Couser, W. G., & Rosenstock, L. (1988). Occupational solvent exposure and glomerulonephritis. *Journal of the American Medical Association, 259,* 2280–2283.

Davies, B., Thorley, A., & O'Connor, D. (1985). Progression of addiction careers in young adult solvent misusers. *British Medical Journal, 290,* 109–110.

Diamond, I. D., Pritchard, C., Choudry, N., Fielding, M., Cox, M., & Bushnell, D. (1988). The incidence of drug and solvent misuse among southern English normal comprehensive schoolchildren. *Public Health, 102,* 107–114.

Dinwiddie, S. H. (1996). Volatile Substances. In H. Rommelspacher & M. Schuckit (Eds.), *Balliere's clinical psychiatry* (pp. 501–516). London: Balliere Tindall.

Dinwiddie, S. H., Zorumski, C., & Rubin, E. H. (1987). Psychiatric correlates of chronic solvent abuse. *Journal of Clinical Psychiatry, 48,* 334–337.

Dinwiddie, S. H., Reich, T., & Cloninger, C. R. (1990). Solvent use and psychiatric comorbidity. *British Journal of Addiction, 85,* 1647–1656.

Dinwiddie, S. H., Reich, T., & Cloninger, C. R. (1991a). The relationship of solvent use to other substance use. *American Journal of Drug and Alcohol Abuse, 17,* 173–186.

Dinwiddie, S. H., Reich, T., & Cloninger, C. R. (1991b). Solvent abuse as a precursor to intravenous drug abuse. *Comprehensive Psychiatry, 32,* 133–140.

Duque, L. F., Rodriguez, E., & Huertas, J. (1995). Use of inhalants in Colombia. In N. Kozel, Z. Sloboda, & M. De La Rosa (Eds.), *Epidemiology of inhalant abuse: An international perspective* (NIDA Research Monograph No. 148, pp. 79–99). Rockville, MD: National Institute on Drug Abuse.

Edwards, R. W., & Oetting, E. R. (1995). Inhalant use in the United States. In N. Kozel, Z. Sloboda, & M. De La Rosa (Eds.), *Epidemiology of inhalant abuse: An international perspective* (NIDA Research Monograph No. 148, pp. 8–28). Rockville, MD: National Institute on Drug Abuse.

Epstein, M. H., & Wieland, W. F. (1978). Prevalence survey of inhalant abuse. *International Journal of the Addictions, 13,* 271–284.

Escobar, A., & Aruffo, C. (1980). Chronic thinner intoxication: Clinico-pathologic report of a human case. *Journal of Neurology, Neurosurgery and Psychiatry, 43,* 986–994.

Flanagan, R. J., Ruprah, M., Meredith, T. J., & Ramsey, J. D. (1990). An introduction to the clinical toxicology of volatile substances. *Drug Safety, 5,* 359–383.

Frank, B. (1995). Gathering epidemiologic information on inhalant abuse: Some methodological issues. In N. Kozel, Z. Sloboda, & M. De La Rosa (Eds.), *Epidemiology of inhalant abuse: An international per-*spective (NIDA Research Monograph No. 148, pp. 260–273). Rockville, MD: National Institute on Drug Abuse.

Frank, B., Marel, R., & Schmeidler, J. (1988). The continuing problem of youthful solvent abuse in New York State. In R. A. Crider & B. A. Rouse (Eds.), *Epidemiology of inhalant abuse: An update* (NIDA Research Monograph No. 85, pp. 77–105). Rockville, MD: National Institute on Drug Abuse.

Garriott, J. C. (1992). Death among inhalant abusers. In C. W. Sharp, F. Beauvais & R. Spence (Eds.), *Inhalant abuse: A volatile research agenda* (NIDA Monograph No. 129, pp. 181–192). Rockville, MD: National Institute on Drug Abuse.

Goldings, A. S., & Stewart, R. M. (1982). Organic lead encephalopathy: Behavioral change and movement disorder following gasoline inhalation. *Journal of Clinical Psychiatry, 43,* 70–72.

Grabski, D. A. (1961). Toluene sniffing producing cerebellar degeneration. *American Journal of Psychiatry, 118,* 461–462.

Hansen, W. B., & Rose, L. A. (1995). Recreational use of inhalant drugs by adolescents: A challenge for family physicians. *Family Medicine, 27,* 383–387.

Hersh, J. H. (1989). Toluene embryopathy: Two new cases. *Journal of Medical Genetics, 26,* 333–337.

Hersh, J. H., Podurch, P. E., Rogers, G., & Weisskopf, B. (1985). Toluene embryopathy. *Journal of Pediatrics, 106,* 922–927.

Herskowitz, A., Ishii, N., & Schaumburg, H. (1971). N-hexane neuropathy. *New England Journal of Medicine, 285,* 82–85.

Hormes, J. T., Filley, C. M., & Rosenberg, N. L. (1986). Neurologic sequelae of chronic solvent vapor abuse. *Neurology, 36,* 698–702.

Jacobs, A. M., & Ghodse, A. H. (1988). Delinquency and regular solvent abuse: An unfavourable combination? *British Journal of Addiction, 83,* 965–968.

Johns, A. (1991). Volatile solvent abuse and 963 deaths. *British Journal of Addiction, 86,* 1053–1056.

Johnston, L. D., O'Malley, P. M., & Bachman, J. G. (1992). *Smoking, drinking, and illicit drug use among American secondary school students, college students, and young adults, 1975–1991* (DHHS Publication No. (ADM)93-3480). Washington, DC: U.S. Government Printing Office.

Jumper-Thurman, P., & Beauvais, F. (1992). Treatment of volatile solvent abusers. In C. W. Sharp, F. Beauvais, & R. Spence (Eds.), *Inhalant abuse: A volatile research agenda* (NIDA Monograph No. 129, pp. 203–213). Rockville, MD: National Institute on Drug Abuse.

Katona, E. (1995). Inhalant abuse: A Hungarian review. In N. Kozel, Z. Sloboda, & M. De La Rosa (Eds.), *Epidemiology of inhalant abuse: An international perspective* (NIDA Research Monograph No. 148, pp. 100–120). Rockville, MD: National Institute on Drug Abuse.

Keane, J. R. (1978). Toluene optic neuropathy. *Annals of Neurology, 4,* 390.

Kelly, T. W. (1975). Prolonged cerebellar dysfunction associated with paint-sniffing. *Pediatrics, 56,* 605–606.

Kin, F., & Navaratnam (1995). An overview of inhalant abuse in selected countries of Asia and the Pacific region. In N. Kozel, Z. Sloboda, & M. De La Rosa (Eds.), *Epidemiology of inhalant abuse: An international perspective* (NIDA Research Monograph No. 148, pp. 29–49). Rockville, MD: National Institute on Drug Abuse.

King, M. D., Day, R. E., Oliver, J. S., Lush, M., & Watson, J. M. (1981). Solvent encephalopathy. *British Medical Journal, 283,* 663–665.

Knox, J. W., & Nelson, J. R. (1966). Permanent encephalopathy from toluene inhalation. *New England Journal of Medicine, 275,* 1494–1496.

Kramer, J. P. (1972). The adolescent addict. *Clinical Pediatrics, 11,* 382–385.

Langrod, J. (1970). Secondary drug use among heroin users. *International Journal of the Addictions, 5,* 611–635.

Lazar, R. B., Ho, S. U., Melen, O., & Daghestani, A. N. (1983). Multifocal central nervous system damage caused by toluene abuse. *Neurology, 33,* 1337–1340.

Linden, C. H. (1990). Volatile substances of abuse. *Emergency Medicine Clinics of North America, 8,* 559–578.

Lockhart, W. H., & Lennox, M. (1983). The extent of solvent abuse in a regional secure unit sample. *Journal of Adolescence, 6,* 43–55.

Lolin, Y. (1989). Chronic neurological toxicity associated with exposure to volatile substances. *Human Toxicology, 8,* 293–300.

Marjot, R., & McLeod, A. A. (1989). Chronic non-neurological toxicity from volatile substance abuse. *Human Toxicology, 8,* 301–308.

Mata, A. G., & Andrew, S. R. (1988). Inhalant abuse in a small rural south Texas community: A social epidemiological overview. In R. A. Crider & B. A. Rouse (Eds.), *Epidemiology of inhalant abuse: An update* (NIDA Research Monograph No. 85, pp. 49–76). Rockville, MD: National Institute on Drug Abuse.

McSherry, T. M. (1988). Program experiences with the solvent abuser in Philadelphia. In R. A. Crider & B. A. Rouse (Eds.), *Epidemiology of inhalant abuse: An update* (NIDA Research Monograph No. 85, pp. 106–120). Rockville, MD: National Institute on Drug Abuse.

Medina-Mora, M. E., & Berenzon, S. (1995). Epidemiology of inhalant abuse in Mexico. In N. Kozel, Z. Sloboda, & M. De La Rosa (Eds.), *Epidemiology of inhalant abuse: An international perspective* (NIDA Research Monograph No. 148, pp. 136–174). Rockville, MD: National Institute on Drug Abuse.

Merry, J. (1967). Glue sniffing and heroin abuse. *British Medical Journal, 2,* 360.

Metrick, S. A., & Brenner, R. P. (1982). Abnormal brainstem auditory evoked potentials in chronic paint sniffers. *Annals of Neurology, 12,* 553–556.

Narvarte, J., Saba, S. R., & Ramirez, G. (1989). Occupational exposure to organic solvents causing chronic tubulointerstitial nephritis. *Archives of Internal Medicine, 149,* 154–158.

Obot, I. S. (1995). Epidemiology of inhalant abuse in Nigeria. In N. Kozel, Z. Sloboda, & M. De La Rosa (Eds.), *Epidemiology of inhalant abuse: An international perspective* (NIDA Research Monograph No. 148, pp. 175–190). Rockville, MD: National Institute on Drug Abuse.

Oetting, E. R., & Webb, J. (1992). Psychosocial characteristics and their links with inhalants: A research agenda. In C. W. Sharp, F. Beauvais, & R. Spence (Eds.), *Inhalant abuse: A volatile research agenda* (NIDA Monograph No. 129, pp. 59–97). Rockville, MD: National Institute on Drug Abuse.

Oetting, E. R., Edwards, R. W., & Beauvais, F. (1988). Social and psychological factors underlying inhalant abuse. In R. A. Crider & B. A. Rouse (Eds.), *Epidemiology of inhalant abuse: An update* (NIDA Research Monograph No. 85, pp. 172–203). Rockville, MD: National Institute on Drug Abuse.

Padilla, E. R., Padilla, A. M., Morales, A., Olmedo, E. L., & Ramirez, R. (1979). Inhalant, marijuana, and alcohol abuse among barrio children and adolescents. *International Journal of the Addictions, 14,* 945–964.

Press, E., & Done, A. K. (1967). Physiologic effects and community control measures for intoxication from the intentional inhalation of organic solvents: I. *Pediatrics, 39,* 451–461.

Prockop, L. D., Alt, M., & Tison, J. (1974). "Huffer's" neuropathy. *Journal of the American Medical Association, 229,* 1083–1084.

Ramsay, A. W. (1982). Solvent abuse: An educational perspective. *Human Toxicology, 1,* 265–270.

Ramsey, J., Anderson, H. R., Bloor, K., & Flanagan, R. J. (1989). An introduction to the practice, prevalence and chemical toxicology of volatile substance abuse. *Human Toxicology, 8,* 261–269.

Ramsey, J., Taylor, J., Anderson, H. R., & Flanagan, R. J. (1995). Volatile substance abuse in the United Kingdom. In N. Kozel, Z. Sloboda, & M. De La Rosa (Eds.), *Epidemiology of inhalant abuse: An international perspective* (NIDA Research Monograph No. 148, pp. 205–249). Rockville, MD: National Institute on Drug Abuse.

Reed, B. J., & May, P. A. (1984). Inhalant use and juvenile delinquency: A control study in Albuquerque, New Mexico. *International Journal of the Addictions, 19,* 789–803.

Robinson, R. O. (1978). Tetraethyl lead poisoning from gasoline sniffing. *Journal of the American Medical Association, 240,* 1473–1474.

Ron, M. (1986). Volatile substance abuse: A review of possible long-term neurological, intellectual and psychiatric sequelae. *British Journal of Psychiatry, 148,* 235–246.

Rosenberg, N. L., & Sharp, C. W. (1992). Solvent toxicity: A neurological focus. In C. W. Sharp, F. Beauvais, & R. Spence (Eds.), *Inhalant abuse: A volatile research agenda* (NIDA Monograph No. 129, pp. 117–171). Rockville, MD: National Institute on Drug Abuse.

Rosenberg, N. L., Spitz, M. C., Filley, C. M., Davis, K. A., & Schaumburg, H. H. (1988). Central nervous system effects of chronic toluene abuse—Clinical, brainstem evoked response and magnetic resonance imaging studies. *Neurotoxicology and Teratology, 10,* 489–495.

Schutz, C. G., Chilcoat, H. D., & Anthony, J. C. (1994). The association between sniffing inhalants and injecting drugs. *Comprehensive Psychiatry, 35,* 99–105.

Shepherd, R. T. (1989) Mechanism of sudden death associated with volatile substance abuse. *Human Toxicology, 8,* 287–292.

Silva, M. T., Barros, R. S., & de Magalhaes, M. P. (1994). Use of marijuana and other drugs by college students of Sao Paulo, Brazil. *The International Journal of the Addictions, 29,* 1045–1056.

Skuse, D., & Burrell, S. (1982). A review of solvent abusers and their management by a child psychiatric out-patient service. *Human Toxicology, 1,* 321–329.

Streicher, H. Z., Cabow, P., Moss, A., Kono, D., & Kaehny, W. D. (1981). Syndromes of toluene sniffing in adults. *Annals of Internal Medicine, 94,* 758–762.

Taher, S. M., Anderson, R. J., McCartney, R., Popovtzer, M. M., & Schrier, R. W. (1974). Renal tubular acidosis associated with toluene "sniffing." *New England Journal of Medicine, 290,* 765–768.

Tsushima, W. T., & Towne, W. S. (1977). Effects of paint sniffing on neuropsychological test performance. *Journal of Abnormal Psychology, 86,* 402–407.

Vega, W. A., Zimmerman, R. S., Warheit, G. J., Apospori, E., & Gil, A. G. (1993). Risk factors for early adolescent drug use in four ethnic and racial groups. *American Journal of Public Health, 83,* 185–189.

Wada, K., & Fukui, S. (1993). Prevalence of volatile solvent inhalation among junior high school students in Japan and background life style of users. *Addiction, 88,* 89–100.

Whitehead, P. C. (1974). Multidrug use: Supplementary perspectives. *International Journal of the Addictions, 9,* 185–204.

Wodka, R. M., & Jeong, E. W. (1989). Cardiac effects of inhaled typewriter correction fluid. *Annals of Internal Medicine, 110,* 91–92.

VII

Nicotine

19

Pharmacology of Nicotine

NEAL L. BENOWITZ

Introduction

Nicotine has been consumed in the form of tobacco and other plants for many hundreds of years. The compulsive use of tobacco has been observed in nearly every culture into which tobacco has been introduced. About 25% of adult Americans smoke despite, in most cases, a desire to quit and common knowledge of the health hazards (Centers for Disease Control, 1987). Their failure to quit smoking is attributable in large part to the addictive properties of nicotine. Nicotine is also available as a pharmaceutical agent, marketed as chewing gum, transdermal delivery systems, nasal spray, and inhaler to help people stop smoking. This chapter examines the mechanisms of action and pharmacologic properties of nicotine in humans, the role of nicotine in determining cigarette-smoking behavior, and the use of nicotine as medication for diseases other than tobacco addiction. The reader is also referred to the 1987 Surgeon General's Report, *The Health Consequences of Cigarette Smoking: Addiction,* for a detailed review of the pharmacology and toxicology of nicotine and its role in tobacco addiction (U.S. Department of Health and Human Services, 1988). Treatment of tobacco addiction, including the use of nicotine replacement medications, is discussed elsewhere in this volume.

Mechanisms of Action

Nicotine is a tertiary amine consisting of a pyridine and a pyrrolidine ring. (S)-Nicotine, found in tobacco, binds stereoselectively to nicotinic cholinergic receptors. (R)-Nicotine, found in small quantities in cigarette smoke due to racemization during the pyrolysis process, and commonly used in pharmacologic studies, is a weak agonist at cholinergic receptors.

Nicotinic cholinergic receptors are found in the brain, autonomic ganglia, and the neuromuscular junction. The neuromuscular nicotinic cholinergic receptor has been well characterized to be a ligand-gated ion channel composed of five subunits (Changeux, Galzi, Devillers-Thiery, & Betrand, 1992).

Most relevant to nicotine addiction are the neuronal nicotinic acetylcholine receptors. These receptors are found throughout the brain, with the greatest number of binding sites in the cortex, thalamus, and interpeduncular nucleus, and substantial binding in the amygdala, septum, and brain stem motor nuclei and locus ceruleus (Clarke, Schwartz, Paul, Pert, & Pert, 1985). Neuronal acetylcholine receptors are composed of alpha and beta subunits. There is much diversity in nicotinic cholinergic receptors with alpha-2 through alpha-9 and beta-2 through beta-4 subunits identified in brain tissues (McGehee

NEAL L. BENOWITZ • Departments of Medicine, Psychiatry, and Biopharmaceutical Sciences, University of California at San Francisco, San Francisco, California 94143.

Handbook of Substance Abuse: Neurobehavioral Pharmacology, edited by Tarter *et al.* Plenum Press, New York, 1998.

& Role, 1995). The predominant neuronal receptor is alpha-4, beta-2, which accounts for more than 90% of high-affinity binding in the rat brain. The alpha-7–containing receptors are most likely responsible for α-bungaratoxin and low-affinity nicotine binding (Seguela, Wadiche, Dineley-Miller, Dani, & Patrick, 1993). Different nicotinic cholinergic receptors are found in different areas of the brain and have different chemical conductances for sodium and calcium and different sensitivity to different nicotinic agonists, and result in correspondingly different pharmacologic actions (for review, see McGehee & Role, 1995). Diversity of nicotinic cholinergic receptors may explain the multiple effects of nicotine in humans, and may present targets for specific nicotinic agonists or antagonist therapies.

When nicotine binds to nicotine receptors, allosteric changes occur, such that there are several different functional states. These include the resting state, an activated state (channel open), and two desensitized states (channel closed) (Lena & Changeux, 1993). The transition and persistence of receptors in the desensitized state is believed to explain tachyphylaxis and perhaps the observation that tolerance to nicotine is associated with an increased number of nicotinic cholinergic receptors (i.e., similar to a response to an antagonist in other receptor systems) (Wonnacott, 1990). An increased number of nicotine receptors has been observed both in experimental animals during nicotine treatment and in human smokers at autopsy (Benwell, Balfour, & Anderson, 1988; Collins, Luo, Selvaag, & Marks, 1994).

Nicotinic receptors appear to be located both on cell bodies and at nerve terminals. All nicotine receptors are permeable to calcium ions. Nicotinic receptor activation works, at least in part and possibly in the main, by facilitating the release of neurotransmitters, including acetylcholine, norepinephrine, dopamine, serotonin, beta endorphin, glutamate, and others. Nicotine also releases growth hormone, prolactin, and ACTH. Behavioral rewards from nicotine and perhaps nicotine addiction as well appear to be linked to dopamine release, particularly in the nigrostriatal region (Corrigall, Coen, & Adamson, 1994). Most of the behavioral effects of nicotine in people are believed to be mediated by actions on central nervous system receptors. However, activation of the brain by afferent receptors may also contribute. Activation of nicotinic cholinergic receptors in the adrenal medulla releases epinephrine and beta endorphin.

Two issues are particularly relevant in understanding the pharmacodynamics of nicotine: a complex dose–response relationship and the development of tolerance produced by exposure to nicotine. In experimental preparations, nicotine in low doses causes ganglionic stimulation, but in high doses it causes ganglionic blockade after brief stimulation. This biphasic response pattern is observed in the intact organism as well, although the mechanisms are far more complex. At very low doses, similar to those seen during cigarette smoking, the cardiovascular effects appear to be mediated by the central nervous system, either through activation of chemoreceptor afferent pathways or by direct effects on the brain stem (Comroe, 1960; Su, 1982). The net result is sympathetic neural discharge with an increase in blood pressure and heart rate. At higher doses, nicotine may act directly on the peripheral nervous system, producing ganglionic stimulation and the release of adrenal catecholamines. With extremely high doses, nicotine produces hypotension and slowing of the heart rate, mediated by either peripheral ganglionic blockade, vagal afferent nerve stimulation, or direct depressor effects mediated by effects on the brain.

A second pharmacologic issue of importance is development of tolerance. Tolerance is usually defined as a state in which, after repeated doses, a given dose of a drug produces less effect than before, or in which increasing doses are required to achieve the effect observed with the first dose. Pharmacodynamic tolerance can be further defined as a state in which a particular concentration of a drug at a receptor site (in the intact organism this is approximated by the concentration in blood) produces a lesser effect than it did after a previous exposure.

Studies in animals demonstrate rapid development of tolerance to many effects of nicotine, although tolerance may not be complete (Marks, Stitzel, & Collins, 1985). Smokers know that tolerance develops to some effects of smoking. The first cigarette one smokes as a teenager commonly produces dizziness, nausea, and vomiting, effects to which the smoker rapidly becomes tolerant. Tolerance to subjective effects and acceleration of the heart rate develop within a day in regular smokers (West & Russell, 1987). Tolerance may develop to toxic effects, such as nausea, vomiting, and pallor, even during the 8-hr course of an accidental nicotine poisoning, despite the persistence of nicotine in the blood in extremely high concentrations (200–300 ng/ml) (Benowitz, Lake, Keller, & Lee, 1987).

Absorption of Nicotine from Tobacco and Nicotine Medications

Nicotine is distilled from burning tobacco and is carried proximally on tar droplets (0.1–1.0 μM) which are inhaled and deposited in the small airways and alveoli. The absorption of nicotine across biologic membranes depends on pH. The pH of smoke from flue-cured tobaccos found in most cigarettes is acidic (pH 5.5). At this pH, the nicotine is primarily ionized. In this state, it does not cross membranes rapidly. Consequently, there is little buccal absorption of nicotine from cigarette smoke, even when it is held in the mouth (Gori, Benowitz, & Lynch, 1986). The pH of smoke from air-cured tobaccos, such as those in pipes, cigars, and in a few European cigarettes, is alkaline (pH 8.5), and nicotine is primarily un-ionized. Nicotine from such products is absorbed well through the mouth.

When tobacco smoke reaches the small airways and alveoli of the lung, the nicotine is absorbed rapidly, regardless of the pH of the smoke. Blood concentrations of nicotine rise quickly during cigarette smoking and peak at its completion (Figure 1). Presumably, the rapid absorption of nicotine from cigarette smoke through the lung is the result of the huge surface area of the alveoli and small airways and the dissolution of nicotine into fluid of physiologic pH, which facilitates transfer across cell membranes.

Chewing tobacco, snuff, and nicotine gum are buffered to an alkaline pH to facilitate the absorption of nicotine through the mucous membranes. Concentrations of nicotine in the blood rise gradually with use of smokeless tobacco and tend to reach a plateau after about 30 min, with the levels persisting and declining only slowly over 2 hr or more (Figure 1).

Transdermal nicotine systems deliver 5–22 mg over 16–24 hr, depending on the patch. Nicotine is absorbed slowly, resulting in a relatively steady level of nicotine, substantial development of tolerance, and little, if any, psychological effect (Benowitz, 1995). Nicotine gum results in the systemic absorption of 1 or 2 mg from the 2- or 4-mg nicotine gums, respectively, over 20–30 min. This results in moderate subjective effects, but less than that of smoking a cigarette. Blood levels of nicotine rise with each piece of nicotine gum and fall between pieces, and blood levels of nicotine with typical levels of use are substantially less than those derived from cigarette smoking (Benowitz, Jacob, & Savanapridi, 1987). Nicotine nasal spray delivers 1.0 mg nicotine to the nostrils, of which 0.5 mg is absorbed systemically (Johansson, Olsson, Bende, Carlsson, & Gunnarsson, 1991). Nasal nicotine is very rapidly absorbed and results in more intense subjective effects than other types of nicotine replacement therapy. Nicotine nasal spray is initially perceived as irritating and unpleasant, but after a few days tolerance develops to these noxious effects. The nicotine inhaler is a plastic device that resembles a cigarette and contains a refillable nicotine cartridge. The inhaler is puffed or sucked for 20–30 min. The nicotine inhaler delivers nicotine as an aerosol to the mouth and upper airway (Molander, Lunell, Andersson, & Kuylenstierna, 1996). Virtually none of the nicotine from the inhaler is delivered to the lungs. Use of the inhaler results in a dose of nicotine and an absorption profile similar to that of nicotine gum.

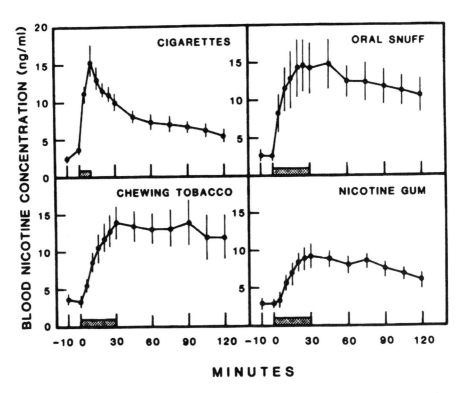

FIGURE 1. Mean (± SEM) blood concentrations of nicotine in 10 subjects who smoked cigarettes for 9 minutes (1¹/₃ cigarettes), used oral snuff (2.5 g), used chewing tobacco (mean, 7.9 g), and chewed nicotine gum (two 2-mg pieces). Shaded bars above the time axis indicate the period of exposure to tobacco or nicotine gum. From "Nicotine Absorption and Cardiovascular Effects of Smokeless Tobacco Use: Comparison With Cigarettes and Nicotine Gum," by N. L. Benowitz, H. Porchet, L. Scheiner, and P. Jacob, III, 1988, *Clinical Pharmacology & Therapeutics, 44*, p. 24. Copyright 1988 by Mosby, Inc. Reprinted with permission of the publisher.

The process of cigarette smoking is complex and the smoker can manipulate the dose of nicotine on a puff-by-puff basis. Thus, the intake of nicotine from a given product depends on the puff volume, the depth of inhalation, the extent of dilution with room air, the rate of puffing, and intensity of puffing (Herning, Jones, Benowitz, & Mines, 1983). For certain "low-tar" cigarettes, intake depends on whether ventilation holes in the filter are occluded by the smoker (Zacny, Stitzer, & Yingling, 1986).

Because of the complexity of the smoking process and of the use of smokeless tobacco products, the dose of nicotine taken in by the tobacco user cannot be predicted from the nicotine content of the tobacco or its absorption characteristics. To determine the dose, one needs to measure blood levels and know how fast the smoker eliminates nicotine. One study of 22 cigarette smokers who smoked an average of 36 cigarettes a day (range, 20–62) found an average daily intake of 37 mg, with a wide range of 10–79 mg nicotine (Benowitz & Jacob, 1984). The intake of nicotine per cigarette averaged 1.0 mg, but ranged from 0.37 to 1.56 mg. Similar results have been reported in other studies (Armitage *et al.*, 1975; Feyerabend, Ings, & Russell, 1985). A study of nicotine intake from smokeless tobacco reported an average of 3.6 mg nicotine from 2.5 g of oral snuff and 4.6 mg from an average of 7.9 g of chewing tobacco, when both were kept in the mouth for 30 min (Benowitz, Porchet, Sheiner, & Jacob, 1988).

Pharmacokinetics and Metabolism of Nicotine

Distribution

Smoking is a unique form of systemic drug administration, in that nicotine enters the circulation through the pulmonary rather than the portal or systemic venous circulations. It takes 10–19 s for nicotine to pass through the brain (Benowitz, 1990). The lag time between smoking and the entry of nicotine into the brain is shorter than that observed when nicotine is injected intravenously. Nicotine enters the brain quickly, but brain levels decline rapidly thereafter, as the drug is distributed to other body tissues.

Nicotine levels then fall due to uptake by peripheral tissues, then later due to elimination from the body. Arteriovenous differences during cigarette smoking are substantial, with arterial levels exceeding venous levels 6–10-fold (Henningfield, Stapleton, Benowitz, Grayson, & London, 1993). The pharmacologic relevance of this observation is that rapid delivery of nicotine results in a more intense pharmacologic response, owing both to higher arterial levels entering the brain and effects occurring rapidly, before there is adequate time for the development of tolerance (Porchet, Benowitz, Sheiner, & Copeland, 1987). Nicotine levels in the brain decline between cigarettes, providing an opportunity for resensitization of receptors, so that positive reinforcement can, to some extent, occur with successive cigarettes despite the development of tolerance.

Nicotine crosses the placenta freely and has been found in amniotic fluid and the umbilical cord blood of neonates (Luck & Nau, 1984). It is found in breast milk and in the breast fluid of nonlactating women (Luck & Nau, 1987; Petrakis, Gruenke, Beelen, Castagnoli, & Craig, 1978). Its concentration in breast milk is so low that the dose of nicotine consumed by an infant is small and unlikely to be of physiologic consequence.

Elimination

Nicotine is rapidly and extensively metabolized, primarily in the liver, but also to a small extent in the lung. The level of renal excretion depends on urinary pH and urine flow, and accounts for 2%–35% of total elimination (Benowitz & Jacob, 1985).

Approximately 70%–80% of nicotine is metabolized to cotinine, and about 4% to nicotine N′-oxide (Benowitz & Jacob, 1994; Benowitz, Jacob, Fong, & Gupta, 1994; Byrd, Chang, Greene, & deBethizy, 1992). Cotinine is extensively metabolized to 3′-hydroxycotinine, which is the most abundant metabolite of nicotine found in the urine. Nicotine and cotinine and 3′-hydroxycotinine are further metabolized by glucuronidation. Nicotine and cotinine undergo N-glucuronidation, while 3′-hydroxycotinine undergoes O-glucuronidation. There is considerable individual variability in the metabolism of nicotine.

One individual with deficient C-oxidation of nicotine has been identified (Benowitz, Jacob, & Sachs, 1995). This woman converted only 8% of nicotine to cotinine. As the metabolism of nicotine to cotinine is a rate-limiting step of nicotine metabolism, this individual with deficient C-oxidation had an unusually long half-life of nicotine. The metabolism of nicotine to cotinine is a two-step process via an intermediate, the nicotine iminium ion. The first step is metabolism by a CYP-450 enzyme, most likely CYP2A6, while the second step is metabolized by aldehyde oxidase. The enzyme that is deficient in the case with deficient nicotine oxidation has not yet been identified.

The half-life of nicotine averages 2 hr, although there is considerable individual variability (range 1–4 hr) (Benowitz, Jacob, Jones, & Rosenberg, 1982). Nicotine's primary metabolites are cotinine and nicotine-N-oxide (Figure 2), neither of which appears to be pharmacologically active. Cotinine, because of its long half-life (16–20 hr) (Benowitz, Kuyt,

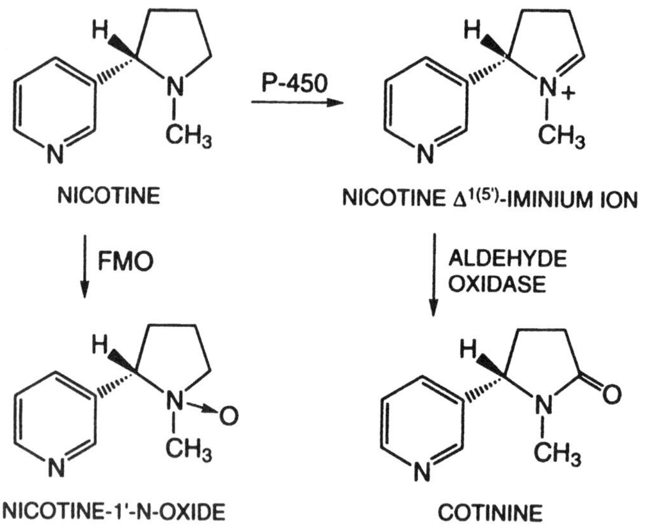

FIGURE 2. Chemical structure of nicotine and major pathways of nicotine metabolism. From "Cotinine Disposition and Effects," by N. L. Benowitz, F. Kuyt, P. Jacob, III, R. T. Jones, and A. L. Osman, 1983, *Clinical Pharmacology & Therapeutics, 309*, p. 605. Copyright 1983 by Mosby, Inc. Reprinted with permission of the publisher.

Jacob, Jones, & Osman, 1983), is commonly used in surveys and treatment studies as a marker of nicotine intake.

Time-Course of Nicotine in the Body during Daily Smoking

Smoking is commonly considered to be a process of intermittent dosing of nicotine, which is in turn rapidly eliminated from the body. There is considerable peak-to-trough oscillation in levels from cigarette to cigarette. However, in a manner consistent with a half-life of 2 hr, nicotine accumulates over 6–8 hr of regular smoking and persists overnight, even as the smoker sleeps (Figure 3) (Benowitz, Kuyt, & Jacob, 1982). Thus, smoking results not in intermittent exposure but in exposure to nicotine that lasts 24 hr of each day.

Nicotine Addiction

Most people who smoke cigarettes would like to quit (Orleans, 1985). Many of these people, who make up a group familiar to health care providers, either have a tobacco-related illness or recognize the threat posed by such illnesses, but still cannot stop smoking. Their behavior is described well by a recent World Health Organization definition of drug dependence as "a behavioral pattern in which the use of a given psychoactive drug is given a sharply higher priority over other behaviors which once had a significantly higher value" (Edwards, Arif, & Hodgson, 1982, p. 19). In other words, the drug has come to control behavior to an extent that is considered detrimental to the individual or society. Cigarette smoking and tobacco use meet primary and additional criteria for drug dependence that are presented in the recent Surgeon General's report, *The Health Consequences of Smoking* (see Table 1; U.S. Department of Health and Human Services, 1988).

Recent studies in animals and humans have enhanced our understanding of nicotine addiction. Animals of several species, including rats and squirrel monkeys (as well as humans), will self-administer intravenous nicotine. Nicotine is self-administered by animals at dose levels comparable to those taken in by human smokers. Self-administration occurs for other addicting drugs, and provides a method for exploring mechanisms of reinforcement. Studies in the rat suggest that the mesolimbic dopamine system is central to the reinforcing effects of nicotine (Corrigall *et al.*, 1994). The mesolimbic system projects from the ventral tegmental area of the midbrain to the nucleus accumbens, and is known to be involved in reinforcement for other drugs of abuse such as cocaine. High-

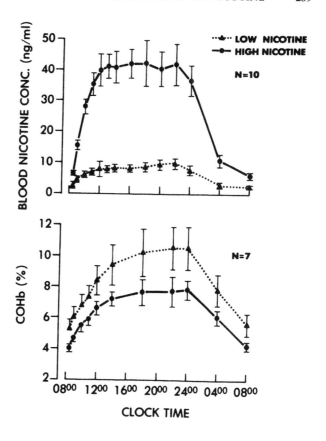

FIGURE 3. Mean (± SEM) blood nicotine and carboxyhemoglobin concentrations in cigarette smokers. Subjects smoked cigarettes every half hour from 8:30 A.M. to 11:00 P.M., for a total of 30 cigarettes a day. The cigarettes were research cigarettes that were high or low in nicotine content (as distinguished from commercial cigarettes which differ in yield but not in nicotine content). COHb denotes carboxyhemoglobin. From "Circadian Blood Nicotine Concentrations During Cigarette Smoking," by N. L. Benowitz, F. Kuyt, and P. Jacob, III, 1982, *Clinical Pharmacology & Therapeutics, 32,* p. 759. Copyright 1982 by Mosby, Inc. Adapted with permission of the publisher.

affinity binding of labeled nicotine to cell bodies and terminal fields of the mesolimbic neurons and expression of mRNAs for α_3, α_4, α_5, and $\beta 2$ subunits in mesolimbic neurons has been demonstrated (Clarke & Pert, 1985). Nicotine increases firing of ventral tegmental area neurons and facilitates release of neurotransmitters in this system. Supporting the role of dopaminergic neurons in sustaining self-administration are studies with dopamine antagonists and chemical lesions of the dopaminergic system using 6-hydroxydopamine, both of which abolish self-administration (Corrigall, Coen, Franklin, & Clarke, 1992). In addition, nicotine antagonists such as chlorosondamine infused directly into the ventral segmental area or the nucleus accumbens reduce self-administration.

Humans have been shown to like and self-administer intravenous nicotine, and the reinforcing effects and the self-administration is blocked by pretreatment with the nicotine antagonist mecamylamine (Henningfield, 1984). In smokers, nicotine self-administration appears to be motivated both by positive reinforcement and negative reinforcement. Positive reinforcing effects reported include relaxation, reduced stress, enhanced vigilance, improved cognitive function, mood modulation, and lower body weight. Negative reinforcement refers to the relief of nicotine withdrawal symptoms in the context of physical dependence. Withdrawal symptoms are well documented to include nervousness, restlessness, irritability, anxiety, impaired concentration, impaired cognitive function, increased appetite, and weight gain (Hughes & Hatsukami, 1986). It is difficult to separate reported positive reinforcement from relief of withdrawal symptoms in smokers. Recent studies of nonsmokers, however, indicate some enhancement of cognitive function and less decrement in performance with repetitive tasks after nicotine (LeHouezec *et al.,* 1994).

TABLE 1. Criteria for Drug Dependence[a]

Primary criteria	Highly controlled or compulsive use
	Psychoactive effects
	Drug-reinforced behavior
Additional criteria	Addictive behavior often involves the following
	Stereotypical patterns of use
	Use despite harmful effects
	Relapse following abstinence
	Recurrent drug cravings
	Dependence-producing drugs often produce the following
	Tolerance
	Physical dependence
	Pleasant (euphoriant) effects

[a] From *The Health Consequences of Smoking: Nicotine Addiction. A Report of the Surgeon General* (DHHS [CDC] Publication No. 88-8406), by U.S. Department of Health and Human Services, P. H. S., 1988, Washington, DC: U.S. Government Printing Office. Copyright 1988 by U.S. DHHS.

Of note is that performance of smokers (compared with deprived smokers) in a complex behavioral task has also been reported to be impaired by nicotine (Spilich, June, & Renner, 1992).

Some smokers report that smoking helps relieve depression and other affective disorders and, conversely, some smokers become severely depressed after stopping smoking (Covey, Glassman, & Stetner, 1990). Neurochemical effects of nicotine, including release of dopamine, norepinephrine, and serotonin, resemble effects of some antidepressant medications. Conceivably, nicotine is self-administered by some smokers to treat affective disorders. In addition to nicotine-related effects, there is evidence that sensory stimulation induced by nicotine contributes to the satisfaction from smoking (Rose, Behm, & Levin, 1993). This, however, may be a short-term conditioned response, and is not likely to maintain nicotine self-administration in the long term.

In smokers, nicotine produces electroencephalographic activation including increased beta power, decreased alpha and theta power, and increased alpha frequency (Pickworth, Herning, & Henningfield, 1989). Changes in the opposite direction are seen during tobacco abstinence, and these changes are rapidly reversed by nicotine in any form. Nicotine has been shown to increase regional cerebral glucose metabolism in areas that are also shown to have high-affinity nicotine binding, possibly representing a neuroanatomical correlate of nicotine effects (McNamara, Larson, Rapoport, & Soncrant, 1990).

The addiction to nicotine depends on the rate and route of nicotine dosing. Inhalation of nicotine via cigarette smoking appears to be the most addictive method of dosing. After inhalation, nicotine passes rapidly into the arterial bloodstream and then into the brain, resulting in a transient exposure of the brain to high levels of nicotine. This exposure results in relatively intense central nervous system effects that occur in close temporal proximity to smoking, an ideal situation for behavioral reinforcement. As discussed previously, arterial levels of nicotine are several-fold higher than venous levels after smoking, and arterial levels far exceed those that would be tolerated with nicotine dosing via a systemic route. Transiently high nicotine levels in the brain, which subsequently fall between cigarettes, allow time for resensitization of brain nicotinic receptors. Thus, nicotine from sequential cigarettes is capable of overcoming tolerance to produce further pharmacologic effects. Finally, rapid delivery of nicotine to the brain allows the smoker to titrate the dose of nicotine from a cigarette to achieve a particular desired effect without toxicity.

In contrast to cigarette smoking, slow release of nicotine, such as via transdermal nicotine, produces little or no behavioral reinforcement. Blood levels of nicotine rise gradually, allowing tolerance to develop. Peak arterial levels are much lower with transdermal nicotine compared with cigarette smoking, even with a similar daily nicotine dose. Not surprisingly, smokers do not rate transdermal nicotine as reinforcing, whereas cigarette smoking and intravenous nicotine are highly reinforcing (Pickworth, Bunker, & Henningfield, 1994). Other nicotine delivery systems, such as nicotine chewing gum and nicotine nasal spray, are absorbed more rapidly than transdermal nicotine, and have some behavioral reinforcing effects, although much less than those of cigarette smoking. In summary, the delivery system, which controls the route and rate of nicotine dosing, is a critical determinant of the development of nicotine addiction.

Many features of nicotine dependence resemble those seen in people dependent on other frequently abused drugs—heroin, alcohol, and cocaine (U.S. Department of Health and Human Services, 1988). First, many such drugs produce physiologic dependence, also called neuroadaptation, with long-term use. This means that tolerance develops to the effects of the drug and withdrawal or abstinence symptoms develop when consumption of the drug ceases. The development of tolerance to nicotine and the tobacco abstinence syndrome have been described. Second, smoking even a few cigarettes may result in the development of tobacco dependence. After smoking begins, cigarette consumption gradually escalates over several years (Henningfield, 1986), a pattern similar to those observed in heroin use. Third, once a person has become a habitual smoker, it is difficult to stop. When smokers try to quit, the relapse rate is high, averaging 70% in 3 months. This relapse rate is similar to that observed in heroin addicts and alcoholics (Hunt

& Barnett, 1971). Finally, substitution therapy such as use of nicotine medications is similar to the detoxification, maintenance, and tapering schemes used in the treatment of heroin addicts with methadone.

Cardiovascular, Endocrine, and Metabolic Effects of Nicotine

Nicotine is well known to affect cardiovascular function via sympathetic neural stimulation. Sympathomimetic effects of nicotine are mediated by several mechanisms. Central nervous system–mediated sympathetic stimulation can occur via activation of peripheral chemoreceptors, direct effect on the brainstem, effects on more caudal portions of the spinal cord, or a combination (Comroe, 1960; Su, 1982). Intrapulmonary chemoreceptors may also contribute to brain-mediated sympathetic arousal. The site that appears to be most sensitive to low levels of nicotine is the carotid chemoreceptor (Comroe, 1960). Peripheral mechanisms include catecholamine release from the adrenal and direct release or enhancement of release of catecholamines from vascular nerve endings.

Sympathetic neural stimulation results in heart rate acceleration and a transient increase in blood pressure, associated with an increase in cardiac output. Blood flow to various vascular beds is differentially affected, with constriction of blood vessels in the skin and dilation of skeletal muscle blood vessels. The coronary blood vessels appear to be constricted by nicotine as evidenced by a smaller increase in coronary blood flow than anticipated with a given increase in heart rate produced either by exercise or pacing, and directly observed coronary vasoconstriction, particularly in coronary arteries with atherosclerotic disease (Kaijser & Berglund, 1985; Quillen et al., 1993; Winniford et al., 1986). The effects of cigarette smoking on coronary arterial tone can be blocked by phentolamine, supporting a catecholamine-mediated mechanism.

Substantial, although not complete, tolerance develops to the heart rate accelerating and other cardiovascular effects of nicotine. Tolerance has been studied in detail using pharmacokinetic-pharmacodynamic modeling, as described in previous publications (Porchet, Benowitz, & Sheiner, 1988). Of note is that tolerance develops fairly rapidly with a half-life of about 30 min, and even with full development of tolerance there is a persistent effect that is about 20% of the effect that would be expected without the development of tolerance.

Thrombosis is an important mechanism of smoking-induced cardiac events. Therefore, there has been considerable interest in whether nicotine promotes thrombosis, particularly via platelet activation. Nicotine does not appear to have direct effects on platelets *in vitro* (Pfueller, Burns, Mak, & Firkin, 1988). However, one study in dogs showed that high doses of intravenous nicotine could induce platelet aggregation as measured by phasic flow in partially occluded coronary arteries (Folts & Bonebrake, 1982). When platelets are activated, they release thromboxane A2, and stable metabolites of thromboxane A2 may be measured in the urine as an index of *in vivo* platelet activation in humans. Cigarette smokers show enhanced thromboxane A2 metabolite excretion compared with nonsmokers and with snuff users, even though the latter have similar daily intake of nicotine compared with smokers (Nowak, Murray, Oates, & FitzGerald, 1987; Wennmalm *et al.*, 1991). In addition, cigarette smokers show enhanced platelet activation, based on thromboxane A2 excretion as well as plasma beta thromboglobulin and platelet factor 4 while smoking, compared with treatment with nicotine or placebo patches (Benowitz, Fitzgerald, Wilson, & Zhang, 1993). Furthermore, nicotine gum chewing does not activate platelets (Mundal, Hjemdahl, & Gjesdal, 1995). Thus, in humans the role of nicotine in enhancing platelet activity has not been demonstrated, although it is still possible that transient high levels of nicotine such as those that develop after cigarette smoking could activate platelets, while slower release of nicotine, as from transdermal systems, does not.

Some *in vitro* studies have suggested that nicotine reduces vascular synthesis of prostacyclin, an endothelial cell-derived local vasodilator and antiplatelet hormone (Chahine, Calderone, & Navarro-Delmasure, 1990). Reduced prostacyclin synthesis could aggravate tissue ischemia. Recent studies measuring stable metabolites of prostacyclin in the urine, however, find no evidence of a decrease with cigarette smoking, no difference comparing snuff users versus nontobacco users, and no change when switching from cigarette smoking to transdermal nicotine or placebo patches (Benowitz *et al.*, 1993; Nowak *et al.*, 1987; Wennmalm *et al.*, 1991). Thus, it does not appear that nicotine suppresses prostacyclin synthesis in humans.

Metabolic effects of nicotine are of interest in regard to effects on body weight and serum lipids, the latter of which could affect cardiovascular disease risk. On average, cigarette smokers weigh 4 kg less than nonsmokers and, when a smoker quits, body weight increases that amount on average (Williamson *et al.*, 1991). Lower body weight seems to be maintained primarily by an increase in metabolic rate, with concomitant appetite suppression that is evidenced by the absence of a compensatory increase in caloric intake that would be expected when metabolic rate increases (Perkins, 1992). Both cigarette smoking and intravenous nicotine have been shown to increase the metabolic rate (Arcavi, Jacob, Hellerstein, & Benowitz, 1994). Smoking cessation is associated with an increase in appetite and caloric intake, particularly of sweet foods, with a resultant increase in body weight over 6–12 months (Perkins, 1992). Subsequently, caloric intake is reduced and returns to baseline, indicating a new set point for body weight. The mechanism for the nicotine-mediated increase in metabolic rate has not been fully elucidated. Catecholamine release is most likely involved, as the increase in metabolic rate is inhibited by beta blockers (Wahren, 1990).

Nicotine, via release of catecholamines, induces lipolysis and releases free fatty acids into the plasma. Cigarette smoking in humans and nicotine administration in animals has been shown to substantially enhance free fatty acid turnover (Hellerstein *et al.*, 1994). Fatty acids are primarily taken up by the liver, which might be expected to increase the synthesis of very low-density lipoproteins. Increased low-density lipoproteins and very low-density lipoproteins and decreased high-density lipoprotein levels have been reported in smokers (Craig, Palomaki, & Haddow, 1989). It is conceivable that the effects of nicotine could contribute to the lipid abnormalities of cigarette smoking. Such abnormalities have not, however, been seen in individuals using nicotine replacement therapies (Quensel, Agardh, & Nilsson-Ehle, 1989).

Nicotine has a variety of endocrine effects that are of biological interest. The release of neurotransmitters that could influence the psychotropic effects and addiction to nicotine have been discussed previously. Cigarette smoking, presumably via effects of nicotine, has been shown to increase ACTH and cortisol release (Baron, Comi, Cryns, Brinck-Johnsen, & Mercer, 1995; Seyler, Pomerleau, Fertig, Hunt, & Parker, 1986). Excessive cortisol release could have effects on mood and could contribute to osteoporosis.

Nicotine can release beta endorphins (Seyler *et al.*, 1986). Nicotine has been shown to have antinociceptive effects in animals and possibly in humans as well; these effects could be mediated, at least in part, by endorphin release (Pomerleau, Turk, & Fertig, 1984; Rogers & Iwamoto, 1993), although there is also evidence for antinociception via spinal and brainstem neural pathways. Release of catecholamines and endorphins may also contribute to the effects of nicotine in reducing the fluid extravasation response to bradykinin from the synovium in joints of rats (Miao, Dallman, Benowitz, Basbaum, & Levine, 1993). Inhibition of synovial fluid extravasation suggests that nicotine might contribute to inflammatory arthritis.

Cigarette smoking is a risk factor for osteoporosis (Hopper & Seeman, 1994). The mechanism is not clear but is likely to involve the lower body weight of smokers (which is mediated by nicotine, as discussed previously), and

possibly by the antiestrogenic effects of cigarette smoking (Baron, LeVecchia, & Levi, 1990). Recent studies have indicated that estrogen and steroid levels in smokers are normal, although estrogen levels in postmenopausal women on estrogen replacement who smoke cigarettes are lower than those of nonsmokers (Cassidenti, Pike, Vijod, Stanczyk, & Lobo, 1992; Kiel, Baron, Anderson, Hannan, & Felson, 1992). The eliminiation of the protective effect of oral estrogens for hip fracture by smoking may be an effect of cigarette smoking and resulting enzyme induction on estrogen metabolism rather than an effect of nicotine. However, animal studies indicate that nicotine can reduce bone mass, although the mechanism has not been determined (Broulik & Jarab, 1993). Corticosteroids reduce the sensitivity to nicotine in mice, at least in part by reducing nicotinic binding, and nicotine-mediated corticosteroid release has been speculated to contribute to nicotine tolerance (Pauly & Collins, 1993).

Pharmacology of Nicotine Metabolites

Nicotine metabolism results in the generation of a number of metabolites, as discussed previously. Some of these metabolites have pharmacologic activities that could contribute to the effects of nicotine in people. Cotinine is the primary proximate metabolite of nicotine. Cotinine has a much longer half-life than nicotine (average 16 hr vs. 2 hr for nicotine), and cotinine levels are on average 15-fold higher than levels of nicotine during regular smoking or nicotine replacement therapy (Benowitz & Jacob, 1994; Benowitz *et al.*, 1995). Cotinine has no effect on nicotinic cholinergic receptors (Abood, Grassi, & Costanza, 1983). However, cotinine does have effects on the release of some neurotransmitters in the brain and affects a number of enzymes, including those involved in steroidogenesis (Barbieri, York, Cherry, & Ryan, 1987; Fuxe, Everitt, & Hokfelt, 1979; Yeh, Barbieri, & Friedman, 1989). Cotinine decreases vascular resistance and decreases blood pressure in animals, although this occurs at relatively high concentrations (Dominiak, Fuchs, von Toth, & Grobecker, 1985). It has been suggested that cotinine may contribute to the lower blood pressure seen in cigarette smokers at times when they are not smoking compared with nonsmokers (Benowitz & Sharp, 1989). One recent study with humans reported that cotinine modifies the symptoms of tobacco withdrawal, although it does so in a way that is dissimilar to the effects of nicotine (Keenan, Hatsukami, Pentel, Thompson, & Grillo, 1994). Cotinine appeared to produce some stimulant-like effects and reduced overall withdrawal score. Thus, cotinine could be of considerable importance in understanding the pharmacology of nicotine and nicotine addiction. Cotinine could contribute to withdrawal symptoms after smoking cessation, and could contribute to some of the cardiovascular and endocrine effects of nicotine, as discussed previously.

ACKNOWLEDGMENTS

I thank Kaye Welch for editorial assistance. Preparation of this review supported in part by National Institute on Drug Abuse, National Institutes of Health, Grants DA02277 and DA01696.

References

Abood, L. G., Grassi, S., & Costanza, M. (1983). Binding of optically pure (–)-[³H]nicotine to rat brain membranes. *Federation of European Biochemical Societies Letters, 157,* 147–149.

Arcavi, L., Jacob, P., Hellerstein, M., & Benowitz, N. L. (1994). Divergent tolerance to metabolic and cardiovascular effects of nicotine in smokers with low and high levels of cigarette consumption. *Clinical Pharmacology & Therapeutics, 56,* 55–64.

Armitage, A. K., Dollery, C. T., George, C. F., Houseman, T. H., Lewis, P. J., & Turner, D. M. (1975). Absorption and metabolism of nicotine from cigarettes. *British Medical Journal, 4,* 313–316.

Barbieri, R. L., York, C. M., Cherry, M. L., & Ryan, K. J. (1987). The effects of nicotine, cotinine and anabasine on rat adrenal 11β-hydroxylase and 21-hydroxylase. *Journal of Steroid Biochemistry and Molecular Biology, 28,* 25–28.

Baron, J. A., LeVecchia, C., & Levi, F. (1990). The antiestrogenic effect of cigarette smoking in women. *American Journal of Obstetrics and Gynecology, 162,* 502–514.

Baron, J. A., Comi, R. J., Cryns, V., Brinck-Johnsen, T., & Mercer, N. G. (1995). The effect of cigarette smoking on adrenal cortical hormones. *Journal of Pharmacology and Experimental Therapeutics, 272,* 151–155.

Benowitz, N. L. (1990). Clinical pharmacology of inhaled drugs of abuse: Implications in understanding nicotine dependence. In C. N. Chiang & R. L. Hawks (Eds.), *Research findings on smoking of abused substances* (NIDA Research Monograph No. 99, pp. 12–29). Washington, DC: Superintendent of Documents.

Benowitz, N. L. (1995). Clinical pharmacology of transdermal nicotine. *European Journal of Pharmaceutics and Biopharmaceutics, 41,* 168–174.

Benowitz, N. L., & Jacob, P., III. (1984). Daily intake of nicotine during cigarette smoking. *Clinical Pharmacology & Therapeutics, 35,* 499–504.

Benowitz, N. L., & Jacob, P., III. (1985). Nicotine renal excretion rate influences nicotine intake during cigarette smoking. *Journal of Pharmacology and Experimental Therapeutics, 234,* 153–155.

Benowitz, N. L., & Jacob, P., III. (1994). Metabolism of nicotine to cotinine studied by a dual stable isotope method. *Clinical Pharmacology & Therapeutics, 56,* 483–493.

Benowitz, N. L., & Sharp, D. S. (1989). Inverse relationship between serum cotinine concentration and blood pressure in cigarette smokers. *Circulation, 80,* 1309–1312.

Benowitz, N. L., Jacob, P., III, Jones, R. T., & Rosenberg, J. (1982). Interindividual variability in the metabolism and cardiovascular effects of nicotine in man. *Journal of Pharmacology and Experimental Therapeutics, 221,* 368–372.

Benowitz, N. L., Kuyt, F., & Jacob, P., III. (1982). Circadian blood nicotine concentrations during cigarette smoking. *Clinical Pharmacology & Therapeutics, 32,* 758–764.

Benowitz, N. L., Kuyt, F., Jacob, P., III, Jones, R. T., & Osman, A. L. (1983). Cotinine disposition and effects. *Clinical Pharmacology & Therapeutics, 309,* 139–142.

Benowitz, N. L., Jacob, P., III, & Savanapridi, C. (1987). Determinants of nicotine intake while chewing nicotine polacrilex gum. *Clinical Pharmacology & Therapeutics, 41,* 467–473.

Benowitz, N. L., Lake, T., Keller, K. H., & Lee, B. L. (1987). Prolonged absorption with development of tolerance to toxic effects following cutaneous exposure to nicotine. *Clinical Pharmacology & Therapeutics, 42,* 119–120.

Benowitz, N. L., Porchet, H., Sheiner, L., & Jacob, P., III. (1988). Nicotine absorption and cardiovascular effects with smokeless tobacco use: Comparison with cigarettes and nicotine gum. *Clinical Pharmacology & Therapeutics, 44,* 23–28.

Benowitz, N. L., Fitzgerald, G. A., Wilson, M., & Zhang, Q. (1993). Nicotine effects on eicosanoid formation and hemostatic function: Comparison of transdermal nicotine and cigarette smoking. *Journal of the American College of Cardiology, 22,* 1159–1167.

Benowitz, N. L., Jacob, P., III, Fong, I., & Gupta, S. (1994). Nicotine metabolic profile in man: Comparison of cigarette smoking and transdermal nicotine. *Journal of Pharmacology and Experimental Therapeutics, 268,* 296–303.

Benowitz, N. L., Jacob, P., III, & Sachs, D. P. L. (1995). Deficient C-oxidation of nicotine. *Clinical Pharmacology & Therapeutics, 57,* 590–594.

Benwell, M. E. M., Balfour, D. J. K., & Anderson, J. M. (1988). Evidence that tobacco smoking increases the density of (–)-[³H]nicotine binding sites in human brain. *Journal of Neurochemistry, 50,* 1243–1247.

Broulik, P. D., & Jarab, J. (1993). The effect of chronic nicotine administration on bone mineral content in mice. *Hormone and Metabolic Research, 25,* 219–221.

Byrd, G. D., Chang, K., Greene, J. M., & deBethizy, J. D. (1992). Evidence for urinary excretion of glucuronide conjugates of nicotine, cotinine, and trans-3'-hydroxycotinine in smokers. *Drug Metabolism and Disposition, 20,* 192–197.

Cassidenti, D. L., Pike, M. C., Vijod, A. G., Stanczyk, F. Z., & Lobo, R. A. (1992). A reevaluation of estrogen status in postmenopausal women who smoke. *American Journal of Obstetrics and Gynecology, 166,* 1444–1448.

Centers for Disease Control. (1987). Cigarette smoking in the United States, 1986. *Morbidity and Mortality Weekly Report, 36,* 581–585.

Chahine, R., Calderone, A., & Navarro-Delmasure, C. (1990). The in vitro effects of nicotine and cotinine on prostacyclin and thromboxane biosynthesis. *Prostaglandins Leukotrienes and Essential Fatty Acids, 40,* 261–266.

Changeux, J. P., Galzi, J. L., Devillers-Thiery, A., & Betrand, D. (1992). The functional architecture of the acetylcholine nicotinic receptor explored by affinity labeling and site-directed mutatgenesis. *Quarterly Review of Biophysics, 25,* 395–432.

Clarke, P. B. S., & Pert, A. (1985). Autoradiographic evidence for nicotine receptors on nigrostriatal and mesolimbic dopaminergic neurons. *Brain Research, 348,* 355–358.

Clarke, P. B. S., Schwartz, R. D., Paul, S. M., Pert, C. B., & Pert, A. (1985). Nicotinic binding in rat brain: Autoradiographic comparison of [³H]acetylcholine, [³H]nicotine and [¹²⁵I]α-bungarotoxin. *Journal of Neuroscience, 5,* 1307–1315.

Collins, A. C., Luo, Y., Selvaag, S., & Marks, M. J. (1994). Sensitivity to nicotine and brain nicotinic receptors are altered by chronic nicotine and mecamylamine infusion. *Journal of Pharmacology and Experimental Therapeutics, 271,* 125–133.

Comroe, J. H. (1960). The pharmacological actions of nicotine. *Annals of the New York Academy of Science, 90,* 48–51.

Corrigall, W. A., Coen, K. M., Franklin, K. B. J., & Clarke, P. B. S. (1992). The mesolimbic dopamine system is implicated in the reinforcing effects of nicotine. *Psychopharmacology, 107,* 285–289.

Corrigall, W. A., Coen, K. M., & Adamson, K. L. (1994). Self-administered nicotine activates the mesolimbic dopamine system through the ventral tegmental area. *Brain Research, 653,* 278–284.

Covey, L. S., Glassman, A. H., & Stetner, F. (1990). Depression and depressive symptoms in smoking cessation. *Comprehensive Psychiatry, 31,* 350–354.

Craig, W. Y., Palomaki, G. E., & Haddow, J. E. (1989). Cigarette smoking and serum lipid and lipoprotein concentrations: An analysis of published data. *British Medical Journal, 298,* 784–788.

Dominiak, P., Fuchs, G., von Toth, S., & Grobecker, H. (1985). Effects of nicotine and its major metabolites on blood pressure in anaesthetized rats. *Klinische Wochenschrift, 63,* 90–92.

Edwards, G., Arif, A., & Hodgson, R. (1982). Nomenclature and classification of drug and alcohol-related problems: a shortened version of a WHO memorandum. *British Journal of Addiction, 77,* 3–20.

Feyerabend, C., Ings, R. M. J., & Russell, M. A. H. (1985). Nicotine pharmacokinetics and its application to intake from smoking. *British Journal of Clinical Pharmacology, 19,* 239–247.

Folts, J. D., & Bonebrake, F. C. (1982). The effects of cigarette smoke and nicotine on platelet thrombus formation in stenosed dog coronary arteries: Inhibition with phentolamine. *Circulation, 65,* 465–469.

Fuxe, K., Everitt, B. J., & Hokfelt, T. (1979). On the action of nicotine and cotinine on central 5-hydroxytryptamine neurons. *Pharmacology, Biochemistry and Behavior, 10,* 671–677.

Gori, G. B., Benowitz, N. L., & Lynch, C. J. (1986). Mouth versus deep airways absorption of nicotine in cigarette smokers. *Pharmacology, Biochemistry and Behavior, 25,* 1181–1184.

Hellerstein, M. K., Benowitz, N. L., Neese, R. A., Schwartz, J., Hoh, R., Jacob, P., III, Hsieh, J., & Faix, D. (1994). Effects of cigarette smoking and its cessation on lipid metabolism and energy expenditure in heavy smokers. *Journal of Clinical Investigation, 93,* 265–272.

Henningfield, J. E. (1984). Behavioral pharmacology of cigarette smoking. In T. Thompson, P. B. Dews, & J. E. Barrett (Eds.), *Advances in behavioral pharmacology* (pp. 131–210). New York: Academic Press.

Henningfield, J. E. (1986). How tobacco produces drug dependence. In J. K. Ockene (Eds.), *The pharmacologic treatment of tobacco dependence: Proceedings of the World Congress, November 4–5, 1985* (pp. 19–31). Nashua, NH: Puritan.

Henningfield, J. E., Stapleton, J. M., Benowitz, N. L., Grayson, R. F., & London, E. D. (1993). Higher levels of nicotine in arterial than in venous blood after cigarette smoking. *Drug and Alcohol Dependence, 33,* 23–29.

Herning, R. I., Jones, R. T., Benowitz, N. L., & Mines, A. H. (1983). How a cigarette is smoked determines nicotine blood levels. *Clinical Pharmacology & Therapeutics, 33,* 84–90.

Hopper, J. L., & Seeman, E. (1994). The bone density of female twins discordant for tobacco use. *New England Journal of Medicine, 330,* 387–392.

Hughes, J. R., & Hatsukami, D. (1986). Signs and symptoms of tobacco withdrawal. *Archives of General Psychiatry, 43,* 289–294.

Hunt, W. A., & Barnett, L. W. (1971). Relapse rates in addiction programs. *Journal of Clinical Psychology, 27,* 455–456.

Johansson, C. J., Olsson, P., Bende, M., Carlsson, T., & Gunnarsson, P. O. (1991). Absolute bioavailability of nicotine applied to different nasal regions. *European Journal of Clinical Pharmacology, 41,* 585–588.

Kaijser, L., & Berglund, B. (1985). Effect of nicotine on coronary blood-flow in man. *Clinical Physiology, 5,* 541–552.

Keenan, R. M., Hatsukami, D. K., Pentel, P. R., Thompson, T. N., & Grillo, M. A. (1994). Pharmacodynamic effects of cotinine in abstinent cigarette smokers. *Clinical Pharmacology & Therapeutics, 55,* 581–590.

Kiel, D. P., Baron, J. A., Anderson, J. J., Hannan, M. T., & Felson, D. T. (1992). Smoking eliminates the protective effect of oral estrogens on the risk for hip fracture among women. *Annals of Internal Medicine, 116,* 716–721.

LeHouezec, J., Halliday, R., Benowitz, N. L., Callaway, E., Naylor, H., & Herzig, K. (1994). A low dose of subcutaneous nicotine improves information processing in nonsmokers. *Psychopharmacology, 114,* 628–634.

Lena, C., & Changeux, J.-P. (1993). Allosteric modulations of the nicotinic acetylcholine receptor. *Trends in Neurosciences, 16,* 181–186.

Luck, W., & Nau, H. (1984). Exposure of the fetus, neonate, and nursed infant to nicotine and cotinine from maternal smoking. *New England Journal of Medicine, 311,* 672.

Luck, W., & Nau, H. (1987). Nicotine and cotinine concentrations in the milk of smoking mothers: Influence of cigarette consumption and diurnal variation. *European Journal of Pediatrics, 146,* 21–26.

Marks, M. J., Stitzel, J. A., & Collins, A. C. (1985). Time course study of the effects of chronic nicotine infusion on drug response and brain receptors. *Journal of Pharmacology and Experimental Therapeutics, 235,* 619–628.

McGehee, D. S., & Role, L. W. (1995). Physiological diversity of nicotinic acetylcholine receptors expressed by vertebrate neurons. *Annual Review of Physiology, 57,* 521–546.

McNamara, D., Larson, D. M., Rapoport, S. I., & Soncrant, T. T. (1990). Preferential metabolic activation of subcortical brain areas by acute administration of nicotine to rats. *Journal of Cerebral Blood Flow and Metabolism, 10,* 48–56.

Miao, F. J., Dallman, M. F., Benowitz, N. L., Basbaum, A. I., & Levine, J. D. (1993). Adrenal medullary modulation of the inhibition of bradykinin-induced plasma extravasation by intrathecal nicotine. *Journal of Pharmacology and Experimental Therapeutics, 53,* 6–14.

Molander, L., Lunell, E., Andersson, S-B, & Kuylenstierna, F. (1996). Dose released and absolute bioavailability of nicotine from a nicotine vapor inhaler. *Clinical Pharmacology & Therapeutics, 59,* 394–400.

Mundal, H. H., Hjemdahl, P., & Gjesdal, K. (1995). Acute effects of low dose nicotine gum on platelet function in nonsmoking hypertensive and normotensive men. *European Journal of Clinical Pharmacology, 47,* 411–416.

Nowak, J., Murray, J. J., Oates, J. A., & FitzGerald, G. A. (1987). Biochemical evidence of a chronic abnormality in platelet and vascular function in healthy individuals who smoke cigarettes. *Circulation, 76,* 6–14.

Orleans, C. T. (1985). Understanding and promoting smoking cessation: Overview and guidelines for physician intervention. *Annual Review of Medicine, 36,* 51–61.

Pauly, J. R., & Collins, A. C. (1993). An autoradiographic analysis of alterations in nicotinic cholinergic receptors following 1 week of corticosterone supplementation. *Neuroendocrinology, 57,* 262–271.

Perkins, K. A. (1992). Metabolic effects of cigarette smoking. *Journal of Applied Physiology, 72,* 401–409.

Petrakis, N. L., Gruenke, L. D., Beelen, T. C., Castagnoli, N., & Craig, J. C. (1978). Nicotine in breast fluid of nonlactating women. *Science, 199,* 303–305.

Pfueller, S. L., Burns, P., Mak, K., & Firkin, B. G. (1988). Effects of nicotine on platelet function. *Haemostasis, 18,* 163–169.

Pickworth, W. B., Herning, R. I., & Henningfield, J. E. (1989). Spontaneous EEG changes during tobacco abstinence and nicotine substitution in human volunteers. *Journal of Pharmacology and Experimental Therapeutics, 251,* 976–982.

Pickworth, W. B., Bunker, E. B., & Henningfield, J. E. (1994). Transdermal nicotine: Reduction of smoking with minimal abuse liability. *Psychopharmacology, 115,* 9–14.

Pomerleau, O. F., Turk, D. C., & Fertig, J. B. (1984). The effects of cigarette smoking on pain and anxiety. *Addictive Behaviors, 9,* 265–271.

Porchet, H. C., Benowitz, N. L., Sheiner, L. B., & Copeland, J. R. (1987). Apparent tolerance to the acute effect of nicotine results in part from distribution kinetics. *Journal of Clinical Investigation, 80,* 1466–1471.

Porchet, H. C., Benowitz, N. L., & Sheiner, L. B. (1988). Pharmacodynamic model of tolerance: Application to nicotine. *Journal of Pharmacology and Experimental Therapeutics, 244,* 231–236.

Quensel, M., Agardh, C.-D., & Nilsson-Ehle, P. (1989). Nicotine does not affect plasma lipoprotein concentrations in healthy men. *Scandinavian Journal of Clinical and Laboratory Investigation, 49,* 149–153.

Quillen, J. E., Rossen, J. D., Oskarsson, H. J., Minor, R. L., Jr., Lopez, J. A. G., & Winniford, M. D. (1993). Acute effect of cigarette smoking on the coronary circulation: Constriction of epicardial and resistance vessels. *Journal of the American College of Cardiology, 22,* 642–647.

Rogers, D. T., & Iwamoto, E. T. (1993). Multiple spinal mediators in parenteral nicotine-induced antinociception. *Journal of Pharmacology and Experimental Therapeutics, 267,* 341–349.

Rose, J. E., Behm, F. M., & Levin, E. D. (1993). Role of nicotine dose and sensory cues in the regulation of smoke intake. *Pharmacology, Biochemistry and Behavior, 44,* 891–900.

Seguela, P., Wadiche, J., Dineley-Miller, K., Dani, J. A., & Patrick, J. W. (1993). Molecular cloning, functional properties, and distribution of rat brain α_7: A nicotinic cation channel highly permeable to calcium. *Journal of Neuroscience, 13,* 596–604.

Seyler, L. E., Pomerleau, O. F., Fertig, J. B., Hunt, D., & Parker, K. (1986). Pituitary hormone response to cigarette smoking. *Pharmacology, Biochemistry and Behavior, 24,* 159–162.

Spilich, G. J., June, L., & Renner, J. (1992). Cigarette smoking and cognitive performance. *British Journal of Addiction, 87,* 1313–1326.

Su, C. (1982). Actions of nicotine and smoking on circulation. *Pharmacology and Therapeutics, 17,* 129–141.

U.S. Department of Health and Human Services, P. H. S. (1988). *The health consequences of smoking: Nicotine addiction. A Report of the Surgeon General* (DHHS [CDC] Publication No. 88-8406). Washington, DC: U.S. Government Printing Office.

Wahren, J. (1990). *Nicotine, cigarette smoking and energy expenditure in humans* [Abstract]. In European Chemical Society Conference on Nicotine, Visby, Sweden.

Wennmalm, A., Benthin, G., Granström, E. F., Persson, L., Peterson, A., & Winell, S. (1991). Relation between tobacco use and urinary excretion of thromboxane A_2 and prostacyclin metabolites in young men. *Circulation, 83,* 1698–1704.

West, R. J., & Russell, M. A. H. (1987). Cardiovascular and subjective effects of smoking before and after 24 h of abstinence from cigarettes. *Psychopharmacology, 92,* 118–121.

Williamson, D. F., Madans, J., Anda, R. F., Kleinman, J. C., Giovino, G. A., & Byers, T. (1991). Smoking cessation and severity of weight gain in a national cohort. *New England Journal of Medicine, 324,* 739–745.

Winniford, M. D., Wheelan, K. R., Kremers, M. S., Ugolini, V., Van Den Berg, E., Jr., Niggemann, E. H., Jansen, D. E., & Hillis, L. D. (1986). Smoking-induced coronary vasoconstriction in patients with atherosclerotic coronary artery disease: Evidence for adrenergically mediated alterations in coronary artery tone. *Circulation, 73,* 662–667.

Wonnacott, S. (1990). The paradox of nicotinic acetylcholine receptor upregulation by nicotine. *Trends in Pharmacological Sciences, 11,* 216–219.

Yeh, J., Barbieri, R. L., & Friedman, A. J. (1989). Nicotine and cotinine inhibit rat testis androgen biosynthesis in vitro. *Journal of Steroid Biochemistry and Molecular Biology, 33,* 627–630.

Zacny, J. P., Stitzer, M. L., & Yingling, J. E. (1986). Cigarette filter vent blocking: Effects on smoking topography and carbon monoxide exposure. *Pharmacology, Biochemistry and Behavior, 25,* 1245–1452.

20

Behavioral Pharmacology of Nicotine

KENNETH A. PERKINS AND MAXINE STITZER

This chapter focuses on nicotine reinforcement, highlighting basic research that demonstrates its reinforcing efficacy along with subjective mood and performance effects that may be responsible for reinforcement. Because our major area of interest is to improve understanding of nicotine reinforcement in humans, research on humans is emphasized. The environmental context surrounding nicotine intake can play a critical role in modulating its effects and thus its reinforcing value. Clearer understanding of nicotine reinforcement, including factors that modulate reinforcement, will lead to new insights about the conditions that promote initiation and maintenance of tobacco use and facilitate development of new behavioral and pharmacological interventions for smoking cessation.

Nicotine Reinforcement: Self-Administration

One definition of drug reinforcement is the degree to which the drug will be self-adminis-

tered, or the amount and frequency of behavior an organism will engage in to obtain the drug. As described in more detail later, recent research clearly indicates that animals and humans will self-administer nicotine in the absence of tobacco. These observations provide strong evidence that nicotine per se is reinforcing.

Animal Studies

Until fairly recently, there was some question as to whether nicotine was reinforcing in animals because of difficulty demonstrating robust self-administration. Although animals could be trained to respond for iv nicotine administration, the rate of responding was generally quite low unless extensive training conditions were imposed, such as substantial food deprivation to reduce body weight or lengthy, complex schedules of reinforcement (see Corrigall, 1992). Since there are select drugs that are self-administered by humans but not by animals (e.g., most hallucinogens), it seemed possible that the mechanisms of nicotine reinforcement in humans might not be present in animals.

However, identification of the important pharmacological factors of dose, dose delivery speed, and dose spacing allowed for development of a rodent model demonstrating robust responding for nicotine by rapid iv infusion (Corrigall, 1992). Not only will ani-

KENNETH A. PERKINS • Department of Psychiatry, University of Pittsburgh School of Medicine, Pittsburgh, Pennsylvania 15213. MAXINE STITZER • Department of Psychiatry, Division of Behavioral Biology, Johns Hopkins University, Baltimore, Maryland 21224.

Handbook of Substance Abuse: Neurobehavioral Pharmacology, edited by Tarter et al. Plenum Press, New York, 1998.

mals reliably self-administer nicotine under proper conditions, they will also alter response rate to maintain consistent nicotine intake following changes in reinforcement schedule. For example, Corrigall has shown a five-fold increase in responding among rats following a five-fold increase in the response requirement for each nicotine infusion. This model has since been replicated in other laboratories (e.g., Donny, Caggiula, Brown, & Knopf, 1995; Shoaib, Swanner, Schindler, & Goldberg, 1996). Reliable nicotine self-administration in primates has also been reported (Wakasa, Takada, & Yanagita, 1995). Additional evidence of nicotine reinforcement in animals comes from early research by Yanagita, Ando, Kato, and Takada (1983) showing that primates will self-administer high numbers of puffs on nicotine-containing tobacco cigarettes, while nicotine-free cigarettes result in extinction of puffing behavior.

Human Studies

Self-administration of nicotine by tobacco smoking is one of the most widely observed examples of drug taking in humans. As with animal research, there were questions about the degree to which nicotine was essential to maintaining smoking behavior in humans until the late 1970s (M. A. H. Russell, 1979). However, similar to Yanagita and colleagues' monkeys, humans have been shown to reject nicotine-free tobacco cigarettes when they have been introduced into the marketplace (Jaffe, 1990) and to adjust intake when nicotine content of tobacco smoke is altered (Zacny, Stitzer, Brown, Yingling, & Griffiths, 1987). Nevertheless, the degree to which nicotine per se, isolated from tobacco smoke, will be self-administered has been less certain. Henningfield and Goldberg (1983) demonstrated that humans with other drug use histories self-administer iv nicotine significantly more often than iv saline, showing that nicotine is reinforcing. Although rate of acquisition of this self-administration behavior was variable, all subjects eventually self-administered nicotine when given extended access (e.g., seven daily sessions of exposure).

Pure nicotine can be administered by a variety of routes. Each route produces a different pharmacokinetic profile that may be expected to influence the likelihood of self-administration (see the following discussion), but some routes have successfully sustained self-administration. In particular, low-dose nicotine nasal spray has been shown to be self-administered significantly more often than placebo nasal spray among smokers during the first week of smoking cessation, further demonstrating reinforcement due to nicotine (Perkins, Grobe, D'Amico, Wilson, & Stiller, 1996). However, this effect was observed only in men and not in women, consistent with other evidence supporting a sex difference in nicotine reinforcement (Perkins, 1996). An acute laboratory study showed that choice of active nicotine nasal spray increased relative to choice of placebo spray following overnight abstinence from smoking; this observation is consistent with nicotine's reinforcing properties (Perkins, Grobe, Weiss, Fonte, & Caggiula, 1996). In a study by Hughes and colleagues (J. R. Hughes et al., 1989), self-administration behavior was not greater for nicotine versus placebo gum in briefly abstinent smokers not trying to quit smoking who were blind to gum contents. This finding suggests a limit to the reinforcing properties of nicotine. Although nicotine is clearly self-administered by humans under some circumstances, an important issue in interpreting these studies concerns whether the drug acts to relieve withdrawal, thereby producing negative reinforcement, or produces direct pleasurable effects (positive reinforcement), or both.

Role of Administration Speed and Dose

While recent research clearly indicates that animals and humans will self-administer nicotine via various routes, a more relevant question is whether nicotine intake via the inhalation route from tobacco smoking (the most common means of consumption in humans) is reinforcing. Evidence has accumulated indicating that speed of drug delivery is an important parameter that determines in part the reinforcing effects of a drug. In the case of nicotine, recent research in animals has shown that speed of infusion is directly associated with degree of reinforcing efficacy. Wakasa and colleagues (1995) found high rates of responding for intravenous nicotine over an 8-day period among rhesus monkeys when the infusion speed was 5.2 μg/kg/s but reduced responding over a subsequent 8-day period when the infusion speed was 1.3 μg/kg/s and almost no responding at 0.3 μg/kg/s, despite the total dose per infusion being identical (30 μg/kg) under each condition. Since inhalation delivers nicotine to the brain within 10–20 s, compared with at least 30 s via iv infusion (Henningfield & Keenan, 1993), iv infusion studies most likely underestimate the reinforcing efficacy of nicotine inhalation from smoking. In any case, speed of uptake is a critical element in explaining why tobacco smoke inhalation is extremely reinforcing, while nicotine intake by buccal (e.g., polacrilex; approximately 30 min to peak plasma nicotine levels) or transdermal (patch; approximately 4 hr to peak plasma nicotine) absorption is generally not (Henningfield & Keenan, 1993).

Dose is a second pharmacological factor that is very important for understanding nicotine reinforcement. The nicotine dosing ranges typically self-administered by animals and humans are narrow but similar, approximately 3–30 μg/kg (Corrigall, 1992; Donny et al., 1995; Goldberg, Spealman, Risner, & Henningfield, 1983; Henningfield & Goldberg, 1983; Wakasa et al., 1995), although differences in bioavailability across administration methods and species make direct comparisons difficult (Plowchalk & deBethizy, 1992). Notably, these doses are comparable to typical cigarette yields (U.S. DHHS, 1988). Doses below this range result in extinction of responding (Donny et al., 1995; Henningfield & Goldberg, 1983), while doses exceeding this range can produce sharp reductions in responding among animals (Corrigall, 1992) and toxic side effects such as nausea and lethargy in humans (U.S. DHHS, 1988). A similar inverted-U dose–response relationship has been observed between nicotine content of cigarettes and rated "desirability" after smoking

them (Herskovic, Rose, & Jarvik, 1986), and also in the effect of nicotine dose on brain-stimulation responding, another marker of reinforcement in animals (Huston-Lyons & Kornetsky, 1992). Thus, it is the effects of relatively low to moderate doses of nicotine that appear to support self-administration, and therefore are reinforcing, while the effects of higher doses appear to be aversive. Dose-dependent effects of nicotine that may explain this inverted-U relationship with reinforcement will be discussed later.

Environmental Modulation

Discussion of nicotine self-administration has thus far been presented as if the only important modulating factor were the particular formulation of the product, specifically dose and speed of administration. However, as with any drug self-administration, or indeed any other reinforcing behavior, environmental context can also alter the strength of nicotine reinforcement. For example, food deprivation has been shown to enhance self-administration of nicotine (and other drugs) in several animal species (e.g., de la Garza & Johanson, 1989). There is suggestive evidence of a similar effect on smoking behavior in humans, as acute (several days; Cheskin et al., 1994) and long-term (several months; Niaura, Clark, Raciti, Pera, & Abrams, 1992) reductions in food intake have been associated with increased smoking consumption. Conversely, increased weight has been associated with sustained abstinence from smoking after quitting (Perkins, 1994).

The mechanism for this inverse relationship between food consumption and smoking is not clear. However, a broader concept that may be applicable is the notion that restrictions placed on access to alternative reinforcers (e.g., food) often lead to increased consumption of other available reinforcers (e.g., smoking) and vice versa (Vuchinich & Tucker, 1988). This is readily demonstrated in animals (e.g., Carroll, 1993) but is usually difficult to test in humans because of the typical lack of control over all available reinforcers during an extended period of time. However, human research has shown that manipulating monetary reward as an alternative to smoking can influence smoking behavior, with the amount of smoking reduction related to the amount of money offered as an alternative (Stitzer & Bigelow, 1983, 1984). This relationship is seen particularly when access to money and smoking are mutually exclusive choices (Perkins, Epstein, Grobe, & Fonte, 1994), although the relationship may not always be apparent when access to money is unilaterally altered and smoking is always readily available (deGrandpre, Bickel, Higgins, & Hughes, 1994).

Various chronic manipulations besides food availability may also alter nicotine reinforcement. Chronic pretreatment with caffeine has been shown to enhance acquisition of nicotine self-administration in rats (Shoaib et al., 1996). Notably, chronic pretreatment with nicotine (or amphetamine) has been shown to enhance acquisition of cocaine self-administration (Horger, Giles, & Schenk, 1992), implying that frequent use of one drug may facilitate onset of dependence on another. Chronic stress may similarly increase intake of nicotine, as has been observed with consumption of other drugs, such as ethanol (Pohorecky, 1990).

Similarly, acute manipulations of the context surrounding nicotine intake, other than availability of money, can influence nicotine self-administration. For example, smoking-reinforced responding (responses on a computer task) has been shown to increase in the presence of a lit cigarette "cue" versus no cue when the schedule of reinforcement is lean (Perkins, Epstein, et al., 1994). Moreover, in a series of studies with potentially important clinical implications, J. R. Hughes, Pickens, Spring, and Keenan (1985) demonstrated that instructions regarding the contents of nicotine or placebo gum controlled whether nicotine gum was self-administered more than placebo; that is, whether or not it was reinforcing in smokers trying to quit smoking. Expectations of drug contents of products and their effects ("expectancy") have been repeatedly demonstrated to influence drug self-administration (Marlatt, Baer, Donovan, & Klivahan, 1988). This effect clearly calls into question the simple notion that reinforcement is an inherent property of the drug itself and demonstrates that drug reinforcement cannot be evaluated in the absence of the environmental context surrounding its use.

Nicotine Reinforcement: Subjective Effects

As outlined above, nicotine alone, isolated from tobacco smoke, has been shown to be reinforcing in animals and humans (Henningfield & Goldberg, 1983; Perkins, Grobe, D'Amico, et al., 1996). Nevertheless, it has been difficult to ascertain clearly the mechanisms that explain why nicotine is reinforcing. In smokers, nicotine may enhance performance on certain behavioral and cognitive tasks, as discussed later in this chapter. However, these effects are unlikely to play a major role in the onset of nicotine dependence (Heishman, Taylor, & Henningfield, 1994). Other research indicates that nicotine may act to modulate existing dysphoric mood states. Importantly, like most other substances of abuse, nicotine also produces direct interoceptive stimulus effects in the brain that are positively reinforcing (Henningfield, Miyasato, & Jasinski, 1985; C. S. Pomerleau & Pomerleau, 1992; U.S. DHHS 1988). Since a drug's interoceptive stimulus effects are likely to be critical in understanding its reinforcing efficacy (Jasinski & Henningfield, 1989), a key to determining nicotine's reinforcing efficacy in humans lies in greater knowledge of its relatively subtle interoceptive effects and factors that modulate their magnitude (Henningfield et al., 1985; Perkins, Sanders, et al., 1997; U.S. DHHS, 1988).

Methodological Issues

There are significant methodological obstacles in examining the effects of nicotine on subjective or other measures that may be related to reinforcement in humans. Several are related to manipulation of nicotine, the independent variable. First, findings from laboratory studies manipulating acute exposure to tobacco smoking are often reported as reflecting the effects of nicotine, and "tobacco smoking" and "nicotine" effects are often used interchangeably. Tobacco smoke contains at least 4,000 other compounds besides nicotine (Gori & Lynch, 1985); some of these may be psychoactive or have reinforcing stimulus effects (Rose & Levin, 1991). Thus, manipulation of smoking exposure involves manipulation of much more than simply nicotine intake.

Second, nicotine dose is very difficult to manipulate if administered by tobacco smoking (O. F. Pomerleau, Pomerleau, & Rose, 1989). Subtle variations in depth and duration of inhalation, as well as differences in number of puffs, can result in widely differing nicotine delivery to the body from cigarettes containing a given amount of nicotine (U.S. DHHS, 1988; Zacny et al., 1987). Technology has been developed to allow measured amounts of tobacco smoke to be delivered (e.g., Gilbert, Jensen, & Meliska, 1989), but this technology can be expensive and is not in widespread use. Methods of administering measured doses of pure nicotine, isolated from smoke, can potentially overcome the difficulties of eliminating nonnicotine constituents of smoke and controlling nicotine exposure. These methods include intravenous nicotine and nasal spray nicotine (O. F. Pomerleau et al., 1989). Intravenous nicotine allows the greatest control and, along with subcutaneous or intraperitoneal administration, is common in animal research. However, in humans, iv nicotine can produce serious safety risks. Nasal spray carries fewer risks, may be less expensive, and is portable, but because of sensory effects specific to the spray (e.g., nasal irritation), may elicit subjective responses due to factors other than nicotine (Perkins, Sexton, Reynolds, et al., 1994; Sutherland, Russell, Stapleton, Feyerabend, & Ferno, 1992). Obviously, this issue of control over exposure to nicotine itself is critical to research on nicotine reinforcement; without clear control over the independent variable to be manipulated, observed responses of subjects are extremely difficult to interpret (Perkins, 1995).

A third methodological issue in human research is potentially even more perplexing. This issue concerns whether responses to nicotine in smokers constitute true effects of the drug or may reflect relief of withdrawal (normalization of subjective state from atypical baseline due to nicotine deprivation). In other words, "true" effects would reflect positive reinforcement, while withdrawal-relief would constitute negative reinforcement. While withdrawal relief may be very important for maintenance of regular tobacco smoking (Schuh & Stitzer, 1995), it would be less likely to explain onset of nicotine self-administration. There is some debate as to what the "baseline" state of a smoker should be in examining acute reinforcing effects of nicotine or smoking. Is it following ad-lib smoking (i.e., absence of any smoking deprivation) or following brief abstinence from smoking (so that basal blood nicotine levels are minimal)? If smokers are allowed to smoke ad lib during baseline, prior to the manipulation of nicotine exposure, they should not experience withdrawal and resulting responses to nicotine should not be complicated by relief of withdrawal. The disadvantage of this approach is that responses to subsequent nicotine exposure may be greatly affected by existing blood levels of nicotine, for example, by acute tolerance (Perkins, Grobe, Fonte, et al., 1994), which could vary across subjects due to variable amounts of smoking prior to the session. The advantage and disadvantage is reversed if smokers are required to abstain for some period of time prior to manipulation of nicotine exposure; that is, there is little blood nicotine to influence subsequent responses to nicotine, but some of the observed effect of that nicotine manipulation may be due to relief of withdrawal resulting from smoking abstinence. Either approach may be appropriate, depending on the particular topic of study, and researchers should take care to select the method most relevant to their topic and explain their rationale clearly. A compromise procedure sometimes used is to have smokers abstain overnight so that blood levels are low but withdrawal is not pronounced during baseline (Perkins, Grobe, Fonte, et al., 1994). For example, we often find no significant difference in self-reported withdrawal after overnight abstinence versus ad-lib smoking in smokers who do not want to quit permanently and who typically smoke at least 15 cigarettes a day (unpublished observations). Note, though, that onset of certain withdrawal symptoms can occur within a few hours of the last cigarette (Schuh & Stitzer, 1995). Use of comparison groups of never-smokers and ex-smokers, those who do not experience withdrawal since they have no recent nicotine use, also may clarify interpretation of observed nicotine effects (J. Hughes, 1991). Yet, this approach also is not as clear as it may seem, as discussed in the"Tolerance" section.

Studies of Subjective Effects

Because they are often assumed to be synonymous with subjective effects, interoceptive effects of nicotine and other drugs have typically been assessed in humans with various standardized or study-specific self-report measures (e.g., paper-and-pencil questionnaires). The two most common standard measures used have been the Profile of Mood States (POMS) and the Addiction Research Center Inventory (ARCI). In addition, investigators may utilize Visual Analog Scale (VAS) items that tap known or plausible direct effects of nicotine. For the POMS and ARCI, scores are added across items within a subscale to arrive at a score for a particular subjective effect (e.g., POMS "tension," ARCI "euphoria" scale). VAS items usually entail marking on a scale from 0 to 100 the degree to which subjective state is described by the item (e.g., "lightheaded," "dizzy," "head rush," "jittery," "tired").

Smoking, and nicotine in particular, has commonly been found to acutely increase subjective stimulation and reduce fatigue, among other effects (U.S. DHHS, 1988). However, of particular interest in assessing nicotine's abuse liability is to understand what subjective effects may be associated with nicotine self-administration. Notably, greater behavioral activation following nicotine exposure is associated with nicotine place preference in mice (Shechter, Meehan, & Schechter, 1995), indicating that "stimulating" effects of nicotine may be critical to reinforcement. Because there have been very few human studies of

self-administration of nicotine per se, as previously noted, there is little information addressing this issue. Two studies showed that the intensity of several specific positive subjective effects from nicotine during initial exposure predicted subsequent self-administration of nicotine both in a choice procedure (Perkins, Grobe, Weiss, *et al.*, 1996) and in ad-lib spray use (Perkins, Grobe, Caggiula, Wilson, & Stiller, 1997). The predictive subjective effects in each study included VAS items of "pleasant," "relaxed," and "satisfied," and POMS scales of vigor and arousal. Aversive effects (e.g., "jittery," POMS-Tension), and effects of nicotine on "liking" and "decrease in urge to smoke" were *not* related to self-administration in either study. Because the smokers in these studies were overnight abstinent, it is not clear whether these positive subjective effects are true drug effects or reflect withdrawal relief due to abstinence. However, the study of ad-lib spray use also included assessment of nicotine spray effects on withdrawal and found no relationship between withdrawal relief provided by nicotine spray and its self-administration (Perkins *et al.*, 1997). A third study also found no association between attenuation of withdrawal and amount of ad-lib spray use in the natural environment during the week after quitting smoking (Perkins, Grobe, D'Amico, *et al.*, 1996).

The degree to which these results with nicotine spray generalize to nicotine via other means, including smoking, is unknown. As discussed previously under nicotine self-administration, the speed of uptake of nicotine or any drug can have a clear effect on the degree to which it will be self-administered. Not surprisingly, rate of uptake can have a similar mpact on self-reported subjective effects following drug administration. Slow methods of nicotine gum and patch have very mild subjective effects, compared with sharper increases in these measures following other forms of nicotine administration (deWit & Zacny, 1995; Henningfield & Keenan, 1993).

Finally, it should be acknowledged that this is a relatively cursory overview of the subjective effects of nicotine, and that other, more specific subjective effects may also contribute to reinforcement. For example, smoking (and perhaps nicotine) enhances and prolongs the decline in hunger following a meal (i.e., enhances satiety), which for some smokers may be very reinforcing (Perkins, Epstein, Fonte, Mitchell, & Grobe, 1995). However, it has little effect on hunger in the fasting state and is thus not a straightforward "anorectic" drug. In addition, smoking and nicotine may have very modest effects on reducing self-reported sensitivity to pain stimuli which could also be reinforcing (Perkins, Grobe, Stiller, *et al.*, 1994).

Tolerance

Acute tolerance with repeated exposure over the course of a day as well as chronic tolerance with regular intake over years can be demonstrated for subjective and other effects of nicotine. Although definitions of acute versus chronic tolerance are not always clear-cut, acute tolerance can be demonstrated by comparing responses to a nicotine challenge following recent exposure (earlier in the day) to nicotine versus placebo. Acute tolerance is demonstrated when reduced responding to the challenge is observed following recent exposure to nicotine (Kalant & Khanna, 1990). Acute tolerance has in fact been observed for subjective responses including "head rush," "jittery," and "relaxed," as well as POMS scales of tension and confusion; these tolerance effects have been demonstrated in smokers and nonsmokers (Perkins, Grobe, Fonte, *et al.*, 1994). Acute tolerance to subjective effects has been shown to persist for at least 2 hr between nicotine exposures (Perkins, Grobe, *et al.*, 1995) and probably persists for longer than 6 hr (Fant, Schuh, & Stitzer, 1995). These observations suggest that acute tolerance plays an important role in modifying subjective effects of smoking over the course of a normal smoking day.

Chronic tolerance, on the other hand, is not as easily studied in humans. Chronic tolerance can be defined as differential response to a drug challenge as a function of chronic exposure to that drug versus no exposure (Kalant & Khanna, 1990). Thus, direct comparison of responses to nicotine between those with versus those without a chronic history of exposure (i.e., regular smokers vs. never smokers) should provide data on chronic tolerance to nicotine. Differences have been demonstrated such that smokers show less response than nonsmokers on the same measures as described previously for acute tolerance (e.g., "head rush," "jittery," POMS-tension) (Perkins, Grobe, Fonte, *et al.*, 1994). The similarity in responses affected by acute versus chronic tolerance suggests that similar mechanisms may be operating. Moreover, nicotine dose appears to produce changes in subjective arousal in an inverted-U fashion—increased arousal with low doses and no change or decreased arousal with high doses, with the dose–response curve of smokers shifted to the right, indicating tolerance. This nonlinear dose effect is similar to other effects of nicotine in animals, for example, locomotion (Clarke, 1990), and may help explain the narrow range of doses that are self-administered by animals and humans.

However, it is possible that any difference due to smoking status may be mediated by other factors specific to smokers (e.g., personality, genetics), and that nicotine might have different effects in those individuals who do and do not go on to become regular smokers even before chronic exposure has become a factor (Heath, Madden, Slutske, & Martin, 1995). Unlike the situation with animal research, those studying humans cannot ethically or practically randomize their subjects to different exposure histories (e.g., chronic nicotine vs. chronic saline); humans self-select their drug histories. Thus, it cannot be ascertained whether differences in responding to nicotine in smokers versus never smokers represents chronic tolerance or a more fundamental and static individual difference. Use of ex-smokers and very light smokers for additional comparison may allow for clarification of the source of differential responding, but these groups may differ significantly from smokers in other ways besides nicotine exposure history (J. Hughes, 1991). A strong argument in favor of the view that differences in nicotine response between smokers and nonsmokers reflect chronic tolerance is that chronic tolerance to other effects of nicotine (cardiovascular and some behavioral responses) have been found in both animals (e.g., Collins, Burch, de Fiebre, & Marks, 1988; Collins, Luo, Selvaag, & Marks, 1994), where self-selection is not a factor, and in humans, where it is a factor (Perkins, Grobe, Fonte, et al., 1994). In any case, researchers need to be aware of possible limitations in interpreting differences in response to nicotine as a function of self-selected smoking histories.

Environmental Modulation

Virtually all of the findings on subjective effects of nicotine or smoking described earlier, were found in quiescent subjects under resting laboratory conditions. Most laboratory research on drug effects attempts to minimize variability in biological and behavioral activity of subjects by having them remain at quiet rest, so that changes in measures of interest will be more readily observable. In contrast, however, much tobacco smoking (as well as other drug use) occurs in the context of various environmental conditions and in combination with other influences on mood and behavior. For example, smoking often occurs in conjunction with other drug consumption (e.g., alcohol and caffeine intake) and during light physical activity of some kind in the course of typical daily tasks. Smokers are more likely to drink alcohol or coffee and to consume greater amounts of each, compared with nonsmokers (Istvan & Matarazzo, 1984). Furthermore, much of smoking occurs while smokers are busy with tasks such as work, driving, walking, or leisure activities. It is estimated that these types of activities constitute a majority of the waking hours of adults (McArdle, Katch, & Katch, 1986). Smoking is also known to be more likely during periods characterized by stress or boredom (Gilbert, 1979). Thus, a better understanding of the subjective effects of nicotine may require examination of these effects in conjunction with environmental situations commonly found when smokers smoke.

Although environmental modulation of subjective effects of nicotine has received very little specific research attention, several studies suggest that these effects can be altered by environmental and other concurrent influences. For example, alcohol pretreatment enhanced responses to nicotine nasal spray on measures of "dizzy" and POMS scales of Vigor and Arousal in women smokers but tended to attenuate responses in men (Perkins, Sexton, et al., 1995). Perhaps analogously, in animals, chronic alcohol pretreatment can produce cross-tolerance (i.e., reduced responding) to some effects of nicotine (Collins et al., 1988), while acute alcohol pretreatment has been shown to enhance other behavioral effects of nicotine (Lapin, Maker, & Bhardwaj, 1995).

Unlike these mixed effects due to pretreatment with other drugs, light physical activity (standardized by having subjects pedal a stationary bike at a light workload) has been shown to eliminate or even reverse the increase in POMS Arousal and Vigor due to nicotine typically observed at rest (Perkins, Sexton, Stiller, et al., 1994). This attenuating effect of activity was observed only for nicotine and not for caffeine, suggesting specificity of environmental modulation and that simple distraction is not the likely mechanism. These observations suggest that smokers would require a larger nicotine dose to experience the subjectively "stimulating" effect of nicotine when smoking occurs during other activities compared with smoking at rest.

A more general notion subsuming all of these observations is that pre-drug baseline subjective state may determine subjective response to nicotine (and other drugs), such that low baseline levels of arousal may produce substantial increases following nicotine intake whereas high baseline levels produce no change or even a decrease in arousal following nicotine intake (Perkins, Grobe, Epstein, Caggiula, & Stiller, 1992). Manipulations of other subjective states, such as stress or tension, may also result in similar differential effects of nicotine (Gilbert, 1979). Smoking has been shown to acutely reduce subjective distress during a challenging task but not during a nonchallenging task (Perkins, Grobe, Fonte, & Breus, 1992). Furthermore, smoking and nicotine gum have been shown to reduce detection of muscle tension (Epstein, Dickson, McKenzie, & Russell, 1984; P. O. Russell, Epstein, Sittenfield, & Block, 1986), which increases with greater stress, perhaps helping to explain the influence of nicotine on subjective stress (see the following discussion on mood modulation effects).

These observations are consistent with a well-known and venerable concept in behavioral pharmacology, the rate-dependency hypothesis, which states that a drug will increase behavior when pre-drug behavioral activity is low but decrease behavior when pre-drug behavioral activity is high (Dews & Wenger, 1977). This is a very important concept, since it essentially states that an observed "drug" effect is based not only on its specific pharmacological action but also on the environmental context of its consumption. Environmental modulation of drug effects is an important factor that should be taken into consideration in future research, as it may provide orderly explanations for apparent variability in reported effects of nicotine.

Discriminative Stimulus Effects

Subjective measures may provide an imprecise characterization of a drug's interoceptive stimulus effects. The relationship between subjective self-reports and interoceptive stimulus effects is unclear and may not be straightforward (Preston & Bigelow, 1991). Moreover, many of these subjective measures lack sensitivity at low doses (as noted later), require good comprehension of language, use terms not familiar to some study volunteers, are lengthy to complete, and have other shortcomings that prevent them from completely describing the interoceptive stimulus effects of nicotine, including the idiosyncratic experimenter-based method of deriving items for inclusion in subjective report measures which could result in omission of features of the drug effect. These problems can be circumvented at least in part by using a supplemental assessment method that does not rely on subjective report.

Since interoceptive effects are not independently observable, a method of assessing these effects that may complement traditional subjective measures is the behavioral drug discrimination procedure. This procedure relies on observable behavioral responses to determine whether a drug's stimulus effects have been perceived by the subject (Preston & Bigelow, 1991). Widely used in animal studies, this method has shown that animals can discriminate nicotine from saline and can discriminate among different doses of nicotine, and that mecamylamine, a central and peripheral nicotinic cholinergic antagonist, can block nicotine's discriminative stimulus effects, while blockers that act only peripherally do not (e.g., Rosecrans, 1989; Stolerman, 1987). Recently, animals have been shown to discriminate nicotine analogs from placebo (e.g., ABT-418; Brioni, Kim, O'Neill, Williams, & Decker, 1994). The discriminative stimulus effects of nicotine in animals also appear to generalize to amphetamine and cocaine but not diazepam, caffeine, or other drugs (Rosecrans, 1989; Stolerman, 1987; Yanagita et al., 1983), providing some indication of the specificity of nicotine's stimulus effects.

Nicotine discrimination is also very important to study in humans; such studies can determine the extent to which findings from animal research apply to humans. In addition, since drug discrimination is sometimes viewed as an animal model of subjective effects in humans, direct comparison between discriminative stimulus and subjective effects is necessary and can be done only with humans (Preston & Bigelow, 1991). Smokers have been shown to be sensitive to differences among cigarettes varying in nicotine content (Kallman, Kallman, Harry, Woodson, & Rosecrans, 1982; Rose, 1984). However, as noted previously, administering nicotine by tobacco smoking makes it very difficult to control dosing and to clearly distinguish discrimination of nicotine from other sensory effects of smoking (e.g., harshness, taste) that may differ between cigarettes (Kallman et al., 1982).

In one study, smokers learned to reliably discriminate active nicotine nasal spray (12 μg/kg dose) from placebo, and generalization of responding was linear across intermediate doses (Perkins, DiMarco, Grobe, Scierka, & Stiller, 1994). Subjective responses associated with behavioral discrimination included increases in visual analog scales of "head rush," "jittery," and "stimulated"; no POMS scores were associated with discrimination. However, a gender difference was noted in that this association of discrimination with subjective effects was found in women but not men, whose discrimination behavior was unrelated to any subjective measure. Notably, this behavioral discrimination procedure appeared to be much more sensitive than traditional subjective measures to low doses of nicotine. The ED_{50} for discrimination (dose at which 50% of subjects are able to discriminate) was 3 µg/kg, while dose–response curves for the VAS and POMS scales were flat across generalization doses 0–8 µg/kg, increasing only at the training dose of 12 µg/kg. Similarly, research with other drugs has shown that humans will reliably self-administer drug versus placebo at doses that produce no significant subjective effects over placebo (Lamb et al., 1991), further supporting the sensitivity of behavioral measures at low drug doses. Thus, discrimination research may lead to clues about additional subjective and/or physiological dimensions of drug effects that have not previously been identified.

Other research demonstrates comparability of results in humans with findings from animal studies. For example, as in animals, nicotine discrimination in humans (by nasal spray) is attenuated by pretreatment with the central and peripheral antagonist mecamylamine (Sanders et al., 1996), but not with the peripheral antagonist trimethaphan (Perkins et al., 1998). Magnitude of dose used to train initial discrimination also influences subsequent nicotine discrimination behavior in smokers (Perkins, D'Amico, et al., 1996), as previously demonstrated in animals (Stolerman, 1987). This is important because it shows that nicotine discrimination is not an inherent characteristic of the drug but can be altered by training conditions. Interestingly, smokers self-administering iv nicotine versus saline verbally identified the drug as "cocaine" when asked if they knew what drug they were receiving (Henningfield & Goldberg, 1983). This is similar to animal studies showing generalization of nicotine discrimination to cocaine (Yanagita et al., 1983). Also consistent with some animal research and the demonstration of chronic tolerance to nicotine's subjective effects, noted previously, there is evidence that smokers are tolerant to the discriminative stimulus effects of nicotine, compared with nonsmokers (Perkins, Sanders, D'Amico, & Wilson, 1997).

It remains to be seen whether environmental modulation of nicotine's discriminative stimulus effects parallels modulations observed with subjective effects and those demonstrated in animals. Several animal studies show that nicotine discrimination is altered by pretreatment with other drugs; these findings are consistent with altered subjective effects of nicotine produced by ethanol treatment (Perkins, Sexton, et al., 1995). Ethanol, as well as diazepam, pretreatment attenuates nicotine discrimination by more than 50% in rats (Kim & Brioni, 1995), while nicotine pretreatment can enhance ethanol discrimination (Signs & Schechter, 1986). In addition, nicotine discrimination training has been found to be impaired when conducted in the presence of other drugs, such as midazolam or morphine; stimulus overshadowing (stimulus effects of one drug overwhelming the effects of another) may be the explanation (Stolerman, Mariathasan, & Garcha, 1991). Finally, concurrent clozapine (Brioni et al., 1994) and haloperidol have been shown to attenuate nicotine discrimination in animals, perhaps helping to explain increased nicotine intake from smoking that has been observed in humans given haloperidol or clozapine during experimental procedures (George, Sernyak, Ziedonis, & Woods, 1995; McEvoy, Freudenreich, Levin, & Rose, 1995).

Mood Modulating Effects of Nicotine

In addition to producing direct subjective effects (positive reinforcement) and alleviating withdrawal-induced dysphoria (negative reinforcement), nicotine may also produce its reinforcing effects in part by modulating pre-existing negative affect. A strong link between smoking and negative affect has been clearly established in epidemiological research. The first association detected was that between depression and smoking. The key findings were that depressed individuals are more likely to smoke while smokers with depression are less likely to quit (Anda *et al.*, 1990; Glassman *et al.*, 1990). Further analysis has revealed that negative affect, including neuroticism and general emotional distress, is more prominent among individuals who meet criteria as dependent smokers (Breslau, Kilbey, & Andreski, 1993). Further, the link between negative affect and smoking is clearly present even in adolescent smokers, particularly females (Patton *et al.*, 1996). These observed associations raise the possibility that nicotine is serving a functional role, at least in certain smokers, as a modulator of preexisting negative affect. Consistent with this view is the recent report that brains of smokers (assessed with PET using a radiotracer) contain 40% less MAO-B than brains of nonsmokers or former smokers (Fowler *et al.*, 1996). MAO-B is involved in the breakdown of dopamine, a neurotransmitter implicated in brain reward mechanisms and mood regulation. Further, inhibition of MAO-B is the primary mechanism of action for an entire class of effective antidepressant medications (tricyclic antidepressants). This observation lends further credence to a mood modulatory effect of nicotine, tobacco smoke, or both.

Direct evidence demonstrating a mood modulatory role for nicotine is presently limited. Research examining affect during a normal day of smoking has demonstrated that subjective reports of stressful affect are high before smoking each cigarette and decrease reliably after smoking (Parrot & Joyce, 1993). However, this could reflect cyclic patterns of withdrawal onset and relief during a day of regular smoking rather than modulation of preexisting mood. Direct experimental evidence supporting a mood-modulating effect for nicotine and/or tobacco smoking has been obtained primarily in studies where negative affect has been manipulated by exposing subjects to stress-inducing performance tasks (Payne, Share, Levis, & Coletti, 1991; C. S. Pomerleau & Pomerleau, 1987). These studies have generally shown that smoking urges and actual smoking behaviors increase more during stressful than nonstressful situations and that smoking during a stressful situation generally results in decreased reports of stress. Given the strong link between smoking and negative affect as well as the strongly implicated role of negative affect in relapse (Shiffman, 1986), additional research is warranted to further illuminate the potential role played by mood modulation (including depression, anxiety, and subclinical emotional distress) in the reinforcing effects of nicotine.

Nicotine Reinforcement: Performance Effects

Nicotine reinforcement may also derive from its effects on response domains other than interoceptive stimuli. Nicotine is known to improve performance on selective behavioral or cognitive tasks, although the robustness of these effects and their relationship to initiation of smoking has been questioned (Heishman *et al.*, 1994). Many of the same methodological issues discussed previously concerning interpretation of nicotine's subjective effects also apply to its performance effects. For example, if nicotine improves performance in abstinent smokers but not in nonabstinent smokers, this could reflect restoration of performance from adverse effects due to withdrawal in abstinent smokers, acute tolerance to nicotine's effects in the nonabstinent smokers, or both. Moreover, there is the additional complication that repeated performance testing can lead to either improvement over trials because of practice effects or impairment over trials because of fatigue, necessitating use of placebo controls. A comprehensive examination of nicotine effects on human behavior and performance is beyond the scope of this chapter. A more general overview follows.

Animals

The dose–response relationship of nicotine's effects on many behavioral measures in animals is nonlinear. Small doses typically increase locomotion and various nonspecific behaviors, while large doses usually decrease these behaviors (Clarke, 1990). Tolerance develops quickly such that nicotine pretreated animals show a shift to the right in this nonlinear nicotine challenge dose–response curve, relative to saline pretreated animals (Stolerman, Mirza, & Shoaib, 1995). Nicotine's influence on more complex behaviors is not as clear, but nicotine has been shown to improve visual tracking (Evenden, Turpin, Oliver, & Jennings, 1993) and radial maze memory (Levin, Briggs, Christopher, & Rose, 1992). Nicotine also reverses behavioral deficits in animals resulting from aging (Stolerman *et al.*, 1995), chronic consumption of a choline-deficient diet (Sasaki *et al.*, 1991), and scopolamine pretreatment (Terry, Buccafusco, & Jackson, 1993). Recent research has extended many of these findings to the effects of nicotine analogs. For example, ABT-418, a selective nicotine acetylcholine receptor agonist, restores normal performance in septal-lesioned animals, enhances matching-to-sample performance, and reduces inhibitory avoidance (Garvey *et al.*, 1994).

Humans: Direct Performance Enhancement

As suggested previously, it is important to separate effects of nicotine in abstinent smokers, where withdrawal relief may be an explanation, from effects in the absence of withdrawal (e.g., in nonsmokers). The most reliable performance effect of nicotine observed in the absence of withdrawal is increased speed of finger tapping and simple cognitive processing (e.g., reaction time), while effects on more complex tasks do not appear to be consistent or robust (Heishman *et al.*, 1994). For example, iv nicotine improves speed but not accuracy of simple choice reaction-time performance in nonsmokers (Le Houzec *et al.*, 1994). Similar to the nonlinear dose effects of nicotine on behavior in animals, nicotine by nasal spray has been shown to improve memory recognition (correct identification of words presented 10 min earlier) and speed fin-

ger tapping in an inverted-U fashion, with improvement at small doses and no change or decline at moderate doses (Perkins, Grobe, Fonte, *et al.*, 1994). An inverted-U relationship between nicotine yield of acutely smoked cigarette and memory performance has also been reported (Krebs, Petros, & Beckwith, 1994). Other research has also shown that smoking and nicotine (by gum) can prevent performance decline on vigilance tasks (e.g., identifying a designated stimulus pattern of consecutive odd numbers within a larger array of numbers presented over headphones continuously for 1 hr) (Parrott & Winder, 1989; see also Heishman *et al.*, 1994). On other performance measures (e.g., learning and other cognitive abilities), there is no evidence that nicotine improves performance.

Studies with nonsmokers may be particularly useful in evaluating the influence of nicotine on performance; since withdrawal relief cannot explain their slightly improved performance at low doses, this influence may reflect a true drug effect (J. Hughes, 1991). To the extent that improved performance on these simple cognitive and psychomotor tasks may be reinforcing, observing improvement only at small or moderate doses may further explain the narrow range of doses self-administered by humans. However, it is important to emphasize that nicotine improves performance only on a small number of relatively simple tasks. It has been argued (Heishman *et al.*, 1994) that nicotine's ability to enhance and maintain performance may not be critical to smoking initiation or dependence because most smokers are not frequently faced with the kinds of simple performance tasks improved by nicotine, nor do they face serious consequences for sub-par performance on these tasks. However, other research has shown that, when performance on specific tasks is emphasized, choice of drug is altered substantially in order to improve or prevent impaired performance (Silverman, Kirby, & Griffiths, 1994). Thus, in selected smokers who may benefit from specific performance effects of nicotine, or who experience deficits in performance of important tasks due to abstinence, these performance effects may be important in maintaining smoking behavior.

Reversal of Withdrawal-Induced Performance Impairment

In contrast with the limited evidence for improvements in performance in the absence of withdrawal, the evidence that nicotine restores performance impaired by nicotine withdrawal is somewhat more consistent (Heishman *et al.,* 1994). Snyder and Henningfield (1989), for example, clearly showed that nicotine gum dose-dependently reversed the adverse effects of tobacco abstinence on attention and cognitive processing tasks such as letter searching and speed (but not accuracy) of arithmetic problem completion. Similarly, Petrie and Deary (1989) examined the effects of smoking on a variety of cognitive processing tasks in briefly abstinent smokers and found that smoking improved performance only on measures involving a motor component, consistent with the notion that simple psychomotor performance, but not more complex cognitive functions, is facilitated by nicotine. Other research has shown that nicotine gum reverses abstinence-induced impairment of performance on psychomotor tracking tasks and critical flicker fusion threshold, a measure of cortical arousal (Sherwood, Kerr, & Hindmarch, 1992). However, reversal of abstinence-induced performance impairment is not universal; Snyder and Henningfield (1989) found no effect of nicotine gum on speed or accuracy of logical reasoning or on immediate or delayed recall. Overall, existing data support reversal of withdrawal-induced impairment primarily on tasks involving motor speed and attention (Heishman *et al.,* 1994). Nevertheless, the degraded task performance induced by smoking abstinence may be quite salient to smokers, and avoidance of withdrawal-induced performance deficits provides a plausible mechanism that may account at least in part for maintenance of nicotine intake by regular smokers.

The specific mechanism for nicotine's effects in reversing these selective abstinence-induced impairments is not known with certainty, but may involve amelioration of concentration deficits typically experienced during abstinence (Rusted & Warburton, 1992) as well as more direct enhancing effects on cognitive processing. Two mechanisms other than withdrawal relief may also contribute to nicotine-induced restoration of impaired performance caused by smoking abstinence. First, repeated performance of specific tasks in conjunction with nicotine intake by smoking can lead to smoking becoming a conditioned stimulus for the task; eliminating smoking can thus disrupt performance by disrupting the conditioned association of smoking with the task (Payne, Etscheidt, & Corrigan, 1990). Also, smoking has been shown to produce state-dependent learning (SDL) (Lowe, 1991). In SDL, performance on a task learned in one drug state (e.g., presence of nicotine) is impaired when tested in another drug state (e.g., absence of nicotine). Performance of a word-recall memory task has been shown to be best when learning and testing, conducted on separate days, are both done in the same state (i.e., smoking before both or not smoking before both) than when done in different states (smoking before one or the other, but not both; Peters & McGee, 1982). Comparable results have been found in studies combining drug states, such as nicotine in combination with alcohol (Lowe, 1991).

Environmental Modulation of Performance Effects

As with nicotine's effects on subjective measures, it may be critical to consider environmental context and other factors in evaluating nicotine's influence on performance tasks. The research on state-dependent learning demonstrates that effects of nicotine on performance during testing can depend on the state in which learning occurred and is not simply based on the pharmacological actions of nicotine. As discussed previously, the rate-dependency hypothesis would predict that nicotine increases responding when pre-drug level is low but decrease responding when pre-drug level is high. Specific task demands producing high or low response rates would be expected to be differentially influenced by nicotine intake. Nicotine has been shown to have such an effect on behavior in animals, increasing behavior in those with low baseline rates and decreasing behavior in those with high baseline rates (Rosecrans, 1971).

Performance Effects in Neuropsychiatric Disorders

Finally, an area with exciting potential for advancing basic and clinical research is the study of nicotine's effects on performance and cognitive processing in patients with neuropsychiatric disorders. Evidence from studies of relatively short-term dosing indicates that nicotine (gum, patch, iv) may improve sensory gating (filtering out irrelevant stimuli) in schizophrenia (Freedman *et al.*, 1994), attenuate verbal learning errors and improve long-term recall in Alzheimer's disease (Newhouse, Potter, & Lenox, 1993), reduce tremor and disorganized thinking and improve depression in patients with Parkinson's disease (Fagerstrom, Pomerleau, Giordani, & Stelson, 1994), and potentiate the effects of neuroleptics in reducing motor and vocal tics in Tourette's syndrome (Silver & Sanberg, 1993). Recently, Levin and colleagues (1996) found that transdermal nicotine improved reaction time and time estimation (measure of inattention) in adults with attention-deficit/hyperactivity disorder. Improvements were stronger among nonsmokers versus smokers, indicating a true drug effect. Nicotine has also been shown to reverse memory deficits in humans due to scopolamine pretreatment (Riedel *et al.*, 1995).

In summary, nicotine produces modest improvement in performance of relatively simple psychomotor tasks in those not experiencing nicotine withdrawal (e.g., nonsmokers), but few other direct performance-enhancing effects have been reliably observed. Thus, it is questionable whether direct performance enhancement is a component of nicotine's positive reinforcement effect. Nicotine does restore performance impaired due to tobacco abstinence, however, suggesting a source of negative reinforcement that may be a factor in promoting continued smoking among regular smokers. Finally, nicotine may have previously unrecognized medical utility for restoring impaired cognitive and motor deficits in certain neuropsychiatric disorders. As with nicotine's interoceptive effects, its influence on task performance may depend on the environmental context of nicotine intake, prior performance of the task in conjunction with nicotine, and other contextual factors beyond its direct pharmacological actions. There is a need to take these factors into account in further exploring the features and clinical implications of nicotine's performance effects.

ACKNOWLEDGMENTS

Preparation of this chapter was supported by NIDA grants DA05807 (KAP), DA08578 (KAP), and DA03893 (MLS).

References

Anda, R. F., Williamson, D. F., Escobedo, L. G., Mast, E. E., Giovino, G. A., & Remington, P. L. (1990). Depression and the dynamics of smoking: A national perspective. *Journal of the American Medical Association, 26,* 1541–1545.

Breslau, N., Kilbey, M., & Andreski, P. (1993). Vulnerability to psychopathology in nicotine-dependent smokers: An epidemiologic study of young adults. *American Journal of Psychiatry, 150,* 941–946.

Brioni, J. D., Kim, D. J. B., O'Neill, A. B., Williams, J. E. G., & Decker, M. W. (1994). Clozapine attenuates the discriminative stimulus properties of -nicotine. *Brain Research, 643,* 1–9.

Carroll, M. E. (1993). The economic context of drug and non-drug reinforcers affects acquisition and maintenance of drug-reinforced behavior and withdrawal effects. *Drug and Alcohol Dependence, 33,* 201–210.

Cheskin, L. J., Wiersema, L., Hess, J., Goldsborough, D., Tayback, M., Henningfield, J. E., & Gorelick, D. A. (1994). Caloric restriction increases nicotine consumption in cigarette smokers. *Problems of Drug Dependence 1994* (NIDA Research Monograph No. 153, p. 262). Washington, DC: U.S. Public Health Service.

Clarke, P. B. S. (1990). Dopaminergic mechanisms in the locomotor stimulant effects of nicotine. *Biochemical Pharmacology, 40,* 1427–1432.

Collins, A. C., Burch, J. B., de Fiebre, C. M., & Marks, M. J. (1988). Tolerance to and cross-tolerance between ethanol and nicotine. *Pharmacology, Biochemistry and Behavior, 29,* 365–373.

Collins, A. C., Luo, Y., Selvaag, S., & Marks, M. J. (1994). Sensitivity to nicotine and brain nicotinic receptors are altered by chronic nicotine and mecamylamine infusion. *Journal of Pharmacology and Experimental Therapeutics, 271,* 125–133.

Corrigall, W. A. (1992). A rodent model for nicotine self-administration. In A. Boulton, G. Baker, & P. H. Wu (Eds.), *Neuromethods: Vol. 24. Animal models of drug addiction* (pp. 315–344). Clifton, NJ: Humana.

deGrandpre, R. J., Bickel, W. K., Higgins, S. T., & Hughes, J. R. (1994). A behavioral economic analysis of concurrently available money and cigarettes. *Journal of the Experimental Analysis of Behavior, 61,* 191–201.

de la Garza, R., & Johanson, C. E. (1989). The effects of food deprivation on the self-administration of psychoactive drugs. *Drug and Alcohol Dependence, 19,* 17–27.

deWit, H., & Zacny, J. (1995). Abuse potential of nicotine replacement therapies. *CNS Drugs, 4,* 456–468.

Dews, P. B., & Wenger, G. R. (1977). Rate-dependency of the behavioral effects of amphetamine. In T. Thompson & P. B. Dews (Eds.), *Advances in behavioral pharmacology* (Vol. 1, pp. 167–227). New York: Academic Press.

Donny, E., Caggiula, A. R., Knopf, S., & Brown, C. (1995). Nicotine self-administration in rats. *Psychopharmacology, 122,* 390–394.

Epstein, L. H., Dickson, B. E., McKenzie, S., & Russell, P. O. (1984). The effect of smoking on perception of muscle tension. *Psychopharmacology, 83,* 107–113.

Evenden, J. L., Turpin, M., Oliver, L., & Jennings, C. (1993). Caffeine and nicotine improve visual tracking by rats: A comparison with amphetamine, cocaine, and apomorphine. *Psychopharmacology, 110,* 169–176.

Fagerstrom, K. O., Pomerleau, O., Giordani, B., & Stelson, F. (1994). Nicotine may relieve symptoms of Parkinson's disease. *Psychopharmacology, 116,* 117–119.

Fant, R. V., Schuh, K. J., & Stitzer, M. L. (1995). Response to smoking as a function of prior smoking amounts. *Psychopharmacology, 119,* 385–390.

Fowler, J. S., Volkow, N. D., Wang, G. J., Pappas, N., Logan, J., MacGregor, R., Alexoff, D., Shea, C., Schlyer, D., Wolf, A., Warner, D., Zezulkova, I., & Cilento, R. (1996). Inhibition of monoamine oxidase B in the brains of smokers. *Nature, 379,* 733–736.

Freedman, R., Adler, L. E., Bickford, P., Byerley, W., Coon, H., Cullum, C. M., Griffith, J. M., Harris, J. G., Leonard, S., Miller, C., Myles-Worsley, M., Nagamoto, H. T., Rose, G., & Waldo, M. (1994). Schizophrenia and nicotinic receptors. *Harvard Review of Psychiatry, 2,* 179–192.

Garvey, D. S., Wasicak, J. T., Decker, M. W., Brioni, J. D., Sullivan, J. P., Carrera, G. M., Holladay, M., Arneric, S., & Williams, M. (1994). Novel isoxazoles which interact with brain cholinergic channel receptors have intrinsic cognitive enhancing and anxiolytic activities. *Journal of Medicinal Chemistry, 37,* 1055–1059.

George, T. P., Sernyak, M. J., Ziedonis, D. M., & Woods, S. W. (1995). Effects of clozapine on smoking in chronic schizophrenic outpatients. *Journal of Clinical Psychiatry, 56,* 344–346.

Gilbert, D. G. (1979). Paradoxical tranquilizing and emotion-reducing effects of nicotine. *Psychological Bulletin, 86,* 643–661.

Gilbert, D. G., Jensen, R. A., & Meliska, C. J. (1989). A system for administering quantified doses of tobacco smoke to human subjects: Plasma nicotine and filter pad validation. *Pharmacology, Biochemistry and Behavior, 31,* 905–908.

Glassman, A. H., Helzer, J. E., Covey, L. S., Cottler, L. B., Stetner, F., Tipp, J. E., & Johnson, J. (1990). Smoking, smoking cessation, and major depression. *Journal of the American Medical Association, 264,* 1546–1549.

Goldberg, S. R., Spealman, R. D., Risner, M. E., & Henningfield, J. E. (1983). Control of behavior by intravenous nicotine injections in laboratory animals. *Pharmacology, Biochemistry and Behavior, 19,* 1011–1020.

Gori, G. B., & Lynch, C. J. (1985). Analytical cigarette yields as predictors of smoke bioavailability. *Regulatory Toxicology and Pharmacology, 5,* 314–326.

Heath, A. C., Madden, P. A., Slutske, W. S., & Martin, N. G. (1995). Personality and the inheritance of smoking behavior: A genetic perspective. *Behavior Genetics, 25,* 103–117.

Heishman, S. J., Taylor, R. C., & Henningfield, J. E. (1994). Nicotine and smoking: A review of effects on human performance. *Experimental and Clinical Psychopharmacology, 2,* 345–395.

Henningfield, J. E., & Goldberg, S. R. (1983). Control of behavior by intravenous nicotine injections in human subjects. *Pharmacology, Biochemistry and Behavior, 19,* 1021–1026.

Henningfield, J. E., & Keenan, R. (1993). Nicotine delivery kinetics and abuse liability. *Journal of Consulting and Clinical Psychology, 61,* 743–750.

Henningfield, J. E., Miyasato, K., & Jasinski, D. R. (1985). Abuse liability and pharmacodynamic characteristics of intravenous and inhaled nicotine. *Journal of Pharmacology and Experimental Therapeutics, 234,* 1–12.

Herskovic, J. E., Rose, J. E., & Jarvik, M. E. (1986). Cigarette desirability and nicotine preference in smokers. *Pharmacology, Biochemistry and Behavior, 24,* 171–175.

Horger, B. A., Giles, M. K., & Schenk, S. (1992). Preexposure to amphetamine and nicotine predisposes rats to self-administer a low dose of cocaine. *Psychopharmacology, 107,* 271–276.

Hughes, J. (1991). Distinguishing withdrawal relief and direct effects of smoking. *Psychopharmacology, 104,* 409–410.

Hughes, J. R., Pickens, R. W., Spring, W., & Keenan, R. M. (1985). Instructions control whether nicotine will serve as a reinforcer. *Journal of Pharmacology and Experimental Therapeutics, 235,* 106–112.

Hughes, J. R., Strickler, G., King, D., Higgins, S. T., Fenwick, J. W., Gulliver, S. B., & Mireault, G. (1989). Smoking history, instructions, and the effects of nicotine: Two pilot studies. *Pharmacology, Biochemistry and Behavior, 34,* 149–155.

Huston-Lyons, D., & Kornetsky, C. (1992). Effects of nicotine on the threshold for rewarding brain stimulation in rats. *Pharmacology, Biochemistry and Behavior, 41,* 755–759.

Istvan, J., & Matarazzo, J. D. (1984). Tobacco, alcohol and caffeine use: A review of their interrelationships. *Psychological Bulletin, 95,* 301–326.

Jaffe, J. H. (1990). Tobacco smoking and nicotine dependence. In S. Wonnacott, M. A. H. Russell & I. P. Stolerman (Eds.), *Nicotine psychopharmacology: Molecular, cellular, and behavioural aspects* (pp. 1–37). New York: Oxford University Press.

Jasinski, D. R., & Henningfield, J. E. (1989). Human abuse liability assessment by measurement of subjective and physiological effects. In M. W. Fischman & N. K. Mello (Eds.), *Testing for abuse liability of drugs in humans* (NIDA Research Monograph No. 92, pp. 73–100). Washington, DC: U.S. Government Printing Office.

Kalant, H., & Khanna, J. M. (1990). Methods for the study of tolerance. In M. Adler & A. Cowan (Eds.), *Modern methods in pharmacology* (Vol. 6, pp. 43–66). New York: Wiley-Liss.

Kallman, W. M., Kallman, M. J., Harry, G. J., Woodson, P. P., & Rosecrans, J. A. (1982). Nicotine as a discriminative stimulus in human subjects. In F. C. Colpaert & J. L. Slangen (Eds.), *Drug discrimination: Applications in CNS pharmacology* (pp. 211–218). Amsterdam: Elsevier Biomedical Press.

Kim, D. J. B., & Brioni, J. D. (1995). Modulation of the discriminative stimulus properties of (–)nicotine by diazepam and ethanol. *Drug Development Research, 34,* 47–54.

Krebs, S. J., Petros, T. V., & Beckwith, B. E. (1994). Effects of smoking on memory for prose passages. *Physiology & Behavior, 56,* 723–727.

Lamb, R. J., Preston, K. L., Schindler, C. W., Meisch, R. A., Davis, F., Katz, J. L., Henningfield, J. E., & Goldberg, S. R. (1991). The reinforcing and subjective effects of morphine in post-addicts: A dose–response study. *Journal of Pharmacology and Experimental Therapeutics, 259,* 1165–1173.

Lapin, E. P., Maker, H. S., & Bhardwaj, A. (1995). Ethanol enhancement of the motor-stimulating effect of nicotine in the rat. *Alcohol, 12,* 217–220.

Le Houzec, J., Halliday, R., Benowitz, N. L., Callaway, E., Naylor, H., & Herzig, K. (1994). A low dose of subcutaneous nicotine improves information processing in non-smokers. *Psychopharmacology, 114,* 628–634.

Levin, E. D., Briggs, S. J., Christopher, N. C., & Rose, J. E. (1992). Persistence of chronic nicotine-induced cognitive facilitation. *Behavioral and Neural Biology, 58,* 152–158.

Levin, E. D., Conners, C. K., Sparrow, E., Hinton, S. C., Erhardt, D., Meck, W. H., Rose, J. E., & March, J. (1996). Nicotine effects on adults with attention-deficit/hyperactivity disorder. *Psychopharmacology, 123,* 55–63.

Lowe, G. (1991). State-dependent learning with social drugs. In R. A. Glennon, T. U. C. Jarbe & J. Frankenheim (Eds.), *Drug discrimination: Applications to drug abuse research* (NIDA Research Monograph No. 116, pp. 267–276). Washington, DC: U.S. Government Printing Office.

Marlatt, G. A., Baer, J. S., Donovan, D. M., & Klivahan, D. R. (1988). Addictive behaviors: Etiology and treatment. *Annual Review of Psychology, 39,* 223–252.

McArdle, W. D., Katch, F. I., & Katch, V. L. (1986). *Exercise physiology* (2nd ed.). New York: Lea & Fibiger.

McEvoy, J. P., Freudenreich, O., Levin, E. D., & Rose, J. E. (1995). Haloperidol increases smoking in patients with schizophrenia. *Psychopharmacology, 119,* 124–126.

Newhouse, P. A., Potter, A., & Lenox, R. H. (1993). The effects of nicotinic agents on human cognition: Possible therapeutic applications in Alzheimer's and Parkinson's diseases. *Medicinal Chemistry Research, 2,* 628–642.

Niaura, R., Clark, M. M., Raciti, M. A., Pera, V., & Abrams, D. B. (1992). Increased saliva cotinine concentrations in smokers during rapid weight loss. *Journal of Consulting and Clinical Psychology, 60,* 985–987.

Parrott, A. C., & Joyce, C. (1993). Stress and arousal rhythms in cigarette smokers, deprived smokers, and non-smokers. *Human Psychopharmacology, 8,* 21–28.

Parrott, A. C., & Winder, G. (1989). Nicotine chewing gum (2 mg, 4 mg) and cigarette smoking: Comparative effects upon vigilance and heart rate. *Psychopharmacology, 97,* 257–261.

Patton, G. C., Hibbert, M., Rosier, M. J., Carlin, J. B., Caust, J., & Bowes, G. (1996). Is smoking associated with depression and anxiety in teenagers? *American Journal of Public Health, 86,* 225–230.

Payne, T. J., Etscheidt, M., & Corrigan, S. A. (1990). Conditioning arbitrary stimuli to cigarette smoke intake: A preliminary study. *Journal of Substance Abuse, 2,* 113–119.

Payne, T. J., Share, M. L., Levis, D. J., & Coletti, G. (1991). Exposure to smoking-relevant cues: Effects on desire to smoke and topographical components of smoking behavior. *Addictive Behaviors, 16,* 467–479.

Perkins, K. A. (1994). Issues in the prevention of weight gain after smoking cessation. *Annals of Behavioral Medicine, 16,* 46–52.

Perkins, K. A. (1995). Individual variability in response to nicotine. *Behavior Genetics, 25,* 119–132.

Perkins, K. A. (1996). Sex differences in nicotine vs. non-nicotine reinforcement as determinants of tobacco smoking. *Experimental and Clinical Psychopharmacology, 4,* 166–177.

Perkins, K. A., Grobe, J. E., Epstein, L. H., Caggiula, A. R., & Stiller, R. L. (1992). Effects of nicotine on subjective arousal may be dependent on baseline subjective state. *Journal of Substance Abuse, 4,* 131–141.

Perkins, K. A., Grobe, J. E., Fonte, C., & Breus, M. (1992). "Paradoxical" effects of smoking on subjective stress versus cardiovascular arousal in males and females. *Pharmacology, Biochemistry and Behavior, 42,* 301–311.

Perkins, K. A., DiMarco, A., Grobe, J. E., Scierka, A. C., & Stiller, R. L. (1994). Nicotine discrimination in male and female smokers. *Psychopharmacology, 116,* 407–413.

Perkins, K. A., Epstein, L. H., Grobe, J. E., & Fonte, C. (1994). Tobacco abstinence, smoking cues, and the reinforcing value of smoking. *Pharmacology, Biochemistry and Behavior, 47,* 107–112.

Perkins, K. A., Grobe, J. E., Fonte, C., Goettler, J., Caggiula, A. R., Reynolds, W. A., Stiller, R. L., Scierka, A., & Jacob, R. (1994). Chronic and acute tolerance to subjective, behavioral, and cardiovascular effects of nicotine in humans. *Journal of Pharmacology and Experimental Therapeutics, 270,* 628–638.

Perkins, K. A., Grobe, J. E., Stiller, R. L., Scierka, A., Goettler, J., Reynolds, W., & Jennings, J. R. (1994). Effects of nicotine on thermal pain detection in humans. *Experimental and Clinical Psychopharmacology, 2,* 95–106.

Perkins, K. A., Sexton, J. E., Reynolds, W. A., Grobe, J. E., Fonte, C., & Stiller, R. L. (1994). Comparison of acute subjective and heart rate effects of nicotine intake via tobacco smoking vs. nasal spray. *Pharmacology, Biochemistry and Behavior, 47,* 295–299.

Perkins, K. A., Sexton, J. E., Stiller, R. L., Fonte, C., DiMarco, A., Goettler, J., & Scierka, A. (1994). Subjective and cardiovascular responses to nicotine combined with caffeine during rest and casual activity. *Psychopharmacology, 113,* 438–444.

Perkins, K. A., Epstein, L. H., Fonte, C., Mitchell, S.L., & Grobe, J. E. (1995). Gender, dietary restraint, and smoking's influence on hunger and the reinforcing value of food. *Physiology & Behavior, 57,* 675–680.

Perkins, K. A., Grobe, J. E., Mitchell, S. L., Goettler, J., Caggiula, A., Stiller, R. L., & Scierka, A. (1995). Acute tolerance to nicotine in smokers: Lack of dissi-

pation within 2 hours. *Psychopharmacology, 118,* 164–170.

Perkins, K. A., Sexton, J. E., DiMarco, A., Grobe, J., Scierka, A., & Stiller, R. L. (1995). Subjective and cardiovascular responses to nicotine combined with alcohol in male and female smokers. *Psychopharmacology, 119,* 205–212.

Perkins, K. A., D'Amico, D., Sanders, M., Grobe, J. E., Wilson, A., & Stiller, R. L. (1996). Influence of training dose on nicotine discrimination in humans. *Psychopharmacology, 126,* 132–9.

Perkins, K. A., Grobe, J. E., D'Amico, D., Fonte, C., Wilson, A. S., & Stiller, R. L. (1996). Low-dose nicotine nasal spray use and effects during initial smoking cessation. *Experimental and Clinical Psychopharmacology, 4,* 157–165.

Perkins, K. A., Grobe, J. E., Weiss, D., Fonte, C., & Caggiula, A. (1996). Nicotine preference in smokers as a function of smoking abstinence. *Pharmacology, Biochemistry and Behavior, 55,* 257–263.

Perkins, K. A., Grobe, J. E., Caggiula, A., Wilson, A. S., & Stiller, R. L. (1997). Acute reinforcing effects of low-dose nicotine nasal spray in humans. *Pharmacology, Biochemistry and Behavior, 56,* 235–241.

Perkins, K. A., Sanders, M., D'Amico, D., & Wilson, A. (1997). Nicotine discrimination and self-administration in humans as a function of smoking status. *Psychopharmacology, 131,* 361–370.

Perkins, K. A., Sanders, M., Fonte, C., Wilson, A. S.,White, W., Stiller, R. L., & McNamara, D. (1998). Effects of central and peripheral nicotinic blockade on human nicotine discrimination. Unpublished manuscript.

Peters, R., & McGee, R. (1982). Cigarette smoking and state dependent memory. *Psychopharmacology, 76,* 232–235.

Petrie, R. X. A., & Deary, I. J. (1989). Smoking and human information processing. *Psychopharmacology, 99,* 393–396.

Plowchalk, D. R., & deBethizy, J. D. (1992). Interspecies scaling of nicotinic concentration in the brain. In P. M. Lippiello, A. C. Collins, J. A. Gray, & J. H. Robinson (Eds.), *The biology of nicotine: Current research issues* (pp. 55–70). New York: Raven.

Pohorecky, L. A. (1990). Interaction of ethanol and stress: research with experimental animals—An update. *Alcohol & Alcoholism, 25,* 263–276.

Pomerleau, C. S., & Pomerleau, O. F. (1987). The effects of a psychological stressor on cigarette smoking and subsequent behavioral and physiological reponses. *Psychophysiology, 24,* 278–285.

Pomerleau, C. S., & Pomerleau, O. F. (1992). Euphoriant effects of nicotine in smokers. *Psychopharmacology, 108,* 460–465.

Pomerleau, O. F., Pomerleau, C. S., & Rose, J. E. (1989). Controlled dosing of nicotine: A review of problems and progress. *Annals of Behavioral Medicine, 11,* 158–163.

Preston, K. L., & Bigelow, G. E. (1991). Subjective and discriminative effects of drugs. *Behavioural Pharmacology, 2,* 293–313.

Riedel, W., Hogervorst, E., Leboux, R., Verhey, F., van Praag, H., & Jolles, J. (1995). Caffeine attenuates scopolamine-induced memory impairment in humans. *Psychopharmacology, 122,* 158–168.

Rose, J. E. (1984). Discriminability of nicotine in tobacco smoke: Implications for titration. *Addictive Behaviors, 9,* 189–193.

Rose, J. E., & Levin, E. D. (1991). Inter-relationships between conditioned and primary reinforcement in the maintenance of cigarette smoking. *British Journal of Addiction, 86,* 605–609.

Rosecrans, J. A. (1971). Effects of nicotine on behavioral arousal and brain 5-hydroxytryptamine function in female rats selected for differences in activity. *European Journal of Pharmacology, 14,* 29–37.

Rosecrans, J. A. (1989). Nicotine as a discriminative stimulus: A neurobiological approach to studying central cholinergic mechanisms. *Journal of Substance Abuse, 1,* 287–300.

Russell, M. A. H. (1979). Tobacco dependence: Is nicotine rewarding or aversive? In N. Krasnegor (Ed.), *Cigarette smoking as a dependence process* (NIDA Research Monograph No. 23, pp. 100–122). Washington, DC: U.S. Government Printing Office.

Russell, P. O., Epstein, L. H., Sittenfield, S. L., & Block, D. R. (1986). The effects of nicotine chewing gum on the sensitivity to muscle tension. *Psychopharmacology, 89,* 230–233.

Rusted, J. M., & Warburton, D. M. (1992). Facilitation of memory by post-trial administration of nicotine: Evidence for an attentional explanation. *Psychopharmacology, 108,* 452–455.

Sanders, M., D'Amico, D., Perkins, K. A., Wilson, A. S., Stiller, R. L., Heesch, C., & McNamara, D. (1996, March). *Effects of mecamylamine on human nicotine discrimination.* Paper presented at the 2nd annual meeting of the Society for Research on Nicotine and Tobacco, Washington, DC.

Sasaki, H., Yanai, M., Meguro, K., Sekizawa, K., Ikarashi, Y., Maruyama, Y., Yamamoto, M., Matsuzaki, Y., & Takishima, T. (1991). Nicotine improves cognitive disturbance in rodents fed with a choline-deficient diet. *Pharmacology, Biochemistry and Behavior, 38,* 921–925.

Schechter, M. D., Meehan, S. M., & Schechter, J. B. (1995). Genetic selection for nicotine activity in mice correlates with conditioned place preference. *European Journal of Pharmacology, 279,* 59–64.

Schuh, K. J., & Stitzer, M. L. (1995). Desire to smoke during spaced smoking intervals. *Psychopharmacology, 120,* 289–295.

Sherwood, N., Kerr, J. S., & Hindmarch, I. (1992). Psychomotor performance in smokers following single and repeated doses of nicotine gum. *Psychopharmacology, 108,* 432–436.

Shiffman, S. (1986). A cluster analytic classification of smoking relapse episodes. *Addictive Behaviors, 11,* 295–307.

Shoaib, M., Swanner, L. S., Schindler, C. W., & Goldberg, S. R. (1996, March). *Genetic and environmental factors in nicotine self-administration.* Paper presented at the 2nd annual meeting of the Society for Research on Nicotine and Tobacco, Washington, DC.

Signs, S. A., & Schechter, M. D. (1986). Nicotine-induced potentiation of ethanol discrimination. *Pharmacology, Biochemistry and Behavior, 24,* 769–771.

Silver, A. A., & Sanberg, P. R. (1993). Transdermal nicotine patch and potentiation of haloperidol in Tourette's syndrome. *Lancet, 342,* 182.

Silverman, K., Kirby, K. C., & Griffiths, R. R. (1994). Modulation of drug reinforcement by behavioral requirements following drug ingestion. *Psychopharmacology, 114,* 243–247.

Snyder, F. R., & Henningfield, J. E. (1989). Effects of nicotine administration following 12 h of tobacco deprivation: Assessment on computerized performance tasks. *Psychopharmacology, 97,* 17–22.

Stitzer, M. L., & Bigelow, G. E. (1983). Contingent payment for carbon monoxide reduction: Effects of pay amount. *Behavior Therapy, 14,* 647–656.

Stitzer, M. L., & Bigelow, G. E. (1984). Contingent reinforcement for carbon monoxide reduction: Within-subject effects of pay amount. *Journal of Applied Behavior Analysis, 17,* 477–483.

Stolerman, I. P. (1987). Psychopharmacology of nicotine: Stimulus effects and receptor mechanisms. In L. Iversen, S. D. Iverson, & S. H. Snyder (Eds.), *Handbook of psychopharmacology* (Vol. 19, pp. 421–465). New York: Plenum.

Stolerman, I. P., Mariathasan, E. A., & Garcha, H. S. (1991). Discriminative stimulus effects of drug mixtures in rats. In R. A. Glennon, T. U. C. Jarbe, & J. Frankenheim (Eds.), *Drug discrimination: Applications to drug abuse research* (NIDA Research Monograph No. 116, pp. 277–306). Washington, DC: U.S. Government Printing Office.

Stolerman, I. P., Mirza, N. R., & Shoaib, M. (1995). Nicotine psychopharmacology: Addiction, cognition, and neuroadaptation. *Medicinal Research Reviews, 15,* 47–72.

Sutherland, G., Russell, M. A. H., Stapleton, J., Feyerabend, C., & Ferno, O. (1992). Nasal nicotine spray: A rapid nicotine delivery system. *Psychopharmacology, 108,* 512–518.

Terry, A. V., Buccafusco, J. J., & Jackson, W. J. (1993). Scopolamine reversal of nicotine enhanced delayed matching-to-sample performance in monkeys. *Pharmacology, Biochemistry and Behavior, 45,* 925–929.

U.S. Department of Health and Human Services. (1988). *The health consequences of smoking: Nicotine addiction.* A report of the Surgeon General. Washington, DC: U.S. Government Printing Office.

Vuchinich, R. E., & Tucker, J. A. (1988). Contributions from behavioral theories of choice to an analysis of alcohol abuse. *Journal of Abnormal Psychology, 97,* 181–195.

Wakasa, Y., Takada, K., & Yanagita, T. (1995). Reinforcing effect as a function of infusion speed in intravenous self-administration of nicotine in rhesus monkeys. *Japanese Journal of Psychopharmacology, 15,* 53–59.

Yanagita, T., Ando, K., Kato, S., & Takada, K. (1983). Psychopharmacological studies on nicotine and tobacco smoking in rhesus monkeys. *Psychopharmacology Bulletin, 19,* 409–412.

Zacny, J. P., Stitzer, M. L., Brown, F. J., Yingling, J. E., & Griffiths, R. R. (1987). Human cigarette smoking: Effects of puff and inhalation parameters on smoke exposure. *Journal of Pharmacology and Experimental Therapeutics, 240,* 554–564.

21

Psychological and Psychiatric Consequences of Nicotine

JANET BRIGHAM

Introduction

Most reports about nicotine begin with an explanation of the numerous health risks and horrific death toll of smoking. Perhaps no more powerful statement can be made about the psychoactive and addictive effects of nicotine than a reminder that most of the millions of persons in the United States who use nicotine are aware of the health risks and yet continue to use tobacco. In some populations, notably among adolescents, nicotine use is increasing rather than decreasing, despite legislative, educational, and societal efforts to the contrary. Among U.S. youth, smokeless tobacco use is now so common that one fourth of white high-school-age males report current use (Centers for Disease Control and Prevention [CDC], 1996b). Some factors such as education influence nicotine use; nearly 46% of U.S. males who did not graduate from high school are smokers. Nearly one third of women with comparable education are smokers. Nonetheless, more than 1 in 10 adults with a college education are smokers (CDC, 1996a). Why, when the risks are so great, do so many people start smoking and keep smoking?

An easy, noncomprehensive answer points in at least two directions, toward addiction and toward the psychology of nicotine use. The addictive properties of nicotine have been identified and established for at least a decade (U.S. Department of Health and Human Services [USDHHS], 1988). Do smokers as a group avoid the cognitive dissonance of engaging in a behavior they know to be dangerous by denying or dismissing the dangers of smoking (Lee, 1989)? Research has shown that young smokers (ages 10–18) have objective awareness of risk, though they focus more on immediate consequences (e.g., breathlessness during strenuous exercise) than on long-term health risks (e.g., cancer or heart trouble) (Hansen & Malotte, 1986). A more comprehensive explanation, however, must go far beyond the concepts of addiction and denial.

To nonusers of tobacco, tobacco use may appear uncomplicated; that is, common wisdom would explain that someone takes up "the habit" and then just keeps smoking because it is a habit. According to this somewhat simplistic explanation, when the person wants to quit, he or she has to summon willpower, and if he or she has enough willpower, cessation is possible, if not certain. The reality, however, is that tobacco use is a complex activity in which psychological and biobehavioral factors intertwine and interact. For most users, it is an addiction as persistent as that associated with

JANET BRIGHAM • SRI International, Menlo Park, California 94025.

Handbook of Substance Abuse: Neurobehavioral Pharmacology, edited by Tarter *et al.* Plenum Press, New York, 1998.

heroin, alcohol, or cocaine (Hughes, Higgins, & Bickel, 1994; USDHHS, 1988). Smoking is not solely a habit, although some aspects of it are indeed habitual. Tobacco use is not a univariate behavior, and success in cessation is not merely a matter of willpower.

Characterization of Nicotine Use

Tobacco use has been a challenging behavior to describe etiologically, psychologically, and behaviorally. Gilbert (1995; also Gilbert & Gilbert, 1995) has argued for a more complex approach to nicotine use than is typically utilized in research protocols (see USDHHS 1988, 1990). He also has called for greater examination of psychosocial and personality variables related to patterns of nicotine use. These variables are particularly difficult to study since tobacco use does not occur in a behavioral vacuum. Not only does nicotine use co-occur with psychiatric morbidity (Resnick, 1993), but nicotine use frequently accompanies the use of other substances (Breslau, 1995), and nicotine users report a variety of reasons for continued use (Carton, Jouvent, & Widlöcher, 1994; Hatsukami, Anton, Callies, & Keenan, 1991). The interactive effects of nicotine and other substances have only recently been examined; for example, see a report by Pritchard, Robinson, deBethizy, Davis, and Stiles (1995) on subjective, performance, and psychophysiological effects of caffeine and smoking.

Considerable evidence supports the hypothesis that specific psychoactive effects of nicotine are related to its titration, which depends in large measure on the nature of the delivery system. Early research in nicotine titration (e.g., Russell, Jarvis, Iyer, & Feyerabend, 1980; West, Russell, Jarvis, & Feyerabend, 1984) indicated that smokers control nicotine levels, and presumably also affect the psychoactive impact of nicotine, by varying the intensity and rapidity of inhalation. This line of inquiry also has shown nicotine titration differences among smoking, smokeless tobacco use, and chewing of polacrilex gum (Benowitz, Porchet, Sheiner, & Jacob, 1988). These differences in titration and, conse-

quently, in blood levels, also have been identified in smokeless tobacco products, including oral snuff and chewing tobacco (Benowitz, 1992; Benowitz et al., 1988).

Three psychophysiological measures have been employed most often to study the effects of nicotine on the central nervous system: heart rate (HR), event-related potentials (ERP), and EEG. As would be expected, the three measures yield different types of information that illuminate various aspects of nicotine's psychophysiological effects. HR studies (e.g., Domino & Matsuoka, 1994; Domino, Riskalla, Zhang, & Kim, 1992; Hasenfratz, Nil, & Battig, 1990; Hori et al., 1994; Kadoya, Domino, & Matsuoka, 1994; Robinson, Pritchard, & Davis, 1992) indicate a direct relationship between nicotine dose and cardiovascular effect, such that the more nicotine used, the greater the increase in heart rate. ERP studies (e.g., Knott, 1986) suggest that nicotine enhances attention and information processing. EEG research has found with some consistency that the administration of nicotine through smoking affects alpha1 and alpha2 frequencies differentially according to dose, and increases beta power (Domino & Matsuoka, 1994; Foulds et al., 1994; Hasenfratz et al., 1990; Shikata, Fukai, Ohya, & Sakaki, 1995). Several researchers have noted the lateralization of nicotine dose effects (Brigham & Herning, 1990; Golding, 1988; Hasenfratz et al., 1990; Norton, Brown, & Howard, 1992; Pritchard, 1991; Roth & Battig, 1991) and have linked this to specific anxiolytic and affective effects (Balfour, 1991; Gilbert, Robinson, Chamberlin, & Spielberger, 1989; Pritchard, 1991). Similarly, nicotine's modulating effect on input from the reticular activating system (Pritchard et al., 1995) has been noted. Several lines of research have indicated that nicotine's specific psychoactive effects depend on variables such as depth of inhalation (Pritchard, 1991), and relation to other activities such as eating a meal or drinking alcohol (Hasenfratz, Pfiffner, Pellaud, & Battig, 1989).

Researchers generally agree that the most prominent addictive and psychoactive agent in tobacco is nicotine, although metabolites of nicotine may also have a psychoactive affect (Schuh *et al.*, 1997). Nicotine has been found to enhance memory, alleviate anxiety and tension, increase intensity of certain sensory experiences, raise pain threshold, and moderate appetite (US-DHHS, 1988; see Jarvik and Henningfield, 1988). It also is believed to have possible antidepressant effects (Breslau, 1995; Breslau, Davis, & Andreski, 1991; Breslau, Kilbey, & Andreski, 1991, 1992, 1993a, 1993b, 1994; Carton *et al.*, 1994; Edmundsen, Glover, Holbert, Alston, & Schroeder, 1988; Gilbert, 1994; Gilbert & Gilbert, 1995; Gilbert, Meliska, Welser, & Estes, 1994; Glassman, 1993; Glassman *et al.*, 1993; Hall, Muñoz, Reus, & Sees, 1993; Hall, Muñoz, & Reus, 1994).

These reinforcing effects are easily obtained, as well. The nicotine delivery system (e.g., a cigarette, a cigar, or a packet of snuff) is portable, easy to use, and devised to deliver nicotine through rapid absorption. Thus the effects are immediately available and are associated psychologically and behaviorally with the circumstances in which they are experienced. Such immediate, dependable delivery enables nicotine to control behavior efficiently (Pomerleau & Pomerleau, 1984). An anecdote related by a family physician exemplifies this. One of his patients quit smoking after many years of heavy use. This patient could not smoke at work, so he timed his smoking such that he lit up his final cigarette just as he drove by a prominent road sign near his work. This allowed him just enough time to smoke the cigarette and extinguish it before he arrived at work. After he quit smoking, he found himself experiencing intense cravings whenever he approached that road sign; consequently, he had to find a new route to work.

Nicotine is more than reinforcing; it is a substance of dependence, with abstinence effects commencing perhaps several hours after a dose is missed. These effects, which do not occur in all smokers and do not occur with equal reliability (Hughes, Higgins, & Hatsukami, 1990), include the following: anxiety, irritability, difficulty concentrating, restlessness, impatience, hunger, tremor, racing heart, sweating, dizziness, craving for nicotine, insomnia, drowsiness, headaches, digestive disturbances, and depression (USDHHS, 1988). The effects typically begin to fade within minutes of readministration of nicotine.

The cognition-enhancing effects of nicotine encourage tobacco users to depend on nicotine for what they perceive and experience as normal mental functioning (USDHHS, 1988), and to use it in a consistent context (e.g., Gilbert, 1995; Warburton, Wesnes, Shergold, & James, 1986). The cognitive and performance debilitation associated with abstinence effects is quickly reversed with administration of nicotine, thus increasing the likelihood of rapid relapse (Snyder & Henningfield, 1989; Snyder, Davis, & Henningfield, 1989). Similarly, the pleasurable affect associated by many tobacco users with nicotine's pharmacologic action is not only reinforcing, but is absent in abstinence but quickly reinstated with relapse, thus weaving tobacco use into the "fabric of daily life" (Pomerleau & Pomerleau, 1984).

Psychiatric Comorbidity

Among psychiatric patients, tobacco use is common (Hughes, Hatsukami, & Mitchell, 1986); between 50% and 80% of psychiatric patients are smokers (Hughes, 1993), compared to roughly one fourth of the general adult population. A compilation of articles and scientific meeting presentations related to psychiatric patients' smoking behaviors (Hughes, 1993) indicated that smoking is prevalent among depressed and psychotic patients. This is in concordance with findings (Breslau *et al.*, 1994) that both males and females with nicotine dependence have greater incidence of alcohol and illegal drug use disorders, major depression, and anxiety disorders. The researchers also found that the more dependent the smoker, the greater the likelihood of illegal drug use. Other research has found that smoking cessation programs are possible with this population, provided that treatment is sufficiently intense (Ziedonis & George, 1997).

Since some psychiatric inpatient units are now smoke-free, some psychiatric patients experience abstinence effects that could be misdiagnosed because of physiologic and behavioral changes resulting in false positive or false negative conclusions. For example, abstinence effects could mask the tachycardia of alcohol or drug withdrawal or anxiety disorders. Sleep disturbances, irritability, anger, anxiety, impatience, and restlessness are also common abstinence effects that could be diagnostically and behaviorally problematic in an inpatient setting. Smokers with a history of depression are more prone to abstinence-related depression than are smokers with no history of depression (Covey, Glassman, & Stetner, 1990), thus complicating the diagnostic and clinical picture for these patients. The restlessness associated with abstinence effects also could be confused with akathisia, resulting in a confusing treatment situation for patients on neuroleptics. All of these situations could be compounded by a clinician's mistaken belief that abstinence effects are clinically insignificant. Consequently, Hughes (1993) recommends that clinicians be aware of the physiologic, behavioral, and subjective effects of nicotine abstinence, and realize that they might worsen some disorders or result in incorrect diagnoses and treatment. An additional complication is that some antipsychotic medications work differently when nicotine is present, as well as when a dependent smoker quits using nicotine while remaining on the medication (Ziedonis & George, 1997).

Glassman (1993), noting that "[p]sychiatry has been essentially uninterested in cigarette smoking and nicotine" (p. 546), counters the field's obliviousness with his insistence that the relationships between nicotine and psychiatric disorders indicate "profound implications" (p. 551) for psychiatry. He raises the caveat that successful nicotine cessation may risk exacerbating psychopathology. The brighter aspect to the picture is that a greater comprehension of nicotine's cellular-level association with psychiatric disorders may open new therapeutic avenues.

A Gateway Drug

One consequence of tobacco use, specifically cigarette smoking, is that it is both a precursor to other substance use and is linked to other substance use. Some 80% to 95% of alcohol and drug abusers are also smokers (DiFranza & Guerrera, 1990; Istvan & Matarazzo, 1984). Also, tobacco is believed to be a "gateway" or "stepping-stone" drug; that is, a substance the early use of which leads to later use of illicit drugs. This belief has been reinforced by recent research in the United States and Australia (e.g., Blaze-Temple & Lo, 1992; Crundall, 1992). As Breslau and colleagues (1994) explain, the relationship between smoking and use of illicit drugs is strongest among adolescents and young adults. Their findings are concordant with previous work describing the typical course of substance use, in which high use of alcohol, marijuana, and nicotine tends to be followed by use of harder drugs (e.g., Kandel, Marguilies, & Davies, 1978; Huba, Wingard, & Bentler, 1981; O'Donnell & Clayton, 1982).

Smokeless Tobacco: Differing Mechanisms?

The prevalence of smoking, the most common nicotine-delivery system, has leveled off and even diminished in some populations; on the other hand, the use of smokeless tobacco has increased dramatically (CDC, 1994). The increase among young persons and continuing use as young users become adults has reflected the nationwide expanding popularity of smokeless tobacco products, primarily moist oral snuff (CDC, 1993), since about 1980. While the use of smokeless tobacco products has risen, research characterizing smokeless tobacco use has not shown the same dramatic increase, perhaps because of lingering perceptions that smokeless tobacco use is an outdated practice conducted only by the rural elderly, or a practice with negligible health risk. As a result, differences between the profiles of smoking and smokeless tobacco are being examined (Boyle, Jensen, Hatsukami, & Severson, 1995; Hatsukami, Anton, Keenan, & Callies, 1992; Severson, 1993), and specific biochemical markers of smokeless tobacco are being identified (Holiday, McLarty, Yanagihara, Riley, &

Shepherd, 1995; Jacob, Yu, Liang, Shulgin, & Benowitz, 1993). To date, only the cardiovascular effects of smokeless tobacco have been measured (Benowitz, 1992; Benowitz et al., 1988), leaving numerous threads yet to be pursued in a systematic biological and psychological characterization of smokeless tobacco use.

Since the effects of cigarette smoking appear to vary considerably according to dose and titration, and since the absorption and titration patterns of smokeless tobacco use differ from those of smoked tobacco, it is reasonable to expect that psychophysiological effects of smokeless tobacco will differ from those of cigarettes. Also, it is possible that psychophysiological data will corroborate subjective findings and speculations about the specific arousal effects of smokeless tobacco. Such research investigations have not yet been conducted or reported, however.

It is unclear whether smokeless tobacco use might, like smoking, have a demonstrable link to depressive sympoms, or whether its effects relate more to general arousal than to specific antidepressant effects. To the extent that its use does appear related to depressive symptoms (Foreyt et al., 1993; Hatsukami et al., 1991; Jacobs, Neufeld, Sayers, Spielberger, & Weinberg, 1988; Landers, Crews, Boutcher, Skinner, & Gustafsen, 1992), this may reflect an attempt by smokeless tobacco users to compensate for a state of underarousal associated with depression. What remains is for these lines of research to be linked to the specific, distinct titration and arousal patterns of smokeless tobacco use. It is likely that such findings can open new avenues for cessation efforts.

Cessation and Relapse

As the health consequences of tobacco use have been publicized and even integrated into public initiatives, smoking rates have declined among some groups. Nonetheless, there is no shortage of tobacco users who need or desire to quit, and who find quitting to be one of the more difficult tasks they have confronted. The Year 2000 Objectives Supplement of the National Health Interview Survey for 1994 indicated that approximately 32% of U.S. males and 28% of U.S. women ages 25–44 reported smoking to some degree (CDC, 1996a). These numbers indicate the massive public-health effort that would need to be undertaken to educate and assist these individuals in nicotine cessation, if such an effort would be an effective deterrent. The overall numbers, however, are less meaningful on an individual level. It is the individual, after all, who will most likely experience abstinence effects, and then will face the possibility of relapse throughout his or her lifetime.

Tobacco researchers are not entirely united in the use of the term *relapse,* but a task force of the National Working Conference on Smoking Relapse (Shumaker & Grunberg, 1986) defined relapse as 7 consecutive days of smoking at least one puff per day. This may or may not involve a return to baseline smoking rate. It is not only difficult or impossible to determine how many smokers quit, but it is even more difficult to assess relapse in them. This is because the majority of cessation efforts occur outside a formal smoking research study or formal intervention program. In addition, self-quitters do not appear to be necessarily more successful than those utilizing formal programs (Cohen et al., 1989). However, it is commonly noted among researchers that both lapse (reexposure) and relapse (continued reexposure) are common in cessation attempts, and may occur within a year at a rate of 70% to 80%. The more hopeful and optimistic approaches encourage viewing lapse and relapse as part of a process in which the tobacco user is learning to quit. The cessation phase is probably best seen as a process, or as a transition within a process, which influences whether a smoker will relapse (Brownell et al., 1986).

Both anecdotal and statistical data underscore the power of situational factors in nudging a former smoker toward relapse. Marlatt (1985) included among relapse risk factors the expectation of a lapse being a positive experience (e.g., the ex-smoker anticipates enjoying a cigarette), the actual reinforcement of the lapse experience (e.g., the smoker does enjoy the cigarette), and the pressures edging the ex-smoker toward lapsing. In some cases, this might be social contact with friends who smoke, contact with environmental reminders of smoking, or unexpected stressors. On the other hand, work by Kenford and colleagues (1994) has shown that abstinence during the first 2 weeks of cessation is a powerful predictor of success. Also, realistically negative expectations of the difficulty of cessation predict success in quitting (Wetter *et al.,* 1994).

A former smoker's life circumstances may contribute to the tendency toward relapse. Many smokers whose spouses or other family members also smoke report difficulty quitting in such a home environment (Baer & Lichtenstein, 1988). Individuals whose friends or work associates build smoking into social activities also find quitting difficult and relapse a temptation (Mermelstein, Cohen, Lichtenstein, Baer, & Kamarck, 1986; Morgan, Ashenberg, & Fisher, 1988). Additional factors found to be related to relapse include degree of dependence, amount of smoking, life stressors (e.g., financial, health), motivation, cravings for a cigarette, urges to smoke, treatment factors, and coping skills (USDHHS, 1988). The availability of nicotine replacement therapy demonstrably improves the likelihood of success (Henningfield, 1995; USDHHS, 1996). Other pharmacotherapies also appear promising (e.g., Hurt *et al.,* 1997). These possibilities are particularly important since only a small percentage of successful quitters use formal stop-smoking programs. Such programs are continually being adapted, as well. For example, efficacious treatment modalities from other substance programs are adapted for use with nicotine, such that some intervention programs now match patients with treatment plans on relevant dimensions, in an effort to maximize individual success at cessation (e.g., Finney, 1995; Hall *et al.,* 1993; Jorenby, Keehn, & Fiore, 1995; Niaura, Goldstein, & Abrans, 1994; Schmitz & Tate, 1994).

Conclusion

Tobacco use can and must be approached from a variety of perspectives for a comprehen-sion of the complexity of the behavior and the idiosyncratic challenges that smokers face in quitting. Prevention efforts, while at times effective, evidently are failing to stop or even slow the initiation of nicotine use of millions of young persons. Tobacco use is not associated with immediate functional impairment and may, in fact, facilitate one's perception of his or her cognitive enhancement. As young tobacco users age, tobacco-related behaviors become ingrained in their lives and routines, as part of their social functioning, coping strategies, and emotional maintenance. Consequently, many tobacco users will die of causes related to their tobacco use. Of those who quit, cessation is likely to require multiple attempts. Viewing cessation and the possibility of relapse as learning processes may help these individuals develop skills and attitudes that will enable them to become and remain tobacco-free.

References

Baer, J. S., & Lichtenstein, E. (1988). Classification and prediction of smoking relapse episodes: An exploration of individual differences. *Journal of Consulting and Clinical Psychology, 56,* 104–110.

Balfour, D. J. (1991). The influence of stress on psychopharmacological responses to nicotine. *British Journal of Addiction, 86,* 489–493.

Benowitz, N. L. (1992). Pharmacology of smokeless tobacco use: Nicotine addiction and nicotine-related health consequences. In *Smokeless tobacco or health: An international perspective* (NIH Publication No. 92-3461, pp. 219–228). Washington, DC: U.S. Department of Health and Human Services.

Benowitz, N. L., Porchet, H., Sheiner, L., & Jacob P. (1988). Nicotine absorption and cardiovascular effects with smokeless tobacco use: Comparison with cigarettes and nicotine gum. *Clinical Pharmacology & Therapeutics, 44,* 23–8.

Blaze-Temple, D., & Lo, S. K. (1992). Stages of drug use: A community servey of Perth teenagers. *British Journal of Addiction, 87,* 215–225.

Boyle, R. G., Jensen, J., Hatsukami, D. K., & Severson, H. H. (1995). Measuring dependence in smokeless tobacco users. *Addictive Behaviors, 20,* 443–450.

Breslau, N. (1995). Psychiatric comorbidity of smoking and nicotine dependence. *Behavior Genetics, 25,* 95–101.

Breslau, N., Davis, G. C., & Andreski, P. (1991). Migraine, psychiatric disorders, and suicide attempts: An epidemiological study of young adults. *Psychiatry Research, 37,* 11–23.

Breslau, N., Kilbey, M. M., & Andreski, P. (1991). Nicotine dependence, major depression, and anxiety in young adults. *Archives of General Psychiatry, 48,* 1069–1074.

Breslau, N., Kilbey, M. M., & Andreski, P. (1992). Nicotine withdrawal symptoms and psychiatric disorders: Findings from an epidemiologic study of young adults. *American Journal of Psychiatry, 149,* 464–469.

Breslau, N., Kilbey, M. M., & Andreski, P. (1993a). Nicotine dependence and major depression: New evidence from a prospective investigation. *Archives of General Psychiatry, 50,* 31–35.

Breslau, N., Kilbey, M. M., & Andreski, P. (1993b). Vulnerability to psychopathology in nicotine-dependent smokers: An epidemiologic study of young adults. *American Journal of Psychiatry, 150,* 941–946.

Breslau, N., Kilbey, M. M., & Andreski, P. (1994). DSM-III-R nicotine dependence in young adults: Prevalence, correlates and associated psychiatric disorders. *Addiction, 89,* 743–754.

Brigham, J., & Herning, R. I. (1990). *Nicotine effects in EEG spectral data in male smokers vs. nonsmokers* (NIDA Research Monograph No. 105, p. 607). Rockville, MD: National Institute on Drug Abuse.

Brownell, K. D., Glynn, T. J., Glasgow, R., Lando, H., Rand, C., Gottlieb, A., & Pinney, J. M. (1986). Task Force 5: Interventions to prevent relapse. *Health Psychology, 5* (Suppl.), 53–68.

Carton, S., Jouvent, R., & Widlöcher, D. (1994). Nicotine dependence and motives for smoking in depression. *Journal of Substance Abuse, 6,* 67–76.

Centers for Disease Control and Prevention. (1993). Use of smokeless tobacco among adults, United States. *Morbidity and Mortality Weekly Report, 42,* 263–266.

Centers for Disease Control and Prevention. (1994). Reasons for tobacco use and symptoms of nicotine withdrawal among adolescent and young adult tobacco users—United States, 1993. *Morbidity and Mortality Weekly Report, 43,* 745–750.

Centers for Disease Control and Prevention. (1996a). Cigarette smoking among adults—United States, 1994. *Morbidity and Mortality Weekly Report, 45,* 588–590.

Centers for Disease Control and Prevention. (1996b). Tobacco use and usual source of cigarettes among high school students—United States, 1995. *Morbidity and Mortality Weekly Report, 45,* 413–418.

Cohen, S., Lichtenstein, E., Prochaska, J. O., Rossi, J. S., Gritz, E. R., Carr, C. R., Orleans, C. T., Schoenbach, V. J., Biener, L., Abrams, D., DiClemente, C., Curry, S., Marlatt, G. A., Cummings, K. M., Emont, S. L., Giovino, G., & Ossip-Klein, D. (1989). Debunking myths about self-quitting: Evidence from 10 prospective studies of persons who attempt to quit smoking by themselves. *American Psychologist, 44,* 1355–1365.

Covey, L. S., Glassman, A. H., & Stetner, F. (1990). Depression and depressive symptoms in smoking cessation. *Comprehensive Psychiatry, 31,* 350–354.

Crundall, I. A. (1992). Student perceptions of the danger of drug use: A factor analysis. *Journal of Drug Education, 22,* 147–153.

DiFranza, J. R., & Guerrera, M. P. (1990). Alcoholism and smoking. *Journal of Studies on Alcohol, 51,* 130–135.

Domino, E. F., & Matsuoka, S. (1994). Effects of tobacco smoking on the topographic EEG-I. *Progress in Neuro-Psychopharmacology & Biological Psychiatry, 18,* 879–889.

Domino, E. F., Riskalla, M., Zhang, Y., & Kim, E. (1992). Effects of tobacco smoke on the topographic EEG II. *Progress in Neuro-Psychopharmacology & Biological Psychiatry, 16,* 463–482.

Edmundson, E. W., Glover, E. D., Holbert D., Alston, P. P., & Schroeder, K. L. (1988). Personality profiles associated with smokeless tobacco use patterns. *Addictive Behaviors, 13,* 219–223.

Finney, J. W. (1995). Enhancing substance abuse treatment evaluations: Examining mediators and moderators of treatment effects. *Journal of Substance Abuse, 7,* 135–150.

Foreyt, J. P., Jackson, A. S., Squires, W. G., Jr., Hartung, G. H., Murray, T. D., & Gotto, A. M., Jr. (1993). Psychological profile of college students who use smokeless tobacco. *Addictive Behaviors, 18,* 107–116.

Foulds, J., McSorley, K., Sneddon, J., Feyerabend, C., Jarvis, M. J., & Russell, M. A. (1994). Effect of subcutaneous nicotine injections of EEG alpha frequency in non-smokers: A placebo-controlled pilot study. *Psychopharmacology, 115,* 163–166.

Gilbert, D. G. (1994). Why people smoke: Stress-reduction, coping enhancement, and nicotine. *Recent Advances in Tobacco Science, 20,* 106–161.

Gilbert, D. G. (1995). *Smoking: Individual differences, psychopathology, and emotion.* Washington, DC: Taylor & Francis.

Gilbert, D. G., & Gilbert, B. O. (1995). Personality, psychopathology, and nicotine response as mediators of the genetics of smoking. *Behavior Genetics, 25,* 133–147.

Gilbert, D. G., Robinson, J. H., Chamberlin, C. L., & Spielberger, C. D. (1989). Effects of smoking/nicotine on anxiety, heart rate, and lateralization of EEG during a stressful movie. *Psychophysiology, 26,* 311–320.

Gilbert, D. G., Meliska, C. J., Welser, R., & Estes, S. L. (1994). Depression, personality, and gender influence EEG, cortisol, beta-endorphin, heart rate, and subjective responses to smoking multiple cigarettes. *Personality and Individual Differences, 16,* 247–264.

Glassman, A. H. (1993). Cigarette smoking: Implications for psychiatric illness. *American Journal of Psychiatry, 150,* 546–553.

Glassman, A. H., Covey, L. S., Dalack, G. W., Stetner, F., Rivelli, S. K., Fleiss, J., & Cooper, T. B. (1993). Smoking cessation, clonidine, and vulnerability to nicotine among dependent smokers. *Clinical Pharmacology & Therapeutics, 54,* 670–679.

Golding, J. F. (1988). Effects of cigarette smoking on resting EEG, visual evoked potentials and photic driving. *Pharmacology, Biochemistry and Behavior, 29,* 23–32.

Hall, S. M., Muñoz, R. F., Reus, V. I., & Sees, K. L. (1993). Nicotine, negative affect, and depression. *Journal of Consulting and Clinical Psychology, 61,* 761–767.

Hall, S. M., Muñoz, R. F., & Reus, V. I. (1994). Cognitive-behavioral intervention increases abstinence rates for depressive-history smokers. *Journal of Consulting and Clinical Psychology, 62,* 141–146.

Hansen, W. B., & Malotte, C. K. (1986). Perceived personal immunity: The development of beliefs about susceptibility to the consequences of smoking. *Preventive Medicine, 15,* 363–372.

Hasenfratz, M., Pfiffner, D., Pellaud, K., & Battig, K. (1989). Postlunch smoking for pleasure seeking or arousal maintenance? *Pharmacology, Biochemistry and Behavior, 34,* 631–639.

Hasenfratz, M., Nil, R., & Battig, K. (1990). Development of central and peripheral smoking effects over time. *Psychopharmacology, 101,* 359–365.

Hatsukami, D. K., Anton, D., Callies, A., & Keenan, R. (1991). Situational factors and patterns associated with smokeless tobacco use. *Journal of Behavioral Medicine, 14,* 383–396.

Hatsukami, D. K., Anton, D., Keenan, R., & Callies, A. (1992). Smokeless tobacco abstinence effects and nicotine gum dose. *Psychopharmacology, 106,* 60–66.

Henningfield, J. E. (1995). Nicotine medications for smoking cessation. *New England Journal of Medicine, 333,* 1196–1203.

Holiday, D. B., McLarty, J. W., Yanagihara, R. H., Riley, L., & Shepherd, S. B. (1995). Two biochemical markers effectively used to separate smokeless tobacco users from smokers and nonusers. *Southern Medical Journal, 88,* 1107–1113.

Hori, T., Hayashi, M., Oka, M., Agari, I., Kawabe, K., & Takagi, M. (1994). Re-examination of arousing and de-arousing effects of cigarette smoking. *Perceptual & Motor Skills, 78,* 787–800.

Huba, G. J., Wingard, J. A., & Bentler, P. M. (1981). A comparison of two latent variable causal models for adolescent drug use. *Journal of Personality and Social Psychology, 40,* 180–193.

Hughes, J. R. (1993). Possible effects of smoke-free inpatient units on psychiatric diagnosis and treatment. *Journal of Clinical Psychiatry, 54,* 109–114.

Hughes, J. R., Hatsukami, D. K., & Mitchell, J. E. (1986). Prevalence of smoking in psychiatric outpatients. *American Journal of Psychiatry, 143,* 993–997.

Hughes, J. R., Higgins, S. T., & Hatsukami, D. K. (1990). Effects of abstinence from tobacco: A critical review. In L. T. Kozlowski, H. Annis, & H. D. Cappell (Eds.) *Research Advances in Alcohol and Drug Problems* (Vol. 10, pp. 317–398). New York: Plenum.

Hughes, J. R., Higgins, S. T., & Bickel, W. K. (1994). Nicotine withdrawal versus other drug withdrawal syndromes: Similarities and dissimilarities. *Addiction, 89,* 1461–1470.

Hurt, R. D., Sachs, D. P., Glover, E. D., Offord, K. P., Johnston, J. A., Dale, L. C., Khayrallah, M. A., Schroeder, D. R., Glover, P. N., Sullivan, C. R., Croghan, I. T., & Sullivan, P. M. (1997). A comparison of sustained-release bupropion and placebo for smoking cessation. *New England Journal of Medicine, 337,* 1195–1202.

Istvan, J., & Matarazzo, J. D. (1984). Tobacco, alcohol and caffeine use: A review of their interrelationships. *Psychological Bulletin, 95,* 301–326.

Jacob, P., Yu, L., Liang, G., Shulgin, A. T., & Benowitz, N. L. (1993). Gas chromatographic-mass spectrometric method for determination of anabasine, anatabine and other tobacco alkaloids in urine of smokers and smokeless tobacco users. *Journal of Chromatography, 619,* 49–61.

Jacobs, G. A., Neufeld, V. A., Sayers, S., Spielberger, C. D., & Weinberg, H. (1988). Personality and smokeless tobacco use. *Addictive Behaviors, 13,* 311–318.

Jarvik, M. E., & Henningfield, J. E. (1988). Pharmacological treatment of tobacco dependence. *Pharmacology, Biochemistry and Behavior, 30,* 279–294.

Jorenby, D. E., Keehn, D. S., & Fiore, M. (1995). Comparative efficacy and tolerability of nicotine replacement therapies. *CNS Drugs, 3,* 227–236.

Kadoya, C., Domino, E. F., Matsuoka, S. (1994). Relationship of electroencephalographic and cardiovascular changes to plasma nicotine levels in tobacco smokers. *Clinical Pharmacology & Therapeutics, 55,* 370–377.

Kandel, D. B., Marguilies, R. Z., & Davies, M. (1978). Analytic stragteies for studying transitions into developmental stages. *Sociology of Education, 52,* 162–176.

Kenford, S. L., Fiore, M. C., Jorenby, D. E., Smith, S. S., Wetter, D., & Baker, T. B. (1994). Predicting smoking cessation: Who will quit with and without the nicotine patch. *Journal of the American Medical Association, 271,* 589–594.

Knott, V. J. (1986). Tobacco effects on cortical evoked potentials to task stimuli. *Addictive Behaviors, 11,* 219–223.

Landers, D. M., Crews, D. J., Boutcher, S. H., Skinner, J. S., & Gustafsen, S. (1992). The effects of smokeless tobacco on performance and psychophysiological response. *Medicine & Science in Sports & Exercise, 24,* 895–903.

Lee, C. (1989). Perceptions of immunity to disease in adult smokers. *Journal of Behavioral Medicine, 12,* 267–277.

Lewis, S. F., & Fiore, M. C. (1995). Smoking cessation: What works? What doesn't? *Journal of Respiratory Diseases, 16,* 497–510.

Marlatt, G. A. (1985). Relapse prevention: Theoretical rationale and review of the model. In G. A. Marlatt &

J. R. Gordon (Eds.*), Relapse prevention: Maintenance strategies in the treatment of addictive behaviors*, pp. 3–70. New York: Guilford.

Mermelstein, R., Cohen, S., Lichtenstein, E., Baer, J. S., & Kamarck, T. (1986). Social support and smoking cessation and maintenance. *Journal of Consulting and Clinical Psychology, 54*, 447–453.

Morgan, D. G., Ashenberg, Z. S., & Fisher, E. B., Jr. (1988). Abstinence from smoking and the social environment. *Journal of Consulting and Clinical Psychology, 56*, 298–301.

Nelson, D. E., Emong, S. L., Brackbill, R. M., Cameron, L. L., Peddicord, J., & Fiore, M. C. (1994). Cigarette smoking prevalence by occupation in the United States: A comparison between 1978 to 1980 and 1987 to 1990. *Journal of Occupational Medicine, 36*, 516–525.

Niaura, R., Goldstein, M. G., & Abrams, D. B. (1994). Matching high- and low-dependence smokers to self-help treatment with or without nicotine replacement. *Preventive Medicine, 23*, 70–77.

Norton, R., Brown, K., & Howard, R. (1992). Smoking, nicotine dose and the lateralization of electrocortical activity. *Psychopharmacology, 108*, 473–479.

O'Donnell, J. A., & Clayton, R. R. (1982). The stepping stone hypothesis—Marijuana, heroin, and causality. *Chemical Dependencies, 4*, 229–241.

Pomerleau, O. F., & Pomerleau, C. S. (1984). Neuroregulators and the reinforcement of smoking: Towards a biobehavioral explanation. *Neuroscience and Biobehavioral Reviews, 8*, 503–513.

Pritchard, W. S. (1991). Electroencephalographic effects of cigarette smoking. *Psychopharmacology, 104*, 485–490.

Pritchard, W. S., Robinson, J. H., deBethizy, J. D., Davis, R. A., & Stiles, M. F. (1995). Caffeine and smoking: Subjective, performance, and psychophysiological effects. *Psychophysiology, 32*, 19–27.

Resnick, M. P. (1993). Treating nicotine addiction in patients with psychiatric co-morbidity. In C. T. Orleans & J. Slade (Eds.), *Nicotine addiction: Principles and management* (pp. 327–336). New York: Oxford University Press.

Robinson, J. H., Pritchard, W. S., & Davis, R. A. (1992). Psychopharmacological effects of smoking a cigarette with typical "tar" and carbon monoxide yields but minimal nicotine. *Psychopharmacology, 108*, 466–472.

Roth, N., & Battig, K. (1991). Effects of cigarette smoking upon frequencies of EEG alpha rhythm and finger tapping. *Psychopharmacology, 105*, 186–190.

Russell, M. A. H., Jarvis, M., Iyer, R., & Feyerabend, C. (1980). Relation of nicotine yield of cigarettes to blood nicotine concentrations in smokers. *British Medical Journal, 280*, 972–976.

Schmitz, J. M., & Tate, J. C. (1994). Treatment session frequency and smoking cessation. *Journal of Substance Abuse, 6*, 77–85.

Schuh, L., Henningfield, J., Fant, R., Pickworth, W., Rothman, R., Ohuoha, D., & Keenan, R. (1997.) *Pharmacodynamic effects of cotinine* (NIDA Research Monograph No. 174, p. 67). Rockville, MD: National Institute on Drug Abuse.

Severson, H. H. (1993). Smokeless tobacco: Risks, epidemiology, and cessation. In C. T. Orleans & J. Slade (Eds.), *Nicotine addiction: Principles and management* (pp. 262–278). New York: Oxford University Press.

Shikata, H., Fukai, H., Ohya, I., & Sakaki, T. (1995). Characterization of topographic EEG changes when smoking a cigarette. *Psychopharmacology, 119*, 361–367

Shumaker, S. A., & Grunberg, N. E. (1986). Proceedings of the national working conference on smoking relapse. *Health Psychology, 5* (Suppl.), 1–99.

Snyder, F. R., & Henningfield, J. E. (1989). Effects of nicotine administration following 12 h of tobacco deprivation: Assessment on a computerized performance tasks. *Psychopharmacology, 97*, 17–22.

Snyder, F. R., Davis, F. C., & Henningfield, J. E. (1989). The tobacco withdrawal syndrome: Performance decrements assessed on a computerized test battery. *Drug and Alcohol Dependence, 23*, 259–266.

U.S. Department of Health and Human Services. (1988*). The health consequences of smoking: Nicotine addiction.* Washington, DC: U.S. Government Printing Office.

U.S. Department of Health and Human Services. (1990*). The health benefits of smoking cessation: A report of the surgeon general.* Washington, DC: U.S. Government Printing Office.

U.S. Department of Health and Human Services. (1996). *Smoking cessation.* Clinical Practice Guideline No. 18, Agency for Health Care Policy and Research. Washington, DC: U.S. Government Printing Office.

Warburton, D. M., Wesnes, K., Shergold, K., & James, M. (1986). Facilitation of learning and state dependency with nicotine. *Psychopharmacology, 89*, 55–59.

West, R. J., Russell, M. A. H., Jarvis, M. J., & Feyerabend, C. (1984). Does switching to an ultra-low nicotine cigarette induce nicotine withdrawal effects? *Psychopharmacology, 84*, 120–123.

Wetter, D. W., Smith, S. S., Kenford, S. L., Jovenby, D. E., Fiore, M. C., Hurt, R. D., Offord, K. P., & Baker, T. P. (1994). Smoking outcome expectancies: Factor structure, predictive validity, and discriminant validity. *Journal of Abnormal Psychology, 103*, 801–811.

Ziedonis, D., & George, T. (1997). Schizophrenia and nicotine use: Report of a pilot smoking cessation program and review of neurobiological and clinical issues. *Schizophrenia Bulletin, 23*, 247–254.

VIII

Opiates

22

Pharmacology of Opiates

LISA BORG AND MARY JEANNE KREEK

Introduction

There are three major opioid receptors in the central nervous system: mu, kappa, and delta, the genes for which have been cloned. There are also possible subtypes within each class, although separate genes have not yet been cloned for any subtypes. Opioids are both the natural opiates and their synthetic congeners which are the class of agonist and antagonist drugs with primarily morphine-like activity mostly at the mu opioid receptor, and also the other naturally occurring endogenous and synthetic opioid peptides, which act also at the other receptor types.

In general, opioids are well absorbed from the gastrointestinal tract after oral dosing, with a longer duration of action than following parenteral administration. However, most opioids (but not all, e.g., methadone) have reduced systemic bioavailability and thus reduced effect after oral versus parenteral administration, due to first-pass metabolism in the liver (Reisine & Pasternak, 1996). Natural opiates and their synthetic congeners are also well absorbed after subcutaneous or intramuscular injection and, depending on degree of lipophilicity, may be administered through the nasal or buccal mucosa (Weinberg *et al.,* 1988) or transdermally (Portenoy *et al.,* 1993). This chapter reviews the disposition, metabolism, pharmacokinetics, and excretion of four opioids that are particularly important in the area of illicit opioid abuse and its treatment: heroin, morphine, methadone, and levo-alpha-acetylmethadol (LAAM).

Diacetylmorphine or heroin is a synthetic derivative of a natural opiate which has a rapid onset of action and a very short half-life which has greatly contributed to its popularity as a drug of abuse. Heroin is increasingly abused intranasally, both due to recent concerns regarding risk of HIV-1 transmission with the more potent but less safe intravenous route, and also due to the recent increased availability of higher-purity street heroin (about 70% purity in some geographic regions, compared with less than 30% in the recent past years). Heroin is rapidly metabolized first to monoacetylmorphine and then primarily metabolized to morphine, an opioid with a somewhat longer half-life that is used primarily for pain relief.

Methadone is an orally administered long-acting opioid that was developed in the 1960s as an effective treatment for heroin addiction, and levo-alpha-acetylmethadol (LAAM) is a longer-acting and also orally effective opioid which was recently also approved for clinical use in the United States by the Food and Drug Administration as a treatment for opioid addiction.

Heroin

Diacetylmorphine was originally synthesized in 1874 and marketed in 1898 by the Bayer company under the name "Heroin," and

LISA BORG AND MARY JEANNE KREEK • Laboratory on the Biology of Addictive Diseases, The Rockefeller University, New York, New York 10021.

Handbook of Substance Abuse: Neurobehavioral Pharmacology, edited by Tarter *et al.* Plenum Press, New York, 1998.

331

is more water soluble and potent than morphine (Sawynok, 1986). Heroin is derived from morphine by acetylation of morphine both at the 3 and 6 position. When catabolized, heroin is deacetylated to 6-mono-acetylmorphine and then, mostly in the liver, metabolized to morphine. Heroin is not available for therapeutic use in the United States.

To date, there have been only a few well-designed studies of heroin pharmacokinetics. Kaiko, Wallenstein, Rogers, Grabinski, and Houde (1981) used visual analog scales to measure pain relief in comparing intramuscular heroin to intramuscular morphine in cancer patients, and found that heroin was about twice as potent as morphine (on average 4.8 mg of heroin was equivalent to 10 mg of morphine) with faster onset (average 1.2 vs. 1.5 hr, respectively) but more transient effects. Inturrisi and colleagues (1983) performed opiate binding studies using rat brain to determine the relative abilities of heroin, 6-acetylmorphine, and morphine to displace tritiated (^{3}H-naltrexone) from opiate binding sites. Heroin did not bind to the rat brain opiate receptor, while morphine and 6-acetylmorphine clearly did, suggesting that heroin lacks intrinsic opioid activity, and is actually a lipid soluble prodrug with two active metabolites.

In a later clinical study extending these earlier findings, Inturrisi and colleagues (1984) observed the pharmacokinetics of heroin in 11 patients with chronic pain, using high-performance liquid chromatography (HPLC) to measure differences in the areas under the curve after parenteral (intravenous bolus, continuous infusion, and intramuscular) heroin versus oral heroin administration. Heroin and morphine given orally were also compared. The time-course of appearance of heroin and its metabolites, 6-acetylmorphine and morphine, in venous blood was measured in relation to the onset of pain relief and sedation. The authors found that with intravenous administration, heroin has a mean half-life of 3.0 min. Steady state blood levels were achieved with continuous infusion of heroin, with doubling of blood levels when the infusion rate was double, thus demonstrating that elimination kinetics remain

linear with infusion rates given up to 333 μg/min. Oral heroin was found to have complete first-pass metabolism to morphine, but morphine itself given orally at the same dose as heroin yielded 20% higher blood levels of morphine than heroin. However, both heroin and morphine have very low systemic bioavailability with oral administration, as compared with methadone and LAAM. The blood clearance rate of heroin (2,134 ml/min) was greater than the maximal rate of hepatic blood flow (1,500 ml/min) in humans. Thus, it is likely that other organs besides the liver are involved in the biotransformation and elimination of heroin, such as the gastrointestinal wall and the kidney. The onset of pain relief between 15 and 45 min after the start of the heroin infusion was coincident with the presence of heroin and 6-acetylmorphine in the blood prior to the appearance of morphine. The half-life of 6-acetylmorphine has not been precisely determined in humans, but appears to be around 2 hr. Weinberg and colleagues (1988) used high-performance liquid chromatography to compare sublingual versus oral absorption of selected opioid analgesics in normal subjects, subtracting the percentage of opioid recovered from the oral cavity (upon expectoration after 10 min) from 100%. The more lipid-soluble drugs (buprenorpine, fentanyl, methadone, and heroin) were absorbed to the greatest degree. Drug absorption was independent of concentration of opioid, with greater absorption permitting greater potential systemic bioavailability of the opioid. However, in comparison with morphine sulfate with 18% absorption, heroin was not significantly better absorbed via the sublingual route.

Further work needs to be done in order to better determine the contribution of 6-acetylmorphine to the pharmacokinetics of parenteral heroin, particularly in terms of its faster onset of action and greater potency compared with morphine.

Morphine

Morphine, relatively selective for the mu opioid receptor, is the opioid agonist with which other opioid and nonopioid analgesics are generally compared. Since morphine is difficult to synthesize in the laboratory, it is still usually obtained from opium from the poppy plant. Morphine is an alkaloid of the phenanthrene class and comprises 10% of opium (Reisine & Pasternak, 1996).

The pharmacokinetics of morphine and its two glucuronidated metabolites, the major metabolite morphine-3-glucuronide (M3G), and the minor but biologically active morphine-6-glucuronide (M6G) metabolite, vary depending on the route of administration. Neumann, Henriksen, Grosman, and Christensen (1982) used radioimmunoassay (RIA) to analyze the plasma concentration of morphine orally administered every 4 hr to 16 cancer patients with chronic pain. They found a significant, linear correlation between dose and mean plasma level, using a radioimmunoassay with a sensitivity of 0.25 ng morphine/ml and with cross reactivity between morphine and M3G <0.3%. However, there was much variation in individual plasma levels of morphine during the same dose intervals, possibly due to rapid absorption and brief elimination half-life.

In a study by Osborne, Joel, Trew, and Slevin (1990), single doses of morphine via five different routes were given to 10 normal volunteers, with the finding that M6G plasma levels and AUC were greater than morphine (ratio 1.4:1) with intravenous administration. Oral administration of morphine produced M6G and M3G mean AUC ratios to morphine of 9.7:1 and 56:1 respectively, findings that suggest that most of the clinical effects of morphine after oral administration and many of the effects of intravenous morphine may be due to the active metabolite M6G. Delayed morphine absorption was the main effect of sublingual, buccal, and sustained-release buccal morphine. The half-life of orally administered morphine was measured as 1.4 ± 0.44 hr in this study, and 1.7 ± 0.8 hr when given intravenously, comparable to the 2-hr plasma half-life of morphine when given by the intramuscular or subcutaneous route (Reisine & Pasternak, 1996).

Hasselström and Säwe (1993) studied morphine and its metabolites with high-perfor-

mance liquid chromatography (HPLC) in plasma and urine after 72 hr in 7 healthy volunteers who were given single doses of morphine (20 mg orally and 5 mg intravenously), and found that the systemic plasma clearance of morphine was on average 21.1 ± 3.4 ml/min/kg, the volume of distribution was 2.9 ± 0.8 l/kg, and the oral bioavailability was 29.2% ± 7.2%. The terminal half-life of morphine given orally was 2.2 ± 0.8 hr, and 1.8 ± 0.4 hr when morphine was given intravenously. Morphine clearance to the formation of M3G and M6G was 57.3% and 10.4%, respectively, and renal clearance was 10.9% of total systemic plasma clearance; thus the remaining 20.8% was unidentified residual clearance. Using the plasma AUC after oral and intravenous doses, the ratios of M6G:morphine were 3.6 ± 1.2 and 0.7 ± 0.3 respectively, and M3G:morphine was 29.9 ± 6.8 and 7.7 ± 1.4 (ratios which are about half the amounts measured in the Osborne et al., 1990, study). In this study, the differences in the metabolic ratios with the different routes of administration were probably due to differences in circulating morphine concentrations, as shown by plasma and urine concentrations. The authors speculated that an oral:parenteral potency ratio of 1:3 may be due to differences in circulating amounts of morphine, since they found that the ratios of M6G:M3G for a dose given by either route were the same. The authors also found that there was a very slowly declining terminal phase over 12 hr of morphine and metabolites in both plasma and urine excretion curves (which they refer to as the $t_{1/2\gamma3}$), with the greater part of morphine and metabolites excreted during this phase after the oral dose (vs. the intravenous dose), suggesting enterohepatic cycling. Most studies have shown that over 90% of morphine is excreted in urine within 24 hr. However, in the setting of renal disease, less than 10% of morphine and morphine metabolites are excreted in feces.

The mechanism of enterohepatic cycling has also been suggested by others. Westerling, Frigen, and Hogland (1993) studied morphine pharmacokinetics using high-performance liquid chromatography in a complete crossover design in which morphine (10 mg intravenous, 20 mg oral, and 30 mg controlled release tablets) was administered to 10 healthy volunteers on three separate occasions. Using a two-compartment model to calculate pharmacokinetic parameters, the absolute systemic bioavailability was somewhat greater on average (21.6% vs. 17.1%) for the oral solution of morphine as compared with the controlled release tablet, with secondary peaks in plasma concentration curves indicating an enterohepatic circulation of morphine.

Extrahepatic metabolism of morphine was suggested in another study using a radioimmunoassay method (Mazoit, Sandouk, Scherrmann, & Roche, 1990) in which intravenous morphine was given to 6 patients, and samples were obtained from arterial and venous (mesenteric, hepatic, and peripheral) blood, with dye infusion to measure hepatic blood flow. There were no differences found in morphine concentration between the peripheral artery and superior mesenteric vein, suggesting an absence of gut wall metabolism of morphine in these patients. Total body clearance of morphine was 38% greater than hepatic clearance, with the kidney as the most likely site of extrahepatic, extraintestinal morphine clearance. Hasselström and Säwe (1993) also found that the renal clearance of M6G and morphine was greater than creatinine clearance, and postulated the presence of an "active secretion process."

Renal aspects of morphine pharmacokinetics have also been addressed in a review article by Chan and Matzke (1987) on renal insufficiency and opioids, noting that the presence of an effect of renal failure on morphine disposition has been reported by investigators using less specific radioimmunoassay techniques that measure morphine as well as its glucuronides, and has not been observed by those investigators using specific chromatography assays. Got, Baud, Sandouk, Diamant-Berger, and Scherrmann (1994) studied plasma morphine disposition in opiate-intoxicated patients comparing a highly morphine-specific radioimmunoassay with a nonspecific morphine

radioimmunoassay, and found that the nonspecific assay gave a 3- to 16-fold higher concentration than the specific morphine assay. Thus, it can be seen that the use of a specific assay is important in order to study morphine metabolism accurately.

Additional studies have been performed to examine differences in morphine pharmacokinetics by route of administration. Transdermal versus intravenous morphine in 10-mg doses was given to 12 healthy subjects (Westerling, Höglund, Lundin, & Svedman, 1994), with lower plasma concentrations of both M6G and M3G, as measured by high-performance liquid chromatography after transdermal administration and a delay up to 1 hr before metabolites were detectable. AUC ratios, however, were similar for both intravenous and transdermal routes of administration for M6G and M3G relative to morphine. Oral versus rectal disposition of morphine and its metabolites was assessed using a radioimmunoassay for morphine and high-performance liquid chromatography for morphine metabolites in 6 normal volunteers (Babul & Darke, 1993). The rectal route produced a lower concentration of metabolites, probably due to bypassing of hepatic biotransformation. However, there was also greater intersubject variability of absorption per rectum, attributed to the probable differences in the extent of first-pass metabolism related to anatomic placement of the suppository in relation to portal and systemic venous drainage. Sublingual absorption of morphine, as derived by measuring the amount of drug not absorbed from the oral cavity after 10 min, has been estimated to range on average from 18%–22%, with an apparent mean systemic bioavailability of 9% in the same subjects (as measured by comparing the plasma area under the curve[AUC] for sublingual morphine over 6 hr to that of morphine given via the intramuscular route), a difference that could be explained by local biotransformation of morphine or a possible local depot in the oral cavity (Weinberg et al., 1988).

Studies of the pharmacokinetics of the minor metabolite M6G have demonstrated the important contribution of this metabolite to the analgesic properties of morphine. Osborne, Joel, Trew, and Slevin (1988) used visual analog scales to assess the analgesic activity of M6G given directly to 6 cancer patients, with pain relief demonstrated in 5 of the 6 patients; this study thus suggests that most of morphine analgesia may be due to this metabolite, and in fact there may be therapeutic plasma levels of M6G. Pharmacokinetics in 2 of these patients, one with chronic renal failure, also demonstrated that the elimination of M6G was closely related to renal function (AUC 370 vs. 1319).

Portenoy, Thaler, Inturrisi, Friedlander-Klar, and Foley (1992) found that higher ratios of M6G/morphine as measured by HPLC correlated with greater average and peak pain relief in 14 patients with chronic pain and normal renal function (thus ruling out effects of accumulation of metabolite) given morphine infusions.

Receptor binding studies of mouse brain tissue homogenates (Paul, Standifer, Inturrisi, & Pasternak, 1989) have shown that M6G and morphine strongly compete for two likely subtypes of opioid receptors, mu_1 (supraspinal) and mu_2 (spinal and gastrointestinal), with a greater affinity for both subtypes demonstrated by morphine. The metabolite M3G and its possible analgesic effects and binding characteristics were not assessed in this study. Since *in vivo* studies have shown that M6G demonstrates a much greater potency than morphine, this contrast may be explained by a number of differences between binding studies and physiological conditions.

The effect of aging on morphine pharmacokinetics has also been examined. Owen and colleagues (1983) looked at age-related morphine kinetics in 13 young versus 7 older subjects after one intravenous dose morphine (10 mg/70 kg), and found that the total apparent volume of distribution at steady state in the elderly was half that of younger adults due to reduced central and peripheral kinetic compartment volumes. They also found higher calculated peripheral compartment morphine concentrations in elderly, maintained for about 1.5 hr, suggesting that the increased sensitivity of the elderly to the analgesic effects of morphine may be due in part to altered pharmacokinetics.

Methadone

Methadone was first synthesized for the indication of analgesia in Germany in the late 1930s but was not developed fully until after WW II. In the 1960s it was studied in the United States as a possible treatment for heroin addiction and was found to be very effective, because of its oral efficacy due to high systemic bioavailability after oral administration and long apparent half-life when administered on a chronic basis. At this time there are more than 120,000 former illicit opioid addicts in long-term methadone maintenance treatment programs in the United States and in similar numbers in Europe, with programs in many other countries. Methadone is also used increasingly as a treatment for chronic pain.

Pharmacokinetic studies of methadone were performed in the early 1970s when gas chromatography techniques with adequate sensitivity were developed. These studies showed that methadone has a very slow onset of action after oral administration, with peak plasma level reached between 2 and 4 hr, and with a sustained plasma level over a 24-hr dosing interval (Änggård *et al.*, 1974; Dole & Kreek, 1973; Inturrisi & Verebely, 1972a, 1972b; Kreek, 1973a, 1973b; Kreek *et al.*, 1974; Kreek, Oratz, & Rothschild, 1978). It was also shown that the average plasma apparent terminal half-life of methadone was about 24 hr in study subjects. Inturrissi and Verebely (1972a, 1972b) studied methadone blood levels over a 24-hr period in 5 dose-stabilized patients (maintained on 100 or 120 mg of methadone for 6 weeks to 1 year), and found that the peak plasma level occurred at 4 hr, with a slow decline so that at 24 hr the mean plasma level was about equal to the predose level, with a mean apparent half-life of 24 hr. Kreek (1973b) also used gas chromatography to measure plasma methadone levels in 9 stabilized methadone patients and found peak methadone levels occurred 2 hr after drug ingestion and were relatively low, usually less than twice the pre-dose or sustained plasma level, with substantial levels remaining 24 hr after dosing, and an apparent half-life of about 24 hr.

Methadone is stored in tissue where it accumulates, mostly in the liver. In the course of methadone maintenance with persistent oral dosing, these hepatic reservoirs keep methadone plasma levels relatively constant, thus extending the apparent terminal half-life. A further analysis of the Kreek 1973b study by Dole and Kreek (1973) hypothesized that, since the ratios of the peak to trough levels of methadone in plasma were 1:6 and the half-life was approximately 24 hr, there must be a reservoir of drug outside the plasma to account for both the relatively low plasma concentrations after absorption of a large dose and the presence of relatively high plasma levels after 24 hr. This hypothesis was confirmed in later animal studies (Harte, Gutjahr, & Kreek, 1976; Kreek, Oratz, & Rothschild, 1978). Studies in humans have also demonstrated that methadone is over 90% plasma protein-bound with binding to both albumin and all globulin fractions (Kreek, Gutjahr, Garfield, Bowen, & Field, 1976; Kreek, Oratz, & Rothschild, 1978; Pond, Kreek, Tong, Raghunath, & Benowitz, 1985). Thus, the hepatic reservoir allows for later release of unmetabolized methadone into the circulation, with buffering of the free or unbound plasma methadone.

These pharmacokinetic findings support earlier pharmacodynamic observations of patients in studies of methadone as a pharmacotherapy for heroin addiction (Dole, Nyswander, & Kreek, 1966). At this time, studies have been inconclusive that attempt to correlate oral methadone dose with methadone serum levels and symptoms of opioid abstinence in the small subset of methadone maintenance patients who experience such symptoms in the setting of use of apparently adequate doses of methadone (Borg, Ho, Peters, & Kreek, 1995; Wolff, Hay, & Raistrick, 1991; Wolff, Hay, Raistrick, & Calvert, 1993). These symptoms in otherwise well-stabilized patients are probably due to pharmacodynamic factors not yet fully understood.

Methadone is metabolized primarily in two N-demethylation steps by hepatic microsomal enzymes, first to form its major pyrollidine metabolite, and then to form a pyrolline, both of which are inactive metabolites which then require hepatic p450-related enzymes for further oxidative metabolism (Änggård et al., 1974; Kreek, Garfield, Gutjahr, & Giusti, 1976; Kreek, Gutjahr, et al., 1976; Sullivan, Smits, Due, Booher, & McMahon, 1972). Methadone is excreted almost equally in urine and, after biliary secretion, in feces, and in the presence of renal compromise may be secreted essentially entirely by the fecal route, which prevents accumulation and thus potential toxicity, in contrast to many other opiate drugs (Bowen, Smit, & Kreek, 1978; Kreek, Gutjahr, et al., 1976; Kreek, Gutjahr, Bowen, & Field, 1978; Kreek, Bencsath, & Field, 1980; Kreek, Kalisman, Irwin, Jaffery, & Scheflan, 1980; Kreek, Bencsath, Fanizza, & Field, 1983). In the setting of dialysis, less than 1% of the unchanged methadone is removed, probably due to both the extensive plasma protein binding and the small amount of methadone actually present in the total blood volume at any given time (Kreek, Schecter, Gutjahr, & Hecht, 1980).

Using selective stable isotope labeling, deuterium in different amounts has been placed at different sites in the methadone molecule, and pharmacokinetic studies in patients have been performed (Hachey, Kreek, & Mattson, 1977; Kreek, Hachey, & Klein, 1979; Nakamura, Hachey, Kreek, Irving, & Klein, 1982). These studies have shown that in patients receiving methadone chronically for treatment of addiction, the half-life of the active l-(R[–])enantiomer is approximately 48 hr, and the half-life of the inactive d (S[+]) enantiomer is approximately 16 hr, further demonstrating that methadone has both a slow onset of action and a sustained pharmacokinetic profile in humans. This sharply differs from the pharmacokinetic activity of heroin and morphine, both of which have a very rapid onset and brief duration of action, with rapidly declining effect. When initiating methadone treatment, however, the long half-life can result in accumulation in plasma with sedation and respiratory depression.

Cerebrospinal fluid (CSF) levels of methadone range from 2% to 73% of concurrently measured plasma levels, with peak methadone levels in CSF appearing about 3–8 hr after methadone administration, in contrast to peak plasma levels at 2–4 hr after methadone dosing; thus, the highest levels of CSF methadone may occur when plasma levels are declining toward steady state (Rubenstein et al., 1978). In contrast to morphine, methadone has more than 90% systemic bioavailability after oral administration (Hachey et al., 1977; Nakamura et al., 1982). Methadone is relatively lipid soluble, with sublingual absorption of 34% for methadone at pH 6.5, which increases to 75% under alkaline (pH 8.5) conditions due to predominance of the un-ionized form at a more alkaline pH, which also favors sublingual absorption pH 6.5 (Weinberg et al., 1988). Sublingual absorption has been shown to be contact time dependent for methadone, perhaps related to tissue reservoir formation (Weinberg et al.).

Methadone metabolism can be affected by a number of factors. Research on the effects of hepatic compromise on methadone metabolism have shown that patients with severe chronic liver disease have slower methadone metabolism due to the hepatic impairment, and thus have retarded metabolic clearance of methadone. However, these patients with severe liver compromise tend to have lower than expected plasma methadone levels, probably due to decreased hepatic stores of methadone in the setting of a poorly functioning liver, a reduced liver size, or both. In the setting of mild to moderate liver disease, methadone disposition is essentially normal (Kreek, Oratz, & Rothschild, 1978; Kreek, Bencsath, & Field, 1980; Kreek, Kalisman, et al., 1980; Kreek, Bencsath, et al., 1983; Novick et al., 1981; Novick et al., 1985).

Drug interactions with methadone can occur, with studies demonstrating accelerated metabolism of methadone with the concurrent administration of rifampin and phenytoin, in the setting of increased hepatic enzyme activity (Kreek, Garfield, et al., 1976; Kreek, Gutjahr, et al., 1976; Tong, Pond, Kreek, Jaffery, & Benowitz, 1981), an effect that also probably occurs with the use of barbiturates. Ethanol effects on methadone biotransformation are bimodal: there is enhanced methadone biotransformation several hours following chronic heavy alcohol intake (when ethanol is no longer present) and thus lowered methadone blood levels; however, there is possibly reduced methadone biotransformation, due to hepatic enzyme competition, following similar excessive ethanol intake when blood levels of ethanol are still very high (greater than 150 mg/dl). Methadone levels are generally unchanged in the presence of regular, "social" drinking (four or fewer drinks a day) (Kreek, 1978a, 1981, 1984, 1988, 1990).

In the second half of pregnancy there appears to be accelerated methadone metabolism, probably due to enhancement of hepatic microsomal P450-related enzymes by high levels of progestins (Kreek 1979, 1981–1982, 1983; Kreek et al., 1974; Pond et al., 1985). Also, it has been suggested recently that methadone may alter the biotransformation of medications, such as zidovudine, used to treat HIV-1 and its complications (Borg & Kreek, 1995).

LAAM

Acetyl-methadol, which is the racemic mixture of the opioid active or "l" form and the nonopioid active "d" form, was synthesized and first studied for its potential analgesic activity and addiction possibilities in the late 1940s and early 1950s (Bockmuhl & Erhart, 1948; Eddy, May, & Mosettig, 1952; Fraser & Isbell, 1951, 1952; Keats & Beecher, 1952; Sung & Way, 1954). LAAM was approved in 1993 by the Food and Drug Administration to be used as a treatment for heroin addiction following a period of more than 12 years after most of the clinical studies documenting the actions, pharmacokinetics, and efficacy of LAAM were completed, and 41 years after the first studies in humans of its opioid properties. This hiatus was due to earlier, mostly administrative, problems with the preclinical drug testing results (Abramowic, 1994; ORLAAM™ drug information. 1993).

L-alpha-acetyl-methadol (LAAM) is an acetylated, single enantiomeric congener of methadone that is longer acting in man (48 hr as contrasted to 24 hr for methadone) and also orally effective, thus like methadone meeting the two major criteria for a pharmacotherapy for treatment of an addictive disease (Kaiko & Inturrisi, 1973; Kreek, 1973b, 1978b; Levine, Zaks, Fink, & Freedman, 1973). Like methadone, LAAM is a pure opioid agonist directed primarily at the mu type opioid receptor, and thus pharmacologically effective as a treatment for opioid addiction. Also like methadone with its long duration of action, LAAM maintains steady-state perfusion of these specific opioid receptors. LAAM differs from methadone, however, in that LAAM undergoes extensive oxidative metabolism by hepatic P450-type enzymes to two major active metabolites produced via n-demethylation: noracetylmethadol (norLAAM) produced after the first n-demethylation, dinoracetylmethadol (dinorLAAM), produced after a second demethylation, and also very small amounts of three other active metabolites resulting from deacetylation: methadol, nor-methadol, and dinor-methadol, all of which are present in urine along with the parent compound (Billings, McMahon, & Blake, 1974; Kiang, Campos-Flor, & Inturrisi, 1981; Sullivan, Due, & McMahon, 1973; Sung & Way, 1954).

Plasma levels of LAAM show a biexponential plasma decay curve after acute or chronic administration, with norLAAM and dinorLAAM plasma levels increased 5- to 10-fold, respectively, after chronic administration. The long duration of action of LAAM is probably due to the accumulation of these two active metabolites, as well as binding of LAAM and its metabolites to tissue proteins (Henderson, Wilson, & Lau, 1976). Pharmacological studies suggest that norLAAM has a clearance similar to that of LAAM, with the clearance of dinorLAAM at a rate even longer than that of the parent compound. However, pharmacokinetics studies of these two metabolites in man

have not yet been done since these compounds have not been administered directly to man.

A number of pharmacokinetic studies of LAAM in humans have been performed and have been accepted by the FDA; these studies have demonstrated that the apparent beta terminal half-life for LAAM is 2.6 days, for norLAAM, 2 days, and for dinorLAAM, 4 days (Abramowic, 1994; Blaine & Renault, 1976; Henderson et al., 1976; Kaiko & Inturrisi, 1975; Misra & Mule, 1975; ORLAAM™ package insert, 1993). However, one study (Kaiko & Inturrisi, 1975) in patients maintained on a stable dose of medication found that the plasma levels of LAAM itself peaked at 4 hr and were barely detectable at 24 hr with a mean apparent half-life of 7 hr (range 2–12 hr), a half-life less than the FDA-accepted value. NorLAAM levels peaked at 4–8 hr and slowly declined over the next 40 hr with a mean apparent half-life of 48 hr (range 13–78 hr), and dinorLAAM plasma levels remained essentially constant over 48 hr (thus the half-life could not be calculated). However, the peak pharmacologic effect of LAAM as measured by degree of pupillary constriction occurred at 8 hr, then declined at a rate intermediate between that of the parent compound and its active metabolites, but closest to that of norLAAM.

A unique type of potential clinical pharmacotherapeutic problem with LAAM could result from the fact that the long-acting properties of LAAM are due to its metabolism by the hepatic P450-related enzyme system to these two other biologically active and long-acting compounds. For example, with the use of medications that tend to accelerate the hepatic P450-related enzyme system (including rifampin, phenytoin, phenobarbital, or carbamazepine), or with chronic alcohol abuse once ethanol itself has been metabolized, LAAM may be metabolized more quickly than in healthy subjects with no other medication use or heavy use of ethanol, as studies have demonstrated does occur with methadone (Kreek, 1990; Kreek, Garfield, et al., 1976; Kreek, Gutjahr, et al., 1976; Tong et al., 1981). This increased rate of biotransformation could lead to rapid production of the active metabolites norLAAM and dinorLAAM, although it is unknown how this might potentially affect the overall steady state of perfusion of critical opioid receptors. It may also be possible that in the presence of impaired hepatic drug metabolism, such as occurs during the ingestion of very large amounts of either ethanol or possibly with the use of high doses of benzodiazepines, or with the use of cimetidine, the metabolism of LAAM could, in theory, be retarded. The actual occurrences of such possible drug interactions and their effects have not yet been determined.

References

Abramowic, M. (1994). LAAM: a long-acting methadone for treatment of heroin addiction. *Medical Letter on Drugs and Therapeutics, 36,* 52.

Änggård, E., Gunne, L-M., Holmstrand, J., McMahon, R. E., Sandberg, C-G., & Sullivan, H. R. (1974). Disposition of methadone in methadone maintenance. *Clinical Pharmacology & Therapeutics, 17,* 258–266.

Babul, N., & Darke, A. C. (1993). Disposition of morphine and its glucuronide metabolites after oral and rectal administration: Evidence of route specificity. *Clinical Pharmacology & Therapeutics, 54,* 286–292.

Billings, R. E., McMahon, R. E., & Blake, D. A. (1974). L-acetylmethadol (LAAM) treatment of opiate dependence: Plasma and urine levels of two pharmacologically active metabolites. *Life Sciences, 14,* 1437–1446.

Blaine, J. D., & Renault, P. (Eds.). (1976). *RX 3x a Week LAAM: Alternative to methadone* (DHEW–NIDA Research Monograph Series No. 8). Rockville, MD: National Institute on Drug Abuse.

Bockmühl, M., & Erhart, G. (1948) *Justus Liebigs Annalen der Chemie, 561,* 52–85.

Borg, L., & Kreek, M. J. (1995). Clinical problems associated with interactions between methadone pharmacotherapy and medications used in the treatment of HIV-positive and AIDS patients. *Current Opinion in Psychiatry, 8,* 199–202.

Borg, L., Ho, A., Peters, J. E., & Kreek, M. J. (1995). Availability of reliable serum methadone determination for management of symptomatic patients. *Journal of Addictive Diseases, 14,* 83–96.

Bowen, D. V., Smit, A. L. C., & Kreek, M. J. (1978). Fecal excretion of methadone and its metabolites in man: Application of GC-MS. In N. R. Daly (Ed.,) *Advances in mass spectrometry* (pp. 1634–1639). Philadelphia: Heyden.

Chan, G. L. C., & Matzke, G. R. (1987). Effects of renal insufficiency on the pharmacokinetics and pharma-

codynamics of opioid analgesics. *Drug Intelligence and Clinical Pharmacy, 21,* 773–783.

Dole, V. P., & Kreek, M. J. (1973). Methadone plasma level: Sustained by a reservoir of drug in tissue. *Proceedings of the National Academy of Sciences, USA, 70,* 10.

Dole, V. P., Nyswander, M. E., & Kreek, M. J. (1966). Narcotic blockade. *Archives of Internal Medicine, 118,* 304–309.

Eddy, N. B., May, E. L., & Mosettig, E. (1952). Chemistry and pharmacology of the methadols and acetylmethadols. *Journal of Organic Chemistry, 17,* 321–326.

Fraser, H. F., & Isbell, H. (1951). Addiction potentialities of isomers of 6-di-methylamino-4-4-diphenyl-3 acetyoxy-heptane (acetylmethadol). *Journal of Pharmacology and Experimental Therapeutics, 101,* 12.

Fraser, H. F., & Isbell, H. (1952). Actions and addiction liabilities of alpha-acetylmethadols in man. *Journal of Pharmacology and Experimental Therapeutics, 105,* 210–215.

Got, P., Baud, F. J., Sandouk, P., Diamant-Berger, O., & Scherrmann, J. M. (1994). Morphine disposition in opiate-intoxicated patients: Relevance of nonspecific opiate immunoassays. *Journal of Analytical Toxicology, 18,* 189–194.

Hachey, D. L., Kreek, M. J., & Mattson, D. H. (1977). Quantitative analysis of methadone in biological fluids using deuterium-labelled methadone and GLC-chemical-ionization mass spectrometry. *Journal of Pharmaceutical Sciences, 66,* 1579–1582.

Harte, E. H., Gutjahr, C. L., & Kreek, M. J. (1976). Long-term persistence of dl-methadone in tissues. *Clinical Research, 24,* 623A.

Hasselström, J., & Säwe, J. (1993). Morphine pharmacokinetics and metabolism in humans: Enterohepatic cycling and relative contribution of metabolites to active opioid concentrations. *Clinical Pharmacokinetics, 24,* 344–354.

Henderson, G. L., Wilson, K., & Lau, D. H. M. (1976). Plasma l-α-acetylmethadol (LAAM) after acute and chronic administration. *Clinical Pharmacology & Therapeutics, 21,* 16–25.

Inturrisi, C. E., & Verebely, K. (1972a). A gas–liquid chromatographic method for the quantitative determination of methadone in human plasma and urine. *Journal of Chromatography, 65,* 361–369.

Inturrisi, C. E., & Verebely, K. (1972b). The levels of methadone in the plasma in methadone maintenance. *Clinical Pharmacology & Therapeutics, 13,* 633–637.

Inturrisi, C. E., Schultz, M., Shin, S., Umans, J. G., Angel, L., & Simon, E. J. (1983). Evidence from opiate binding that heroin acts through its metabolites. *Life Sciences, 33* (Suppl. 1), 773–776.

Inturrisi, C. E., Max, M. B., Foley, K. M., Schultz, M., Shin, S-U., & Houde, R. W. (1984). The pharmacokinetics of heroin in patients with chronic pain. *New England Journal of Medicine, 310,* 1213–1217.

Kaiko, R. F., & Inturrisi, C. E. (1973). A gas–liquid chromatographic method for the quantitative determination of acetylmethadol and its metabolites in human urine. *Journal of Chromatography, 82,* 315–321.

Kaiko, R. F., & Inturrisi, C. E. (1975). Disposition of acetylmethadol in relation to pharmacologic action. *Clinical Pharmacology & Therapeutics, 18,* 96–103.

Kaiko, R. F., Wallenstein, S. L., Rogers, A. G., Grabinski, P. Y., & Houde, R. W. (1981). Analgesic and mood effects of heroin and morphine in cancer patients with postoperative pain. *New England Journal of Medicine, 304,* 1501–1505.

Keats, A. S., & Beecher, H. K. (1952). Analgesic activity and toxic effects of acetylmethadol isomers in man. *Journal of Pharmacology and Experimental Therapeutics, 105,* 210–215.

Kiang, C-H., Campos-Flor, S., & Inturrisi, C. E. (1981). Determination of acetylmethadol and metabolites by use of high-performance liquid chromatography. *Journal of Chromatography, 222,* 81–93.

Kreek, M. J. (1973a). Medical safety and side effects of methadone in tolerant individuals. *Journal of the American Medical Association, 223,* 665–668.

Kreek, M. J. (1973b). Plasma and urine levels of methadone. *New York State Journal of Medicine, 73,* 2773–2777.

Kreek, M. J. (1978a): Effects of drugs and alcohol on opiate disposition and action. In M. W. Adler, L. Manara, & R. Samnin (Eds.), *Factors affecting the action of narcotics* (pp. 717–739). New York: Raven.

Kreek, M. J. (1978b). Medical complications in methadone patients. *Annals of the New York Academy of Sciences, 311,* 110–134.

Kreek, M. J. (1979). Methadone disposition during the perinatal period in humans. *Pharmacology, Biochemistry and Behavior, 11,* 1–7.

Kreek, M. J. (1981). Metabolic interactions between opiates and alcohol. *Annals of the New York Academy of Sciences, 362,* 36–49.

Kreek, M. J. (1981–1982). Disposition of narcotics in the perinatal period. *Publication of AMERSA and The Career Teacher Program in Alcohol and Drug Abuse, 3,* 7–10.

Kreek, M. J. (1983). Discussion on clinical perinatal and developmental effects of methadone. In J. R. Cooper, F. Altman, B. S. Brown, & D. Czechowicz (Eds.), *Research in the treatment of narcotic addiction: State of the art* (NIDA Monograph, DHHS Publication No. [ADM] 83-1281, pp. 444–453). Rockville, MD: National Institute on Drug Abuse.

Kreek, M. J. (1984). Opioid interactions with alcohol. *Journal of Addictive Diseases, 3,* 35–46.

Kreek, M. J. (1988). Opiate–ethanol interactions: Implications for the biological basis and treatment of combined addictive diseases. In L. S. Harris (Ed.), *Problems of drug dependence, 1987; Proceedings of the 49th annual scientific meeting of the committee on problems of drug dependence* (NIDA Research Monograph Series, DHHS Publication No. [ADM]

88-1564, 81, pp. 428–439). Rockville MD: National Institute on Drug Abuse.

Kreek, M. J. (1990). Drug interactions in humans related to drug abuse and its treatment. *Modern Methods in Pharmacology, 6,* 265–282.

Kreek, M. J., Schecter, A., Gutjahr, C. L., Bowen, D., Field, F., Queenan, J., & Merkatz, I. (1974). Analyses of methadone and other drugs in maternal and neonatal body fluids: Use in evaluation of symptoms in a neonate of mother maintained on methadone. *American Journal of Drug and Alcohol Abuse, 1,* 409–419.

Kreek, M. J., Garfield, J. W., Gutjahr, C. L., & Giusti, L. M. (1976). Rifampin-induced methadone withdrawal. *New England Journal of Medicine, 294,* 1104–1106.

Kreek, M. J., Gutjahr, C. L., Garfield, J. W., Bowen, D. V., & Field, F. H. (1976). Drug interactions with methadone. *Annals of the New York Academy of Science, 281,* 350–374.

Kreek, M. J., Gutjahr, C. L., Bowen, D. V., & Field, F. H. (1978). Fecal excretion of methadone and its metabolites: A major pathway of elimination in man. In A. Schecter, H. Alksne, & E. Kaufman (Eds.), *Critical concerns in the field of drug abuse: Proceedings of the 3rd National Drug Abuse Conference* (pp. 1206–1210). New York: Dekker.

Kreek, M. J., Oratz, M., & Rothschild, M. A. (1978). Hepatic extraction of long- and short-acting narcotics in the isolated perfused rabbit liver. *Gastroenterology, 75,* 88–94.

Kreek, M. J., Hachey, D. L., & Klein, P. D. (1979). Stereoselective disposition of methadone in man. *Life Sciences, 24,* 925–932.

Kreek, M. J., Bencsath, F. A., & Field, F. H. (1980). Effects of liver disease on urinary excretion of methadone and metabolites in maintenance patients: Quantitation by direct probe chemical ionization mass spectrometry. *Biomedical Mass Spectrometry, 7,* 385–395.

Kreek, M. J., Kalisman, M., Irwin, M., Jaffery, N. F., & Scheflan, M. (1980). Biliary secretion of methadone and methadone metabolites in man. *Research Communications in Chemical Pathology and Pharmacology, 29,* 67–78.

Kreek, M. J., Schecter, A., Gutjahr, C. L., & Hecht, M. (1980). Methadone use in patients with chronic renal disease. *Drug and Alcohol Dependence, 5,* 197–205.

Kreek, M. J., Bencsath, F. A., Fanizza, A., & Field, F. H. (1983). Effects of liver disease on fecal excretion of methadone and its unconjugated metabolites in maintenance patients: Quantitation by direct probe chemical ionization mass spectrometry. *Biomedical Mass Spectrometry, 10,* 544–549.

Levine, R., Zaks, A., Fink, M., Freedman, A. M. (1973). Levomethadyl acetate: Prolonged duration of opioid effects, including cross tolerance to heroin in man. *Journal of the American Medical Association, 226,* 316–318.

Mazoit, J. X., Sandouk, P., Scherrmann, J-P., & Roche, A. (1990). Extrahepatic metabolism of morphine occurs in humans. *Clinical Pharmacology & Therapeutics, 4,* 613–618.

Misra, A. L., & Mule, S. J.(1975). L-alpha-acetylmethadol (LAAM) pharmacokinetics and metabolism: Current status. *American Journal of Drug and Alcohol Abuse, 2,* 301–305.

Nakamura, K., Hachey, D. L., Kreek, M. J., Irving, C. S., & Klein, P. D. (1982). Quantitation of methadone enantiomers in humans using stable isotope-labeled [2H3]-[2H5]-, and [2H8] methadone. *Journal of Pharmaceutical Sciences, 71,* 39–43.

Neumann, P. B., Henriksen, H., Grosman, N., & Christensen, C. B. (1982). Plasma morphine concentrations during chronic oral administration in patients with cancer pain. *Pain, 13,* 247–252.

Novick, D. M., Kreek, M. J., Fanizza, A. M., Yancovitz, S. R., Gelb, A. M., & Stenger, R. J. (1981). Methadone disposition in patients with chronic liver disease. *Clinical Pharmacology & Therapeutics, 30,* 353–362.

Novick, D. M., Kreek, M. J., Arns, P. A., Lau, L. L., Yancovitz, S. R., & Gelb, A. M. (1985). Effect of severe alcoholic liver disease on the disposition of methadone in maintenance patients. *Alcoholism, Clinical and Experimental Research, 9,* 349–354.

ORLAAM™ drug information. (1993). *Levomethadyl acetate hydrochloride oral solution* [Package insert]. Author.

Osborne, R., Joel, S., Trew, D., & Slevin, M. (1988). Analgesic activity of morphine-6-glucuronide [Letter]. *Lancet, 1,* 828.

Osborne, R., Joel, S., Trew, D., & Slevin, M. (1990). Morphine and metabolite behavior after different routes of morphine administration: Demonstration of the importance of the active metabolite morphine-6-glucuronide. *Clinical Pharmacology & Therapeutics, 47,*12–19.

Owen, J. A., Sitar, D. S., Berger, L., Brownell, L., Duke, P. C., & Mitenko, P. A. (1983). Age-related morphine kinetics. *Clinical Pharmacology & Therapeutics, 34,* 364–368.

Paul, D., Standifer, K. M., Inturrisi, C. E., & Pasternak, G. W. (1989). Pharmacological characterization of morphine-6β-glucuronide, a very potent morphine metabolite. *Journal of Pharmacology and Experimental Therapeutics, 251,* 477–483.

Pond, S. M., Kreek, M. J., Tong, T. G., Raghunath, J., & Benowitz, N. L. (1985). Altered methadone pharmacokinetics in methadone-maintained pregnant women. *Journal of Pharmacology and Experimental Therapeutics, 233,* 1–6.

Portenoy, R. K., Thaler, H. T., Inturrisi, C. E., Friedlander-Klar, H., & Foley, K. M. (1992). The metabolite morphine-6-glucuronide contributes to the analgesia produced by morphine infusion in patients with pain and normal renal function. *Clinical Pharmacology & Therapeutics, 51,* 422–431.

Portenoy, R. K., Southam, M. A., Gupta, S. K., Lapin, J., Layman, M., Inturrisi, C. E., & Foley, K. M. (1993). Transdermal fentanyl for cancer pain. *Anesthesiology, 78,* 36–43.

Reisine, T., & Pasternak, G. (1996). Opioid analgesics and antagonists. In J. G. Hardman, A. G. Gilman, & L. E. Limbird (Eds.), *Goodman and Gilman's the pharmacological basis of therapeutics* (9th ed., pp. 521–555). New York: McGraw-Hill,

Rubenstein, R. B., Kreek, M. J., Mbawa, N., Wolff, W. I., Korn, R., & Gutjahr, C. L. (1978). Human spinal fluid methadone levels. *Drug and Alcohol Dependence, 3,* 103–106.

Sawynok, J. (1986). The therapeutic use of heroin: A review of the pharmacological literature. *Canadian Journal of Physiology and Pharmacology, 64,* 1–6.

Sullivan, H. R., Smits, S. E., Due, S. L., Booher, R. E., & McMahon, R. E. (1972). Metabolism of *d*-methadone: Isolation and identification of analgesically active metabolites. *Life Sciences, 11,* 1093–1104.

Sullivan, H. R., Due, S. L., & McMahon, R. E. (1973). Metabolism of alpha-l-methadol: N-acetylation, a new metabolic pathway. *Research Communications in Chemical Pathology and Pharmacology, 6,* 1072–1078.

Sung, C-Y., & Way, E. L. (1954). The fate of the optical isomers of alpha-acetylmethadol. *Journal of Pharmacology and Experimental Therapeutics, 110,* 260–270.

Tong, T. G., Pond, S. M., Kreek, M. J., Jaffery, N. F., & Benowitz, N. L. (1981). Phenytoin-induced methadone withdrawal. *Annals of Internal Medicine, 94,* 349–351.

Weinberg, D. S. A., Inturrisi, C. E., Reidenberg, B., Moulin, D. W., Nip, T. J., Wallenstein, S., Houde, R. W., & Foley, K. M. (1988). Sublingual absorption of selected opioid analgesics. *Clinical Pharmacology & Therapeutics, 44,* 335–342.

Westerling, D., Frigen, L., & Hogland, P. (1993). Morphine pharmacokinetics and effects on salivation and continuous reaction times in healthy volunteers. *Therapeutic Drug Monitoring, 15,* 364–374.

Westerling, D., Höglund, P., Lundin, S., & Svedman, P. (1994). Transdermal administration of morphine to healthy subjects. *British Journal of Clinical Pharmacology, 37,* 571–576.

Wolff, K., Hay, A., & Raistrick, D. (1991). High-dose methadone and the need for drug measurements. *Clinical Chemistry, 37,* 1651–1654.

Wolff, K., Hay, A. W. M., Raistrick, D., & Calvert, R. (1993). Steady-state pharmacokinetics of methadone in opioid addicts. *European Journal of Clinical Pharmacology, 44,* 189–194.

23

Behavioral Pharmacology of Opiates

JAMES P. ZACNY AND ELLEN A. WALKER

Introduction

The purpose of this chapter is to describe and discuss what is currently known about the behavioral pharmacology of opioids in infrahumans and humans. This is a daunting task, given the breadth and depth of research that has been conducted during the past 50 years. Several reviews on the behavioral pharmacology of opioids cover certain areas in much greater detail than what can be covered here; the reader is encouraged to refer to these reviews, some of which appear yearly as an "update" (see Appendix for review bibliography).*

Behavioral pharmacologists employ several methods to examine the effects of drugs on behavior. These methods include the assessment of the subjective, discriminative stimulus, and reinforcing effects of drugs. This chapter de-

scribes what behavioral pharmacologists have learned about opioids using these methodologies. The specific areas of opioid behavioral pharmacology that are addressed in this chapter are (1) experimental studies of motivational and reinforcing effects of opioids, and (2) characterization of the interoceptive effects of opioids, including their discriminative stimulus and subjective effects.

Before discussing these two areas, we briefly review the terminology that we use throughout this chapter when discussing opioids. Opioids are believed to produce their pharmacological effects through μ, κ, and δ opioid receptors (Lord, Waterfield, Hughes, & Kosterlitz, 1977; W. R. Martin, Eades, Thompson, Huppler, & Gilbert, 1976). Drugs that interact with these receptors are either agonists (i.e., morphine and heroin) or antagonists (i.e., naloxone and naltrexone). Antagonists have no effects of their own and block the effects of agonists. Agonists are further differentiated on a continuum by how strong a biological effect (intrinsic efficacy) they produce once bound to a pharmacological receptor. Agonists that produce a strong or full effect at the receptor are termed full- or high-efficacy agonists. Other agonists (i.e., buprenorphine, nalbuphine, butorphanol) produce full or partial agonist effects under some conditions and antagonist effects under other conditions. These agonists can produce agonist and antagonist effects by

*Other areas of opioid behavioral pharmacology that have been studied in detail and have an extensive literature include the role of opioids in schedule-controlled behavior, feeding and drinking, sexual behavior, learning, memory, psychomotor performance, and classical conditioning.

JAMES P. ZACNY • Department of Anesthesia and Critical Care, The University of Chicago, Chicago, Illinois 60637. ELLEN A. WALKER • Department of Psychology, University of North Carolina at Chapel Hill, Chapel Hill, North Carolina 27599.

Handbook of Substance Abuse: Neurobehavioral Pharmacology, edited by Tarter *et al.* Plenum Press, New York, 1998.

either interacting with more than one opioid receptor or simply not producing strong biological signals at the receptor. These drugs are termed partial agonists, low-efficacy agonists, or mixed agonist–antagonists.

Experimental Studies of Motivational and Reinforcing Effects of Opioids

Infrahuman Studies

Opioid Self-Administration: Assessment of Reinforcing Effects

One of the major characteristics of opioids is their capacity to promote self-administration and drug-seeking behavior. Opioid self-administration has been observed across a range of species, procedures, response requirements, and routes of administration. Generally in opioid self-administration studies, rats or monkeys are prepared with indwelling venous catheters and drugs are delivered directly into the veins. Drug delivery can be contingent on performance under various schedules of reinforcement such as fixed ratio, variable ratio, progressive ratio, and multiple schedules. Usually in self-administration experiments, the rates of responding and the number of infusions are the dependent measures. Drugs are considered reinforcers if response rate increases and remains higher for the drug solution than the response rate observed for the vehicle solutions. Typically when measuring rates of responding, low doses are not self-administered. As the dose of an agonist is increased, a dose-dependent increase is observed for response rates. High doses of agonists, however, can suppress response rates directly so that the final dose–response curve for self-administration is an inverted U-shaped function (Pickens, Meisch, & Thompson, 1978).

A number of μ opioids, full and mixed agonists–antagonists, are self-administered by monkeys and rats. For example, full agonists such as morphine, fentanyl, heroin, methadone, levorphanol, codeine, and etorphine maintain intravenous (iv) self-administration behavior (Woods, Young, & Herling, 1982; Young,

Swain, & Woods, 1981). Oral fentanyl and etonitazene in rats and rhesus monkeys, respectively, also maintain self-administration behavior (Carroll & Meisch, 1978; Colpaert, Meert, De Witte, & Schmitt, 1982; Kupers & Gybels, 1995; Meisch, 1995). The mixed agonists–antagonists nalbuphine (Collins, Weeks, Cooper, Good, & Russell, 1984; Lukas, Griffiths, & Brady, 1983; Winger, Skjoldager, & Woods, 1992; Young, Stephens, Hein, & Woods, 1984), butorphanol (Butelman, Winger, Zernig, & Woods, 1995; Lukas, Brady, & Griffiths, 1986) and pentazocine (Yanagita, Katoh, Wakasa, & Oinuma, 1982) are self-administered by animals and these effects appear to be predominantly mediated through μ opioid receptor mechanisms. Rates of responding for mixed agonists–antagonists are sometimes lower than rates for full agonists and this result has been attributed to lower reinforcing efficacy of these compounds (Balster & Lukas, 1985; Woods, France, & Winger, 1992). However, the observation of lower rates of responding for mixed agonists–antagonists clearly depends on the mixed agonist–antagonist, species, and procedure studied (Aigner & Balster, 1979; Slifer & Balster, 1983; Winger, Woods, & Hursh, 1996).

An interesting compound in self-administration is buprenorphine. Buprenorphine is self-administered in monkeys (Mello, Bree, & Mendelson, 1981; Woods, 1977). However, in baboons, buprenorphine self-administration was characterized by a shallow dose–response curve across a wide range of doses and overall did not meet the criterion for self-administration (Lukas et al., 1986). Interestingly, buprenorphine blocks the effects of opioid (Mello, Bree, & Mendelson, 1983; Winger & Woods, 1996) as well as cocaine-maintained responding (Mello et al., 1992; Mello, Mendelson, Bree, & Lukas, 1989).

Opioid antagonists such as naloxone and naltrexone do not maintain self-administration responding (Lukas et al., 1986; Winger et al., 1992). While morphine-dependent monkeys respond to administer iv morphine (Thompson & Schuster, 1964), morphine-dependent as well as nondependent monkeys respond to escape or avoid administration of opioid antagonists such as naloxone (Downs & Woods,

1975, 1976). Competitive antagonist administration can alter agonist self-administration in two ways. Competitive antagonists can either produce rightward displacements of the agonist dose–response curves (Bertalmio & Woods, 1989; Winger *et al.,* 1992) or produce suppression of behavior so that self-administration of an agonist may be blocked and patterns of extinction behavior become evident (Koob, 1992; Negus, Burke, Medzihradsky, & Woods, 1993). For example, the opioid antagonist quadazocine dose-dependently blocks the ascending limb of μ agonist dose–response curves in a parallel, rightward fashion (Bertalmio & Woods, 1989). However, when quadazocine is administered prior to access to butorphanol, no dose of butorphanol is self-administered and the butorphanol dose–response curve is flat (Butelman *et al.,* 1995). Similarly, the selective, insurmountable μ antagonist β-funaltrexamine produced an extinction-like pattern of responding as well as a long-lasting antagonism of heroin self-administration (T. J. Martin, Dworkin, & Smith, 1995; Negus *et al.,* 1993).

The κ agonists do not appear to produce reinforcing effects (Bals-Kubik, Herz, & Shippenberg, 1989; Mucha & Herz, 1985; Woods & Winger, 1987). For example, U50,488 fails to maintain self-administration in rats (A. Tang & Collins, 1985). Also, under some conditions, the κ mixed agonists–antagonists cyclazocine and nalorphine maintain avoidance or escape behavior (Hoffmeister, 1979). The selective κ antagonist nor-binaltorphimine fails to alter self-administration of heroin, morphine, or cocaine in rats (Glick, Maisonneve, Raucci, & Archer, 1995; Negus *et al.,* 1993) suggesting that the κ receptors do not play a role in self-administration of these compounds. However, the κ agonists U50,488 and spiradoline produced long-lasting antagonism of both morphine and cocaine self-administration in rats, suggesting that perhaps pharmacological activation of the κ opioid receptor may modulate self-administration of opioid, stimulant, or both in some manner (Glick *et al.,* 1995).

Effects of δ receptor activation have also led to mixed results regarding self-administration.

For example, the δ agonist BW383U86 is not self-administered in rhesus monkeys (Negus *et al.,* 1994; Negus, Mello, Portoghese, Lukas, & Mendelson, 1995) whereas the δ agonist DPDPE ([D-Pen^2, D-Pen^3]-enkephalin) is self-administered when delivered intracerebroventricularly (icv) in rats (Devine & Wise, 1994). The δ antagonist naltrindole antagonized self-administration of heroin in rats, suggesting that perhaps a component of heroin self-administration might be mediated via δ receptors (Negus *et al.,* 1993). Naltrindole, however, has been observed to have μ antagonist effects at high doses (Comer *et al.,* 1993; Kitchen & Kennedy, 1990).

Opioid Conditioned Place Preference or Aversion: Assessment of Motivational Effects

Another common procedure used to measure the reinforcing effects of drugs is the conditioned place preference or aversion technique (Carr, Fibiger, & Phillips, 1989; Hoffman, 1989). The conditioned place preference apparatus is usually a box with two separate chambers. In this procedure a drug injection is paired over several training sessions with one of the novel chambers. After the training sessions, the subject is placed back into the apparatus without the drug and subsequent approach, preference, or avoidance of the two chambers is measured. Approach and preference suggests that the chamber is paired with a reinforcing drug and avoidance suggests that the chamber is paired with an aversive drug. The conditioned place preference experiment is novel in that the rats are tested in the absence of the training drug. Therefore, the direct effect of drugs on behavior is not a consideration when interpreting the results.

Overall, the results in the conditioned place preference procedure are similar to the results from the operant self-administration procedure described earlier. Compounds with significant μ opioid activity such as morphine, DAMGO ([D-Ala^2, *N*-Me-Phe^4, Gly^3-ol]-enkephalin), sufentanil, and fentanyl produce preference for an environment previously paired with the drug (Hoffman, 1989; Mucha & Herz, 1985).

This effect is blocked by the μ selective antagonist CTOP (D-Phe-Cys-Tyr-D-Trp-Orn-Thr-Pen-Thr-NH$_2$), but not by a δ antagonist (Bals-Kubik, Shippenberg, & Herz, 1990b). The κ agonists, such as U50,488 and U69,593, generally produce conditioned place aversions (Mucha & Herz, 1985; Shippenberg & Bals-Kubik, 1991). Other studies have demonstrated that κ antagonists produce conditioned place preferences. This observation suggests that blocking κ receptor activity produces positive approach and preference for the paired environment (Bechara & van der Kooy, 1987).

In conditioned place preference procedures (unlike operant self-administration), δ agonists such as DPDPE consistently produce conditioned place preferences that are blocked by the δ antagonist ICI 174,864 but not the μ antagonist CTOP (Bals-Kubik *et al.*, 1990b; Shippenberg, Bals-Kubik, & Herz, 1987). β-endorphin appears to produce conditioned place preference by activating both μ and δ receptors. However, neither μ nor δ antagonists could completely block the conditioned place preference produced by β-endorphin, suggesting that μ and δ receptors are involved perhaps at separate recognition sites in the reinforcement process (Almaric, Cline, Martinez, Bloom, & Koob, 1987; Bals-Kubik, Shippenberg, & Herz, 1990a).

Human Studies

A number of studies over the past 30 years have assessed the reinforcing effects of opioids in humans, using a range of different subpopulations and a number of different methodologies. Although there have been far fewer studies conducted with humans than with infrahumans, the human studies have produced results which are for the most part concordant with the infrahuman studies.

In the human studies, opioids have typically been self-administered via the oral, intramuscular, or intravenous route. The first studies to assess the reinforcing effects of opioids were conducted at the Addiction Research Center when it was located in Lexington, Kentucky. In two studies opioid abusers first sampled an opioid, later on rank-ordered the drug in terms of preference relative to other drugs they had sampled in the same study, and then finally chose whether they wanted to participate in a subsequent 7-day direct addiction test with that drug, in which ascending doses of the drug would be given across successive days. Drugs examined in the first study were morphine, codeine, and *d*-propoxyphene (Fraser, Martin, Wolbach, & Isbell, 1961); drugs examined in the second study were intravenous morphine and pentazocine (Fraser & Rosenberg, 1964). In the first study, 5, 3, and 2 of 7 subjects chose and finished the morphine, codeine, and *d*-propoxyphene trial. In the second study, 5 and 0 subjects out of a total of 5 subjects chose and finished the morphine and pentazocine trial. These two early studies using a pseudochoice paradigm demonstrated the reinforcing efficacy of morphine and the lack of such efficacy with pentazocine.

Another early study used a rather novel dependent measure as an index of reinforcing efficacy: The number of times subjects would come back to the clinic to receive medication (Schuster, Smith, & Jaffe, 1971). In this study, subjects who had recently been through a heroin detoxification program that involved methadone tapering were divided into three groups. The groups could self-administer up to 40 mg of methadone, 400 mg of codeine or pentazocine, or placebo per day for 10 days. During the first 5 days, subjects were given $2 for simply coming to the clinic, regardless of whether they used the study drug or not. The major findings of the study were that as time progressed, fewer people from all four groups attended the clinic, but the greatest attrition rate was in the placebo and pentazocine groups. Greater attendance was generated in the methadone and codeine groups, indicative of greater reinforcing efficacy of these two drugs. Perhaps not surprisingly, the greatest divergence between groups occurred during the last 5 days of the study, when clinic attendance was not reinforced. An ancillary study was also conducted by this group of investigators (Schuster, 1976). Inpatients who had undergone methadone detoxification were offered over a 4-day period the same doses of codeine, pentazocine, or placebo as in the outpatient study. Pentazocine and codeine choices were both high and differed significantly from placebo choice. Thus pentazocine functioned as a reinforcer in a situation that imposed minimal response effort on the part of the subject (the inpatient study), but under more effortful conditions (Schuster *et al.,* 1971) it did not. Such a discrepancy in results between the inpatient and outpatient studies could be due to other factors besides differences in response effort, but behavioral pharmacologists early on recognized the modulatory role that the environment can have on the degree to which a drug functions as a reinforcer.

Several more recent studies of opioid abusers have used more traditional self-administration or choice procedures. Mello and her associates developed a self-administration procedure in which 18 completions of a second-order schedule of reinforcement (fixed ratio [FR] 300, fixed interval [FI] 1 sec:S) on one manipulandum resulted in the availability of 10 mg of intravenous heroin, and identical responding on a second manipulandum yielded $1.50. A maximum of four heroin injections could be self-administered each day, each injection separated from the others by 6 hr. Subjects were opioid abusers who had recently been detoxified; they were divided into two groups: One group was tested with a pretreatment of oral naltrexone (50 mg) and the other group was tested with placebo pretreatment. Subjects in the placebo pretreatment group self-administered 57.5%–100% of the total heroin available. Although heroin functioned as a reinforcer in all 9 subjects in this group, there was some variability in responding: 5 subjects responded almost exclusively for heroin, and 4 subjects often self-administered less heroin than was available each day. In contrast, heroin did not function as a reinforcer in the subjects who were pretreated each day with naltrexone; these subjects self-administered 2%–7.5% of the total heroin available (Mello, Mendelson, Kuehnle, & Sellers, 1981). In a second study similar in design, subjects who were pretreated with placebo-saline self-administered 93%–100% of all the heroin

available (7 or 13.5 mg per injection with three possible injections per day) over a 10-day period of availability. Buprenorphine pretreatment (8 mg a day, subcutaneous) significantly reduced heroin use by 69%–98% (Mello, Mendelson, & Kuehnle, 1982). This attenuation of heroin use provided early support for the use of buprenorphine as a pharmacotherapeutic agent for heroin abuse.

In a study using a choice procedure (Preston, Bigelow, & Liebson, 1985), methadone maintenance patients underwent a detoxification regimen during which patients were divided into three groups and were given exposure to one of the following drugs and placebo on separate days: clonidine (0.3 mg, po), oxazepam (30 mg, po), or hydromorphone (3 mg, po). After the 2 sampling days, 2 choice days commenced in which patients could choose between placebo and the active drug they had sampled previously (as well as the dose of drug they wished to administer). Throughout the detoxification regimen, this procedure (sampling and choice days) was enacted six times. Hydromorphone self-administration rate was significantly higher than that of placebo, indicating its reinforcing efficacy. In contrast, clonidine and oxazepam, drugs that are sometimes given as ancillary medication during opioid withdrawal or detoxification, did not engender choice rates higher than that of placebo.

In the most recent study using nondependent users, Lamb and his associates used a second-order schedule of reinforcement (FR 30 [FR100:s]) in which 30 completions of the FR 100 schedule resulted in intramuscular administration of a single exposure to morphine (Lamb *et al.,* 1991). Subjects were exposed to each dose of morphine for 7 days, at which time another dose was tested. Placebo did not maintain responding in any of the 5 subjects, but morphine generally at a low dose (3.75 mg) and always at higher doses (7.5, 15, and 30 mg) maintained robust responding. Self-administration was maintained by the 3.75-mg dose, although this dose did not generate any apparent subjective effects. This last finding suggests that subjective effects are not a necessary condition for a drug to function as a rein-forcer, and that the drug self-administration paradigm may be the more valid test of the abuse liability of a drug.

The reinforcing effects of methadone, or the ability of methadone to reduce the reinforcing effects of other opioids, have been assessed in physically dependent patients. In one of the earlier studies, methadone maintenance pa-tients had the opportunity to respond for 100 methadone reinforcements per session (Angle, Knowles, Marrazzi, & Sletten, 1973). The total dose that could be obtained was equal to their normal daily medication dose (25–100 mg). During the five session study, subjects were exposed to four different schedules of drug re-inforcement (fixed interval, variable interval, fixed ratio, differential reinforcement of low rates). Patterns of responding differed between the different schedules in a fashion fairly con-sistent with what has been obtained with other consummatory reinforcers in human operant studies. In another study, male prisoners who were heroin addicts were allowed to work for hydromorphone (4 mg, iv) or saline prior to and during methadone maintenance (100 mg/day, po) (Jones & Prada, 1975). Prior to methadone maintenance, hydromorphone self-administration was robust. During the mainte-nance period, hydromorphone continued to maintain self-administration behavior, but at reduced levels. The authors concluded that methadone reduced the reinforcing efficacy of hydromorphone.

Stitzer and her colleagues have conducted several studies determining whether additional methadone, relative to a patient's normal daily medication dose, can function as a reinforcer. In the first study, subjects self-administered the additional methadone reliably when they were informed that the drug available was methadone (Stitzer, Bigelow, & Liebson, 1979). In a related study, subjects were in-formed of the amount of extra methadone available, which varied across conditions, and they could choose this or an alternative mone-tary reinforcer (Stitzer, McCaul, Bigelow, & Liebson, 1983). Methadone functioned as a re-inforcer but the size of the alternative mone-tary reinforcer modulated methadone choice rates. In the next study, a double-blind proce-dure was used to determine whether dose in-formation was a necessary condition for the extra methadone to function as a reinforcer. Using a two-option choice procedure, metha-done-maintenance patients could choose be-tween 50 mg of methadone and 50, 60, 75, and 100 mg of methadone (Bickel, Higgins, & Stitzer, 1986). With patients blind to the dos-ing conditions, drug choice was systematically related to dose with the higher dose engender-ing higher choice rates.

Finally, in the most recent study examining methadone maintenance patients, the effects of methadone dose (0.05, 0.27, 1.1 mg) and re-sponse requirement to obtain the drug (fixed ratio 32, 64, 128) on self-administration were examined (Spiga, Grabowski, Silverman, & Meisch, 1996). All doses maintained respond-ing higher than that for vehicle, and the self-administration of the two lower methadone doses was inversely related to response re-quirement.

One study has assessed the reinforcing ef-fects of opioids in non-drug-abusing volun-teers. In that study, the reinforcing effects of fentanyl (50 mcg, iv) were examined in 10 healthy volunteers (Zacny et al., 1996). In each of three sessions, volunteers could self-admin-ister the drug three times via a patient-con-trolled analgesia (PCA) infusion pump, after having been exposed to the drug and saline in two sampling trials that preceded the three choice trials. What differed across the three sessions was the temperature of the water that subjects had to immerse one of their forearms in 5 min after administration of fentanyl or saline (2, 10, and 37° C). Results indicated that fentanyl functioned as a reinforcer in the cold-water (painful) conditions, but did not exceed chance responding in the nonpainful condition (37° C). Thus, it was established that the rein-forcing effects of 50 mcg of fentanyl could be modulated by the presence of a painful stimu-lus in non-drug-abusing volunteers. These re-sults complement those studies conducted in non-drug-abusing patients who self-administer small amounts of opioids, intermittently, for postoperative pain relief, using infusion pumps. PCA, as has been mentioned before (Bigelow & Preston, 1995), is a clinical form of opioid self-administration. A number of studies using the PCA methodology have demonstrated that rate of self-administration of opioids is directly related to pain; that is, greater use of the PCA pump when pain is higher than when it is lower (e.g., Berman *et al.,* 1990; Graves, Arrigo, Foster, Baumann, & Batenhorst, 1985; Parker, Holtmann, & White, 1991; Schechter, Berrien, & Katz, 1988). Further studies need to be conducted in non-opioid abusers to determine to what extent other μ opioids, such as morphine and meperidine, and mixed agonist–antagonists, such as nalbuphine and butorphanol, can function as reinforcers. The reinforcing efficacy of these compounds should be tested both in the absence and in the presence of pain or other stressful stimuli to determine whether a stressor is a necessary condition for opioids to function as a reinforcer in this population.

Characterization of the Interoceptive Effects of Opioids

Drug Discrimination

Opioids, like other psychoactive drugs, can readily serve as discriminative stimuli in humans and infrahumans. In drug discrimination experiments, subjects are trained to discriminate between the presence and absence of a given dose of opioid by arranging the conditions so that one behavior (e.g., responding on the right lever) is reinforced in the presence of the dose of opioid and a second behavior (e.g., responding on the left lever) is reinforced in the absence of the opioid.

Infrahuman Studies

The drug discrimination procedure has a number of advantages as a behavioral pharmacology procedure. The drug discrimination procedure is a sensitive procedure (i.e., the dose required for a given effect is low) and therefore both low- and high-efficacy agonists produce agonist-like responding (Koek & Woods, 1989; Paronis & Holtzman, 1994;

Young, Masaki, & Geula, 1992). In general, the drug discrimination is also a highly selective procedure in that only compounds that share a common pharmacological receptor mechanism produce drug-appropriate responding (Holtzman & Locke, 1988; Young, 1991).

Since the initial characterization of opioids such as morphine and fentanyl as discriminative stimuli (e.g., Colpaert, 1977), a number of investigators have demonstrated that opiate discriminative stimuli are centrally mediated (Locke & Holtzman, 1985, 1986; Ukai & Holtzman, 1988), stereoselective (Bertalmio, Herling, Hampton, Winger, & Woods, 1982; Jarbe, 1978; Picker, Negus, & Dykstra, 1989; Schaefer & Holtzman, 1977; Teal & Holtzman, 1980b), and susceptible to antagonism by opiate antagonists such as naloxone, naltrexone, and quadazocine (Bertalmio & Woods, 1987; H. E. Shannon & Holtzman, 1976; Walker, Makhay, House, & Young, 1994).

A number of studies have demonstrated that opiate discriminative stimuli are pharmacologically selective for one of three opioid receptors: μ, κ, and δ. Drug discrimination procedures have been particularly useful in distinguishing between agonist effects mediated by μ and κ receptors. In drug discrimination paradigms, μ and κ agonists have been distinguished in monkeys (Dykstra, Gmerek, Winger, & Woods, 1987; Young & Stephens, 1984), pigeons (Picker, 1995; Picker & Dykstra, 1987) and rats (Shearman & Herz, 1982). The κ agonists U50,488, bremazocine, and spiradoline (Holtzman & Steinfels, 1994; Holtzman, Cook, & Steinfels, 1991) have been successfully established as discriminative stimuli. The profile of discriminative stimulus effects for bremazocine, for example, is not similar to that of morphine or fentanyl (France & Woods, 1990; Picker, 1994; Picker & Dykstra, 1989). In subjects trained to discriminate the μ opiates etorphine, morphine, or fentanyl, κ agonists fail to produce significant agonist-like responding (France, Medzihradsky, & Woods, 1994; Holtzman *et al.,* 1991; Young *et al.,* 1984). Furthermore, bremazocine fails to antagonize the fentanyl discriminative stimulus suggesting that bremazocine does not interact with the μ opioid receptor at least at the training doses used in these studies. Additionally, the selective μ receptor antagonist, β-funaltrexamine, blocks the discriminative stimulus effects of μ but not κ agonists (France & Woods, 1987; Locke & Holtzman, 1986; Picker & Dykstra, 1989) whereas the selective κ antagonist nor-binaltorphimine blocks the discriminative stimulus effects of κ but not μ agonists (Bergman & Carey, 1996). Taken together, these data suggest that μ and κ opioid receptor actions can be differentiated in the drug discrimination procedure.

More recently, δ receptor agonists have been investigated as discriminative stimuli. Whereas δ and κ agonists are generally distinguished in drug discrimination (e.g., Picker, 1995), δ and μ agonists may produce partial cross-substitution depending on the species and agonist used to establish the discriminative stimulus. For example, when BW373U86, a nonpeptide agonist selective for the δ opioid receptor is established as a discriminative stimulus, some μ agonists produce partial BW383U86-like discriminative stimulus effects in pigeons and BW373U86 produces partial substitution in pigeons trained to discriminate morphine (Comer et al., 1993). In rhesus monkeys trained to discriminate the μ agonist alfentanil or the κ agonist ethylketocyclazocine, BW373U86 failed to produce any drug-appropriate responding (Negus et al., 1994). Whereas it might appear that rhesus monkeys discriminate δ agonists better than pigeons, the discriminative stimulus effects of the δ peptide DPDPE in pigeons appears selective for δ receptors. In this discrimination established by the icv route of administration in pigeons, the δ peptides DPDPE, deltorphin II, and DSLET ([D-Ser^2, L-Leu^5]enkephalyl-Thr) produced DPDPE-like discriminative stimulus effects whereas BW373U86 produced partial substitution. The μ agonists DAMGO and morphine, κ agonist U69,593, as well as cocaine did not produce DPDPE-like stimulus effects (Jewett, Mosberg, & Woods, 1996).

An interesting group of compounds that have been established as discriminative stimuli are the opioid mixed agonist–antagonists. Earlier predictions suggested that discriminations established by a mixed agonist–antagonist might be less selective than discriminations established by a full agonist. First, it was found that lower training doses of morphine and fentanyl appeared less selective than higher training doses (Colpaert, Niemegeers, & Janssen, 1980; H. Shannon & Holtzman, 1979). Second, a number of mixed agonist–antagonists trained as discriminative stimuli had opiate as well as nonopiate receptor actions. Indeed, early drug discrimination experiments with NANM (Balster, 1989; Picker, 1991; H. E. Shannon, 1983), pentazocine (G. H. White & Holtzman, 1982), and cyclazocine (Teal & Holtzman, 1980a) indicated the discriminative stimulus profile of these compounds have both an opioid and a nonopioid component. The opioid selectivity of these discriminative stimuli has been improved, however, by using a three-choice drug discrimination procedure in which a subject discriminates between saline and two drugs (France & Woods, 1985; J. M. White & Holtzman, 1983) or two doses of the same drug (Gauvin & Young, 1989; Vanecek & Young, 1995). Such three-choice drug discrimination procedures are used to separate the opiate from the nonopiate component or the μ opiate from the κ opiate component of a discriminative stimulus. For example, cross-substitution between cyclazocine and morphine is reduced if these compounds are trained in a three-choice discrimination of cyclazocine, morphine, and saline (J. White & Holtzman, 1981; J. M. White & Holtzman, 1983).

More recently, discriminative stimuli have been established using mixed agonists–antagonists such as nalbuphine and butorphanol that appear to produce their stimulus effects through the μ opioid receptor without nonopioid receptor effects. In subjects trained to discriminate nalbuphine (Gerak & France, 1996; Walker & Young, 1993) or butorphanol (Picker et al., 1996), high- and low-efficacy agonists produced nalbuphine-like or butorphanol-like effects whereas κ agonists and nonopioids produced saline-like effects. The discriminative stimulus effects of these low-efficacy agonists also were antagonized by μ selective antagonists.

The training dose in a drug discrimination assay determines selectivity as well as the intensity or efficacy requirement of the assay. If the training dose of a high-efficacy agonist is low, mixed agonists–antagonists may produce full substitution. For example, the mixed agonist–antagonist nalbuphine produces morphine-like discriminative stimulus effects if the training dose of morphine is low (Colpaert *et al.*, 1980; Holtzman, 1982). However, if the training dose of a high-efficacy agonist is high, mixed agonist–antagonists fail to fully substitute. The mixed agonist–antagonist may now antagonize the effects of the high-efficacy agonists because the mixed agonist–antagonist is still interacting with the opioid receptor but does not have enough intrinsic efficacy to produce full effects under these high training dose conditions. For example, if the morphine training dose is increased from 3.2 to 5.6 mg/kg, nalbuphine fails to produce morphine-like stimulus effects, but antagonizes the morphine-like stimulus effects of morphine (Young *et al.*, 1992).

Although species differences have been observed to occur for opioid interactions at the κ receptor (Holtzman, 1983; Holtzman & Steinfels, 1994; Picker, 1994), these differences may be due to differences in the training doses of the drugs used to establish the discrimination. Ethylketocyclazocine and ketocyclazocine produce κ opioid-like stimulus effects in rats and monkeys but μ opioid-like stimulus effects in pigeons (Herling, Coale, Valentino, Hein, & Woods, 1980; Picker *et al.*, 1989; Shearman & Herz, 1981). Low-efficacy agonists (−)-NANM, (−)-cyclazocine, nalorphine, and levallorphan produce opioid-like stimulus effects in pigeons (Koek & Woods, 1989; Picker *et al.*, 1989; Picker *et al.*, 1993) but κ opioid-like stimulus effects in rats and monkeys (Hein, Young, Herling, & Woods, 1981; Shearman & Herz, 1981; A. H. Tang & Code, 1983). Initially these observations led investigators to suggest that pigeons lacked κ receptors. However, more recently, parametric studies with training doses in pigeons and rats have suggested that both species can discriminate κ and μ agonists (Picker, 1994; Picker &

Dykstra, 1987; Young *et al.*, 1992). Parametric studies with training doses in rhesus monkeys are limited; perhaps the species differences for κ receptors are more dependent on the training dose of the κ agonists available for study at the time.

Tolerance to the discriminative stimulus effects of opiates has been observed in a number of studies by suspending discrimination training and giving the training drug or another μ agonist noncontingently for an extended period of time (Young, 1991). Tolerance to the discriminative stimulus effects of opiates appears to be pharmacologically selective in that only repeated treatment with opioid agonists produces tolerance to these effects. For example, repeated treatment with morphine produces tolerance to the discriminative stimulus effects of opiates such as morphine (Miksic & Lal, 1977; Young, Kapitsopoulos, & Makhay, 1991), fentanyl (Emmett-Olgesby, Shippenberg, & Herz, 1988), and methadone (H. E. Shannon & Holtzman, 1976). In addition, repeated treatment with other opiate agonists such as fentanyl (Emmett-Olgesby *et al.*, 1988) and meperidine (Paronis & Holtzman, 1994) can also produce tolerance and cross-tolerance to the discriminative stimulus effects of opiates under some conditions. Tolerance to morphine or fentanyl was not observed after repeated treatment with pentobarbital (Emmett-Oglesby *et al.*, 1988; Miksic & Lal, 1977; H. E. Shannon & Holtzman, 1976).

Dependence has also been studied using the drug discrimination procedure. Rats dependent on morphine can be trained to discriminate between an opiate antagonist (presumed to be a withdrawal cue) and saline. These discriminative stimulus effects can be reversed by μ agonists but not by κ agonists and nonopioids (France & Woods, 1987; Holtzman, 1985). Interestingly, the ability of mixed agonists–antagonists to reverse antagonist-like stimulus effects in morphine-dependent subjects is dependent on the intrinsic efficacy of the mixed agonist–antagonist tested as well as the degree of drug dependence (France, DeCosta, Jacobson, Rice, & Woods, 1990; Villarreal, 1973). Drug discrimination procedures have been used to study opioid withdrawal and dependence in experiments in which pigeons are treated with morphine and trained to discriminate morphine, saline, and naltrexone. In these subjects, the discriminative stimulus effects of naltrexone appear to be based on the capacity of naltrexone to precipitate withdrawal since withholding the daily morphine injection produces naltrexone-like stimulus effects (France *et al.*, 1990; France & Woods, 1987; Holtzman, 1985). Morphine and other high-efficacy μ agonists produce morphine-like stimulus effects and reversed naltrexone-like stimulus effects; buprenorphine produces partial morphine-like stimulus effects and reverses naltrexone-like stimulus effects; the mixed agonist–antagonist nalbuphine produces considerable naltrexone-like stimulus effects (France & Woods, 1990). This procedure in essence provides an animal model of the subjective effects of opioid withdrawal in morphine-dependent subjects. By the use of this model, novel compounds can be tested for their ability to produce or block the subjective effects of withdrawal.

Human Studies

Over the past 10 years, Bigelow, Preston, and their colleagues have conducted a number of drug discrimination studies in both nondependent and dependent opioid abusers. The discrimination procedure is roughly parallel to that used in infrahumans: A saline-drug (two-choice discrimination) or saline-drug-drug discrimination (three-choice discrimination) is trained between a drug and saline or two drugs and saline and then test sessions are run, in which the doses of the training drugs or different drugs are tested. The studies are elegant, among other reasons, because most of the studies involve the successful training of a three-choice discrimination, and all of the studies involve concurrent assessment of subjective, psychomotor, and physiological effects. The advantages of training a three-choice discrimination is that it increases the selectivity of the drug discrimination methodology. For example, when nondependent users were trained to discriminate between hydromorphone and saline, drugs with lower efficacy at the μ receptor sub-

stituted fully for the hydromorphone cue, including buprenorphine, butorphanol, pentazocine, and nalbuphine (Preston, Liebson, & Bigelow, 1992). This was in spite of subjects reporting differential subjective effects between the training and test opioids. In contrast, when subjects were trained to discriminate between hydromorphone, butorphanol, and saline, buprenorphine substituted for hydromorphone (the two drugs also had similar subjective effects), nalbuphine substituted for butorphanol (the two drugs had similar subjective effects), and pentazocine substituted for neither training drug (pentazocine differed in subjective effects from that of the two training drugs) (Preston & Bigelow, 1994). Thus, the three-choice drug discrimination procedure enhanced selectivity of the drug discrimination methodology in humans, and the results were consistent with the action of these drugs in humans using other assays (e.g., buprenorphine has a subjective effects profile similar to that of hydromorphone and nalbuphine has a subjective effects profile similar to that of butorphanol).

Drug discrimination studies have also been conducted in dependent opioid users. Training drugs in methadone-maintained volunteers have included hydromorphone, naloxone, and saline (Preston, Bigelow, Bickel, & Liebson, 1987). Test drugs have included hydromorphone, nalbuphine, and butorphanol. Hydromorphone can function as a discriminative stimulus in dependent volunteers, albeit at higher training and test doses than those used in nondependent users. Drugs with lower efficacy at the μ receptor substitute for naloxone (Preston, Bigelow, & Liebson, 1990), which is consistent with the fact that these same drugs precipitate withdrawal in methadone-maintained patients (Preston, Bigelow, & Liebson, 1988, 1989; Strain, Preston, Liebson, & Bigelow, 1993). This drug discrimination preparation can be used to examine potential pharmacotherapies that are designed to attenuate opioid withdrawal.

Subjective Effects

The profile of mood-altering effects of a drug can be assessed only in humans, because of their ability to verbalize their experiences. The profile of mood effects of a drug is important because it may tell us something about the underlying receptor mechanisms of the drug and is also used in characterizing the abuse liability of the drug. Studies have been conducted with non-opioid-abusing volunteers, nondependent opioid-abusing volunteers, and dependent opioid-abusing volunteers. The research conducted in this area is voluminous (cf. Preston & Jasinski, 1991), but certain conclusions can be drawn, in part because many of the studies use the same methodology to assess subjective effects. The assessment techniques were developed in large part by scientists at the Addiction Research Center and include the Single Dose Effect Questionnaire (SDEQ) (Fraser, van Horn, Martin, Wolbach, & Isbell, 1961) and variants thereof (e.g., Preston, Bigelow, Bickel, & Liebson, 1989; Strain, Preston, Liebson, & Bigelow, 1992) and the Addiction Research Center Inventory (ARCI; Haertzen, 1966; W. R. Martin, Sloan, Sapira, & Jasinski, 1971). The SDEQ is composed of scales that assess self-reports of strength of drug effect, identification of the drug from a list of possible drugs, drug symptomatology, and drug liking. The ARCI is a true–false questionnaire designed to differentiate among different classes of psychoactive drugs (Haertzen, 1966). A short form of the ARCI (W. R. Martin et al., 1971) typically has been used in most abuse liability studies; this form consists of 49 items and yields scores for five different scales: Pentobarbital-Chlorpromazine-Alcohol Group (PCAG), sensitive to sedative effects; Benzedrine Group (BG) and Amphetamine (A), sensitive to amphetamine-like effects; Lysergic Acid Diethylamide (LSD), sensitive to somatic and dysphoric changes; and Morphine-Benzedrine Group (MBG), sensitive to euphoric effects. Other popularly used assessment tools include the visual analog scale (VAS) and observer rating checklists.

Most of the high-efficacy μ agonists that are available for clinical use today, such as morphine, hydromorphone, meperidine, and fentanyl, have been subjected to subjective effects testing in all of the aforementioned subpopulations of volunteers. In general, opioid abusers, both dependent and nondependent, report increased scores on the MBG scale of the ARCI, indicative of euphoric effects, increased scores on the agonist scale of revised versions of the SDEQ, and increased "good drug effects" ratings (Gorodetzky & Martin, 1966; Greenwald, June, Stitzer, & Marco, 1996; Jasinski & Preston, 1986; W. R. Martin & Fraser, 1961; Strain et al., 1992). Non-opioid-abusing volunteers tend to show inconsistent effects on these measures of "positive" effects (Zacny, Lichtor, Zaragoza, & de Wit, 1992; Zacny et al., 1993; Zacny, Lichtor, Flemming, Coalson, & Thompson, 1994), bolstering the claim made many years ago that this population is likely to show more variability in their affective response to high-efficacy agonists, including the degree to which they like the effects, than opioid-abusing populations (Lasagna, von Felsinger, & Beecher, 1955). Further, in non-opioid-abusing volunteers, the constellation of subjective effects often includes increased PCAG and LSD scores, and increased adjective ratings of "drowsiness" and "drunk." These effects induced by μ opioids in non-opioid-abusing volunteers are typically not noted in opioid abusers. The differences in subjective effects between the two groups might be due to tolerance development to these effects in the opioid-abusing group.

Partial μ agonists, such as buprenorphine and dezocine, tend to be identified as "dope," and produce a profile of "positive" subjective effects, similar to that of higher-efficacy agonists, in nondependent opioid abusers (Jasinski & Preston, 1985; Preston, Bigelow, Bickel, & Liebson, 1989). The one difference between partial and full μ agonists is that the effects of partial agonists tend to plateau, or show a ceiling effect, unlike that of high-efficacy agonists (Walsh, Preston, Bigelow, & Stitzer, 1995). In dependent methadone maintenance volunteers, buprenorphine tends to produce no subjective effects, and in some cases produces subjective effects indicative of withdrawal. When volunteers were maintained on a low dose of methadone (30 mg, po), buprenorphine challenges (0.5–8.0 mg, sl) delivered 20 hr after the patient's daily methadone dose did not induce agonist or antagonist-like effects (Strain et al., 1992) but did precipitate withdrawal in volunteer patients maintained on a higher dose of methadone (60 mg) (Walsh, June, et al., 1995). Further, when buprenorphine challenges (0.5–8 mg, im) occurred only 2 hr after the daily methadone dose (30 mg, po) was administered, withdrawal was precipitated (Strain, Preston, Liebson, & Bigelow, 1995).

Opioid agonists that are considered mixed agonist–antagonists, nalbuphine, butorphanol, and pentazocine, tend to elicit a different picture of opioid effects than do high-efficacy agonists in all of the subpopulations listed. For example, in non-opioid-abusing volunteers, butorphanol (2 mg/70 kg, iv) increased VAS ratings of "confused," "floating," and "difficulty concentrating," but in the same sample an equianalgesic dose of morphine (10 mg/70 kg, iv) did not (Zacny, Lichtor, Thapar, et al., 1994). In nondependent opioid-abusing volunteers, butorphanol was compared to equianalgesic doses of hydromorphone, and while the latter drug showed euphorigenic effects and was identified as "dope," butorphanol increased both ARCI LSD scores (indicative of dysphoria) and VAS ratings of "bad effects," and tended to be identified as a drug from the class of benzodiazepines or barbiturates (Preston, Bigelow, Bickel, & Liebson, 1989). In another study, pentazocine was compared with morphine, and while morphine had prototypic "positive" effects, pentazocine presented a mixed profile: increased VAS "liking" and "good effects," but also increased VAS "bad effects" and increased ARCI LSD and PCAG scores, indicative of both dysphoria and sedation (Preston, Bigelow, & Liebson, 1987). In dependent volunteers, subjective effects of these drugs resembled that produced by naloxone (Preston et al., 1988, Preston, Bigelow, & Liebson, 1989; Strain et al., 1993).

Several studies have examined the subjective effects of opioid agonists that appear to have a stronger κ-like component than do the mixed agonist–antagonist drugs. These drugs have included cyclazocine (Haertzen, 1970; Jasinski, Martin, & Sapira, 1968; Kumor, Haertzen, Johnson, Kocher, & Jasinski, 1986), nalorphine (Haertzen, 1970; Hamilton, Dundee, Clarke, Loan, & Morrison, 1967), ketocyclazocine (Kumor et al., 1986), spiradoline (Chappell et al., 1993), enadoline (Pande et al., 1996) and a benzomorphan, MR 2033 and its isomers, MR 2034 and MR 2035 (Pfeiffer, Branti, Herz, & Emrich, 1986). Subjects tested have been opioid abusers as well as non-drug-abusing volunteers. Based on the overall profile of subjective effects these agents engender, it does not appear that selective k agonists will be used for pain therapy anytime soon in humans. There are clear psychotomimetic effects with these drugs regardless of the drug or population in which they are tested. The psychotomimesis can include depersonalization, derealization, hallucinations, bad dreams, and loss of self-control. It should be noted that some mixed agonist–antagonists, including nalbuphine and pentazocine, can, especially at high doses, induce these effects (Bellville & Green, 1965; Boccuni, Cangi, Fusco, Curradi, & Sicuteri, 1987; Hamilton et al., 1967; Jasinski & Mansky, 1972; Jasinksi, Martin, & Haeldke, 1970). It is also interesting that a low dose of naltrexone given with pentazocine altered the profile of this drug so that greater κ activity manifested itself (Preston & Bigelow, 1993). In this study, subjects were pretreated with saline or naltrexone (12.5 or 25 mg) and then were injected, using a cumulative dosing procedure, with increasing doses of hydromorphine (0–3 mg) or pentazocine (0–60 mg). Both doses of naltrexone blocked hydromorphine's subjective effects, but only the high dose of naltrexone blocked pentazocine's effects. At the low naltrexone dose, subjects reported increased LSD scores and increased "bad effects" ratings after having received pentazocine. These dysphoric effects from pentazocine were not reported after saline pretreatment; rather, μ-like effects were reported. It was concluded that the low dose of naltrexone blocked the μ receptors while sparing the κ receptor, and hence the κ-like subjective effects of pentazocine became magnified. This study suggests that opioid antagonists can be used in human studies to better understand the neurochemical mechanisms of action of full, partial and mixed agonist–antagonist opioids.

Summary

In this chapter, we have given a brief overview of the reinforcing and interoceptive effects of opioids both in infrahumans and in humans. There is an excellent concordance between infrahuman and human research on the reinforcing effects of full μ agonists. In animals and in opioid abusers, these opioids reliably function as reinforcers. One avenue of research that remains relatively unexplored is the degree to which opioids such as morphine, meperidine, and methadone function as reinforcers in non-opioid-abusing volunteers. Such research may have clinical implications in that many individuals are given these opioids for pain relief, most often on an acute basis (for postoperative pain) but in some situations on a chronic basis (for cancer pain). The drugs are taken for pain relief, but it would be interesting to know the relative importance of pain in modulating the reinforcing effects of opioids in non-opioid abusers. That is, is pain a necessary condition for opioids to function as reinforcers in this particular subject population? Another avenue of research that remains to be developed is assessing the reinforcing effects of partial and mixed agonist–antagonist opioids in several different human volunteer populations (non-opioid abusers, nondependent opioid abusers, and dependent opioid abusers). These opioids do function as reinforcers in infrahumans. Although there are only scattered reports of "street" abuse of such drugs as butorphanol and pentazocine, this may be because of the ready availability of full μ agonists in the drug abuser's environment.

The interoceptive effects of opioids in infrahumans and humans have been extensively studied so that comparisons and contrasts can be made, at least with μ and κ agonists. Κ agonists in infrahumans tend to exhibit a different discriminative stimulus profile than that of μ agonists, and in humans, the subjective effects of the two subtypes of opioids differ. Full μ agonists tend to substitute for one another in infrahuman drug discrimination studies, and these agonists tend to share similar subjective effects profiles at least in opioid abusers. Mixed agonist–antagonists tend to substitute for full μ agonists in infrahumans and opioid abusers. However, a three-choice discrimination between a full μ agonist, a mixed agonist–antagonist, and saline can be trained in humans, and further, mixed agonist–antagonists are likely to share discriminative stimulus effects with the mixed agonist–antagonist training drug than with the full μ agonist. This suggests that the discriminative stimulus effects of mixed agonist–antagonists in humans may not be mediated by μ receptors, or that mixed agonist–antagonists share more stimulus effects with other mixed agonist–antagonists (i.e., low efficacy) than with full μ agonists.

In conclusion, a great deal has been learned about the interoceptive and reinforcing effects of opioids in the past 40 years. The knowledge gleaned over this time has significantly enhanced our understanding of the complex interplay between opioids and the organism, the environment, and behavior. Such research from a clinical standpoint has established new pharmacotherapies for opioid addiction (e.g., buprenorphine) and developed sound methodologies to test the abuse liability of newly developed opioid compounds. It is anticipated that continued research of the type described in this chapter will enable us to develop even more effective pharmacotherapies both for pain management and for opioid addiction.

ACKNOWLEDGMENTS

Preparation of this manuscript was supported by NIDA grants DA08573 (JPZ) and DA07947 (EAW).

References

Aigner, B., & Balster, R. L. (1979). Rapid substitution procedure for iv drug self-administration studies in rhesus monkeys. *Pharmacology, Biochemistry and Behavior, 10,* 105–112.

Almaric, M., Cline, E., Martinez, J., Jr., Bloom, F. E., & Koob, G. (1987). Rewarding properties of beta-endorphin as measured by conditioned place preference. *Psychopharmacology, 91,* 14–19.

Angle, H. V., Knowles, R. R., Marrazzi, A. S., & Sletten, I. W. (1973). Method for self-administering methadone by the heroin addict. *International Journal of the Addictions, 8,* 435–441.

Bals-Kubik, R., Herz, A., & Shippenberg, T. (1989). Evidence that the aversive effects of opioid antagonists and k-agonists are centrally mediated. *Psychopharmacology, 98,* 203–206.

Bals-Kubik, R., Shippenberg, T. S., & Herz, A. (1990a). Involvement of central mu and delta opioid receptors in mediating the reinforcing effects of beta-endorphin in the rat. *European Journal of Pharmacology, 175,* 63–69.

Bals-Kubik, R., Shippenberg, T. S., & Herz, A. (1990b). Neuroanatomical substrates mediating the motivational effects of opioids. In J. van Ree, A. Mulder, V. Wiegart, & T. van Wimersma-Geidarus (Eds.), *New Leads in Opioid Research. Proceedings of the International Narcotics Research Conference* (pp. 11–12). Amsterdam: Exerpta Medica.

Balster, R. L. (1989). Substitution and antagonism in rats trained to discriminate (+)-n-allylnormetazocine from saline. *Journal of Pharmacology and Experimental Therapeutics, 249,* 749–756.

Balster, R. L., & Lukas, S. E. (1985). Review of self-administration. *Drug and Alcohol Dependence, 14,* 249–261.

Bechara, S., & van der Kooy, D. (1987). Kappa receptors mediate the peripheral aversive effects of opiates. *Pharmacology, Biochemistry and Behavior, 28,* 227–233.

Bellville, J. W., & Green, J. (1965). The respiratory and subjective effects of pentazocine. *Clinical Pharmacology & Therapeutics, 6,* 152–159.

Bergman, J., & Carey, G. (1996). Antagonism of the discriminative stimulus effects of enadoline. In L. S. Harris (Ed.), *Problems of drug dependence 1996* (NIDA Research Monograph No. 174, p. 312). Washington, DC: U.S. Government Printing Office.

Berman, M. L., Briggs, G. G., Bogh, P., Mannel, R., Manetta, A., & DiSaia, P. J. (1990). Simplified postoperative patient-controlled analgesia on a gynecology-oncology service. *Gynecologic Oncology, 38,* 55–58.

Bertalmio, A. J., & Woods, J. H. (1987). Differentiation between mu and kappa receptor-mediated effects in opioid drug discrimination: Apparent pA₂ analysis. *Journal of Pharmacology and Experimental Therapeutics, 243,* 591–597.

Bertalmio, A. J., & Woods, J. H. (1989). Reinforcing effect of alfentanil is mediated by mu opioid receptors: Apparent pA₂ analysis. *Journal of Pharmacology and Experimental Therapeutics, 251,* 455–460.

Bertalmio, A. J., Herling, S., Hampton, R., Winger, G., & Woods, J. H. (1982). A procedure for rapid evaluation of the discriminative stimulus effects of drugs. *Journal of Pharmacological Methods, 7,* 289–299.

Bickel, W. K., Higgins, S. T., & Stitzer, M. L. (1986). Choice of blind methadone dose increases by methadone maintenance patients. *Drug and Alcohol Dependence, 18,* 165–171.

Bigelow, G. E., & Preston, K. L. (1995). Opioids. In F. E. Bloom & D. J. Kupfer (Eds.), *Psychopharmacology: The fourth generation of progress* (pp. 1731–1744). New York: Raven.

Boccuni, M., Cangi, F., Fusco, B. M., Curradi, C., & Sicuteri, F. (1987). Pentazocine in migraine: Subjective and pupillary abnormal effects. *Headache, 27,* 503–508.

Butelman, E. R., Winger, G., Zernig, G., & Woods, J. H. (1995). Butorphanol: Characterization of agonist and antagonist effects in rhesus monkey. *Journal of Pharmacology and Experimental Therapeutics, 272,* 845–853.

Carr, G., Fibiger, H., & Phillips, A. (1989). Conditioned place preference as a measure of drug reward. In J. Liebman & S. Cooper (Eds.), *The neuropharmacological basis of reward* (pp. 264–319). New York: Oxford University Press.

Carroll, M. E., & Meisch, R. A. (1978). Etonitazene as a reinforcer: Oral intake of etonitazene by rhesus monkeys. *Psychopharmacology, 59,* 225–229.

Chappell, P. B., Leckman, J. F., Scahill, L. D., Hardin, M. T., Anderson, G., & Cohen, D. J. (1993). Neuroendocrine and behavioral effects of the selective κ agonist spiradoline in Tourette's syndrome: A pilot study. *Psychiatry Research, 47,* 267–280.

Collins, R., Weeks, J., Cooper, M., Good, P., & Russell, R. (1984). Prediction of abuse liability of drugs using IV self-administration by rats. *Psychopharmacology, 82,* 6–13.

Colpaert, F. C. (1977). Drug-produced cues and states: Some theoretical and methodological inferences. In H. Lal (Ed.), *Discriminative stimulus properties of drugs* (pp. 5–21). New York: Amsterdam.

Colpaert, F. C., Niemegeers, C., & Janssen, P. A. (1980). Factors regulating drug cue sensitivity: The effect of training dose in fentanyl-saline discrimination. *Neuropharmacology, 19,* 705–713.

Colpaert, F. C., Meert, T., De Witte, P., & Schmitt, P. (1982). Further evidence validating adjuvant arthritis as an experimental model of chronic pain in the rat. *Life Sciences, 31,* 67–75.

Comer, S. D., McNutt, R., Chang, K., DeCosta, B. R., Mosberg, H., & Woods, J. H. (1993). Discriminative stimulus effects of BW373U86: A nonpeptide ligand with selectivity for delta opioid receptors. *Journal of Pharmacology and Experimental Therapeutics, 267,* 866–874.

Devine, D. P., & Wise, R. A. (1994). Self-administration of morphine, DAMGO, and DPDPE into the ventral tegmental area of the rat. *Journal of Neuroscience, 14,* 1978–1984.

Downs, D. A., & Woods, J. H. (1975). Fixed-ratio escape and avoidance-escape from naloxone in morphine-dependent monkeys: Effects of naloxone dose and morphine pretreatment. *Journal of Experimental Analysis of Behavior, 23,* 415–427.

Downs, D. A., & Woods, J. H. (1976). Naloxone as a negative reinforcer in rhesus monkeys: Effects of dose, schedule, and narcotic regimen. *Pharmacological Reviews, 27,* 397–406.

Dykstra, L. D., Gmerek, D. E., Winger, G., & Woods, J. H. (1987). Kappa opioids in rhesus monkeys: II. Analysis of the antagonistic actions of quadazocine and B-funaltrexamine. *Journal of Pharmacology and Experimental Therapeutics, 242,* 421–427.

Emmett-Olgesby, M., Shippenberg, T., & Herz, A. (1988). Tolerance and cross-tolerance to the discriminative stimulus properties of fentanyl and morphine. *Journal of Pharmacology and Experimental Therapeutics, 245,* 17–23.

France, C. P., & Woods, J. H. (1985). Opiate agonist–antagonist interactions: Application of a three-key drug discrimination procedure. *Journal of Pharmacology and Experimental Therapeutics, 234,* 81–89.

France, C. P., & Woods, J. H. (1987). β-Funaltrexamine antagonizes the discriminative stimulus effects of morphine but not naltrexone in pigeons. *Psychopharmacology, 91,* 213–216.

France, C. P., & Woods, J. H. (1990). Discriminative stimulus effects of opioid agonists in morphine-dependent pigeons. *Journal of Pharmacology and Experimental Therapeutics, 254,* 626–632.

France, C. P., de Costa, B. R., Jacobson, A. E., Rice, K. C., & Woods, J. H. (1990). Apparent affinity of opioid antagonists in morphine-treated rhesus monkeys discriminating between saline and naltrexone. *Journal of Pharmacology and Experimental Therapeutics, 252,* 600–604.

France, C. P., Medzihradsky, F., & Woods, J. H. (1994). Comparison of kappa opioids in rhesus monkeys: Behavioral effects and receptor binding affinities. *Journal of Pharmacology and Experimental Therapeutics, 268,* 47–58.

Fraser, H. F., & Rosenberg, D. E. (1964). Studies on the human addiction liability of 2′-hydroxy-5,9-dimethyl-2-(3,3-dimethylallyl)-6,7-benzomorphan (WIN 20,228): A weak narcotic antagonist. *Journal of Pharmacology and Experimental Therapeutics, 143,* 149–156.

Fraser, H. F., Martin, W. R., Wolbach, A. B., & Isbell, H. (1961). Addiction liability of an isoquinoline analgesic, 1-(p-chlorophenetyl)-2-methyl-6,7-dimethoxy-1,2,3,4-tetrahydrois oquinoline. *Clinical Pharmacology & Therapeutics, 2,* 287–299.

Fraser, H. F., van Horn, G. G., Martin, W. R., Wolbach, A. B., & Isbell, H. (1961). Methods for evaluating abuse liability. (A) "Attitude" of opiate addicts towards opiate-like drugs. (B) A short-term "direct" addiction test. *Journal of Pharmacology and Experimental Therapeutics, 133,* 371–387.

Gauvin, D., & Young, A. M. (1989). Effects of prior saline-morphine discrimination by pigeons on three-

way discrimination including two morphine doses. *Psychopharmacology, 98,* 222–230.

Gerak, L. R., & France, C. P. (1996). Discriminative stimulus effects of nalbuphine in rhesus monkeys. *Journal of Pharmacology and Experimental Therapeutics, 276,* 523–531.

Glick, S. D., Maisonneve, I. M., Raucci, J., & Archer, S. (1995). Kappa opioid inhibition of morphine and cocaine self-administration in rats. *Brain Research, 681,* 147–152.

Gorodetzky, C. W., & Martin, W. R. (1966). A comparison of fentanyl, droperidol, and morphine. *Clinical Pharmacology & Therapeutics, 6,* 731–739.

Graves, D. A., Arrigo, J. M., Foster, T. S., Baumann, T. J., & Batenhorst, R. L. (1985). Relationship between plasma morphine concentrations and pharmacologic effects in postoperative patients using patient-controlled analgesia. *Clinical Pharmacy, 4,* 41–47.

Greenwald, M. K., June, H. L., Stitzer, M. L., & Marco, A. P. (1996). Comparative pharmacology of short-acting mu opioids in drug abusers. *Journal of Pharmacology and Experimental Therapeutics, 277,* 1228–1236.

Haertzen, C. A. (1966). Development of scales based on patterns of drug effects, using the Addiction Research Center Inventory (ARCI). *Psychological Reports, 18,* 163–194.

Haertzen, C. A. (1970). Subjective effects of narcotic antagonists cyclazocine and nalorphine on the Addiction Research Center Inventory (ARCI). *Psychopharmacologia, 18,* 366–377.

Hamilton, R. C., Dundee, J. W., Clarke, S. J., Loan, W. B., & Morrison, J. D. (1967). Studies of drugs given before anaesthesia: XIII. Pentazocine and other opiate antagonists. *British Journal of Anaesthesia, 39,* 647–656.

Hein, D. W., Young, A. M., Herling, S., & Woods, J. H. (1981). Pharmacological analysis of the discriminative stimulus characteristics of ethylketazocine in the rhesus monkey. *Journal of Pharmacology and Experimental Therapeutics, 218,* 7–15.

Herling, S., Coale, E., Jr., Valentino, R. J., Hein, D. W., & Woods, J. H. (1980). Narcotic discrimination in pigeons. *Journal of Pharmacology and Experimental Therapeutics, 214,* 139–146.

Hoffman, D. (1989). The use of place conditioning in studying the neuropharmacology of drug reinforcement. *Brain Research Bulletin, 23,* 373–387.

Hoffmeister, F. (1979). Progressive-ratio performance in the rhesus monkey maintained by opiate infusions. *Psychopharmacology, 62,* 181–186.

Holtzman, S. G. (1982). Discriminative stimulus properties of opioids in the rat and squirrel monkey. In F. C. Colpaert & J. Slangen (Eds.), *Drug discrimination: Applications in CNS pharmacology* (pp. 17–36). Amsterdam: Elsevier Biomedical Press.

Holtzman, S. G. (1983). Discriminative stimulus properties of opioid agonists and antagonists. In S. Cooper

(Ed.), *Theory in psychopharmacology* (Vol. 2, pp. 1–45). London: Academic Press.

Holtzman, S. (1985). Discriminative stimulus effects of morphine withdrawal in the morphine-dependent rat: Suppression by opiate and nonopiate drugs. *Journal of Pharmacology and Experimental Therapeutics, 233,* 80–86.

Holtzman, S. G., & Locke, K. W. (1988). Neural mechanisms of drug stimuli: Experimental approaches. Transduction mechanisms of drug stimuli. In F. Colpaert & R. Balster (Eds.), *Psychopharmacology* (pp. 139–153). Berlin: Springer-Verlag.

Holtzman, S. G., & Steinfels, G. F. (1994). Antagonism of the discriminative stimulus effects of the kappa-opioid agonist spiradoline. *Psychopharmacology, 116,* 243–248.

Holtzman, S. G., Cook, L., & Steinfels, G. F. (1991). Discriminative stimulus effects of spiradoline, a kappa-opioid agonist. *Psychopharmacology, 105,* 447–452.

Jarbe, T. (1978). Discriminative effects of morphine in the pigeon. *Pharmacology, Biochemistry and Behavior, 9,* 411–416.

Jasinski, D. R., & Mansky, P. A. (1972). Evaluation of nalbuphine for abuse potential. *Clinical Pharmacology & Therapeutics, 13,* 78–90.

Jasinski, D. R., & Preston, K. L. (1985). Assessment of dezocine for morphine-like subjective effects and miosis. *Clinical Pharmacology & Therapeutics, 38,* 544–548.

Jasinski, D. R., & Preston, K. L. (1986). Evaluation of tilidine for morphine-like subjective effects and euphoria. *Drug and Alcohol Dependence, 18,* 273–292.

Jasinski, D. R., Martin, W. R., & Sapira, J. D. (1968). Antagonism of the subjective, behavioral, pupillary, and respiratory depressant effects of cyclazocine by naloxone. *Clinical Pharmacology & Therapeutics, 9,* 215–222.

Jasinski, D. R., Martin, W. R., & Haeldke, R. D. (1970). Effects of short- and long-term administration of pentazocine in man. *Clinical Pharmacology & Therapeutics, 11,* 385–403.

Jewett, D. C., Mosberg, H., & Woods, J. H. (1996). Discriminative stimulus effects of a centrally administered, delta-opioid peptide (D-Pen²-D-Pen⁵-enkephalin in pigeons. *Psychopharmacology, 127,* 225–229.

Jones, B. E., & Prada, J. A. (1975). Drug-seeking behavior during methadone maintenance. *Psychopharmacologia* (Berlin), *41,* 7–10.

Kitchen, I., & Kennedy, A. (1990). Effects of δ-opioid receptor antagonist naltrindole on opioid induced in vivo release of corticosterone. In J. van Ree, A. Mulder, V. Wiegant, & T. van Wimersma Griedanus (Eds.), *New leads in opioid research* (pp. 2321–2322). Amsterdam: Excerpta Medica.

Koek, W., & Woods, J. H. (1989). Partial generalization in pigeons trained to discriminate morphine from saline: Applications of receptor theory. *Drug Development Research, 16,* 169–181.

Koob, G. F. (1992). Neural mechanisms of drug reinforcement. *Annals of the New York Academy of Sciences, 654,* 171–191.

Kumor, K. M., Haertzen, C. A., Johnson, R. E., Kocher, T., & Jasinski, D. R. (1986). Human psychopharmacology of ketocyclazocine as compared with cyclazocine, morphine and placebo. *Journal of Pharmacology and Experimental Therapeutics, 238,* 960–968.

Kupers, R., & Gybels, J. (1995). The consumption of fentanyl is increased in rats with nociceptive but not with neuropathic pain. *Pain, 60,* 137–141.

Lamb, R. J., Preston, K. L., Schindler, C. W., Meisch, R. A., Davis, F., Katz, J. L., Henningfield, J. E., & Goldberg, S. R. (1991). The reinforcing and subjective effects of morphine in post-addicts: A dose–response study. *Journal of Pharmacology and Experimental Therapeutics, 259,* 1165–1173.

Lasagna, L., von Felsinger, J. M., & Beecher, H. K. (1955). Drug-induced mood changes in man. *Journal of the American Medical Association, 157,* 1006–1020.

Locke, K. W., & Holtzman, S. G. (1985). Characterization of the discriminative stimulus effects of centrally-administered morphine in the rat. *Psychopharmacology, 87,* 1–6.

Locke, K. W., & Holtzman, S. G. (1986). Behavioral effects of opioid peptides selective for mu or delta receptors: I. Morphine-like discriminative stimulus effects. *Journal of Pharmacology and Experimental Therapeutics, 238,* 900–906.

Lord, J. A. H., Waterfield, A. A., Hughes, J., & Kosterlitz, H. W. (1977). Endogenous opioid peptides: Multiple agonists and receptors. *Nature, 267,* 495–499.

Lukas, S. E., Griffiths, R. R., & Brady, J. V. (1983). Buprenorphine self-administration by the baboon: Comparison with other opioids. In L. S. Harris (Ed.), *Problems of drug dependence 1982* (NIDA Monograph Series No. 43, pp. 178–183). Washington, DC: U.S. Government Printing Office.

Lukas, S. E., Brady, J. V., & Griffiths, R. R. (1986). Comparison of opioid self-injection and disruption of schedule-controlled performance in the baboon. *Journal of Pharmacology and Experimental Therapeutics, 238,* 924–931.

Martin, T. J., Dworkin, S. I., & Smith, J. E. (1995). Alkylation of mu opioid receptors by β-funaltrexamine in vivo: Comparison of the effects on in situ binding and heroin self-administration in rats. *Journal of Pharmacology and Experimental Therapeutics, 272,* 1135–1140.

Martin, W. R., & Fraser, H. F. (1961). A comparative study of physiological and subjective effects of heroin and morphine administered intravenously in postaddicts. *Journal of Pharmacology and Experimental Therapeutics, 133,* 388–399.

Martin, W. R., Sloan, J. W., Sapira, J. D., & Jasinski, D. R. (1971). Physiologic, subjective, and behavioral effects of amphetamine, methamphetamine, ephedrine, phenmetrazine, and methylphenidate in man. *Clinical Pharmacology & Therapeutics, 12,* 245–258.

Martin, W. R., Eades, C. G., Thompson, J. A., Huppler, R. E., & Gilbert, P. E. (1976) The effects of morphine- and nalorphine-like drugs in the non-dependent and morphine-dependent chronic spinal dog. *Journal of Pharmacology and Experimental Therapeutics, 197,* 517–532.

Meisch, R. A. (1995). Oral self-administration of etonitazene in rhesus monkeys: Use of a fading procedure to establish etonitazene as a reinforcer. *Pharmacology, Biochemistry and Behavior, 50,* 571–580.

Mello, N. K., Bree, M., & Mendelson, J. (1981). Buprenorphine self-administration by rhesus monkeys. *Pharmacology, Biochemistry and Behavior, 15,* 215–225.

Mello, N. K., Mendelson, J. H., Kuehnle, J. C., & Sellers, M. S. (1981). Operant analysis of human heroin self-administration and the effects of naltrexone. *Journal of Pharmacology and Experimental Therapeutics, 216,* 45–54.

Mello, N. K., Mendelson, J. H., & Kuehnle, J. C. (1982). Buprenorphine effects on human heroin self-administration: an operant analysis. *Journal of Pharmacology and Experimental Therapeutics, 223,* 30–39.

Mello, N. K., Bree, M., & Mendelson, J. (1983). Comparison of buprenorphine and methadone effects on opiate self-administration. *Journal of Pharmacology and Experimental Therapeutics, 225,* 378–386.

Mello, N. K., Mendelson, J., Bree, M., & Lukas, S. E. (1989). Buprenorphine suppresses cocaine self-administration by rhesus monkeys. *Science, 245,* 859–862.

Mello, N. K., Lukas, S. E., Kamien, J. B., Mendelson, J. H., Drieze, J., & Cone, E. J. (1992). The effects of chronic buprenorphine treatment on cocaine and food self-administration by rhesus monkeys. *Journal of Pharmacology and Experimental Therapeutics, 260,* 1185–1193.

Miksic, L., & Lal, H. (1977). Tolerance to morphine-produced discriminative stimuli and analgesia. *Psychopharmacology, 54,* 217–211.

Mucha, R., & Herz, A. (1985). Motivational properties of kappa and mu opioid receptor agonists studied with place and taste preference conditioning. *Psychopharmacology, 86,* 274–280.

Negus, S. S., Burke, T. F., Medzihradsky, F., & Woods, J. H. (1993). Effects of opioid agonists selective for mu, kappa, and delta opioid receptors on schedule-controlled responding in rhesus monkeys: Antagonism by quadazocine. *Journal of Pharmacology and Experimental Therapeutics, 267,* 896–902.

Negus, S. S., Butelman, E. R., Chang, K., DeCosta, B., Winger, G., & Woods, J. H. (1994). Behavioral effects of the systemically active delta opioid agonist BW373U86 in rhesus monkeys. *Journal of Pharmacology and Experimental Therapeutics, 270,* 1025–1034.

Negus, S. S., Mello, N. K., Portoghese, P. S., Lukas, S. E., & Mendelson, J. H. (1995). Role of delta opioid receptors in the reinforcing and discriminative stimulus effects of cocaine in rhesus monkeys. *Journal of Pharmacology and Experimental Therapeutics, 273,* 1245–1256.

Pande, A. C., Pyke, R. E., Greiner, M., Wideman, G. L., Benjamin, R., & Pierce, M. W. (1996). Analgesic efficacy of enadoline versus placebo or morphine in postsurgical pain. *Clinical Neuropharmacology, 19,* 451–456.

Parker, R. K., Holtmann, B., & White, P. F. (1991). Patient-controlled analgesia: Does a concurrent opioid infusion improve pain management after surgery? *Journal of the American Medical Association, 266,* 1947–1952.

Paronis, C. A., & Holtzman, S. G. (1994). Sensitization and tolerance to the discriminative stimulus effects of mu-opioid agonists. *Psychopharmacology, 114,* 601–310.

Pfeiffer, A., Branti, V., Herz, A., & Emrich, H. M. (1986). Psychotomimesis mediated by opiate receptors. *Science, 233,* 774–776.

Pickens, R., Meisch, R. A., & Thompson, T. (1978). Drug self-administration: An analysis of the reinforcing effects of drugs. In L. L. Iversen, D. Iversen, & S. Snyder (Eds.), *Handbook of psychopharmacology* (pp. 1–7). New York: Plenum.

Picker, M. J. (1991). Discriminative stimulus properties of (+)- and (–)-n-allylnormetazocine: The role of training dose in the stimulus substitution patterns produced by PCP/sigma and mixed action opioid compounds. *Behavioural Pharmacology, 2,* 497–511.

Picker, M. J. (1994). Kappa agonist and antagonist properties of mixed action opioids in a pigeon drug discrimination procedure. *Journal of Pharmacology and Experimental Therapeutics, 268,* 1190–1198.

Picker, M. J. (1995). Assessment of the kappa agonist and antagonist properties of mixed action opioids, mu opioids, and a delta opioid in pigeons. *Experimental and Clinical Psychopharmacology, 3,* 240.

Picker, M. J., & Dykstra, L. A. (1987). Comparison of the discriminative stimulus properties of U50,488 and morphine in pigeons. *Journal of Pharmacology and Experimental Therapeutics, 243,* 938–945.

Picker, M. J., & Dykstra, L. A. (1989). Discriminative stimulus effects of mu and kappa opioids in the pigeon: Analysis of the effects of full and partial mu and kappa agonists. *Journal of Pharmacology and Experimental Therapeutics, 249,* 557–566.

Picker, M. J., Negus, S. S., & Dykstra, L. A. (1989). Opioid-like discriminative stimulus properties of benzomorphans in the pigeon: Stereospecificity and differential substitution patterns. *Life Sciences, 45,* 1637–1645.

Picker, M. J., Yarbrough, J., Hughes, C. E., Smith, M. A., Morgan, D., & Dykstra, L. A. (1993). Agonist and antagonist effects of mixed action opioids in the pigeon drug discrimination procedure: Influence of training dose, intrinsic efficacy and interanimal differences. *Journal of Pharmacology and Experimental Therapeutics, 266,* 756–767.

Picker, M. J., Benyas, S., Horwitz, J., Thompson, K., Mathewson, C., & Smith, M. A. (1996). Discriminative stimulus effects of butorphanol: Influence of training dose on the substitution patterns produced by mu, kappa, and delta opioids. *Journal of Pharmacology and Experimental Therapeutics, 279,* 1130–1141.

Preston, K. L., & Bigelow, G. E. (1993). Differential naltrexone antagonism of hydromorphine and pentazocine effects in human volunteers. *Journal of Pharmacology and Experimental Therapeutics, 264,* 813–823.

Preston, K. L., & Bigelow, G. E. (1994). Drug discrimination assessment of agonist–antagonist opioids in humans: a three-choice saline-hydromorphone-butorphanol procedure. *Journal of Pharmacology and Experimental Therapeutics, 271,* 48–60.

Preston, K. L., & Jasinski, D. R. (1991). Abuse liability studies of opioid agonist–antagonists in humans. *Drug and Alcohol Dependence, 28,* 49–82.

Preston, K. L., Bigelow, G. E., & Liebson, I. A. (1985). Self-administration of clonidine, oxazepam, and hydromorphone by patients undergoing methadone detoxification. *Clinical Pharmacology & Therapeutics, 38,* 219–227.

Preston, K. L., Bigelow, G. E., Bickel, W., & Liebson, I. A. (1987). Three-choice drug discrimination in opioid-dependent humans: Hydromorphone, naloxone and saline. *Journal of Pharmacology and Experimental Therapeutics, 243,* 1002–1009.

Preston, K. L., Bigelow, G. E., & Liebson, I. A. (1987). Comparative evaluation of morphine, pentazocine and ciramadol in postaddicts. *Journal of Pharmacology and Experimental Therapeutics, 240,* 900–910.

Preston, K. L., Bigelow, G. E., & Liebson, I. A. (1988). Butorphanol-precipitated withdrawal in opioid-dependent human volunteers. *Journal of Pharmacology and Experimental Therapeutics, 246,* 441–448.

Preston, K. L., Bigelow, G. E., Bickel, W. K., & Liebson, I. A. (1989). Drug discrimination in human postaddicts: Agonist–antagonist opioids. *Journal of Pharmacology and Experimental Therapeutics, 250,* 184–196.

Preston, K. L., Bigelow, G. E., & Liebson, I. A. (1989). Antagonist effects of nalbuphine in opioid-dependent human volunteers. *Journal of Pharmacology and Experimental Therapeutics, 248,* 929–937.

Preston, K. L., Bigelow, G. E., & Liebson, I. A. (1990). Discrimination of butorphanol and nalbuphine in opioid-dependent humans. *Pharmacology, Biochemistry and Behavior, 37,* 511–522.

Preston, K. L., Liebson, I. A., & Bigelow, G. E. (1992). Discrimination of agonist–antagonist opioids in humans trained on a two-choice saline-hydromorphone discrimination. *Journal of Pharmacology and Experimental Therapeutics, 261,* 62–71.

Schaefer, G. J., & Holtzman, S. G. (1977). Discriminative effects of morphine in the squirrel monkey. *Journal of Pharmacology and Experimental Therapeutics, 201,* 67–75.

Schechter, N. L., Berrien, F. B., & Katz, S. M. (1988). The use of patient-controlled analgesia in adolescents with sickle cell crisis pain: A preliminary report. *Journal of Pain and Symptom Management, 2,* 109–113.

Schuster, C. R. (1976). Drugs as reinforcers in monkey and man. *Pharmacological Reviews, 27,* 511–521.

Schuster, C. R., Smith, B. B., & Jaffe, J. H. (1971). Drug abuse in heroin users: An experimental study of self-administration of methadone, codeine, and pentazocine. *Archives of General Psychiatry, 24,* 359–362.

Shannon, H., & Holtzman, S. G. (1979). Morphine training dose: A determinant of stimulus generalization to narcotic antagonists in the rat. *Psychopharmacology, 61,* 239–244.

Shannon, H. E. (1983). Pharmacological evaluation of n-allylnormetazocine (SKF 10,047) on the basis of its discriminative stimulus properties in the rat. *Journal of Pharmacology and Experimental Therapeutics, 225,* 144–152.

Shannon, H. E., & Holtzman, S. G. (1976). Evaluation of the discriminative stimulus effects of morphine in the rat. *Journal of Pharmacology and Experimental Therapeutics, 198,* 54–65.

Shearman, G., & Herz, A. (1981). Discriminative stimulus properties of bremazocine in the rat. *Neuropharmacology, 20,* 1209–1213.

Shearman, G., & Herz, A. (1982). Evidence that the discriminative stimulus properties of fentanyl and ethylketocyclazocine are mediated by an interaction with different opiate receptors. *Journal of Pharmacology and Experimental Therapeutics, 221,* 735–739.

Shippenberg, T. S., & Bals-Kubik, R. (1991). Motivational aspects of opioids: Neurochemical and neuroanatomical substrates. In O. Almedia & T. S. Shippenberg (Eds.), *The neurobiology of opioids* (pp. 331–350). New York: Springer-Verlag.

Shippenberg, T. S., Bals-Kubik, R., & Herz, A. (1987). Motivational properties of opioids: Evidence that an activation of delta-receptors mediates reinforcement processes. *Brain Research, 436,* 234–239.

Slifer, B., & Balster, R. L. (1983). Reinforcing properties of stereoisomers of the putative sigma agonists N-allylnormetazocine and cyclazocine in rhesus monkeys. *Journal of Pharmacology and Experimental Therapeutics, 225,* 522–528.

Spiga, R., Grabowski, J., Silverman, P. B., & Meisch, R. A. (1996). Human methadone self-administration: Effects of dose and ratio requirement. *Behavioural Pharmacology, 7,* 130–137.

Stitzer, M., Bigelow, G., & Liebson, I. (1979). Supplementary methadone self administration among methadone maintenance clients. *Addictive Behaviors, 4,* 61–66.

Stitzer, M. L., McCaul, M. E., Bigelow, G. E., & Liebson, I. A. (1983). Oral methadone self-administration: Effects of dose and alternative reinforcers. *Clinical Pharmacology & Therapeutics, 34,* 29–35.

Strain, E. C., Preston, K. L., Liebson, I. A., & Bigelow, G. E. (1992). Acute effects of buprenorphine, hydromorphone and naloxone in methadone-maintained volunteers. *Journal of Pharmacology and Experimental Therapeutics, 261,* 985–993.

Strain, E. C., Preston, K. L., Liebson, I. A., & Bigelow, G. E. (1993). Precipitated withdrawal by pentazocine in methadone-maintained volunteers. *Journal of Pharmacology and Experimental Therapeutics, 267,* 624–634.

Strain, E. C., Preston, K. L., Liebson, I. A., & Bigelow, G. E. (1995). Buprenorphine effects in methadone-maintained volunteers: Effects at two hours after methadone. *Journal of Pharmacology and Experimental Therapeutics, 272,* 628–638.

Tang, A., & Collins, R. (1985). Behavioral effects of a novel kappa opioid analgesic, U-50,488, in rats and rhesus monkeys. *Psychopharmacology, 85,* 309–314.

Tang, A. H., & Code, R. A. (1983). Discriminative stimulus properties of nalorphine in the rhesus monkeys. *Journal of Pharmacology and Experimental Therapeutics, 227,* 563–569.

Teal, J. J., & Holtzman, S. G. (1980a). Discriminative stimulus effects of cyclazocine in the rat. *Journal of Pharmacology and Experimental Therapeutics, 212,* 368–376.

Teal, J. J., & Holtzman, S. G. (1980b). Stereoselectivity of the stimulus effects of morphine and cyclazocine in squirrel monkeys. *Journal of Pharmacology and Experimental Therapeutics, 215,* 369–376.

Thompson, T., & Schuster, C. R. (1964). Morphine self-administration, food-reinforced, and avoidance behaviors in rhesus monkeys. *Psychopharmacologia, 5,* 87–94.

Ukai, M., & Holtzman, S. G. (1988). Morphine-like discriminative stimulus effects of opioid peptides: Possible modulatory role of D-Ala^2-D-Leu^5-enkephalin (DADL) and dynorphin A(1-13). *Psychopharmacology, 94,* 32–37.

Vanecek, S., & Young, A. (1995). Pharmacological characterization of an operant discrimination among two doses of morphine and saline in pigeons. *Behavioural Pharmacology, 6,* 669–681.

Villarreal, J. E. (1973). The effects of morphine agonists and antagonists on morphine-dependent rhesus monkeys. In H. Kosterlitz, H. Collier, & J. Villarreal (Eds.), *Agonist and antagonist actions of analgesic drugs* (pp. 73–83). Baltimore: University Park Press.

Walker, E. A., & Young, A. M. (1993). Discriminative-stimulus effects of the low efficacy mu agonist nalbuphine. *Journal of Pharmacology and Experimental Therapeutics, 267,* 322–330.

Walker, E. A., Makhay, M. M., House, J. D., & Young, A. M. (1994). In vivo apparent pA$_2$ analysis for naltrexone antagonism of discriminative stimulus and analgesic effects of opiate agonists in rats. *Journal of Pharmacology and Experimental Therapeutics, 271,* 959–968.

Walsh, S. L., June, H. L., Schuh, K. J., Preston, K. L., Bigelow, G. E., & Stitzer, M. L. (1995). Effects of buprenorphine and methadone in methadone-maintained subjects. *Psychopharmacology, 119,* 268–276.

Walsh, S. L., Preston, K. L., Bigelow, G. E., & Stitzer, M. L. (1995). Acute administration of buprenorphine in humans: Partial agonist and blockade effects. *Journal of Pharmacology and Experimental Therapeutics, 274,* 361–372.

White, G. H., & Holtzman, S. G. (1982). Properties of pentazocine as a discriminative stimulus in the squirrel monkey. *Journal of Pharmacology and Experimental Therapeutics, 223,* 396–401.

White, J., & Holtzman, S. G. (1981). Three-choice drug discrimination in the rat: Morphine, cyclazocine and saline. *Journal of Pharmacology and Experimental Therapeutics, 217,* 254–262.

White, J. M., & Holtzman, S. (1983). Three-choice drug discrimination: Phencyclidine-like stimulus effects of opioids. *Psychopharmacology, 80,* 1–9.

Winger, G., & Woods, J. H. (1996). Effects of buprenorphine on behavior maintained by heroin and alfentanil in rhesus monkeys. *Behavioural Pharmacology, 7,* 155–159.

Winger, G., Skjoldager, P., & Woods, J. H. (1992). Effects of buprenorphine and other opioid agonists and antagonists on alfentanil- and cocaine-reinforced responding in rhesus monkeys. *Journal of Pharmacology and Experimental Therapeutics, 261,* 311–317.

Winger, G., Woods, J. H., & Hursh, S. R. (1996). Behavior maintained by alfentanil or nalbuphine in rhesus monkeys: Fixed-ratio and time-out changes to establish demand curves and relative reinforcing effectiveness. *Experimental and Clinical Psychopharmacology, 4,* 131–140.

Woods, J. H. (1977). Narcotic-reinforced responding: A rapid screening procedure. In *Proceedings of the 39th meeting of the Committee on Problems of Drug Dependence* (pp. 420–437). Cambridge, MA: National Academy of Sciences.

Woods, J. H., & Winger, G. (1987). Behavioral characterization of opioid mixed agonist–antagonists. *Drug and Alcohol Dependence, 20,* 303–315.

Woods, J. H., Young, A. M., & Herling, S. (1982). Classification of narcotics on the basis of their reinforcing, discriminative, and antagonist effects in rhesus monkeys. *Federation Proceedings, 41,* 221–227.

Woods, J. H., France, C. P., & Winger, G. D. (1992). *Behavioral pharmacology of buprenorphine: Issues relevant to its potential in treating drug abuse* (NIDA Research Monograph Series No. 121, pp. 12–27). Rockville, MD: National Institute on Drug Abuse.

Yanagita, T., Katoh, S., Wakasa, Y., & Oinuma, N. (1982). Drug dependence liability of pentazocine evaluated in the rhesus monkey. *Central Institute Experimental Animal Preclinical Report, 1,* 51–57.

Young, A. M. (1991). Discriminative stimulus profiles of psychoactive drugs. In N. K. Mello (Ed.), *Ad-*

vances in substance abuse, behavioral and biological research (Vol. 4, pp. 139–203N). London: Kingsley.

Young, A. M., & Stephens, K. (1984). Antagonism of the discriminative stimulus effects of ethylketazocine, cyclazocine, and nalorphine in macaques. Psychopharmacology, 84, 356–361.

Young, A. M., Swain, H. H., & Woods, J. H. (1981). Comparison of opioid agonists in maintaining responding and in suppressing morphine withdrawal in rhesus monkeys. Psychopharmacology, 74, 329–335.

Young, A. M., Stephens, K. R., Hein, D. W., & Woods, J. H. (1984). Reinforcing and discriminative stimulus properties of mixed agonists–antagonist opioids. Journal of Pharmacology and Experimental Therapeutics, 229, 118–126.

Young, A. M., Kapitsopoulos, G., & Makhay, M. (1991). Tolerance to morphine-like stimulus effects of mu opioid agonists. Journal of Pharmacology and Experimental Therapeutics, 257, 795–805.

Young, A. M., Masaki, M. A., & Geula, C. (1992). Discriminative stimulus effects of morphine: Effects of training dose on agonist and antagonist effects of mu opioids. Journal of Pharmacology and Experimental Therapeutics, 261, 246–257.

Zacny, J. P., Lichtor, J. L., & de Wit, H. (1992). Subjective, behavioral, and physiologic responses to intravenous dezocine in healthy volunteers. Anesthesia and Analgesia, 74, 523–530.

Zacny, J. P., Lichtor, J. L., Zaragoza, J. G., & de Wit, H. (1992). Subjective and behavioral responses to intravenous fentanyl in healthy volunteers. Psychopharmacology, 107, 319–326.

Zacny, J. P., Lichtor, J. L., Binstock, W., Coalson, D. W., Cutter, T., Flemming, D. C., & Glosten, B. (1993). Subjective, behavioral and physiological responses to intravenous meperidine in healthy volunteers. Psychopharmacology, 111, 306–314.

Zacny, J. P., Lichtor, J. L., Flemming, D., Coalson, D. W., & Thompson, W. K. (1994). A dose–response analysis of the subjective, psychomotor, and physiological effects of intravenous morphine in healthy volunteers. Journal of Pharmacology and Experimental Therapeutics, 268, 1–9.

Zacny, J. P., Lichtor, J. L., Thapar, P., Coalson, D. W., Flemming, D., & Thompson, W. K. (1994). Comparing the subjective, psychomotor, and physiological effects of intravenous butorphanol and morphine in healthy volunteers. Journal of Pharmacology and Experimental Therapeutics, 270, 579–588.

Zacny, J. P., McKay, M. A., Toledano, A. Y., Marks, S., Young, C. J., Klock, P. A., & Apfelbaum, J. L. (1996). The effects of a cold-water immersion stressor on the reinforcing and subjective effects of an opioid in healthy volunteers. Drug and Alcohol Dependence, 42, 133–142.

Appendix

Review Articles on the Behavioral Pharmacology of Opioids

Bigelow, G. E., & Preston, K. L. (1995). Opioids. In F. E. Bloom, & D. J. Kupfer (Eds.), Psychopharmacology: The fourth generation of progress (pp. 1731–1744). New York: Raven.

Childress, A. R., Hole, A. V., Ehrman, R. N., Robbins, S. J., McLellan, A. T., & O'Brien, C .P. (1993). Cue reactivity and cue reactivity interventions in drug dependence (NIDA Research Monograph Series No. 137, pp. 73–95). Washington, DC: U.S. Government Printing Office.

de Zwaan, M., & Mitchell, J. E. (1992). Opiate antagonists and eating behavior in humans: A review. Journal of Clinical Pharmacology, 32, 1060–1072.

Di Chiara, G., & North, R. A. (1992). Neurobiology of opiate abuse. Trends in the Pharmacological Sciences, 13, 185–193.

Dykstra, L. A. (1996). Opioid analgesics. In C. R. Schuster & M. J. Kuhar (Eds.), Pharmacological aspects of drug dependence (pp. 197–232). Berlin: Springer.

Morley, J. E., Levine, A. S., Yim, G. K., & Lowy, M. T. (1983) Opioid modulation of appetite. Neuroscience & Biobehavioral Reviews, 7, 281–305.

Olson, G. A., Olson, R. D., & Kastin, A. J. (1995). Endogenous opioids: 1994. Peptides, 16, 1517–1555. [Note: this is one of a series of articles that date back to 1979 that summarize research from a given year or years on a number of opioid effects on behavior.]

Pfaus, J. G., & Gorzalka, B. B. (1987). Opioids and sexual behavior. Neuroscience & Biobehavioral Reviews, 11, 1–34.

Preston, K. L., & Jasinski, D. R. (1991). Abuse liability studies of opioid agonist–antagonists in humans. Drug and Alcohol Dependence, 28, 49–82.

Schaefer, G. J. (1992). Opiate antagonists and rewarding brain stimulation. Neuroscience & Biobehavioral Reviews, 12, 1–17.

Spanagel, R. (1995). Modulation of drug-induced sensitization processes by endogenous opioid systems. Behavioural Brain Research, 70, 37–49.

Stewart, J., de Wit, H., & Eikelboom, R. (1984). Role of unconditioned and conditioned drug effects in the self-administration of opiates and stimulants. Psychological Review, 91, 251–268.

Young, A. M., & Sannerud, C. A. (1989). Tolerance to drug discriminative stimuli. In A. Goudie & M. Emmett-Oglesby (Eds.), Psychoactive drugs (pp. 221–278). Clifton, NJ: Humana.

Zacny, J. P. (1995). A review of the effects of opiates on psychomotor and cognitive functioning in humans. Experimental and Clinical Psychopharmacology, 3, 432–466.

24

Psychological and Psychiatric Consequences of Opiates

MARK S. GOLD AND CHRISTOPHER R. JOHNSON

History

The powerful effects of opiates have been well known from the dawn of human existence. The poppy art of Assyria from 4000 B.C. to the increasing popularity of heroin in present times illustrates the tenacious hold opiates have on our lives. *Opium,* the Latin derivation of the Greek *opos,* meaning juice, has long been associated with sleep. Opiates are the natural alkaloids of the opium poppy (*Papaver somniferum*). They include such substances as codeine and morphine. Narcotics are a broader group of opiate-like drugs which include synthesized substances like methadone, fentanyl, heroin, and meperidine. However, "narcotics" is often loosely used in common parlance to refer to any illicit drug.

The bulk of human experience with opiates lay mainly in eating or smoking raw opium. The era of patent medicines (late 19th and early 20th centuries) brought us new concoctions such as "laudanum," a mixture of opium and alcohol. Such medicines were widely available and unregulated before the Pure Food

and Drug and the Harrison Narcotic Control Acts were passed by the U.S. Congress early in the 20th century. Compared with other medical treatments at the time (bloodletting, high doses of laxatives, calomel, and radium water), "[t]he sweet effect of opium in fevers, inflammatory disease, delirium tremens, insanity, depression, convulsions, poisoning, hemorrhages, and venereal disease must thus have appeared in many cases superior to [these alternatives]" (Musto, 1987, p. 198). These tonics were popularized and are frequently associated with noted individuals such as Elizabeth Barrett Browning, Samuel Taylor Coleridge, and Thomas DeQuincey. DeQuincey, who describes his experience with opium in *Confessions of an English Opium Eater,* was an avid supporter of opium use and at one time used more than 20 grams of opium per day (Karch, 1989).

Three momentous events during late 19th century brought new dimensions to our experience of opiates: (1) the invention of the hypodermic syringe, (2) isolation of specific alkaloids from raw opium, and (3) the synthesis of heroin from morphine. These events brought us the ability to isolate pure alkaloids, synthesize more potent drugs from them, and directly administer these drugs into the circulation, bypassing both digestion and "first-pass" metabolism. The ability to rapidly deliver a large amount of potent opiate drug to

MARK S. GOLD • University of Florida Brain Institute, Gainesville, Florida 32610. CHRISTOPHER R. JOHNSON • Department of Psychiatry, Baylor University, Houston, Texas 77030.

Handbook of Substance Abuse: Neurobehavioral Pharmacology, edited by Tarter *et al.* Plenum Press, New York, 1998.

the brain by injection greatly increases addiction liability.

Even though regular opiate use leaves the user anxious, dysphoric, and at risk for the so-called pains of withdrawal, the powerful reinforcing effects of opiates in spite of the many risks of use encourage continued self-administration (Gold, 1995). Public health concerns began to mount as the numbers of persons addicted to opiates rose in the late 19th century. Our recent experience with crack cocaine parallels the American experience with opiates 100 years ago. Today, we have seen a time of toleration of cocaine use during the 1970s and early 1980s when cocaine users were mainly young professionals using the drug "recreationally" or to "enhance performance." The invention of crack cocaine brought our association of the drug to poor, inner-city African Americans. When this occurred, public opinion of cocaine came to view cocaine as a public anathema. Opiate use similarly grew rapidly in the United States during a time of drug toleration.

Pharmacology

Use in Medicine

The use of opiates as a therapeutic agent is as old as the drug itself. Opiates have probably always been used for their analgesic and anesthetic qualities. Laudanum was an invention of Paracelsus in the early 16th century; he knew that sleep and analgesia are part of curing disease. Freud was initially a popular supporter of opium as a near-panacea; he later advocated cocaine (see Karch, 1989). The most important property of opium and its alkaloids is their unparalleled ability to relieve pain. They have contributed significantly to the progress of modern medicine by allowing patients to tolerate otherwise painful procedures and to live with previously crippling illnesses. They also have been and still are used as antitussive, antidiarrheal and antiemetic agents. Modern research in molecular biology has elucidated the important role that opioids play in homeostasis. Discovery of opioid receptor antagonists allows us to study the role that opioids

play in regulation of rewarding activities including eating, drinking, and copulation. In addition, the expanding list of opioid receptor subtypes has increased our understanding of the role that opioids have in the mechanisms of drug reinforcement. Opioids are postulated to modulate reward in continued self-administration of cocaine, marijuana, nicotine, alcohol, PCP, and other drugs.

Mechanism of Action

Opiates bind to specific sites in the brain and body that cause the numerous and seemingly diverse effects (Hughes, 1975; Pert & Snyder, 1973; Simon, Hiller, & Edelman, 1973). The effects of opiates on diarrhea, cough, mood, and pain can now be explained as a result of binding to specific sites in central and peripheral locations known to involve control of these events (Watson, Akil, Khachaturian, Young, & Lewis, 1984). Identification of these receptors led to the discovery of naturally occurring endogenous substances that possess opiate activity (Childers, 1991; Cox, Goldstein, & Li, 1976; Mains, Eipper, & Ling, 1977). The first substances discovered were called endorphins, a contraction of "endogenous morphine." Discovery of endorphins led many to question why every vertebrate and some invertebrates possess opioid receptors, whether endorphins are neurotransmitters or hormones (Mains *et al.*, 1977), and why authentic morphine and codeine have been found in the mammalian nervous systems (Donnerer, Oka, Brossi, Rice, & Spector, 1986).

Opioid drugs exert their actions by binding to receptors on cell membranes of neurons and other cells (Koob & Bloom, 1988). These opiate receptors are diverse in type and function. They have been divided into mu, kappa, delta, and lambda subtypes. These receptors are thought to be a part of the G-protein receptor super-family. These receptors, when activated, stimulate GTPase activity and are naloxone sensitive. Both GTP and sodium have been demonstrated to decrease agonist but not antagonist binding. The agonists inhibit adenylyl cyclase; a GTP-dependent and pertussis-toxin-sensitive effect. A summary of the purported

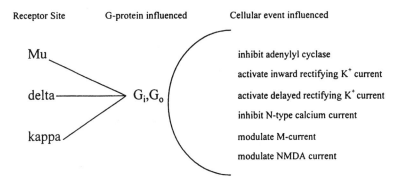

FIGURE 1. Opioid receptor mediated G-protein dependent effects on second messenger systems. Precise effect depends on cell type. From "Neuropharmacology of Endogenous Opioid Peptides," by J. J. Wagner and C. I. Charkin, in *Psychopharmacology: The Fourth Generation of Progress* (pp. 519–529), edited by F. E. Bloom and D. J. Kupfer, 1995, New York: Raven. Copyright 1995 by Raven Press. Adapted with permission.

molecular effects of opiate agonist binding to these receptors is listed in Figure 1.

In summary, all opiate drugs stimulate opiate receptors which are apparently coupled to molecular effector systems involving the so-called G-proteins. Opiate inhibition of adenylate cyclase results in changes in structure and function of intracellular proteins which may form the basis for neuroadaptation to opiates. Many effects on the neurons appear to result in changes in gene expression which cause gradual but persistent shift in cell function. Long-term and even permanent changes may be mediated by opiates through these shifts (Nestler, 1992).

A number of important differences among these opiate receptor subtypes have been identified. Kappa receptors are found in the dorsal horn and deep cortical areas. Activation of these kappa receptors by agonists such as ketocyclazocine produce analgesia, miosis, and sedation. Unlike mu and delta agonists, kappa agonists are not self-administered by laboratory animals. Consistent with this self-administration data, it now appears that the kappa agonists are dysphoric rather than euphoric. Mu agonists such as morphine or heroin are generally administered by injection or smoking. The opiate intoxication state is described as an intense, almost "orgasmic" sense of well-being referred to as a "high" or "rush." This euphoric state appears re-sponsible for the continuation of self-administration and the inability to think logically, to appreciate the imminent risk of drug-taking, or to deter it. Whether the dose of mu agonist also causes nausea and vomiting is not related to the user's feeling of well-being and interest in repeating the experience. Mu agonists inhibit the activity of the locus coeruleus (LC) which appears essential in the development of the most pronounced features of the abstinence syndrome. Mu opioids also suppress cough, slow the passage of food through the gastrointestinal system, inhibit diarrhea, decrease urinary voiding, decrease respiration, decrease pulse and blood pressure, decrease anxiety, and create an overwhelming sense of indifference to physical or psychic "pain" that is taken by addicts for the sense of euphoria or "high." These effects can be blocked by pretreatment with opiate antagonists and withdrawal provoked in tolerant humans by antagonists as well.

Twenty or so drugs are known to have opioid activity (see Table 1). These drugs are defined and categorized in terms of their binding profile or activity at each receptor as agonists, antagonists, and partial antagonist–agonists. The opiate antagonist naloxone reverses electrical brain stimulation analgesia, acupuncture (Pomeranz & Chiu, 1976) and electroacupuncture analgesia (Akil, Mayer, & Liebeskind, 1976), and even placebo-induced analgesia

TABLE 1. Opiate Agonists, Antagonists, and Mixed Antagonists

Agonists	Morphine
	Methadone
	Meperidine (Demerol)
	Oxycodone (Percodan)
	Propoxyphene (Darvon)
	Heroin
	Hydromorphone (Dilaudid)
	Fentanyl (Sublimaze)
	Codeine
Antagonists	Naloxone (Narcan)
	Naltrexone (Trexan)
Mixed antagonists	Pentazocine (Talwin)
	Nalbuphine (Nubain)
	Buprenorphine (Buprenex)
	Butorphanol (Stadol)

(Levine, Gordon, & Fields, 1978). These and other studies have led to the widespread belief that all of the three major receptor types for the naturally occurring opioid peptides are involved in analgesia but that the mu receptor is most closely related to the actions of morphine; the dissociation of physical dependence and abstinence from analgesic effect is a major pharmaceutical goal of this work.

Since tolerance and physical dependence could be demonstrated to pharmacological administration of opioid peptides (Wei & Loh, 1976), with cross-tolerance between synthetic and natural opiates, it was a natural extension to believe that many of the symptoms of opiate withdrawal could be understood by analysis of the interactions between the mu opioid system and other important neurotransmitter systems such as the noradrenergiclocus coeruleus.

The neural substrates underlying behavioral sensitization to cocaine and other drugs involve the mesolimbic dopamine system which arises from the ventral tegmental area to the ventral tegmentum. With repeated cocaine administration mesolimbic dopamine (DA) neurotransmission changes with increased DA firing rate and increases in DA release with subsequent cocaine challenges. Kappa opioid agonists inhibit the firing rate of mesolimbic DA neurons and decrease DA release within the ventral striatum possibly through a tonically active kappa opioid system located within the stria-

tum regulating DA release. Increases in kappa opioid receptor number and tissue levels of the endogenous ligand for kappa system dynorphin are reported to occur with repeated cocaine administration. Compensatory increases in the activity of the kappa opioid system produced by drug self-administration may in turn increase DA levels and lead to sensitization and consequent tendency to repeat administration of rewarding drugs. Thus, opioid systems may play a critical role in all compulsive drug use and relapse on the basis of a progressive and extremely persistent hypersensitivity. This neural sensitization increases the ability of a drug to elicit a marked effect and to capture and monopolize an organism's attention. Once induced, neural sensitization is extremely persistent, lasting for up to a year in some studies. Finally, this links opioid systems to the development of sensitization controlled by associative learning or Pavlovian conditioning so that stimuli associated with the drug can then stimulate or enhance the drug state. It is important to note that the opioid antagonist naltrexone has been approved for use in the treatment of opioid dependence and alcohol dependence and has been recently tried in nicotine dependence. Opioidergic neurons inhibit the activity of hypothalamic LHRH neurons and decrease the secretion of LH. Nicotine causes increased release of endogenous opioids in various brain regions increasing B-endorphin from the pituitary and decreases LH secretion. Both are attenuated by naltrexone.

Typically the effects of the opiate analgesics are morphine-like and attributed to the stimulation of mu opioid receptors. Mixed agonists, kappa agonists, antagonists, and now meperidine are understood to have additional important pharmacological effects and receptor interactions. Differences between the pharmacology of meperidine and other mu opioid agonists have been suspected and documented. Chronic exposure to meperidine produces stimulant effects, including tremor and convulsions, hyperreflexia, and increased startle. These effects do not occur with morphine. Haloperidol is a meperidine with some analgesic activity of its own in addition to dopamine antagonism. Meperidine intoxication itself shares certain features with cocaine intoxication. Equivalent morphine and meperidine miosis-producing and "liking" doses has allowed researchers to observe striking differences with meperidine producing hyper drive for the drug, nervousness, and "drunkenness." Many of the effects of meperidine are not reversible by opiate antagonists. High doses of meperidine and morphine produce seizures antagonized by naloxone but meperidine reversal is minimal. Some studies had suggested that the nonopioid effects of meperidine might be due to inhibition of serotonin uptake but now research has demonstrated that these effects are due to cocaine-like effects of meperidine at the dopamine transporter (Izenwasser, Newman, Cox, & Katz, 1996).

Feedback inhibition is a well-described and commonplace feature of neurotransmitter system regulation. Stimulation of presynaptic autoreceptors by excessive release of dopamine by cocaine led to the dopamine hypothesis's predictions of decreased release and biosynthesis for dopamine (Dackis & Gold, 1985). Similar hypotheses have been presented for opiates. In this model opiate self-administration would through feedback inhibition decrease the release and biosynthesis of endogenous opioids (Gold, Pottash, Extein, & Kleber, 1980; Goldstein, 1975). This hypothesized decrease could contribute to the development of tolerance, dependence, and withdrawal. Until recently this hypothesis was without consistent support (Trujillo, Bronstein, & Akil, 1993). Trujillo and colleagues have recently demonstrated that chronic infusion or repeated injection of morphine increases prodynorphin peptides. Since opiates appear to regulate both prodynorphin and proopiopiomelancortin (POMC), changes in these systems are more likely to be important in chronic opiate self-administration than are changes in other systems (Trujillo, Bronstein, Sanchez, & Akil, 1995).

Epidemiology

The opioids include natural opioids (e.g., morphine), semisynthetics (e.g., heroin), and synthetics with morphine-like action (e.g., codeine, hydromorphone, methadone, oxycodone, meperidine, fentanyl). Medications such as pentazocine and buprenorphine that have both opiate agonist and antagonist effects are also included in this class because their agonist properties produce similar physiological and behavioral effects. Opioids are prescribed as analgesics, anesthetics, antidiarrheal agents, or cough suppressants. Heroin is one of the most commonly abused drugs of this class and is usually taken by injection, although it can be smoked or "snorted" when very pure heroin is available. Fentanyl is injected, whereas cough suppressants and antidiarrheal agents are taken orally (*DSM-IV;* American Psychiatric Association, 1994).

The 1993 National Household Survey on Drug Abuse reported a lifetime prevalence of 1.1% for use of heroin among the 26,489 persons surveyed. This survey estimated that there were 2.3 million persons in 1993 who had used heroin in their lifetime. Reports of heroin use were higher among those who did not graduate from high school and in the West and the South. The results of this study indicate that up to that time heroin use had not increased significantly, but the Drug Abuse Warning Network (DAWN) reported increased heroin-related emergency department visits, from 48,000 in 1992 to 63,200 in 1993. Between 1988 and 1992, the most recent years available for analysis, the numbers of heroin sniffers requiring treatment at an emergency room increased by 470%. Heroin injection increases were also reported to increase by 31%. Heroin-related visits to an emergency room had been increasing: 38,100 in 1988, 48,000 in 1992, and 63,000 in 1993. Most recently, there has been a resurgence in smoking and sniffing heroin and opium as use becomes more widespread and new users try to avoid the risks of intravenous use.

Heroin addiction is a disease with considerable associated morbidity and mortality. Even when treated, this disease is not associated with longevity. In a recent study, of all heroin addicts registered for methadone treatment, 1,019 patients in 1969–1971 were subjects of follow-up. The authors located 776, dead or alive. At least one third of the original group had died during the 22-year period; standard mortality ratios were 4.0 for males and 6.8 for females. Drug overdose, violence, alcohol, or suicide accounted for nearly all deaths. Despite availability of treatment criminality and heroin use continued. Of the survivors, 48% were currently enrolled in a methadone program; they were using less heroin, alcohol, and other drugs. Heroin addiction is a chronic, lifelong, relapsing disease with a high fatality rate (Goldstein & Herrera, 1995). A number of experts and clinicians throughout the United States have reported increases in heroin and opium sniffing and smoking.

The UM/NIDA Monitoring the Future Study reported a statistically significant increasing trend of heroin use, especially among younger persons in the eighth grade, from 1.4% to 2.0% between 1993 and 1994 ($p < 0.001$). The study also reports a trend of increasing heroin use among 10th- and 12th-grade students as well. This trend is also reflected among other opiates. The study reports that the noncontinuation rate for heroin is 50% and that for other opiates is 42% suggesting that these drugs have considerable ability to cause dependence and addiction.

While the overall use of heroin and other opiates is relatively low, history has taught that depressant drugs such as heroin often make a "comeback" following a period of stimulant use (e.g. crack, Ecstasy). The increasing trend of heroin abuse despite the low overall rate is particularly troubling when considered in conjunction with the risk of becoming infected with HIV or hepatitis B. Intravenous drug use remains the second most common route of acquiring HIV and 35.3% of all AIDS cases are attributable to intravenous drug use. Opiates continue to represent an increasingly disproportionate percentage of drug-related deaths, from 45.8% of the 5,628 deaths reported by the DAWN in 1990 to 57.7% of the 7,485 deaths reported in 1993.

Diagnosis of Opioid Addiction

The diagnosis of opioid addiction is made by using criteria similar to those employed for the diagnosis of other drug addictions. The criteria include a preoccupation with the acquisition of the opioid, compulsive use in spite of adverse consequences, an inability to reduce the amount of use, and a pattern of relapse to opioids after a period of abstinence. The pursuit of opioid drugs is particularly dramatic in the typical addict who first needs to find the money or barter, then must with regularity find and use the drug. Physical examination with special reference to commonly related medical illnesses of the skin and evidence of parenteral use is essential. Table 2 lists the signs and symptoms of opiate withdrawal.

Laboratory diagnosis is available and reliable when the physician chooses the correct

TABLE 2. Signs and Symptoms Useful in Identifying Opiate Withdrawal

	Common to opiate and sedative-hypnotic withdrawal	Specific to opiate withdrawal
Signs	hypertension tachycardia hyperreflexia tremor vomiting diarrhea diaphoresis hyperthermia	lacrimation mydriasis rhinorrhea fasciculation yawning pilomotor erection decreased light reflex
Symptoms	irritability anxiety insomnia nausea panic	craving opiates bone pain muscle aches orgasm hot and cold flashes

methodology and the correct body fluid for the particular opioid being abused. Thin-layer chromatography (TLC) testing, the most inexpensive and most commonly ordered comprehensive testing, will detect high-dose, current use of some opioids. While TLC is usually adequate to detect morphine quinine (a diluent of heroin), methadone, codeine, dextromethorphan, and propoxyphene used within 12 hr, another screen, the enzyme-linked immunoassays (EIA), has technical and detection advantages for routine screening (Vereby, 1991). These advantages make EIA comparable in many respects to screening 25–40 drugs in a single analysis by capillary gas–liquid chromatography–mass spectrometry (GC/MS). EIA screens can detect opiates (e.g., morphine, codeine, heroin metabolite, hydrocodone), methadone, and propoxyphene, even in the microgram or even picogram per milliliter range. EIA tests have gained popularity over the TLC because no extraction or centrifugation is required and the system for comprehensive testing can be automated. Although EIA screening is more costly than TLC, the screens are more sensitive for most drugs and thereby detect lower drug concentrations. For example TLC sensitivity for opiates is 2,000 ng/ml, EIA is 300 ng/ml, and GC/MS is 20 or less. Detectability of opiates like morphine can be increased to 1–2 days by use of EIA or GC/MS. While only GC/MS operating in the scanning mode, looking at the full range of fragmentation, is considered absolute identification, the expense of this test makes it suitable only for forensic identification or corroboration of a positive by TLC or EIA (Vereby, 1991).

When drug screens are ordered, the physician should be aware that false negative results occur more frequently than false positives due to the lack of sensitivity of TLC (Vereby Gold, & Mule, 1986). A negative test for opiates or drugs by TLC alone is not reliable. Also a screening test by EIA or radio immune assays (RIA) may not be totally reliable, if the laboratory set the cutoff for detecting and reporting positives too high or if the sample was taken too late after the drug was used. Finally, some opioids such as fentanyl occur in such small amounts for short periods that diagnosis can be made only with suspicion and blood testing for the specific opiate in question.

Naloxone challenge tests can also be used to discover opiate dependence. Inducement of withdrawal symptoms after administration of naloxone (Narcan), a short-acting opioid receptor antagonist, is virtually pathognomic of opiate dependence. Note that if the patient is a multiple drug abuser naloxone will not reverse the effects of nonopiate drugs. It is also not uncommon for drug abusers to use over-the-counter (OTC) and prescription drugs such as Benadryl or clonidine to prolong the high and mask withdrawal symptoms. The test is typically administered as follows:

1. 0.2–0.4 mg iv over 5 min or bolus im/sq
2. Observe patient for signs of withdrawal
3. If no response is observed over 30 min give a second iv dose of 0.4 mg or 0.4–0.8 mg im/sq
4. No response after two doses excludes diagnosis of opiate dependence

Diagnostic criteria for opioid intoxication includes (1) recent use of an opioid; (2) clinically significant maladaptive behavioral or psychological changes (e.g., initial euphoria followed by apathy, dysphoria, psychomotor agitation or retardation, impaired judgment, or impaired social or occupational functioning) that developed during, or shortly after, opioid use; and (3) pupillary constriction (or pupillary dilation due to anoxia from severe overdose) and one or more of the three signs (drowsiness or coma, slurred speech, or impairment in attention or memory), developing during or shortly after opioid use.

The *DSM-IV* (American Psychiatric Association, 1994) criteria for opioid withdrawal includes most individuals who are dependent on short-acting drugs such as heroin; withdrawal symptoms occur within 6–24 hr after the last dose. Symptoms may take 2–4 days to emerge in the case of longer-acting drugs such as methadone or LAAM (L-alphacetylmethadol). Acute withdrawal symptoms for a short-acting opioid such as heroin usually peak within 1–3 days and gradually subside over a period of

5–7 days. Less acute withdrawal symptoms can last for weeks to months. These more chronic symptoms include anxiety, dysphoria, anhedonia, insomnia, and drug craving.

Treatment

Acute Toxicity (Overdose)

Opiate toxicity is a medical emergency. Patients are typically found unconscious with shallow respiration and pinpoint pupils (miosis). Severe toxicity may also result in bradycardia and hypotension. Typical procedure for any unconscious patient brought into emergency centers, especially when no obvious cause is noted, is to administer naloxone. Treatment includes airway support and 0.4–0.8 mg naloxone iv. Naloxone may also be administered im while waiting for intravenous access. Since the half-life of naloxone is shorter than many opiates the patient must be continuously observed for signs of opiate toxicity. It has not been an uncommon occurrence to see addicts treated for acute intoxication and discharged only to return soon afterward after the naloxone has been cleared.

Treatment of Opiate Withdrawal

Treatment for opiate dependence follows an assessment of the nature and duration of drug use and addiction. After a medical evaluation, inpatient or outpatient detoxification, methadone maintenance, or naltrexone maintenance are considered. Long-term residential treatment in a therapeutic community is also considered where available. Matching a particular patient to a specific program is difficult given the lack of random-assigned treatment data.

In general, the "detoxification only" approach is not appropriate; it is followed by relapse in most cases in which the patient is not willing or amenable to follow the Narcotics Anonymous or other 12-step self-help programs with close urine monitoring. However, notable exceptions have been reported from Vietnam War veterans, addicts treated in the corrections systems, and those who adopt a new religion and lifestyle. Methadone maintenance is a major treatment option for the opi-

ate-dependent person. Individual methadone programs differ greatly in the degree of other services provided to help the addict stop using intravenous drugs, all drugs, and alcohol, find a job, and stop antisocial activities. Many patients have benefited from long-term methadone maintenance and others have used methadone for a short period to stop intravenous drug use and change many other aspects of their lives. For those patients who are maintained on methadone for many years and who now have stable non-drug-using home environments with no criminality and a stable work history, detoxification followed by naltrexone or abstinence and close urine monitoring can be very successful. On the other hand, long-term residential treatment placements have little appeal to addicts with stable home environments and current employment. Adolescent or young opiate addicts with chaotic home environments, criminality, and other antisocial attitudes and behavior do quite well as therapeutic community residents. Finally, with the advent of reliable urine drug testing the addict can be treated as part of an outpatient drug-free program with family and other therapy while attending NA. Slips and relapses can, with a good patient–therapist relationship, be minimized, and alternative, more intensive treatment can be prescribed when indicated.

Nonopiate Pharmacological Management of Opiate Withdrawal

Ideally, a nonaddicting maintenance medication would make the addict immune to exogenous opioids and would act to first reduce and then eliminate drug-seeking behavior by "deconditioning" the addict's linkage of drug with euphoria. Unfortunately, results have been less dramatic than hoped.

Naltrexone

Generally, naltrexone is an effective treatment for addicts with high motivation to recover and with the social supports that eventually encourage total abstinence (Gold & Roehrich, 1987). Naltrexone is taken orally three times weekly in doses of 100 mg weekdays and 150 mg on weekends. Naltrexone acts as an opiate antagonist by indiscriminately binding with opiate receptors and thereby blocking the affects of heroin, methadone, or exogenous opiates. This medication has been used effectively as an interim phase between opioid addiction and total abstinence in those patients actively engaged in psychotherapy and AA and NA.

Before the advent of clonidine-assisted therapy, a period of 7–10 days after last opiate needed to elapse before starting naltrexone. One large double-blind study of public clinics using naltrexone found the dropout rate with this medication was so great that it questioned whether naltrexone had any beneficial effects. Since this multicenter study was completed before clonidine-assisted detoxification, many of the dropouts could have been a result of the problems in switching patients from opioid addiction to naltrexone without clonidine. Naltrexone is not addicting and has been reported to produce few, if any, side effects. It is a unique and important option for patients desiring a nonaddicting treatment and total abstinence from all mood-altering drugs. Naltrexone has the obvious advantage of allowing the recovering addict to discontinue treatment without withdrawal and the obvious "disadvantage" of not stimulating its own taking. Supervised administration and the use of blood or urine testing of naltrexone and its metabolites, as monitors of compliance, may prove useful to the physician managing an addict with naltrexone.

Clonidine

Before the discovery of clonidine's efficacy in human opioid withdrawal and facilitating naltrexone administration were made, a number of important discoveries in divergent fields occurred:

1. Since the first human clonidine protocol was based upon the investigators' formulating an LC hyperactivity theory, such a theory was supported by the literature.
2. Since clonidine was an approved medication that had been widely studied in humans and animals, the existing literature on clonidine's specific actions and side effects supported the LC hyperactivity hypothesis and clonidine's morphine-like effects without being an opioid.
3. Physicians treating opiate addicts had reason to believe that addicts could be treated and that naltrexone maintenance or abstinence were possible for some patients.
4. An antiwithdrawal or anti-LC dose of clonidine which would be effective in man could be extrapolated from single rodent LC cell studies.
5. LC electrical stimulation or chemical activation in nonhuman primates produced behaviors which were similar to those observed in human opiate addicts in withdrawal rather than a model for human anxiety or mania.
6. Divergent and complex opiate withdrawal signs and symptoms could be localized to a neurotransmitter system (NE) and the actual behavior of a neuroanatomic cell body (LC) and viewed with the assumption that withdrawal effects were the opposite of the drug's effects and with extrapolations from what was known about LC neuroanatomy.

The convergence of the aforementioned conditions led Gold, Redmond, and Kleber (1978b) to suggest that clonidine could suppress opiate withdrawal by replacing opiate-mediated inhibition in the LC (Gold, Redmond, & Kleber, 1978a). Even though the antihypertensive clonidine was an imadazoline derivative, alpha receptor–stimulating medication in widespread worldwide use, many experts were quite critical of this hypothesis and clinical findings and believed that clonidine was an opiate drug like morphine, heroin, or methadone. The fact that clonidine when taken for high blood pressure could not be abruptly discontinued without a rebound or withdrawal syndrome of its own added to the controversy. Actually this effect suggested that the LC hyperactivity theory of opioid withdrawal was correct since alpha-2 and opioid receptors both inhibited the LC when taken acutely or chronically, and since withdrawal phenomena would be expected to occur after abrupt discontinuation of chronic use. Since withdrawal phenomena are generally the exact opposite of acute effects, clonidine at the alpha-2 receptor and heroin at the opioid mu receptor would chronically inhibit the LC.

Withdrawal from either substance would produce a release from inhibition or rebound hyperactivity; therefore it follows that clonidine would reverse opioid withdrawal.

It is now nearly 20 years after the original discovery of clonidine's efficacy in alleviating withdrawal symptoms. Research and clinical experiences since the original discoveries have

1. supported the notion of LC hyperactivity as the neural substrate for the opioid withdrawal syndrome;
2. supported the efficacy of clonidine and established clonidine detoxification as a standard treatment for adult opiate addicts and extended it to application to neonates and to alcohol and other drug withdrawal that share a preponderance of behaviors with the opioid withdrawal syndrome;
3. demonstrated that abstinence could be maintained by some opioid addicts and others could benefit from antagonist therapy with naltrexone with clonidine or accelerated clonidine-naltrexone detoxification;
4. led to considerable progress in the understanding of the critical cellular events causing LC hyperactivity in opioid withdrawal and hypoactivity in the presence of clonidine or opioid agonists;
5. led to the rapidly expanding clinical armamentarium available to treat addicts on the basis of rodent and primate studies. Clonidine's efficacy and the longevity of the LC hyperactivity hypothesis have provided convincing evidence for basic neuroscientific studies relevance to clinical medication development and understanding;
6. identified other medications that suppress withdrawal by a similar mechanism, such as lofexidine, and by independent mechanisms through effects at the LC.

While the initial treatment protocol for clonidine eliminated the 10-day wait period when switching from methadone to naltrexone, more recent protocols have achieved accelerated detoxification by combining clonidine and naltrexone. Charney, Heninger, and Kleber (1986) used clonidine and naltrexone in combination to shorten the entire detoxification period to 6 days, with little loss in success rate. More recently O'Connor and colleagues (1995) looked at two protocols for ambulatory opioid detoxification developed that are applicable to primary care practice. Clonidine, an alpha-2 adrenergic agonist, has been shown to effectively suppress signs and symptoms of opioid withdrawal, with rates of successful detoxification ranging from 36% to 80%. A newer protocol using naltrexone, a long-acting narcotic antagonist, in combination with clonidine (clonidine-naltrexone) has been shown to effectively promote withdrawal in a more rapid detoxification regimen. The two methods (clonidine and clonidine-naltrexone) have been evaluated with considerable success in primary care settings (Farrell & Strang, 1995; Kosten & McCance, 1996; Vining, Kosten, & Kleber, 1988).

The dihydropyridine L-type calcium channel blockers reduce the magnitude of naloxone-precipitated withdrawal in rats and mice. Central noraderergic systems play an important modulatory role in the expression of opiate withdrawal. Opiates acutely inhibit the locus coeruleus and activation of this region during withdrawal is associated with the display of withdrawal behaviors that are increased by alpha-2 antagonists and decreased by alpha-2 adrenergic agonists in animals and humans. Nimodipine pretreatment reduces norepinephrine turnover and release in the cortex during precipitated withdrawal and decreases opiate withdrawal with a time-course similar to its effects on the locus coeruleus (Krystal, Compere, Nestler, & Rasmussen, 1996). Nimodipine suppression of opiate withdrawal in rats at a dose of 10 mg/kg, like clonidine and lofexidine, also inhibits LC neurons but not through alpha-2 receptor stimulation. This approach may be an important addition to detoxification treatment and the beginning of a greater understanding of opiate addiction and withdrawal.

Buprenorphine

More recently, buprenorphine, the opioid mixed agonist–antagonist that has some methadone-like effects and some naltrexone-like effects, has been tried in the treatment of out-patients (Jasinski, Pevnick, & Griffith, 1978). Buprenorphine appears to combine the patient acceptance and cross-tolerance that make the agonist methadone clinically effective as a maintenance treatment with the narcotic-blocking ability of naltrexone (Johnson, Fudala, & Jaffe, 1992). In addition, little physical dependence has been shown for buprenorphine. Doses of 4–8 mg a day of buprenorphine are adequate for opiate blockade and in addition appear to block the effects of cocaine when taken by these patients (Kosten, Kleber, & Morgan, 1989). Kosten, Schottenfeld, Morgan, Falcioni, and Ziedonis (1991) reported comparison of buprenorphine to methadone in 130 opioid-dependent patients who also used cocaine and found that buprenorphine had better efficacy than 65 mg of methadone a day. Gastfriend, Mendelson, Mello, and Teoh (1991) reported beneficial effects of sublingual daily buprenorphine in users of opiates and cocaine. In animals buprenorphine produced a dose-dependent protection against the lethal effects of cocaine (Grayson, Witkin, Katz, Cowan, & Rice, 1991). The ultimate abuse potential of buprenorphine will be determined in the ongoing clinical trials but Cone, Holicky, Pickworth, and Johnson, (1991) recently reported long-acting behavioral effects and abuse liability of intravenous buprenorphine. Furthermore, a study of 50 drug addicts admitted to Marseille hospital found that 18% (9) tested positive for the presence of buprenophrine or its metabolite, confirming the abuse of this medication (Arditti *et al.,* 1992).

Oral naltrexone can help to shorten the opiate withdrawal syndrome in combination with anesthetics, benzodiazepines, and clonidine. The shortening of the withdrawal time is the most important aspect of combined naltrexone and clonidine use. Naloxone-precipitated withdrawal shortens withdrawal itself but does not appear to eliminate the protracted withdrawal syndrome, though it is possible that it shortens protracted abstinence as well (Farrell & Strang, 1995). Recent 3-day studies starting with a single first-day naltrexone dose of 12.5 mg produced only mild withdrawal symptoms when patients are also given clonidine. Starting with 12.5 mg naltrexone, clonidine was needed for 4 days with a total dose of 1.7 mg and peak dose of 0.6 mg on Day 1. While Vining and colleagues (1988) showed that more than 90% of patients could be detoxified and placed on naltrexone, they showed only half remained on naltrexone for even 14 days.

Opioid Maintenance Medications

Three maintenance pharmacotherapies are currently in use—methadone, naltrexone, and LAAM. Naltrexone has been quite effective in physicians and other highly motivated addicts but others have reported dysphoric effects. Poor compliance is common for opiate addicts (Shippenberg & Kubik-Bals, 1995). Opioid antagonists' aversive side effects appear to be independent of mesolimbic DA neurons. Side effects and compliance problems appear to be much more common in opiate addicts than in alcoholics treated with naltrexone suggesting a role for opiates in endorphin dysregulation and persistent abstinence in these problems encountered in opioid relapse prevention maintenance with antagonists. Buprenorphine is also becoming available (Kosten & McCance, 1996). Johnson and colleagues' (1992) study of buprenorphine 8 mg per day demonstrated equivalence for 65 mg per day of methadone, with the 8 mg buprenorphine having 37% positive urine for opiates and the 65 mg methadone patients having 50% positive opiate urine. Doses of 16 mg buprenorphine appear more effective in retaining patients and reducing positive urine. However, buprenorphine may itself have intravenous abuse potential.

Methadone

Methadone maintenance with adjunctive counseling is considered by many experts in the field to be the treatment of choice (Fulco, Liverman, & Earley, 1995; McLellan, Arndt, Metzger, Woody, & O'Brien, 1993). Methadone programs are generally available throughout the United States. While there are an estimated 650 methadone programs in the United States they have not grown to meet the needs of the addict population. In 1993 it was estimated that 117,000 of the 500,000 opiate-addicted people in the United States received methadone (Harwood, Thomson, & Nesmith, 1994). A typical program has a nursing function with methadone dispensing, counseling offices, medical examining room, and clerical-administrative area. Patients are usually given their methadone dose at the dispensing office with take-home doses considered a privilege that comes to those who follow the program and are abstinent. Patients in such a program are monitored with urine tests for drugs of abuse. They are given counseling in a group and may receive additional services depending on the clinic and their needs. Methadone treatment is considered long-term treatment with an average stay for an addict approximately 1 year. Some patients stay in the program indefinitely. It is reported that 80% of the patients admitted for methadone have had prior opiate treatment episodes with and average of 1.4 in the past year (Batten *et al.*, 1993). A large body of evidence suggests that methadone works (McLellan *et al.*, 1993) as long as doses are adequate and other services administered. Treatment is effective in reducing opiate use, criminality, intravenous drug use, medical problems, mental health problems and problems in global functioning. After a person has become abstinent relapse can occur at any time. Relapse can occur after successful medical treatment and psychosocial treatment for psychological and social problems. Relapse can be triggered by factors that initially led to drug use but often relapse is unrelated to these or any identifiable factors. Relapse can be described as automatic, involuntary, or of unknown origin. Addiction is thus a disease characterized by compulsive use of drugs, tolerance, dependence, craving, and relapse. Of these we provide the best services for medical detoxification and are having the most difficulty in relapse prevention.

Diagnostic criteria for opioid withdrawal is characterized by dysphoric mood; nausea or vomiting; muscle aches; lacrimation or rhinorrhea; pupillary dilation, piloerection, or sweating; diarrhea; yawning; fever; or insomnia, or some combination of these symptoms. The symptoms typically cause clinically significant distress or impairment in social, occupational, or other important areas of functioning.

Opioid use and dependence are important public health problems. Use of opioids by the intranasal route and by smoking has increased the numbers of experimental and chronic users. Opiates have important effects on endogenous opioid systems, nucleus accumbens, the locus coeruleus, and elsewhere. Once established, opiate addiction is accompanied by numerous social, addictive, and medical problems which compromise survival. Heroin addiction is a chronic, lifelong, relapsing disease with a high fatality rate. Current treatment approaches should be multimodal and not overly focused on detoxification as an end point for all patients (O'Brien & McLellan, 1996). Addictions are chronic disorders, not acute conditions like a broken leg. Addiction does not end when the drug is removed from the body (detoxification) or when the acute post-drug-taking illness dissipates (withdrawal). Rather, the underlying addictive disorder persists, and this persistence produces a tendency to relapse to active drug taking. Detoxification does not address the underlying disorder and thus is not adequate treatment. Treatment works and can be improved by focusing on the improvement in areas of social, employment, medical, addiction, and psychological function over time and with psychosocial and medical treatment. Research into the molecular mechanisms of exogenous opiates' acute and prolonged effects, neuroadaptation and the locus coeruleus, release from chronic inhibition that accompanies withdrawal, and long-term compromise of endogenous opioid systems by opiate self-administration is necessary.

Opiate self-administration would through feedback inhibition decrease the release and biosynthesis of endogenous opioids (Gold *et al.*, 1980; Goldstein, 1975). This hypothesized decrease could contribute to the development of tolerance, dependence, and withdrawal, and is supported by Trujillo and colleagues (1995) who have recently demonstrated that chronic infusion or repeated injection of morphine increases prodynorphin peptides. These results are supported by other observations in the field (Nylander, Vlaskovska, & Terenius, 1995). Since their discovery, the endogenous opioid peptides have been postulated to be altered by opiate dependence and tolerance mechanisms with the assumption that exogenous administration of opiates would downregulate endogenous opioid peptide systems, leading to a deficit, which in opiate withdrawal contributed to the abstinence syndrome. Others have suggested that such changes are persistent, redefining normal for the organism, and involved in the high recidivism and need for long-term treatment and treatment with agonists. Naturally, just taking opiates is not addiction; neuroadaptive changes may be accelerated and require a critical pairing with volitional motivated behavior directed at acquiring and taking the drug to produce euphoria.

References

Akil, H., Mayer, D. J., & Liebeskind, J. C. (1976). Antagonism of stimulation-produced analgesia by naloxone, a narcotic antagonist. *Science, 191,* 961–962.

American Psychiatric Association. (1994). *Diagnostic and statistical manual of mental disorders* (4th ed.). Washington, DC: Author.

Arditti J, Bourdon, J. H., Jean, P., Landi, H., Nasset, D., Jouglard, J., & Thirion, X. (1992). Buprenorphine abuse in a group of 50 drug-use abusers admitted to Marseille Hospital. *Therapie, 47,* 561–562.

Batten, H., Prottas, J., Horgan, C. M., Simon, L. J., Larson, M. J., Elliot, E. A., & Marsden, M. E. (1993). *Drug services research survey final report: Phase II.* Waltham, MA: Bigel Institute for Health Policy, Brandeis University. Contract 271-90-8319/1. Submitted to National Institute on Drug Abuse, February 22, 1993.

Charney, D. S., Heninger, G. R., & Kleber, H. D. (1986). The combined use of clonidine and naltrexone as a rapid, safe, and effective treatment of abrupt withdrawal from methadone. *American Journal of Psychiatry, 143,* 831–837.

Childers, S. R. (1991). Minireview: Opioid receptor-coupled second messenger systems. *Life Science, 48,* 1991–2003.

Cone, E., Holicky, B., Pickworth, W., & Johnson, R. E. (1991, June). *Pharmacologic and behavioral effects of high doses of intravenous buprenorphine.* Report of the Committee on Problems of Drug Dependence, 53rd annual scientific meeting, Palm Beach, FL.

Cox, B. M., Goldstein, A., & Li, C. H. (1976). Opioid activity of a peptide, B-lipotropin (61-91) derived from B-lipotropin. *Proceedings of the National Academy of Sciences, 73,* 1821–1823.

Dackis, C. A., & Gold, M. S. (1985). New concepts in cocaine addiction: The dopamine depletion hypothesis. *Neuroscience and Biobehavioral Reviews, 9,* 469–477.

Donnerer, J., Oka, K., Brossi, A., Rice, K. C., & Spector, S. (1986). Presence and formation of codeine and morphine in the rat. *Proceedings of the National Academy of Sciences, 83,* 4566–4567.

Farrell, M., & Strang, J. (1995). Compressed opiate withdrawal syndrome and naltrexone. *Journal of Psychopharmacology, 94,* 383–385.

Fulco, C. E., Liverman, C. T., & Earley, L. E. (Eds.). (1995). *The development of medications for the treatment of opiate and cocaine addictions.* Washington, DC: Institute of Medicine, National Academy Press.

Gastfriend, D. R., Mendelson, J. H., Mello, N. K., & Teoh, S. K. (1991, June). *Preliminary results of an open trial of buprenorphine in the outpatient treatment of combined heroin and cocaine dependence.* Paper presented to the Committee on Problems of Drug Dependence, 53rd annual scientific meeting, Palm Beach, FL.

Gold, M. S. (1995). *Principles of addiction medicine,* Section 2, Chap. 4 (First official manual for American Society of Addiction Medicine: Opioids, pharmacology of addictive drugs). Chevy Chase, MD: ASAM.

Gold, M. S. (Ed.). (1993). The facts about tobacco, alcohol, and other drugs, *4,* University of Florida, Drug Abuse Warning Network.

Gold, M. S., & Roehrich, H. (1987). Treatment of opiate withdrawal with clonidine. *ISI: Atlas of Science: Pharmacology, 1741,* 29–32.

Gold, M. S., Redmond, D. E., & Kleber, H. D. (1978a). Clonidine blocks acute opiate withdrawal symptoms. *Lancet, 2,* 599–602.

Gold, M. S., Redmond, D. E., & Kleber, H. D. (1978b). Clonidine in opiate withdrawal. *Lancet, 1,* 929–930.

Gold, M. S., Pottash, A. L., Extein, I., & Kleber, H. D. (1980). Anti endorphin effects of methadone. *Lancet, 2,* 972–973.

Goldstein, A. (1975). Are opiate tolerance and dependence reversible? In H. D. Cappell & A. E. LeBlanc (Eds.), *Biological and behavioral approaches to drug dependence* (pp. 27–41). Toronto, Ontario, Canada: Addiction Research Foundation.

Goldstein, A., & Herrera, J. (1995). Heroin addicts and methadone treatment in Albuquerque: A 22 year follow-up. *Drug and Alcohol Dependence, 40,* 139–150.

Grayson, N. A., Witkin, J. M., Katz, J. L., Cowan, A., & Rice, K. C. (1991, June). *Actions of buprenorphine on cocaine and opiate mediated effects.* Paper presented to the Committee on Problems of Drug Dependence, 53rd annual scientific meeting, Palm Beach, FL.

Harwood, H. J., Thomson, M., & Nesmith, T. (1994). *Healthcare reform and substance abuse treatment: The cost of financing under alternative approaches.* Fairfax, VA: Lewin-VHI.

Hughes, J. (1975). Isolation of an endogenous compound from the brain with properties similar to morphine. *Brain Research, 88,* 295–308.

Izenwasser, S., Newman, A. H., Cox, B. M., & Katz, J. L. (1996). The cocaine-like behavioral effects of meperidine are mediated by activity at the dopamine transporter. *European Journal of Pharmacology, 297,* 9–17.

Jasinski, D. R., Pevnick, J. S., & Griffith, J. D. (1978). Human pharmacology and abuse potential of the analgesic buprenorphine. *Archives of General Psychiatry, 35,* 501–516.

Johnson, R. E., Fudala, P. J., & Jaffe, J. H. (1992). A controlled trial of buprenorphine for opioid dependence. *Journal of the American Medical Association, 267,* 2750–2755.

Johnston, L. M. (1995). *The UM/NIDA Monitoring the Future Study.* Ann Arbor, MI: University of Michigan.

Karch, S. B. (1989). The history of cocaine toxicity. *Human Pathology, 20*(11), 1037–1039.

Koob, G. F., & Bloom, F. E. (1988). Cellular and molecular mechanisms of drug dependence. *Science, 242,* 715–723.

Kosten, T. R., & McCance, E. A. (1996). review of pharmacotherapies for substance abuse. *American Journal on Addictions, 5,* 58–65.

Kosten, T. R., Kleber, H. D., & Morgan, C. (1989). Role of opioid antagonists in treating intravenous cocaine abuse. *Life Science, 44,* 887–892.

Kosten, T. R., Schottenfeld, R. S., Morgan, C., Falcioni, J., & Ziedonis, D. (1991, June). *Buprenorphine vs. methadone for opioid and cocaine dependence.* Paper presented to the Committee on Problems of Drug Dependence, 53rd annual scientific meeting, Palm Beach, FL.

Krystal, J. H., Compere, S., Nestler, E. J., & Rasmussen, K. (1996). Nimodipine reduction of Naltrexone-precipitated locus coeruleus activation and abstinence behavior in morphine-dependent rats. *Physiology and Behavior, 52,* 863–866.

Levine, J. D., Gordon, N. C., & Fields, H. L. (1978). The mechanism of placebo analgesia. *Lancet, 2,* 654–657.

Mains, R. E., Eipper, B. A., & Ling, N. (1977). Common precursor to corticotropins and endorphins. *Proceedings of the National Academy of Sciences, 74,* 3014–3018.

McLellan, A. T., Arndt, I. O., Metzger, D. S., Woody, G. E., & O'Brien, C. P. (1993). The effects of psychosocial services in substance abuse treatment. *Journal of the American Medical Association, 269,* 1953–1959.

Musto, D. (1987). *The American disease: Origins of narcotic control.* New York: Oxford University Press.

National Household Survey on Drug Abuse: Main Findings. (1993). 73–74.

Nestler, E. J. (1992). Molecular mechanisms of drug addiction. *Journal of Neuroscience, 12,* 2439–2450.

Nylander, I., Vlaskovska, M., & Terenius, L. (1995). The effects of morphine treatment and morphine withdrawal on the dynorphin and enkephalin systems in Sprague-Dawley rats. *Psychopharmacology, 118,* 391–400.

O'Brien, C. P., & McLellan, A. T. (1996). Myths about the treatment of addiction. *Lancet, 347,* 237–240.

O'Connor, P. G., Waugh, M. E., Carroll, K. M., Rounsaville, B. J., Diagkogiannis, I. A., & Schottenfeld, R. D. (1995). Primary care-based ambulatory opioid detoxification: The results of a clinical trial. *Journal of General Internal Medicine, 10,* 255–260.

Pert, C. B., & Snyder, S. H. (1973). Opiate receptor demonstration in nervous tissue. *Science, 179,* 1011–1014.

Pomeranz, B., & Chiu, D. (1976). Naloxone blockade of acupuncture analgesia: Endorphin implicated. *Life Science, 19,* 1757–1762.

Shippenberg, T. S., & Kubik-Bals, R. (1995). Involvement of the mesolimbic dopamine system in mediating the aversive effects of opioid antagonists in the rat. *Behavioral Pharmacology, 6,* 99–106.

Simon, E. J., Hiller, J. M., & Edelman, I. (1973). Stereospecific binding of the potent narcotic analgesic 3H-etorphine to rat brain homogenate. *Proceedings of the National Academy of Science, 70,* 1947–1949.

Trujillo, K. A., Bronstein, D. M., & Akil, H. (1993). Regulation of opioid peptides by self-administration drugs. In R. P. Hammer, Jr. (Ed.), *The neurobiology of opiates* (pp. 223–256). Boca Raton, FL: CRC.

Trujillo, K. A., Bronstein, D. M., Sanchez, I. O., & Akil, H. (1995). Effects of chronic opiate and opioid antagonist treatment on striatal opioid peptides. *Brain Research, 698,* 69–78.

Vereby, K. (1991). Laboratory methods for drug and alcohol addiction. In N. S. Miller, *Comprehensive handbook of drug and alcohol addiction* (pp. 809–842). New York: Dekker.

Vereby, K., Gold, M. S., & Mule, S. J. (1986). Laboratory testing in the diagnosis of marijuana intoxication and withdrawal. In M. S. Gold (Ed.), *Psychiatric Annals, 16,* 235–241.

Vining, E., Kosten, T. R., & Kleber, H. D. (1988). Clinical utility of rapid clonidine-naltrexone detoxification for opioid abusers. *British Journal of Addiction, 83,* 567–575.

Wagner, J. J., & Chavkin, C. I. (1995). Neuropharmacology of endogenous opioid peptides. In F. E. Bloom & D. J. Kupfer, (Eds.), *Psychopharmacology: The fourth generation of progress* (pp. 519–529). New York: Raven.

Watson, S., Akil, H., Khachaturian, H., Young, E., & Lewis, M. E. (1984). Opioid systems: Anatomical, physiological and clinical perspectives. In J. Hughes, H. O. Collier, M. J. Rance, & M. B. Tyers (Eds.), *Opi-oids past, present and future* (pp. 145–178). London: Taylor & Francis.

Wei, E., & Loh, H. H. (1976). Physical dependence on opiate-like peptides. *Science, 193,* 1262–1263.

25

Medications of Abuse

Opioids

ANDREA C. KING AND NORMAN S. MILLER

Introduction

Opioid drugs are commonly used for the relief of pain. The standard medications for severe pain are the derivatives of the opium poppy (opiates) and synthetic drugs that activate the same receptors (opioids). In addition to alleviating perception of pain, however, many opioids also produce a state of well-being or euphoria through central nervous system (CNS) mediated effects. Some individuals may be susceptible to abuse or addiction to the opioids because of these mood-altering effects. Recent research efforts focus on separating the mechanisms underlying analgesia and euphoria in order to develop analgesic medications that do not produce mood-altering effects, and therefore have less abuse liability (O'Brien, 1996). Currently, opioid-related drugs are the standard treatment for severe, acute, and chronic pain associated with cancer, trauma, headache, or other injury. In this chapter we review opioid pharmacology and opioid medications commonly used in analgesia, issues of addiction, including tolerance, withdrawal, and physical dependence, and finally, relevant clinical issues related to the incidence of iatrogenic addiction and individual differences in susceptibility to opioid abuse and addiction.

Opioids and Opioid Receptors: A Brief Review

Opioid Receptors

Since the discovery of opioid receptors over 20 years ago (Pert & Snyder, 1973; Simon, Hiller, & Edelman, 1973; Terenius, 1973), ongoing research has supported the existence of multiple opioid receptors (Zaki et al., 1996). The three types of known opioid receptors are the μ, κ, and δ, each identified by their different selectivities for various naturally occurring peptide and alkaloid opioid ligands, as well as selective synthetic ligands (Goldstein & Naidu, 1989). In addition, the existence of various subtypes of each of these three opioid receptor types has been suggested from different pharmacological studies (Mattia, Vanderah, Mosberg, & Porreca, 1991; Paul, Bodnar, Gistrak, & Pasternak, 1989; Sofulglu, Portoghese, & Takemori, 1991; Zukin, Eghbali, Olive, Unterwald, & Tempel, 1988).

The majority of the clinically used opioids (endogenous prototype β-endorphin and exogenous prototype morphine) bind to μ-opioid

ANDREA C. KING • Laboratory of the Biology of Addictive Diseases, The Rockefeller University, New York, New York 10021; present address: Department of Psychiatry, The University of Chicago, Chicago, Illinois 60637. NORMAN S. MILLER • Department of Psychiatry, The University of Illinois at Chicago, Chicago, Illinois 60612.

Handbook of Substance Abuse: Neurobehavioral Pharmacology, edited by Tarter et al. Plenum Press, New York, 1998.

receptors (Markenson, 1996). The μ-opioid receptors have two subtypes (Wood, Richard, & Thakur, 1982) including the μ_1 receptor, which is responsible for analgesia, and μ_2 receptor, which mediates respiratory depression, bradycardia, and inhibition of gastrointestinal motility. Although the majority of the therapeutic opioid-based agents bind primarily to μ receptors, at high enough doses, many opioids will also bind to additional receptor subtypes, leading to possible changes in their pharmacological properties. In addition, some opioid drugs interact with more than one receptor class even at usual clinical doses.

In addition to μ opioid receptors, there are the κ and δ opioid receptors. Activation of κ and δ causes spinal analgesia. Binding assay and pharmacological studies have suggested several κ-receptor subtypes, including κ_1 receptors, which produce spinal analgesia and have Dynorphin A as the endogenous ligand; κ_3 receptors, which relieve pain via supraspinal mechanisms; and κ_2 receptors, which are presently not well understood in terms of pharmacological properties. The δ receptors include δ_1 and δ_2-opioid receptor subtypes based on differential response to novel antagonists (Portoghese, Sultana, Nagase, & Takemori, 1992; Sofulglu et al., 1991). Enkephalins are the endogenous ligands for δ-opioid receptors, and appear to produce both spinal and supraspinal analgesia, although the spinal system appears more robust.

Opioid Medications: Analgesics

Opioid analgesics include substances in three general pharmacologic classifications, including morphine-like agonists, partial agonists, or mixed agonist–antagonists. The most commonly prescribed for pain relief are in the first category, including morphine, methadone, codeine, oxycodone (Percocet), meperidine (Demerol), hydromorphone (Dilaudid), propoxyphene (Darvon), oxymorphone, and levorphanol. The second category includes the partial μ agonists, such as buprenorphine (Buprenex). Finally, the third general category includes the mixed agonist–antagonists which differ in analgesic action from morphine and the full opioid agonists at all opioid receptor subtypes. These drugs include nalorphine, cyclazocine, and nalbuphine (Nubain) which are competitive μ antagonists, but exert analgesic actions primarily by working as agonists at κ receptors (Reisine & Pasternak, 1996). Pentazocine (Talwin) and butorphanol, in contrast, have κ agonist properties but may be weaker μ antagonists or partial μ agonists.

In general, opioid medications provide pain relief by their action at selective binding of opioid receptors distributed throughout the central

TABLE 1. Some Oral Nonopioid and Opioid Analgesics Indicated for Mild to Moderate Pain

	Equianalgesic dose (mg)[a]	Duration (hr)	Plasma half-life (hr)	Comments
Aspirin	650	4–6	3–5	Standard for nonnarcotic comparisons.
Acetaminophen	650	4–6	104	Weak anti-inflammatory; safer than aspirin.
Propoxyphene (Darvon)	65	4–6	12	Used in combination with nonopioid analgesics; metabolite norpropoxyphene may be toxic.
Codeine	32	4–6	3	Available in combination with nonopioid analgesics; biotransformed to morphine.
Meperidine (Demerol)	50	4–6	3–4	Biotransformed to active toxic metabolite normeperidine; associated with myoclonus and seizures.
Pentazocine (Talwin)	30	4–6	2–3	Only available in combination with naloxone, aspirin, or acetaminophen (U.S.); psychotomimetic effects with dose escalation.

[a]Relative potency of drugs, as compared with that of aspirin, for mild to moderate pain. Adapted in part from Foley (1985).

nervous system (CNS), with highest concentrations in the limbic system, thalamus, striatum, hypothalamus, midbrain, and spinal cord (Reisine & Pasternak, 1996). In addition, opioid drugs alter the release and action of several neurotransmitters, such as serotonin and acetylcholine, which are intricately involved in pain perception. Although the primary effect of opioid drugs is sedation, there is some support for opioid interactions with dopamine activity, which may be in part associated with the euphoric and addictive properties of opioids (Miller & Gold, 1993). Opioid receptors are abundant in regions that have been suggested as "reinforcement" centers in the brain acting on the natural reward system (Wise, 1989), the pathway implicated in other drugs of abuse, including cocaine, alcohol, and amphetamines.

The action of opioids is complex and may ultimately result in either depression or stimulation, depending on the dose administered, site of action, and individual susceptibility (Tucker, 1990). In the following section, we briefly review the effects and onset of action of several commonly prescribed opioid medications, such as morphine, meperidine, methadone, and codeine, and compare these effects to the illicit short-acting opioid heroin (see Tables 1 and 2).

The two most commonly used postoperative narcotic analgesics are morphine and meperi-

TABLE 2. Some Oral and Parenteral Opioid Analgesics Indicated for Severe Pain[a]

	Route	Equianalgesic dose (mg)	Duration (hr)	Plasma half-life (hr)	Comments
			Agonist		
Morphine	IM	10	4–6	2–3.5	Standard for comparison; available in
	PO	60	4–7	2–3.5	slow-release tablets.
Codeine	IM	130	4–6	3	Biotransformed to morphine; useful
	PO	200	4–6	2–3.5	as initial narcotic.
Meperidine	IM	75	4–5	3–4	Contraindicated in patients with renal
(Demerol)	PO	300	4–6	12–16 (normeperidine)	disease; normeperidine (toxic metabolite) accumulation produces CNS excitation.
Oxycodone	IM	15		—	Short acting; available alone or as
(Percocet)	PO	30	3–5		5 mg dose in combination with aspirin and acetaminophen.
Hydromorphone	IM	1.5	4–5	2–3	Available in high-potency injectable
(Dilaudid)	PO	7.5	4–6	2–3	form; more soluble than morphine.
Heroin	IM	5	4–5	0.5	*Illegal* in United States; high solubility for parenteral administration.
	PO	60	4–5	0.5	
			Mixed Agonist-Antagonists		
Pentazocine	IM	60	4–6	2–3	Psychotomimetic effects with dose
(Talwin)	PO	180	4–7	2–3	escalation; available with naloxone, aspirin, or acetaminophen; may precipitate withdrawal in dependent persons.
Nalbuphine	IM	10	4–6	5	Not available orally; less severe
(Nubain)					psychotomimetic effects than pentazocine; may precipitate withdrawal in dependent persons.
			Partial Agonist		
Buprenorophine	IM	0.4	4–6	?	Not available in the U.S.; no psychoto-
(Temgesic)	SL	0.8	5–6		mimetic effects; may precipitate withdrawal in dependent persons.

[a] Adapted in part from Foley (1985).

dine (Tucker, 1990). The CNS effects of morphine include analgesia, dysphoria or euphoria, drowsiness, respiratory depression, cough suppression, and clouding of mental abilities (Reisine & Pasternak, 1996). When morphine is given to a normal, pain-free individual, the experience can be unpleasant and nausea and vomiting may occur. In patients experiencing acute or chronic pain, however, the relief of pain from morphine is relatively selective in that other major sensory modalities are not altered. Morphine continues to be the major treatment for moderate-to-severe pain and is usually administered subcutaneously or intramuscularly (approximate dose 10mg/70kg body weight), although in selected situations it can be administered epidurally and intrathecally (Foley, 1993). Duration of action for morphine is relatively short, reported at approximately 4–6 hr in both oral and parenteral administrations (McCaffrey & Beebe, 1989); however, sustained release oral preparations are available for administrations at 8–10 hr intervals (Reisine & Pasternak, 1996).

Meperidine (Demerol) produces rapid analgesic effects, with onset of analgesia occurring within 10 min with subcutaneous or intramuscular administration and 15 min after oral administration. Meperidine is similar to morphine but is not as effective an analgesic and has a shorter duration of action, approximately 2–4 hr, therefore, more frequent injections may be needed for pain relief. Unlike morphine and its congeners, the major use of meperidine is for analgesia and not for cough or diarrhea. The pattern and incidence of unpleasant side effects with meperidine is similar to that of equianalgesic doses of morphine, with the exception of less incidence of constipation and urinary retention. In contrast to morphine, toxic doses of meperidine can produce CNS excitation, characterized by mood changes, tremors, muscle twitches, and seizures (McCaffrey, 1987; Reisine & Pasternak, 1996). These effects are believed to be due to the accumulation of the metabolite normeperidine, which has a much longer half-life than the parent compound.

In contrast to morphine and most of the opioids, codeine is approximately 60% as effective orally as parenterally, both as an analgesic and as a respiratory depressant. The other opioids that share such a high oral–parenteral potency ratio are methadone, oxycodone, and levorphanol (Reisine & Pasternak, 1996). The plasma half-life of codeine is 2–4 hr. Codeine has a very low affinity for opioid receptors and its analgesic effect is most likely due to the small fraction of codeine that is converted to morphine. The antitussive effects of codeine most likely involve distinct receptors that bind to codeine itself (Reisine & Pasternak, 1996).

Methadone is an opioid with effective analgesic properties and is effective by the oral route of administration with a slow onset; it has an extended duration of action (Kreek, 1973, 1978). It is, therefore, a preferred treatment of chronic pain, and is also used to prevent withdrawal symptoms, postoperatively, in patients with a substance abuse history. The structure of methadone is quite different from morphine, but their actions are similar. Methadone can be administered every 6–8 hr for analgesia. Chronic use extends the plasma half-life from 17–24 hr to 2–3 days (McCaffrey & Beebe, 1989; Twycross & McQuay, 1989). When discontinued, low concentrations are maintained in plasma by slow release from extravascular binding sites (Kreek, 1979) which may account for the typical mild but prolonged withdrawal symptoms.

In contrast to the slow-onset opioids mentioned earlier, heroin is not available for therapeutic use in the United States. Heroin has a relatively rapid onset with maximal blood levels reached within minutes of administration (Inturrisi et al., 1984). Heroin is biotransformed to its two active metabolites, morphine and 6-acetylmorphine; however, it is an inefficient means of providing morphine to the systemic circulation. It has been suggested that heroin might have unique analgesic properties for the treatment of severe pain, but data from double-blind trials comparing heroin with other parenteral opioids have not supported this theory (O'Brien, 1996). In light of the fact that there is a much higher abuse and addiction liability with heroin, it is obvious that heroin has no discernible therapeutic advantage over the available opioids (Inturrisi *et al.,* 1984; Kaiko, Wallenstein, Rogers, Grabinski, & Houde, 1981; Sawynok, 1986).

Opioid Side Effects, Toxicity, and Withdrawal

Nausea occurs in 10% to 40% of patients given opioid substances, but tolerance develops rapidly and prophylactic antiemetics are usually not necessary (Manion, 1995); however, if vomiting and nausea persist, prochlorperazine or metoclopramide can be effective. Opioids can also produce sedation, which persists for only several days before the evidence of tolerance to this effect. When opioid doses are elevated, the adjunct treatment with dextroamphetamine or methylphenidate may be used to counteract sedation. The most serious potential side effect, respiratory depression, is rare in patients chronically treated with stable doses of opioids.

Opioid intoxication is characterized by signs of sedation, clouded sensorium, hypotension, bradycardia, depressed respirations, hyporeflexia, pupillary constriction (e.g., "pinpoint pupils"), and slowed motor movements (Miller, 1991). During acute intoxication, the individual reports intense euphoria or "high," sleepiness, relaxation, depression, and analgesia. Depending on the half-life of the opioid, the signs and symptoms of opioid intoxication may last for several hours. Overdose of an opioid may lead to stupor, coma, or both, with the respiratory rate sometimes as low as 2 to 4 breaths per minute, and cyanosis may also be present (Reisine & Pasternak, 1996). In general, signs of pinpoint pupils, coma, and depressed respiration indicate opioid poisoning. Death resulting from this condition is usually due to respiratory failure or complications related to coma, such as pneumonia or shock. In addition to establishing an airway and ventilating the patient, treatment often also involves use of an opioid antagonist, usually naloxone, administered in a dosing regimen sufficient to reverse the respiratory depression effects without precipitating withdrawal in dependent patients.

Due to tolerance and pharmacological dependence, the chronic opioid user reports less intense euphoria and increased anxiety and depression with repeated administration. Use of short-acting opioids (i.e., heroin) results in the user spending little time in the "straight" state, due to rapid metabolism (Kreek, 1992), and therefore the initial sensation of a "rush" is quickly followed by the relaxing "nod," followed by the appearance of classic withdrawal symptoms. The withdrawal state can best be understood as the opposite of the initial drug effects, such as occur with μ-agonist withdrawal or rebound hyperactivity. Withdrawal signs and symptoms include hypertension, increased heart rate and respirations, nausea, diarrhea, dysphoria, yawning, rhinorrhea, lacrimation, piloerection ("goose flesh"), anxiety, perspiration, and sleep difficulties. The opioid withdrawal syndrome varies in duration and intensity, according to the duration of action of the particular opioid (Miller, 1991). For example, heroin has a very rapid onset of action, and therefore withdrawal signs and symptoms can occur within a few hours and peak at approximately 3 days after discontinuation. In contrast, for the longer-acting opioid methadone, withdrawal may not occur for days and peaks at 7–10 days. In general, the more potent the narcotic, the more severe the ensuing withdrawal state.

Nonopioid Medications

Controversies have arisen in the use of opioid-based analgesics, including the choice of analgesic to be used (e.g., morphine, methadone, oxycodone, meperidine), the route and schedule of administration (fixed or as needed), and the risk of psychological dependence with long-term use (Foley, 1981, 1985). The analgesic used depends on many factors related to the particular patient, treatment condition, and situational or environmental factors, and may include a series of different opioid and nonopioid agents across patients or within the same patient. The nonopioid analgesics, such as aspirin or nonsteroidal anti-inflammatory drugs (NSAIDs) and adjuvant analgesics, may be used alone or in conjunction with opioids. For example, agents such as aspirin, acetaminophen, and NSAIDS may be sufficient for relief of mild to moderate pain (Manion, 1995). The World Health Organization has outlined an approach to the selection of these drugs, otherwise known as the "WHO analgesic ladder" (Stambaugh, 1993; World Health Organization, 1990). Briefly, this ladder recommends a sequential movement initiating with NSAIDS, possibly in combination with an adjuvant analgesic for mild-to-moderate pain. The next rung consists of "weak" opioids such as codeine or oxycodone in combination with an NSAID, hydrocodone, and propoxyphene, also in combination products, for those patients with moderate pain or those who fail to achieve relief with NSAIDS. Finally, treatment with "strong" opioids such as morphine, levorphanol, methadone, hydromrorphone, and oxycodone (not in combination products), alone or possibly co-administered with an NSAID or adjuvant analgesic, is suggested for moderate-to-severe pain or for those patients who do not achieve analgesia from the second rung of the analgesic ladder.

Since the nonopioids and adjuvant analgesics affect a different component of the pain pathway with less central nervous system effect than opioids, combinations of analgesics may provide improved analgesia at lower doses of each drug and with fewer side effects (Buck & Paice, 1994). For example, it has been suggested that the combination of an opioid with an amphetamine may enhance the opioid analgesic effects while reducing sedation. However, nonopioid preparations also produce side effects; for example, the action of NSAIDS in inhibition of prostaglandins also produces its adverse effects (Buck & Paice, 1994), including gastrointestinal irritation or bleeding, platelet aggregation abnormalities, and renal and hepatic toxicity, especially at very high doses.

The only NSAID available for intramuscular as well as oral use is Ketorolac (Toradol) (Buck & Paice, 1994). Ketorolac given intramuscularly has been found to be comparable to buprenorphine (partial opioid agonist) in analgesic potency and onset of action (Canadell-Carafi, Moreno-Londono, & Gonzalez-Caudevilla, 1991). However, keterolac is not a substitute for opioid medications, but may be an option when opioids are contraindicated, or used in conjunction with opioids for optimal effect.

Adjuvant analgesics are ancillary analgesics developed originally for purposes other than pain relief; yet they have pain-relieving properties that may be utilized for treating patients with pain. Examples of adjuvant analgesics include corticosteroids, tricyclic antidepressants, anticonvulsants, antihistamines, anxiolytics, and neuroleptics. These medications produce analgesia in certain painful states by mechanisms not clearly established or directly related to the opioid receptor system (Foley, 1985). The mechanism of intravenous or intramuscular corticosteroids providing pain relief is through reduction of swelling pressure on nerves and reduction of edema, which is often observed in postoperative inflammation or from tumors on surrounding organs. The tricyclic antidepressants inhibit the transmission of pain sensation in the spinothalamic tract through augmentation of norepinephrine and serotonin in the pain-modulating descending spinal pathways. The tricyclics also produce improvements in general mood and sleep which may augment analgesia and indirectly affect pain perception (Walsh, 1983).

Prevalence of Opioid Abuse and Addiction

From the results of several epidemiological surveys, including DAWN (Drug Abuse Warning Network), the household survey, and the high-school student survey, it has been estimated that approximately 2 million individuals in the United States have used illicit opioids, with about 1 million reporting using heroin either recently or frequently. The actual numbers are most likely higher than those reported, given some of the inherent difficulties with surveys. Although it is difficult to know the percise number of heroin addicts, current reports from overdose deaths, arrest records, and treatment program enrollment statistics estimate the number to be around 750,000 to 1 million (O'Brien, 1996).

A recent community survey in the United States showed an estimated 6% of the population sampled or used analgesics for nonmedical purposes and that 2.5% had used them within the previous year (Gold & Miller, 1997). In medical settings, it has been estimated that approximately 3% of patients misuse medications or seek psychoactive drugs for the purpose of intoxication (Drug Enforcement Administration, 1987). Comorbidity with other drugs of abuse and alcohol is not uncommon. A survey by the National Institute on Drug Abuse showed that more than half of patients who sought treatment for or died of drug-related medical problems were also abusing prescription drugs (Wilford, 1987).

Patient compliance surveys have indicated that as many as half of all patients deviate from the physician's directions. Noncompliant behaviors include never obtaining or taking the prescribed drug, taking the drug improperly (i.e., incorrect quantity per dose, incorrect number of doses per day, omitting or "doubling up" doses, discontinuing prematurely), and/or taking discontinued medications or nonprescribed drugs and alcohol in addition to or in place of the prescribed drug (Cohen, 1980). Although compliance issues are important for any prescribed medication, they become even more pertinent when the drug in question has abuse or addiction potential.

Addiction, Tolerance, and Dependence

The term *addiction,* or *substance dependence* as defined in the *DSM-IV* (American Psychiatric Association, 1994), refers to a constellation of symptoms marked by compulsive drug use, drug seeking, and the continued use of the substance despite significant substance-related social, familial, and occupational problems. *Substance abuse* is a less severe disorder

which involves a pattern of adverse consequences from repeated use of a substance. *Tolerance* refers to the need for greater amounts of a drug to achieve the desired or usual effect or a markedly diminished effect with continued use of the same amount of the substance. *Withdrawal* is a maladaptive behavioral change that occurs when blood or tissue concentrations of a substance decline after heavy use of the substance.

Evidence of tolerance and withdrawal are included in the list of symptoms of substance dependence, but neither tolerance nor withdrawal is necessary or sufficient for a diagnosis of substance dependence (O'Brien, 1996). Physical dependence is a state that develops as a result of tolerance and is a natural biological phenomenon. It is produced by a homeostatic resetting of the body in response to repeated administration of a substance and the symptoms do not imply that the individual is involved in abuse or addiction. Physical dependence is defined by the occurrence of an abstinence syndrome, that is, withdrawal, subsequent to an abrupt dose reduction or administration of an antagonist (Dole, 1972; Jaffe, 1985; Martin & Jasinski, 1969; Redmond & Krystal, 1984). Patients treated with substances in a medically supervised manner may still show tolerance, physical dependence, and withdrawal symptoms if the drug is stopped abruptly rather than gradually (O'Brien, 1996). Therefore, the occurrence of tolerance and dependence do not imply an addiction, but derive from basic physiological adaptations of the body to the presence of a drug and, as such, can occur in response to regular use of both addictive and nonaddictive drugs (Jaffe, 1990; Miller & Gold, 1993).

The distinction between physical dependence and addiction has been demonstrated in animal studies of opioid self-administration, which have shown persistence of drug-taking behavior even in the absence of physical dependence (Dai, Corrigal, Coen, & Kalant, 1989). Studies have shown that once initial tolerance has developed, animals continue to self-administer fixed doses of morphine and if self-administration is interrupted, the signs and symptoms of withdrawal appear. However, long after the resolution of tolerance and dependence, self-administration has been shown to be rapidly reinstated, indicating the animals have become addicted (Bozarth & Wise, 1983; Deneu, Hangita, & Seevers, 1969).

Clinical Issues Relevant for Opioid Medications

There are two major clinical issues relevant for this chapter on the use of potentially addictive opioid medications. The first important issue relates to the addictive properties of opioids and the consequent need for proper diagnosis and assessment of presenting symptoms of addiction in those afflicted patients. The second related issue is on the other end of the continuum, that of the underprescribing of opioids when they are clearly medically indicated, resulting in some patients suffering unjustifiably. Common to both issues is the need for physicians' increased awareness and understanding of the signs and symptoms of the disorder, careful clinical management, and thorough follow-up of patients who are prescribed opioids.

Iatrogenic addiction refers to the abuse or addictive use of a substance following initiation by a treating physician. Similarly, the term "medical addict" has been coined to refer to the patient who, in the course of treatment for a medical disorder, has become addicted to the medication. The prototypical behaviors include obtaining prescriptions from multiple doctors, visiting emergency rooms with high frequency to obtain the drug, taking the drug in a manner that is unsupervised by appropriate medical care workers, or a combination of these behaviors. There are several published case reports on iatrogenic or medically induced opiate addiction (Portnow & Strassman, 1985; Twerski, 1978; Walker, 1978; Wilford, 1990). The majority of these reports describe the need for specialized treatment, dose tapering, or methadone induction for patients in whom previously treating physicians indiscriminately doled out percodan or morphine, or prescribed opioids without assessing concomitant alcohol or other drug abuse.

Although the DEA reports that 3% of the U.S. population misuses psychoactive medications, research is lacking on the extent, nature, and course of iatrogenic opioid addiction. At present, the etiology for the development and maintenance of opioid abuse and addiction in medical patients is unclear, but may relate to both patient- and clinician-related factors. The paucity of research in this area limits our understanding of the neurophysiologic and clinical relationships among addictive disease, pain management, and individual differences or inherent vulnerability to abuse and addiction. Current estimates of the extent and incidence of opioid addiction are largely based on speculation, case studies, and a few well-controlled studies and general household surveys (Savage, 1993).

Obvious evidence of abuse or addiction in the treated patient includes compulsive use of illicit drugs or illegal behaviors, such as prescription forgery, drug acquisition from nonmedical sources, drug sales of prescribed opioids, or the use of an illicit opioid to supplement therapy (Portenoy & Payne, 1992). It is important for physicians to assess thoroughly compulsive use and other aberrant drug-seeking behavior. Some addicts feign illness to obtain drugs for diversion or personal use (Wilford, 1990). In other cases, it may be that the patient has a genuine medical illness, but seeks opioid drugs to sustain an addiction rather than treat the presenting symptom.

The practitioner needs to be keenly aware of the risk for addiction and the difficult distinction between appropriate and inappropriate drug-taking behavior. For example, drug-seeking behavior may be solely in the context of inadequate pain relief. Some cancer patients have been termed "pseudoaddicts" in that they express intense concern and psychological distress about opioid availability, but this is related to inadequate pain relief; the behaviors are completely resolved when adequate pain relief is achieved (Weissman & Haddox, 1989).

In addition to the more obvious signs of abuse or addiction in medically treated patients, there are some more subtle signs of compulsive use such as unsanctioned dose escalation, use of the drug to treat symptoms other than those targeted by the therapy, frequent visits to emergency rooms, and hoarding of drugs obtained from routine prescriptions (Portenoy & Payne, 1992). Also, the addicted patient may show signs of relapse after withdrawal, which is a very common feature of substance dependence. The skillful clinician should properly assess the circumstances of the relapse and view it as an opportunity to provide intervention and introduce the patient to treatment for opioid abuse or addiction.

On the other end of the continuum is the physician's reluctance either to prescribe or use adequate doses of opioid analgesic medications when they are clearly indicated to alleviate pain. For example, one common problem in treating cancer patients is that physicians underestimate the level of pain that the patient may be experiencing and are often reluctant to prescribe opiate medications. This is most likely due to lack of knowledge about tolerance and physical dependence, which normally occur with repeated use of drugs from many different categories (O'Brien, 1996). Tolerance and physical manifestations of dependence do not imply addiction or abuse, which are behavioral sequelae involving compulsive use and lack of control. As a consequence of this common misunderstanding, patients experiencing pain are often denied adequate treatment. If pain is not controlled, the patient may have to undergo potentially unnecessary or repeated diagnostic procedures, additional incurred costs, attempts at cessation, and treatment for additional conditions such as anxiety or depression (Gold, 1989).

Case review data suggest that, with proper medical management, only a very few patients with no history of addiction who are prescribed opioids begin their drug addiction via misuse of prescription medications (Perry & Heidrich, 1982; Porter & Hick, 1980). However, it is unclear how many patients are receiving appropriate treatment, and therefore, the number of patients becoming addicted might be higher than current estimates. Also,

given that 3%–16% of the population have addictive disorders (Regier, Meyers, & Kramer, 1984; Vailliant, 1983) and other individuals are at high risk based on genetic and other factors (Cloninger, Bohman, & Sivardsson, 1981; Goodwin, Schulsinger, Hermansen, Guze, & Winokur, 1983), patient-related characteristics must be taken into account before any conclusions regarding narcotic abuse and addiction are drawn. In light of this issue, it is imperative that physicians assess each patient individually in terms of presenting symptoms of pain and potential vulnerability for addiction. Patients must be taught that opiate drugs provide easy but incomplete pain relief and that behavior and lifestyle changes are needed for both adequate pain management and addiction recovery (Miotto, Compton, Ling, & Conolly, 1996). Opioids can continue to be a legitimate and successful adjunct in the treatment of chronic pain even in those individuals with addictive disease.

Pain Management and Addictive Disease

General Issues

The major risk for abuse or addiction occurs in patients complaining of pain with no clear physical explanation or with evidence of a chronic non-life-threatening disorder such as chronic headache, backache, or peripheral neuropathy (O'Brien, 1996). In these cases, a treating physician might consider an opioid as a brief emergency treatment, but long-term treatment with opioids is not advisable.

Pain is often viewed as an entity characterized in terms of intensity, with little understanding of the nature and etiology of both acute and chronic pain. The different types of pain may involve separate pathophysiological mechanisms that differ in susceptibility to analgesic drugs (Arnér & Meyerson, 1988; Foley & Intrurrisi, 1986). Other dimensions of pain, such as character and site, are not fully taken into account when response to medication is assessed (Kaiko, Wallenstein, Rogers, Grabinski, & Houde, 1986). Unfortunately, this confusion may result in the prescribing of analgesics and opioid medications on the mere reporting of "pain" without further specification. One double-blind study showed that primary nociceptive pain but not neuropathic pain was effectively alleviated with morphine or equivalent doses of other opioids (Arnér & Meyerson, 1988). This finding highlights the importance of recognizing different neurobiological mechanisms of pain and differences in responsiveness to analgesic drugs. Although there are some studies in animals (Dennis & Melzack, 1980; Schmauss & Yaksh, 1984) and clinical trials in humans (Arnér & Arnér, 1985; Arnér & Meyerson, 1988; Bloomfield, Barden, & Mitchell, 1976), there is still a great need for research in pain classification, pathophysiologic mechanisms, and differential response to analgesic drugs.

The management of pain associated with major trauma is especially relevant to the addictive disease population, given that alcohol and drug abusers experience a higher incidence of accidents, injuries, and medical disorders and therefore may be targeted for short- or long-term opioid management at a higher rate than the general nonaddicted population (Cameron, 1964; Sapiro, 1968). In a study of nearly 400 consecutive admissions to a community hospital for traumatic injury, 40% were intoxicated with alcohol at the time of injury (Reyna, Hollis, & Hulsebus, 1985). Although the prevalence of addiction has also been documented to be higher (i.e., 19%–25%) in general surgical and medical patients than in the general population (Graham, 1991; Moore *et al.*, 1989), lack of proper screening and assessment results in undiagnosed or underdiagnosed addiction in pain management patients and therefore improper pain management strategies. Treatment for pain associated with injury or trauma can usually proceed using the WHO analgesic ladder as a general guideline, with an initial trial of an NSAID or mild opioid analgesic, along with careful assessment of patient characteristics and frequent compliance inquiries.

Headache is the pain syndrome for which doctors in the United States are most fre-quently consulted (Ziegler, 1994). Oral opiate drugs such as codeine, oxycodone, and propoxyphene are the most commonly prescribed medication for headache. Although the etiology of headache syndromes is not well understood, one often-cited theory for migraine headaches is that they derive from stimulation of pain endings in blood vessel walls. Migraine pain could therefore be classified as nociceptive and a rationale could be given for its relief by opioid medications (Ziegler, 1994). However, other types of headache, such as "tension headache," are most idiopathic in origin and, therefore, treatment with opioid medications has been called into question (Ziegler, 1994).

Cancer pain most often arises secondarily from tumor growth invasion of soft tissues, nerves, bone, and muscles (Conroy & Harvey, 1996). Management of the pain is often successful with pharmacologic strategies using opiate medications such as morphine, hydromorphone, or methadone, perhaps in conjunction with nonopioid pain relievers (National Institute of Health, 1987; World Health Organization, 1986). Cancer pain specialists have accumulated much evidence in support of the opioid management of pain, especially in the more advanced stage of the disease (Portenoy & Payne, 1992) with dose escalations indicated when the level of pain increases due to tumor growth (Conroy & Harvey, 1996). Conversely, treatment response or disease remission requires careful medical management and dose tapering and reduction.

Another clinically relevant issue is that clinicians should avoid treating pain as an isolated entity, as patients often suffer from concomitant anxiety or emotional distress (Cherny & Portenoy, 1993). Depression is present in one fourth of cancer patients (Bukberg, Penman, & Holland, 1984; Conroy & Harvey, 1996; Massie & Holland, 1990; Plumb & Holland, 1977), with the depressive symptoms possibly interacting with and altering the general perception of and reaction to pain. In addition, suicidal thoughts may occur with the other signs and symptoms of clinical depression or as a result of improperly managed or uncontrolled pain (Breitbart, 1987). Psychotherapy, support groups, cognitive-behavioral techniques of imagery or relaxation training, acupuncture, acupressure, and the use of heat, cold, massage, or vibration may enable the patient to have an active role in symptom management and counter the sense of loss of control.

Pain Management in Patients with Histories of Substance Abuse

Clinical experience suggests three major subgroups for treatment of pain in patients with past or ongoing opioid dependence: patients who are active opioid addicts (i.e., engaging in drug-seeking behavior and not currently in treatment), patients in methadone maintenance treatment, and patients who are former opioid abusers (Foley, 1985). Unfortunately, there have been no adequate studies to address the needs and problems posed by these patient types during pain management. However, such distinctions have been generated from clinical practice and might identify patients with potential pain management problems, which in turn might facilitate assessment and therapeutic strategies (Portenoy & Payne, 1992). A further subclassification of this general scheme for pain management has been suggested; this includes a category for those patients who have either past or current alcohol or nonopioid drug abuse or addiction (Portenoy & Payne, 1992). The medical and psychological needs of patients in any of these subgroups can be properly managed, but individualized assessment and consultation with specialists in chemical dependency is strongly recommended (Fultz & Senay, 1975).

Selection of an appropriate drug includes initial selection of nonopioid versus opioid, choice of pure opioid agonist versus partial agonists or agonist–antagonist, choice of "weak" versus "strong" opioid, route of administration, dosing guidelines, side effects, and use of adjuvant analgesics. The first subgroup (active users) represents perhaps the most difficult to treat for pain management, given drug interactions, poor compliance, and denial of substance abuse problems and consequences. Pain

assessment can be complicated by the fact that symptoms may resemble drug-seeking behavior (Foley, 1985) and therefore opioid analgesics may be underprescribed. On the other hand, patients with a history of substance abuse might be at risk for noncompliance and thus undermine the efficacy of opioid therapy. This is most likely due to patients' fear of these medications as mood-altering drugs and a fear of risk for relapse to the drug of choice or to opioids or related drugs. However, in the context of a good therapeutic relationship, these issues can be discussed appropriately and the possibility of relapse also should be explored in terms of risks associated with unmanaged pain symptomatology. Thus, optimal treatment of people with former addictive disorders should incorporate careful, ongoing assessment of drug-taking behavior and the recognition that successful treatment may be compromised by attitudes of both clinicians and patients.

The final general category includes those patients in methadone maintenance programs. One of the most egregious errors in incorporating pain treatment in this population is the assumption that a single daily dose of methadone, which is used for the management of the addiction, is also adequate for pain management (Portenoy & Payne, 1992). This view is in contrast to the clinical data in cancer pain management indicating sustained analgesia maintained by at least three doses of the medication daily (Sawe *et al.,* 1981). Another perceived problem with this group is that a stabilized methadone maintenance patient may return to aberrant drug-taking behaviors or may lose control given therapeutic regimen of opioids. Again, careful ongoing management and an ongoing positive therapeutic alliance with the patient decreases the likelihood of the return to addictive use of opioid drugs. Finally, another potential complication in this subgroup of patients is failure of the staff to recognize potential for tolerance. Although there are no data to confirm that tolerance might reduce the efficacy of opioid treatment in methadone patients, it is possible that the typical initial dose might not produce relief of pain, and the continued report of pain might be perceived as manipulative or addictive behavior rather than inadequate dosing; this would result in erosion of trust in the relationships between the patient and treatment staff.

Summary

It is strongly suggested that additional research focus on the incidence of and the initiation, maintenance, and relapse to opioid abuse or addiction in the medically treated patient. Future investigations should emphasize patient subgroups, past substance abuse history, individual differences in vulnerability to addiction, and the qualifications and expertise of treating physicians as important potential factors that may each play a role in opioid abuse and addiction liability.

References

American Psychiatric Association. (1994). *Diagnostic and statistical manual of mental disorders* (4th ed.). Washington, DC: Author.

Arnér, S., & Arnér, B. (1985). Differential effects of epidural morphine in the treatment of cancer-related pain. *Acta Anaesthesiologica Scandinavica, 29,* 332–336.

Arnér, S., & Meyerson, B. A. (1988). Lack of analgesic effect of opioids on neuropathic and idiopathic forms of pain. *Pain, 33,* 11–23.

Bloomfield, S. S., Barden, T. P., & Mitchell, J. (1976). Aspirin and codeine in two postpartum pain models. *Clinical Pharmacology & Therapeutics, 24,* 499–503.

Bozarth, M. A., & Wise, R. A. (1983). Dissociation of the rewarding and physical dependence-producing properties of morphine. In L. S. Harris (Ed.), *Problems of drug dependence* (NIDA Research Monograph Series No. 43, pp. 171–177). Washington, DC: U.S. Government Printing Office.

Breitbart, W. (1987). Suicide in cancer patients. *Oncology Review, 1,* 49–55.

Buck, M., & Paice, J. A. (1994). Pharmacologic management of acute pain in the orthopaedic patient. *Orthopaedic Nursing, 13,* 14–23.

Bukberg, J., Penman, D., & Holland, J. (1984). Depression in hospitalized cancer patients. *Psychosomatic Medicine, 46,* 199–212.

Cameron, A. J. (1964). Heroin addicts in a casualty department. *British Medical Journal, 1,* 594.

Canadell-Carafi, J., Moreno-Londono, A., & Gonzalez-Caudevilla, B. (1991). Ketorolac, a new non-opioid analgesic: A single-blind trial versus buprenorphine in pain after orthopaedic surgery. *Current Medical Research & Opinion, 12,* 343–349.

Cherny, N. I., & Portenoy, R. K. (1993). Cancer pain management. *Cancer, 72,* 3393–3415.

Cloninger, C., Bohman, M., & Sivardsson, S. (1981). Inheritance of alcohol abuse: Cross fostering analysis of adopted men. *Archives of General Psychiatry, 38,* 861–868.

Cohen, S. (1980). Drug abuse and the prescribing physician. In S. Cohen, D. Katz, C. Buchwald, & V. Solomon (Eds.), *Frequently prescribed and abused drugs: Their indications, efficacy and rational prescribing* (NIDA Monograph Series No. 2, pp. 1–6). Rockville, MD: National Institute on Drug Abuse.

Conroy, J. M., & Harvey, S. C. (1996). Management of cancer pain. *Southern Medical Journal, 89,* 744–760.

Dai, S., Corrigal, W. A., Coen, K. M., & Kalant, H. (1989). Heroin self-administration by rats: Influence of dose and physical dependence. *Pharmacology, Biochemistry and Behavior, 32,* 1009–1015.

Deneu, G., Hangita, T., & Seevers, M. H. (1969). Self-administration of psychoactive substances by the monkey. *Psychopharmacology, 16,* 30–48.

Dennis, S. G., & Melzack, R. (1980). Pain modulation by 5-hydroxytrytaminergic agents and morphine as measured by three pain tests. *Experimental Neurology, 69,* 260–270.

Dole, V. P. (1972). Narcotic addiction, physical dependence and relapse. *New England Journal of Medicine, 286,* 988–992.

Drug Enforcement Administration. (1987). *Guidelines for prescribers of controlled substances.* Washington, DC: U.S. Department of Justice.

Foley, K. M. (1981). *Current controversies in the management of cancer pain* (NIDA Research Monograph Series No. 36, pp. 169–181). Rockville, MD: National Institute on Drug Abuse.

Foley, K. M. (1985). The treatment of cancer pain. *New England Journal of Medicine, 313,* 84–95.

Foley, K. M. (1993). Opioid analgesics in clinical pain management. In A. Herz (Ed.), *Handbook of experimental pharmacology: Vol. 104/II. Opioids II* (pp. 697–743). Berlin: Springer-Verlag.

Foley, K. M., & Inturrisi, C. E. (1986). *Opioid analgesics in management of clinical pain. Advances in pain research and therapy* Vol. 8. New York: Raven.

Fultz, J. M., & Senay, E. C. (1975). Guidelines for management of hospitalized narcotic addicts. *Annals of Internal Medicine, 82,* 815–818.

Gold, M. S. (1989). Opiates. In A. E. Slaby & J. A. Giannini (Eds.), *Drugs of abuse* (pp. 127–144). Oradell, NJ: Medical Economics Publishing Group.

Gold, M. S., & Miller, N. S. (1997). Intoxication and withdrawal from opiates and inhalants. In N. S. Miller, M. S. Gold, & D. E. Smith (Eds.), *Manual of therapeutics for addictions* (pp. 72–85). New York: Wiley.

Goldstein, A., & Naidu, A. (1989). Multiple opioid receptors: Ligand selectivity profiles and binding site signatures. *Molecular Pharmacology, 36,* 265–272.

Goodwin, D. W., Schulsinger, F., Hermansen, L., Guze, S. B., & Winokur, G. (1983). Alcohol problems in adoptees raised apart from alcoholic biological parents. *Archives of General Psychiatry, 28,* 238–243.

Graham, A. W. (1991). Screening for alcoholism by lifestyle risk assessment in a community hospital. *Archives of Internal Medicine, 121,* 958–963.

Inturrisi, C. E., Mitchell, B. M., Foley, K. M., Schultz, M., Shin, S. U., & Houde, R. W. (1984). The pharmacokinetics of heroin in patients with chronic pain. *New England Journal of Medicine, 310,* 1213–1217.

Jaffe, J. H. (1985). Drug addiction and drug abuse. In A. G. Gilman, L. S. Goodman, T. W. Rall, & F. Murad (Eds.), *The pharmacological basis of therapeutics* (7th ed., pp. 532–581). New York: Macmillan.

Jaffe, J. H. (1990). Drug addiction and drug abuse. In A. G. Gilman, T. W. Rall, A. S. Nies, & P. Taylor (Eds.), *The pharmacological basis of therapeutics* (8th ed., pp. 522–573). New York: Macmillan.

Kaiko, R. F., Wallenstein, S. L., Rogers, A. G., Grabinski, P. Y., & Houde, R. W. (1981). Analgesic and mood effects of heroin and morphine in cancer patients with postoperative pain. *New England Journal of Medicine, 304,* 1501–1505.

Kaiko, R. F., Wallenstien, S. L., Rogers, A. G., Grabinski, P. Y., & Houde, R. W. (1986). Clinical analgesic studies and sources of variation in analgesic responses to morphine. In K. M. Foley & C. E. Inturrisi (Eds.), *Opioid analgesics in management of clinical pain: Advances in pain research and therapy* (Vol. 8, pp. 13–23). New York: Raven.

Kreek, M. J. (1973). Medical safety and side effects of methadone in tolerant individuals. *Journal of the American Medical Association, 223,* 665–668.

Kreek, M. J. (1978). Medical complications in methadone patients. *Annals of the New York Academy of Sciences, 311,* 110–134.

Kreek, M. J. (1979). Methadone in treatment: Physiological and pharmacological issues. In R. I. Dupont, A. Goldstein, & J. O'Donnell (Eds.), *Handbook on drug abuse* (pp. 57–86). Washington, DC: U.S. Government Printing Office.

Kreek, M. J. (1992). Rationale for maintenance pharmacotherapy of opiate dependence. In C. P. O'Brien & J. H. Jaffe (Eds.), *Addictive states, association for research in nervous and mental disease* (Vol. 70, pp. 205–230). New York: Raven.

Manion, J. C. (1995). Cancer pain management in the hospice setting. *Minnesota Medicine, 78,* 25–28.

Markenson, J. A. (1996). Mechanisms of chronic pain. *American Journal of Medicine, 101,* 6S–18S.

Martin, W. R., & Jasinski, D. R. (1969). Physiological parameters of morphine dependence in man—Tolerance, early abstinence, protracted abstinence. *Journal of Psychiatric Research, 7,* 9–17.

Massie, M. J., & Holland, J. C. (1990). Depression and the cancer patient. *Journal of Clinical Psychiatry, 7,* 12–17.

Mattia, A., Vanderah, T., Mosberg, H. I., & Porreca, F. (1991). Lack of antinociceptive cross-tolerance between [D-Pen2, D-Pen5]enkephalin and [D-Ala2]del-

torphin II in mice: Evidence for delta receptor subtypes. *Journal of Pharmacology and Experimental Therapeutics, 258,* 583–587

McCaffrey, M. (1987). Giving meperidine for pain: Should it be so mechanical? *Nursing, 17,* 61–64.

McCaffrey, M., & Beebe, A. (1989). Pharmaceutical control of pain. In *Pain: Clinical manual for nursing practice* (pp. 42–128). St. Louis: C. V. Mosby.

Miller, N. S. (1991). Special problems of the alcohol and multiple-drug dependent: Clinical interactions and detoxification. In R. J. Frances & S. I. Miller (Eds.), *Clinical textbook of addictive disorders* (pp. 194–218). New York: Guilford.

Miller, N. S., & Gold, M. S. (1993). A neurochemical basis for alcohol and other drug addiction. *Journal of Psychoactive Drugs, 25,* 121–128.

Miotto, K., Compton, P., Ling, W., & Conolly, M. (1996). Diagnosing addictive disease in chronic pain patients. *Psychosomatics, 37,* 223–235.

Moore, R. D., Bone, L. R., Geller, G., Mamon, J. A., Stokes, E. J., & Levine, D. M. (1989). Prevalence, detection and treatment of alcoholism in hospitalized patients. *Journal of the American Medical Association, 261,* 403–407.

National Institute of Health Consensus Development Conference. (1987). The integrated approach to the management of pain. *Journal of Pain and Symptom Management, 2,* 35–44.

O'Brien, C. P. (1996). Drug addiction and drug abuse. In J. G. Hardman, L. E. Limbird, P. B. Molinoff, R. W. Rudden, & A. G. Gilman (Eds.). *The pharmacological basis of therapeutics* (9th ed., pp. 557–577). New York: McGraw Hill.

Paul, D., Bodnar, R. J., Gistrak, M. A., & Pasternak, G. W. (1989). Different mu receptor subtypes mediate spinal and supraspinal analgesia in mice. *European Journal of Pharmacology, 168,* 307–314.

Perry, S., & Heidrich, G. (1982). Management of pain during débridement: A survey of U.S. burn units. *Pain, 13,* 267–280.

Pert, C. B., & Snyder S. H. (1973). Opiates receptor: Demonstration in nervous tissue. *Science, 179,* 1011–1014.

Plumb, M. M., & Holland, J. C. (1977). Comparative studies of psychological function in patients with advanced cancer. *Psychosomatic Medicine, 39,* 264–176.

Portenoy, R. K., & Payne, R. (1992). Acute and chronic pain. In J. H. Lowinson, P. Ruiz, R. B. Millman, & J. G. Langrod (Eds.), *Substance abuse: A comprehensive textbook* (2nd ed., pp. 691–721). Baltimore, MD: Williams & Wilkins.

Porter, J., & Hick, H. (1980). Addiction rare in patients treated with narcotics [Letter]. *New England Journal of Medicine, 302,* 123.

Portnow, J. M., & Strassman, H. D. (1985). Medically induced drug addiction. *International Journal of the Addictions, 20,* 605–611.

Portoghese, P. S., Sultana, M., Nagase, H., & Takemori, A. E. (1992). A highly selective delta-1 opioid receptor antagonist: 7-benzylidenenaltroxone. *European Journal of Pharmacology, 218,* 195–196.

Redmond, D. E., & Krystal, J. H. (1984). Multiple mechanisms of withdrawal from opioid drugs. *Annual Review of Neuroscience, 7,* 443–478.

Regier, D., Meyers, J. K., & Kramer, M. (1984). The NIMH epidemiological catchment area study. *Archives of General Psychiatry, 41,* 934–958.

Reisine, T., & Pasternak, G. (1996). Opioid analgesics and antagonists. In J. G. Hardman, L. E. Limbird, P. B. Molinoff, R. W. Ruddon, & A. G. Gilman (Eds.), *The pharmacological basis of therapeutics* (9th ed., pp. 521–555). New York: McGraw Hill.

Reyna, T. M., Hollis, H., & Hulsebus, R. C. (1985). Alcohol related trauma. *Annals of Surgery, 201,* 194–199.

Sapiro, J. D. (1968). The narcotic addict as a medical patient. *American Journal of Medicine, 45,* 555–588.

Savage, S. R. (1993). Addiction in the treatment of pain: Significance, recognition, and management. *Journal of Pain and Symptom Management, 8,* 265–278.

Sawe, J., Hansen, J., Ginman, C., Hartvig, P., Jakobsson, P., Nilsson, M., Rane, A., & Anggard, E. (1981). A patient-controlled dose regimen of methadone in chronic cancer pain. *British Medical Journal, 282,* 771–773.

Sawynok, J. (1986). The therapeutic use of heroin: A review of the pharmacological literature. *Canadian Journal of Physiology and Pharmacology, 64,* 1–6.

Schmauss, C., & Yaksh, T. (1984). In vivo studies on spinal opiate receptor systems mediating antinociception: II. Pharmacological profiles suggesting a differential association of mu, delta and kappa receptors with visceral chemical and cutaneous termal stimuli in the rat. *Journal of Pharmacology and Experimental Therapeutics, 228,* 1–12.

Simon, E. J., Hiller, J. M., & Edelman, I. (1973). Stereospecific binding of the potent narcotic analgesic [3H]Etorphine to rat brain homogenate. *Proceedings of the National Academy of Sciences, 70,* 1947–1949.

Sofulglu, M., Portoghese, P. S., & Takemori, A. E. (1991). Differential antagonism of delta opioid agonists by naltrindole and its benzofuran analog (NTB) in mice: Evidence for delta opioid receptor subtypes. *Journal of Pharmacology and Experimental Therapeutics, 257,* 676–680.

Stambaugh, J. E. (1993). Role of nonsteroidal anti-inflammatory drug. In R. B. Patt (Ed.), *Cancer pain* (pp. 105–117). Philadelphia: Lippincott.

Terenius, L. (1973). Stereospecific interaction between narcotic analgesics and a synaptic plasma membrane

fraction of rat cerebral cortex. *Acta Pharmacologica et Toxicologica, 32,* 317–320.

Tucker, C. (1990). Acute pain and substance abuse in surgical patients. *Journal of Neuroscience Nursing, 22,* 339–350.

Twerski, A. J. (1978). Iatrogenic addiction no less devastating because it's legal. *Pennsylvania Medicine,* December, 21–24.

Twycross, R. G., & McQuay, H. J. (1989). Opioids. In P. Wall & R. Melzack (Eds.), *Textbook of pain* (pp. 686–724). New York: Churchill Livingstone.

Vailliant, G. E. (1983). *The natural history of alcoholism.* Cambridge, MA: Harvard University Press.

Walker, L. (1978). Iatrogenic addiction and its treatment. *International Journal of the Addictions, 13,* 461–473.

Walsh, T. D. (1983). Antidepressants in chronic pain. *Clinical Neuropharmacology, 6,* 271–295.

Weissman, D. E., & Haddox J. D. (1989). Opioid pseudoaddiction—An iatrogenic syndrome. *Pain, 36,* 363–366.

Wilford, B. B. (1987). *Prescribing controlled drugs.* Chicago: American Medical Association.

Wilford, B. B. (1990). Abuse of prescription drugs. *Western Journal of Medicine, 152,* 609–612.

Wise, R. A. (1989). The brain and reward. In J. M. Liedban & S. J. Cooper (Eds.), *The neuropharmacological basis of reward.* Oxford, England: Oxford University Press.

Wood, P. L., Richard, J. W., & Thakur, M. (1982). Mu opiate iso receptors: Differentiation with kappa agonists. *Life Sciences, 31,* 2313–2317.

World Health Organization. (1986). *Cancer pain relief.* Geneva, Switzerland: Author.

World Health Organization. (1990). *Technical report series. Cancer pain relief and palliative care.* Geneva, Switzerland: Author.

Zaki, P. A., Bilsky, E. J., Vanderah, T. W., Lai, J., Evans, C. J., & Porreca, F. (1996). Opioid receptor types and subtypes: The delta receptor as a model. *Annual Review of Pharmacology & Toxicology, 36,* 379–401.

Ziegler, D. K. (1994). Opiate and opioid use in patients with refractory headache. *Cephalalgia, 14,* 5–10.

Zukin, R. S., Eghbali, M., Olive, D., Unterwald, E. M., & Tempel, A. (1988). Characterization and visualization of rat and guinea pig brain kappa opioid receptors: Evidence for kappa 1 and kappa 2 opioid receptors. *Proceedings of the National Academy of Sciences of the United States of America, 85,* 4061–4065.

IX

Sedatives, Hypnotics, and Anxiolytics

Pharmacology of Sedatives, Hypnotics, and Anxiolytics

JEWELL W. SLOAN AND ELZBIETA P. WALA

Introduction

This chapter is concerned with the pharmacology of agents that are used therapeutically for the treatment of a variety of disorders including anxiety, sleep, and psychosomatic disorders, and for sedation, skeletal muscle relaxation, and for the treatment of epilepsy. The distinct classification of these agents as sedatives, hypnotics, and anxiolytics is clouded since they have overlapping pharmacologic activities. For example, some agents, particularly certain benzodiazepines, can be used therapeutically either to treat the aforementioned conditions or achieve the effects mentioned to one degree or another. The drugs that are discussed include the benzodiazepines (full and partial agonists, full and partial inverse agonists, and antagonists), buspirone, zolpidem, selected barbiturates, and other sedative-hypnotics of diverse chemical structures.

The sedative-hypnotics have central nervous system (CNS) depressant properties at higher doses and anxiety-relieving properties at lower doses. Although various unreliable concoc-

tions have been used since earliest times for these purposes, it was not until the mid 1800s that bromide, the first agent to be specifically used as a sedative-hypnotic, was introduced. Chloral hydrate, paraldehyde, sulfonal, and urathane were the only additional ones introduced until the 20th century ushered in the barbiturate era. After barbital and phenobarbital were introduced in the early 1900s, these drugs were so much in demand that by the 1970s 2,500 barbiturates had been synthesized and tested, more than 50 of which were in commercial use. The barbiturates were so popular that there was practically no interest in the development of other classes of drugs such as sedative-hypnotics, and consequently less than a dozen were successfully marketed prior to the 1960s. Eventually the need to separate the anticonvulsive from the sedative properties of phenobarbital in the treatment of epilepsy led to the introduction of two anticonvulsants (phenytoin and trimethadione) that had markedly reduced sedative properties. In the early 1950s chlorpromazine and meprobamate were introduced. These agents that have "taming" or "tranquilizing" properties have had an enormous impact on the field of psychiatry. Efforts in this direction continued and resulted in the synthesis of the benzodiazepines. Chlordiazepoxide (CDZ) was introduced into clinical medicine in 1961 followed by diazepam in

JEWELL W. SLOAN AND ELZBIETA P. WALA • Department of Anesthesiology, University of Kentucky College of Medicine, Lexington, Kentucky 40536.

Handbook of Substance Abuse: Neurobehavioral Pharmacology, edited by Tarter *et al.* Plenum Press, New York, 1998.

1963. These drugs introduced the benzodiazepine era of safer and more effective treatment of a wide variety of anxiety states, epilepsy, sleep disorders, muscle tension, and safer adjunct drug use in surgical anesthesia. The benzodiazepines gained popularity rapidly, mainly because they have a low propensity to produce fatal central nervous system (CNS) and respiratory depression, a greater dose margin between anxiolysis and sedation, and a reduced abuse potential compared with barbiturates. Currently, more than 3,000 benzodiazepines have been synthesized and approximately 35 are used clinically throughout the world. The benzodiazepines are now the drugs of choice for the previously mentioned conditions to such an extent that at present the barbiturates have become obsolescent but not obsolete as sedative-hypnotics.

Drugs that Act through Benzodiazepine Receptor(s)

Mechanism of Action

Electrophysiological Studies

Investigations into the actions of benzodiazepines at the spinal motoneuron level with regard to the phenomenon of presynaptic inhibition were aggressively pursued in the 1960s. The results of these early studies with diazepam (Schmidt, Vogel, & Zimmermann, 1967) were later explained by the role γ-aminobutyric acid (GABA) plays as neurotransmitter in the axo-axonal synapses on primary afferent endings (Bell & Anderson, 1972; Curtis, Duggan, Felix, & Johnson, 1971). In most studies, the local or systemic administration of benzodiazepines depressed the spontaneous or evoked electrical activity of the major neurons in all regions of the brain and spinal cord that release a variety of monoamines. These large neurons are regulated mainly by small inhibitory GABAergic interneurons arranged in both feedback and feedforward circuits. The application of GABA to this region of the neuron induces an increase in chloride conductance and prevents neuronal discharge, an effect that is prolonged by benzodiazepines and reversed by bicuculline. Further, repetitive afterdischarges produced by a single shock applied, for example, to a single neuron in the limbic system are depressed by benzodiazepines, a phenomenon which may be associated with antiseizure and antiepileptic activity. Benzodiazepines also depress posttetanic potentiation in doses that have no effect on transmission, an effect that may relate to antiseizure and muscle relaxant effects of benzodiazepines (Smith, 1992).

Discovery of Benzodiazepine Receptor(s)

Receptors with specificity for this class of drugs were first identified within the CNS by [^{3}H]-diazepam binding studies (cf. Braestrup, 1981). The high correlation between binding and pharmacologic activity led to the conclusion that these binding sites represented the primary site of action. At least two types of central benzodiazepine receptors (CBR) were originally identified, a high-affinity CBR1, accounting for most CBR in the cerebellum for which CL, 218872, zolpidem, and some β-carbolines show selectivity (Arbilla, Depoortere, George, & Langer, 1985; Klepner, Lippa, Benson, Sano, & Beer, 1979; Williams, 1984) and a low-affinity CBR2, the predominant receptor in the spinal cord. The largest functional difference that was identified between CBR1 and CBR2 was the strong sedative action of selective agonists for CBR1. Autoradiographic mapping of the rat CNS indicated that CBR1 are predominant in lamina IV of the cerebral cortex, the molecular layer of the cerebellum, the substantia nigra pars reticulata, ventral pallidum, and globus pallidus, whereas CBR2 are predominant in the molecular layer of the dentate gyrus, pyramidal cell layer of the hippocampus CA1, the basolateral amygdala, the nucleus accumbens, superior colliculus, the ventromedial hypothalamic nucleus, the caudate-putamen, and the dorsal horn of the spinal cord (cf. Niddam, Dubois, Scatton, Arbilla, & Langer, 1987; Richards, Möhler, & Haefely, 1986). Although there are some species differences in the regional distribution of the CBR subtypes, in humans, primates, and rats, CBR1 and CBR2 are preferentially localized in the sensorimotor and the limbic regions respectively (Dennis, Dubois, Benavides, & Scatton, 1988).

$GABA_A$ Receptors and Benzodiazepine Receptor Systems

The $GABA_A$ receptor contains an integral binding site for the CBR (a physiologic target structure for CBR ligands) located at some distance from the GABA binding site. The exact composition of the $GABA_A$ receptor is unknown; however, 5 subunits and their isoforms have been cloned and sequenced (6 α, 4 β, 3 γ, δ, and ρ) [cf. Persohn, Malherbe, & Richards, 1992, for review]. The binding site for GABA is associated mainly with the β subunit whereas the α subunit containing the binding site for benzodiazepines appears to require the presence of a γ subunit for benzodiazepine receptor-mediated modulatory effects. The $GABA_A$ receptor provides allosteric binding sites for the benzodiazepines, steroids, barbiturates, and possibly the γ-buterolactones, agents that can induce a positive or negative modulation of GABergic transmission (Sieghart, 1995). The $GABA_A$ receptor is known to have two benzodiazepine recognition sites, one that interacts with anxiolytic benzodiazepines and enhances GABA binding and another that interacts with anxiogenic beta-carbolines (inverse agonists) and depresses the function of the $GABA_A$ receptor channel. The binding of an agonist ligand (GABA, muscimol) to the $GABA_A$ receptor enhances benzodiazepine ligand binding to the anxiolytic CBR site. The CBR has been shown to be an allosteric modulatory site that can adjust the affinity and/or number of GABA-binding sites in either direction and may also bring about the coupling of GABA receptor activation to Cl^- channel opening (Haefely, Martin, & Schoch, 1990). Radio- and immunochemical mapping indicate that CBR are localized in CNS regions which have GABAergic innervation and where benzodiazepines have an electrophysiological effect. The highest densities of both GABAergic nerve terminals and CBR are found in the olfactory bulb. The distribution of $GABA_A$ and CBR correlate well in some laminae of the cerebral cortex; the pallidum has a dense GABAergic innervation and a high density of CBR and GABA receptors. The CBR are localized in the basolateral nucleus of the amygdala and in the substantia nigra, an area that receives major projections from the striatum (which is partly GABAergic) and from the globus pallidus (which is almost exclusively GABAergic). CBR1 and CBR2 are localized post- and presynaptically, respectively. The CBR and GABA receptors are concentrated in the superficial superior and inferior colliculus and in the cerebellum where $GABA_A$ and CBR receptors are concentrated in the molecular layers, but CBR are absent in GABAergic Purkinje cells. In the hippocampus, the distribution of GABA is related to the dendritic array of pyramidal and granule cells where the density of the CBR is lower in comparison with the density in the molecular layer. The CBR are localized in the lateral preoptic, ventromedial, lateral mammary, and subthalamic nuclei of the hypothalamus but not in the median eminence which has a GABAergic innervation; the thalamic GABAergic cells and nerve terminals are localized in the reticular nucleus. GABA receptors are concentrated in the dorsomedial part of the geniculate nuclei which corresponds with a moderate density of CBR, and, in the spinal cord, CBR and GABA receptors are concentrated in the dorsal horn (Richards *et al.*, 1986).

Although early binding studies showed the existence of at least two CBR receptors, the molecular cloning of $GABA_A$ receptor subunits and recombinant coexpression of these subunits have shown that an even greater number of $GABA_A$ receptor subtypes may exist *in vivo*. Experiments with both photolabeled and recombinant receptors suggest that the α_1 subunit expressed together with the β_1, γ_2 subunits mimics the native CBR1 subtype, whereas the CBR2 subtype consists of a heterogenous population of sites containing at least 3 different α subunits, α_2, α_3, and α_5 subunits. In most cases, activation of CBR associated with α_3 subunits causes a greater potentiation of the GABA-induced increase in Cl^- permeability than the receptors bearing α_1 or α_5 subunits

(Doble & Martin, 1992; Levitan *et al.*, 1988; Pritchett *et al.*, 1988; Schofield *et al.*, 1987; Verdoorn, 1994; Verdoorn, Draguhn, Ymer, Seeburg, & Sakmann, 1990).

Another important discovery that has enhanced our understanding of the CBR system was that of flumazenil, a benzodiazepine derivative that was found to be a specific CBR antagonist (Hunkeler *et al.*, 1981). It does not enhance GABAergic transmission and its binding to CBR is not enhanced by GABA. Agonists for the anxiogenic site (inverse agonists) inhibit GABAergic transmission and their effects are also inhibitable by flumazenil (Bianchi & Steiner, 1992). Thus, although the structure of the CBR\GABA$_A$ receptor complex *in vivo* is still elusive, our knowledge of the functioning of this system has shown rapid advances in recent years.

Peripheral Benzodiazepine Receptors

At about the same time as the CBR were identified, it was found that [^{3}H]-diazepam bound with high affinity to several rat peripheral tissues including kidney, adrenal glands, liver, and testes. These binding sites were found to be pharmacologically distinct from CBR1 and CBR2, were thought not to be connected to any GABA-regulated chloride channel, and were called the "peripheral benzodiazepine receptors" (PBR). This terminology is not exactly appropriate since the PBR are located in large part on the outer mitochondrial membrane and are widely distributed in tissues including the CNS. Effects of PBR on mitochondrial functions include the mediation of intermembrane cholesterol transport and of mitochondrial respiration thereby producing many cellular effects including alterations in cell growth and differentiation. The PBR can alter the rate of steroidogenesis by altering the rate of cholesterol transport to the mitochondrial cytochrome P-450$_{SCC}$ enzyme and may modulate the production of endogenous brain steroids by glial cells as well (Gavish, Bar-Ami, & Weitzman, 1992; Hertz, 1993; Krueger & Papadopoulos, 1993; Saano, 1993; Whitehouse, 1992). The P-450$_{SCC}$ enzyme is responsible for catalyzing the conversion of cholesterol to pregnenolone, the rate-controlling step in steriodogenesis. Further, several steroid metabolites alter GABA$_A$ receptor function (Morrow, Pace, Purdy, & Paul, 1990). These data suggest a possible indirect link between the CBR/GABA complex and PBR neuronal peripheral sites although the details for such an interaction are unknown. In this regard several benzodiazepines stimulate steroid production. There appear to be some inconsistencies with these findings, however, in that under some conditions benzodiazepines have also been found to inhibit steroidogenesis (Whitehouse, 1992). These inconsistencies may be related to differences in the concentration of the benzodiazepine ligand (Thomson, Fraser, & Kenyon, 1995).

It has been shown in a range of CNS pathologies that the PBR are markers of macrophage and microglial reactions to injury in the CNS and that the presence of high densities of PBR is indicative of tissue damage. Although the PBR are ubiquitous, their density is under a number of control systems, including hormonal (autocrine, paracrine, and endocrine) regulation; PBR-specific ligands produce different effects in different organs and up- or downregulation has been postulated to be one of the main mechanisms of regulating the function of the PBR. The PBR has two ligand-binding domains, one for an isoquinoline site, identified by high-affinity binding of the specific peripheral antagonist, PK 11195, and a benzodiazepine site identified by binding of the specific PBR agonist, Ro 5-4864 (4′-chlorodiazepam). The PBR density is high in the mitochondria of endocrine tissues such as the anterior pituitary, adrenal cortex, testes, ovaries, and uterus. The density of PBR in the ovary is increased during estrus, whereas treatment of male rats with estrogen for 10 days decreases PBR-binding sites in the testes but upregulates binding in the kidney (cf. Gavish, Bar-Ami, & Weitzman, 1993). Within the brain, the PBR are found mainly on glial cells, depending on the species. In the rat brain, the ventricular walls, choroid plexus, and the olfactory bulb have the highest density of PBR, followed by the brain stem, hypothalamus, cerebellum, cortex, striatum, and hippocampus (cf. Gavish *et al.*, 1993; Hertz, 1993). In the human brain, the PBR are heterogeneously distributed but limited to the gray matter with the highest densities in the forebrain structures (Doble *et al.*, 1987). The commonly used benzodiazepines have varying degrees of selectivity for the PBR.

Overview of Biochemical and Molecular Actions

Effective CBR agonists enhance GABA-ergic transmission but do not act as GABA agonists or antagonists nor do they alter the synthesis, release, or metabolism of GABA. The effectiveness of a given CBR agonist at a given central site depends on the structure of the GABA$_A$ receptor with relation to its subunit components. The consequence of this is that CBR agonists do not bind to all GABA$_A$ receptors and therefore the extent of benzodiazepine agonist potentiation of GABA will vary greatly at different synapses. Further, if no GABA is released within a synapse, or if the concentration of GABA is high enough to saturate all the GABA$_A$ receptors and produce a maximal effect, CBR agonists will produce no effect (Haefely, 1990; J. R. Martin & Haefely, 1995). The major effects of acute therapeutic doses of benzodiazepines appear to be the consequence of highly selective interactions with their receptor(s) on the GABA$_A$ complex. However, virtually no drug shows absolute specificity for one target site and the benzodiazepines are no exception. Evidence indicates that mechanisms other than the GABA$_A$ system are also involved. One example is in hippocampal neurons where the depressant effects of low concentrations of benzodiazepines are not blocked by the GABA antagonists bicuculline and picrotoxin (Polc, 1988). Further, neither bicuculline nor picrotoxin prevents the induction of sleep by benzodiazepines, whereas flumazenil is effective in this regard (Mendelson, 1992). Some benzodiazepine receptor ligands inhibit the uptake of adenosine and some, particularly in high doses, produce a depressant effect on voltage-dependent channels for Na$^+$ and Ca^{2+} (Polc, 1988). If the benzodiazepine ligands interact with the GABA receptor systems to exert their anxiolytic and anticonvulsant effects, the mechanism is unclear since the affected GABA systems are not involved in anxiety or seizures; serotonergic and other neurotransmitter systems appear to be more likely candidates. There may be endogenous ligand(s) for benzodiazepine receptors that are anxiogenic. In this regard, β-carbolines have been found to be elevated in conditions associated with high levels of anxiety. Additional evidence that benzodiazepines act through receptors that are not directly associated with the GABA$_A$ receptor came with the discovery of the PBR. Relative affinities of many CBR ligands are markedly different for the PBR than for those receptors associated with the GABA$_A$ complex. A wider range of selective drugs for the different receptors are needed, however, to convincingly equate pharmacologic effects with receptor subtypes.

Chemistry

Basic Structure and Some General Consequences of Its Modification

Table 1 shows the structure, half-life, main clinical use, and dosing regimen for drugs used clinically as anxiolytics, sedatives, and hypnotics in the United States. A few drugs that act through benzodiazepine receptors but are not approved for clinical use (indicated in Table 1) are also included since they have been studied extensively. The structures of the first benzodiazepines introduced into clinical medicine, chlordiazepoxide and diazepam, illustrate the basic benzodiazepine structure that includes a benzene ring (ring A) fused to a 7-membered ring with nitrogen atoms in the 1 and 4 positions (ring B). The benzodiazepines shown in Table 1 are all substituted in position 7 and the nitrogen in position 1 carries an alkyl substituent (such as a methyl group) in many benzodiazepines. The carbon atom in position 2 carries a methylamino group in chlordiazepoxide, but usually carries a C = O. Ring B can be fused to a five-membered heteroaromatic cycle at positions 1 and 2. A substituent on carbon 3 usually decreases activity, except

TABLE 1. Drugs that Produce (or Antagonize) Sedative, Hypnotic, or Anxiolytic Effects and Act through the Benzodiazepine Receptor(s)

	Generic name (trade name)	Mean or median half-life (hr) (range)	Main therapeutic use (representative dosing regimen)[a]
	Alprazolam (Xanax)	~12	Anxiety disorders (oral: 07.5–1.5 mg/day to a maximal 4 mg/day, dosage should be individualized)
	Chlordiazepoxide (Librium, others)	~10 (24–48)	Anxiety disorders; alcohol withdrawal; anesthetic premedication (oral: 15–40 mg up to maximum of 100 mg/day; IM, IV: dosage and administration varies according to indication 25–200 mg/day, maximum of 300 mg/day)
	Clonazepam (Klonopin)	~23 (18–50)	Antiepileptic (oral: 1.5–10 mg/day, maximum of 20 mg/day dosage must be individualized)
	Clorazepate (Tranxene, others) [parent drug] [active metabolite nordiazepam]	~2.0 (0.5–1.5) (40–50)	Anxiety disorders, antiepileptic (oral: 7.5–30 mg/day as anxiolytic, 15 mg at bedtime, initial dose 22.5 mg/day up to maximum 90 mg/day as anticonvulsant)

TABLE 1. *(Continued)*

Generic name (trade name)	Mean or median half-life (hr) (range)	Main therapeutic use (representative dosing regimen)[a]
Diazepam (Valium, others)	~43 (20–70)	Anxiety disorders, anticonvulsant, sedative, skeletal muscle relaxation, anesthetic premedication (oral: 4–40 mg/day IM, IV: dosage and administration varies according to indication)
Estazolam (Prosom)	(10–24)	Hypnotic (oral: 1–2 mg at bedtime)
Flunitrazepam[b] (Rohypnol)	~15 (9–25)	Hypnotic, anesthetic (oral: 0.5–2 mg at bedtime IM, IV: dosage and administration varies according to indication)
Flurazepam (Dalmane) [parent drug] [active metabolite desalkylflurazepam]	~74 (1.5–2.3) (47–100)	Hypnotic (oral: 15–30 mg at bedtime)

(continued)

TABLE 1. (*Continued*)

	Generic name (trade name)	Mean or median half-life (hr) (range)	Main therapeutic use (representative dosing regimen)[a]
	Halazepam[b] (Paxipam) [parent drug] [active metabolite nordiazepam]	~14 (9–28) (76–90)	Anxiety disorders (oral: 80–120 mg/day)
	Lorazepam (Ativan)	~14 (10–20)	Anxiety disorders; preanesthetic medication (oral, sublingual: 2–6 mg maximal 10 mg/day IM, IV: dosage and administration varies according to indication)
	Midazolam (Versed)	~1.9 (1.2–12.3)	Preanesthetic and intraoperative medication (oral: 7.5–15 mg at bedtime IM, IV: dosage and administration varies according to indication; should be closely monitored)
	Nordiazepam[b] (Desmethyl-diazepam; Nordiazepam; Nordaz)	~73 (30–100)	Tranquilizer (oral: 5–15 mg as divided daily dose)
	Oxazepam (Serex)	~8.0	Anxiety disorders (oral: 30–60 mg/day maximal 120 mg/day dosage should be individualized)

TABLE 1. (*Continued*)

Generic name (trade name)	Mean or median half-life (hr) (range)	Main therapeutic use (representative dosing regimen)[a]
Quazepam (Doral)	~39 (27–53)	Hypnotic (oral: 7.5–15 mg at bedtime)
Temazepam (Restoril)	~11 (3.5–18.4)	Hypnotic (oral: 7.5–30 mg at bedtime)
Trizolam (Halcion)	~2.9 (1.5–5.5)	Hypnotic (oral: 0.125–0.25 mg at bedtime; maximal 0.5 mg)
Zolpidem[c] (Ambien)	~2.2 (1.4–4.5)	Hypnotic (oral: 10–20 mg at bedtime dose should be individualized)

(*continued*)

TABLE 1. (*Continued*)

Generic name (trade name)	Mean or median half-life (hr) (range)	Main therapeutic use (representative dosing regimen)[a]
4'-Chlordiazepam[b] (Ro5-4864)	?	Specific peripheral agonist
Flumazenil (Romazicon)	~0.9 (0.7–1.3)	BZ central antagonist (IV: dosage and administration varies according to indication)
PK 11195[b,c]	~3.7	BZ peripheral antagonists

[a] The information contained in the above table is a compilation from extensive sources collected in healthy adults. The daily doses are given in mg/day assuming they are divided into 2–4 portions/day unless indicated otherwise. The information regarding doses and usage is for general comparative purposes and should not be used as a basis for medical decisions with regard to individual patients.
[b] Not approved for clinical use in the United States.
[c] Not a benzodiazepine.

for an OH group which can be acetylated to form an ester or a carbamate. The carboxyl group on carbon 3 allows chemically unstable water soluble salts to be made (clorazepate). Substituents in position 3 introduce a chirality center with only the S-enantomer able to interact with the benzodiazepine receptor(s). The nitrogen in position 4 is not usually oxidized (except for chlordiazepoxide) and is usually connected to C_5 by a double bond. Most benzodiazepines have a phenyl substitution in position 5. The phenyl ring is substituted by a carbonyl function in flumazenil (Haefely, Kyburz, Gerecke, & Mohler, 1985). Diazepam and flunitrazepam are potent PBR ligands, but the removal of the N-methyl group from their structure leads to a dramatic loss of affinity for the PBR whereas shifting fluorane from 2′ of flunitrazepam to a chlorine at the 4′ position of ring C or the addition of chlorine to the 4′ position of ring C of diazepam produced the first selective agonist for the PBR (4′chlordiazepam). PK 11195 is a potent and selective PBR antagonist chemically unrelated to the benzodiazepines (Bourguignon, 1993).

Pharmacology

General Effects

Within the therapeutic range, the benzodiazepines and other drugs that act as agonists at CBR receptors have a broad spectrum of reproducible pharmacologic effects, which have been thought to be due mainly to their selective action on the CNS. Depending on the drug, these effects range from full agonistic effects, such as those produced by diazepam with relatively low fractional occupancy of receptor sites; to partial agonistic effects (brought about by agonists that require relatively high fractional receptor occupancy to produce a maximal effect less intense than the full agonistic effect produced by diazepam); and to inverse agonistic or partial inverse agonistic effects (brought about by compounds that produce effects opposite to diazepam in the absence of benzodiazepinelike agonists). Most of these effects can be prevented or reversed by flumazenil, which suggests that they are principally mediated by one or more CBR subtypes (Hobbs, Rall, & Verdoorn, 1996).

Although there are often marked individual differences in the effects of a given dose of a specific benzodiazepine agonist there are many dose-related reproducible actions. These actions include the relief of anxiety, the calming of a hyperexcited state, the production of sedation, amnesia, drowsiness, and the impairment of cognitive functioning. Some patients feel both intoxicated and relaxed while others have dysphoric feelings. Some appear relaxed and free of anxiety; some are talkative, sleepy, have slurred speech, ataxia, and muscle incoordination, feel dizzy, have a headache, become nervous, nauseous, have unclear thought processes, and may become disinhibited and increasingly aggressive and hostile.

Therapeutic Treatment of Anxiety Disorders with Benzodiazepine Agonists

General Description of Anxiety

Anxiety is a subjective experience that is difficult to quantitate. It may be defined as a pervading feeling of apprehension or dread that often contains a fear component that may or may not be based on reality. Anxiety can take on harmful and medically meaningful effects when translated into behaviors and symptoms such as muscle tension, restlessness, tremors, headache, fatigue, tachypnea, tachycardia, chest pains, and other signs of a hyperactivated autonomic system.

Types of Anxiety Disorders

Anxiety, other than the generalized anxiety syndrome, is associated with many psychiatric disorders, including depression and schizophrenia. The different manifestations of anxiety include phobia (e.g., agoraphobia, simple phobias, social phobia), panic disorder, posttraumatic stress syndrome, and obsessive-compulsive disorder. In addition, anxiety has been shown to be produced by a wide variety of drugs including indomethacin, theophylline, caffeine, cocaine, and propranolol, as well as by a number of diseases such as hyperthyroidism, hypoglycemia, and coronary heart disease. Anxiolytic drugs can effectively relieve the anxiety associated with many of these syndromes. Drugs acting as full CBR agonists provide the predominant drug therapy of these disorders (see Table 1). The major group of drugs used for this purpose are the benzodiazepines. The most prevalent documented use of benzodiazepines in the literature is for the treatment of generalized anxiety disorders and by far the largest volume of studies pertains to diazepam. Comparisons of diazepam with barbiturates clearly showed that diazepam was consistently superior and safer for the therapeutic treatment of patients with anxiety and depression and this has contributed to the shift in prescribing from barbiturates to diazepam and other benzodiazepines (Hollister, Müller-Oerlinghausen, Rickels, & Shader, 1993).

Panic Disorders

One type of anxiety, panic disorder, has been distinguished from generalized anxiety disorder. It was found that high doses of alprazolam produced a clear antipanic effect. This has been confirmed, but there is a question as to whether this antipanic effect is specific for alprazolam among the benzodiazepines (Hollister & Csernansky, 1990; Judd, Norman, & Burrows, 1990).

Phobias

Few studies of the use of benzodiazepines for the treatment of phobias have been reported. The benzodiazepines alleviate acute anxiety in many patients to a level where they can begin desensitization therapy (Hollister *et al.*, 1993).

Posttraumatic Stress Syndrome and Obsessive-Compulsive Disorders

The benzodiazepines have been reported to be effective in the treatment of posttraumatic stress and obsessive-compulsive disorders. However, selective serotonin uptake inhibitors and clomipramine are the agents of choice for these purposes.

Efficacy in Long-Term Treatment of Anxiety

Many studies of animals suggest that tolerance develops to the effects of benzodiazepines (cf. File, 1990; File & Baldwin, 1989). This does not appear to be the case in humans where existing evidence supports the assumption that, contrary to prevalent opinions, benzodiazepines remain effective over long periods of use. Well-designed studies to test the long-term effects of these drugs in the treatment of anxiety disorders are lacking (Hollister *et al.*, 1993). Nevertheless, benzodi-

azepines should be prescribed with some degree of caution in the treatment of anxiety, and only in situations where they have been proven effective. A careful evaluation of the patient's lifestyle, eating habits, and medication regimen may suggest alternative nondrug methods of treatment.

Therapeutic Uses for Benzodiazepine Agonists as Sedatives and Hypnotics

Description of Sedative and Hypnotic States

The term "sedation" is an ambiguous one. It can refer to a normalization of an abnormally aroused state or it can refer to a reduction from a normal to a subnormal level of CNS function. Sedation results in a calming effect and a decrease in activity and excitement. The benzodiazepines produce amnesia that is patchy and generally not recognized by the patient. This amnesia can be retrograde, where past events are not remembered, but more frequently is anterograde, where the events taking place after benzodiazepine administration are lost to recall at a later time. This is a favorable effect in the management of surgical procedures but can be disastrous in the workplace or in elderly patients who have memory problems. Sedation is a side effect of many drugs that produce specific dose-related therapeutic effects at doses lower than those producing CNS depression. A hypnotic drug produces drowsiness and facilitates and maintains a state of sleep that resembles natural sleep with regard to the EEG.

Use in Surgical Anesthesia

Benzodiazepines are frequently used the night before surgery to relieve anxiety and apprehension and to help the patient sleep, and on the day of surgery to aid in the induction of anesthesia. The ability of benzodiazepines to potentiate the effects of general anesthesia is advantageous in maintenance (or balanced) anesthesia since this effect allows a reduction in the amount of opioids and other induction agents, thus reducing cardiorespiratory depressant effects. Benzodiazepine agonists, however, do not produce complete surgical anesthesia; therefore, analgesics must be given if there is a need to control pain. Diazepam and midazolam are the two benzodiazepines most frequently used for this purpose.

Sleep Disorders

Insomnia frequently occurs in situations where excitement, anxiety, fear, depression, pain, or discomfort are present and is estimated to affect about one third of the general population. In women and the elderly the prevalence is even higher (J. R. Martin & Haefely, 1995). Situational insomnia occurs in most people at one time or another and may be the result of a large spectrum of life stresses, environmental factors, lifestyle, the ingestion of certain drugs such as caffeine, amphetamines, and diet pills, and disease states that produce pain. Insomnia also appears to be a paradoxical effect of some drugs and situations including alcohol, benzodiazepines or hypnotics, antihistamines, and alcohol or drug dependence and withdrawal. Before prescribing a hypnotic for sleep, the nature of the sleep disturbance should be carefully assessed to determine the cause of the problem (Smith, 1992). The main reason for using these drugs as hypnotics is to prevent the disabling discomfort that can be produced by insomnia. Benzodiazepines acting as full CBR agonists are among the drugs predominantly used for sleep disorders (flurazepam, triazolam, temazepam, quazepam). In addition, a nonbenzodiazepine that acts as a full CBR agonist (zolpidem) has recently been added to the list. Drugs that have a short half-life are generally preferred as hypnotics to avoid daytime sleepiness. Flurazepam was the first benzodiazepine promoted as a hypnotic drug in the United States and for many years was the drug most often prescribed for insomnia. Although flurazepam has a short half-life in plasma, its major metabolite has a long half-life and may lead to daytime "hangover" and impaired mental function, particularly in the elderly. Short-acting drugs, such as triazolam, are not likely to produce hangover effects the next day but

can produce early morning awakening or rebound insomnia the next night (Smith, 1992).

Tolerance to the hypnotic effect has been reported to develop during even short-term administration of benzodiazepines. However, Hollister and colleagues (1993) in a comprehensive review of the literature found no consistent agreement on this issue, although some investigators found significant hypnotic effects after prolonged periods of nightly administration of benzodiazepines.

EEG Effects

Benzodiazepines administered in acute doses share certain common features in their effects on the EEG: decrease in the alpha (α) frequency band (8.5–12 Hz), increase in beta (β) activity (12–30 Hz) and occasional bursts of delta (δ) waves (0.5–3.5 HZ) (cf. Herrmann & Schaerer, 1986). A good correlation exists between blood concentration, anticonvulsant effect, and change in β activity produced by flunitrazepam, midazolam, oxazepam, and clobazam in rats (cf. Mandema & Danhof, 1992). In humans, diazepam blood levels correlate well with the increase in β frequency waves (Fink, Irwin, Weinfeld, Schwartz, & Conney, 1976; Friedman *et al.*, 1992) and the dose of midazolam correlates well with the increase in frontal β and decrease in occipital lobe α activity (Domino, French, Pohorecki, Galus, & Pandit, 1989).

The intensity of EEG effects produced by benzodiazepine agonists, partial agonists, antagonists, and inverse agonists differs significantly (Mandema, Sansom, Dios-Vièitez, Hollander-Jansen, & Danhof, 1991; Mandema, Kuck, & Danhof, 1992a, 1992b). Ligands with different selectivities for benzodiazepine receptors have different EEG profiles. In rabbits and rats, single doses of diazepam and flunitrazepam (CBR1, CBR2, PBR), clonazepam (CBR1, CBR2), and zolpidem (CBR1) induce spindle bursts in the EEG recorded from the neocortex. However, the largest increase in the power of β waves occurs after diazepam and clonazepam with a lesser effect observed after flunitrazepam and only a slight increase in β

waves after zolpidem. This suggests the involvement of CBR2 in the genesis of β activity (Longo, Massotti, DeMedici, & Valerio, 1988). Single and multiple doses of benzodiazepines have different effects on the EEG. After chronic treatment, changes in the EEG vary with the benzodiazepine (Valerio & Massotti, 1988). The rapid tolerance (2–5 days) that develops to the sedative effects of diazepam and flunitrazepam is accompanied by concomitant changes in the EEG consisting of replacement of the low-frequency spindles with high-frequency β waves (Iwaya, Morita, & Miyoshi, 1989; Massotti, Mele, & De Luca, 1990; Mele, Sagratella, & Massotti, 1984; Valerio & Massotti, 1988); however, the administration of much higher doses of diazepam and flunitrazepam can restore the EEG. Discontinuation of chronic benzodiazepines in humans results in a gradual decrease in fast waves toward the baseline (Hallstrom & Lader, 1981; Manmaru & Matsuura, 1990; Pétursson & Lader, 1981). The CBR antagonist, flumazenil, reverses the EEG produced by CBR agonists (cf. Mandema & Danhof, 1992) and with increasing concentrations produces a parallel shift to the right in the midazolam concentration-EEG effect relationship indicating a competitive CBR agonist–antagonist interaction (Briemer *et al.,* 1991; Mandema, Tukker, & Danhof, 1992). Interestingly, signs of EEG-manifested tolerance to the sedative effect of diazepam can be abolished by the PBR antagonist, PK 11195, and prevented by the concomitant administration of the PBR agonist, Ro 5-4864, during chronic treatment with clonazepam. This suggests that the increase in β activity that accompanies tolerance to the sedative effect of some benzodiazepines may be related to repeated and concurrent activation of CBR2 and PBR (Massotti *et al.,* 1990; Valerio & Massotti, 1988).

Multilead topical EEG recordings have shown that benzodiazepine effects on different EEG frequency bands in rats (Dimpfel, Spüller, & Nickel, 1986) and humans vary from one brain structure to another (Buchsbaum *et al.,* 1985; Kinoshita, Michel, Yagyu, Lehmann, & Saito, 1994; Yamedera, Kato,

Ueno, Tsukahara, & Okuma, 1993) suggesting that differences in the effect of benzodiazepines on sleep changes in the EEG are due to differences in the regional distribution of benzodiazepine receptor subtypes (Scheuler, 1990–1991).

Skeletal Muscle Relaxation

Muscle tone is known to be reduced by benzodiazepine agonists after a variety of experimental procedures in animals. Skeletal muscle relaxation has generally been attributed to a unique effect of diazepam and neither the active metabolites of diazepam nor most other benzodiazepines, including chlordiazepoxide, have been thought to be clinically useful for this purpose. However, despite the frequent use of diazepam to treat acute muscle spasm and the favorable clinical impressions of the effects, there have been few controlled studies in this regard and the findings have been inconsistent (Hollister *et al.,*1993).

Anticonvulsant Activity

Diazepam, nitrazepam, and clonazepam are among the CBR full agonists that are useful as antiepileptics (see Table 1). Benzodiazepines are indicated in all convulsive states of any cause. There are, however, differences among the benzodiazepines with regard to relative effective doses for their anticonvulsant as well as for their intoxicating activities (Chiu & Rosenberg, 1995). In spite of the fact that benzodiazepines are drugs of choice for status epilepticus, they are not preferred anticonvulsants for chronic treatment for two reasons: (1) tolerance develops to the anticonvulsant effects; and (2) in effective therapeutic doses, oversedation and impairment of cognitive functions make them undesirable.

Detoxification during Withdrawal from Alcohol and Other Drugs

Chlordiazepoxide and diazepam have been the benzodiazepine agonists most frequently used for acute alcohol withdrawal but others, including oxazepam, chlorazepate, alprazolam, and halazepam, have also been used. They all seem to be equally effective. Chlordiazepoxide and other benzodiazepine agonists have been shown to be effective in treating the psychiatric symptoms after acute withdrawal from alcohol; however, due to the dependence-producing properties of benzodiazepines, most physicians avoid their long-term use in patients who are at high risk of dependence. There is also some evidence that the benzodiazepine agonists may be useful in detoxification from heroin, for treating cocaine poisoning, and for ameliorating the effects of intoxication from LSD and other hallucinogens (Hollister *et al.*, 1993).

Mood, Psychosomatic, and Psychotic Symptoms and Disorders

Due to the diversity of depressive disorders, it is difficult to make general statements about the effectiveness of benzodiazepines for their treatment. Alprazolam has been thought to be the benzodiazepine of choice for this purpose but treatment in each case must be individualized. Current data suggest that benzodiazepines should be the drugs of choice. Midazolam and lorazepam are being promoted for the management of aggressive and violent patients either alone or in combination with antipsychotic agents (Smith, 1992). Benzodiazepines are also preferred for treating cardiovascular, respiratory, uriogenital, and gastrointestinal (GI) disorders where psychogenic factors cannot be eliminated by other treatments.

Pharmacokinetics: Benzodiazepine Agonists

Benzodiazepine agonists as well as available nonbenzodiazepine agonists have an overall poor water solubility except for some salts (chlorazepate dipotassium salt, chlordiazepoxide hydrochloride, flurazepam hydrochloride, midazolam hydrochloride, oxazepam hemisuccinate). All the benzodiazepines have high lipid:water distribution coefficients in the nonionized form although lipophilicity varies from about 50 to 10,000 according to the polarity and electronegativity of various substituents. Oral effectiveness varies markedly among the benzodiazepines. Diazepam, flurazepam, and nordiazepam (the active meta-

bolite formed in the stomach from the prodrug clorazepate) are among the most rapidly absorbed whereas oxazepam is one of the most slowly absorbed. Diazepam and chlordiazepoxide should not be administered intramuscularly (im) due to their poor and erratic absorption by this route. Midazolam and lorazepam are marketed for both im and intravenous (iv) use and diazepam is available for iv administration. Most benzodiazepines, however, are not available for iv use because of their poor water solubility. All the benzodiazepines in therapeutic use are highly bound to plasma proteins (70%–99%) and share the same binding site as tryptophan and aspirin, thus accounting for the competition that occurs. Their distribution to brain and other tissues is correlated with lipid solubility. The high lipid solubility leads to a large tissue distribution which principally determines the duration of therapeutic action rather than elimination half-life for many benzodiazepines. Diazepam is more rapidly absorbed from the intestine and has a higher lipid solubility and a more rapid distribution to the CNS than chlordiazepoxide. Diazepam and its metabolites, nordiazepam and oxazepam, accumulate in fat. Benzodiazepines and their metabolites can cross the placenta and accumulate in fetal circulation. The benzodiazepines are metabolized mainly through N-dealkylation or hydroxylation by liver microsomal systems followed by glucuronidation to form inactive compounds that are excreted in the urine. For benzodiazepines that are substituted in positions 1 of the B ring (with the exception of triazolam, estazolam, alprazolam, and midazolam which have either a fused triazolo or imidazolo ring [Table 1]), the first phase of metabolism involves modification and/or removal of the substituent (Table 2), eventually resulting in biologically active N-desalkylated compounds. Nordiazepam is the major metabolite common to diazepam, chlorazepate, halazepam, and chlordiazepoxide. Corresponding desalkyl derivatives occur after the administration of flurazepam and quazepam. Because the desalkyl derivatives have long half-lives, they accumulate when benzodiazepines are given once a

TABLE 2. Common Metabolic Pathways for Some Benzodiazepines

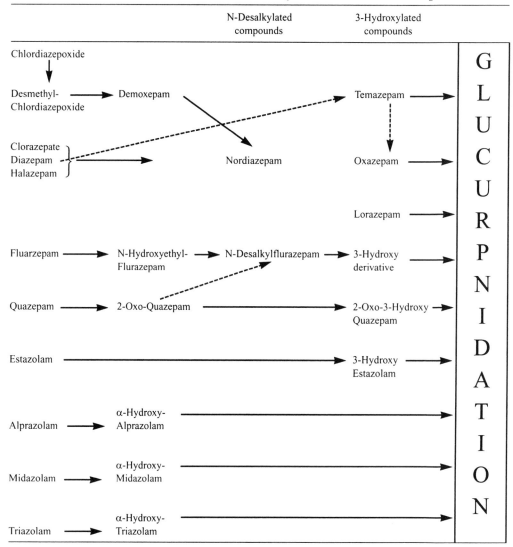

day or more frequently and consequently the pharmacologic effects of both the parent drug and the metabolite will most likely contribute to the overall clinical effect, the time-course for reversal of drug effect, and the emergence and severity of withdrawal effects. The second phase of metabolism involves hydroxylation at position 3 which usually yields an active metabolite such as oxazepam. Alprazolam, midazolam, and triazolam are metabolized initially by the hydroxylation of the methyl group on the fused ring to active α-hydroxylated compounds that are rapidly metabolized. Microsomal enzymes are not induced by benzodiazepines in therapeutic doses to any major extent. The third major phase of metabolism is conjugation of the 3-hydroxyl compounds, principally with glucuronic acid. With the exception of benzodiazepines such as oxazepam that undergo glucuronidation, the elimination rate of benzodiazepines is usually prolonged in geriatric patients and in patients with hepatic dysfunction. The pharmacokinetics of lorazepam, oxazepam, zolpidem, and their respective metabolites are altered in the presence of renal disease (cf. Hobbs *et al.,* 1996; J. R. Martin & Haefely, 1995; Smith, 1992).

Pharmacology of a Nonbenzodiazepine CBR Agonist: Zolpidem

Zolpidem, a nonbenzodiazepine sedative-hypnotic drug that shows selectivity for the CBR1/GABA$_A$ receptor, has been approved for clinical use as a hypnotic in the United States (Table 1). It is absorbed readily from the GI tract and its oral bioavailability is about 70% due to a liver first-pass effect, a value that is reduced when the drug is ingested with food. Zolpidem is distributed throughout the body with the lowest concentrations in the CNS and the highest in glandular tissues and fat. It is highly bound to plasma proteins and is eliminated mainly by conversion to inactive carboxylic acid metabolites in the liver, with no unchanged zolpidem eliminated in the urine in humans under normal conditions (Hobbs *et al.,* 1996). Studies in males with histories of sedative abuse showed that some tolerance develops and that it has a likelihood of abuse in this group (Evans, Funderburk, & Griffiths, 1990). Most human studies have shown little evidence of tolerance or withdrawal effects although the details of having looked for dependence are missing (Langtry & Benfield, 1990).

Pharmacology of Benzodiazepine Receptor Antagonists

PK11195

The PBR antagonist, PK 11195, is not approved for clinical use; however, due to its specificity as an antagonist of the PBR, it is a key drug for the study of peripheral effects of the benzodiazepines. Paradoxically, it appears to be a potent agonist at some sites, suggesting that there are at least two different PBR sites: one where PK 11195 acts as an agonist and one where it acts as an antagonist. The response of a particular tissue may depend on the dominance of the PBR receptor type (Hertz, 1993).

Pharmacology of Flumazenil

Flumazenil is the established reference neuronal CBR antagonist as well as the only one approved for clinical use. For these reasons it is the only CBR antagonist that is discussed in depth. Flumazenil has a high affinity for and blocks all the effects of the CBR/GABA$_A$ agonists and inverse agonists but does not bind to the peripheral (PBR) site. Its efficacy at the CBR site is extremely weak although it is not devoid of activity and can show both antagonistic and agonistic actions, depending on the dose (File & Pellow, 1986; Sloan, Martin, & Wala, 1990). Chronic exposure to flumazenil in drug-naive rats upregulated benzodiazepine receptors in the cerebral cortex and hippocampus (Medina, Novas, & de Robertis, 1983), increased exploratory activity, and produced a long-lasting anxiolytic effect after its withdrawal (Urbancic, Gadek, & Marczynski, 1990). Effects of agonists requiring high functional receptor occupancy (e.g., sedation) are antagonized with smaller doses of flumazenil than those requiring only low fractional receptor occupancy (anticonvulsant and anxiolytic effects) which means that lower doses of flumazenil are required to reverse the effects induced by high doses of CBR agonists than are required to reverse the effects induced by low doses (J. R. Martin & Haefely, 1995; Sloan, Martin, & Wala, 1993a). The administration of flumazenil to benzodiazepine-dependent animals very rapidly blocks the agonistic actions of benzodiazepine at CBR sites. Depending on the experimental condition, flumazenil can produce a dramatic abstinence syndrome in a variety of benzodiazepine-dependent animal species including the rat, cat, baboon, monkey, and dog (cf. File, 1990; Grant *et al.,* 1985; cf. Haefely, 1986; J. R. Martin, Moreau, & Jenck, 1995; W. R. Martin, Sloan, & Wala, 1993; Rosenberg & Chiu, 1982; Sloan, Martin, & Wala, 1990; 1991a, 1991b, 1993a; cf. Woods, Katz, & Winger, 1992). The level of dependence revealed by flumazenil-precipitated abstinence has been shown to increase with both the dose and duration of benzodiazepine administration (Lukas

& Griffiths, 1984; Sloan *et al.,* 1993a). The repeated administration of flumazenil at 1- or 2-week intervals over long periods of chronic administration of benzodiazepines did not diminish the precipitated abstinence syndrome across time in dogs (Sloan *et al.,* 1991a, 1991b, 1993a; cf. Woods *et al.,* 1992), and in squirrel monkeys (J. R. Martin *et al.,* 1995). The periodic injection of flumazenil did not alter tolerance to the anticonvulsant effect of clobazepam during subchronic treatment in the kindled-rat (Löscher & Runfeldt, 1989) or tolerance to the sedative effects of chronic diazepam or triazolam administration to baboons (Lamb & Griffiths, 1985), nor was tolerance to the anxiolytic effects of lorazepam or oxazepam administered daily for 7 days to normal human subjects reversed by a low dose of flumazenil (Cittadini & Lader, 1991). Not all data are consistent in this regard. Persisting attenuation of tolerance to diazepam's effect on GABAergic sensitivity was seen in dorsal raphe neurons of the rat (Gonsalves & Gallager, 1988); a slight attenuation of tolerance to sedative effects was observed in baboons after several doses of midazolam (Sannerud, Cook, & Griffiths, 1989); decreased withdrawal effects were seen in rhesus monkeys treated 13 days with diazepam (Gallager, Heninger, & Heninger, 1986), and in baboons infused continuously with diazepam or triazolam (Lamb & Griffiths, 1985) when flumazenil was administered every third day. In summary, the inconsistencies in the studies just mentioned may be due in part to differences in experimental design, including duration of benzodiazepine treatment, flumazenil dosing intervals, species, sex, and the signs of abstinence measured.

Pharmacokinetics of Flumazenil

Flumazenil (Table 1) is rapidly and well absorbed from the GI tract although a liver first-pass effect markedly reduces its bioavailability. This is the reason it is administered iv for clinical purposes. Following iv injection, plasma concentration rapidly declines, reflecting redistribution throughout the body. Metabolism to the free acid by hepatic microsomal oxidation and its corresponding glucuronide is also rapid and complete after iv administration. These inactive metabolites are excreted by the kidney with less than 0.2% of the drug appearing unchanged in the urine. The pharmacokinetic profile of flumazenil is susceptible to changes in both functional liver cell mass and hepatic blood flow as seen in liver disease. This may prolong clinical effects and require dosage adjustments.

Therapeutic Uses of Flumazenil

Flumazenil is used clinically to reverse overdose with CBR agonists in nondependent subjects but should not be used in chronic users of CBR agonists due to the danger of precipitating a withdrawal syndrome. It is also used to reduce sedation due to CBR agonists during and after surgery, and it appears to initiate a modest improvement in the EEG and clinical grade of hepatic encephalopathy (Cadranel *et al.,* 1995).

Adverse Effects and Toxicity of Flumazenil

Flumazenil is usually well tolerated and the majority of adverse effects are mild and self-limiting. Side effects include nausea, vomiting, dizziness, headache, anxiety, and confusion. Because flumazenil has a relatively short elimination half-life compared with benzodiazepines, benzodiazepine effects can recur after initial antagonism has subsided but can be prevented by the repeated administration of flumazenil. In addition to the danger of precipitating a severe abstinence syndrome in chronic benzodiazepine users, patients with mixed overdoses of benzodiazepines and convulsant agents may be placed in a high-risk situation by the administration of flumazenil. Flumazenil-induced seizures have been reported in association with mixed overdoses of benzodiazepines and tricyclic antidepressants and could result from flumazenil administration with mixed overdoses of other convulsants such as cocaine and benzodiazepines. Flumazenil is used by cocaine abusers to suppress overt cocaine-induced seizures. In the rat, flumazenil unmasked seizures and produced death in 90% of the animals with combined cocaine-diazepam intoxication (Derlet & Albertson, 1994; Spivey, 1992).

Pharmacology of Benzodiazepine Partial Agonists, Antagonists, and Inverse Agonists Not Approved for Clinical Use

Space does not permit a comprehensive review of these compounds which have helped to increase our understanding of the CBR/GABA$_A$ receptor and offer hope for the development of benzodiazepines that have specificity in producing the desired pharmacologic effects without the undesired side effects. The reader is directed to Gardner, Tully, and Hedgecock (1993) for a comprehensive review of research involving a wide range of benzodiazepine receptor ligands. Several partial agonists and agents with benzodiazepine receptor subtype selectivity have been developed and show some promise for therapeutic use. These include bretazenil, RU 32698, and abecarnil.

Adverse Effects and Toxicity of Benzodiazepines

Therapeutic Doses

The most frequently encountered adverse effects are due to excessive depression of CNS functions. In relatively low therapeutic doses these effects range from reduced attention and slow mentation, drowsiness, mental confusion, disorientation, slurred speech, amnesia, aggravation of symptoms of dementia, nystagmus, and ataxia to paradoxical effects such as aggressive behavior, hyperactivity, delirium, insomnia, and serious depression. Thus therapeutic doses of benzodiazepines can impair the patient's driving ability as well as judgment in assessing his or her impairment of function. In doses used to promote sleep, short-acting benzodiazepines such as triazolam, oxazepam, and temazepam may cause rebound insomnia. The administration of benzodiazepines can precipitate or exacerbate hepatic encephalophy in patients with poor hepatocellular function (Bakti, Fisch, Karlaganis, Minder, & Bircher, 1987; Branch, Morgan, Jones, & Read, 1976). In this

regard, endogenous PBR ligands are thought to be implicated in the ammonia-induced astrocyte swelling that accompanies hepatic encephalopathy (Basile, Jones, & Skolnick, 1991), an effect that is enhanced by PBR ligands and diminished by the PBR antagonist, PK 11195, in primary astrocyte cultures prepared from cerebral cortices of 1–2-day-old rats (Norenberg & Bender, 1994).

Drug Interactions

The benzodiazepines can have serious interactions with other CNS depressants such as ethanol, barbiturates, antidepressants, antipsychotics, opioid analgesics, and antihistamines. The CNS depressant interaction is at least additive and usually synergistic and may be more pronounced in the elderly. Death from overdoses is usually associated with the combined effects of benzodiazepines with alcohol and other CNS depressants that have the potential for altering the metabolism of other drugs, including benzodiazepines. Although the biotransformation of benzodiazepines may be affected by other drugs that induce hepatic enzymes, they have no significant ability themselves to induce these enzymes.

Respiration

Benzodiazepines have no effect on respiration in normal subjects in hypnotic doses, whereas in very high doses they can produce alveolar hypoxia and/or CO_2 narcosis in patients with chronic obstructive pulmonary disease. Apnea can result from the benzodiazepines during anesthesia, or when combined with opioids, but this usually does not present a major problem unless the patient has ingested other CNS-depressant drugs such as alcohol. Respiratory depression and apnea can occur after iv administration, especially in asthmatic patients. Further, benzodiazepines in hypnotic doses may worsen sleep-related breathing disorders such as obstructive sleep apnea and should be given with caution or not at all to these patients.

Risk Factors in the Elderly

Benzodiazepines are a major, independent risk factor for falls leading to femur fractures.

The increased risk is probably explained by prescribing doses to the elderly that are too high (Herings, Stricker, de Boer, Bakker, & Sturmans, 1995).

Liver Toxicity

In therapeutic doses, the benzodiazepines are generally safe. Caution should be exercised when administered chronically in therapeutic, or very high, doses. Studies of benzodiazepine dependence have shown that high chronic doses of either diazepam or halazepam (Sloan, Martin, Wala, & Dickey, 1991) produce changes in liver function tests and hepatotoxicity in dogs. Preliminary studies indicate that diazepam produces dose- and time-related changes in liver function tests, dose-related changes in liver histology, and liver and spleen hypertrophy in rats (Sloan, Wala, Jing, Holtman, & Lee, 1994). There are circumstances in which the effects of benzodiazepines on the liver may assume clinical importance in humans. These include the use of high doses therapeutically for an extended period of time, when abused, when administered with other drugs that impair liver function, and when administered to cirrhotic patients or patients with hepatic encephalopathy (Basile et al., 1991). Jaundice has been reported in patients receiving chlordiazepoxide chronically (Abbruzzese & Swanson, 1965; Cacioppo & Merlis, 1961; Lo, Eastwood, & Eidelman., 1967); hepatitis, after the chronic administration of diazepam (Cunningham, 1965; Tedesco & Mills, 1982) and alprazolam (Judd, Norman, Marriott, & Burrows, 1986; Roy-Byrne, Vittone, & Uhde, 1983). A fatal intrahepatic cholestasis was associated with the chronic administration of triazolam (Cobden, Record, & White, 1981). Patients receiving clozapine and other benzodiazepines together had greater elevations in gamma glutamyltransferase, SGOT, and SGPT than when receiving clozapine alone (Sassim & Grohmann, 1988).

Carcinogenic Potential

Benzodiazepines have not been associated with marked carcinogenic potential in humans. Studies in the past with some benzodiazepines in animals have presented some evidence of increased liver neoplasia which has been largely unsubstantiated. Temazepam caused a slight increase in liver adenomas in mice (Robinson, Van Ryzin, Stoll, Jensen, & Bagdon, 1984) as did diazepam (De la Iglesia et al., 1981) and oxazepam (Fox & Lahcen, 1974). In a more recent study, it has been shown that oxazepam is carcinogenic in mice based on increased incidences of hepatic neoplasia as well as increased incidences of hyperplasia of thyroid gland follicular cells and of follicular cell adenomas (Bucher et al., 1994).

Consequences of Prenatal Exposure to Benzodiazepines

Benzodiazepines are highly lipid-soluble agents and pass rapidly from maternal to fetal blood where they circulate in higher concentrations than in the maternal blood. Benzodiazepines are retained in fetal tissues for long periods since excretion is slow. Benzodiazepines such as diazepam are used in pregnancy as anticonvulsants, muscle relaxants, anxiolytics, for eclampsia, preeclampsis, threatened abortion, and during labor. Withdrawal symptoms have been reported in neonates born to mothers treated with diazepam for long periods (Rementeria & Bhatt, 1977). The "floppy infant syndrome," characterized by hypotonia, unresponsiveness, hypothermia, reluctance to feed, and apneic episodes, has also been reported after chronic maternal treatment with diazepam or nitrazepam (Speight, 1977).

Teratogenic effects of benzodiazepines have not been reported with great frequency in humans. In an extensive review (Hines, 1981) it was concluded that reported teratogenic effects in humans and animals were unsubstantiated and that the results of postnatal evaluation of prenatal exposure to diazepam in rats were conflicting. However, more recently it was found that children born to mothers who used oxazepam, diazepam or diazepam plus lorazepam in therapeutic doses during pregnancy had craniofacial malformations (Laegreid, Olegard, Wahlstrom, & Conradi, 1989). Reports of developmental alterations due to prenatal exposure to benzodiazepines are numerous in animals (Tucker, 1985). A single oral dose of nitrazepam on day 12 of gestation in rats (but not in mice) produced a significant degree of malformations (Takeno, Hirano, Kitamura, & Sakai, 1993). Mice treated prenatally with diazepam from the 6th to the 15th day of gestation showed histological changes in the lung, kidney, placenta, heart, cerebral cortex, and liver, as well as ultrastructural changes in the heart, placenta, and retina (cf. M. C. Márquez-Orozco, Márquez-Orozco, & Gazca-Ramírez, 1993). Histological changes were also observed in the tibia (A. Márquez-Orozco, Márquez-Orozco, & Gazca-Ramírez, 1993), ovary (Hernández-Alvarez, Márquez-Orozco, Márquez-Orozco, & Hicks, 1991), and testes (Mata-Santibánez, Márquez-Orozco, & Márquez-Orozco, 1993). Mice treated prenatally with diazepam had a delay in differentiation and migration of cerebellar cells (Andrada-Mártinez, Márquez-Orozoco, & Márquez-Orozco, 1993), a reduction in sexual performance in males (A. Márquez-Orozco, Hernández-Alvarez, & Márquez-Orozco, 1994), and enhancement of the lordodotic index and intensity of lordosis (Hernández-Alvarez, Márquez-Orozco, & Márquez-Orozco, 1994). Gestational exposure to diazepam increased the sensitivity to convulsants that act at the GABA/benzodiazepine receptor complex (Bitran, Primus, & Kellogg, 1991) and altered motor activity and pentylenetetrazole-induced seizure threshold in mice at the onset of maturity at 6 weeks and up to 12 months after prenatal exposure to lorazepam (Byrnes & Miller, 1993; Chesley et al., 1991; Koff & Miller, 1995). Prenatal exposure to diazepam in rats produced enduring reductions in brain receptors and deep slow wave sleep (Livezey, Radulovacki, Isaac, & Marczynski, 1985); decreased pain sensitivity, startle response, and cortical benzodiazepine receptors (Shibuya, Watanabe, Hill, & Salafsky, 1986); and decreased PBR on splenic macrophages (Schlumpf, Parmar, & Lichtensteiger, 1993). Prenatal exposure to diazepam altered stressor-induced changes in GABA$_A$ receptor function in the cerebral cortex of adult rats (Kellogg, Taylor, Rodriguez-Zafra, & Pleger, 1993) and impaired the immune system in the rat that was shown to involve the PBR site (Schlumpf, Parmar, Ramseier, & Lichtensteiger, 1990; Schlumpf, Lichtensteiger, & van Loveren, 1994).

Although a teratogenic effect of benzodiazepines has not been conclusively proven, prenatal exposure to benzodiazepines has been repeatedly associated with a specific developmental syndrome in both humans and animals, factors that should be considered in the prescribing of benzodiazepines to women of childbearing age.

Tolerance, Dependence, and Abuse

Since their introduction into clinical use, the benzodiazepines have been the most commonly prescribed psychotropic drugs and are among the most commonly prescribed of any class of drugs. Approximately 12% of the population use a prescribed benzodiazepine during the course of a year. Benzodiazepines were among the most commonly mentioned drugs in the DAWN report for emergency room admissions and accounted for about 5% of all medical examiner mentions (National Institute on Drug Abuse, 1994a, 1994b). The fear of addicting patients has led to a decline in their prescribed use during the last decade resulting sometimes in the withholding of warranted therapy.

Tolerance

Chronic exposure to benzodiazepine receptor agonists can result in the development of tolerance (a loss of efficacy) to some of the drug's effects. Both functional and metabolic tolerance are known to develop to the benzodiazepines, but, unlike the barbiturates, metabolic tolerance develops to such a limited extent that it has no clinical significance (Yanagita, 1981). Tolerance is undesirable if it reduces the therapeutic effectiveness of the drug, but it can be beneficial if it develops to some of the drug's unwanted effects such as sedation. Tolerance to the motor impairment effects (such as muscle incoordination) and to the anticonvulsant effects induced by benzodiazepines is clearly observable during chronic treatment whereas these agents remain effective in a large percentage of patients with regard to their hypnotic and anxiolytic properties (cf. Chiu & Rosenberg, 1995; Hollister *et al.*, 1993). Studies of cross-tolerance between benzodiazepines and other sedative hypnotics in animals and humans have been limited, and, in general, only partial tolerance has been demonstrated. For a more detailed report of these studies, the reader is directed to other reviews (Chiu, Tietz, & Rosenberg, 1987; Gallager & Primus, 1993; Woods *et al.*, 1992; Yanagita, 1981).

Dependence, Abuse, and the Consequences

A major problem associated with long-lasting treatment with benzodiazepine receptor agonists even at therapeutic doses is the development of dependence. This is manifested as a withdrawal syndrome following discontinuation of drug treatment. The nature of the withdrawal syndrome is a function of the drug, duration of exposure, duration of action of the drug, and personality of the patient (Woods *et al.*, 1992). Several extensive summaries of the signs and symptoms of benzodiazepine withdrawal have been published (Ashton, 1984; Hallstrom & Lader, 1981; Juergens, 1993; Ladewig, 1984; Pétursson, 1994; Pétursson & Lader, 1981). The signs and symptoms fall into five categories: (1) autonomic signs, (2) sensory and perceptual disturbances, (3) affective and cognitive aberrations, (4) convulsive phenomena and impairment of motor function, and (5) nausea, vomiting, and anorexia (W. R. Martin, Sloan, & Wala, 1990). The most common signs and symptoms of withdrawal consist of at least three patterns, the first of which is the short-lived (2–3 days) "rebound" anxiety and insomnia phase having an onset within 1–4 days after discontinuation. The second pattern is a florid withdrawal syndrome, usually lasting 10–14 days. Finally, a third pattern emerges which may represent a return of the symptoms in a more intense form than were originally treated. This latter pattern probably persists until therapy is instituted. Persistence of the original disorder during abstinence may lead to subsequent chronic drug use and abuse (J. R. Martin & Haefely, 1995). Although prolonged, daily benzodiazepine self-administration does not necessarily escalate to high, nontherapeutic dose levels (Woods *et al.*, 1992). The proportion of long-term benzodiazepine users who do escalate their dose is, however, not insignificant (cf. Barnas, Whitworth, & Fleischacker, 1993; Griffiths, 1995; King, Gabe, Williams, & Rodrigo, 1990; Romach *et al.*, 1991). The nonmedical use of benzodiazepines represents a significant problem among polydrug abusers such as alcoholics, cocaine and other drug abusers generally, and methadone maintenance patients in particular (Griffiths & Wolf, 1990; Iguchi, Handelsman, Bickel, & Griffiths, 1993; Lader, 1995). In contrast to normal subjects who demonstrate little preference or liking for benzodiazepines (Woods *et al.*, 1992), polydrug abusers show a clear preference for benzodiazepines, barbiturates, and opiates but not for other nonabused psychotropic compounds such as buspirone and chlorpromazine (de Wit & Griffiths, 1991; Troisi, Critchfield, & Griffiths, 1993). The data are unclear concerning the relative dependence liability of short- versus long-acting benzodiazepine receptor agonists. However, laboratory studies of subjective reinforcing effects, epidemilogic studies, and interviews with drug abusers all indicate that diazepam has a greater abuse liability than many other benzodiazepines and that lorazepam and alprazolam also have high abuse liability whereas oxazepam, halazepam, and possibly chlordiazepoxide have low abuse liability. It is thought that the differences in abuse liability of benzodiazepines among drug abusers is related to the speed of onset of effects. Among the marketed benzodiazepines, diazepam has one of the most rapid oral onset of effects whereas oxazepam and halazepam are among the benzodiazepines with the slowest onset (Greenblatt & Shader, 1985; Griffiths & Wolf, 1990; Jaffe, Ciraulo, Nies, Dixon, & Monroe 1983). The more rapid onset and severity of withdrawal with the shorter-acting benzodiazepines than with the longer-acting ones such as diazepam is probably related to the pharmacokinetics of the benzodiazepine (Fialip *et al.*, 1987; Rickels, Schweizer, Case, &

Greenblatt, 1991). This wide variance in onset of abstinence is not seen in flumazenil-precipitated abstinence (animal studies). The withdrawal syndrome may be managed in mild cases with slow tapering of the drug over a period of a few weeks whereas dependence produced by some of the shorter-acting benzodiazepines may be best managed by the substitution of a longer-acting benzodiazepine in gradually reduced doses.

Studies of withdrawal as well as flumazenil- or PK 11195-precipitated abstinence suggest that different benzodiazepines or their metabolites produce dependencies that differ both qualitatively and quantitatively (W. R. Martin et al., 1990; Martinez, Fargeas, & Bueno, 1992; Rosenberg, 1995; Sanger, et al., 1994; Scherkl & Frey, 1986; Sloan et al., 1991). Further, after chronic treatment with diazepam, iontophoretic and microinjection studies of different areas of the rat CNS show major differences in sensitivity to GABA and to the flumazenil-evoked signs and intensity of precipitated abstinence (cf. Gallager, Jacobs, Crais, During, & Hernandez, 1991; Sloan, Martin, & Wala, 1993b; Sloan, Wala, & Jing, 1994, 1995a, 1995b; Sloan, Jing, Wala, & Milliken, 1996; Wala, Sloan, & Jing, 1994, 1997a; Wala, Sloan, Martin, & Jing, 1994; Wala, Sloan, Jing, & Holtman, 1996). Studies have shown that the dorsal raphe nucleus (DRN) of the benzodiazepine-dependent rat develops a subsensitivity to GABA and to the benzodiazepine agonists with regard to their ability to enhance GABA sensitivity along with an increased GABA sensitivity to flumazenil whereas in the substantia nigra (SN), the sensitivity to applied GABA, benzodiazepine agonists, or flumazenil is unaltered. The cerebral cortex in the benzodiazepine-dependent rat, like the DRN, shows a decreased sensitivity to GABA in that there is a reduced ability of GABA to stimulate chloride influx; it develops a decrease in muscimol-stimulated chloride uptake, a decrease in the ability of GABA to enhance benzodiazepine agonist binding, and in the ability to decrease inverse agonist binding. The cerebellum, like the SN, shows no change in GABA sensitivity and the GABA-

stimulated CL influx is unchanged (cf. Gallager & Primus, 1993; Gallager, Marley, & Hernandez, 1991; Primus & Gallager, 1992). Several studies have shown downregulation of CBR during chronic benzodiazepine treatment whereas others have shown that not all benzodiazepines decrease benzodiazepine binding after chronic administration (for review see Gallager & Primus, 1993; Miller et al., 1990). Using autoradiographic studies, regional variations were found in the degree and rate of downregulation of CBR during chronic flurazepam treatment suggesting that some areas may be more important than others for the development of tolerance and dependence (Tietz, Rosenberg, & Chiu, 1986).

While numerous studies have suggested that multiple types of benzodiazepine receptors exist, molecular cloning of $GABA_A$ receptor subunits and recombinant coexpression of these subunits have further confirmed the diversity of $GABA_A$ receptor subtypes in vivo. Taking advantage of one of the baculovirus Sf9 expression systems (a system devoid of neuronal elements) it was shown that the allosteric uncoupling of the α_1, β_2, and γ_2; α_2, β_3, and γ_2; and α_5, β_3, and γ_2; GABA receptor subtypes after chronic benzodiazepine exposure replicates coupling changes measured in rat cortical membranes in in vivo studies. This uncoupling was time-related with the magnitude of the uncoupling dependent on the efficacy of the ligand at a given receptor subtype. Flumazenil reversed the uncoupling, and the uncoupling was not accompanied by changes in benzodiazepine receptor number or affinity at any expressed $GABA_A$ receptor examined. These studies suggested that during chronic benzodiazepine exposure, the agonistic effects of benzodiazepines are responsible for changes in the $GABA_A$ receptor complex rather than the surrounding neuronal environment and that drug efficacy is more important than affinity in determining uncoupling and most likely in the development of tolerance and dependence (Primus et al., 1996).

The PBR site may also play a significant role in the production of tolerance and dependence as well as in the development of some of the toxic effects of chronic benzodiazepines. Several agents that exert their effects through the benzodiazepine receptor bind both to the CBR and the PBR; among them are Ro 5-4864 (prototypical ligand for PBR and a proconvulsant), diazepam, flunitrazepam, and alpidem (a drug that has been removed from the European market due to its liver toxicity). Some CBR agonists (such as nordiazepam, clonazepam, zolpidem) do not bind (or show very low affinity) for the PBR. Little is known so far concerning the effect of the long-term administration of benzodiazepines on PBR. One study reported that chronic treatment with low doses of diazepam produced a slight increase in cerebral cortical and cardiac PBR (Weizman & Gavish, 1989). More recent studies in the rat have shown that chronic diazepam produces downregulation of [^{3}H]-Ro 5-4864 binding in the cerebral cortex (Diana & Massotti, 1992), an upregulation of PBR in the kidney and heart, and a downregulation of testicular PBR (Calvo & Medina, 1992) whereas in female rates chronic diazepam produced an upregulation of ovarian and adrenal [^{3}H]-PK 11195 binding with no change in ovarian and adrenal hormonal levels (Weizman, Leschiner, Schlegel, & Gavish, 1997). These studies suggest that chronic diazepam exposure differentially regulates PBR in peripheral organs and that chronic diazepam may produce some gender-related differences in these effects that are not correlated with steroidogenesis. A growing body of evidence suggests that the peripheral receptor is involved in many of the undesirable effects resulting from the indiscriminate or long-term use of high-dose benzodiazepines. Regan and colleagues (1990) have shown that the pathogenesis of teratogenic effects arise from disturbances in the fundamental phases of development such as mitosis and cell differentiation, phases that have been shown to be at least partially controlled by the PBR and altered by benzodiazepines (see the section "Prenatal Exposure to Benzodiazepines and Developmental Effects") (Andersson, Lehto, Stenman, Badley, & Virtanen, 1981; Ober, 1974). Further, evidence that the PBR is involved in tolerance and/or dependence has been demonstrated in

the rat where the coadministration of the PBR antagonist PK 11195 prevented the development of tolerance to the EEG effects of chronically administered diazepam (Massotti et al., 1990); where precipitated abstinence was evoked by the administration of PK 11195 in diazepam-dependent rats (Martinez et al., 1992; Sloan, Wala, & Jing, 1997a, 1997b; Wala, Sloan, & Jing, 1997b, c); where the coadministration of PK 11195 attenuated behavioral tolerance, receptor downregulation, and the withdrawal syndrome induced by chronic lorazepam; and where specificity was demonstrated when the administration of the PBR agonist Ro 5-4864 antagonized the actions of PK (Miller & Koff, 1994).

Although the benzodiazepines are effective drugs when their use is limited to the therapeutic indications for which they are prescribed, they are not without risk factors, particularly during chronic use and in situations of abuse. For these reasons short-term or intermittent prescriptions are desirable to prevent some of the attendant problems of chronic administration such as tolerance, dependence, and withdrawal. There are instances, however, when the benefits outweigh the consequences of long-term treatment. These are judgments the clinician must make.

Drugs that Do Not Act through Benzodiazepine Receptors

Serotonin Partial Agonist: Buspirone

Buspirone, approved for the treatment of anxiety symptoms, does not produce CNS depression. Also there is little sedation, drowsiness, or amnesia. Buspirone neither antagonizes nor potentiates the effects of other antianxiety or hypnotic agents (see Table 3). Unlike all previously discussed anxiolytics, buspirone does not affect the CBR/GABA$_A$ receptor system directly but appears to act as a partial agonist at the serotonin-1A class of receptors, although it may also have activity as a dopamine receptor antagonist. Given in divided daily doses of 15–30 mg, it shows few side effects, and is less likely to be abused due to its potential to induce dysphoria. Reported side effects include nausea, dizziness, headache, nervousness, and lightheadness. It is well absorbed, but due to extensive first-pass metabolism, bioavailibility is only about 4%. It is highly protein bound. It is rapidly eliminated, predominantly by hepatic metabolism and renal excretion. This mechanism of action proscribes its use in patients with severe hepatic or renal impairment (J. R. Martin & Haefely, 1995; Smith, 1992).

Antihistamines: Diphenhydramine and Hydroxazine

At low concentrations these H_1-receptor antagonists block the effect of histamine at this receptor (Table 3). They are two of the first antihistamines discovered with side effects that include sedative and hypnotic properties and are therefore still used for these purposes. Diphenhydramine is frequently prescribed as a hypnotic and is also available as an over-the-counter drug. Hydroxyzine is occasionally used as an antianxiety agent. H_1-receptor antagonists are reasonably well absorbed when administered by mouth and reach peak serum concentrations in about 2 hr. They are metabolized by the P-450 system and have an apparent large volume of distribution. Children have shorter serum elimination half-life values than adults. The elderly may have prolonged values compared with young adults. These agents have not been studied in humans as extensively as the benzodiazepines and, therefore, their place in the treatment of anxiety is uncertain (cf. Smith, 1992).

Barbiturates and Primidone

General Pharmacology

Although the barbiturates (see Table 3) were once widely prescribed as sedative-hypnotics, they have been largely replaced by benzodiazepines, due mainly to their poor separation of anxiolytic and sedative effects. Consequently, this topic is not reviewed here. For reviews, the reader is directed to the literature (Glaser, Penry, & Woodbury, 1980; Haefely, 1977; Ho, 1987; Ho & Harris, 1981; MacDonald &

McLean, 1986; Nicoll, 1980; Okamoto, 1978; Richter & Holtman, 1982; Saunders & Ho, 1990). Barbiturates have been shown to be effective against all kinds of experimentally induced epileptiform activities in animals. At nonsedative doses, the long-acting agent phenobarbital is an effective anticonvulsant. The barbiturates produce dose-related depression of CNS function ranging from mild sedation, to sleep, to coma accompanied by respiratory depression, and ultimately death. The deoxy barbiturate, primidone, is converted to two active metabolites, phenobarbital and phenylethylmalonamide, and, like phenobarbital, is effective against tonic-clonic and partial seizures. It is used as an adjunct to other antiepileptic drugs.

The division of the barbiturates according to their time-course of action has correlated with their therapeutic use. The short-acting barbiturates have been used therapeutically primarily as hypnotic agents. When given in recommended doses to promote sleep at bedtime, they present little risk except grogginess that persists into the next day. They can, however, impair memory, reasoning, and higher cognitive integrative functions. Secobarbital, pentobarbital, and amobarbital continue to be used for this purpose (Hobbs *et al.*, 1996; J. R. Martin & Haefely, 1995; Smith, 1992). For further information pertaining to the effects of barbiturates on sleep the reader is referred to reviews by Kay, Blackburn, Buckingham, and Karacan (1976) and Mendelson, Gillin, & Wyatt (1977).

Mechanism of Action

The mechanism of action of the barbiturates on $GABA_A$ receptors appears to be different from those of either the benzodiazepines or GABA, thus resulting in pharmacologic effects different in part from those of benzodiazepine receptor ligands. The barbiturate modulatory sites are poorly characterized and none have been demonstrated to mediate bidirectional modulation like the benzodiazepine receptor. The barbiturates, like the benzodiazepines, enhance the binding of GABA to $GABA_A$ receptors in a chloride-dependent and picro-

TABLE 3. Drugs that Produce Sedative, Hypnotic, or Anxiolytic Effects but Do Not Act through the Benzodiazepine Receptor(s)

Generic name (trade name)	Mean or median half-life (hr) (range)	Main therapeutic use (representative dosing regimen)[a]
		Serotonin Agonists
Buspirone (Buspar)	~2.5 2–3	Anxiolytic (oral: 15–30 mg/day maximum 60 mg/day)
		Antihistamines (H$_1$-Receptor Antagonists)
Diphenhydramine (Benadryl)	~8.5	Hypnotic (oral: 50 mg at bedtime)
Hydroxyzine (Atarax)	~20	Hypnotic; sedative (oral: 25–100 mg/day IM: 25–100 mg as a preanesthetic)
		Barbiturates and Primidone
Amobarbital (Amytal)	(10–40)	Hypnotic, sedative, anticonvulsant preanesthetic (oral: 65–200 mg at bedtime as hypnotic; 50–300 mg/day as sedative IV: 65–200 mg as anticonvulsant)

	Arprobarbital (Alurate)	(14–34)	Hypnotic (oral: 40–200 mg at bedtime as hypnotic)
	Butabarbital (Butisol, others)	(35–50)	Hypnotic, preanesthetic (oral: 50–100 mg at bedtime as hypnotic; 50–100 mg 60 to 90 min before surgery as a preanesthetic; 45–120 mg/day as sedative)
	Mephobarbital (Mebaral)	(10–70)	Anticonvulsant, sedative (oral: 400–600 mg/day as an anticonvulsant; 96–400 mg/day as sedative)
	Methohexital (Brevital)	(3–5)	Induction and/or maintenance of anesthesia (IV: individualized dosage)

(continued)

TABLE 3. (*Continued*)

Generic name (trade name)	Mean or median half-life (hr) (range)	Main therapeutic use (representative dosing regimen)[a]
Pentobarbital (Nembutal)	(15–50) (dose-dependent)	Preoperative anesthetic; anticonvulsant; sedative; hypnotic (oral: 100 mg preoperative; 60–120 mg/day as a sedative; 100 mg at bedtime as hypnotic; IM, IV: 100 mg or more as an anticonvulsant)
Phenobarbital (Luminal, others)	~90 (80–120)	Antiepileptic; sedative, hypnotic (oral: 60–200 mg/day as an antiepileptic; 30–120 mg/day as sedative; 100–200 mg at bedtime as hypnotic)
Secobarbital (Seconal)	~28 (15–40)	Sedative; hypnotic; preanesthetic; anticonvulsant (oral: 50–100 mg at bedtime as hypnotic; 200–300 mg 1–2 hr before surgery; 90–200 mg/day as sedative; IV: 5.5 mg/kg repeated as needed as anticonvulsant)
Thiopental (Pentothal)	~9 (8–10)	Induction and/or maintenance of anesthesia; preanesthetic; antiepileptic (IV: individualized doses the usual 50 mg test dose is followed by 100–200 mg, maximum 1,000 mg/day)

	Primidone (Mysoline)	~15 (5–15)	Anticonvulsant (oral: 750–1,500 mg/day, maximum 2,000 mg/day)
			Piperidindiones
	Glutethimide (Doriden)	(7–15)	Sedative; hypnotic (oral: 200–500 mg at bedtime as hypnotic)
	Methyprylon (Noludar)	(3–6)	Sedative; hypnotic (oral: 150–400 mg/day as sedative; 200–400 mg at bedtime as hypnotic)
			Propandiole
$NH_2COOCH_2CCH_2OOCNH_2$ with CH_3 and $CH_2CH_2CH_3$	Meprobamate (Miltown)	(6–17) (dose-dependent)	Anxiolytic; sedative hypnotic (oral: 800–1,600 mg/day as anxiolytic; 800 mg at bedtime as hypnotic)

[a]The information contained in the above table is a compilation from extensive sources collected in healthy adults. The daily doses are given in mg/day assuming they are divided into 2–4 portions/day unless indicated otherwise. The information regarding doses and usage is for general comparative purposes and should not be used as a basis for medical decisions with regard to individual patients.

toxin-sensitive fashion; they enhance but do not displace the binding of benzodiazepines. It has been demonstrated that the potentiating action of the barbiturates results in an increase in the relative frequency of the occurrence of long versus short bursts of chloride channel opening and prolongation of the open state. At the electrophysiologic level, barbiturates prolong GABA-mediated presynaptic and postsynaptic inhibition and, at sufficiently high doses, mimic GABA effects at the subsynaptic membranes. These direct effects on chloride conductance may be the mechanism whereby increasing doses of barbiturates, unlike the benzodiazepines, progress from anesthesia, to coma, and to death. The GABA subunits required for barbiturate action differ from the benzodiazeines in that only α and β (not γ) are required; barbiturate-induced increases in chloride conductance are not affected by the removal of the tyrosine and threonine residues in the β subunit that govern the sensitivity of GABA receptors to activation by agonists (Amin & Weiss, 1993).

Tolerance and Dependence

Barbiturates are subject to abuse and can produce both tolerance and dependence. The short-acting agents such as pentobarbital and secobarbital are more prone to abuse than longer-acting agents such as phenobarbital. This rapid onset and offset of action is probably related to reinforcing drug-seeking behavior. The tolerance associated with barbiturate use is both metabolic and functional. Metabolic tolerance is due to the ability of the barbiturates to induce hepatic enzyme formation that results in faster metabolism and shortening of their duration of action. With functional tolerance, tolerance develops to the "usual" doses but not to the effects of higher doses. Physical dependence may result in an abstinence syndrome when the drug is abruptly withdrawn, and its rate of appearance is related to the degree of dependence as well as to the pharmacokinetics of the drug (Boisse & Okamoto, 1978a,1978b). The abstinence syndrome can be very severe after the chronic ingestion of high doses (Essig, 1967; Isbell & Fraser, 1950).

Undesirable Side Effects

A profound central and peripheral nervous system depression, combined with impairment of function of most peripheral tissues including the cardiovascular system, is a consequence of the acute toxicity of barbiturates. Adverse effects most commonly observed include confusion, hangover, drowsiness, skin rash, and nausea. Overdose symptoms include profound sleep, coma, marked respiratory depression, and possibly death. Barbiturate effects are potentiated by alcohol and other CNS depressants. They can competitively inhibit as well as accelerate the metabolism of many drugs.

Piperidindiones

Glutethimide

The pharmacologic actions of glutethimide are similar to those of the barbiturates, but in addition include pronounced anticholinergic activity. It is erratically absorbed from the GI tract. More than 95% of the drug is metabolized in the liver. Its active metabolites, including 4-hydroxyglutethimide, accumulate after repeated administration and after high doses. Therapeutic doses seldom produce toxic side effects, which consist of "hangover," headache, excitement, gastric irritation, blurred vision, and, rarely, skin rash, thrombocytopenia, aplastic anemia, and leukopenia. The respiratory depression associated with acute intoxication is less severe than seen with barbiturates. Patients given glutethimide chronically in moderate doses may develop symptoms resembling abstinence, probably because it induces hepatic microsomal enzymes which may result in faster disappearance of the drug.

Methyprylon

Methyprylon has a structure similar to glutethimide (Table 3) and is also sometimes used as a sedative and a hypnotic. About 97% of the drug is metabolized, almost entirely by the liver with the urinary excretion of both free and conjugated metabolites. It stimulates the microsomal enzyme system and δ-ALA synthatase which proscribes its use with intermittent porphyria. Untoward effects are not usually encountered, but include "hangover," headache, nausea, vomiting, diarrhea, and esophagitis. With acute intoxication, hypotension, shock, and pulmonary edema are more obvious than respiratory depression. Tolerance and physical dependence can occur.

Propandiole: Meprobamate

The only approved use for meprobamate (Table 3) in the United States is as an anxiolytic. It became popular as a sedative-hypnotic agent, however, and is still used for this purpose. It resembles the benzodiazepines in that it can cause behavioral disinhibition in doses that cause little impairment of locomotor activity, and cannot produce anesthesia although it can cause widespread depression of the CNS. Unlike the benzodiazepines, in high doses, it can cause severe or fatal respiratory depression, hypotension, shock, and heart failure. It is well absorbed when administered orally; however, with intoxicating doses, gastric compacted masses of undissolved tablets form and may need to be removed mechanically. The drug is mainly metabolized in the liver to a side-chain hydroxy derivative and to a glucuronide. Chronic administration may prolong the half-life even though the drug can induce some hepatic microsomal enzymes. The major untoward effects of therapeutic sedative doses are drowsiness and ataxia with larger doses producing impairment of motor coordination and learning, enhancement of the CNS depression produced by other drugs, and dependence after long-term use. In spite of its decline in clinical use, its abuse continues; it is preferred over benzodiazepines by subjects who abuse drugs (Hobbs *et al.*, 1996; Smith, 1992).

Miscellaneous Sedative Hypnotics

In addition to the drugs shown in Tables 1 and 3, other agents are sometimes used. Chloral hydrate is used acutely (but not chronically, since it produces dependence and hepatic damage) as a sedative as well as a hypnotic. Adrenergic β blockers (propanolol in particular) have been used as anxiolytics to attenuate stage fright. The tricyclic antidepressants have

been used as anxiolytics and as hypnotics. They are, however, slow in onset and can produce adverse cardiovascular effects. Haloperidol had been employed, mostly in the elderly as an anxiolytic, but is limited in use because of its extrapyramidal effects.

References

Abbruzzese, A., & Swanson, J. (1965). Jaundice after therapy with chlordiazepoxide hydrochloride. *New England Journal of Medicine, 273*, 321–322.

Amin, J., & Weiss, D. S. (1993). GABA$_A$ receptor needs two homologous domains of the β-subunit for activation by GABA but not by pentobarbital. *Nature, 366,* 565–569.

Andersson, L. C., Lehto, V. P., Stenman, S., Badley, R. A., & Virtanen, I. (1981). Diazepam induces mitotic arrest at prometaphase by inhibiting centriolar separation. *Nature, 291,* 247–248.

Andrada-Martínez, R., Márquez-Orozco, M. C., & Márquez-Orozco, A. (1993). Cerebellar histological changes produced by diazepam. *Proceedings of the Western Pharmacology Society, 36,* 219–225.

Arbilla, S., Depoortere, H., George, P., & Langer, S. Z. (1985). Pharmacological profile of the imidazopyridine zolpidem at benzodiazepine receptors and electrocorticogram in rats. *Archives of Pharmacology, 330,* 248–251.

Ashton, H. (1984). Benzodiazepine withdrawal: An unfinished story. *British Medical Journal, 288,* 1135–1140.

Bakti, G., Fisch, H. U., Karlaganis, G., Minder, C., & Bircher, J. (1987). Mechanism of the excessive sedative response of cirrhotics to benzodiazepines: Model experiments with triazolam. *Hepatology, 7,* 629–638.

Barnas, C., Whitworth, A. B., & Fleischhacker, W. W. (1993). Are patterns of benzodiazepines use predictable? *Psychopharmacology, 111,* 301–305.

Basile, A. S., Jones, E. A., & Skolnick, P. (1991). The pathogenesis and treatment of hepatic encephalopathy: Evidence for the involovement of benzodiazepine receptor ligands. *Pharmacological Reviews, 43,* 27–71.

Bell, J. A., & Anderson E. G. (1972). The influence of semicarbazide-induced depletion of γ-aminobutyric acid on presynaptic inhibition. *Brain Research 43,* 161–169.

Bianchi, G., & Steiner, P. (1992). A clinical double-blind study of flumazenil, antagonist of benzodiazepines in loco-regional anesthesia. *Acta Anesthesthesiologica Belgica, 43,* 121–129.

Bitran, D., Primus, R. J., & Kellogg, C. K. (1991). Gestational exposure to diazepam increases sensitivity to convulsants that act at the GABA/benzodiazepine receptor complex. *European Journal of Pharmacology, 196,* 223–231.

Boisse, N. R., & Okamoto, M. (1978a): Physical dependence to barbital compared to pentobarbital: I.

"Chronically equivalent" dosing method. *Journal of Pharmacology and Experimental Therapeutics, 204,* 497–506.

Boisse, N. R., & Okamoto, M. (1978b). Physical dependence to barbital compared to pentobarbital: IV. Influence of elimination kinetics. *Journal of Pharmacology and Experimental Therapeutics, 204,* 526–540.

Bourguignon, J. (1993). Endogenous and synthetic ligands of mitochondrial benzodiazepine receptors: Structure-affinity relationships. In E. Geisen-Crouse (Ed.), *Peripheral benzodiazepine receptors* (pp. 59–82). New York: Academic Press.

Braestrup, C. (1981). Biochemical effects of anxiolytics. In F. Hoffmeister & G. Stille (Eds.), *Handbook of experimental pharmacology* (Vol. 55/II, pp. 293–319). Berlin: Springer-Verlag.

Branch, R. A., Morgan, M. H., Jones, J., & Read, A. E. (1976). Intravenous administration of diazepam in patients with chronic liver disease. *Gut, 17,* 975–983.

Briemer, L. T. M., Burm, A. G. L., Danhof, M., Hennis, P. J., Vletter, A. A., de Voogt, J. H., Spierdijk, J., & Bovill, J. G. (1991). Pharmacokinetic-pharmacodynamic modelling of the interaction between flumazenil and midazolam in volunteers by aperiodic EEG analysis. *Clinical Pharmacokinetics, 20* (6), 497–508.

Bucher, J. R., Shackelford, C. C., Haseman, J. K., Johnson, J. D., Kurtz, P. J., & Persing, R. L. (1994). Carcinogenicity studies of oxazepam in mice. *Fundamental and Applied Toxicology, 23,* 280–297.

Buchsbaum, M. S., Hazlett, E., Sicotte, N., Stein, M., Wu, J., & Zetin, M. (1985). Topographic EEG changes with benzodiazepine administration in generalized anxiety disorder. *Biological Psychiatry, 20,* 832–842.

Byrnes, J. J., & Miller, L. G. (1993). Prenatal benzodiazepine exposure: III. Lorazepam exposure is associated with a shift toward inverse agonist efficacy. *Journal of Psychopharmacology, 7,* 39–42.

Cacioppo, J., & Merlis, S. (1961). Chlordiazepoxide hydrochloride (librium) and jaundice: Report of a case. *American Journal of Psychiatry, 117,* 1040–1041.

Cadranel, J. F., Younsi, M. E., Pidoux, B., Zylberberg, P., Benhamou, Y., Valla, D., & Opolon, P. (1995). Flumazenil therapy for hepatic encephalopathy in cirrhotic patients: A double-blind pragmatic randomized, placebo study. *European Journal of Gastroenterology and Hepatology, 7,* 325–329.

Calvo, D. J., & Medina, J. H. (1992). Regulation of peripheral-type benzodiazepine receptors following repeated benzodiazepine administration. *Functional Neurology, 7,* 227–230.

Chesley, S., Lumpkin, M., Schatzki, A., Galpern, W. R., Greenblatt, D. J., Shader, R. I., & Miller, L. G. (1991). Prenatal exposure to benzodiazepine: I. Prenatal exposure to lorazepam in mice alters open-field activity and GABA$_A$ receptor function. *Neuropharmacology, 30,* 53–58.

Chiu, T. H., Tietz, E. I., & Rosenberg, H. C. (1987). Benzodiazepines. In I. K. Ho (Ed.), *Toxicology of CNS depressants* (pp. 1–32). Boca Raton, FL: CRC.

Chiu, T. H., & Rosenberg, H. C. (1995). Barbiturates and benzodiazepines: Effects and mechanisms. In L. W. Chang & R. S. Dyer (Eds), *Handbook of neurotoxicology* (pp. 739–767). New York: Dekker.

Cittadini, A., & Lader, M. (1991). Lack of effect of a small dose of flumazenil in reversing short-term tolerance to benzodiazepines in normal subjects. *Journal of Psychopharmacology, 5,* 220–227.

Cobden, I., Record, C. O., & White, R. W. B. (1981). Fatal interhepatic choleostasis associated with triazolam. *Postgraduate Medical Journal, 57,* 730–731.

Cunningham, M. L. (1965). Acute hepatic necrosis following treatment with amitriptyline and diazepam. *American Journal of Psychiatry, 111,* 1107–1109.

Curtis, D. R., Duggan, A. W., Felix D., & Johnston, G. A. R. (1971). Bicuculline, an antagonist of GABA and synaptic inhibition in the spinal cord. *Brain Research, 32,* 69–96.

De la Iglesia, A., Barsoum, N., Gough, A., Mitchell, L., Martin, R. A., di Fonzo, C., & McGuire, E. J. (1981). Carcinogenesis bioassay of prazepam (Verstran) in rats and mice. *Toxicology & Applied Pharmacology, 57,* 39–54.

Dennis, T., Dubois, A., Benavides, J., & Scatton, B. (1988). Distribution of central ω_1 (Benzodiazepine$_1$) and ω_2 (Benzodiazepine$_2$) receptor subtypes in the monkey and human brain. An autoradiographic study with [^{3}H]Flunitrazepam and the ω_1 selective ligand [^{3}H]Zolpidem. *Journal of Pharmacology and Experimental Therapy, 247,* 309–322.

Derlet, R. W., & Albertson, T. E. (1994). Flumazenil induces seizures and death in mixed cocaine-diazepam intoxications. *Annals of Emergency Medicine, 23,* 494–498.

de Wit, H., & Griffiths, R. R. (1991). Testing the abuse liability of anxiolytic and hypnotic drugs in humans. *Drug and Alcohol Dependence, 28,* 83–111.

Diana, G., & Massotti, M. (1992). Repeated administration of diazepam reduces [^{3}H]Ro 5-4864 binding in cerebral cortex of rats. *Pharmacology, Biochemistry and Behavior, 42,* 297–300.

Dimpfel, W., Spüler, M., Nickel, B. (1986). Radioelectroencephalography (tele-stereo-EEG) in the rat as a pharmacological model to differentiate the central action of flupirtine from that of opiates, diazepam and phenobarbital. *Neuropsychobiology, 16,* 163–168.

Doble, A., & Martin, I. L. (1992). Multiple benzodiazepine receptors: No reason for anxiety. *TiPS, 13,* 76–78.

Doble, A., Malgouris, C., Daniel, M., Daniel, N., Imbault, F., Basbaum, A., Uzan, A., Guérémy, C., & Le Fur, G. (1987). Labelling of peripheral-type benzodiazepine binding sites in human brain with [^{3}H]PK 11195: Anatomical and subcellular distribution. *Brain Research Bulletin, 18,* 49–61.

Domino, E. F., French, J., Pohorecki, R., Galus, C. F., & Pandit, S. K. (1989). Further observations on the effects of subhypnotic doses of midazolam in normal volunteers. *Psychopharmacology, 25,* 460–465.

Essig, C. F. (1967). Clinical and experimental aspects of barbiturate withdrawal convulsions. *Epilepsia, 8,* 21–30.

Evans, S. M., Funderburk, F. R., & Griffiths, R. R. (1990). Zolpidem and triazolam in humans: Behavioral and subjective effects and abuse liability. *Journal of Pharmacology and Experimental Therapeutics, 255,* 1246–1255.

Fialip, J., Aumaitre, O., Eschalier, A., Maradeix, B., Dordain, G., & Lavarenne, J. (1987). Benzodiazepine withdrawal seizures: Analysis of 48 case reports. *Clinical Neuropharmacology, 6,* 536–544.

File, S. E. (1990). The history of benzodiazepine dependence: A review of animal studies. *Neuroscience and Biobehavioral Review, 14,* 135–146.

File, S. E., & Baldwin, H. A. (1989). Changes in anxiety in rats tolerant to, and withdrawn from, benzodiazepines: Behavioural and biochemical studies. In P. Tyrer, (Ed.), *Psychopharmacology of anxiety* (pp. 28–51). Oxford, England: Oxford University Press.

File, S. E., & Pellow, S. (1986). Intrinsic actions of the benzodiazepine receptor antagonist Ro 15-1788. *Psychopharmacology, 88,* 1–11.

Fink, M., Irwin, P., Weinfeld, R. E., Schwartz, M. A., & Conney, A. H., (1976). Blood levels and electroencephalographic effects of diazepam and bromazepam. *Clinical Pharmacology & Therapeutics, 20,* 184–191.

Fox, K. A., & Lahcen, R. B. (1974). Liver-cell adenomas and peliosis hepatis in mice associated with oxazepam. *Research Communications in Chemical Pathology and Pharmacology, 8,* 481–488.

Friedman, H., Greenblatt, D. J., Peters, G. R., Metzler, C. M., Charlton, M. D., Harmatz, J. S., Antal, E. J., Sanborn, E. C., & Francom, S. F. (1992). Pharmacokinetics and pharmacodynamics of oral diazepam: Effects of dose, plasma concentration, and time. *Clinical Pharmacology & Therapeutics, 52,* 139–150.

Gallager, D. W., & Primus, R. J. (1993). Benzodiazepine tolerance and dependence: GABA$_A$ receptor complex locus of change. In S. Wonnacott & G. Glunt (Eds.), *Neurochemistry of drug dependence* (pp. 135–151). London: Portland.

Gallager, D. W., Heninger, K., & Heninger, G. (1986). Periodic benzodiazepine antagonist administration prevents benzodiazepine withdrawal symptoms in primates. *European Journal of Pharmacology, 132,* 31–38.

Gallager, D. W., Jacobs, A. A., Crais, J. S., During, M. J., & Hernandez, T. D. (1991). Chronic treatments that produce reversible and irreversible changes in gamma-aminobutyric acid sensitivity. In E. A. Bernard & E. Costa (Eds.), *Transmitter amino acid receptors, structures, transactions and model* (pp. 113–128). New York: Raven.

Gallager, D. W., Marley, R. J., & Hernandez, T. D. (1991). Biochemical and electrophysiological mechanisms underlying benzodiazepine tolerance and dependence. In J. Pratt (Ed.), *The biological bases of drug tolerance and dependence* (pp. 49–70). London: Academic Press.

Gardner, C. R., Tully, W. R., & Hedgecock, C. J. R. (1993). The rapidly expanding range of neuronal benzodiazepine receptor ligands. *Progress in Neurobiology 40,* 1–61.

Gavish, M., Bar-Ami, S., & Weitzman, R. (1992). The endocrine system and mitochondrial benzodiazepine receptors. *Molecular and Cellular Endocrinology 88,* 1–13.

Gavish, M., Bar-Ami, S., & Weitzman, R. (1993). Pathophysiological and endocrinological aspects of peripheral-type benzodiazepine receptors. In E. Giesen-Crouse (Ed.), *Peripheral benzodiazepine receptors* (pp. 210–227). London: Academic Press.

Glaser, G. H., Penry, J. K., & Woodbury, D. M. (1980). *Antiepileptic drugs: Mechanisms of action.* New York: Raven.

Gonsalves, S. F., & Gallager, D. W. (1988). Persistent reversal of tolerance to anticonvulsant effects and GABAergic subsensitivity by a single exposure to benzodiazepine antagonist during chronic benzodiazepine administration. *Journal of Pharmacology and Experimental Therapy, 244,* 79–83.

Grant, S. J., Galloway, M. P., Mayor, R., Fenerty. J. P., Finkelstein, M. F., Roth, R. H., & Redmond, D. E., Jr. (1985). Precipitated diazepam withdrawal elevates noradrenergic metabolism in primate brain. *European Journal of Pharmacology, 107,* 127–132.

Greenblatt, D. J., & Shader, R. I. (1985). Clinical pharmacokinetics of the benzodiazepines. In D. E. Smith & D. R. Wesson (Eds.), *The benzodiazepines: Current standards for medical practice* (pp. 43–64). Lancaster, England: MTP.

Griffiths, R. R. (1995). Commentary on review by Woods and Winger. Benzodiazepines: Long-term use among patients is a concern and abuse among polydrug abusers is not trivial [Letter to the editor]. *Psychopharmacology, 118,* 116–117.

Griffiths, R. R., & Wolf, B. (1990). Relative abuse liability of different benzodiazepines in drug abusers. *Journal of Clinical Psychopharmacology, 10*(4), 237–243.

Haefely, W. E. (1977). Synaptic pharmacology of barbiturates and benzodiazepines. *Agents Actions, 7,* 353–359.

Haefely, W. (1986). Biological basis of drug induces tolerance, rebound, and dependence. Contribution of recent research on benzodiazepines. *Pharmacopsychiatria* (Stuttgart), *19,* 353–361.

Haefely, W. E. (1990). The GABA$_A$-benzodiazepine receptor: Biology and pharmacology. In G. D. Brown, M. Ruth, & R. Noyer (Eds.), *Handbook of anxiety: Vol. 3 The neurobiology of anxiety* (pp. 165–188). Amsterdam: Elsevier.

Haefely, W., Kyburz, E., Gerecke, M., & Möhler, H. (1985). Recent advances in the molecular pharmacology of benzodiazepine receptors and in the structure–activity relationships of their agonists and antagonists. In B.Testa (Ed.), *Advances in drug research* (Vol.14, pp.165–322). London: Academic Press.

Haefely, W., Martin, J. R., & Schoch, P. (1990). Novel anxiolytics that act as partial agonists at benzodiazepine receptors. *TiPS, 11*, 452–456.

Hallstrom, C., & Lader, M. (1981). Benzodiazepine withdrawal phenomena. *International Pharmacopsychiatry, 16*, 235–244.

Herings, R. M. C., Stricker, B. H., de Boer, A., Bakker, A., & Sturmans, F. (1995). Benzodiazepines and the risk of falling leading to femur fractures. *Archives of Internal Medicine, 155*, 1801–1807.

Hernández-Alvarez, L. A. I., Márquez-Orozco, M. C., Márquez-Orozco, A., & Hicks, J. J. (1991). Efectos teratológicos de las benzodiazepinas. *Ginecologia y Obstetricia de Mexico, 59*, 195–201.

Hernández-Alvarez, L. A. I., Márquez-Orozco, M. C., & Márquez-Orozco, A. (1994). Mating behavior of female mice treated prenatally with diazepam. *Proceedings of the Western Pharmacology Society, 37*, 69–71.

Herrmann, W. M., & Schaerer, E. (1986). Pharmaco-EEG: Computer EEG analysis to describe the projection of drug effects on a functional cerebral level in humans. In F. H. Lopes da Silva, W. Storm van Leevwen, & A. Redmond (Eds.), *Handbook of electroencephalography and clinical neurophysiolog: Vol. 2. Clinical applications of computer analysis of EEG and other neurophysiological signals* (pp. 385–445). Amsterdam: Elsevier.

Hertz, L. (1993). Binding characteristics of the receptor and coupling to transport proteins. In E. Giesen-Crouse (Ed.), *Peripheral benzodiazepine receptors* (pp. 27–57). London: Academic Press.

Hines, L. R. (1981). Toxicology and side-effects of anxiolytics. In F. Hoffmeister & G. Stille (Eds.), *Handbook of experimental pharmacology* (Vol. 55/II, pp. 359–393). Berlin: Springer-Verlag.

Ho, I. K. (1987). Barbiturate sedative-hypnotics. In I. K. Ho (Ed.), *Toxicology of CNS depressants* (pp. 33–55). Boca Raton, FL: CRC.

Ho, I. K., & Harris, R. A. (1981). Mechanism of action of barbiturates. *Annual Review of Pharmacology and Toxicology,21*, 83–111.

Hobbs, W. R., Rall, T. W., & Verdoorn, T. A. (1996). Hypnotics and sedatives; Ethanol. In J. G. Hardman, L. E. Limbird, P. B. Molinoff, R. W. Ruddon, & A. Goodman Gillman (Eds.), *Goodman & Gilman's the pharmacological basis of therapeutics* (pp. 361–430). New York: McGraw-Hill..

Hollister, L. E. (1985). Principles of therapeutic applications of benzodiazepines. In D. E. Smith & D. R. Wesson (Eds.), *The benzodiazepines current standards for medical practice* (pp. 87–96). Lancaster, England: MTP.

Hollister, L. E., & Csernansky, J. G. (1990). *Clinical pharmacology of psychotherapeutic drugs* (3rd ed.). New York: Churchill Livingstone.

Hollister, L. E., Muller-Oerlinghausen, B., Rickels, K., & Shader, R. I. (1993). Clinical uses of benzodiazepines. *Journal of Clinical Psychopharmacology, 13*, 1–169.

Hunkeler, W., Möhler, H., Pieri, L., Polc, P., Bonetti, E. P., Cumin-Schaffner, R., & Haefely, W. (1981). Selective antagonists of benzodiazepines. *Nature, 290*, 514–516.

Iguchi, M. Y., Handelsman, L., Bickel, W. K., & Griffiths, R. R. (1993). Benzodiazepine and sedative use/abuse by methadone maintenance clients. *Drug and Alcohol Dependence, 32*, 257–266.

Isbell, H., & Fraser, H. F., (1950). Addiction to analgesics and barbiturates. *Journal of Pharmacology and Experimental Therapeutics, Part II, 99*, 355–397.

Iwaya, N., Morita, Y., & Miyoshi, K. (1989). Determination of pharmoco-dynamics of diazepam by quantitative pharmaco-EEG. *Japanese Journal of Psychiatry and Neurology, 43*, 675–684.

Jaffe, J. H., Ciraulo, D. A., Nies, A., Dixon, R. B., & Monroe, L. L. (1983). Abuse potential of halazepam and of diazepam in patients recently treated for acute alcohol withdrawal. *Clinical Pharmacology & Therapeutics, 34*, 623–630.

Judd, F. K., Norman, T. R., Marriott, P. F., & Burrows, G. D. (1986). A case of alprazolam-related hepatitis. *American Journal of Psychiatry, 143*, 388–389.

Judd, F. K., Norman, T. R., & Burrows, G. D. (1990). Pharmacotherapy of panic disorder. *International Review of Psychiatry, 2*, 399–409.

Juergens, S. M. (1993). Benzodiazepines and addiction. *Psychiatric Clinics of North America, 16*, 75–86.

Kay, D. C., Blackburn, A. B., Buckingham, J. A., & Karacan, I. (1976). Human pharmacology of sleep. In R. L. Williams & I. Karacan (Eds.), *Pharmacology of sleep* (pp. 83–210). New York: Wiley.

Kellogg, C. K., Taylor, M. K., Rodriguez-Zafra, M., & Pleger, G. L. (1993). Altered stressor-induced changes in GABA$_A$ receptor function in the cerebral cortex of adult rats exposed in utero to diazepam. *Pharmacology, Biochemistry and Behavior, 44*, 267–273.

King, M. B., Gabe, J., Williams, P., & Rodrigo, E. K. (1990). Long term use of benzodiazepines: The views of patients. *British Journal of General Practice, 40*, 194–196.

Kinoshita, T., Michel, C. M., Yagyu, T., Lehmann, D., & Saito, M. (1994). Diazepam and sulpiride effects on frequency domain EEG source locations. *Neuropsychobiology, 30*, 126–131.

Klepner, C. A., Lippa, A. S., Benson, D. I., Sano, M. C., & Beer, B. (1979). Resolution of two biochemically and pharmacologically distinct benzodiazepine receptors. *Pharmacology, Biochemistry and Behavior, 11*, 457–462.

Koff, J. M., & Miller, L. G. (1995). Prenatal lorazepam exposure: 4. Persistent alterations in pentylenetetrazole-induced seizure threshhold and GABA-dependent chloride uptake after prenatal lorazepam exposure. *Pharmacology, Biochemistry and Behavior, 51,* 721–724.

Krueger, K. E., & Papadopoulos, V. (1993). The role of mitochondrial benzodiazepine receptors in steriodogenesis. In E. Giesen-Crouse (Ed.), *Peripheral benzodiazepine receptors* (pp. 89–109). London: Academic Press.

Lader, M. (1995). Commentary on review by Woods and Winger entitled "Current benzodiazepine issues" [Letter to the editor]. *Psychopharmacology, 118,* 118.

Ladewig, D. (1984). Dependence liability of the benzodiazepines. *Drug and Alcohol Dependence, 13,* 139–149.

Laegreid, L., Olegard, R., Wahlstrom, J., & Conradi, N. (1989). Teratogenic effects of benzodiazepine use during pregnancy. *Journal of Pediatrics, 114,* 126–131.

Lamb, R. J., & Griffiths, R. R. (1985). Effects of repeated Ro 15-1788 administration in benzodiazepine-dependent baboons. *European Journal of Pharmacology, 110,* 257–261.

Langtry, H. D., & Benfield, P. (1990). Zolpidem. A review of its pharmacodynamic and pharmacokinetic properties and therapeutic potential. *Drugs, 40,* 291–313.

Levitan, E. S., Schofield, P. R., Burt, D. R., Rhee, L. M., Wisen, W., Kohler, M., Fujita, N., Rodriguez, H. F., Stephenson, A., Darlison, M. G., Barnard, E. A., & Seeburg, P. H. (1988). Structural and functional basis for GABA$_A$ receptor heterogeneity. *Nature* (London), *335,* 76–70.

Livezey, G. T., Radulovacki, M., Isaac, L., & Marczynski, T. J. (1985). Prenatal exposure to diazepam results in enduring reductions in brain receptors and deep slow wave sleep. *Brain Research, 334,* 361–365.

Lo, K. J., Eastwood, I. R., & Eidelman, S. (1967). Cholestatic jaundice associated with chlordiazepoxide hydrochloride (librium). *American Journal of Digest Diseases, 12,* 845–849.

Longo, V. G., Massotti, M., DeMedici, D., & Valerio, A. (1988). Modifications of brain electrical activity after activation of the benzodiazepine receptor types in rats and rabbits. *Pharmacology, Biochemistry and Behavior, 29,* 785–790.

Löscher, W., & Rundfeldt, C. (1989). Intermittent flumazenil and benzodiazepine tolerance: Discouraging findings in rats. *Lancet, I,* 1386.

Lukas, S. E., & Griffiths, R. R. (1984). Precipitated diazepam withdrawal in baboons: Effects of dose and duration of diazepam exposure. *European Journal of Pharmacology, 100,* 163–171.

Macdonald, R. L., & McLean, M. J. (1986). Anticonvulsant drugs: Mechanisms of action. *Advances in Neurology, 44,* 713–736.

Mandema, J. W., & Danhof, M. (1992). Electroencephalogram effect measures and relationships between pharmacokinetics and pharmacodynamics of centrally acting drugs. *Clinical Pharmacokinetics, 23,* 191–215.

Mandema, J. W., Sansom, L. N., Dios-Vièitez, M. C., Hollander-Jansen, M., & Danhof, M. (1991). Pharmacokinetic-pharmacodynamic modeling of the electroencephalographic effects of benzodiazepines. Correlation with receptor binding and anticonvulsant activity. *Journal of Pharmacology and Experimental Therapeutics, 257,* 472–478.

Mandema, J. W., Kuck, M. T., & Danhof, M. (1992a). Differences in intrinsic efficacy of benzodiazepines are reflected in their concentration-EEG effect relationship. *British Journal of Pharmacology, 105,* 164–170.

Mandema, J. W., Kuck, M. T., & Danhof, M. (1992b). In vivo modeling of the pharmacodynamic interaction between benzodiazepines which differ in intrinsic efficacy. *Journal of Pharmacology and Experimental Therapeutics, 26,* 56–61.

Mandema, J. W., Tukker, E., & Danhof, M. (1992). In vivo characterization of the pharmacodynamic interaction of a benzodiazepine agonist and antagonist: Midazolam and flumazenil. *Journal of Pharmacology and Experimental Therapeutics, 260,* 36–44.

Manmaru, S., & Matsuura, M., (1990). Two kinds of spatiotemporal EEG changes after discontinuation of benzodiazepine, medazepam. *Japanese Journal of Psychiatry and Neurology, 44,* 85–90.

Márquez-Orozco, A., Márquez-Orozco, M. C., & Gazca-Ramírez, M. V. (1993). Histological changes in the tibia of the mouse fetus exposed to diazepam. *Proceedings of the Western Pharmacology Society,36,* 107–112.

Márquez-Orozco, A., Hernandez-Alvarez, L. A. I., & Márquez-Orozco, M. C. (1994). Sexual activity in male mice treated prenatally with diazepam. *Proceedings of the Western Pharmacology Society, 37,* 65–68.

Márquez-Orozco, M. C., Márquez-Orozco, A., & Gazca-Ramírez, M. V. (1993). Effects of diazepam on the ultrastructure of fetal mice hepatocytes. *Proceedings of the Western Pharmacology Society, 36,* 113–116.

Martin, J. R., & Haefely, W. E. (1995). Drugs used for the treatment of anxiety and sleep disorders. In P. L. Munson, R. A. Mueller, & G. R. Briese, (Eds.), *Principles of pharmacology, basic concepts & clinical practice* (pp. 243–277). New York: Chapman & Hall.

Martin, J. R., Moreau, J. L., & Jenck, F. (1995). Precipitated withdrawal in squirrel monkeys after repeated daily oral administration of alprazolam, diazepam, flunitrazepam or oxazepam. *Psychopharmacology, 118,* 273–279.

Martin, W. R., Sloan, J. W., & Wala, E. (1990). Precipitated abstinence in orally dosed benzodiazepine-dependent dogs. *Journal of Pharmacology and Experimental Therapeutics, 255,* 744–755.

Martin, W. R., Sloan, J. W., & Wala, E. P. (1993). Precipitated abstinence in the diazepam-dependent rat.

Pharmacology, Biochemistry and Behavior, 46, 683–688.

Martinez, J. A., Fargeas, M. J., & Bueno, L. (1992). Physical dependence on diazepam: Precipitation of abstinence syndromes by peripheral and central benzodiazepine receptor antagonists. *Pharmacology, Biochemistry and Behavior, 41,* 461–464.

Massotti, M., Mele, L., & De Luca, C. (1990). Involvement of the "peripheral" benzodiazepine receptor type (ω_3) in the tolerance to the electroencephalographic effects of benzodiazepines in rats: Comparison of diazepam and clonazepam. *Pharmacology, Biochemistry and Behavior, 35,* 933–936.

Mata-Santibánez, M. V., Márquez-Orozco, M. C., & Márquez-Orozco, A. (1993). Testicular histological changes in mice after prenatal administration of diazepam. *Proceedings of the Western Pharmacology Society, 36,* 177–121.

Medina, J. H., Novas, M. L., & de Robertis, E. (1983). Chronic Ro 15-1788 treatment increases the number of benzodiazepine receptors in rat cerebral cortex and hippocampus. *European Journal of Pharmacology, 90,* 125–128.

Mele, L., Sagratella, S., & Massotti, M. (1984). Chronic administration of diazepam to rats causes changes in EEG patterns and in coupling between GABA receptors and benzodiazepine binding sites in vitro. *Brain Research, 323,* 93–102.

Mendelson, W. B. (1992). Neuropharmacology of sleep induction by benzodiazepines. *Critical Reviews in Neurobiology, 6,* 221–232.

Mendelson, W. B., Gillin, J. C., & Wyatt, R. J. (1977). *Human sleep and its disorders.* New York: Plenum.

Miller, L G., & Koff, J. M. (1994). Interaction of central and peripheral benzodiazepine sites in benzodiazepine tolerance and discontinuation. *Progress in Neuro-Psychopharmacology & Biological Psychiatry, 18,* 847–857.

Miller, L. G., Greenblatt, D. J., Lopez, F., Schatzki, A., Heller, J., Lumpkin, M., & Shader, R. I. (1990). Chronic benzodiazepine administration: Effects *in vivo* and *in vitro.* In G. Biggio & E. Costa (Eds.), *GABA and benzodiazepine receptor subtypes* (pp. 167–175). New York: Raven.

Morrow, A. L., Pace, J. R., Purdy, R. H., & Paul, S. M. (1990). Characterization of steriod interactions with GABA receptor-gated chloride ion channels. *Molecular Pharmacology, 37,* 262–270.

National Institute on Drug Abuse. (1994a). *Data from the Drug Abuse Warning Network (DAWN): Annual emergency room data 1992* (NIDA Statistical Series I, No. 12-A, p. 37). Rockville, MD: Author.

National Institute on Drug Abuse. (1994b). *Data from the Drug Abuse Warning Network (DAWN): Annual medical examiner data 1992* (NIDA Statistical Series I, No. 12-B, p. 21). Rockville, MD: Author.

Nicoll, R. A. (1980). Sedative-hypnotics: Animal pharmacology. In L. L. Iversen, S. D. Iversen, & S. H. Snyder (Eds.), *Handbook of psychopharmacology: Vol. 12. Drugs of abuse* (pp. 187–234). New York: Plenum.

Niddam, R., Dubois, A., Scatton, B., Arbilla, S., & Langer, S. Z. (1987). Autoradiographic localization of [^{3}H]Zolpidem binding sites in the rat CNS: Comparison with the distribution of [^{3}H]Flunitrazepam binding sites. *Journal of Neurochemistry, 49,* 890–899.

Norenberg, M. D., & Bender, A. S. (1994). Astrocyte swelling in liver failure: Role of glutamine and benzodiazepines. *Acta Neurochirurgica 60,* (Suppl.), 24–27.

Ober, K. (1974). Effects of diazepam on cell division rates and productivity of *Scenedesmus obliquus* in synchronous cultures. *Archives of Microbiology, 99,* 369–378.

Okamoto, M. (1978). Barbiturates and alcohol: Comparative overviews on neurophysiology and neurochemistry. In M. A. Lipton, A. DiMascio, & K. F. Killam (Eds.), *Psychopharmacology: A generation of progress* (pp. 1575–1590). New York: Raven.

Persohn, E., Malherbe, P., & Richards, J. G. (1992). Comparative molecular neuroanatomy of cloned GABA$_A$ receptor subunits in the rat CNS. *Journal of Comparative Neurology, 326,* 193–216.

Pétursson, H. (1994). The benzodiazepine withdrawal syndrome. *Addiction, 89,* 1455–1459.

Pétursson, H., & Lader, M. H. (1981). Withdrawal from long-term benzodiazepine treatment. *British Medical Journal, 283,* 643–645.

Polc, P. (1988). Electrophysiology of benzodiazepine receptor ligands: Multiple mechanisms and sites of action. *Progress in Neurobiology, 31,* 349–423.

Primus, R. J., & Gallager, D. W. (1992). GABA$_A$ receptor subunit mRNA levels are differentially influenced by chronic FG 7142 and diazepam exposure. *European Journal of Pharmacology—Molecular Pharmacology Section, 226,* 21–28.

Primus, R. J., Yu, J., Xu, J., Hartnett, M., Meyyappan, M., Kostas, C., Ramabhadran, T. V., & Gallager, D. W. (1996). Allosteric uncoupling after chronic benzodiazepine exposure of recombinant γ-aminobutyric acid$_A$ receptors expressed in Sf9 cells: Ligand efficacy and subtype selectivity. *Journal of Pharmacology and Experimental Therapeutics, 276,* 882–890.

Pritchett, D. B., Sontheimer, H., Gorman, C. M., Kettenmann, H., Seeburg, P. H., & Schofield, P. R. (1988). Transient expression shows ligand gating and allostericpotentiation of GABA$_A$ receptor subunits. *Science* (Washington, DC), *242,* 1306–1308.

Regan, C. M., Gorman, A. M. C., Larsson, O. M., Maguire, C., Martin, M. L., Schousboe, A., & Williams, D. C. (1990). *In vitro* screening for anticonvulsant-induced teratogenesis in neural primary cultures and cell lines. *International Journal of Developmental Neuroscience, 8,* 143–150.

Rementeria, J. L., & Bhatt, K. (1977). Withdrawal symptoms in neonates from intrauterine exposure to diazepam. *Journal of Pediatrics, 90,* 123–126.

Richards, G., Möhler, H., & Haefely, W. (1986). Mapping benzodiazepine receptors in the CNS by radiohistochemistry and immunohistochemistry. In P. Panula, H. Paivarinta, & S. Soinila (Eds.), *Neurohistochemistry: Modern methods and applications* (pp. 629–677). New York: Liss.

Richter, J. A., & Holtman, J. R., Jr. (1982). Barbiturates: Their in vivo effects and potential biochemical mechanisms. *Progress in Neurobiology, 18,* 275–319.

Rickels, K., Schweizer, E., Case, W. G., & Greenblatt, D. J. (1991). Long term therapeutic use of benzodiazepines: I. Effects of abrupt discontinuation. *Archives of General Psychiatry, 47,* 899–907.

Robinson, R. L., Van Ryzin, R. J., Stoll, R. E., Jensen, R. D., & Bagdon, R. E. (1984). Chronic toxicity/carcinogenesis study of temazepam in mice and rats. *Fundamentals and Applied Toxicology, 4,* 394–405.

Romach, M. K., Busto, U. E., Sobell, L. C., Sobell, M. B., Somer, M. A., & Sellers, E. M. (1991). Long-term alprazolam use: Abuse, dependence or treatment. *Psychopharmacology Bulletin, 27,* 391–395.

Rosenberg, H. C. (1995). Differential expression of benzodiazepine anticonvulsant cross-tolerance according to time following flurazepam or diazepam treatment. *Pharmacology, Biochemistry and Behavior, 51,* 363–368.

Rosenberg, H. C., & Chiu, T. H. (1982). An antagonist-induced benzodiazepine abstinence syndrome. *European Journal of Pharmacology, 81,* 153–157.

Roy-Byrne, P., Vittone, B. J., & Uhde, T. W. (1983). Alprazolam-related hepatotoxicity. *Lancet, 2,* 786–787.

Saano, V. (1993). Effects of peripherally acting benzodiazepines on cell growth and differentiation. In E. Giesen-Crouse (Ed.), *Peripheral benzodiazepine receptors* (pp. 111–124). London: Academic Press.

Sanger, D. J., Benavides, J., Perrault, G., Morel, E., Cohen, C., Joly, D., & Zivkovic, B. (1994). Recent developments in the behavioral pharmacology of benzodiazepine (ω) receptors: Evidence for the functional significance of receptor subtypes. *Neuroscience and Biobehavioral Reviews, 18,* 355–372.

Sannerud, C. A., Cook, J. M., & Griffiths, R. R. (1989). Behavioral differentiation of benzodiazepine ligands after repeated administration in baboons. *European Journal of Pharmacology, 167,* 333–343.

Sassim, N., & Grohmann, R. (1988). Adverse drug reactions with clozapine and simultaneous application of benzodiazepines. *Pharmacopsychiatry, 21,* 306–307.

Saunders, P. A., & Ho, I. K. (1990). Barbiturates and the GABA$_A$ receptor complex. *Progress in Drug Research, 34,* 261–286.

Scherkl, R., & Frey, H. (1986). Physical dependence on clonazepam in dogs. *Pharmacology, 32,* 18–24.

Scheuler, W. (1990–1991). EEG sleep activities react topographically different to GABAergic sleep modulation by flunitrazepam: Relationship to regional distribution of benzodiazepine receptor subtypes? *Neuropsychobiology, 23,* 213–221.

Schlumpf, M., Parmar, R., Ramseier, H. R., & Lichtensteiger, W. (1990). Prenatal benzodiazepine immunosuppression: Possible involvement of peripheral benzodiazepine site. *Developmental Pharmacology Therapeutics, 15,* 178–185.

Schlumpf, M., Parmar, R., & Lichtensteiger, W. (1993). Prenatal diazepam induced persisting downregulation of peripheral (ω3) benzodiazepine receptors on rat splenic macrophages. *Life Sciences, 52,* 927–934.

Schlumpf, M., Lichtensteiger, W., & van Loveren, H. (1994). Impaired host resistance to *Trichinella spiralis* as a consequence of prenatal treatment of rats with diazepam. *Toxicology, 94,* 223–230.

Schmidt, R. F., Vogel, M. E., & Zimmerman, M. (1967). Die wirkung von diazepam auf die präsynaptische hemmung und andere rückenmarksreflexe. *Naunyn-Schmiedebergs Archives of Pharmacology, 258,* 69–82.

Schofield, P. R., Darlison, M. G., Fugita, N., Burt, D. R., Stephenson, F. A., Rodriguez, H., Rhee, L. M., Ramachandran, J., Reale, V., Glencorse, T. A., Seeburg, P. H., & Barnard, E. A. (1987). Sequence and functional expression of the GABA$_A$ receptor shows a ligand-gated receptor super-family. *Nature* (London), *328,* 221–227.

Shibuya, T., Watanabe, Y., Hill, H. F., & Salafsky, B. (1986). Developmental alterations in maturing rats caused by chronic prenatal and postnatal diazepam treatments. *Japanese Journal of Pharmacology, 40,* 21–29.

Sieghart, W. (1995). Structure and pharmacology of γ-aminobutyric acid$_A$ receptor subtypes. *Pharmacological Reviews, 47,* 181–234.

Sloan, J. W., Martin, W. R., & Wala, E. P. (1990). Dependence-producing properties of alprazolam in the dog. *Pharmacology, Biochemistry and Behavior, 35,* 651–657.

Sloan, J. W., Martin, W. R., & Wala, E. P. (1991a). A comparison of the physical dependence inducing properties of flunitrazepam and diazepam. *Pharmacology, Biochemistry and Behavior, 39,* 395–405.

Sloan, J. W., Martin, W. R., & Wala, E. (1991b). Duration of diazepam (DZ) treatment and the intensity of flumazenil precipitated abstinence (FPA) in dogs [Abstracts]. *Federation of the American Society for Experimental Biology Journal, 3,* Part I, A703.

Sloan, J. W., Martin, W. R., Wala, E., & Dickey, K. M. (1991). Chronic administration of and dependence on halazepam, diazepam, and nordiazepam in the dog. *Drug and Alcohol Dependence, 28,* 249–264.

Sloan, J. W., Martin, W. R., & Wala, E. (1993a). Effect of the chronic dose of diazepam on the intensity and characteristics of the precipitated abstinence syndrome in the dog. *Journal of Pharmacology and Experimental Therapeutics, 265,* 1152.

Sloan, J. W., Martin, W. R., & Wala, E. P. (1993b). Effects of flumazenil (F) and DMSO vehicle (V) microinjected (MI) into 4 brain sites in diazepam (D) dependent rats [Abstracts]. *Pharmacologist, 35,* 132.

Sloan, J. W., Wala, E. P., & Jing, X. (1994). Comparison of the response of 4 hippocampal (H) sites in diazepam (DZ) dependent rats to flumazenil (F) microinjections. *Society for Neuroscience Abstracts, 20,* 1604.

Sloan, J. W., Wala, E. P., Jing, X., Holtman, J., Jr., & Lee, E. (1994). Chronic graded doses of diazepam capsule implants alter rat liver function tests [Abstracts]. *Federation of the American Society for Experimental Biology Journal, 8*(4), Part I, 381.

Sloan, J. W., Wala, E. P., & Jing, X. (1995a). Comparison of precipitated abstinence (PA) induced by focally injected flumazenil (FL) into different cerebellar (CB) loci in diazepam (DZ) dependent rats [Abstracts]. *Federation of the American Society for Experimental Biology Journal, 9,* A407.

Sloan, J. W., Wala, E. P., & Jing, X. (1995b). The effect of intra-amygdaloid administration of flumazenil in diazepam-dependent rats. *Society for Neuroscience Abstracts, 21,* 2098.

Sloan, J. W., Jing, X., Wala, E., & Milliken, B. (1996). The focal injection of flumazenil (FLU) into the CA$_1$ of hippocampus (Hi) of diazepam (DZ)-dependent rats produces a dose-related precipitated abstinence [Abstracts]. *Federation of the American Society for Experimental Biology Journal 10*(3), A713.

Sloan, J. W., Wala, E. P., & Jing, X. (1997a). PK 11195 (PK)-evoked withdrawal in diazepam (DZ)-dependent rats: Effect of dose of PK, DZ and gender. *Neuroscience Abstracts, 23*(2), 2392.

Sloan, J. W., Wala, E. P., & Jing, X. (1997b). The effect of focal injections of graded doses of flumazenil (FLU) and PK 11195 (PK) into the CA1 of the hippocampus (HI) of diazepam (DZ)-dependent rats. *Pharmacologist, 39*(1), 90.

Smith, C. M. (1992). Antianxiety drugs. In C. M. Smith, & A. M. Reynard, (Eds.), *Textbook of pharmacology* (pp. 271–297). Philadelphia: Saunders.

Speight, A. N. (1977). Floppy-infant syndrome and maternal diazepam and/or nitrazepam. *Lancet, 2,* 878.

Spivey, W. H. (1992). Flumazenil and seizures: Analysis of 43 cases. *Clinical Therapeutics, 14,* 292–305.

Takeno, S., Hirano, Y., Kitamura, A., & Sakai, T. (1993). Comparative developmental toxicity and metabolism of nitrazepam in rats and mice. *Toxicology & Applied Pharmacology, 121,* 233–238.

Tedesco, F. J., & Mills, L. R. (1982). Diazepam (valium) hepatitis. *Digestive Diseases and Sciences, 27,* 470–472.

Thomson, I., Fraser, R., & Kenyon, C. J. (1995). Regulation of adrenocortical steroidogenesis by benzodiazepines. *Journal of Steroid Biochemistry and Molecular Biology, 53,* 75–79.

Tietz, E. I., Rosenberg, H. C., & Chiu, T. H. (1986). Autoradiographic localization of benzodiazepine receptor downregulation. *Journal of Pharmacology and Experimental Therapeutics, 236,* 284–292.

Troisi, I. I., Jr., Critchfield, T. S., & Griffiths, R. R. (1993). Buspirone and lorazepam abuse liability in humans: Behavioral effects, subjective effects and choice. *Behavioral Pharmacology, 4,* 217–230.

Tucker, J. C. (1985). Benzodiazepines and the developing rat: A critical review. *Neuroscience and Biobehavioral Reviews, 9,* 101–111.

Urbancic, M., Gadek, M. A., & Marczynski, T. J. (1990). Chronic exposure to flumazenil: Anxiolytic effect and increased exploratory behavior. *Pharmacology, Biochemistry and Behavior, 35,* 503–509.

Valerio, A., & Massotti, M. (1988). Electroencephalographic changes after short-term exposure to agonists of benzodiazepine receptors in the rat. *Pharmacology, Biochemistry and Behavior, 29,* 791–795.

Verdoorn, T. A. (1994). Formation of heteromeric γ-aminobutyric acid type A receptors containing two different α subunits. *Molecular Pharmacology, 45,* 475–480.

Verdoorn, T. A., Draguhn, A., Ymer, S., Seeburg, P. H., & Sakmann, B. (1990). Functional properties of recombinant rat GABA$_A$ receptors depend upon subunit composition. *Neuron, 4,* 919–928.

Wala, E. P., Sloan, J. W., & Jing, X. (1994). Intra-stratial administration of flumazenil (FL) to diazepam (DZ) dependent rats. *Society for Neuroscience Abstracts 20,* 1612.

Wala, E. P., Sloan, J. W., Martin, W. R., & Jing, X. (1994). Abstinence syndrome following focal administrations of flumazenil (FL) into the cerebellum (CB) and fourth ventricle (4V) in diazepam (DZ) dependent rats. *Canadian Journal of Physiology and Pharmacology, Abstracts XII International Congress of Pharmacology* (Vol. 72, Suppl. 1), 391.

Wala, E. P., Sloan, J. W., Jing, X., & Holtman, P. H. (1996). Intrathecally administed flumazenil and PK 11195 precipitate abstinence syndrome in diazepam dependent rats. *Drug and Alcohol Dependence, 43,* 169–177.

Wala, E. P., Sloan, J. W., & Jing, X. (1997a). Dorsal raphe and substantia nigra response to flumazenil in diazepam-dependent rats. *Pharmacology, Biochemistry and Behavior, 58*(1), 221–229.

Wala, E. P., Sloan, J. W., & Jing, X. (1997b). Comparison of abstinence syndromes precipitated by flumazenil and PK 11195 in female diazepam-dependent rats. *Psychopharmacology, 133*(3), 214–223.

Wala, E. P., Sloan, J. W., & Jing, X. (1997c). Substantia nigra: The involvement of the central and peripheral benzodiazepine receptors in physical dependence on diazepam in rats. *Society for Neuroscience Abstracts, 231*(2), 2401.

Weitzman, R., & Gavish, M. (1989). Chronic diazepam treatment induces an increase in peripheral benzodiazepine binding sites. *Clinical Neuropharmacology, 12,* 346–351.

Weizman, R., Leschiner, S., Schlegel, W., & Gavish M. (1997). Peripheral-type benzodiazepine receptor ligands and serum steroid hormones. *Brain Research, 772,* 203–308.

Whitehouse, B. J. (1992). Benzodiazepines and steroidogenesis. *Journal of Endocrinology 134,* 1–3.

Williams, M. (1984). Molecular aspects of the action of benzodiazepines and non-benzodiazepine anxiolytics: A hypothetical allosteric model of the benzodiazepine receptor complex. *Progress in Neuro-Psychopharmacology and Biological Psychiatry, 8,* 209–247.

Woods, J. H., Katz, J. L., & Winger, G. (1992). Benzodiazepines: Use, abuse, and consequences. *Pharmacological Reviews, 44,* 151–347.

Yamadera, H., Kato, M., Ueno, T., Tsukahara, Y., & Okuma, T. (1993). Pharmaco-EEG mapping of diazepam effects using different references and absolute and relative power. *Pharmacopsychiatry, 26,* 254–258.

Yanagita, T. (1981). Dependence-producing effects of anxiolytics. In F. Hoffmeister & G. Stille (Eds.), *Psychotropic agents* (pp. 395–406). Berlin: Springer-Verlag.

Behavioral Pharmacology of Sedatives, Hypnotics, and Anxiolytics

CRAIG R. RUSH, CATHERINE A. HAYES, AND STEPHEN T. HIGGINS

The purpose of this chapter is to review the behavioral pharmacology and abuse liability of commonly prescribed anxiolytics and hypnotics. More specifically, this chapter reviews the behavioral pharmacology and abuse liability of commonly prescribed benzodiazepines (e.g., alprazolam, diazepam, estazolam, lorazepam, temazepam, and triazolam) and nonbenzodiazepine anxiolytics-hypnotics (e.g., buspirone and zolpidem). The behavioral pharmacology and abuse liability of the benzodiazepines is not exhaustively reviewed since such a review is beyond the scope of this chapter, and comprehensive reviews have previously been published (Woods, Katz, & Winger, 1987, 1992). Instead, this chapter focuses on studies that attempted to determine putative differences between benzo-diazepines. This chapter then reviews the behavioral pharmacology and abuse liability of two nonbenzodiazepine compounds marketed for the treatment of anxiety and sleep disorders: buspirone and zolpidem, respectively. Buspirone was the first pyrimidinylpiperazine derivative marketed for the treatment of anxiety disorders, while zolpidem was the first imidazopyridine derivative marketed for the treatment of sleep disorders. Only studies that directly compared these drugs with a benzodiazepine are reviewed in an attempt to determine if these nonbenzodiazepine compounds have an improved abuse liability profile. Both nonhuman and human studies are reviewed.

Defining and Characterizing Abuse Liability

Many drugs, including commonly prescribed anxiolytics and hypnotics have liability *for* abuse. That is, commonly prescribed anxiolytics and hypnotics are often taken for nonmedical purposes at supratherapeutic doses. Commonly prescribed anxiolytics and hypnotics also have liability *of* abuse. That is, they produce adverse effects such as physiological dependence and performance impairment. The

CRAIG R. RUSH • Department of Pharmacology and Toxicology, The University of Mississippi Medical Center, Jackson, Mississippi 39216. CATHERINE A. HAYES • Department of Psychiatry and Human Behavior, The University of Mississippi Medical Center, Jackson, Mississippi 39216. STEPHEN T. HIGGINS • Departments of Psychiatry and Psychology, University of Vermont, Burlington, Vermont 05401.

Handbook of Substance Abuse: Neurobehavioral Pharmacology, edited by Tarter *et al.* Plenum Press, New York, 1998.

relative abuse liability of a drug is an interactive function of its liability *for* and *of* abuse (Brady & Ator, 1990; R. R. Griffiths, Lamb, Ator, Roache, & Brady, 1985).

Preclinical studies with nonhuman laboratory animals typically assess a drug's liability *for* abuse by determining whether it maintains self-administration (Brady & Ator, 1990; R. R. Griffiths *et al.*, 1985). In a typical self-administration experiment, nonhuman laboratory animals receive oral or intravenous administrations of drug or vehicle (i.e., placebo) contingent on emitting a response (e.g., lever press). Drugs that maintain rates of self-administration greater than those observed with vehicle are deemed to be reinforcers. Importantly, there is a high degree of concordance between drugs that maintain self-administration and function as reinforcers in nonhuman laboratory animals and those that are abused by humans (Fischman & Mello, 1989). Preclinical laboratory studies also characterize a drug's interoceptive or discriminative stimulus effects using drug-discrimination procedures (Glennon, Jarbe, & Frankenheim, 1991). In a typical drug-discrimination experiment, a subject learns one response (e.g., press right lever) following the injection of drug and a different response (e.g., press left lever) following the injection of vehicle. Following training, novel drugs can be substituted for the training drug to determine whether they share discriminative stimulus effects. A drug is inferred to have at least some liability *for* abuse if it substitutes for a drug known to be abused (Preston & Bigelow, 1991). Finally, preclinical studies determine a drug's ability to produce physiological dependence by chronically treating animals and then abruptly terminating drug administration and observing the animal for symptoms of withdrawal, or by administering an appropriate antagonist to determine whether it precipitates withdrawal.

Self-administration and drug-discrimination procedures adapted for use with human subjects are being used more frequently to determine the liability *for* abuse of commonly prescribed anxiolytics and hypnotics (R. R. Griffiths, Bigelow, & Liebson, 1979; Kamien, Bickel, Hughes, Higgins, & Smith, 1993).

Human laboratory studies also often assess liability *for* abuse using subject ratings of drug liking, euphoria, and mood (de Wit & Griffiths, 1991; Roache & Griffiths, 1989a). Drugs of abuse typically increase subject ratings of drug liking and euphoria, or produce positive-mood changes. Clinical studies most typically determine a drug's ability to produce physiological dependence by chronically treating patients, discontinuing treatment, and then observing the patient for symptoms of withdrawal. Human laboratory experiments further determine a drug's liability *of* abuse (i.e., adverse effects) using tasks that measure various aspects of human performance (e.g., recall).

Benzodiazepine Compounds

Benzodiazepines are indicated in the treatment of anxiety, sleep problems, and musculoskeletal disorders, and are among the most widely prescribed psychoactive drugs (Hollister, Muller-Oerlinghausen, Rickels, & Shader, 1993). While their abuse liability is low compared to other abused drugs (Katz, Winger, & Woods, 1990; Rifkin, Doddi, Karajgi, Hasan, & Alvarez, 1989; Woods *et al.*, 1987, 1992), there is sufficient evidence documenting that benzodiazepines have some liability *for* abuse (i.e., they maintain self-administration) and significant liability *of* abuse (i.e., adverse effects). The nonmedical use of benzodiazepines at supratherapeutic doses is common among individuals with histories of ethanol, opioid, and sedative dependence (Bigelow *et al.*, 1980; Darke, Ross, & Hall, 1995; DuPont, 1988; R. R. Griffiths & Wolf, 1990; Iguchi, Handelsman, Bickel, & Griffiths, 1993; Miller & Giannini, 1991; Navaratnam & Foong, 1990a, 1990b; Sellers *et al.*, 1993; Stitzer, Griffiths, McLellan, Grabowski, & Hawthorne, 1981). Benzodiazepines produce a myriad of adverse effects including physiological dependence and performance impairment (Bowen & Larson, 1993; Curran, 1991; Rush, Higgins, Bickel, & Hughes, 1993a).

Some evidence suggests that the available benzodiazepines may be distinguishable in terms of their abuse liability. First, individuals with histories of ethanol and opiate abuse report preferring alprazolam, diazepam, and lorazepam to other benzodiazepines such as chlordiazepoxide, clorazepate, and oxazepam, and that the former compounds produce a greater "high" (R. R. Griffiths & Wolf, 1990; Iguchi *et al.,* 1993; Wolf & Griffiths, 1991). Second, 91% of drug-abuser-experienced physicians surveyed believe there are meaningful differences among available benzodiazepines regarding their liability for abuse (R. R. Griffiths & Wolf, 1990). Alprazolam, diazepam, and lorazepam were cited as having a relatively high liability *for* abuse, while clonazepam, clorazepate, and oxazepam were cited as having a relatively low liability *for* abuse (R. R. Griffiths & Wolf, 1990). Third, 84% of physicians surveyed reported that they thought high-potency benzodiazepines (e.g., alprazolam) were more problematic with regard to the severity of the withdrawal syndrome than low-potency benzodiazepines (e.g., diazepam) (Wolf & Griffiths, 1991). Fourth, reports of impairment of recall are up to 99 times more common with triazolam than other benzodiazepines (Bixler, Kales, Brubaker, & Kales, 1987; Wise, 1990; Wysowski & Barash, 1991).

Interestingly, prospective, controlled studies generally do not support the position that the available benzodiazepines differ significantly in terms of their abuse liability. In the following sections we review studies with laboratory animals and humans that attempted to discern differences between available benzodiazepines in terms of their abuse liability.

Liability *for* Abuse

Preclinical Studies

Self-Administration

Several studies with laboratory animals have shown that intravenous administrations of benzodiazepines maintain rates of self-administration greater than vehicle (for a review see Ator & Griffiths, 1987). Between-benzodiazepine differences are small. For the sake of brevity, this section reviews a series of experiments by the same group of investigators that compared the number of daily intravenous self-administrations of 11 benzodiazepines in separate groups of baboons ($N = 2$–6/group): alprazolam (0.01–3.2 mg/kg/injection), bromazepam (0.032–3.2 mg/kg/injection), chlordiazepoxide (0.032–3.2 mg/kg/injection), clonazepam (0.01–10 mg/kg/injection), clorazepate (0.01–5.6 mg/kg/injection), diazepam (0.032–17.8 mg/kg/injection), flurazepam (0.1–30 mg/kg/injection), lorazepam (0.001–3.0 mg/kg/injection), medazepam (0.01–10 mg/kg/injection), midazolam (0.032–10 mg/kg/injection) and triazolam (0.0001–0.32 mg/kg/injection) (R. R. Griffiths, Lamb, Sannerud, Ator, & Brady, 1991; R. R. Griffiths, Lukas, Bradford, Brady, & Snell, 1981). Baboons could self-administer a maximum of 8 injections per day. All benzodiazepines maintained greater self-administration at some dose than vehicle, but there was considerable overlap between all the benzodiazepines tested. The average number of injections per day across the previous 5 days for the dose maintaining the greatest number of self-administrations was 4.1 for alprazolam (range = 2.0–6.5), 3.1 for bromazepam (range = 2.2–4.9), 4.3 for chlordiazepoxide (range = 3.2–5.1), 4.0 for clonazepam (range = 3.5–4.5), 5.0 for clorazepate (range = 5.0–5.0), 3.0 for diazepam (range = 1.6–4.6), 4.0 for flurazepam (range = 3.9–4.1), 4.8 for lorazepam (range = 2.0–7.0), 3.2 for medazepam (range = 2.8–4.0), 5.2 for midazolam (range = 2.2–7.5), and 5.6 for triazolam (range = 4.5–6.6) and 1.5 for vehicle (range = 0.3–3.3). Thus, benzodiazepines with different pharmacokinetic profiles maintain comparable rates of self-administration.

There is only one published study that compared rates of self-administration maintained by different benzodiazepines via the oral route of administration, which may be more analogous to the human situation (Stewart, Lemiaire, Roache, & Meisch, 1994). In this study rates of self-administration maintained by midazolam (0.05–0.8 mg/ml), a short-acting benzodiazepine, and diazepam (0.2–0.8 mg/ml), a long-acting benzodiazepine, were compared in rhesus monkeys with histories of ethanol- and pentobarbital-reinforced behavior. Four monkeys were initially allowed to self-administer midazolam, and diazepam was then substituted. Oral midazolam clearly maintained self-administration in 3 of 4 monkeys, although the concentration that maintained the highest rate of self-administration varied across monkeys. Diazepam readily substituted for midazolam. Rates of self-administration maintained by midazolam and diazepam were comparable despite the pharmacokinetic differences between these two compounds.

Interoceptive Stimulus Effects

The discriminative stimulus effects of various benzodiazepines have been tested in a variety of species trained to discriminate between pentobarbital, a barbiturate anxiolytic-hypnotic known to be abused, and vehicle. Benzodiazepines dose-dependently increase pentobarbital-appropriate responding, which suggest that benzodiazepines and barbiturates have similar liabilities *for* abuse. For example, alprazolam, bromazepam, chlordiazepoxide, diazepam, lorazepam, nordiazepam, temazepam, and triazolam dose-dependently increased pentobarbital-appropriate responding in baboons and rats trained to discriminate between pentobarbital and vehicle (Ator & Griffiths, 1989). There were no discernible between-drug differences in that at least one dose of each drug fully substituted (i.e., occasioned ≥ 80% drug-appropriate responding) for pentobarbital.

Clinical Studies

As noted above, self-administration and drug-discrimination procedures adapted for use with human subjects are being used more frequently to determine the liability *for* abuse of commonly prescribed anxiolytics and hypnotics (R. R. Griffiths *et al.*, 1979; Kamien *et al.*, 1993). Subject-rated drug-effect questionnaires are also often used to assess the liability *of* abuse of drugs in humans (Jasinski & Henningfield, 1989).

Self-Administration

Although studied relatively infrequently, benzodiazepines have been shown to maintain self-administration (i.e., function as rein-

forcers) in individuals with histories of drug and ethanol abuse (Roache & Griffiths, 1989b; Roache *et al.*, 1995), and in at least one study in moderate ethanol drinkers (de Wit & Doty, 1994). Self-administration procedures have been used even more infrequently to determine differences between available benzodiazepines in terms of their liability *for* abuse. We are aware of only two experiments that directly compared the reinforcing effects of two benzodiazepines using self-administration procedures adapted for use with humans (R. R. Griffiths, McLeod, *et al.,* 1984; Roache & Griffiths, 1989b).

In the first study, 16 volunteers with histories of sedative abuse were allowed to choose between varying doses of diazepam (40, 80 and 160 mg) and placebo, or oxazepam (480 mg) and placebo (R. R. Griffiths, McLeod, *et al.,* 1984). Subjects chose diazepam over placebo 100% of the time, regardless of dose. Subjects chose 480 mg oxazepam over placebo approximately 79% of the time. Thus, all doses of drug functioned as reinforcers in that they were chosen over placebo above chance (i.e., 50%) levels. Subjects were also allowed to choose between each dose of diazepam and 480 mg oxazepam. Diazepam (40, 80, and 160 mg) was chosen over 480 mg oxazepam approximately 38%, 63% and 92% of the time, respectively (R. R. Griffiths, McLeod, Bigelow, Liebson, Roache, & Nowowieski, 1984). Thus, the only clear preference for diazepam over oxazepam was at the highest dose of diazepam (160 mg). Worth noting is that the high dose of diazepam (160 mg) and 480 mg oxazepam produced quantitatively different effects on subject ratings of drug effect (i.e., oxazepam < diazepam). Thus, it is unclear whether diazepam and oxazepam differ in terms of their liability *for* abuse since subjects may have chosen diazepam over oxazepam based on quantitative versus qualitative differences.

In the second study, 8 volunteers with histories of sedative abuse were allowed to self-administer diazepam (40 or 80 mg), triazolam (1 or 2 mg), or placebo (Roache & Griffiths, 1989b). After an initial sampling session, volunteers could self-administer a single dose of drug each day for 6 days by completing a progressively increasing bicycle-riding requirement. Order of exposure to diazepam and triazolam was counterbalanced across subjects, and placebo was always tested between the diazepam and triazolam phase. Both diazepam and triazolam maintained self-administration above placebo levels, which means they functioned as reinforcers. There were no discernible differences between diazepam and triazolam in this regard. On the first day of self-administration, 100% of the subjects self-administered diazepam and triazolam. As expected, diazepam and triazolam self-administration decreased as the bicycle-riding requirement was increased. These data suggest that diazepam and triazolam do not differ in terms of their liability *for* abuse.

Interoceptive Stimulus Effects

Human drug-discrimination procedures are being used more frequently to determine similarities and differences between the interoceptive stimulus effects of drugs. Several recent studies have determined that benzodiazepines (e.g., diazepam and triazolam) function as discriminative stimuli (e.g., Bickel, Oliveto, Kamien, Higgins, & Hughes, 1993; Johanson, 1991a; Oliveto, Bickel, Hughes, Higgins, & Fenwick, 1992; Oliveto, Bickel, Kamien, Hughes, & Higgins, 1994). However, to the best of our knowledge, there is only one study that determined that the discriminative stimulus effects of a benzodiazepine in humans are similar to those of pentobarbital, a barbiturate anxiolytic-hypnotic known to be abused (Rush, Madakasira, Goldman, Woolverton, & Rowlett, 1996). In this study, 4 volunteers were trained to discriminate between a hypnotic dose of pentobarbital, 100 mg, and placebo. After acquiring the pentobarbital–placebo discrimination, a range of doses of triazolam, a benzodiazepine hypnotic, and pentobarbital were tested to determine if they shared discriminative stimulus effects with the training dose of pentobarbital. Triazolam (0.063, 0.125, 0.25, and 0.5 mg) on average occasioned 25%, 75%, 75%, and 88% pentobarbital-appropriate responding, respectively. Pentobarbital (25, 50, 100, and 150 mg) on average occasioned 50%, 19%, 85%, and 94% pentobarbital-appropriate responding, respectively. These data suggest that the discriminative stimulus effects of triazolam are similar to those of pentobarbital, which is concordant with preclinical laboratory experiments. To the best of our knowledge, there are no published reports that compared various benzodiazepines in pentobarbital-trained humans, thus it is not known whether other available benzodiazepines (e.g., alprazolam, diazepam, lorazepam, and oxazepam) would differentially engender pentobarbital-appropriate responding.

Subject-Rated Drug Effects

As noted earlier, subject-rated drug-effect questionnaires are often used to assess a drug's liability *for* abuse in humans (Jasinski & Henningfield, 1989). We are aware of four prospective laboratory studies that compared different benzodiazepines to determine putative differences in terms of their liability *for* abuse in individuals with histories of drug and alcohol abuse (Funderburk *et al.*, 1988; R. R. Griffiths, McLeod, Bigelow, Liebson, & Roache, 1984; R. R. Griffiths, McLeod, Bigelow, Liebson, Roache, & Nowowieski, 1984); Jaffe, Ciraulo, Nies, Dixon, & Monroe, 1983). This review is limited to studies that employed subjects with histories of drug or alcohol abuse because these individuals are at increased risk to abuse benzodiazepines and, thus, may represent a more appropriate population to determine between-drug differences in terms of abuse potential (de Wit & Griffiths, 1991; DuPont, 1988; R. R. Griffiths & Wolf, 1990; Miller & Giannini, 1991; Roache & Griffiths, 1989a; Sellers *et al.*, 1993). The experimental methods were similar across these studies: (1) Acute drug effects were assessed before drug administration and periodically after drug administration for 8–24 hours, (2) liability *for* abuse was assessed using subject ratings of drug liking, (3) subject ratings of drug effect and sedation were included to ascertain the comparability of drug effects, and (4) diazepam, a benzodiazepine known to be abused, was included as the standard compound.

One study used an incomplete crossover design to compare the effects of 20 mg diazepam (N = 18), 40 mg diazepam (N = 19), 160 mg halazepam (N = 18), 320 mg halazepam (N = 17), and placebo (N = 18) in volunteers recently treated for acute ethanol withdrawal (Jaffe et al., 1983). Drug effects were measured using subject ratings of drug liking, euphoria, feel the drug, sedation, and drug identification. Diazepam and halazepam increased ratings of drug liking above levels observed with placebo. Peak effects of diazepam were greater than those of halazepam. These doses of diazepam also produced greater increases in subject ratings of sedation than halazepam. By contrast, these doses of halazepam were more often identified as placebo than the doses of diazepam. These findings suggest that halazepam may have less liability *for* abuse than diazepam in patients recently withdrawn from ethanol, but it is unclear whether equivalent doses of halazepam and diazepam were tested.

Two studies compared the abuse potential of diazepam and oxazepam in volunteers with histories of drug abuse (R. R. Griffiths, McLeod, Bigelow, Liebson, & Roache, 1984; R. R. Griffiths, McLeod, Bigelow, Liebson, Roache, & Nowowieski, 1984). The first study compared the effects of diazepam (40, 80, and 160 mg), oxazepam (480 mg), and placebo (R. R. Griffiths, McLeod, Bigelow, Liebson, & Roache, 1984). The second study compared the effects of diazepam (10–160 mg), oxazepam (30–480 mg), and placebo (R. R. Griffiths, McLeod, Bigelow, Liebson, & Roache, 1984). Drug effects were measured using subject ratings of drug effect, drug liking, sleepy, drunken, and relaxed. Analysis of peak-effect data showed that both diazepam and oxazepam increased subject ratings of drug liking as a function of dose, but the effects of 160 mg diazepam were greater than those of 480 mg oxazepam. Similarly, diazepam produced greater effects than oxazepam on subject ratings of drug effect. Thus, findings on subject ratings of drug liking suggest that oxazepam may have less liability *for* abuse than diazepam in subjects with histories of drug abuse, but the fact that diazepam also produced greater effects of subject ratings of drug effect suggests that the doses of diazepam and oxazepam tested were not equivalent.

The final study compared diazepam (0, 10, 20, and 40 mg) and lorazepam (0, 1.5, 3, and 6 mg) in separate groups of volunteers with histories of recreational benzodiazepine use (Funderburk et al., 1988). Diazepam and lorazepam produced comparable dose-related increases in subject ratings of drug liking and drug effect. These findings suggest that diazepam and lorazepam have similar liability *for* abuse. Importantly, these findings raise questions about the differences observed in the other studies. That is, this is the only study in which the compounds were equated for ratings of overall drug effects. Under these conditions the two benzodiazepines did not differ. Whether any between-benzodiazepine differences could be detected under similar conditions is not known.

Liability *of* Abuse

Benzodiazepines produce a myriad of adverse effects. Commonly studied adverse effects include physiological dependence and withdrawal, impairment of performance, and interactions with ethanol. Controlled studies generally do not support the position that benzodiazepines differ in terms of their liability *of* abuse.

Preclinical Studies: Physiological Dependence

Chronically treating laboratory animals with a benzodiazepine results in physiological dependence, and discontinuing treatment results in a recognizable and measurable withdrawal syndrome. Benzodiazepine dependence can also be studied by chronically treating laboratory animals with an agonist and then precipitating withdrawal by administering an antagonist like flumazenil. Putative between-drug differences regarding the severity of the benzodiazepine discontinuation have been most thoroughly studied using the precipitated-withdrawal paradigm. These studies have produced mixed results.

Two reports noted differences between various benzodiazepines in terms of their dependence liability using the precipitated-withdrawal paradigm. The first study examined the precipitated-withdrawal syndrome in dogs ($N = 6$) chronically treated with alprazolam (48 mg/kg/day) (Sloan, Martin, & Wala, 1990). Following at least 1 week of exposure to alprazolam, dogs were challenged with oral administrations of flumazenil (6, 18, or 36 mg/kg). Scores on a modified version of the Nordiazepam-Precipitated-Abstinence Scale and the frequency of seizures were generally an increasing function of flumazenil dose. These data were compared to results from a similar experiment in which dogs were chronically maintained on diazepam (24 or 36 mg/kg/day for at least 2 weeks) and challenged with oral administrations of flumazenil (2, 6, or 18 mg/kg) (McNicholas, Martin, Sloan, & Wala, 1988). Nordiazepam-Precipitated-Abstinence-Scale scores for the alprazolam-treated dogs were significantly less than for the diazepam-treated dogs following the 6 and 18 mg/kg doses of flumazenil. Seizure activity did not differ significantly across drugs.

The second study summarized several experiments from the same laboratory in which dogs were chronically treated with alprazolam (48 mg/kg/day), diazepam (20–36 mg/kg/day), flunitrazepam (7.6 mg/kg/day), halazepam (180–450 mg/kg/day), lorazepam (140 mg/kg/day), oxazepam (270 mg/kg/day), and nordiazepam (18–36 mg/kg/day) and then challenged with flumazenil (2–72 mg/kg) (W. R. Martin, Sloan, & Wala, 1990). Drugs were administered 4–5 times a day for 2–10 weeks followed by oral administrations of flumazenil. Scores on the Benzodiazepine-Precipitated-Abstinence Scale and the frequency of seizures generally were an increasing function of flumazenil dose in all benzodiazepine-treated dogs, while benzodiazepine-naive dogs showed no effect. The benzodiazepines appeared to differ in terms of Benzodiazepine-Precipitated-Abstinence Scale scores (diazepam > flunitrazepam = halazepam > alprazolam = nordiazepam > oxazepam > lorazepam) and the frequency of seizures (flunitrazepam > alprazolam > diazepam > nordiazepam > lorazepam > halazepam = oxazepam) following the administration of high doses of flumazenil. These find-

ings must be viewed tentatively because dose and duration of exposure were not necessarily equivalent across drugs, and these variables are important determinants of the severity of withdrawal (Lukas & Griffiths, 1984).

We are aware of at least two other studies that did not note differences between various benzodiazepines in terms of their dependence liability using the precipitated-withdrawal paradigm (Ator & Griffiths, 1992; J. R. Martin, Moreau, & Jenck, 1995). In the first study, separate groups ($N = 4$–5/group) of squirrel monkeys were treated with orally administered alprazolam (2 mg/kg/day), diazepam (30 mg/kg/day), flunitrazepam (1 mg/kg/day), oxazepam (280 mg/kg/day), or vehicle for 18 consecutive days (J. R. Martin et al., 1995). These doses were selected because they were the lowest doses to consistently induce loss of the righting reflex, which suggests they were behaviorally equivalent. Intravenous flumazenil (10 mg/kg) was administered 5 hr after oral treatment on the 9th and 18th days. The first flumazenil administration precipitated withdrawal (i.e., tremors, vomiting, or convulsions) in 1 alprazolam-, 3 diazepam-, 1 flunitrazepam-, and 2 oxazepam-treated animals. The second flumazenil administration precipitated withdrawal in 3 alprazolam-, 3 diazepam-, 3 flunitrazepam-, and 4 oxazepam-treated animals. Intravenous administration of vehicle did not precipitate withdrawal.

In the second study, baboons ($N = 4$/group) were allowed to orally self-administer triazolam or diazepam for 1 month (Ator & Griffiths, 1992). Intramuscularly administered flumazenil (5 mg/kg) increased the frequency of nose rubbing/scratching, tremor, and retching or vomiting in both the triazolam and diazepam self-administering animals, which suggests a precipitated-withdrawal syndrome. Intrasmucularly administered vehicle did not produce these effects. Triazolam and diazepam did not appear to differ.

Clinical Studies

Physiological Dependence

Terminating treatment in patients chronically maintained on benzodiazepines results in a recognizable discontinuation syndrome. Many clinicians believe the benzodiazepine discontinuation syndrome is more severe when treatment involves a short half-life (SHL) benzodiazepine such as alprazolam or lorazepam versus a long half-life (LHL) benzodiazepine such as clorazepate or diazepam (Wolf & Griffiths, 1991).

Eleven studies compared the withdrawal syndrome following the discontinuation of SHL and LHL benzodiazepines; these studies are summarized in Table 1. This table shows that SHL benzodiazepines produced a more severe withdrawal syndrome than LHL benzodiazepines. This table also shows that most of the studies that compared the severity of the withdrawal syndrome following chronic treatment with SHL and LHL benzodiazepines abruptly discontinued treatment, which is not the medically recommended mode of discontinuation. In three studies that examined the effects of a gradual taper, SHL and LHL benzodiazepines did not differ in terms of the severity of the discontinuation syndrome (Fontaine, Chouinard, & Annable, 1984; Murphy & Tyrer, 1991; Roy-Byrne, Dager, Cowley, Vitaliano, & Dunner, 1989). Similarly, when Schweizer, Rickels, Case, and Greenblatt (1990) combined their data with that from the Rickels, Schweizer, Case, and Greenblatt (1990) study, they noted a statistically significant interaction of half-life and mode of discontinuation across most measures (Rickels *et al.*, 1990; Schweizer *et al.*, 1990). Patients treated with SHL benzodiazepines experienced a more severe discontinuation syndrome than patients treated with LHL benzodiazepines when the drugs were abruptly terminated, but not when they were gradually tapered.

Impairment of Performance

Benzodiazepines dose-dependently impair various aspects of human performance (for reviews see Woods *et al.*, 1987, 1992). Perhaps the most disconcerting performance-impairing effect of benzodiazepines for both the patient and prescribing physician is the impaired recall of information presented after drug administration (i.e., anterograde amnesia).

Numerous studies have compared the recall-impairing effects of various benzodiazepines in an attempt to delineate between-drug differences. These studies have produced mixed results and it remains unclear whether available benzodiazepines differ significantly in terms of their recall-impairing effects.

In the following sections, we review laboratory studies that attempted to discern differences between available benzodiazepines in terms of their recall-impairing effects. For the sake of brevity, only studies that included a standard positive control, triazolam, are reviewed. The recall-impairing effects of triazolam have been characterized across a wide range of doses (Evans, Funderburk, & Griffiths, 1990; Kirk, Roache, & Griffiths, 1990; Roache & Griffiths, 1985; Rush, Higgins, Bickel, & Hughes, 1993b; Rush, Higgins, Hughes, & Bickel, 1993), and, more importantly, some epidemiological studies suggest impaired recall is more common with triazolam than with other benzodiazepines (Bixler *et al.*, 1987; Wise, 1990; Wysowski & Barash, 1991). Thus, the aim of this review is to identify those benzodiazepines for which the recall-impairing potential is less than that of triazolam.

We are aware of 17 published experiments, summarized in Table 2, that directly compared the recall-impairing effects of a benzodiazepine to those of triazolam. Many of the drugs tested produced less impairment than triazolam. However, definitive conclusions are difficult based on these studies because of the methods used. First, many of these studies compared only single doses of the drugs, which often were not chosen to be equivalent on other measures (e.g., subject-rated sedation). Second, studies that tested multiple doses of each drug often used relatively lower doses of the comparison compound than triazolam, which obviously biases the outcome toward finding less impairment. Third, many of the studies assessed recall only one time after drug administration. Thus, between-drug differences observed in these studies in terms of recall-impairing effects are possibly confounded by differences in rate of absorption and time to peak-plasma levels.

TABLE 1. Summary of Studies that Compared the Severity of the Withdrawal Syndrome of Various Benzodiazepines

Authors	Drugs and number of subjects	Mode of discontinuation	Results
Kales et al. (1979)	Diazepam ($N = 4$), flunitrazepam ($N = 28$), flurazepam ($N = 30$), nitrazepam ($N = 14$), and triazolam ($N = 27$)	Abrupt	Rebound insomnia was observed with the short half-life benzodiazepines (flunitrazepam, nitrazepam and triazolam), but not with the long half-life benzodiazepines (diazepam and flurazepam).
Tyrer et al. (1981)	Diazepam ($N = 36$) and lorazepam ($N = 10$)	Abrupt	Severity of the withdrawal syndrome was more severe with the short half-life drug, lorazepam, than the long half-life drug, diazepam.
Fontaine et al. (1984)	Bromazepam ($N = 8$) and diazepam ($N = 8$)	Abrupt and gradual taper	Rebound anxiety was more intense with the short half-life drug, bromazepam, than the long half-life drug, diazepam, when treatment was abruptly discontinued, but not when gradually tapered.
Bixler et al. (1985)	Flurazepam ($N = 6$), lormetazepam ($N = 6$), quazepam ($N = 6$), and triazolam ($N = 7$)	Abrupt	Rebound insomnia was observed with the short half-life drugs, lormetazepam and triazolam, but not with the long half-life drugs, flurazepam and quazepam.
Rickels et al. (1986)	Alprazolam ($N = 15$), clorazepate ($N = 12$), diazepam ($N = 40$), and lorazepam ($N = 36$)	Abrupt	A higher dropout rate was observed in patients treated with the short half-life drugs, alprazolam and lorazepam, than with patients treated with the long half-life drugs, clorazepate and diazepam.
Busto et al. (1986)	Diazepam ($N = 10$), flurazepam ($N = 1$), lorazepam ($N = 5$), and oxazepam ($N = 3$)	Abrupt	Patients withdrawn from the short half-life drugs, lorazepam and oxazepam, had higher dropout rates and used more nonstudy medications than patients withdrawn from the long half-life drugs, diazepam and flurazepam.
Rickels, Fox et al. (1988)	Clorazepate ($N = 32$) and lorazepam (30)	Abrupt	Rebound anxiety was more intense with the short half-life drug, lorazepam, than with the long half-life drug, clorazepate.
Roy-Byrne et al. (1989)	Alprazolam ($N = 13$) and diazepam ($N = 15$)	Gradual taper and abrupt	Following the gradual taper, there were no differences between patients discontinued from the short half-life drug, alprazolam, and the long half-life drug, diazepam, on the Hamilton Anxiety Scale. Following abrupt discontinuation, patients discontinued from alprazolam had higher scores on the Hamilton Anxiety Scale than patients discontinued from diazepam.

(continued)

TABLE 1. (*Continued*)

Authors	Drugs and number of subjects	Mode of discontinuation	Results
Rickels *et al.* (1990)	Alprazolam (*N* = 7), clorazepate (*N* = 19), diazepam (*N* = 16), and lorazepam (*N* = 14)	Abrupt	Patients discontinued from the short half-life drugs, alprazolam and lorazepam, had higher relapse and attrition rates, and higher scores on the Hamilton Anxiety Scale and Physician Withdrawal Checklist, than patients discontinued from the long half-life drugs, clorazepate and diazepam.
Schweizer *et al.* (1990)	Alprazolam (*N* = 15), clorazepate (*N* = 19), diazepam (*N* = 40), and lorazepam (*N* = 36)	Gradual taper	Patients discontinued from the short half-life, alprazolam and lorazepam, had higher relapse and attrition rates than patients discontinued from the long half-life drugs, clorazepate and diazepam. Patients discontinued from the short half-life drugs had lower scores on the Hamilton Anxiety Scale and Physician Withdrawal Checklist than patients discontinued from the short half-life drugs.
Murphy & Tyrer (1991)	Bromazepam (*N* = 23), diazepam (*N* = 22), and lorazepam (*N* = 23)	Gradual taper	There were few differences between the short half-life drugs, bromazepam and lorazepam, and the long half-life drug, diazepam.

TABLE 2. Summary of Studies that Compared the Recall-Impairing Effects of Triazolam and Another Benzodiazepine

Authors	Drugs (dose)	Dosing regimen	Study design	Subjects	Tasks	Results
Baughman et al. (1989)	Triazolam (0.125, 0.25, and 0.5 mg) Diazepam (5 ,10, and 15 mg) Placebo	Acute	Between subject	Surgical patients (N = 11–12/group)	Delayed picture recall	Only 0.5 mg triazolam significantly impaired delayed picture recall.
Bixler et al. (1991)	Triazolam (0.5 mg) Temazepam (30 mg) Placebo	Subchronic	Between subject	Insomniacs (N = 6/group)	Immediate word-list memory and subject-reported rates of next-day memory impairment	Neither triazolam nor temazepam impaired immediate word-list memory. Rates of next-day memory impairment were significantly greater in the triazolam group versus the temazepam and placebo groups.
Greenblatt et al. (1989)	Triazolam (0.25 mg) Temazepam (15 mg) Flurazepam (15 mg) Placebo	Acute	Between subject	Healthy volunteers (N = 11–16/group)	Acquisition and free-recall of word lists	Triazolam produced greater impairment than temazepam, flurazepam, and placebo on delayed free recall of word lists.
Pierce et al. (1990)	Triazolam (0.5 mg) Estazolam (2 mg) Placebo	Acute	Not reported	Adults (N = Not reported)	Immediate and delayed word-list memory	Triazolam, but not estazolam, impaired immediate and delayed work-list memory.
Pinnock et al. (1985)	Triazolam (0.25 mg) Diazepam (10 mg) Placebo	Acute	Between subject	Surgical patients (N = 28–30/group)	Delayed picture recall	Triazolam, but not diazepam, significantly impaired recall to placebo.
Roth et al. (1980)	Triazolam (0.5 mg) Lorazepam (4 mg) Flurazepam (30 mg) Placebo	Acute	Within subject	Healthy volunteers (N = 12/group)	Immediate and delayed recall of a battery of everyday tasks. Subjects had to provide details of these tasks.	All three drugs generally impaired immediate and delayed recall. Impairment was significantly less with flurazepam than triazolam or lorazepam.
Rush & Griffiths (1996)	Triazolam (0.125, 0.25, and 0.5 mg) Temazepam (15, 30, and 60 mg Placebo	Acute	Acute	Healthy volunteers (N = 11)	Repeated acquisition, digit-enter and recall, and picture recall.	Triazolam and temazepam produced comparable dose-related impairment on each of these tasks.

(continued)

TABLE 2. (*Continued*)

Authors	Drugs (dose)	Dosing regimen	Study design	Subjects	Tasks	Results
Rush, Madakasira, & Goldman (1997)	Triazolam (0.125, 0.25, and 0.5 mg) Estazolam (1, 2, and 4 mg) Placebo	Acute	Within subject	Healthy volunteers ($N = 7$)	Repeated acquisition, digit-enter and recall, and picture recall	Triazolam produced greater impairment on the picture recall task, but not the repeated acquisition or digit-enter and recall task, than estazolam.
Rush et al. (1993a)	Triazolam (0.25, 0.5, and 0.75 mg/70 kg Lorazepam (1, 2, 4, and 6 mg/70 kg Placebo	Acute	Within subject	Healthy volunteers ($N = 8$)	Repeated acquisition	Triazolam and lorazepam produce comparable dose-related impairment.
Rush et al. (1993a, Exp. 1)	Triazolam (0.25 and 0.5 mg) Temazepam (15 and 30 mg) Placebo	Acute	Within subject	Healthy volunteers ($N = 8$)	Repeated acquisition, digit-enter and recall, and word-list memory	High doses of triazolam generally produced greater impairment than temazepam on each of these measures.
Rush et al. (1993b, Exp. 2)	Triazolam (0.5 mg) Temazepam (60 mg) Placebo	Acute	Within subject	Healthy volunteers ($N = 6$)	Repeated acquisition, digit-enter and recall, and word-list memory	Temazepam generally produced greater impairment than triazolam on each of these measures.
Scharf et al. (1988)	Triazolam (0.5 mg) Temazepam (30 mg) Placebo	Acute	Between subjects	Insomniacs ($N = 22$, triazolam group) ($N = 30$, temazepam group)	Immediate and delayed word-list memory	Triazolam, but not temazepam, impaired delayed recall of word lists.
Hindmarch et al. (1993)	Triazolam (0.25 and 0.5 mg) Lorazepam (2 mg) Flunitrazepam (1 mg) Lormetazepam (1, 1.5, and 2 mg) Placebo	Acute	Between subjects	Healthy volunteers ($N = 12$/dose)	Short-term memory scanning and retrieval	Flunitrazepam, 0.5 mg triazolam, and 1, 1.5, and 2 mg lormetazepam significantly impaired short-term memory scanning and retrieval relative to placebo. Significant between-drug differences were not mentioned.
Roache & Griffiths (1989b)	Triazolam (1 or 2 mg) Diazepam (40 or 80 mg) Placebo	Subchronic	Within subject	Sedative abusers ($N = 8$)	Immediate and delayed recognition	Triazolam initially produced greater impairment of immediate recognition than diazepam, but tolerance developed so that triazolam and diazepam did not differ. Triazolam and diazepam impaired delayed recognition to a comparable degree.

Study	Drug (dose)		Design	Subjects	Task	Results
Griffiths et al. (1986)	Triazolam (0.25 mg) Lormetazepam (1 mg) Flurazepam (15 mg) Placebo	Acute	Within subject	Healthy volunteers (N = 10)	Memory span	No significant effects of the drugs.
Bickel et al. (1991)	Triazolam (0.375 and 0.75 mg/70 kg) Diazepam (7.5, 15, and 30 mg/70kg) Placebo	Acute	Mixed	Healthy volunteers (N = 3–4/drug)	Repeated acquisition	The high dose of triazolam produced greater impairment than the high dose of diazepam.
Bickel et al. (1990)	Triazolam (0.25, 0.5, and 0.75 mg/70 kg) Diazepam (10, 20, and 30 mg/70 kg) Alprazolam (1, 2, and 3 mg/70 kg) Placebo	Acute	Mixed	Healthy volunteers (N = 2/drug)	Repeated acquisition	The high dose of triazolam produced greater impairment than the high dose of diazepam. High doses of triazolam and alprazolam produced comparable impairment.
Subhan (1984)	Triazolam (0.25 mg) Lormetazapam (1 mg) Flunitrazepam (1 mg) Placebo	Acute	Within subject	Healthy volunteers (N = 10)	Sternberg Memory-Scanning Task	Flunitrazepam produced greater impairment than either triazolam or lormetazepam.
Wickstrøm & Godtlibsen (1988)	Triazolam (0.25 mg) Quazepam (15 mg) Flunitrazepam (1 mg) Placebo	Acute	Within subject	Healthy volunteers (N = 8)	Picture recall and recognition	Triazolam and flunitrazepam, but not quazepam, impaired performance.

While this review is limited to studies that compared the recall-impairing effects of triazolam to another benzodiazepine, it is worth noting that many of the methodological shortcomings noted previously also plague studies that attempted to delineate differences between other benzodiazepines (e.g., lorazepam versus clorazepate). Future studies on this general topic should (1) test a range of doses that have been equated on some behavioral dimension (i.e., subject-rated sedation), (2) administer the recall tasks at multiple times after drug ingestion, and (3) determine whether the drugs differ during peak effect. In the studies summarized in Table 2 that considered these points, differences between triazolam and other benzodiazepines were *not* noted (Rush, Madakasira, & Goldman, 1996; Rush & Griffiths, 1996b; Rush et al., 1993b, 1993).

Interactions with Ethanol

Combined use of ethanol and anxiolytics-hypnotics is widespread and well documented (Grant & Harford, 1990). Moreover, benzodiazepines are often prescribed without adequate information concerning the patient's ethanol use (Graham, Parran, & Jaen, 1992). Combined use of benzodiazepines and ethanol poses increased risk to the individual and society since drug-induced impairment is greater than when comparable doses of the constituent drugs are ingested alone (Hollister, 1990; Linnoila, 1990).

Eight studies directly compared the performance-impairing effects of two benzodiazepines, alone and in combination with ethanol. Table 3 shows that differential interactions with ethanol were observed in most of these studies. However, in those studies that detected differential interactions with ethanol, the drugs alone (i.e., in combination with placebo ethanol) also differentially impaired performance. Discerning differential interactions of benzodiazepines with ethanol requires that the doses or range of doses tested are equivalent when administered alone.

Summary

Commonly prescribed benzodiazepines have some abuse liability, although it is low compared with other abused drugs (Katz et al., 1990; Rifkin et al., 1989; Woods et al., 1987, 1992). Differences between benzodiazepines in terms of abuse liability are small and probably not clinically meaningful. Studies with nonhuman laboratory animals have shown that benzodiazepines with different pharmacokinetic profiles maintain comparable rates of self-administration by the intravenous and oral routes of administration. Benzodiazepines also produce drug-appropriate responding in animals trained to discriminate between pentobarbital and vehicle, and there are no discernible between-drug differences in that all benzodiazepines tested fully substituted for pentobarbital. Studies that used the precipitated-withdrawal paradigm to study the severity of the benzodiazepine discontinuation syndrome have produced mixed results regarding between-drug differences.

Human studies have also found that commonly prescribed benzodiazepines have some abuse liability. Benzodiazepines maintain self-administration and increase ratings of drug liking in volunteers with histories of drug and ethanol abuse. Benzodiazepines also produce drug-appropriate responding in volunteers trained to discriminate between pentobarbital and placebo. Chronically treating patients with a benzodiazepine produces physiological dependence, and discontinuing treatment results in a recognizable discontinuation syndrome. Differences between available benzodiazepines in terms of the severity of the withdrawal syndrome are dependent on the mode of discontinuation. Patients treated with short half-life benzodiazepines experience more severe withdrawal than patients treated with long half-life benzodiazepines when drug is abruptly discontinued, but not when gradually tapered as is medically recommended. Benzodiazepines impair recall and exacerbate the disruptive effects of ethanol. Studies that found differences between the benzodiazepines in terms of their recall-impairing effects often tested only a single dose of each drug and the doses were not chosen to be equivalent on other measures. Finally, studies that found differential interactions with ethanol often tested doses

TABLE 3. Summary of the Studies that Compared the Performance-Impairing Effects of at Least 2 Benzodiazepines in Combination with Ethanol

Authors	Ethanol dose	Drugs and dose	Study design	Subjects	Tasks	Results
Hill et al. (1982)	0.8 g/kg	Flurazepam (30 mg) Triazolam (0.25 mg)	Between subject	Healthy volunteers (N = 48)	Pursuit Rotor Test, Complex Reaction Time, Romberg Test, Tweezer Dexterity Test, Word Association Test, Digit-Symbol Substitution, and Digit Span	The triazolam–ethanol combination produced a higher frequency of ataxia and hiccups, and greater increases in body sway than the flurazepam–ethanol combination. The triazolam–ethanol combination produced less impairment than the flurazepam–ethanol combination on the digit-span and memory tasks.
Hindmarch (1983)	0.5 and 0.8 g/kg	Alprazolam (0.25 and 0.5 mg) Diazepam (5 and 10 mg)	Within subject	Healthy volunteers (N = 10)	Continuous tracking, verbal information processing and verbal memory	Diazepam (10 mg) combined with ethanol impaired performance relative to placebo, but neither dose of alprazolam combined with ethanol did.
Linnoila, Stapleton, Lister, Moss, Lane, Granger, Greenblatt, & Eckardt (1990)	0.8 g/kg	Adinazolam (15 and 30 mg) Diazepam (10 mg)	Within subject	Healthy volunteers (N = 8)	Continuous tracking, verbal and nonverbal information processing, verbal memory, and continuous performance	Ethanol exacerbated the effects of both drugs, but combining adinazolam (30 mg) and ethanol was more deleterious than combining diazepam (10 mg) and ethanol.
Linnoila, Stapleton, Lister, Moss, Lane, Granger, & Eckardt (1990)	0.8 g/kg	Alprazolam (0.5 and 2.0 mg) Diazepam (10 mg)	Within subject	Healthy volunteers (N = 10)	Continuous tracking, verbal information processing and verbal memory	Ethanol exacerbated the effects of both drugs, but combining alprazolam (2 mg) and ethanol was more deleterious than combining diazepam (10 mg) and ethanol.
Funderburk et al. (1989)	0.54 and 1.08 g/kg	Clorazepate (7.5 mg) Diazepam (5 mg) Lorazepam (1 mg)	Mixed	Recreational sedative users (N = 28)	Digit-Symbol Substitution, Circular Lights Test, Recall Test, and Reaction Time	The lorazepam–ethanol combinations generally produced greater impairment than clorazepate–ethanol and diazepam–ethanol combinations.
Aranko et al. (1985)	1 g/kg	Diazepam (10 mg) Lorazepam (2.5 mg)	Within subject	Healthy volunteers (N = 9)	Critical Flicker Fusion, Choice Reaction, Tracking, and Maddox Wing	The lorazepam–ethanol combinations produced greater impairment than the diazepam–ethanol combination across these measures.

(continued)

TABLE 3. (*Continued*)

Authors	Ethanol dose	Drugs and dose	Study design	Subjects	Tasks	Results
Seppala *et al.* (1980)	0.8 g/kg	Diazepam (10 mg) Tofisopam (100 mg)	Within subject	Healthy volunteers (*N* = 12)	Critical Flicker Fusion, Choice Reaction, Tracking, Maddox Wing, Attention Test, Time Anticipation Test, learning and memory tests	The diazepam–ethanol combination produced greater impairment than the tofisopam–ethanol combination across these measures.
Taberner *et al.* (1983)	0.1, 0.2, and 0.4 g/kg	Nitrazepam (5 mg) Temazepam (20 mg)	Within subject	Healthy volunteers (*N* = 10)	Simple reaction time, Critical Flicker Fusion, Digit-Symbol substitution, and Triple-Associate Test	Ethanol alone impaired performance, while neither nitrazepam or temazepam did so. Nitrazepam and temazepam exacerbated the effects of ethanol, but the drugs were comparable in this regard.
Wickstrøm & Godtlibsen (1988)	20 ml of 96% ethanol	Triazolam (0.25 mg) Quazepam (15 mg) Flunitrazepam (1 mg) Placebo	Within subject	Healthy volunteers (*N* = 8)	Picture recall and recognition, tapping rate, card sorting, auditory reaction time, aiming test, cancellation test, digit memory test, visualization test, and visual memory test	The quazepam–ethanol combination generally produced less impairment than the triazolam–ethanol and flunitrazepam–ethanol combinations.

that, when administered alone (i.e., in combination with placebo ethanol), also differentially impaired performance.

Nonbenzodiazepine Compounds

The abuse liability of the benzodiazepines discussed earlier has prompted interest in developing novel anxiolytic-hypnotic compounds with improved abuse liability profiles. We review the behavioral pharmacology and abuse liability of two nonbenzodiazepine compounds that are indicated in the treatment of anxiety and sleep disorders: buspirone and zolpidem, respectively. This review is limited to studies that directly compared the behavioral pharmacology and abuse liability of buspirone or zolpidem to that of a benzodiazepine.

Buspirone

Buspirone (BUSPAR®), a pyrimidinylpiperazine derivative, was the first marketed nonbenzodiazepine compound indicated for the treatment of anxiety disorders. Buspirone is effective in the treatment of anxiety (e.g., Ansseau, Papart, Gerard, Von Frenckell, & Franck, 1990; Enkelmann, 1991; Murphy, Owen, & Tyrer, 1989; Strand et al., 1990), but is pharmacologically distinct from the benzodiazepines in that it acts primarily at the 5-HT$_{1A}$ subtype of the serotonin receptor rather than at the gamma-aminobutyric acid (GABA) receptor complex (Eison & Temple, 1986; Riblet, Taylor, Eison, & Stanton, 1982; Taylor, Eison, Riblet, & Vandermaelen, 1985). Consistent with its different receptor binding profile, buspirone is behaviorally distinct from the benzodiazepines and appears to have less abuse liability.

Liability for Abuse

Preclinical Studies

Self-Administration

Two studies compared the rates of self-administration maintained by buspirone and benzodiazepines in laboratory animals (Balster

& Woolverton, 1982; R. R. Griffiths et al., 1991). In the first study, 4 rhesus monkeys were initially trained to self-administer cocaine (30 g/kg/injection) (Balster & Woolverton, 1982). After self-administration stabilized (< 10% variation in cocaine injections for 3 consecutive days), substitution tests were conducted with buspirone (3–300 g/kg/injection), chlordiazepoxide (30–1,000 g/kg/injection), and clorazepate (30–1,000 g/kg/injection). Cocaine maintained rates of self-administration greater than vehicle in all monkeys under baseline conditions. Buspirone, chlordiazepoxide, and clorazepate generally did not maintain rates of self-administration greater than vehicle in any of the monkeys.

In the second study, rates of self-administration maintained by five benzodiazepines (alprazolam, bromazepam, chlordiazepoxide, lorazepam, and triazolam) and buspirone were assessed in baboons ($N = 3$–4/compound) initially trained to self-administer cocaine (0.32 mg/kg/injection) (R. R. Griffiths et al., 1991). All of the benzodiazepines tested maintained rates of self-administration greater than vehicle at some dose in all baboons. None of the buspirone doses tested, by contrast, maintained rates of self-administration above levels observed with vehicle in any of the baboons (R. R. Griffiths et al., 1991). These studies suggest that buspirone is not likely to be abused since drugs that do not maintain self-administration in laboratory animals usually are not abused by humans (Fischman & Mello, 1989).

Interoceptive Stimulus Effects

The discriminative stimulus effects of buspirone have been compared to benzodiazepines (e.g., lorazepam, midazolam, oxazepam) and barbiturates (e.g., pentobarbital) in pigeons, rats, squirrel monkeys, and baboons trained to discriminate between drug and vehicle (Ator & Griffiths, 1986, 1989; Evans & Johanson, 1989; Hendry, Balster, & Rosecrans, 1983; Spealman, 1985). These studies have consistently shown that the discriminative stimulus effects of buspirone are distinguishable from the benzodiazepines and barbiturates. Across these studies, buspirone occasioned less than 35% drug-appropriate responding. Similarly, midazolam, oxazepam, and pentobarbital occasioned less than 50% drug-appropriate responding in pigeons and rats trained to discriminate between buspirone and vehicle (Hendry *et al.,* 1983; Mansbach & Barrett, 1986).

Clinical Studies

Self-Administration

To the best of our knowledge, there is only one published report that used self-administration procedures to compare the reinforcing effects of buspirone and a benzodiazepine in humans (Troisi, Critchfield, & Griffiths, 1993). After completing a crossover experiment comparing the acute behavioral effects of buspirone, lorazepam, and placebo, 9 subjects with histories of sedative abuse completed a 5-day choice experiment. On the 1st and 3rd days, subjects received a single forced exposure to buspirone (40 mg/70 kg) and lorazepam (4 mg/70 kg), which were identified by arbitrary letter codes. These doses of buspirone and lorazepam produced comparable subject ratings of drug effect in the crossover portion of the study. Subjects were instructed to remember the letter codes because on the 5th day they would be allowed to choose between the two drugs. No drugs were administered on the 2nd and 4th days. On the 5th day, 8 of 9 subjects chose lorazepam. These data are the clearest demonstration that buspirone's liability *for* abuse is less than that of benzodiazepines. This study, unfortunately, did not determine whether subjects would choose buspirone over placebo.

Interoceptive Stimulus Effects

Three reports examined the discriminative stimulus effects of buspirone in humans trained to discriminate between a benzodiazepine and placebo (Frey, Rush, & Griffiths, 1996; Johanson, 1991b; Kamien *et al.,* 1994). Another study examined the discriminative stimulus effects of diazepam in humans trained to discriminate between buspirone and placebo (Johanson, 1993).

In the first study, volunteers were trained to discriminate between 10 mg diazepam and placebo (Johanson, 1991b). Triazolam (0.25 mg) and buspirone (10 mg) were identified as diazepam by at least 70% of the research volunteers. A similar study examined the discriminative stimulus effects of diazepam in volunteers trained to discriminate between 15 mg buspirone and placebo (Johanson, 1993). Diazepam (10 mg) and triazolam (0.25 mg) were identified as buspirone by at least 75% of the volunteers. These findings suggest that the discriminative stimulus effects of buspirone are similar to those of diazepam and triazolam, which is discordant with the preclinical laboratory studies discussed earlier.

Human studies that used other human drug-discrimination arrangements, by contrast, found that buspirone generally does not occasion significant benzodiazepine-appropriate responding (Frey *et al.,* 1996; Kamien *et al.,* 1994). In one study, volunteers were trained to discriminate between 0.32 mg/70 kg triazolam and placebo using a novel-response procedure (Kamien *et al.,* 1994). The novel-response procedure includes an option that allows subjects to indicate whether the test drug was qualitatively distinct from both the training conditions (Bickel *et al.,* 1993). Lorazepam (0.75–3 mg/70 kg) increased triazolam-appropriate responding as a graded function of dose (Kamien *et al.,* 1994). Buspirone (7.5–30 mg/70 kg) occasioned less than 40% triazolam-appropriate responding, but dose-dependently increased novel responding, indicating that its effects were distinct from triazolam's and placebo's (Kamien *et al.,* 1994). In another study, volunteers were trained to discriminate between 15 mg buspirone, 10 mg diazepam, and placebo using a three-choice procedure (Frey *et al.,* 1996). Buspirone dose-dependently increased buspirone-appropriate responding, but did not occasion significant diazepam-appropriate responding. Diazepam dose-dependently increased diazepam-appropriate responding, but did not occasion significant buspirone-appropriate responding. These data suggest that the interoceptive stimulus effects of buspirone are distinguishable from those of benzodiazepines in humans, which is concordant with nonhuman animal studies.

Subject-Rated Drug Effects

Several studies used subject-rated drug-effect questionnaires to assess buspirone's liability *for* abuse relative to a benzodiazepine. Across a range of doses, buspirone produces a different profile of subject-rated drug effects relative to the benzodiazepines (e.g., Goa & Ward, 1986; Lader, 1982; Rush, Critchfield, Troisi, & Griffiths, 1995). We review four studies (Cole, Orzack, Beake, Bird, & Bar-tal, 1982; Griffith, Jasinski, Casten, & McKinney, 1986; Sellers, Schneiderman, Romach, Kaplan, & Somer, 1992; Troisi *et al.,* 1993). Again, this review is limited to studies that employed subjects with histories of drug or alcohol abuse because, as noted above, these individuals are at increased risk to abuse benzodiazepines and may represent a more appropriate population to determine between-drug differences in terms of liability *for* abuse. The experimental methods were generally similar across these studies: (1) Drug effects were assessed before drug administration and periodically after drug administration for 4–24 hours, (2) liability *for* abuse was assessed using subject ratings of drug liking and estimates of street value, and (3) subjects received all possible doses of buspirone and the benzodiazepine in mixed/random order and at least 48 hours separated all sessions to allow adequate drug clearance.

The first study compared the effects of buspirone (10 and 40 mg), methaqualone (300 mg), diazepam (10 and 20 mg), and placebo in 24 volunteers using estimates of street value (Cole *et al.,* 1982). The mean estimated street values of the different dose conditions were $3.50 for 300 mg methaqualone, $1.94 for 20 mg diazepam, $0.68 for 10 mg diazepam, $0.56 for 40 mg buspirone, $0.24 for 10 mg buspirone, and $0.23 for placebo. Diazepam (20 mg) and buspirone (40 mg) produced comparable increases in subject ratings of sedation. The second study compared the effects of buspirone (10 and 20 mg), lorazepam (2 mg), secobarbital (100 mg) and placebo in 15

volunteers using a side-effect checklist (Sellers *et al.,* 1992). Lorazepam, secobarbital, and 10 mg buspirone, but not 20 mg buspirone, increased ratings of drug liking above levels observed with placebo 1, 2, and 4 hr after drug administration. The four active dose conditions produced comparable ratings of drug effect. The third study compared the effects of buspirone (15, 30, 60, and 120 mg/70 kg), lorazepam (1, 2, 4, and 8 mg/70 kg), and placebo in 9 volunteers using measures of drug liking (Troisi *et al.,* 1993). Lorazepam, but not buspirone, dose-dependently increased ratings of drug liking relative to placebo. Lorazepam and buspirone produced comparable dose-related increases in subject ratings of drug strength. The final study compared the effects of buspirone (10, 20, and 40 mg), diazepam (10 and 20 mg), and placebo in 19 volunteers using measures of drug liking (Griffith *et al.,* 1986). Diazepam and buspirone produced comparable ratings of drug liking. The percentage of subjects that reported at least some drug liking was 50 for 10 mg diazepam, 52 for 20 mg diazepam, 39 for 10 mg buspirone, 48 for 20 mg buspirone, 45 for 40 mg buspirone, and 23 for placebo.

Liability *of* Abuse

Preclinical Studies: Physiological Dependence

Only one published report administered buspirone and diazepam chronically to laboratory animals and then assessed withdrawal symptoms following abrupt drug discontinuation or administration of Ro 15-1788, a benzodiazepine antagonist (Eison, 1986). Rats ($N = 30$/group) were randomly assigned to the buspirone, diazepam, or placebo condition. Doses of buspirone and diazepam were increased by 10 mg/kg every day from 50 mg/kg to 100 mg/kg (po, b.i.d.). Rats were then maintained on 100 mg/kg for 21 days prior to initiating the withdrawal phase of the experiment. After 21 days of chronic dosing, rats in each group were assigned to a drug-continuation, drug-discontinuation or benzodiazepine-antagonist group. Body weight was the dependent measure. Animals maintained on drug did not exhibit a significant change in body weight. Diazepam-treated animals in the drug-discontinuation and benzodiazepine-antagonist group showed a significant decrease in body weight during the withdrawal phase. In contrast, buspirone-treated animals in the drug-discontinuation and benzodiazepine-antagonist groups did not lose weight. These data suggest that diazepam, but not buspirone, produced physiological dependence.

Clinical Studies

Physiological Dependence

Six studies, summarized in Table 4, assessed the withdrawal syndrome following abrupt discontinuation of buspirone and a benzodiazepine. This table shows that abrupt discontinuation of buspirone, unlike abrupt discontinuation of the benzodiazepines, generally did not produce a withdrawal syndrome. These data suggest that buspirone's potential to produce physiological dependence is less than that of benzodiazepines.

Impairment of Performance

We are aware of 13 reports, summarized in Table 5, that compared the recall-impairing effects of buspirone to those of a benzodiazepine under similar dosing conditions. This benzodiazepine generally impaired recall relative to placebo. Buspirone also significantly impaired recall in some of these studies (Alford, Bhatti, Curran, McKay, & Hindmarch, 1991; Bourin, Auget, Colombel, & Larousse, 1989; Greenblatt, Harmatz, Gouthro, Locke, & Shader, 1994; Sellers et al., 1992). While the benzodiazepines tested were generally more disruptive than buspirone, it is important to emphasize that buspirone was not devoid of recall-impairing effects.

Interactions with Ethanol

Four studies compared the acute effects of buspirone-ethanol combinations with a benzodiazepine-ethanol combination (Erwin, Linnoila, Hartwell, Erwin, & Guthrie, 1986; M. J. Mattila, Aranko, & Seppala, 1982; Rush &

Griffiths, 1996a; Seppala, Aranko, Mattila, & Shrotriya, 1982). Two studies compared the acute behavioral effects of buspirone (10–20 mg) and lorazepam (2.5 mg), alone and in combination with ethanol (1 g/kg), in healthy volunteers (M. J. Mattila et al., 1982; Seppala et al., 1982). Buspirone, ethanol, and lorazepam alone generally did not impair performance relative to the placebo condition. Combined doses of lorazepam and ethanol significantly impaired performance relative to the placebo condition, while combined doses of buspirone and ethanol did not (M. J. Mattila et al., 1982; Seppala et al., 1982). The third study compared the acute behavioral effects of buspirone (10–20 mg) and diazepam (10 mg), alone and in combination with ethanol (0.8 g/kg), in healthy volunteers (Erwin et al., 1986). Ethanol alone, but not buspirone and diazepam alone, impaired performance. Combined doses of ethanol and diazepam or buspirone 20 mg produced greater impairment than observed with ethanol alone, and no differences between diazepam and buspirone were noted in this regard (Erwin et al., 1986). The final study compared the acute behavioral effects of buspirone (0, 15, and 30 mg/70 kg) and alprazolam (0, 0.75 and 1.5 mg/70 kg), alone and in combination with ethanol (0, 0.3 and 0.6 g/kg), in healthy volunteers (Rush & Griffiths, 1996a). Alprazolam alone, but not ethanol and buspirone alone, dose-dependently impaired performance. The alprazolam-ethanol combinations produced robust performance impairment. The buspirone-ethanol combinations also impaired performance, but not to the extent observed with the alprazolam-ethanol combinations. Considered together, these studies indicate that buspirone-ethanol combinations may produce greater performance-impairing effects than either drug alone, but this effect is generally less than observed when benzodiazepines such as alprazolam, diazepam, and lorazepam are combined with ethanol.

Summary

In summary, buspirone did not maintain rates of self-administration above levels ob-

TABLE 4. Summary of Studies that Compared the Severity of the Withdrawal Syndrome after Chronic Treatment with Buspirone or a Benzodiazepine

Authors	Drugs (dose)	Study design and duration of dosing regimen	Instruments used to assess withdrawal	Subjects	Results
Fontaine et al. (1987)	Buspirone (10–40 mg/day) Diazepam (10–40 mg/day) Placebo	1 week washout, 4 weeks treatment, 3 week withdrawal via placebo substitution. Subjects were randomly assigned to a drug-treatment group.	Hamilton Anxiety Rating Scale (HAM-A) Clinical Global Impression of Mental Illness (CGI) Symptom Checklist CNS Depressant Withdrawal Scale Self-Report Symptoms Inventory (SCL-56)	48 Generalized Anxiety Disorder patients	Placebo substitution resulted in a larger increase in anxiety symptoms in the diazepam group than in the buspirone or placebo groups. During withdrawal the diazepam group had higher HAM-A and CGI scores. The diazepam group also had more symptoms on the CNS Depressant Withdrawal Scale than the buspirone or placebo group. Relative to placebo, diazepam, but not buspirone, reduced anxiety.
Rickels, Schweizer, et al. (1988)	Buspirone (27 mg/day) Clorazepate (33 mg/day)	Patients were treated for 6 months followed by abrupt discontinuation of drug therapy via placebo substitution. Patients were randomly assigned to a drug-treatment group.	Hamilton Anxiety Rating Scale (HAM-A) Physician Checklist of Withdrawal Symptoms (PCWS) Hopkins Symptom Checklist (HSCL) Profile of Mood States (POMS) Daily Benzodiazepine-Withdrawal Checklist (DBWC)	134 Generalized Anxiety Disorder patients and 16 Panic Disorder patients	There were significant between-drug differences on all patient- and physician-rated measures during the first 2 weeks of placebo substitution. The drugs were equally effective in reducing anxiety.
Murphy et al. (1989)	Buspirone (7.5–11.5 mg/day) Diazepam (7.5–11.5 mg/day)	Patients were treated for 6 or 12 weeks followed by abrupt discontinuation of drug therapy via placebo substitution. Patients were randomly assigned to a drug-treatment group.	Comprehensive Psychopathological Scale (CPRS) Brief Scale for Anxiety (BSA) Unusual Symptoms Checklist	40 Generalized Anxiety Disorder patients	Following placebo substitution, diazepam-treated patients, but not buspirone-treated patients, showed a significant increase in symptoms on the CPRS and BSA. Buspirone and diazepam were equally effective in reducing anxiety.

(continued)

TABLE 4. (*Continued*)

Authors	Drugs (dose)	Study design and duration of dosing regimen	Instruments used to assess withdrawal	Subjects	Results
Ansseau et al. (1991)	Buspirone (22 mg/day) Oxazepam (56 mg/day)	Patients were treated for 6 weeks followed by abrupt discontinuation of drug therapy via placebo substitution. Patients were randomly assigned to a drug-treatment group.	Hamilton Anxiety Rating Scale (HAM-A) Hamilton Depression Rating Scale (HAM-D) Association for Methodology and Documentation Hamilton Depression Rating in Psychiatry Clinical Global Impression (CGI)	15 Generalized Anxiety Disorder patients	Patients in either group did not show a significant difference in their changes in clinical ratings on any of the instruments. Buspirone and oxazepam were equally effective in reducing anxiety.
Dimitriou et al. (1992)	Buspirone (15–25 mg/day) Alprazolam (1.5–2.5 mg/day)	Patients were treated for 4 weeks followed by abrupt discontinuation of drug therapy via placebo substitution. Patients were randomly assigned to a drug-treatment group.	Hamilton Anxiety Rating Scale (HAM-A) Physician's Questionnaire (PQ) Zung Anxiety Scale (ZAS) Adverse Reactions Form (ARF)	60 Generalized Physician's Anxiety Disorder patients	Following placebo substitution, significantly more patients in the alprazolam group reported mild or moderate adverse effects (e.g., nervous). Buspirone and alprazolam were equally effective in reducing anxiety.
Bourin & Maling (1995)	Buspirone (15–20 mg/day) Lorazepam (3–4 mg/day) Placebo	Patients were treated for 8 weeks followed by abrupt discontinuation of drug therapy via placebo substitution. Patients were randomly assigned to a drug-treatment group.	Hamilton Anxiety Rating Scale (HAM-A) Visual-Analog Scales Lader Tranquilizer Withdrawal Scale Checklist for Evaluation for Somatic Symptoms	43 Generalized Anxiety Disorder patients	Following placebo substitution, patients in both the buspirone and lorazepam groups experienced withdrawal as measured by the Lader Tranquilizer Withdrawal Scale. Only lorazepam-treated patients experienced withdrawal as measured by the Checklist for Evaluation for Somatic Symptoms. Neither buspirone- nor lorazepam-treated patients experienced withdrawal as measured by the HAM-A.

TABLE 5. Summary of Studies that Compared the Recall-Impairing Effects of Buspirone and a Benzodiazepine

Authors	Drugs (dose)	Dosing regimen	Study design	Subjects	Tasks	Results
Greenblatt et al. (1994)	Buspirone (20 mg) Triazolam (0.25 mg) Placebo	Acute	Within subject	Healthy volunteers (N = 24)	Word-list learning and memory test	Only triazolam impaired learning. Triazolam and buspirone impaired free recall, but impairment was significantly greater with triazolam.
Troisi et al. (1993)	Buspirone (15, 30, 60, and 120 mg/70 kg Lorazepam (1, 2, 4, and 8 mg/70 kg) Placebo	Acute	Within subject	Sedative abusers (N = 9)	Digit-enter and recall task, picture recall and recognition	Lorazepam, but not buspirone, impaired digit-enter and recall performance, immediate and delayed picture recall, and delayed picture recognition.
Sellers et al. (1992)	Buspirone (10 and 20 mg) Lorazepam (2 mg) Placebo	Acute	Within subject	Sedative abusers (N = 15)	Word-list memory test	Lorazepam significantly impaired recall 1, 2, and 4 hr after drug. 20 mg buspirone impaired recall 1 hr after drug. Lorazepam and buspirone did not differ significantly.
Unrug-Neervort et al. (1992)	Buspirone (15 mg) Diazepam (15 mg) Placebo	Acute	Between subject	Healthy volunteers (N = 12/group)	Digit-span, delayed figure recall, and word-list memory test	Neither buspirone nor diazepam impaired digit-span performance. Diazepam, but not buspirone, significantly impaired delayed figure recall. Diazepam was significantly different from buspirone. Diazepam, but not buspirone, impaired delayed recall on the word-list memory Diazepam was significantly different from buspirone.
Barbee et al. (1992)	Buspirone (5 and 10 mg) Alprazolam (0.5 and 1 mg) Placebo	Acute	Between subject	Healthy volunteers (N = 25/group)	Randt Memory Test	Alprazolam, but not buspirone, dose-dependently impaired recall. Alprazolam produced greater impairment than buspirone.
Blom et al. (1992)	Buspirone (5 mg) Chlordiazepoxide (5 mg) Placebo	Acute and chronic (i.e., TID)	Between subject	Healthy volunteers (N = 9)	Sternberg Memory-Scanning Test	No significant drug effects relative to placebo.
Hart et al. (1991)	Buspirone (5 mg) Alprazolam (0.25 mg) Placebo	Chronic (i.e., TID)	Between subject	Elderly volunteers (N = 20/group)	Word-list recall and picture recognition	No significant drug effects relative to placebo.

(continued)

TABLE 5. (Continued)

Authors	Drugs (dose)	Dosing regimen	Study design	Subjects	Tasks	Results
Barbee et al. (1991)	Buspirone (5 and 10 mg) Alprazolam (0.5 and 1 mg) Placebo	Acute	Between subject	Healthy volunteers (N = 25/group)	Randt Memory Test	Buspirone did not significantly impair recall relative to placebo. Alprazolam (0.5 mg) impaired delayed word-list and paired-words recall relative to placebo. Alprazolam (1 mg) impaired delayed word-list, paired-words, and picture recognition relative to placebo. Alprazolam generally differed significantly from both doses of buspirone on these measures.
Boulenger et al. (1989)	Buspirone (10 mg) Diazepam (10 mg) Placebo	Acute	Within subject	Healthy volunteers (N = 12)	Rey Auditory Verbal Learning Task, nonverbal learning and memory task, and Weingartner Cognitive Maps	No significant drug effects relative to placebo.
Lucki et al. (1987)	Buspirone (5 and 10 mg) Diazepam (5 mg) Placebo	Acute	Between subject	Generalized Anxiety Disorder patients (N = 39)	Word-list recall test	None of the drug conditions significantly impaired the immediate recall of word lists relative to placebo. Diazepam, but neither dose of buspirone, significantly impaired the delayed recall of word lists.
Bourin et al. (1989)	Buspirone (10 mg) Bromazepam (3 mg) Clobazam (10 mg) Placebo	Acute	Within subject	Healthy volunteers (N = 20)	Images test	Buspirone, bromazepam, and clobazam impaired free recall 2 hr after drug administration relative to placebo.
Mattila et al. (1986)	Buspirone (15 mg) Diazepam (0.15 and 0.3 mg/kg)	Acute	Within subject	Healthy volunteers (N = 12)	Paired-associate learning task	Diazepam (0.3 mg/kg), but not buspirone, impaired paired-associate learning performance.
Alford et al. (1991, Exp. 1)	Buspirone (5 and 10 mg) Clobazam (10 mg) Lorazepam (1 mg) Placebo	Acute	Within subject	Healthy volunteers (N = 10)	Sternberg Memory-Scanning Test	Lorazepam, but not buspirone or clobazam, significantly impaired performance on the Sternberg Memory-Scanning Test relative to placebo. Buspirone and clobazam differed significantly from lorazepam, but not from each other.
Alford et al. (1991, Exp. 2)	Buspirone (5 and 10 mg) Clobazam (10 mg) Placebo	Chronic (i.e., BID)	Within subject	Healthy volunteers (N = 9)	Sternberg Memory-Scanning Test	Buspirone and clobazam impaired performance on the Sternberg Memory-Scanning Test relative to placebo. Buspirone produced greater impairment than clobazam.

served with vehicle in rhesus monkeys or baboons. Considering the high degree of concordance between drugs that maintain self-administration and function as reinforcers in nonhuman laboratory animals and those that are abused by humans, these results suggest buspirone is not likely to be abused by humans. Buspirone did not occasion significant drug-appropriate responding in animals trained to discriminate between a classic anxiolytic (i.e., benzodiazepines and barbiturates) and saline, nor did benzodiazepines occasion significant drug-appropriate responding in animals trained to discriminate between buspirone and saline, which suggests the interoceptive stimulus effects of buspirone and benzodiazepines are distinguishable. Buspirone did not produce benzodiazepine-like physiological dependence and withdrawal in rats. Studies with human volunteers found that buspirone is not chosen over lorazepam, that it produces discriminative stimulus effects that are distinguishable from benzodiazepines, does not produce benzodiazepine-like physiological dependence and withdrawal, and impairs recall and exacerbates the disruptive effects of ethanol to a lesser extent than benzodiazepines.

Zolpidem

Zolpidem (AMBIEN®) is a rapid-onset, short-duration, quickly eliminated imidazopyridine hypnotic whose actions are mediated at the benzodiazepine recognition site of the $GABA_A$ receptor complex (Sauvanet *et al.,* 1988). The receptor-binding profile of zolpidem is somewhat different from that of classic benzodiazepine agonists. Zolpidem selectively binds to the central BZ_1 receptor subtype, and shows a different pattern of distribution of binding sites *in vitro* and *in vivo* compared with classic benzodiazepine agonists (Arbilla, Depoortere, George, & Langer, 1985; Benavides *et al.,* 1988; Biggio, Concas, Corda, & Serra, 1989; Dennis, DuBois, Benavides, & Scatton, 1988; Lloyd & Zivkovic, 1988). One study using an *in vivo* assay showed that zolpidem did not selectively bind to BZ_1 receptor subtypes, but it did show a unique pattern of

dose–effect relationships across different brain regions (Byrnes, Greenblatt, & Miller, 1992). Despite its unique benzodiazepine-receptor binding profile, controlled studies with nonhumans and humans have shown that zolpidem's abuse liability is not significantly different from prototypical benzodiazepine hypnotics such as triazolam.

Liability *for* Abuse

Preclinical Studies

Self-Administration

Only one published study determined the number of daily self-administrations maintained by zolpidem (0.01–1.0 mg/kg/injection) and triazolam (0.01–0.32 mg/kg/injection) in separate groups of baboons ($N = 8$ and 12/group, respectively) initially trained to self-administer cocaine (0.32 mg/kg/injection) (R. R. Griffiths, Sannerud, Ator, & Brady, 1992). Baboons could self-administer a maximum of 8 injections per day. Zolpidem and triazolam maintained greater self-administration than vehicle at some dose. The average number of injections per day across the previous 5 days for the dose maintaining the greatest number of self-administrations was 6.9 for zolpidem (range = 3.0–7.8) and 5.5 for triazolam (range = 2.1–7.2). Worth noting is that the maximal number of self-administrations maintained by 1 mg/kg/injection zolpidem approached that maintained by 0.32 mg/kg/injection cocaine (mean = 7.5, range = 7–8). The rate of self-administration of zolpidem was also greater than that maintained by 10 other benzodiazepine agonists (i.e., alprazolam, bromazepam, chlordiazepoxide, clonazepam, clorazepate, diazepam, flurazepam, lorazepam, medazepam, and midazolam) under similar laboratory conditions (Griffiths *et al.,* 1981; Griffiths *et al.,* 1991). These data suggest that zolpidem's liability *for* abuse is at least as great as that of benzodiazepines.

Interoceptive Stimulus Effects

Drug-discrimination studies conducted with rodents suggest that the discriminative stimulus effects of zolpidem may be distinguishable from the barbiturates and benzodiazepines (Sanger, 1987; Sanger & Zivkovic, 1986, 1987; Sanger, Perrault, Morel, Joly, & Zivkovic, 1987). First, in rats trained to discriminate between zolpidem (2 mg/kg) and vehicle, high doses of triazolam, pentobarbital and chlordiazepoxide (0.3, 20, and 20 mg/kg, ip, respectively) only partially substituted for zolpidem (i.e., each drug occasioned approximately 70% zolpidem-appropriate responding) (Sanger & Zivkovic, 1986). Second, in rats trained to discriminate chlordiazepoxide (5 or 20 mg/kg, ip) from vehicle, a high dose of zolpidem (3 mg/kg, ip) only partially substituted for chlordiazepoxide (i.e., approximately 55%–70% drug-appropriate responding) (Sanger et al., 1987). Third, in rats trained to discriminate pentobarbital (80 mg/kg, ip), zolpidem (0.5–4 mg/kg, ip) occasioned less than 50% drug-appropriate responding, while triazolam (0.1 and 0.2 mg/kg, ip) occasioned ≥80% drug-appropriate responding (Rowlett & Woolverton, 1996). Fourth, in rats trained to discriminate between 0.32 and 3.2 mg/kg midazolam (sc) from no drug, midazolam (0.032–10 mg/kg), triazolam (0.0032–3.2 mg/kg), and diazepam (0.032–18 mg/kg) produced similar effects: dose-dependent increases first in low-dose (i.e., 0.32 mg/kg midazolam) lever responding and then dose-dependent increases in high-dose (3.2 mg/kg) lever responding (Sannerud & Ator, 1995). Zolpidem (0.032–3.2 mg/kg), by contrast, dose-dependently increased responding only on the low-dose (i.e., 0.32 mg/kg midazolam) lever (Sannerud & Ator, 1995). Fifth, Ro 16-6028 and Ro 17-1812, two mixed agonist–antagonist benzodiazepines, produced drug-appropriate responding in chlordiazepoxide-trained rats, but not zolpidem-trained rats (Sanger, 1987). Finally, CGS 9896, a pyrazoloquinoline, and ZK 91296, a β-carboline, antagonized the discriminative stimulus effects of zolpidem, but not chlordiazepoxide (Sanger & Zivkovic, 1987).

Studies conducted with nonhuman primates, by contrast, suggest that the discriminative stimulus effects of zolpidem are similar to the barbiturates and benzodiazepines (R. R. Griffiths et al., 1992; Rowlett & Woolverton, 1996). Zolpidem (3.2–10 mg/kg, po) completely substituted (i.e., >80% drug-appropriate responding) for the training drug in baboons trained to discriminate between pentobarbital (10 mg/kg, po) or lorazepam (1.8 mg/kg, po) and vehicle (R. R. Griffiths et al., 1992). Similarly, zolpidem (30 mg/kg, ig) completely substituted (i.e., >80% drug-appropriate responding) for pentobarbital in rhesus monkeys trained to discriminate between pentobarbital (10 mg/kg, ig) and vehicle (Rowlett & Woolverton, 1996).

Clinical Studies

Self-Administration and Interoceptive Stimulus Effects

There are no published reports that directly assessed the reinforcing effects of zolpidem relative to those of a benzodiazepine in human research volunteers. Two reports examined the discriminative stimulus effects of zolpidem in humans trained to discriminate between a classic anxiolytic-hypnotic and placebo (Rush et al., 1996; Rush, Madakasira et al., 1997). The first study assessed the discriminative stimulus effects of zolpidem (2.5–20 mg) and pentobarbital (25–150 mg) in 4 healthy volunteers trained to discriminate between a hypnotic dose of pentobarbital, 100 mg, and placebo (Rush, Madakasira et al., 1997). Zolpidem (2.5, 5, 10, and 20 mg) on average occasioned 38, 94, 94, and 77% pentobarbital-appropriate responding, respectively, while pentobarbital (25, 50, 100, and 150 mg) on average occasioned 50, 19, 85, and 94% pentobarbital-appropriate responding, respectively. The second study assessed the discriminative stimulus effects of zolpidem (2.5–20 mg/70 kg) and triazolam (0.063–0.5 mg/70 kg) in 5 healthy volunteers trained to discriminate between a hypnotic dose of triazolam, 0.25 mg/70 kg, and placebo (Rush, Madakasira et al., 1997). Zolpidem (2.5, 5, 10, and 20 mg/70 kg) on average occasioned 0, 25, 75, and 87% triazolam-appropriate responding, respectively, while triazolam (0.063, 0.125, 0.25, and 0.5 mg/70 kg) on average occasioned 25, 46, 92, and 96% triazolam-appropriate responding, respectively. These findings suggest that the discriminative stimulus effects of zolpidem are similar to those of pentobarbital and triazolam.

Subject-Rated Drug Effects

We are aware of one study that assessed zolpidem's (15–45 mg) liability *for* abuse relative to triazolam (0.25–0.75 mg) and placebo using subject ratings of drug liking and estimated street value (Evans *et al.,* 1990). Fifteen volunteers with histories of sedative abuse received each drug condition in mixed order. Across the range of doses tested, zolpidem and triazolam produced comparable increases in subject ratings of drug liking and drug effect. Zolpidem, but not triazolam, significantly increased estimates of street value above levels observed with placebo. These data suggest that zolpidem's liability *for* abuse is at least as great as the benzodiazepine hypnotic triazolam.

Liability *of* Abuse

Preclinical Studies: Physiological Dependence

Two published reports examined whether repeated administrations of zolpidem would produce physiological dependence (R. R. Griffiths *et al.,* 1992; Perrault, Morel, Sanger, & Zivkovic, 1992). In the first study, separate groups of mice were treated with zolpidem or midazolam (30 mg/kg, po, b.i.d.) for 10 consecutive days (Perrault *et al.,* 1992). Flumazenil (5 mg/kg, ip), a benzodiazepine antagonist, was administered 3 and 6 hr after the last administration of zolpidem or midazolam to determine whether a benzodiazepine-like withdrawal syndrome could be precipitated. Spontaneous withdrawal was measured for 67 hr after the last drug administration. Neither precipitated nor spontaneous withdrawal was observed in mice repeatedly treated with zolpidem relative to mice treated with vehicle. By contrast, flumazenil precipitated a benzodiazepine-like withdrawal syndrome (e.g., decreased the latency to convulsions) in mice repeatedly treated with midazolam and spontaneous withdrawal was observed 14 hr after the last administration of midazolam.

Unlike the study conducted with mice, results from experiments in nonhuman primates suggest that repeated administrations of zolpidem produce physiological dependence similar to that observed with benzodiazepines (R. R. Griffiths *et al.,* 1992). When baboons were allowed to self-administer zolpidem (1 mg/kg/injection) for two weeks, substitution of placebo resulted in a time-limited suppression of food intake which suggests a withdrawal effect. That effect was similar to that observed with midazolam (5.6 mg/kg/day) under nearly identical experimental conditions in the same laboratory (Sannerud, Cook, & Griffiths, 1989).

Clinical Studies

Physiological Dependence

There is one published report that compared zolpidem and a benzodiazepine in terms of their liability to produce physiological dependence in humans (Roger, Attali, & Coquelin, 1993). Hospitalized elderly insomniac patients (age = 58–98 years) were randomly assigned to receive 5 mg zolpidem ($N = 70$), 10 mg zolpidem ($N = 74$), or 0.25 mg triazolam ($N = 77$) at bedtime. Active drug treatment was preceded by 3 days of placebo administration. Active drug was then administered nightly for 3 weeks. Active drug treatment was then followed by a 7-day withdrawal period during which time placebo was administered. During the withdrawal period there was no evidence of rebound insomnia in any of the groups. Similarly, there were no signs of agitation or anxiety during the withdrawal period. These findings suggest that physiological dependence does not develop with repeated administrations of zolpidem. However, physiological dependence was not evident with repeated administrations of triazolam, a benzodiazepine hypnotic.

Impairment of Performance

As noted earlier, zolpidem reportedly binds selectively to the BZ_1 receptor subtype (Arbilla *et al.,* 1985; Benavides *et al.,* 1988; Biggio

TABLE 6. Summary of Studies that Compared the Recall-Impairing Effects of Zolpidem and a Benzodiazepine

Authors	Drugs (dose)	Dosing regimen	Study design	Subjects	Tasks	Results
Wesensten et al. (1995)	Zolpidem (5, 10, and 15 mg/70 kg) Triazolam (0.125, 0.25, and 0.5 mg/70 kg) Placebo	Acute	Between subject	Healthy volunteers (N = 10/group)	Restricted-reminding test and paired-associates memory test	Triazolam produced greater impairment than zolpidem.
Rush & Griffiths (1996)	Zolpidem (5, 10, and 20 mg/70 kg) Triazolam (0.125, 0.25, and 0.5 mg/70 kg) Temazepam (15, 30, and 60 mg/70 kg) Placebo	Acute	Within subject	Healthy volunteers (N = 11)	Picture recall and digit-enter and recall	Zolpidem, triazolam, and temazepam produced comparable dose-related impairment.
Roehrs et al. (1994)	Zolpidem (10 and 20 mg) Triazolam (0.25 and 0.5 mg) Placebo	Acute	Within subject	Healthy volunteers (N = 23)	Digit-span and Buschke Selective-Reminding-and-Recognition Task	Zolpidem and triazolam produced comparable impairment.
Berlin et al. (1993)	Zolpidem (10 mg) Triazolam (0.25 mg) Placebo	Acute	Within subject	Healthy volunteers (N = 18)	Paired-associates memory and picture-recall test	Zolpidem and triazolam produced comparable impairment.
Evans et al. (1990)	Zolpidem (15, 30, and 45 mg/70 kg) Triazolam (0.25, 0.5, and 0.75 mg/70 kg) Placebo	Acute	Within subject	Sedative abusers (N = 15)	Picture-recall and digit-enter and recall	Zolpidem, triazolam, and temazepam produced comparable dose-related impairment.
Rush, Madakasira et al. (1997)	Zolpidem (2.5, 5, 10, and 20 mg) Triazolam (0.063, 0.125, 0.25, and 0.5 mg) Placebo	Acute	Within subject	Healthy volunteers (N = 4)	Digit-enter and recall	Zolpidem and triazolam produced comparable dose-related impairment.

et al., 1989; Dennis *et al.,* 1988; Lloyd & Zivkovic, 1988) while benzodiazepines generally bind non-selectively to the BZ_1 and BZ_2 receptor subtypes. Because there is a high concentration of BZ_2 receptors in limbic structures thought to be involved in complex behavioral processes (i.e., recall), zolpidem may be less disruptive than benzodiazepines (Dennis *et al.,* 1988). Six published studies, summarized in Table 6, compared the recall-impairing effects of zolpidem to triazolam. Only one study found that zolpidem produced less impairment of recall than triazolam (Wesensten, Balkin, & Belenky, 1995), while five studies found that zolpidem and triazolam produce comparable impairment of recall (Berlin *et al.,* 1993; Evans *et al.,* 1990; Roehrs, Merlotti, Zorick, & Roth, 1994; Rush & Griffiths, 1996; Rush, Madakasira *et al.,* 1997).

Interactions with Ethanol

As noted earlier, most benzodiazepine agonists bind nonselectively to the BZ_1 and BZ_2 receptor subtype while zolpidem reportedly binds selectively to the BZ_1 receptor subtype (Arbilla *et al.,* 1985; Benavides *et al.,* 1988; Biggio *et al.,* 1989; Dennis *et al.,* 1988; Lloyd & Zivkovic, 1988). Ethanol may also interact with the benzodiazepine receptor (Dar, 1992; Koob, Percy, & Britton, 1989; Suzdak *et al.,* 1986). The unique binding profile of zolpidem, relative to prototypical benzodiazepines such as triazolam, suggests that differential interactions with ethanol might occur.

Only one report examined the effects of zolpidem, alone and in combination with ethanol (Wilkinson, 1995). This study assessed the acute behavioral effects of zolpidem (10 and 15 mg), alone and in combination with ethanol (dose selected on an individual basis to attain a peak blood alcohol concentration of 0.08%), in healthy volunteers. Performance impairment was measured using a divided-attention, visual-backward-masking, vigilance, and Sternberg test. Zolpidem alone (i.e., in combination with placebo ethanol) dose dependently impaired performance on these tests. Ethanol (i.e., in combination with placebo zolpidem) also significantly impaired performance on

most of these tests. Combining zolpidem and ethanol produced greater impairment than observed with either drug alone. The combined effects of zolpidem and ethanol were approximately additive, which is similar to the effects of benzodiazepines in combination with ethanol (Chan, 1984; Linnoila, 1990).

Summary

In summary, studies conducted with rodents suggest that the behavioral pharmacology and abuse liability of zolpidem is different from prototypical benzodiazepines. The discriminative stimulus effects of zolpidem are distinguishable from the barbiturates and benzodiazepines in the rat, and there is no discernible evidence of physiological dependence in mice repeatedly treated with zolpidem. Studies conducted with nonhuman primates, by contrast, suggest that the abuse liability of zolpidem is similar to benzodiazepines. Zolpidem maintained rates of self-administration in baboons above levels observed with vehicle, and above levels observed with several benzodiazepines. Zolpidem occasioned drug-appropriate responding in baboons and monkeys trained to discriminate between a classic anxiolytic (i.e., benzodiazepines and barbiturates) and vehicle. Regarding dependence and withdrawal, substitution of placebo after 2 weeks of zolpidem self-injection resulted in a time-limited suppression of food intake in baboons similar to that observed with midazolam under nearly identical conditions, suggesting a withdrawal effect that is qualitatively similar to that observed with benzodiazepines.

Consistent with studies conducted with nonhuman primates, studies with human volunteers found that zolpidem shares discriminative stimulus effects with the benzodiazepines and barbiturates. Zolpidem and triazolam produced comparable ratings of drug liking in subjects with histories of sedative abuse. Zolpidem and triazolam produced qualitatively and quantitatively similar recall-impairing effects. The combined performance-impairing effects of zolpidem and ethanol are approximately additive, which is similar to the effects of benzodiazepines in combination with ethanol. Neither zolpidem nor triazolam appeared to produce physiological dependence in elderly insomniacs after 3 weeks of nightly dosing.

Overall, these findings suggest that the abuse liability of zolpidem is not significantly different from that of the benzodiazepines. It is important to note, however, that laboratory studies may not accurately predict the relative extent of the abuse of various drugs (Katz, 1990). Postmarketing surveillance and epidemiological studies will be needed to ultimately determine zolpidem's abuse liability.

Final Considerations

Future research with nonhumans and humans should focus on relative reinforcing effects of the various benzodiazepines. Before such studies can be conducted, the procedures used to compare the reinforcing effects of drugs need to be refined (Katz, 1990). The lack of adequate procedures to compare the relative reinforcing effects of drugs may explain the failure to detect significant differences between commonly used benzodiazepines (Griffiths et al., 1991; Griffiths et al., 1981; Stewart et al., 1994). Studies that attempt to determine differences between available benzodiazepines in terms of their relative reinforcing effects must consider important issues such as selecting doses that are equivalent on some measure.

The abuse liability of the benzodiazepines has prompted interest in developing novel anxiolytic/hypnotic componds with improved abuse liability profiles. Buspirone has significantly less abuse liability than the benzodiazepines and does not produce benzodiazepine-like physical dependence and withdrawal in rats. By contrast, zolpidem, an imidazopyridine marketed for the treatment of sleep disorders, does not appear to differ significantly from the benzodiazepines in terms of abuse liability. Studying the relative reinforcing effects of zolpidem and commonly prescribed benzodiazepine hypnotics in individuals with histories of drug and ethanol abuse is important because these individuals are at increased risk to abuse anxiolytics/hypnotics.

Commonly prescribed anxiolytics/hypnotics have some liability *for* abuse and significant liability *of* abuse. The available benzodiazepines do not appear to differ significantly in terms of their abuse liability. Buspirone, but not zolpidem, appears to have significantly less abuse liability than the benzodiazepines. Future studies should attempt to refine the methods currently used to assess the relative abuse liability of drugs.

ACKNOWLEDGMENTS

Preparation of this chapter was supported, in part, by grants from the National Institutes on Health, DA 09841 (C.R.R) and DA 08076 (S.T.H.).

References

Alford, C., Bhatti, J. Z., Curran, S., McKay, G., & Hindmarch, I. (1991). Pharmacodynamic effects of buspirone and clobazam. *British Journal of Clinical Pharmacology, 32,* 91–97.

Ansseau, M., Papart, P., Gerard, M-A., Von Frenckell, R., & Franck, G. (1991). Controlled comparison of buspirone and oxazepam in generalized anxiety. *Neuropsychobiology, 24,* 74–78.

Aranko, K., Seppala, T., Pellinen, J., & Mattila, M. J. (1985). Interaction of diazepam or lorazepam with alcohol. Psychomotor effects and bioassayed serum levels after single and repeated doses. *European Journal of Clinical Pharmacology, 28,* 559–565.

Arbilla, S., Depoortere, H., George, P., & Langer, S. (1985). Pharmacological profile of the imidazopyridine zolpidem at benzodiazepine receptors and electrocorticogram in rats. *Naunyn-Schmiedeberg's Archives Pharmacology, 330,* 248–251.

Ator, N. A., & Griffiths, R. R. (1986). Discriminative stimulus effects of atypical anxiolytics in baboons and rats. *Journal of Pharmacology and Experimental Therapeutics, 237,* 393–403.

Ator, N. A., & Griffiths, R. R. (1987). Self-administration of barbiturates and benzodiazepines: Review. *Pharmacology, Biochemistry and Behavior, 27,* 391–398.

Ator, N. A., & Griffiths, R. R. (1989). Asymmetrical cross-generalization in drug discrimination with lorazepam and pentobarbital training conditions. *Drug Development Research, 16,* 355–364.

Ator, N. A., & Griffiths, R. R. (1992). Oral self-administration of triazolam, diazepam and ethanol in the baboon: Drug reinforcement and benzodiazepine physical dependence. *Psychopharmacology, 108,* 301–312.

Balster, R. L., & Woolverton, W. L. (1982). Intravenous buspirone self-administration in rhesus monkeys. *Journal of Clinical Psychiatry, 43,* 34–37.

Barbee, J. G., Black, F. W., Kehoe, C., & Todorov, A. A. (1991). A comparison of the single-dose effects of alprazolam, buspirone, and placebo upon memory function. *Journal of Clinical Psychopharmacology, 11,* 351–356.

Barbee, J. G., Black, F. W., & Todorov, A. A. (1992). Differential effects of alprazolam and buspirone upon acquisition, retention, and retrieval processes in memory. *Journal of Neuropsychiatry and Clinical Neurosciences, 4,* 308–314.

Baughman, V., Becker, G., Ryan, C., Glaser, M., & Abenstein, J. (1989). Effectiveness of triazolam, diazepam, and placebo as preanesthetic medications. *Anesthesiology, 71,* 196–200.

Benavides, J., Peny, B., DuBois, A., Perrault, G., Morel, E., Zivkovic, B., & Scatton, B. (1988). In vivo interaction of zolpidem with central benzodiazepine (BZD) binding sites (as labeled [3H] Ro 15-1788) in the mouse brain: Preferential affinity of zolpidem for the omega 1 (BZD1) subtype. *Journal of Pharmacology and Experimental Therapeutics, 245,* 1033–1041.

Berlin, I., Warot, D., Hergueta, T., Molinier, P., Bagot, C., Puech, A. J., (1993). Comparison of the effects of zolpidem and triazolam on memory functions, psychomotor performances, and postural sway in healthy subjects. *Journal of Clinical Psychopharmacology, 13,* 100–106.

Bickel, W., Hughes, J., & Higgins, S. (1990). Human behavioral pharmacology of benzodiazepines: Effects on repeated acquisition and performance of response chains. *Drug Development Research, 20,* 53–65.

Bickel, W. K., Higgins, S. T., & Hughes, J. R. (1991). The effects of diazepam and triazolam on repeated acquisition and performance of response sequences with an observing response. *Journal of the Experimental Analysis of Behavior, 56,* 217–237.

Bickel, W. K., Oliveto, A. H., Kamien, J. B., Higgins, S. T., & Hughes, J. R. (1993). A novel-response procedure enhances the selectivity and sensitivity of triazolam discrimination in humans. *Journal of Pharmacology and Experimental Therapeutics, 264,* 360–367.

Bigelow, G., Stitzer, M., Lawrence, C., Krasnegor, N., D'Lugoff, B., & Hawthorne, J. (1980). Narcotics addiction treatment: Behavioral methods concurrent with methadone maintenance. *International Journal of the Addictions, 15,* 427–437.

Biggio, G., Concas, A., Corda, M. G., & Serra, M. (1989). Enhancement of GABAergic transmission by zolpidem, an imidazopyridine with preferential affinity for type I benzodiazepine receptors. *European Journal of Pharmacology, 161,* 173–180.

Bixler, E. O., Kales, J. D., Kales, A., Jacoby, J. A., & Soldatos, C. R. (1985). Rebound insomnia and elimination half-life: Assessment of individual subject response. *Journal of Clinical Pharmacology, 25,* 115–124.

Bixler, E. O., Kales, A., Brubaker, B., & Kales, J. (1987). Adverse reactions to benzodiazepine hypnotics: Spontaneous reporting system. *Pharmacology, 35,* 286–300.

Bixler, E. O., Kales, A., Manfredi, R. L, Vgontzas, A. N., Tyson, K. L. & Kales, J. D. (1991). Next-day memory impairment with triazolam use. *Lancet, 337,* 827–831.

Blom, M. W., Bartel, P. R., Sommers, D. K., Van Der Meyden, C. H., & Becker, P. J. (1992). The comparison of the effects of multi and single doses of buspirone, chlordiazepoxide and hydroxyzine on psychomotor function and EEG. *Fundamentals of Clinical Pharmacology, 6,* 5–9.

Boulenger, J. P., Squillace, K., Simon, P., Herrou, M., Leymarie, P., & Zarifan, E. (1989). Buspirone and diazepam: Comparison of subjective, psychomotor and biological effects. *Neuropsychobiology, 22,* 83–89.

Bourin, M., & Maling, M. (1995). Controlled comparison of the effects and abrupt discontinuation of buspirone and lorazepam. *Progress in Neuro-Psychopharmacology and Biological Psychiatry, 19,* 567–575.

Bourin, M., Auget, J. L., Colombel, M. C., & Larousse, C. (1989). Effects of single oral doses of bromazepam, buspirone and clobazam on performance tasks and memory. *Pharmacopsychiatry, 22,* 141–145.

Bowen, J. D., & Larson, E. B. (1993). Drug-induced cognitive impairment: Defining the problem and finding the solutions. *Drugs and Aging, 3,* 349–357.

Brady, J., & Ator, N. A. (1990). Stimulus functions of drugs and the assessment of abuse liability. *Drug Development Research, 20,* 231–249.

Busto, U., Sellers, E. M., Naranjo, C. A., Cappell, H., Sanchez-Craig, M., & Sykora, K. (1986). Withdrawal reaction after long-term therapeutic use of benzodiazepines. *New England Journal of Medicine, 315,* 854–859.

Byrnes, J., Greenblatt, D., & Miller, L. (1992). Benzodiazepine receptor binding of nonbenzodiazepines in vivo: Alpidem, zolpidem and zopiclone. *Brain Research Bulletin, 29,* 905–908.

Chan, A. W. (1984). Effects of combined alcohol and benzodiazepine: A review. *Drug and Alcohol Dependence, 13,* 315–341.

Cole, J. O., Orzack, M. H., Beake, B., Bird, M., & Bar-tal, Y. (1982). Assessment of the abuse liability of buspirone in recreational sedative users. *Journal of Clinical Psychiatry, 43,* 69–75.

Curran, H. (1991). Benzodiazepines, memory, and mood: A review. *Psychopharmacology, 105,* 1–8.

Dar, M. S. (1992). Selective antagonism of acute ethanol-induced motor disturbances by centrally administered Ro 15-4513 in mice. *Pharmacology, Biochemistry and Behavior, 42,* 473–479.

Darke, S. G., Ross, J. E., & Hall, W. D. (1995). Benzodiazepine use among injecting heroin users. *Medical Journal of Australia, 162,* 645–647.

de Wit, H., & Doty, P. (1994). Preference for ethanol and diazepam in light and moderate social drinkers: A within-subjects study. *Psychopharmacology, 115,* 529–538.

de Wit, H., & Griffiths, R. R. (1991). Testing the abuse liability of anxiolytic and hypnotic drugs in humans [Review]. *Drug and Alcohol Dependence, 28,* 83–111.

Dennis, T., DuBois, A., Benavides, J., & Scatton, B. (1988). Distribution of central w 1 (Benzodiazepine1) and w 2 (Benzodiazepine2) receptor subtypes in the monkey and human brain: An autoradiographic study with [3H]flunitrazepam and the omega 1 selective ligand [3H]zolpidem. *Journal of Pharmacology and Experimental Therapeutics, 247,* 309–322.

Dimitriou, E. C., Parashos, A. J., & Giouzepas, J. S. (1992). Buspirone vs alprazolam: A double-blind comparative study of their efficacy, adverse effects and withdrawal symptoms. *Drug Investigations, 4,* 316–321.

DuPont, R. (1988). Abuse of benzodiazepines: The problems and the solutions. *American Journal of Drug and Alcohol Abuse, 14* (Suppl. 1), 1–69.

Eison, M. S. (1986). Lack of withdrawal signs of dependence following cessation of treatment or Ro-15, 1788 administration to rats chronically treated with buspirone. *Neuropsychobiology, 16,* 15–18.

Eison, A. S., & Temple, D. L. (1986). Buspirone: Review of its pharmacology and current perspectives on its mechanism of action. *American Journal of Medicine, 80,* 1–9.

Enkelmann, R. (1991). Alprazolam versus buspirone in the treatment of outpatients with generalized anxiety disorder. *Psychopharmacology, 105,* 428–432.

Erwin, C. W., Linnoila, M., Hartwell, J., Erwin, A., & Guthrie, S. (1986). Effects of buspirone and diazepam, alone and in combination with alcohol, on skilled performance and evoked potentials. *Journal of Clinical Psychopharmacology, 6,* 199–209.

Evans, S. M., & Johanson, C. E. (1989). Discriminative stimulus properties of midazolam in the pigeon. *Journal of Pharmacology and Experimental Therapeutics, 248,* 29–38.

Evans, S. M., Funderburk, F. R., & Griffiths, R. R. (1990). Zolpidem and triazolam in humans: Behavioral and subjective effects and abuse liability. *Journal of Pharmacology and Experimental Therapeutics, 255,* 1246–1255.

Fischman, M. W., & Mello, N. K. (1989). *Testing for abuse liability of drugs in humans* (National Institute on Drug Abuse Monograph No. 92, Department of Health and Human Services Publication No. [ADM] 89-1613). Washington, DC: U.S. Government Printing Office.

Fontaine, R., Chouinard, G., & Annable, L. (1984). Rebound anxiety in anxious patients after abrupt withdrawal of benzodiazepine treatment. *American Journal of Psychiatry, 141,* 848–852.

Fontaine, R., Beaudry, P., Beauclair, L., & Chouinard, G. (1987). Comparison of withdrawal of buspirone and diazepam: A placebo controlled study. *Progress in Neuro-Psychopharmacology & Biological Psychiatry, 11,* 189–197.

Frey, J. M., Rush, C. R., & Griffiths, R. R. (1996). Discriminative stimulus effects of diazepam and buspirone in a three-choice response paradigm. In L. S. Harris (Ed.), *Problems of drug dependence, 1995* (NIDA Research Monograph Series No. 162, p. 250). Rockville, MD: National Institute on Drug Abuse.

Funderburk, F. R., Griffiths, R. R., McLeod, D. R., Bigelow, G. E., Mackenzie, A., Liebson, I. A., & Nemeth-Coslett, R. (1988). Relative abuse liability of lorazepam and diazepam: An evaluation in "recreational" drug users. *Drug and Alcohol Dependence, 22,* 215–222.

Funderburk, F. R., Bigelow, G. E., Liebson, I. A., Mackenzie, A., McLeod, D., Nemeth-Coslett, R., & Griffiths, R. R. (1989). Behavioral differentiation of anxiolytic medications: Alone and in combination with alcohol. *Current Therapeutic Research, 45,* 21–32.

Glennon, R. A., Jarbe, T. U. C., & Frankenheim, J. (1991). *Drug discrimination: Applications to drug abuse research* (NIDA Research Monograph No. 116, DHHS [ADM] 92-1878). Rockville, MD: National Institute on Drug Abuse.

Goa, K. L., & Ward, A. (1986). Buspirone: A preliminary review of its pharmacological properties and therapeutic efficacy as an anxiolytic. *Drugs, 32,* 114–129.

Graham, A. V., Parran, T. V., & Jaen, C. R. (1992). Physician failure to record alcohol use history when prescribing benzodiazepines. *Journal of Substance Abuse, 4,* 179–185.

Grant, B. F., & Harford, T. C. (1990). Concurrent and simultaneous use of alcohol with sedatives and with tranquilizers: Results of a national survey. *Journal of Substance Abuse, 2,* 1–14.

Greenblatt, D. J., Harmatz, J. S., Engelhardt, N., & Shader, R. I. (1989). Pharmacokinetic determinants of dynamic differences among three benzodiazepine hypnotics. *Archives of General Psychiatry, 46,* 326–332.

Greenblatt, D. J., Harmatz, J. S., Gouthro, T. A., Locke, J., & Shader, R. I. (1994). Distinguishing a benzodiazepine agonist (triazolam) from a nonagonist anxiolytic (buspirone) by electroencephalography: Kinetic-dynamic studies. *Clinical Pharmacology & Therapeutics, 56,* 100–111.

Griffith, J. D., Jasinski, D. R., Casten, G. P., & McKinney, G. R. (1986). Investigation of the abuse liability of buspirone in alcohol-dependent patients. *American Journal of Medicine, 80,* 30–35.

Griffiths, A. N., Jones, D. M., & Richens, A. (1986). Zopiclone produces effects on human performance similar to flurazepam, lormetazepam and triazolam. *British Journal of Clinical Pharmacology, 21,* 647–653.

Griffiths, R. R., & Wolf, B. (1990). Relative abuse liability of different benzodiazepines in drug abusers. *Journal of Clinical Psychopharmacology, 10,* 237–243.

Griffiths, R. R., Bigelow, G., & Liebson, I. A. (1979). Human drug self-administration: Double-blind comparison of pentobarbital, diazepam, chlorpromazine and placebo. *Journal of Pharmacology and Experimental Therapeutics, 210,* 301–310.

Griffiths, R. R., Lukas, S. E., Bradford, L. D., Brady, J. V., & Snell, J. D. (1981). Self-injection of barbiturates and benzodiazepines in baboons. *Psychopharmacology, 75,* 101–109.

Griffiths, R. R., McLeod, D. R., Bigelow, G. E., Liebson, I. A., & Roache, J. D. (1984). Relative abuse liability of diazepam and oxazepam: Behavioral and subjective dose effects. *Psychopharmacology, 84,* 147–154.

Griffiths, R. R., McLeod, D. R., Bigelow, G. E., Liebson, I. A., Roache, J. D., & Nowowieski, P. (1984). Comparison of diazepam and oxazepam: Preference, liking and extent of abuse. *Journal of Pharmacology and Experimental Therapeutics, 229,* 501–508.

Griffiths, R. R., Lamb, R. J., Ator, N. A., Roache, J. D., & Brady, J. V. (1985). Relative abuse liability of triazolam: Experimental assessment in animals and humans. *Neuroscience and Biobehavioral Reviews, 9,* 133–151.

Griffiths, R. R., Lamb, R. J., Sannerud, C. A., Ator, N. A., & Brady, J. V. (1991). Self-injection of barbiturates, benzodiazepines and other sedative-anxiolytics in baboons. *Psychopharmacology, 103,* 154–161.

Griffiths, R. R., Sannerud, C. A., Ator, N. A., & Brady, J. V. (1992). Zolpidem behavioral pharmacology in Baboons: Self-injection, discrimination, tolerance and withdrawal. *Journal of Pharmacology and Experimental Therapeutics, 1992,* 1199–1208.

Hart, R. P., Colenda, C. C., & Hamer, R. M. (1991). Effects of buspirone and alprazolam on the cognitive performance of normal elderly subjects. *American Journal of Psychiatry, 148,* 73–77.

Hendry, J. S., Balster, R. L., & Rosecrans, J. A. (1983). Discriminative stimulus properties of buspirone compared to central nervous system depressants in rats. *Pharmacology, Biochemistry and Behavior, 19,* 97–101.

Hill, S. Y., Goodwin, D. W., Reichman, J. B., Mendelson, W.B., & Hopper, S. (1982). A comparison of two benzodiazepine hypnotics administered with alcohol. *Journal of Clinical Psychiatry, 43,* 408–410.

Hindmarch, I. (1983). Measuring the side-effects of psychoactive drugs: A pharmacodynamic profile of alprazolam. *Alcohol and Alcoholism, 18,* 361–367.

Hindmarch, I., Sherwood, N., & Kerr, J. S. (1993). Amnestic effects of triazolam and other hypnotics. *Progress in Neuro-Psychopharmacology & Biological Psychiatry, 17,* 407–413.

Hollister, L. (1990). Interactions between alcohol and benzodiazepines. *Recent Developments in Alcoholism, 8,* 233–239.

Hollister, L. E., Muller-Oerlinghausen, B., Rickels, K., & Shader, R. I. (1993). Clinical uses of benzodiazepines. *Journal of Clinical Psychopharmacology, 13,* 1S–169S.

Iguchi, M., Handelsman, L., Bickel, W., & Griffiths, R. (1993). Benzodiazepine and sedative use/abuse by methadone maintenance clients. *Drug and Alcohol Dependence, 32,* 257–266.

Jaffe, J. H., Ciraulo, D. A., Nies, A., Dixon, R. B., & Monroe, L. (1983). Abuse potential of halazepam and of diazepam in patients recently treated for acute alcohol withdrawal. *Clinical Pharmacology & Therapeutics, 34,* 623–630.

Jasinski, D. R., & Henningfield, J. E. (1989). Human abuse liability assessment by measurement of subjective and physiological effects. In M. W. Fischman, & N. K. Mello (Eds.), *Testing for abuse liability of drugs in humans* (NIDA Research Monograph No. 92, DHHS publication number [ADM] 89-1613, pp. 73–100). Rockville, MD: National Institute on Drug Abuse.

Johanson, C. E. (1991a). Discriminative stimulus effects of diazepam in humans. *Journal of Pharmacology and Experimental Therapeutics, 257,* 634–643.

Johanson, C. E. (1991b). Further studies on the discriminative stimulus effects of diazepam in humans. *Behavioural Pharmacology, 2,* 357–367.

Johanson, C. E. (1993). Discriminative stimulus effects of buspirone in humans. *Experimental and Clinical Psychopharmacology, 1,* 173–187.

Kales, A., Scharf, M. B., Kales, J. D., & Soldatos, C. R. (1979). Rebound Insomnia. *Journal of the American Medical Association, 241,* 1692–1695.

Kamien, J. B., Bickel, W. K., Hughes, J. R., Higgins, S. T., & Smith, B.T. (1993). Drug discrimination by humans compared to nonhumans: Current status and future directions. *Psychopharmacology, 111,* 259–270.

Kamien, J. B., Bickel, W. K., Oliveto, A. H., Smith, B. J., Higgins, S. T., Hughes, J. R., & Badger, G.J. (1994). Triazolam discrimination by humans under a novel-response procedure: Effects of buspirone and lorazepam. *Behavioural Pharmacology, 5,* 315–325.

Katz, J. (1990). Models of relative reinforcing efficacy of drugs and their predictive utility. *Behavioural Pharmacology, 1,* 283–301.

Katz, J. L., Winger, G., & Woods, J. H. (1990). Abuse liability of benzodiazepines. In I. Hindmarch, G. Beaumount, S. Brandon, & B. Leonard (Eds.), *Benzodiazepines: Current concepts—Biological, clinical, and social perspectives* (pp 181–198). New York: Wiley.

Kirk, T., Roache, J. D., & Griffiths, R. R. (1990). Dose-response evaluation of the amnestic effects of triazolam and pentobarbital in normal subjects. *Journal of Clinical Psychopharmacology, 10,* 160–167.

Koob, G. F., Percy, L., & Britton, K. T. (1989). The effects of Ro 15-4513 on the behavioral actions of ethanol in an operant reaction time task and a conflict test. *Pharmacology, Biochemistry and Behavior, 31,* 757–760.

Lader, M. (1982). Psychological effects of buspirone. *Journal of Clinical Psychiatry, 43,* 62–67.

Linnoila, M. I. (1990). Benzodiazepines and alcohol. *Journal of Psychiatric Research, 24,* 121–127.

Linnoila, M., Stapleton, J. M., Lister, R., Moss, H., Lane, E., Granger, A., & Eckardt, M. J. (1990). Effects of single doses of alprazolam and diazepam, alone and in combination with ethanol, on psychomotor and cognitive performance and on autonomic nervous system reactivity in healthy volunteers. *European Journal of Clinical Pharmacology, 39,* 21–28.

Linnoila, M., Stapleton, J. M., Lister, R., Moss, H., Lane, E., Granger, A., Greenblatt, D. J., & Eckardt, M. J. (1990). Effects of adinazolam and diazepam, alone and in combination with ethanol, on psychomotor and cognitive performance and on autonomic nervous system reactivity in healthy volunteers. *European Journal of Clinical Pharmacology, 38,* 371–377.

Lloyd, K. G., & Zivkovic, B. (1988). Specificity within the GABAA receptor supramolecular complex: A consideration of the new omega 1–receptor selective imidazopyridine hypnotic zolpidem. *Pharmacology, Biochemistry and Behavior, 29,* 781–783.

Lucki, I., Rickels, K., Giesecke, M. A., & Geller, A. (1987). Differential effects of the anxiolytic drugs, diazepam and buspirone, on memory function. *British Journal of Clinical Pharmacology, 23,* 207–211.

Lukas, S. E., & Griffiths, R. R. (1984). Precipitated diazepam withdrawal in baboons: Effects of dose and duration of diazepam exposure. *European Journal of Pharmacology, 100,* 163–171.

Mansbach, R. S., & Barrett, J. E. (1986). Discriminative stimulus properties of buspirone in the pigeon. *Journal of Pharmacology and Experimental Therapeutics, 240,* 364–369.

Martin, J. R., Moreau, J. L., & Jenck, F. (1995). Precipitated withdrawal in squirrel monkeys after repeated daily oral administration of alprazolam, diazepam, flunitrazepam or oxazepam. *Psychopharmacology, 118,* 273–279.

Martin, W. R., Sloan, J. W., & Wala, E. (1990). Precipitated abstinence in orally dosed benzodiazepine-dependent dogs. *Journal of Pharmacology and Experimental Therapeutics, 255,* 744–755.

Mattila, M., Seppala, T., & Mattila, M. J. (1986). Combined effects of buspirone and diazepam on objective and subjective tests of performance in healthy volunteers. *Clinical Pharmacology & Therapeutics, 40,* 620–626.

Mattila, M. J., Aranko, K., & Seppala, T. (1982). Acute effects of buspirone and alcohol on psychomotor skills. *Journal of Clinical Psychiatry, 43,* 56–61.

McNicholas, L. F., Martin, W. R., Sloan, J. W., & Wala, E. (1988). Precipitation of abstinence in nordiazepam- and diazepam- dependent dogs. *Journal of Pharmacology and Experimental Therapeutics, 245,* 221–224.

Miller, N. S., & Giannini, A. J. (1991). Drug misuse in alcoholics. *International Journal of the Addictions, 26,* 851–857.

Murphy, S. M., & Tyrer, P. (1991). A double-blind comparison of the effects of gradual withdrawal of lorazepam, diazepam, and bromazepam in benzodiazepine dependence. *British Journal of Psychiatry, 158,* 511–516.

Murphy, S. M., Owen, R., & Tyrer, P. (1989). Comparative assessment of efficacy and withdrawal symptoms after 6 and 12 weeks' treatment with diazepam or buspirone. *British Journal of Psychiatry, 154,* 529–534.

Navaratnam, V., & Foong, K. (1990a). Adjunctive drug use among opiate addicts. *Current Medical Research and Opinion, 11,* 611–619.

Navaratnam, V., & Foong, K. (1990b). Opiate dependence—The role of benzodiazepines. *Current Medical Research and Opinion, 11,* 620–630.

Oliveto, A. H., Bickel, W. K., Hughes, J. R., Higgins, S. T., & Fenwick, J. W. (1992). Triazolam as a discriminative stimulus in humans. *Drug and Alcohol Dependence, 30,* 133–142.

Oliveto, A. H., Bickel, W. K., Kamien, J. B., Hughes, J. R., & Higgins, S. T. (1994). Effects of diazepam and hydromorphone in triazolam-trained humans under a novel-response drug discrimination procedure. *Psychopharmacology, 114,* 417–423.

Perrault, G., Morel, E., Sanger, D. J., & Zivkovic, B. (1992). Lack of tolerance and physical dependence upon repeated treatment with the novel hypnotic zolpidem. *Journal of Pharmacology and Experimental Therapeutics, 263,* 298–303.

Pierce, M. W., Shu, V. S., & Groves, L. J. (1990). Safety of estazolam: The United States clinical experience. *American Journal of Medicine, 88* (Suppl. 3A), 12S–17S.

Pinnock, C. A., Fell, D., Hunt, P. C., Miller, C. W., & Smith, G. A. (1985). A Comparison of triazolam and diazepam as premedication agents for minor gynecological surgery. *Anaesthesia, 40,* 324–328.

Preston, K., & Bigelow, G. (1991). Subjective and discriminative effects of drugs. *Behavioural Pharmacology, 2,* 293–313.

Riblet, L. A., Taylor, D. P., Eison, M. S., & Stanton, H. C. (1982). Pharmacology and neurochemistry of buspirone. *Journal of Clinical Psychiatry, 43,* 11–16.

Rickels, K., Case, W. G., Schweizer, E. E., Swenson, C., & Fridman, R. B. (1986). Low-dose dependence in chronic benzodiazepine users: A preliminary report on 119 patients. *Psychopharmacology Bulletin, 22,* 407–415.

Rickels, K., Fox, I. L., Greenblatt, D. J., Sandler, K. R., & Schless, A. (1988). Clorazepate and lorazepam: Clinicial improvement and rebound anxiety. *American Journal of Psychiatry, 145,* 312–317.

Rickels, K., Schweizer, E., Csanalosi, I., Case, W. G., & Chung, H. (1988). Long-term treatment of anxiety and risk of withdrawal: Prospective comparison of clorazepate and buspirone. *Archives of General of Psychiatry, 45,* 444–450.

Rickels, K., Schweizer, E., Case, G., & Greenblatt, D. J. (1990). Long-term therapeutic use of benzodiazepines: I. Effects of abrupt discontinuation. *Archives of General Psychiatry, 47,* 899–907.

Rifkin, A., Doddi, S., Karajgi, B., Hasan, N., & Alvarez, L. (1989). Benzodiazepine use and abuse by patients at outpatient clinics. *American Journal of Psychiatry, 146,* 1331–1332.

Roache, J. D., & Griffiths, R. R. (1985). Comparison of triazolam and pentobarbital: Performance impairment, subjective effects and abuse liability. *Journal of Pharmacology and Experimental Therapeutics, 243,* 120-133.

Roache, J. D., & Griffiths, R.R. (1989a). Abuse liability of anxiolytics and sedative/hypnotics: Methods assessing the likelihood of abuse. In M. W. Fischman & N. K. Mello (Eds.), *Testing for abuse liability of drugs in humans* (National Institute on Drug Abuse Monograph No. 92, DHHS Publication No. [ADM] 89-1613, pp. 123–146). Washington, DC: U.S. Government Printing Office.

Roache, J. D., & Griffiths, R. R. (1989b). Diazepam and triazolam self-administration in sedative abusers: Concordance of subject ratings, performance and drug self-administration. *Psychopharmacology, 99,* 309–315.

Roache, J. D., Meisch, R. A., Henningfield, J. E., Jaffe, J. H., Klein, S., & Sampson, A. (1995). Reinforcing effects of triazolam in sedative abusers: Correlation of drug liking and self-administration measures. *Pharmacology, Biochemistry and Behavior, 50,* 171–179.

Roehrs, T., Merlotti, L., Zorick, F., & Roth, T. (1994). Sedative, memory, and performance effects of hypnotics. *Psychopharmacology, 116,* 130–134.

Roger, M., Attali, P., & Coquelin, J. P. (1993). Multicenter, double-blind, controlled comparison of zolpidem and triazolam in elderly patients with insomnia. *Clinical Therapeutics, 15,* 127–136.

Roth, T., Hartse, K. M., Saab, P. G., Piccione, P. M., & Kramer, M. (1980). The effects of flurazepam, lorazepam, and triazolam on sleep and memory. *Psychopharmacology, 70,* 231–237.

Rowlett, J. K., & Woolverton, W. L. (1996). Discriminative stimulus effects of zolpidem in pentobarbital-trained subjects: I. Comparison with triazolam in rhesus monkeys and rats. *Journal of Pharmacology and Experimental Therapeutics* (under review).

Roy-Byrne, P. P., Dager, S. R., Cowley, D. S., Vitaliano, P., & Dunner, D. L. (1989). Relapse and rebound following discontinuation of benzodiazepine treatment of panic attacks: Alprazolam versus diazepam. *American Journal of Psychiatry, 146,* 860–865.

Rush, C. R., & Griffiths, R. R. (1996). Zolpidem, triazolam, and temazepam: Behavioral and subject-rated effects in normal volunteers. *Journal of Clinical Psychopharmacology, 16,* 146–152.

Rush, C. R., & Griffiths, R. R. (1997a). Acute subject-rated and behavioral effects of alprazolam and buspirone, alone and in combination with ethanol, in normal volunteers. *Experimental and Clinical Psychopharmacology, 5,* 28–38.

Rush, C. R., Higgins, S. T., Bickel, W. K., & Hughes, J. R. (1993a). Abuse liability of alprazolam relative to other commonly used benzodiazepines: A review. *Neuroscience and Biobehavioral Reviews, 17,* 277–285.

Rush, C. R., Higgins, S. T., Bickel, W. K., & Hughes, J. R. (1993b). Acute effects of triazolam and lorazepam on human learning, performance and subject ratings. *Journal of Pharmacology and Experimental Therapeutics, 264,* 1218–1226.

Rush, C. R., Higgins, S. T., Hughes, J. R., & Bickel, W. K. (1993). A comparison of the acute behavioral effects of triazolam and temazepam in normals volunteers. *Psychopharmacology, 112,* 407–414.

Rush, C. R., Critchfield, T. S., Troisi, J. R., II, & Griffiths, R. R. (1995). Discriminative stimulus effects of diazepam and buspirone in normal volunteers. *Journal of the Experimental Analysis of Behavior, 63,* 277–294.

Rush, C. R., Mumford, G. K., & Griffiths, R. R. (1996). Discriminative stimulus effects of triazolam, zolpidem, oxazepam, and caffeine in humans. In L. S. Harris (Ed.), *Problems of drug dependence, 1995* (NIDA Research Monograph Series No. 162, pp. 172, 248). Rockville, MD: National Institute on Drug Abuse.

Rush, C. R., Madakasira, S., & Goldman, N. (1997). Acute behavioral effects of estazolam and triazolam in non-drug abusing volunteers. *Experimental and Clinical Psychopharmacology, 4,* 300–307.

Rush, C. R., Madakasira, S., Goldman, N., Woolverton, W. L., & Rowlett, J. (1997). Discriminative-stimulus effects of zolpidem in pentobarbital-trained subjects: II. Comparison with triazolam and caffeine in humans. *Journal of Pharmacology and Experimental Therapeutics, 280,* 174–188.

Sanger, D. J. (1987). Further investigation of the stimulus properties of chlordiazepoxide and zolpidem: Agonism and antagonism by two novel benzodiazepines. *Psychopharmacology, 93,* 365–368.

Sanger, D. J., & Zivkovic, B. (1986). The discriminative stimulus properties of zolpidem, a novel imidazopyridine hypnotic. *Psychopharmacology, 89,* 317–322.

Sanger, D. J., & Zivkovic, B. (1987). Discriminative stimulus properties of chlordiazepoxide and zolpidem: Agonist and Antagonist effects of CGS 9896 and ZK 91296. *Neuropharmacology, 26,* 499–505.

Sanger, D. J., Perrault, G., Morel, E., Joly, D., & Zivkovic, B. (1987). The behavioral profile of zolpidem, a novel hypnotic drug of imidazopyridine structure. *Physiology & Behavior, 41,* 235–240.

Sannerud, C. A., & Ator, N. A. (1995). Drug discrimination analysis of midazolam under a three-lever procedure: I. Dose-dependent differences in generalization and antagonism. *Journal of Pharmacology and Experimental Therapeutics, 272,* 100–111.

Sannerud, C. A., Cook, J. M., & Griffiths, R. R. (1989). Behavioral differentiation of benzodiazepine ligands after repeated administration in baboons. *European Journal of Pharmacology, 167,* 333–343.

Sauvanet, J. P., Maarek, L., Roger, M., Renaudin, J., Louvel, E., & Orofiamma, B. (1988). Open long-term trials with zolpidem in insomnia. In J. P. Sauvanet, S. Z. Lauger, & P. L. Morselli (Eds.), *Imidazopyridines in Sleep Disorders* (pp. 339–349). New York: Raven.

Scharf, M. B., Fletcher, K., & Graham, J. P. (1988). Comparative amnestic effects of benzodiazepine hypnotic agents. *Journal of Clinical Psychiatry, 49,* 134–137.

Schweizer, E., Rickels, K., Case, W. G., & Greenblatt, D. J. (1990). Long-term therapeutic use of benzodiazepines: II. Effects of gradual taper. *Archives of General Psychiatry, 47,* 908–915.

Sellers, E. M., Schneiderman, J., Romach, M., Kaplan, H., & Somer, G. (1992). Comparative drug effects and abuse liability of lorazepam, buspirone, and secobarbital in nondependent subjects. *Journal of Clinical Psychopharmacology, 12,* 79–85.

Sellers, E. M., Ciraulo, D. A., DuPont, R. L., Griffiths, R. R., Kosten, T. R., Romach, M. K., & Woody, G. E. (1993). Alprazolam and benzodiazepine dependence. *Journal of Clinical Psychiatry, 54,* 64–75.

Seppala, T., Palva, E., Mattila, M. J., Korttila, K., & Shrotriya, R. (1980). Tofisopam, a novel 3,4,-benzodiazepine: Multiple-dose effects on psychomotor skills and memory. Comparison with diazepam and interactions with ethanol. *Psychopharmacology, 69,* 209–218.

Seppala, T., Aranko, K., Mattila, M. J., & Shrotriya, R. C. (1982). Effects of alcohol on buspirone and lorazepam actions. *Clinical Pharmacology & Therapeutics., 32,* 201–207.

Sloan, J. W., Martin, W. R., & Wala, E. P. (1990). Dependence-producing properties of alprazolam in the dog. *Pharmacology, Biochemistry and Behavior, 35,* 651–657.

Spealman, R. D. (1985). Discriminative-stimulus effect of midazolam in squirrel Monkeys: Comparison with other drugs and antagonism by Ro 15-1788. *Journal of Pharmacology and Experimental Therapeutics, 235,* 456–462.

Stewart, R. B., Lemiaire, G. A., Roache, J. D., & Meisch, R. A. (1994). Establishing benzodiazepines as oral reinforcers: Midazolam and diazepam self-administration in rhesus monkeys. *Journal of Pharmacology and Experimental Therapeutics, 271,* 200–211.

Stitzer, M. L., Griffiths, R. R., McLellan, A. T., Grabowski, J., & Hawthorne, J. W. (1981). Diazepam use among methadone maintenance patients: Patterns and dosages. *Drug and Alcohol Dependence, 8,* 189–199.

Strand, M., Hetta, J., Rosen, A., Sorensen, S., Malmstrom, R., Fabian, C., Marits, K., Vetterskog, K., Liljestrand, A-G., & Hegen, C. (1990). A double-blind, controlled trial in primary care patients with generalized anxiety: A comparison between buspirone and oxazepam. *Journal of Clinical Psychiatry, 51,* 40–45.

Subhan, Z. (1984). The effects of benzodiazepines on short-term memory and information processing. In I. Hindmarch, H. Ott, & T. Roth (Eds.), *Psychopharmacology* (Suppl. 1, pp. 173–181). Berlin: Springer-Verlag.

Suzdak, P. D., Glowa, J. R., Crawley, J. N., Schwartz, R. D., Skolnick, P., & Paul, S. M. (1986). A selective imidazobenzodiazepine antagonist of ethanol in the rat. *Science, 234,* 1243–1247.

Taberner, P. V., Roberts, C. J. C., Shrosbree, E., Pycock, C. J., & English, L. (1983). An investigation into the interaction between ethanol at low doses and the benzodiazepines nitrazepam and temazepam on psychomotor performance in normal subjects. *Psychopharmacology, 81,* 321–326.

Taylor, D. P., Eison, M. S., Riblet, L. A., & Vandermaelen, C. P. (1985). Pharmacological and clinical effects of buspirone. *Pharmacology, Biochemistry and Behavior, 23,* 687–694.

Troisi, J. R., II, Critchfield, T. S., & Griffiths, R. R. (1993). Buspirone and lorazepam abuse liability in humans: Behavioral effects, subjective effects and choice. *Behavioural Pharmacology, 4,* 217–230.

Tyrer, P., Rutherford, D., & Huggett, T. (1981). Benzodiazepine withdrawal symptoms and propranolol. *Lancet, 1,* 520–522.

Unrug-Neervoort, A., van Luijtelaar, G., & Coenen, A. (1992). Cognition and vigilance: Differential effects of diazepam and buspirone on memory and psychomotor performance. *Neuropsychobiology, 26,* 146–150.

Wesensten, N. J., Balkin, T. J., & Belenky, G. L. (1995). Effects of daytime administration of zolpidem versus triazolam on memory. *European Journal of Clinical Pharmacology, 48,* 115–122.

Wickstrøm, E., & Godtlibsen, O. B. (1988). The effects of quazepam, triazolam, flunitrazepam and placebo, alone and in combination with ethanol, on day-time sleep, memory, mood and performance. *Human Psychopharmacology, 3,* 101–110.

Wilkinson, C. J. (1995). The acute effects of zolpidem, administered alone and with alcohol, on cognitive and psychomotor function. *Journal of Clinical Psychiatry, 56,* 309–318.

Wise, R. (1990). *Increased frequency report (IFR): Triazolam deaths, interactions, with alcohol, CNS depressives.* Washington, DC: Food and Drug Administration, Division of Epidemiology and Surveillance.

Wolf, B., & Griffiths, R. R. (1991). Physical dependence on benzodiazepines: Differences within the class. *Drug and Alcohol Dependence, 29,* 153–156.

Woods, J. H., Katz, J. L., & Winger, G. (1987). Abuse liability of benzodiazepines. *Annual Review of Pharmacology and Toxicology, 39,* 251–413.

Woods, J. H., Katz, J. L., & Winger, G. (1992). Benzodiazepines: Use, abuse, and consequences. *Pharmacological Reviews, 44,* 151–347.

Wysowski, D. K., & Barash, D. (1991). Adverse behavioral reactions attributed to triazolam in the Food and Drug Administration's Spontaneous Reporting System. *Archives of Internal Medicine, 151,* 2003–2008.

28

Psychological and Psychiatric Consequences of Sedatives, Hypnotics, and Anxiolytics

WESLEY SOWERS

Introduction

The use of substances to induce sedation has a long history, even when alcohol is not considered. As early as the mid 19th century, production of agents designed for this purpose began with the introduction of bromide. Paraldehyde, chloral hydrate, urethan, and sulfonyl were also introduced prior to the beginning of the 20th century. Barbiturates dominated the early part of this century after their introduction in 1903, and up to 50 compounds in this class were eventually brought to market (Allgulander, 1986; Janicak, Davis, Preskorn, & Ayd, 1993). The benzodiazepines became available in the 1960s and their use and popularity grew steadily over the next 20 years. The benzodiazepines have now largely replaced barbiturates and other sedatives introduced around mid-century, such as methaqualone, meprobamate, ethchlorvynol, and glutethimide, for most therapeutic uses (Rosenbaum & Gelenburg, 1991; Smith & Seymour, 1991; Stern-

bach, 1993). This has been due largely to their relative safety (high lethal–therapeutic ratio) and an initial perception that they had a lower potential for misuse and physical dependence. It gradually became clear, however, that a dependence syndrome can be produced in some individuals within a short period of time. As these medications have been prescribed more liberally, there has been significant public concern about their level of use and misuse in society (Lader, 1991; Smith & Seymour, 1991).

Despite these concerns, the benzodiazepines have proven to be extremely useful medications for a variety of psychiatric and nonpsychiatric uses, and for the most part, much safer than most of their predecessors. Perhaps the most common use for benzodiazepines is for relief from anxiety symptoms associated with acute stress and anxiety disorders. Insomnia is another common indication for short-term treatment with these agents. Although some benzodiazepines have been promoted primarily for sleep disturbances and others for anxiety symptoms, it is worth noting that these designations are determined more by marketing decisions than by any pharmacologic properties of the agents (Rosenbaum & Gelenburg, 1991). For the remainder of this chapter, use of the term "sedative" will refer to all substances of this class, regardless of whether the primary

WESLEY SOWERS • Center for Addictions Services, St. Francis Medical Center, and Department of Psychiatry, University of Pittsburgh Medical Center, Pittsburgh, Pennsylvania 15201.

Handbook of Substance Abuse: Neurobehavioral Pharmacology, edited by Tarter *et al.* Plenum Press, New York, 1998.

471

use is as an anxiolytic or an hypnotic. It will also refer primarily to the benzodiazepines unless otherwise noted.

In addition to these two primary indications, treatment of muscle tension, seizure disorders, and aggression, and the induction of anesthesia are other uses for the benzodiazepines. They have also become the staple of treatment for detoxification from all cross-tolerant sedative addictions including alcohol and barbiturates (Ballenger, 1995; Meyer, 1993).

As indicated earlier, the benzodiazepines have virtually replaced older sedative agents for most therapeutic uses, although several barbiturates, notably phenobarbital, continue to be produced and are used for limited applications such as seizure disorders. Some of the short-acting barbiturates also continue to be used for sedation in cases of uncontrolled aggression or for anesthesia (Meyer, 1993). For the most part, however, these preparations have seen a drastic reduction in their usage, and many have been taken out of production. There has been a concomitant reduction in their use for nontherapeutic purposes, and barbiturate or other nonbenzodiazepine sedative dependence is, today, quite rare. Benzodiazepines have filled the void created by the demise of these agents and are usually the sedative of choice for persons who misuse this class of substances (Lader, 1991; Morgan, 1990).

Despite concerns about their potential for misuse, benzodiazepines continue to be among the most commonly prescribed medications. Although the number of prescriptions written for the benzodiazepines has recently leveled off, about 60–70 million continue to be issued each year. Diazepam was for many years the most widely prescribed medication in the world. Although some of the newer, shorter-acting preparations have recently overtaken diazepam in popularity, as a class, the benzodiazepines remain the most commonly prescribed medication of any type (Ciraulo, Sands, Shader, & Greenblatt, 1991; Lader, 1991). The wide variety of agents available and the frequency with which they are prescribed make them almost ubiquitous, and,

therefore, easily available. Since they do continue to be widely used as therapeutic agents, their misuse is often perceived by both users and nonusers to be more acceptable than misuse of illicit drugs, such as heroin. The vast majority of these medications are prescribed in the primary care setting, often by practitioners who have limited knowledge of addiction medicine or psychiatry. This may contribute to the prevalence of their misuse, as these practitioners are poorly positioned to adequately monitor their use (Landry, Smith, McDuff, & Baughman, 1992).

Patterns of Use

A variety of methods have been used to estimate the prevalence of sedative use in the general population, and in selected special populations. Estimates of sedative abuse or dependence in the general population have been relatively low. Perhaps the best information available comes from the Epidemiologic Catchment Area study (Regier et al., 1990). Data collected in that study indicated that about 14% of the population used barbiturates at some time in their lives (compared to 86% for alcohol and 33% for cannabis), and that slightly more than 1% developed abuse or dependence at some time during their lives (compared to about 13% for alcohol and 4% for cannabis). These data would suggest that persons who use barbiturates at some time in their lives, have about one half the likelihood of developing problems related to their use as persons who have used alcohol or marijuana. A fairly extensive review of the literature (Ciraulo et al., 1991) over the past 25 years indicated that anywhere from 7.4% to 17.6% of the general population had used sedatives at some time within a year of the sampling. The estimates were about twice this high when sampling psychiatric patients. Of persons in treatment for substance use disorders, up to 9% reported using sedatives along with other substances, but only 0.2% used these substances exclusively.

It does appear that certain segments of the population are more likely than others to develop an addictive disorder involving sedatives. While the numbers of persons who have a primary addiction to sedatives is small, those who are affected are often middle aged or older and frequently female (Finlayson & Davis, 1994; Jinks & Raschko, 1990). They often begin their use through a prescription intended to help control anxiety, other types of emotional distress, somatic symptoms, or sleep problems (Mellinger, Balter, & Uhlenhuth, 1984). Use escalates over time with developing tolerance, reemerging distress, and the development of several sources of supply for the drug. Using several doctors to obtain prescriptions, without informing them of drug use patterns, is a common phenomenon (Kisnad, 1991). Users may not recognize their problem until their pattern of deception and dyscontrol become quite disabling. Even then, it may be difficult for them to seek help.

A second significant pattern that may lead to sedative dependence is that of polysubstance use in persons with established dependence on other substances. It is well known that cocaine and amphetamine users often use sedating drugs or alcohol to take the edge off their stimulant high (Smith & Seymour, 1991). Opiate users often use sedating drugs to enhance the euphoriant effects of the narcotic; this is particularly so when the purity of the opiate they are using declines on the street (Kisnad, 1991). Persons who are in methadone maintenance programs frequently become involved with sedatives in an attempt to replace the high they previously experienced when shooting heroin (Iguchi, Handelsman, Bickel, & Griffiths, 1993; San et al., 1993). Sedatives are also commonly used by persons who are alcohol dependent. They may begin to use sedatives in response to anxiety and discomfort experienced when alcohol withdrawal develops, often unaware or unable to recognize the source of their difficulties. In other instances, the sedatives are used primarily to augment alcohol intoxication. This can be a dangerous and sometimes lethal practice (Greenberg, 1993). Mixed substance use patterns are further discussed later in this chapter, but whatever the impetus to begin using sedatives in this population, gradual escalation of use over time can often lead to an independent syndrome of dependence on the sedating agent.

A third pattern of misuse might be described as bingeing or thrill seeking. This is most common among younger, polysubstance users who may be involved in experimentation with a variety of substances in all imaginable combinations. As with inhalants, the frequent availability of sedatives in the household make them popular and easily obtainable substances for adolescents to include in their repertoire of agents used to produce a high. While this pattern less frequently results in an ongoing or exclusive relationship with sedatives as a primary substance of misuse, it may in some cases lead to heavy use and physical dependence (Kisnad, 1991; Sheehan, Sheehan, Torres, Coppola, & Francis, 1991).

As previously mentioned, these substances may be obtained by users in a variety of ways. They are present in a large number of households as they are often prescribed for "as needed" treatment of stress and insomnia. Small amounts may be diverted by household members either for sale or binge use. Persons who develop dependence and need for higher dosages of these substances often make rounds of several doctors to obtain adequate amounts of the sedative. In many cases, users are able to locate "cooperative" doctors who for a small fee will prescribe as much of the sedative as the user desires (Kisnad, 1991). Some states have attempted to limit the practices of these unscrupulous "pill doctors" by requiring triplicate prescription forms for controlled substances. Although this has been an issue of some controversy, since there has been concern that these triplicate forms would also reduce the frequency with which persons with legitimate need would be adequately treated, it appears that this strategy has been at least partially successful in some locations (Eadie, 1993; Weintraub, Singh, Byrne, Maharaj, & Guttmacher, 1993; Williams, 1993). Another source frequently used by persons with other established addictions is simply to purchase them from local street dealers. These dealers obtain their supplies from a variety of illegal sources and typically sell a mid-range dose sedative pill (e.g., 10 mg diazepam) for about $1 to $3. Diazepam, alprazolam, lorezepam, and clonazepam are preparations that are often available on the street (Wesson, Smith, & Seymour, 1992).

Of available agents, not all are equally attractive to persons with addictions. Agents with quick onset of action (such as diazepam) and short half-lives (such as alprazolam) tend to have the greatest liability for dependence (Mumford, Evans, Fleishaker, & Griffiths, 1995; Roache et al., 1995; Wesson et al., 1992). Agents with a rapid onset give the experience of a rush or at least a pleasant, reinforcing sensation rather quickly following their administration. Agents with a short half-life must be administered more frequently, thus establishing a more frequent reinforcement schedule. Both of these conditions tend to strengthen the behavior pattern. Although their lesser availability limits their use, it is apparent that many of the short-acting barbiturates and several of the now defunct sedative agents have greater abuse liability than do the benzodiazepines (Barnas, Rossmann, Roessler, Riemer, & Fleischhacker, 1992; de Wit & Griffiths, 1991; Sellers, Schneiderman, Romach, Kaplan, & Somer, 1992). In fact, people without histories of substance misuse generally experience very little or no reinforcing effects from benzodiazepines (Cole & Chiarello, 1990; de Wit & Griffiths, 1991; Rush, Higgins, Bickel, & Hughes, 1993).

The method of delivery may also have an effect on the drug use experience and the quality of the dependence. The vast majority of sedatives are administered orally, but some preparations may be injected intravenously, enhancing the intensity of their effect and rapidity of their onset. Some of the barbiturates and diazepam may be administered in this way. In some cases, benzodiazepines have been administered intranasally. This, too, hastens the onset of effects and the intensity of the high (Kisnad, 1991; Sheehan et al., 1991). There have been no reports of smokable forms of sedatives.

The misuse of prescription medications has increased significantly with the advent of benzodiazepines. With a greater margin of safety and relatively few side effects, they have become widely prescribed. Their self-administration has achieved some degree of social sanction and acceptability. Unlike their counterparts, which are illegal to use under any circumstance, their use and problems developed as a result of their use are not subject to the same degree of stigmatization and condemnation (Clinthorne, Cisin, Balter, Mellinger, & Uhlenhuth, 1986). This is particularly so for middle- and upper-class users who are generally treated with more empathy and tolerance when problems develop than are persons who misuse other classes of drugs. While it is fortunate that persons who misuse sedatives are not subjected to some of the negative stereotyping often associated with the use of other substances, in some cases, these attitudes enable ongoing use. The detrimental effects of the use of these substances are often dismissed, and the user's denial is allowed to rule. This pattern has been especially pronounced in the elderly (Finlayson & Davis, 1994).

The progression of use from occasional prescribed or recreational use to uncontrolled use and dependence can be slow and insidious. This is most often the case for persons who have been maintained on benzodiazepines over an extended period of time (Mellinger et al., 1984). While it is possible to induce dependence fairly rapidly at higher than therapeutic doses (1–2 months), the more common pattern is one of slowly escalating doses over the course of several months or years. Persons who begin use for the relief of anxiety or sleep symptoms may begin to increase their dosage if some degree of tolerance develops and symptoms reemerge. Persons using some of the shorter-acting preparations may experience rebound symptoms as the effects of their most recent dose subside, and may increase the frequency of administration in anticipation of these symptoms. Over the course of time, persons using sedatives may begin to experience mild withdrawal symptoms if they miss or reduce their usual dose, increasing the magnitude of their anxiety and their compulsion to read-minister the drug. Although this pattern may vary somewhat depending on the individual and the preparation used, it is not difficult to see how sedative use may become entrenched, with the eventual development of very significant and often dangerous withdrawal symptoms in the absence of the substance (Ciraulo *et al.,* 1991; Herman, Brotman, & Rosenbaum, 1987; Sussman, 1993).

Psychiatric Disorders Associated with Sedative Dependence

Benzodiazepines are used for the treatment of a variety of psychiatric disorders and, as discussed earlier, if this use continues over a long period of time, dependence may develop. In this section, psychiatric disorders that are commonly associated with sedative use are considered with respect to unique issues that may influence the development or pattern of addiction. Psychiatric symptoms induced by sedative use are also considered. It is worth emphasizing at this point that the development of dependence in persons who are prescribed these medications for a legitimate purpose and who are responsibly monitored by the prescribing physician is a rare occurrence. This should be kept in mind lest effective treatment be withheld from a person suffering from anxiety or another disorder for fear of creating a dependency syndrome (Meyer, 1993; Mellinger *et al.,* 1984; Rush *et al.,* 1993).

Anxiety

The treatment of anxiety disorders or symptoms is perhaps the most frequent use of sedatives. While other agents, such as buspirone or some of the antidepressants, may be effective in treating these disorders (Taylor, 1995), their delayed onset make them ineffective when rapid relief is required. That same quality makes their abuse liability quite low compared to sedative anxiolytics. There has recently been a shift in prescribing patterns from longer-acting agents such as diazepam to shorter-acting preparations such as alprazolam. Alprazolam has been shown to be particularly effective in the treatment of panic disorder, but has the disadvantage of perhaps being more addictive due to the rebound anxiety symptoms often associated with its use (Herman *et al.,* 1987). In some cases, persons with anxiety disorders may never obtain care in a medical setting. These persons may begin to self-medicate either with alcohol or with sedatives available in their environment. It is these persons who are perhaps at greatest risk for developing problem use. The presence of a concerned and responsible prescriber to monitor dosage and symptom relief cannot be overemphasized as a means to minimize the development of problem use (Sussman, 1993).

While anxiety disorders may increase a person's vulnerability to becoming dependent on sedatives, their use and subsequent discontinuation may also induce anxiety symptoms. In some cases, users may experience a reduction in their tolerance for anxiety following extended periods of sedative use, making discontinuation difficult. Feelings of anxiety are usually part of the sedative withdrawal syndrome, particularly if some degree of tolerance has developed (Sellers, 1988). This induced anxiety often provides the impetus for the user to readminister the drug and often makes him or her feel overwhelmed by the thought of reducing dosage or discontinuing use. Regardless of whether an anxiety disorder was present prior to the onset of misuse, the masking of anxiety and the lack of practice in managing anxious feelings during periods of extended use may make anxiety encountered upon discontinuation of sedative use more difficult to tolerate (DuPont, 1995). Anxiety is often part of a protracted withdrawal syndrome (Ashton, 1991) that is associated with benzodiazepine withdrawal and may be present for 6 months or more.

Mood Syndromes

Sedative use is commonly associated with depression. In some cases, benzodiazepines may be prescribed to address the anxiety symptoms that often go hand in hand with depression, or they may be self-administered by users to control these symptoms. As with alcohol, sedatives may be used to provide temporary relief from depressed feelings even if significant anxiety symptoms are not present. However, the aftereffects or "hangover" experienced by many users of sedative agents may only compound the preexisting depression, often leading to further misuse and occasionally dependence (Meyer, 1993; Kisnad, 1991).

Some antidepressant effects were demonstrated for the benzodiazepine alprazolam at the time of its introduction, particularly for milder forms of depression. For a brief period, this agent was actively marketed for this condition, but the development of rebound anxiety, and in some cases dependence, has made its use for this purpose uncommon. The introduction of the serotonin reuptake inhibitors has further eroded its utility for depression. Nevertheless, some primary care physicians continue to use alprazolam for mild depression (Warner, Peabody, Whiteford, & Hollister, 1988).

The long-term use of sedating substances, particularly alcohol, has long been associated with increased incidence of depression. Extended use of sedatives may have similar effects on neurotransmitter systems, resulting in alterations that may require an extensive period of abstinence to correct. Depression and irritability are frequently part of protracted withdrawal syndromes commonly experienced after discontinuation of sedatives. In some cases, the use of antidepressants may be helpful in addressing these sedative-induced mood problems and enhancing the user's ability to establish a stable recovery (Geller, 1991).

Bipolar disorder is less frequently associated with sedative use. However, in the depressive phase of the illness, sedatives may be used much as previously described for unipolar depression. While many persons suffering from bipolar disorder use alcohol in the manic phase of their illness, use of sedatives in a similar manner is not well documented (Goodwin & Jamison, 1990). There is little indication, beyond some anecdotal reports mainly involving alprazolam (Cole & Kando, 1993), that sedatives induce manic symptoms in otherwise healthy individuals or that they precipitate a manic phase in persons with bipolar disorder.

Sedatives such as clonazepam and lorazepam are often used, in fact, to bring agitated mania under control (Janicak et al., 1993).

Insomnia

Problems with sleep are frequently associated with depression, anxiety, and substance use. Many persons may experience these problems independently of other psychiatric disturbances. There are a variety of sleeping aids available. Many over-the-counter preparations produce drowsiness and can be helpful for persons who experience difficulty getting to sleep when prescribed properly. Most of these agents have relatively low liability for dependence or disturbance of sleep architecture. The most common treatment for insomnia, however, has become the benzodiazepines.

There is a high degree of variability in approaches taken by the medical community when persons present with sleep disturbances. While most experts in the field recommend limited use of sleep medications over short periods of time and on an intermittent basis according to need (Janicak et al., 1993; Kales, 1990), in practice, these agents are frequently prescribed for extended periods and taken daily. This latter pattern obviously increases the likelihood of developing dependence and disturbing an already disrupted sleep architecture even further. While these agents may provide temporary relief from sleep deprivation, they do not produce the quality of sleep provided by the natural, healthy sleep cycle. In addition, they are not helpful in restoring that natural sleep pattern. It is for this reason that extended use of these agents is not recommended (Kales, 1990; Mendelson, 1993; Nishino, Mlgnot, & Dement, 1995).

Persons who use sedatives regularly for sleep problems may experience some reemergence of these difficulties when some degree of tolerance has developed. This may lead to an escalation of dosage or frequency of use. Often, for those who have established a pattern of daily use, achieving sleep naturally may become nearly impossible, particularly over the short term. It has been observed, for example, that persons using triazolam over periods as short as 7 days may experience rebound insomnia (Greenblatt, Shader, & Abernethy, 1993). It is not difficult to see, then, how easily a pattern of dependence may develop.

As with the use of other drugs, sedative misuse may have a significant effect on the normal sleep-wake cycle of the user. This may cause significant disturbance in sleep architecture and lead to a pattern of continuing or extended use in an attempt to achieve needed rest (Nishino et al., 1995). Sleep disturbances are frequently reported in the early phases of abstinence from many substances, including the sedatives. They may be part of protracted withdrawal syndromes as well (Geller, 1991). While this can cause significant discomfort in the early phases of recovery, clearly, addressing these difficulties with medication may be counterproductive. The treatment of sleep difficulties in persons entering recovery is discussed further toward the end of this chapter.

Substance Use Disorders

As discussed previously, misuse of sedatives may occur predominantly in the context of polysubstance dependence. When this is the case, sedatives are generally not the primary substances of misuse, but significant dependence may develop nonetheless. The coexistence of sedative dependence with other drug dependence may complicate the recovery process, particularly during the withdrawal period (Ciraulo et al., 1991). It may be difficult for the recovering polysubstance user to acknowledge the destructive aspects of all the substances they are using even if they do accept problems related to their primary substance of misuse. When this is the case, they may overtly or covertly expect to be able to continue their use of sedatives during their attempt to abstain from using their primary substance. This is, of course, antithetical to establishing a stable recovery and the denial of this principle must be confronted in treatment.

The sedatives are rarely a "gateway" drug. It is unusual for drug use to begin primarily with sedatives and even more unusual for sedative dependence to lead to the misuse of other classes of addicting substances (Cole &

Chiarello, 1990). One exception to this may be developing a pattern of misuse with a variety of prescription medications. It is not unusual, therefore, to encounter individuals who may be using a variety of pills, usually a mixture of sedatives and opiate-containing agents. Such patterns are commonly associated with pain syndromes, however, and use often begins with opiate-containing agents rather than with sedatives (Hoffmann, Olofsson, Salen, & Wickstrom, 1995).

Maladaptive Personality Traits

The existence of an "addictive" personality has been debated for some time. While there is not currently an independently defined personality disorder associated with addictive behaviors in *DSM-IV* (American Psychiatric Association, 1994), certain character traits may make drug dependence and other addictions more likely. The presence of these traits in the defining criteria for a *DSM-IV* personality disorder diagnosis will make it more likely that both of these diagnoses will be made (Carroll, Ball, & Rounsaville, 1993; Dulit, Fyer, Haas, Sullivan, & Frances, 1990; Gerstley, Alterman, McLellan, & Woody, 1990). A brief consideration of some of the traits commonly associated with addictions is provided in the following discussion.

Mood instability refers to a person's inability to modulate mood in a manner consistent with a broad appraisal of the environment. Mood may shift rapidly and intensely in reaction to transitory events and circumstances. When a person acts out this inner experience, rather than controlling responses until the consequences of action can be considered, they are said to be "impulsive." In some individuals, anger or rage is a predominant emotion that may be triggered by relatively minor environmental provocation, and impulsive aggressivity may be a frequent result. Irresponsible behaviors may be demonstrated in a variety of ways, but they are generally defined in terms of one's ability to fulfill expectations created by social structures such as work, school, family, friendship, and other social or financial contracts. Persons with this trait often see their failure to honor these obligations as lying outside of their control and brought about by environmental circumstances which they are unable to influence. This is sometimes termed an "external locus of control." Dependence and instability of self-concept are also associated with this pattern of externalization. An excessive focus on one's own experience and exclusive motivation to satisfy one's own needs with little regard or understanding of the needs and emotions of others indicates a lack of empathy. Individuals who display this trait may also be grandiose or feel entitled to special treatment or privilege in society.

These are a few of the traits associated with substance use disorders. They are also traits that partially define the *DSM-IV* borderline, antisocial, or narcissistic personality disorders. It does appear that these personality disorders are associated with a higher incidence of substance use than seen in the general population (Vaillant, 1983). It is not clear, however, that any particular set of personality traits or any particular personality disorder leads specifically to the use of sedatives as opposed to the use of other substances.

Although some of the traits defined here may exist prior to the onset of substance use, these traits and others are likely to develop in persons who become drug dependent even if they were not previously present. Traits seen in persons with addiction are often associated with immature defense mechanisms and these mechanisms may be present either because of developmental failures, as in the case of a primary personality disorder, or secondary to regression, as occurs when mature defenses are abandoned and maladaptive personality traits emerge, as commonly occurs in addictions (Walker, 1992). Whatever the case may be, there is again little evidence that sedative use has any greater or lesser association with the induction of these characteristics than any other substance.

Other Psychiatric Disorders Associated with Sedative Dependence

Sedative dependence can be associated with a wide variety of psychiatric disturbances, but are most commonly seen in conjunction with illnesses in which a sedative may be prescribed. In addition to the conditions already described, persons with somatoform disorders (including pain syndromes and somatization disorder), psychotic disorders, and adjustment disorders may be at increased risk for developing sedative dependence. As indicated at the beginning of this section, while exposure through treatment may increase the risk of developing problems, when properly supervised, few patients find these medications so attractive that they escalate their use independently. The development of dependence may be observed with a variety of psychiatric disorders, but those who are most likely to develop this problem may have several concurrent conditions, with anxiety a significant feature of at least one of those disorders. Since the intoxication of the sedatives, particularly the benzodiazepines, is more akin to a peacefulness than a high, those who develop dependence are more often seeking relief rather than euphoria. Here, the concept of the "self-medication" hypothesis is particularly apt (Khantzian, 1985).

Other Sedative-Induced Psychiatric Symptoms

One of the most commonly observed side effects of long-term, high-dose use of benzodiazepines has been cognitive impairment. This usually assumes the form of anterograde amnesia and impaired psychomotor performance during and immediately after the intoxication phase. There is no evidence, however, that cognitive impairments persist for a significant period following the discontinuation of use (Janicak *et al.,* 1993; Mallick, Kirby, Martin, Philp, & Hennessy, 1993). There have been some reports of psychotic symptoms with the discontinuation of benzodiazepines even in the absence of other significant withdrawal symptoms. Triazolam has been primarily associated with these phenomena. Symptoms may consists of confusion, delusions, hallucinations, and delirium. There has been no evidence that these symptoms persist as the period of abstinence is extended (Cole & Kando, 1993; Kales, 1990). Aggression or self-destructive behavior may emerge in some cases with the administration of a benzodiazepine; this would appear to be a paradoxical effect (Dietch & Jennings, 1988). This reaction is thought to be related to the disinhibition that results from in-toxication, more pronounced in some individuals than in others, and it may be enhanced by concurrent use of alcohol (Bond & Silveira, 1993; Cole & Kando, 1993).

Special Issues in Treatment and Prevention

The patterns of use discussed earlier in the chapter provide us with some guidance in considering how the misuse of sedatives might be prevented. Even though the number of persons who are prescribed sedatives and go on to develop problems in using them is quite small relative to the number of persons who are exposed to them, with proper care, physicians could themselves contribute considerably to the elimination of nontherapeutic sedative use (Sussman, 1993).

Adequate education and monitoring are essential aspects of responsible prescribing of sedatives. Many physicians mistakenly believe that discussing the abuse potential of a medication with patients may give them ideas about misuse that they would not otherwise consider. It is clear that many patients who develop dependence problems do so without recognition of the dangers involved in the pattern of their use. Drug dependence, in general, is widely misunderstood and stigmatized in our society, and this state of affairs can only be perpetuated by a lack of candor in confronting the issue whenever it is relevant to do so. We need to recognize that no one chooses to be addicted to any substance, and it is only through adequate education about addiction and addictive substances that persons can recognize dangerous use patterns before dependence and denial become dominant and preclude the possibility of making responsible decisions regarding use (Francis & Borg, 1993).

With this in mind, prescribers should provide complete information to patients about any medication that is considered for treat-ment. The potential for misuse should be part of the information supplied. Patients must be cautioned against self-adjustment of dosage and frequency of use, and the insidious nature of developing dependency problems can be emphasized. Patients must be aware that some degree of tolerance can be expected after the initial phases of use, particularly to the sedating effects of this medication. While modest dosage adjustment may be beneficial in some cases, indefinite escalation of dosage will not, and dosage changes should always be made in consultation with the doctor. Clinicians should always obtain a complete history of substance misuse from patients before making decisions regarding pharmacologic treatment. This should include a history of caffeine and nicotine use. Once a decision has been made to use a benzo-diazepine or other sedative agent, care must be taken to ensure that its use is adequately monitored through periodic discussions with the client and, in some cases, family members, if misuse is suspected or if the client is at high risk for addiction (Francis & Borg, 1993; Sussman, 1993).

Clinicians must also take care in adhering to proper prescribing regimens in the use of sedatives. Prolonged courses of treatment can often be avoided. Attempts to discontinue sedative use are warranted when clients have achieved significant periods of stability. In attempting to discontinue sedative use, clients must be helped in recognizing that they may experience some degree of rebound discomfort initially, but this is often a transient phenomena which will resolve if adequate time is allowed. Alternative methods for tolerating the discomfort can be suggested and may be helpful in establishing drug-free management of the treated condition (Kales, 1990; Zweben & Smith, 1989).

It has recently become common practice to prescribe trazodone, a sedating antidepressant, in low doses in conjunction with newer anti-depressants that may cause sleep disruption early in the course of their use. While there is some evidence of this medication's effectiveness in improving sleep during this period, it is unfortunate that it is often continued indefinitely, and that this may prevent patients from reestablishing normal sleep cycles (Nierenberg, Adler, Peselow, Zornberg, & Rosenthal, 1994; Parrino, Spaggiari, Boselli, DiGiovanni, & Terzano, 1994). In using benzodiazepines and other sedatives as sleeping aids, it is particularly important to avoid extended and consistent use. Their use will not improve sleep over the long term, and the potential for developing dependence on these agents for sleep is relatively high. Clients with sleep problems must be helped in establishing proper sleep hygiene rather than long-term dependence on medication to obtain needed rest (Janicak et al., 1993; Kales, 1990; Mendelson, 1993).

Just as patients cannot be expected to make responsible decisions about use without adequate information, neither can physicians properly inform their clients if they lack an adequate understanding of the use of these medications and of the addiction process. Many of the prescriptions written for sedatives are written by primary care physicians who may have limited training in psychiatry and psychopharmacology. Chances are, they have had even less exposure to training in addiction medicine. Despite the prevalence of these disorders, few training curricula in primary care have developed provisions for adequate attention to addictions. As a result, physicians are often uncomfortable in confronting these issues with their clients and frequently unaware of the role that they can play in reducing the incidence of dependency problems (DuPont, 1995; Smith & Seymour, 1991). General psychiatrists often lack adequate training in addictions as well, and frequently make many of the mistakes discussed here in their prescribing practices. For most persons who are not at high risk for developing dependency problems, management of these medications by a primary care physician or a general psychiatrist should not present problems if a minimal knowledge of addiction is obtained and sensitivity to these issues is maintained.

The use of sedative medications in persons with a history of substance dependence can be a more complicated issue. Most experts agree that the use of these agents in persons who are actively using another substance in a maladaptive manner is contraindicated (Janicak et al., 1993). Until abstinence is achieved for a period of time long enough to rule out significant drug effects, it is extremely difficult to make a determination regarding etiology of psychiatric symptoms. The use of sedatives or other psychoactive medications can only further obscure the situation and make this determination even more difficult. This will only delay the clinician's ability to institute an appropriate treatment regimen (DuPont, 1995; Smith & Seymour, 1991).

Many authors feel that a past history of substance dependence, even without evidence of recent use, is a contraindication for the use of sedative medications (Rosenbaum & Gelenburg, 1991). In fact, there is little evidence to support this position. When adequately monitored and educated, persons in recovery are no more likely than those without a past history of substance dependence to misuse a sedative when prescribed for anxiety or other legitimate indications (Mueller, Goldenberg, Gordon, Keller, & Warshaw, 1996). As a rule of thumb, it is generally sensible to attempt treatment with a nonaddictive anxiolytic such as buspirone or an antidepressant rather than using a sedative as the first line of treatment. When these attempts fail, however, it is usually preferable to initiate treatment with a benzodiazepine than to allow symptoms to continue unabated. This latter course may place the client at greater risk for relapse and reestablishing dependence than the risk posed by the sedative. In these cases, it is prudent to choose agents with slow onset and long duration of action such as clonazepam or chlordiazepoxide to minimize the risk for developing problem use (DuPont, 1995; Francis & Borg, 1993).

Detoxification can often be accomplished on an outpatient basis, particularly if the picture is not complicated by dependence on multiple substances and if there is no significant medical or psychiatric comorbidity (Castaneda & Cushman, 1989; Stockwell et al., 1991). While there are numerous protocols available to accomplish detoxification, several principles should be common to all of them. Long-acting agents are substituted for shorter-acting preparations, and agents with a rapid onset are better avoided. Adequate initial dosing will avoid excessive discomfort and the need for the patient to establish a pattern of asking for more medication. If drowsiness develops, succeeding dosages can be held until this is no longer a problem. A gradual schedule for dosage reduction and discontinuation should be established early on, and clear limits must be placed on any exceptions to the established schedule. A reduction in dosage of 10% daily should be well tolerated, but in outpatient settings a slower taper schedule may be more easily accomplished. Adequate support is an essential ingredient of a successful outpatient detoxification, and it is most helpful if responsible significant others are involved in the treatment and monitoring of the detoxification (Alling, 1992; Janicak *et al.*, 1993). For more complicated detoxification, or when support systems are lacking, inpatient treatment is usually indicated. Monitoring of vital signs can then be accomplished on a 24-hr basis and other symptoms of withdrawal can likewise be observed. Longer-acting agents are, again, generally preferred, and they can be administered on an as-needed basis according to measurable parameters. One advantage of the long-acting agents is the self-tapering effect obtained due to their gradual elimination after an adequate blood level is achieved. The advantage to inpatient medically monitored detoxification is that it can generally be accomplished more rapidly and safely than outpatient regimens which is particularly important when complications exist. After initiating treatment in the inpatient setting, clients can usually be transferred to partial hospital settings rather quickly once the danger of complications is diminished (Alling, 1992).

Summary

Benzodiazepines as a class have become the most widely prescribed medication in the United States and possibly the world. They have largely replaced barbiturates and other older sedatives not only as treatment for anxiety and insomnia, but also as drugs of misuse. Despite their relative safety, dependence on these substances can have serious consequences for the user. The frequency with which these substances are prescribed make them readily available and easily misused. Although the incidence of dependence in persons who have been prescribed a sedative for a valid purpose is quite low, lack of knowledge and attention on the part of the prescriber may contribute to the risk of developing problem use.

These medications may cause a variety of psychiatric symptoms that are usually transient in nature. Considerable confusion and treatment dilemmas may be generated, however, by the coexistence of another psychiatric disorder. Care must be exercised in making diagnostic determinations and initiating treatment for persons with co-occurring disorders. The treatment of sedative dependence, while similar in principle to the treatment of addiction to other substances, may require some unique interventions to facilitate recovery. Chances for a successful recovery are good when timely, well-structured treatment is provided.

References

Allgulander, C. (1986). History and current state of sedative-hypnotic drug use and abuse. *Acta Psychiatrica Scandinavica, 73,* 465–478.

Alling, F. A. (1992). Detoxification and treatment of acute sequelae, from substance abuse. In J. H. Lowinson, P. Ruiz, R. B. Millman, & J. G. Langrod (Eds.), *Substance abuse: A comprehensive textbook* (2nd ed., pp. 402–413). Baltimore: Williams and Wilkens.

American Psychiatric Association. (1994). *Diagnostic and statistical manual of mental disorders* (4th ed.). Washington, DC: Author.

Ashton, H. (1991). Protracted withdrawal syndromes from benzodiazepines. *Journal of Substance Abuse Treatment, 8,* 19–28.

Ballenger, J. C. (1995). Benzodiazepines. In A. F. Schatberg & C. B. Nemeroff (Eds.), *Textbook of psychopharmacology* (pp. 215–225). Washington, DC: American Psychiatric Press.

Barnas, C., Rossmann, M., Roessler, H., Riemer, Y., & Fleischhacker, W. W. (1992). Benzodiazepines and other psychotropic drugs abused by patients in a methadone maintenance program: Familiarity and preference. *Journal of Clinical Psychopharmacology, 12*(6), 397–402.

Bond, A. J., & Silveira, J. C. (1993). The combination of alprazolam and alcohol on behavioral aggression. *Journal of Studies on Alcohol* (Suppl. 11), 30–39.

Carroll, K. M., Ball, S. A., & Rounsaville, B. J. (1993). A comparison of alternate systems for diagnosing antisocial personality disorder in cocaine abusers. *Journal of Nervous Disorders and Mental Disease, 181,* 436–443.

Castaneda, R., & Cushman, P. (1989). Alcohol withdrawal: A review of clinical management. *Journal of Clinical Psychiatry, 50*(8), 278–284.

Ciraulo, D. A., Sands, B. F., Shader, R. I., & Greenblatt, D. J. (1991). Anxiolytics. In D. A. Ciraulo & R. I. Shader (Eds.), *Clinical manual of chemical dependence* (pp. 135–173). Washington, DC: American Psychiatric Press.

Clinthorne, J. K., Cisin, I. H., Balter, M. B., Mellinger, G. D., & Uhlenhuth, E. H. (1986). Changes in popular attitudes and beliefs about tranquilizers. *Archives of General Psychiatry, 43*(6), 527–532.

Cole, J. O., & Chiarello, R. J. (1990). The benzodiazepines as drugs of abuse. *Journal of Psychiatric Research, 24,* 135–44.

Cole, J. O., & Kando, J. C. (1993). Adverse behavioral events reported in patients taking alprazolam and other benzodiazepines. *Journal of Clinical Psychiatry, 54*(10) (Suppl.), 49–61.

de Wit, H., & Griffiths, R. R. (1991). Testing the abuse liability of anxiolytic and hypnotic drugs in humans. *Drug and Alcohol Dependence, 28,* 83–111.

Dietch, J. T., & Jennings, R. K. (1988). Aggressive dyscontrol in patients treated with benzodiazepines. *Journal of Clinical Psychiatry, 49*(5), 184–188.

Dulit, R. A., Fyer, M. R., Haas, G. L., Sullivan, T., & Frances, A. J. (1990). Substance use in borderline personality disorder. *American Journal of Psychiatry, 147*(8), 1002–1007.

DuPont, R. L. (1995). Anxiety and addiction: A clinical perspective on comorbidity. *Bulletin of the Menninger Clinic, 59*(2) (Suppl. A), A53–A73.

Eadie, J. L. (1993). *New York state's triplicate prescription program* (NIDA Research Monograph No. 131, pp. 176–193). Rockville, MD: National Institute on Drug Abuse.

Finlayson, R. E., & Davis, L. J. (1994). Prescription drug dependence in the elderly population: Demographic and clinical features of 100 inpatients. *Mayo Clinic Proceedings, 69,* 1137–1145.

Francis, R., & Borg, L. (1993). The treatment of anxiety in patients with alcoholism. *Journal of Clinical Psychiatry, 54,* 37–43.

Geller, A. (1991). Protracted abstinence. In N. Miller (Ed.), *Comprehensive handbook of drug and alcohol addiction* (pp. 905–913). New York: Dekker.

Gerstley, L. J., Alterman, A. I., McLellan, A. T., & Woody, G. E. (1990). Antisocial personality disorder in patients with substance abuse disorders: A problematic diagnosis? *American Journal of Psychiatry, 146*(4), 508–512.

Goodwin, F. K., & Jamison, K. R. (1990). *Manic-depressive illness.* New York: Oxford University Press.

Greenberg, D. A. (1993). Ethanol and sedatives. *Neurologic Clinics, 11*(3), 523–534.

Greenblatt, D. J., Shader, R. I., & Abernethy, D. R. (1993). Drug therapy: Current state of the benzodiazepines, Part 2. *New England Journal of Medicine, 309,* 410–416.

Herman, J. B., Brotman, A. W., & Rosenbaum, J. F. (1987). Rebound anxiety in panic disorder patients treated with shorter-acting benzodiazepines. *Journal of Clinical Psychiatry 48*(10), 22–26.

Hoffmann, N. G., Olofsson, O., Salen, B., & Wickstrom, L. (1995). Prevalence of abuse and dependency in chronic pain patients. *International Journal of the Addictions, 30,* 919–927.

Iguchi, M. Y., Handelsman, L., Bickel, W. K., & Griffiths, R. R. (1993). Benzodiazepine and sedative use/abuse by methadone maintenance clients. *Drug and Alcohol Dependence, 32,* 257–266.

Janicak, P. G., Davis, J. M., Preskorn, S., & Ayd, F. (1993). *Principles and practice of psychopharmacotherapy* (pp. 357–358, 405–442). Baltimore: Williams and Wilkens.

Jinks, M. J., & Raschko, R. R. (1990). A profile of alcohol and prescription drug abuse in a high-risk community-based elderly population. *Drug Intelligence and Clinical Pharmacology, 24,* 971–975.

Kales, A. (1990). Benzodiazepine hypnotics and insomnia. *Hospital Practice Office Edition, 25* (Suppl. 3), 7–21; discussion 22–23.

Khantzian, E. J. (1985). The self medication hypothesis of addictive disorders: Focus on heroin and cocaine dependence. *American Journal of Psychiatry, 142,* 1259–1264.

Kisnad, H. (1991). Sedatives-hypnotics. In N. Miller (Ed.), *Comprehensive handbook of drug and alcohol addiction* (pp. 405–426). New York: Dekker.

Lader, M. (1991). History of benzodiazepine dependence. *Journal of Substance Abuse Treatment, 8,* 53–59.

Landry, M. J., Smith, D. E., McDuff, D. R., & Baughman, O. L. (1992). Benzodiazepine dependence and withdrawal: Identification and medical management [see comments]. *Journal of the American Board of Family Practice, 5,* 167–175.

Mallick, J. L., Kirby, K. C., Martin, F., Philp, M., & Hennessy, M. J. (1993). A comparison of the amnesic effects of lorazepam in alcoholics and non-alcoholics. *Psychopharmacology, 110,* 181–186.

Mellinger, G. D., Balter, M. B., & Uhlenhuth, E. H. (1984). Prevalence and correlates of the long-term regular use of anxiolytics. *Journal of the American Medical Association, 251*(3), 375–379.

Mendelson, W. B. (1993). Insomnia and related sleep disorders. *Psychiatric Clinics of North America, 16*(4), 841–851.

Meyer, M. (Ed.). (1993). AMA-DE (Drug Evaluations). Chicago: American Medical Association, Division of Drugs and Toxicology.

Morgan, W. W. (1990). Abuse liability of barbiturates and other sedative-hypnotics. *Advances in Alcohol and Substance Abuse, 9,* 67–82.

Mueller, T. I., Goldenberg, I. M., Gordon, A. L., Keller, M. B., & Warshaw, M. G. (1996). Benzodiazepine use in anxiety disordered patients with and without a history of alcoholism. *Journal of Clinical Psychiatry, 57,* 83–89.

Mumford, G. K., Evans, S. M., Fleishaker, J. C., & Griffiths, R. R. (1995). Alprazolam absorption kinetics affects abuse liability. *Clinical Pharmacology & Therapeutics, 57*(3), 356–365.

Nierenberg, A. A., Adler, L. A., Peselow, E., Zornberg, G., & Rosenthal, M. (1994). Trazodone for antidepressant-associated insomnia. *American Journal of Psychiatry, 151,* 1069–1072.

Nishino, S., Mignot, E., & Dement, W. C. (1995). Sedative hypnotics. In A. F. Schatzberg & C. B. Nemeroff (Eds.), *Textbook of psychopharmacology* (pp. 405–413). Washington, DC: APA Press.

Parrino, L., Spaggiari, M. C., Boselli, M., DiGiovanni, G., & Terzano, M. G. (1994). Clinical and polysomnographic effects of trazodone CR in chronic insomnia associated with dysthymia. *Psychopharmacology* (Berlin), *116,* 389–395.

Regier, D. A., Farmer, M. E., Rae, D. S., Locke, B. Z., Keith, S. J., Judd, L. L., & Goodwin, F. K. (1990). Comorbidity and mental disorders with alcohol and other drug abuse. *Journal of the American Medical Association, 264*(19), 2511–2518.

Roache, J. D., Meisch, R. A., Henningfield, J. E., Jaffe, J. H., Klein, S., & Sampson, A. (1995). Reinforcing effects of triazolam in sedative abusers: Correlation of drug liking and self-administration measures. *Pharmacology, Biochemistry and Behavior, 50,* 171–179.

Rosenbaum, J. F., & Gelenburg, A. J. (1991). Anxiety from the practitioners. In A. J. Gelenburg, F. L. Bassak, & S. C. Schoonover (Eds.), *Guide to psychoactive drugs* (pp. 179–218). New York: Plenum.

Rush, C. R., Higgins, S. T., Bickel, W. K., & Hughes, J. R. (1993). Abuse liability of alprazolam relative to other commonly used benzodiazepines: A review. *Neuroscience and Biobehavioral Reviews, 17,* 277–285.

San, L., Tato, J., Torrens, M., Castillo, C., Farre, M., & Cami, J. (1993). Flunitrazepam consumption among heroin addicts admitted for in-patient detoxification. *Drug and Alcohol Dependence, 32,* 281–286.

Sellers, E. M. (1988). Alcohol, barbiturate and benzodiazepine withdrawal syndromes: Clinical management. *Canadian Medical Association Journal, 139,* 113–120.

Sellers, E. M., Schneiderman, J. F., Romach, M. K., Kaplan, H. L., & Somer, G. R. (1992). Comparative drug effects and abuse liability of lorazepam, buspirone, and secobarbital in nondependent subjects. *Journal of Clinical Psychopharmacology, 12*(2), 79–85.

Sheehan, M. F., Sheehan, D. V., Torres, A., Coppola, A., & Francis, E. (1991). Snorting benzodiazepines. *American Journal of Drug and Alcohol Abuse, 17,* 457–468.

Smith, D. E., & Seymour, R. B. (1991). Benzodiazepines. In N. Miller (Ed.), *Comprehensive handbook of drug and alcohol addiction* (pp. 405–426). New York: Dekker.

Sternbach, L. H. (1993). The benzodiazepine story. *Journal of Psychoactive Drugs, 15,* 15–17.

Stockwell, T., Bolt, L., Milner, I., Russell, G., Bolderston, H., & Pugh, P. (1991). Home detoxification from alcohol: Its safety and efficacy in comparison with in-patient care. *Alcohol and Alcoholism, 26,* 645–650.

Sussman, N. (1993). Treating anxiety while minimizing abuse and dependence. *Journal of Clinical Psychiatry, 54,* 44–51.

Taylor, C. B. (1995). Treatment of anxiety disorders. In A. F. Schatzberg & C. B. Nemeroff (Eds.), *Benzodiazepines from textbook of psychopharmacology* (pp. 641–651). Washington, DC: American Psychiatric Press.

Vaillant, G. E. (1983). *The natural history of alcoholism: Causes, patterns, and paths to recovery.* Cambridge, MA: Harvard University Press.

Walker, R. (1992). Substance abuse and B-cluster disorders I and II understanding and treating the dual diagnosis patient. *Journal of Psychoactive Drugs, 24*(3), 223–241.

Warner, P. H., Peabody, C. A., Whiteford, H. A., & Hollister, L. (1988). Alprazolam as an antidepressant. *Journal of Clinical Psychiatry, 49,* 148–150.

Weintraub, M., Singh, S., Byrne, L., Maharaj, K., & Guttmacher, L. (1993). *Consequences of the 1989 New York State triplicate benzodiazepine prescription regulations* (NIDA Research Monograph No. 131, pp. 279–293). Rockville, MD: National Institute on Drug Abuse.

Wesson, D. R., Smith, D. E., & Seymour, M. A. (1992). Sedative, hypnotics and tricyclics. In J. H. Lowinson, P. Ruiz, R. B. Millman, & J. H. Langrod (Eds.), *Substance abuse: A comprehensive textbook* (2nd ed., pp. 271–278). Baltimore: Williams and Wilkens.

Williams, D. H. (1993). Triplicate prescriptions in Washington State (NIDA Research Monograph No. 131, pp. 194–199). Rockville, MD: National Institute on Drug Abuse.

Zweben, J. E., & Smith, D. E. (1989). Considerations in using psychotropic medication with dual diagnosis patients in recovery. *Journal of Psychoactive Drugs, 21*(2), 221–228.

29

Medications of Abuse and Addiction

Benzodiazepines and Other Sedatives/Hypnotics

NORMAN S. MILLER, DEBRA L. KLAMEN,
AND ERMINIO COSTA

Introduction

Most medications with major potential for abuse and addiction belong to the sedative-hypnotic class. This encompasses benzo-diazepines, barbiturates, and the opiates (including natural and synthetic derivations of opium) (Jaffe, 1990; Jaffe & Martin, 1990; Rall, 1990). This chapter is devoted to the sedative-hypnotic class, featuring benzo-diazepines and including other sedative-hypnotic medications. In 1826 bromides were the first sedatives after alcohol to be marketed specifically for the sedative-hypnotic effects. Next, barbituric acid was introduced in 1903 followed by chloral hydrate ("Mickey Finn") in 1932 and meprobamate in 1955. Morphine was discovered in 1806, followed by codeine in 1832, then development of the synthetic derivatives of opiates in the mid 1900s.

The effects of these medications are widespread in the brain and their use consequently affects many aspects of mental functions, including mood, cognition, and behavior. Clinical manifestations of the neurochemical action for benzodiazepines and barbiturates (ethanol) originates on highly specific binding sites on GABA receptors located ubiquitously throughout the central nervous system (CNS). Pharmacological and behavioral tolerance is a regular accompaniment to drug use and is an expected natural adaptation of the nervous system to the presence of a foreign chemical. Pharmacological tolerance reflects a reduction in intrinsic activity of the medication at the identifiable high-affinity binding sites on GABA receptors (Costa & Guidotti, 1996). The absence of the drug is a manifestation of a pharmacologic dependence which reflects the deadaptation to tolerance that is expressed as a withdrawal state (Costa, Thompson, Auta, & Guidotti, 1995). The sedative-hypnotics are discussed in three categories based on their chemical structures: the benzodiazepines, barbiturates, and other sedative-hypnotics as shown in Table 1.

Benzodiazepines

History

In 1960, the first benzodiazepine, chlordiazepoxide, was introduced into clinical prac-

NORMAN S. MILLER, DEBRA L. KLAMEN, AND ERMINIO COSTA • Department of Psychiatry, The University of Illinois at Chicago, Chicago, Illinois 60612.

Handbook of Substance Abuse: Neurobehavioral Pharmacology, edited by Tarter *et al.* Plenum Press, New York, 1998.

TABLE 1. Sedatives/Hypnotics

Benzodiazepines	
Short-acting agents	Triazolam, oxazepam, temazepam, lorazepam, alprazolam
Long-acting agents	Chlordiazepoxide, diazepam, halazepam, clorazepate, prazepam, clonazepam, flurazepam
Nonbenzodiazepines	Zolpidem, buspirone
Barbiturates	Amobarbital, butabarbital, butalbital, pentobarbital, secobarbital, phenobarbital
Glycerol	Meprobamate
Piperidinedione	Glutethimide
Quinazoline	Methaqualone
Chloral derivatives	Chloral hydrate
Ethchlorvynol	Placidyl
Glutethimide	Doriden
Methypryton	Nodular
Paraldehyde	Paral

tice. It was followed by diazepam (Valium), which up to that point was the single most commonly prescribed benzodiazepine. In 1987, it fell second to alprazolam (Salzman, 1993b; Warneke, 1991). At their peak in 1975, 100 million benzodiazepine prescriptions were filled. More than 80 million benzodiazepine prescriptions were filled in 1994 with 1 in 10 Americans reporting the use of a benzodiazepine at least once a year for a medical reason other than insomnia. The popularity of this class of drugs with clinicians and patients is supported by the fact that the first seven of the "top 200 medications of 1993" were benzodiazepines (Gold, Miller, Stennie, & Populla-Vardi, 1995). The widespread use of benzodiazepines appears to be due to actions against the symptoms of anxiety, panic, insomnia, their perceived relative safety, their ability to reinforce consumption, and their propensity to produce pharmacological tolerance and dependence (Miller, Dackis, & Gold, 1987; Salzman, 1993a).

Mechanisms of Action

The hypothesis that benzodiazepine action is mediated by mechanisms involving the neurotransmitter GABA was proposed before a high-affinity binding to brain membranes was reported. The discovery in 1975 of high-affinity binding to the membranes indicated that these drugs were acting on a receptor for an as yet unknown neurotransmitter (Haefely et al., 1975). The hypothesis that benzodiazepines exert their effects by acting on GABA receptors and facilitating GABA action on these receptors was subsequently confirmed by purifying a GABA receptor subunit that included GABA and benzodiazepine binding sites which were saturable and stereospecific on $GABA_A$ receptors (Squires & Braestrup, 1977). This finding was reported at a time when the public and physicians were becoming increasingly alarmed regarding the issues of benzodiazepine abuse and dependence (Paul, Marancos, & Skolnick, 1981; Squires & Braestrup, 1977). The cloning of 13 GABA receptor subunits belonging to four families, α, β, γ, δ, and the expression of various recombinant subtypes of $GABA_A$ receptors have demonstrated that GABA and benzodiazepines have a different intrinsic activity at various GABA receptor subtypes.

Epidemiology

Sources for Evaluating Benzodiazepine Use and Dependence in General Populations

The United States is far from being the world leader in benzodiazepine use. Benzodiazepine use in general populations ranges from 7.4% in the Netherlands to 17% in Belgium, and 25% in selected populations in Iceland (Romach et al., 1992). In the United States, up to 90% of individuals hospitalized for medical care or surgery receive orders for sedative, hypnotic, or anxiolytic medications during their hospital stay, and more than 15% of American adults use these medications (usually by prescription) during one year (Salzman, 1993b). Other countries report high rates of benzodiazepine use, for example, Canada and Chile (Ruiz, Offermanns, Lanctôt, & Busto, 1993). While misuse has not been well studied, one survey conducted in the United States in 1991 reported that about 4% of the population had ever used sedatives for nonmedical purposes; approximately 1% had used in the past year, and 0.4% in the past month (*DSM-IV*, American Psychiatric Association, 1994). However, because the distinction between medical and nonmedical use of benzodiazepines is not always clear and the validity of self-report that require the respondent to distinguish nonmedical from medical use is questionable, actual prevalence rates of nonmedical use may be substantially higher (DuPont, 1988; Miller & Gold, 1991; Miller & Mahler, 1991).

Among the various medications in the anxiolytic and sedative-hypnotic class, the benzodiazepines are the most widely prescribed. The majority of the survey data assess prevalence and patterns of use rather than diagnoses, for example, benzodiazepine addiction. Many surveys, for example, do not report how many of those who used drugs from this class had symptoms that met criteria for *DSM* dependence or abuse. Only one community study, conducted in the United States from 1980 to 1985, used the more narrowly defined *DSM-III* (American Psychiatric Assocation, 1980) criteria. The study found that 1.1% of the population surveyed met criteria for sedative, hypnotic, or anxiolytic abuse or dependence at some time in their lives (Wilford, 1990).

Sources for Evaluating Benzodiazepine Use and Addiction in Medical Populations

The prevalence of benzodiazepine addiction in medical populations is not known. Studies that find low rates of benzodiazepine dependence do not assess for adverse consequences from benzodiazepine use (DuPont, 1988). Symptomatology related to or induced by benzodiazepine use, dependence, and addiction, such as anxiety and depression, are frequently ascribed to other medical and psychiatric illnesses (Juergens, 1994; Miller & Gold, 1991; Shader & Greenblatt, 1993). Because benzodiazepines are used in a medical context, there is a resistance to identifying patients who might have benzodiazepine dependence.

Because of discrepancies in defining addictive use by patients, clinicians, and researchers,

the extent of addictive use in medical populations is not known. However, benzodiazepines are widely prescribed and have the reinforcing potential for self-administration similar to that of other drugs with addictive potential (Roache & Meisch, 1995). The combination of addiction potential, presence of biological vulnerability, and widespread clinical prescribing of benzodiazepines warrants a critical examination of liability to addictive use in medical and nonmedical contexts (Busto, Kaplan, Zawertailo, & Sellers, 1994; Ciraulo *et al.*, 1996).

Sources for Evaluating Benzodiazepine Use and Addiction in Special Populations

Nonmedical use of benzodiazepines is particularly prevalent in people with alcoholism or drug addiction. Individuals with alcohol, drug disorders, or both constitute 25% of general medical populations and 50% of general psychiatry populations (Chan, 1984; Juergens, 1993; Miller & Mirin, 1989). As many as 80% of individuals with alcohol disorders under the age of 30 are addicted to at least one other drug including benzodiazepines (Chan, 1984; Miller & Gold, 1991; Miller & Mirin, 1989). Studies indicate that 30%–50% of individuals with opiate addiction are users of these benzodiazepines (Miller & Mirin, 1989). Cocaine addicts also frequently use benzodiazepines in a compulsive pattern (Miller & Mahler, 1991). It is significant that physicians are the largest source of benzodiazepines for all populations, whether medical or nonmedical (Chan, 1984; Grantham, 1987; Perera, Tulley, & Jenner, 1987; Schuster & Humphries, 1981; Sellers *et al.*, 1981).

Diagnosis of Addiction, Tolerance, and Dependence

Addiction (Anxiolytic Dependence) and *DSM* Criteria

The criteria for dependence in *DSM-IV* may not be sufficiently sensitive and specific to identify adverse consequences from benzodiazepine use in order to make a diagnosis of benzodiazepine (anxiolytic) dependence or addiction. The adverse consequences from benzodiazepines are sometimes subtle (no overt intoxication) and are intermixed with the same clinical symptoms for which physicians make decisions for prescribing benzodiazepines, for example, anxiety, insomnia (*DSM-IV*).

Furthermore, the addictive use of benzodiazepines is not easily determined from the *DSM-IV* criteria because of the confusion between medical and nonmedical use of benzodiazepines. Adverse consequences from benzodiazepine dependence (e.g., impairment in social, occupational, familial, and psychological functions) are not commonly recognized as resulting from addictive use of benzodiazepines, and are often misattributed to the psychiatric problems for which they are prescribed. Adverse consequences from benzodiazepine use with physiological dependence lead to pharmacologically induced anxiety and sleep disorders that are not clearly distinguished from psychiatric and medical indications for anxiolytic prescription use.

Further contributing to the difficulty in applying the criteria for *DSM* diagnoses is that the nosology for Substance Related Disorders fails to clearly distinguish addiction from pharmacological dependence. Inclusion under one diagnosis makes it difficult to interpret reports regarding benzodiazepine dependence (Juergens, 1991; Miller & Mahler, 1991). The distinction between addiction and pharmacological dependence is critical for understanding and assessing liability for addiction as a consequence of benzodiazepine use (American Psychiatric Association, 1994; Busto & Sellers, 1991; Juergens, 1991; Miller & Mahler, 1991). Moreover, studies have not specifically examined the relationship between addictive use (preoccupation with acquiring, compulsive use, and relapse to benzodiazepines) and subsequent development of adverse consequences.

Pharmacological Dependence (Withdrawal)

The criteria for physiological tolerance and physiological dependence in Substance Dependence in *DSM-IV* are (1) a need to markedly increase doses to achieve desired effect, that is, the development of tolerance, and (2) use to avoid withdrawal symptoms. It is important to note that pharmacological tolerance and dependence can develop independently of addictive use. Many chronic users of benzodiazepines show manifestations of pharmacological tolerance and dependence (withdrawal) without the preoccupation, compulsive use, and relapse from addiction to benzodiazepines. On the other hand, pharmacological tolerance and dependence can lead to addictive use because of the regular and chronic course of benzodiazepine use.

Symptoms of substance-induced anxiety similar to those found in anxiety disorders can be expected from acute withdrawal in chronic users of benzodiazepines (Ashton, 1984; Busto & Sellers, 1986; Rosenberg & Chiu, 1985). The contribution of the acute withdrawal symptoms in a state of pharmacological dependence must be excluded before suggesting an independent anxiety disorder as causal of symptoms of anxiety associated with benzodiazepine use. The *DSM-IV* criteria require the exclusion of substance-induced anxiety syndromes; "the anxiety disorder is not due to the direct physiological effects of a substance (e.g., a drug of abuse, a medication)" (American Psychiatric Association, 1994, p. 400).

Controlled studies have provided confirmatory evidence regarding the onset, prevalence, and clinical characteristics of pharmacological dependence (Busto & Sellers, 1986; Juergens, 1993; Lader, 1983; Rickels, Schweizer, Case, & Greenblatt, 1990; Rickels, Schweizer, Weiss, & Zavodnick, 1993; Rosenberg & Chiu, 1985). For clinical practice, pharmacological tolerance and withdrawal follow known pharmacokinetic parameters. Pharmacological dependence to all preparations of benzodiazepines develops within weeks of regular use. Severity is greater in shorter-acting than longer-acting preparations of benzodiazepines, and with higher doses and longer duration of use (Table 1) (Busto & Sellers, 1986; Busto, Simpkins, & Sellers, 1983; Busto *et al.*, 1986; Griffiths & Sannerud, 1987; Juergens, 1993; Lader, 1983; Owen & Tyrer, 1983; Rickels *et al.*, 1990; Rickels *et al.*, 1993; Rosenberg & Chiu, 1985).

Common symptoms of acute withdrawal are anxiety, followed by fear, depression, headache, tremor, sensory disturbances, diaphoresis, insomnia, tension, fatigue, gastrointestinal disturbances, seizures, and delirium (Busto & Sellers, 1986, 1991; U.S. Department of Health and Human Services [USDHHS], 1987; Juergens, 1993; Lader, 1983; Rosenberg & Chiu, 1985). The signs and symptoms of withdrawal can be categorized according to systems (see Table 2). Withdrawal can be separated into acute and protracted states. The acute withdrawal for short-acting preparations peaks in 2–3 days, and has a duration of 5–7 days whereas for long-acting substances the peak period is 4–5 days and the duration is 9–11 days (Alexander & Perry, 1991; Busto & Sellers, 1991; DeVane, Ware, & Lydiard, 1991).

Typically, the onset of symptoms of acute withdrawal from short-acting benzodiazepines begins within hours. With the development of pharmacological dependence, alprazolam (Xanax) produces anxiety symptoms within 2 hr of the last dose, and triazolam (Halcion) produces insomnia within 3 hr of the bedtime dose. The onset of seizure activity is 2–3 days from the last dose, and delirium with hallucinations and delusions may follow in 3–4 days after cessation of use from short-acting preparations. The onset of withdrawal from long-acting benzodiazepines, diazepam (Valium), begins 1–2 days after the last dose, seizures can occur within 5–7 days, and delirium may follow within 8–9 days (Alexander & Perry, 1991; Busto & Sellers, 1991; DeVane et al., 1991).

Following long-term benzodiazepine use, a protracted withdrawal syndrome has been described (Ashton, 1991). Onset begins after the acute withdrawal, and can be viewed as a continuation of acute withdrawal with the addition of other signs and symptoms, particularly neuropsychiatric symptoms. Protracted withdrawal can last for months to years, and can be particularly distressing to the patient. Signs and symptoms of protracted withdrawal are similar to those for anxiety disorders and require exclusionary criteria to be applied as substance-induced (withdrawal) disorders. Treatment should not be additional benzodiazepines, which prolongs the protracted withdrawal, but antidepressants, psychotherapy, and treatment of addiction (Ashton, 1984, 1987).

New Classification for Pharmacological Tolerance and Dependence

The presence of pharmacological tolerance and dependence cannot always be predicted by half-life. A newer classification, based on modification of $GABA_A$ receptor subtypes, may be more informative in understanding the development of tolerance and dependence to benzodiazepines. Full, selective, and partial agonists can be classified according to binding affinity and intrinsic activity at $GABA_A$ receptors. Full agonists bind to most $GABA_A$ receptor subtypes and have high intrinsic activity; selective agonists act only at some receptor subtypes with high intrinsic activity; and partial agonists act at all receptors but with lower intrinsic activity. Full agonists, for example, diazepam and alprazolam, show the greatest liability to develop tolerance, dependence, and addiction. Selective agonists, such as zolpidem, and partial agonists, such as imidazenil and bretazenil, have lower liability for tolerance, dependence, and addiction. Both zolpi-

---

TABLE 2. Signs and Symptoms of Benzodiazepine Withdrawal

Symptoms of hyperexcitability	Agitation, anxiety, hyperactivity, insomnia
Neuropsychiatric symptoms	Ataxia, depersonalization, depression, fasciculations, formication, headache, hyperventilation, malaise, myalgia, paranoid delusions, paresthesias, pruritus, tinnitus, tremor, visual hallucinations
Gastrointestinal symptoms	Abdominal pain, constipation, diarrhea, nausea, vomiting
Cardiovascular symptoms	Chest pain, flushing, palpitations
Genitourinary symptoms	Incontinence, loss of libido, urinary urgency, urinary frequency

dem and triazolam are equally short-acting but zolpidem, a selective agonist, shows less dependence liability than triazolam, a full agonist. A single benzodiazepine may be both a full and selective agonist and have short and long half-lives depending on the pharmacological activity of the metabolites; for example, diazepam is a full agonist with short duration of action but its metabolites are selective agonists with long-lasting duration of action (Table 3).

Behavioral Basis of Addiction

The addiction liability of sedatives, hypnotics, and anxiolytics can be assessed by examining the reinforcing effects of these drugs, based on the assumption that reinforcing effects are correlated with drug self-ingestion (Roache, 1990).

Many animal studies have shown that benzodiazepines function as reinforcers in animals (Ator & Griffiths, 1987; Woods, Katz, & Winger, 1987, 1992). Importantly, reinforcing effects have been demonstrated in several different species including rats, baboons, rhesus monkeys, and humans. Thus, as with other drugs of addiction, there is a broad biological basis for the reinforcing effects of benzodiazepines that is not limited to the human species (Roache & Meisch, 1995).

Benzodiazepines have been shown to be reinforcers in self-administration studies in humans who have histories of sedative, alcohol, or multiple-drug addiction (Ator & Griffiths 1987; Ciraulo, Barnhill, et al., 1988; Ciraulo, Sands, & Shader, 1988; de Wit & Griffiths, 1991; Griffiths & Sannerud, 1987; Roache, 1990; Roache & Griffiths, 1989; Roache et al., 1995; Woods et al., 1987, 1992). In those individuals addicted to other sedative-hypnotics, several benzodiazepines, including diazepam, lorazepam, oxazepam, and triazolam, are self-administered to a greater extent than placebo and other medications (Zawertailo, Busto, Kaplan, & Sellers, 1995). In methadone maintenance patients, diazepam can serve as a reinforcer and has been widely abused by this population. Although alprazolam self-administration has not been examined directly in methadone maintenance patients, it also has high abuse potential in this population (Roache & Meisch, 1995).

Many psychiatric patients find benzodiazepines reinforcing (Ciraulo & Sarid-Segal, 1991). In anxious individuals who seek treatment, diazepam is especially reinforcing (de Wit, McCracken, Uhlenhuth, & Johanson, 1987). Normal volunteers who drink lightly (less than 5 drinks per week) and moderately (an average of 11 drinks per week) (de Wit, Pierri, & Johanson, 1989), abstinent alcoholics and sons of alcoholics (Ciraulo & Sarid-Segal, 1991), and occasional users of sedatives without physical dependence as well as abnormal users (Cole & Chiarello, 1990) show reinforcing responses to benzodiazepines. However, barbiturates, meprobamate, and methaqualone appear to have more euphoric or reinforcing

TABLE 3. Pharmacological Profile Classification of Drugs Acting on Benzodiazepine Recognition Sites

Drug	Occurrence of maximal amplification of GABA action	Cognition impairment	Antagonisms of cognition impairment	Ataxia, sedation, ethanol potentiation	Anxiolytic, anticonvulsant, sleep inducer	Tolerance liability	Classification
Imidazenil	never	No	Yes	No	Yes	No	PAM
Flumazenil	inactive	No	Yes	No	No	No	A
Zolpidem	in some subtypes	?	No	Yes	Weak	Yes	SAM
Alpidem	in some subtypes	?	No	Yes	Weak	?	SAM
Abecarnil	in some subtypes	?	No	Weak	Weak	?	SAM
Diazepam	in many subtypes	Yes	No	Yes	Yes	Yes	FAM
Alprazolam	in many subtypes	Yes	No	Yes	Yes	Yes	FAM
Triazolam	in many subtypes	Yes	No	Yes	Yes	Yes	FAM

A = Antagonist; PAM = partial allosteric modulator; SAM = selective allosteric modulator; FAM = full allosteric modulator properties than benzodiazepines (Ciraulo & Sarid-Segal, 1991).

There appears to be relative abuse and addictive liability of different benzodiazepines among individuals. Diazepam, lorazepam, triazolam, and alprazolam have relatively high liability for abuse and addiction, while oxazepam, halazepam, chlorazepate, and chlordiazepoxide have lower addiction potentials. The speed of onset of drug effects is an important factor in addiction potential as the more rapid the onset, the greater the liability (Ciraulo & Sarid-Segal, 1991).

Absorption and Metabolism

Because all benzodiazepines rapidly enter the brain tissue after entry into the vascular circulation, their onset of action relates to the rate of their absorption from the gastrointestinal tract. The most rapidly absorbed benzodiazepines (such as diazepam) may produce more euphoria and be more reinforcing than those with a slower onset of action (Roache, 1990). The more highly lipophilic benzodiazepines (such as diazepam) also are rapidly distributed to peripheral tissue and have high volumes of distribution. Because of uptake into lipid tissues after single doses, the duration of action is shorter except when active metabolites accumulate, as with diazepam (Cowley, Roy-Byrne, & Greenblatt, 1991).

The accumulation after multiple doses is related to the elimination half-life of the parent drug and its active metabolites (e.g., diazepam). The rate of conversion of benzodiazepines to active metabolites determines the long-lasting action of the compound. In benzodiazepines with a shorter elimination half-life and little accumulation (e.g., lorazepam and alprazolam), there is more intense and noticeable withdrawal or rebound symptoms if doses are missed, spaced too far apart, or abruptly discontinued, so that continued use may be related to this negatively reinforcing quality (Cowley & Dunner, 1991).

Therapeutic Uses

Benzodiazepines are used for a wide variety of indications including alcohol withdrawal.

Their therapeutic efficacy is limited to short-term use. Adverse consequences from addictive use and development of pharmacological tolerance and dependence limit their long-term use.

Benzodiazepines have been used for the treatment of panic disorder, acute and chronic generalized anxiety, and dysphoria. Benzodiazepines also are indicated for severe anxiety from other causes when immediate symptom relief is necessary. Benzodiazepines are best used intermittently during periods when the symptoms are most severe, at the lowest effective dose for the shortest possible time. Patients may do better with antidepressant medications, other anti-anxiety medications such as buspirone, or other forms of psychosocial and behavioral intervention. Benzodiazepines often are combined with antidepressants to achieve initial symptom relief in patients with depression and anxiety. In general, benzodiazepines have not been proved effective as antidepressants (Cowley & Dunner, 1991). The chronically dysphoric or alcohol- or drug-addicted patient may have more difficulty with benzodiazepine addiction and discontinuation of benzodiazepines, so caution is necessary in prescribing to them (American Psychiatric Association, 1990; Rickels et al., 1990; Roy-Byrne & Nutt, 1991; Schweizer, Rickels, Case, & Greenblatt, 1990).

Benzodiazepines are used as an adjunct to the neuroleptics in treating patients with schizophrenia and active psychotic symptomatology who do not respond satisfactorily to neuroleptics alone. They also are useful in treatment of tardive dyskinesia. They are an adjunct to lithium in treating manic bipolar patients (Cohen, 1991). However, the adverse effects from long-term use of benzodiazepines in these populations must be considered.

Zolpidem and benzodiazepine hypnotics are used for transient insomnia, prescribed at the lowest effective dose in a time-limited fashion, usually for 2 to 3 weeks (Pascually, 1991). Tolerance to sedative effects develops within that time, especially with the short half-life agents (American Psychiatric Association, 1990). Rebound insomnia (intense worsening of sleep above baseline levels, following withdrawal of the benzodiazepine) often develops after use of short-term medications. This may lead to patients asking to continue and increase doses of the benzodiazepines for sleep, which should be avoided. Tapering the hypnotic usually attenuates the symptoms of rebound insomnia (Pascually, 1991).

Parasomnias including REM behavior disorder, periodic limb movements during sleep, sleepwalking, and night terrors may be treated with benzodiazepines, but a careful diagnostic workup is needed because treatment is long term and the risk of relapse to the parasomnias on discontinuation of benzodiazepines may be high (Pascually, 1991).

The misuse of benzodiazepines can develop when patients are maintained on higher doses or for a longer term than is necessary. Lack of clear diagnosis without defined measures of benefit and projected time-course of treatment may lead to indiscriminate and pathological use. Once begun, a cycle of addiction, withdrawal, continued use, and further adverse consequences may develop, with many patients unable to withdraw completely from the benzodiazepine (Rickels *et al.*, 1993; Roache, 1990).

Sedative-Hypnotics (Nonbenzodiazepines)

Zolpidem

Zolpidem (Ambien) is a hypnotic with rapid onset, short duration, and quickly eliminated imidazopyridine; its actions are believed to be mediated at selective $GABA_A$ receptors. It is a nonbenzodiazepine. Zolpidem and triazolam were compared over a wide range of doses in subjects who had a history of sedative abuse and addiction; the drugs were found to be similar on a number of subjective ratings of reinforcement and decrements in task-related performance. However, at high doses, triazolam was identified as a barbiturate, benzodiazepine, or alcohol almost twice as often as zolpidem, while more nausea and dysphoria were noted with zolpidem (Evans, Funderburk, & Griffiths, 1990). Thus, use of zolpidem requires caution, as the addiction potential is not clearly established, but still possible.

No information is available on the development of tolerance and dependence following prolonged use of zolpidem. Because the drug is rapidly metabolized by the liver and has a half-life of approximately 2.4 hr, dosage reductions are recommended in patients with hepatic dysfunction and in the elderly patient (Langtry & Benfield, 1990).

Buspirone

Unlike benzodiazepines, buspirone (Buspar) has no hypnotic, anticonvulsant, or muscle relaxant properties. It does not interact directly with GABAergic systems but appears to exert its anxiolytic effects by acting as a partial agonist at $5\text{-}HT_{1A}$ receptors. It is not effective in blocking the withdrawal syndrome resulting from cessation of use of benzodiazepines or other sedative-hypnotics. Buspirone has minimal abuse and addiction liability. It does not potentiate the CNS depressant effects of conventional sedative-hypnotic drugs, ethanol, or tricyclic antidepressants. In contrast to the benzodiazepines, buspirone's anxiolytic effects may take more than a week to become established, making this drug suitable mainly for generalized anxiety states. It is not effective in panic disorders (Rickels, 1990).

Buspirone causes less psychomotor impairment than diazepam and does not affect driving skills. Tachycardia, palpitations, nervousness, gastrointestinal distress, and paresthesias may occur more frequently than with benzodiazepines. Blood pressure may be elevated in patients receiving MAO inhibitors (Rickels, 1990). A number of buspirone analogues have been developed (e.g., ipsapirone, gepirone, tandospirone) and are under study (Taylor & Moon, 1991).

Barbiturates and Nonbarbiturates

The use of barbiturates and other sedative-hypnotic drugs has declined with the advent of benzodiazepines. Except for the anticonvulsant actions of phenobarbital and its congeners, the barbiturates and other barbiturate-like sedative-hypnotics have a low therapeutic index and low degree of selectivity. Compared with the benzodiazepines, barbiturates induce hepatic enzymes, cause more drug interactions, produce more tolerance, physiological impairment, and toxic reactions, have a greater liability for development of addiction and pharmacological dependence (Kisnad, 1991).

Other nonbarbiturate members of the sedative-hypnotic class are chloral hydrate (Notec), ethchlorvynol (Placidyl), glutethimide (Doriden), meprobamate (Miltown), methyprylon (Nodular), paraldehyde (Paral), and triclofos (Triclos). Their pharmacological properties are more alike than distinct. Tolerance and dependence develop rapidly following use of these compounds.

Overall, the patterns of use are varied but adhere to the general principles of use, abuse, and addiction of sedative-hypnotics. They range from regular use for anxiety and insomnia to episodes of gross intoxication, to prolonged, compulsive daily use of large quantities of the drug. A preoccupation with acquisition and maintaining adequate supplies, compulsive use in spite of adverse consequences, and a recurrent pattern of relapse develop. Some users develop tolerance and may not show obvious intoxication in spite of frequent and heavy doses. The original contact with the drug is often through a physician or a "street" vendor.

In the medical patient, the problem may develop gradually over time, whereas use of the drug may accelerate rapidly to addictive use when it is prescribed to the addict. The medical patient begins using the drug for insomnia or anxiety and progresses through increasing doses while the addict requires high doses initially. Eventually, the drug is a major priority of the user's life. Frequently, neither the patient nor the physician may recognize the existence of abuse and addiction. Both assume that the anxiety, tremulousness, and insomnia that emerge when the drug is discontinued is a return of the symptoms for which the drug was initially prescribed. More likely these symptoms represent withdrawal from the drug that may be protracted over weeks and months (Hawthorne, Zabora, & D'Lugolf, 1982).

The subjective effects of the sedative-hypnotics are predictable and stereotypic in the nontolerant individual for a given member of the sedative-hypnotic class. Early drug effects are diminished attention and concentration, impaired recent or short-term memory, euphoria, decreased abstraction, reduced cognitive abilities, and a sensation of intoxication. As the blood level increases, alertness is significantly compromised, mood is depressed, and intellectual function is severely limited. Loss of consciousness occurs in nontolerant individuals at blood levels considerably lower than those observed in tolerant individuals. Changes in personality that resemble significant personality disorders may develop in regular users of sedative-hypnotics. Characteristics of antisocial, histrionic, paranoid, and other personality traits can occur with chronic use of these drugs (Griffiths, Bigelow, & Liehson, 1983).

Treatment of Withdrawal from Benzodiazepines and Other Sedative-Hypnotics

The treatment of withdrawal is necessary to avoid morbidity and mortality from adverse consequences. The signs and symptoms of withdrawal for benzodiazepines are similar to those for sedative-hypnotics and the treatment of withdrawal is similar for benzodiazepines (barbiturates) and for sedative-hypnotics. Withdrawal from benzodiazepines is not usually marked by significant elevations in blood pressure and pulse as with alcohol. Supplemental prn doses are usually not needed for changes in vital signs. The anxiety of withdrawal is usually controlled with a prescribed taper with a long-acting preparation unless objectively it appears that the doses are too low. Caution is urged as drug-seeking behavior must be differentiated from anxiety of withdrawal and anxiety from other disorders. Only the anxiety of withdrawal, or other conditions when severe, need be treated with increased doses of benzodiazepines. Addictive behavior is better treated with specific addiction treatments. Methods other than use of benzodiazepines for treating the anxiety from another disorder are indicated whenever possible. The prescriber must objectively assess the need for benzodiazepines and be in control of the dispensing of the benzodiazepines or other medications used for withdrawal. The addict by definition is out of control in regard to drug use and cannot reliably negotiate the schedule for tapering.

Treatment of withdrawal is aimed at gradually tapering off the depressant drugs or substituting another depressant drug that shares pharmacologic cross-tolerance and dependence to suppress withdrawal symptoms. Benzodiazepines can be substituted for other benzodiazepines and barbiturates and vice versa (Table 4). The conversion for equivalent doses can be calculated if doses are actually known prior to taper. A long-acting benzodiazepine is more effective than short-acting preparations in suppressing withdrawal symptoms and in producing a gradual and smooth transition to the abstinent state. In general, greater patient compliance and less morbidity can be expected from the use of the longer-acting benzodiazepines.

In general, the duration of the tapering schedule is determined by the half-life of the benzodiazepine or barbiturate that is being withdrawn (Table 5). For short-acting benzodiazepines such as alprazolam, 7–10 days of a gradual taper with a long-acting benzodiazepine or barbiturate is often sufficient: 7 days for low-dose and short duration of use and 10 days for high-dose and long duration of benzo-

TABLE 4. Phenobarbital Withdrawal Conversion for Benzodiazepines

Benzodiazepine	Dose (mg)	Phenobarbital withdrawal conversion (mg)
Alprazolam (Xanax)	0.5–1.0	30
Chlordiazepoxide (Librium)	25	30
Clonazepam (Klonopin)	2	30
Chlorazepate (Tranxene)	15	30
Diazepam (Valium)	10	30
Flurazepam (Dalmane)	30	30
Lorazepam (Ativan)	2	30
Temazepam (Restoril)	15	30
Triazolam (Halcion)	0.25–0.50	30
Quazepam (Doral)	15	30
Estazolam (ProSom)	2	30

TABLE 5. Benzodiazepine (Barbiturate) Detoxification

Short-acting:	7- to 10-day taper: Day 1, diazepam 10–20 mg po qid with a gradual decremental reduction in dose to 5–10 mg po qd on last day; avoid prn. Adjustments in dose according to clinical state may be indicated. *Or* 7- to 10-day taper: Calculate barbiturate or benzodiazepine equivalence and taper (if actual dose is known before detoxification). Avoid prn.
Long-acting:	10- to 14-day taper: Day 1, diazepam 10–20 mg po qid with a gradual taper to 5–10 mg po qd on last day. Avoid prn. Adjustments in dose according to clinical state may be indicated. *Or* 10- to 14-day taper: Calculate barbiturate or benzodiazepine equivalence and taper (if actual dose is known before detoxification). Avoid prn.

TABLE 6. Clinical Characteristics

Variable	Inpatients $n = 6,508$	Outpatients $n = 1,572$
Diagnosis of dependence for:		
Alcohol	82	80
Prescription medications	12	5
Marijuana	23	19
Stimulants	7	3
Cocaine	19	15
Opiates	3	1
Number of drugs used at least weekly (alcohol not included):		
1	26	22
2	10	6
3	5	2
Number of substances, including alcohol, used within 24 hr of admission:		
1	32	17
2	9	3
3+	4	1

TABLE 7. One-Year Abstinence by Continuum of Care and
Self-Help Support

Variable	Inpatients (n = 6,508		Outpatients (n = 1,572)	
	% Attending	% Abstinent	% Attending	% Abstinent
Months of continuing care attended in year:				
0	42	53	34	48
1–5	32	55	33	61
6–11	19	71	18	68
12	8	88	14	89
AA attendance:				
Non-attender	54	47	43	49
Regular attender	46	74	57	80

diazepine use. In the case of alprazolam, because of higher rates of withdrawal seizures, the use of phenobarbital substitution is recommended for the taper. For the long-acting benzodiazepines, 10–14 days of a gradual taper with a long-acting benzodiazepine or barbiturate is often sufficient; 10 days for low-dose and short duration and 14 days for high-dose and long duration of use. The doses can be given in qid or tid intervals. The long-acting preparations accumulate during the taper to result in a self-leveling effect of the blood level of the benzodiazepine or barbiturates over time.

Treatment of Addiction to Benzodiazepines and Other Drugs (Including Alcohol)

The treatment of benzodiazepine addiction begins with the detoxification from benzodiazepines and is aimed at the drug-seeking behavior, preoccupation with acquiring, compulsive use, and relapse to benzodiazepines. Many of those who are addicted to benzodiazepines are also addicted to other drugs including alcohol. Standard abstinence-based addiction treatment is effective treatment for benzodiazepine addiction as well as other drug and alcohol addictions (Tables 6 and 7).

Evaluation studies of abstinence-based treatment show abstinence rates of 60% at 1 year and can be increased to 80%–90% with continued treatment and participation in 12-step programs. The abstinence-based methods include group and individual psychosocial therapies, cognitive-behavioral techniques, and strong emphasis on abstinence from addicting drugs including alcohol. Continued long-term involvement in a recovery program is strongly encouraged (e.g., Alcoholics Anonymous or Narcotics Anonymous).

The treatment of benzodiazepine addiction in the absence of other drug addictions is less clearly documented. The prevention of relapse to benzodiazepine use despite recurrence of adverse consequences requires continued monitoring, education, careful assessment and treatment of other psychiatric disorders, and distinguishing drug-seeking from complaints of psychiatric symptoms.

References

Alexander, B., & Perry, P. J. (1991). Detoxification from benzodiazepine: Schedules and strategies. *Journal of Substance Abuse Treatment, 8*, 9–17.

American Psychiatric Association. (1980). *Diagnostic and statistical manual of mental disorders* (3rd ed.). Washington, DC: Author.

American Psychiatric Association. (1990). *Task force report on benzodiazepines.* Washington, DC: Author.

American Psychiatric Association. (1994). *Diagnostic and statistical manual of mental disorders* (4th ed.). Washington, DC: Author.

American Psychiatric Association. (1994). Substance-related disorders. In *Diagnostic and Statistical Man-*

ual of Mental Disorders (4th ed., pp. 393–444). Washington, DC: Author.

Ashton, H. (1984). Benzodiazepine withdrawal: An unfinished story. *British Medical Journal [Clinical Research], 25,* 385–398.

Ashton, H. (1987). Benzodiazepine withdrawal: Outcome in 50 patients. *British Journal of the Addictions, 82,* 665–671.

Ashton, H. (1991). Protracted withdrawal syndromes from benzodiazepines. *Journal of Substance Abuse Treatment, 8,* 19–28.

Ator, N. A., & Griffiths, R. R. (1987). Self-administration of barbiturates and benzodiazepines: A review. *Pharmacology, Biochemistry and Behavior, 27,* 391–398.

Busto, U., & Sellers, E. M. (1986). Pharmacokinetic determinants of drug abuse and dependence: A conceptual perspective. *Clinical Pharmacokinetics, 11,* 144–153.

Busto, U., & Sellers, E. M. (1991). Pharmacologic aspects of benzodiazepine tolerance and dependence. *Journal of Substance Abuse Treatment, 8,* 29–33.

Busto, U., Simpkins, J., & Sellers, E. M. (1983). Objective determination of benzodiazepine use and abuse in alcoholics. *British Journal of the Addictions, 78,* 429–435.

Busto, U., Sellers, E. M., Naranjo, C. A., Cappell, H., Sanchez-Craig, M., & Sykora, K. (1986). Withdrawal reaction after long-term therapeutic use of benzodiazepines. *New England Journal of Medicine, 315,* 854–859.

Busto, U., Kaplan, H. L., Zawertailo, L., & Sellers, E. M. (1994). Pharmacologic effects and abuse liability of bretazenil, diazepam, and alprazolam in humans. *Clinical Pharmacology & Therapeutics, 55,* 451–463.

Chan, A. W. K. (1984). Effects of combined alcohol and benzodiazepines: A review. *Drug and Alcohol Dependence, 13,* 315–341.

Ciraulo, D. A., & Sarid-Segal, O. (1991). Benzodiazepines: Abuse liability. In P. P. Roy-Byrne & D. S. Cowley (Eds.), *Benzodiazepines in clinical practice: Risks and benefits* (pp. 157–174). Washington, DC: American Psychiatric Press.

Ciraulo, D. A., Barnhill, J. G., Greenblatt, D. J., Shader, R. I., Ciraulo, A. M., Tarmey, M. F., Molloy, M. A., & Foti, M. E. (1988). Abuse liability and clinical pharmacokinetics of alprazolam in alcoholic men. *Journal of Clinical Psychiatry, 49,* 333–337.

Ciraulo, D. A., Sands, B. F., & Shader, R. I. (1988). Critical review of liability for benzodiazepine abuse among alcoholics. *American Journal of Psychiatry, 145,* 1501–1506.

Ciraulo, D. A., Sarid-Segal, O., Knapp, C., Ciraulo, A. M., Greenblatt, D. J., & Shader, R. I. (1996). Liability to alprazolam abuse in daughters of alcoholics. *American Journal of Psychiatry, 153,* 956–958.

Cohen, S. (1991). Benzodiazepines in psychotic and related conditions. In P. P. Roy-Byrne & D. S. Cowley (Eds.), *Benzodiazepines in clinical practice: Risks and benefits* (pp. 59–71). Washington, DC: American Psychiatric Press.

Cole, J. O., & Chiarello, R. J. (1990). The benzodiazepines as drugs of abuse. *Journal of Psychiatric Research, 24,* 135–144.

Costa, E., & Guidotti, A. (1996). Benzodiazepines on trial: A research strategy for their rehabilitation. *Trends in Pharmacological Sciences, 17,* 192–200.

Costa, E., Thompson, D. M., Auta, J., & Guidotti, A. (1995). Imidazenil: A potent benzodiazepine partial positive modulator of GABAergic transmission virtually devoid of tolerance liability. *CNS Drug Reviews, 1,* 168–189.

Cowley, D. S., & Dunner, D. L. (1991). Benzodiazepines in anxiety and depression. In P. P. Roy-Byrne & D. S. Cowley (Eds.), *Benzodiazepines in clinical practice: Risks and benefits* (pp. 37–56). Washington, DC: American Psychiatric Press.

Cowley, D. S., Roy-Byrne, P.P., & Greenblatt, D. J. (1991). Benzodiazepines: Pharmacokinetics and pharmacodynamics. In P. P. Roy-Byrne & D. S. Cowley (Eds.), *Benzodiazepines in clinical practice: Risks and benefits* (pp. 21–32). Washington, DC: American Psychiatric Press.

DeVane, C. L., Ware, M. R., & Lydiard, R. B. (1991). Pharmacokinetics, pharmacodynamics, and treatment issues of benzodiazepines: Alprazolam, adinazolam, and clonazepam. *Psychopharmacology Bulletin, 27,* 463–473.

de Wit, H., & Griffiths, R. R. (1991). Testing the abuse liability of anxiolytic and hypnotic drugs in humans. *Drug and Alcohol Dependence, 28,* 83–111.

de Wit, H., McCracken, S. M., Uhlenhuth, E. H., & Johanson, C. E. (1987). *Diazepam preference in subjects seeking treatment for anxiety* (NIDA Research Monograph Series No. 76, pp. 248–254). Rockville, MD: National Institute on Drug Abuse.

de Wit, H., Pierri, J., & Johanson, C. E. (1989). Reinforcing and subjective effects of diazepam in nondrug-abusing volunteers. *Pharmacology, Biochemistry and Behavior, 33,* 205–213.

DuPont, R. L. (Ed.). (1988). Abuse of benzodiazepines: The problems and the solutions: A report of a committee of the Institute for Behavior and Health Inc. *American Journal of Drug and Alcohol Abuse, 14.*

Evans, S. M., Funderburk, F. R., & Griffiths, R. R. (1990). Zolpidem and triazolam in humans: Behavioral and subjective effects and abuse liability. *Journal of Pharmacology and Experimental Therapeutics, 255,* 1246–1255.

Gold, M. S., Miller, N. S., Stennie, K., & Populla-Vardi, C. (1995). Epidemiology of benzodiazepine use and dependence. *Psychiatric Annals, 25,* 146–148.

Grantham, P. (1987). Benzodiazepine abuse. *British Journal of Hospital Medicine, 37,* 999–1001.

Griffiths, R. R., & Sannerud, C. A. (1987). Abuse and dependence on benzodiazepines and other anxiolytic/sedative drugs. In H. Y. Meltzer (Ed.), *Psychopharmacology, the third generation of progress* (pp. 1535–1541). New York: Raven.

Griffiths, R. R., Bigelow, G. E., & Liebson, I. (1983). Differential effects of diazepam and pentobarbital on

mood and behavior. *Archives of General Psychiatry,*
40, 865–873.

Haefely, W., Kulcsár, A., Möhler, H., Pieri, L., Polc, P., &
Schaffner, R. (1975). Possible involvement of GABA
in the central actions of benzodiazepines. In E. Costa
& P. Greengard (Eds.), *Mechanisms of action of ben-*
zodiazepines: Series. Advances in Biochemical Psy-
chopharmacology (Vol. 14, pp. 131–151). New York:
Raven.

Hawthorne, J. W., Zabora, J. R., & D'Lugolf, B. C. (1982).
Outpatient detoxification of patients addicted to seda-
tive/hypnotics and anxiolytics. *Drug and Alcohol De-*
pendence, 9, 143–151.

Jaffe, J. H. (1990). Drug addiction and drug abuse. In
A. G. Gilman, T. W. Rall, A. S. Nies, & P. Taylor
(Eds.), *Goodman and Gilman's the pharmacological*
basis of therapeutics (8th ed., pp. 522–573). New
York: Pergamon.

Jaffe, J. H., & Martin, W. R. (1990). Opioid analgesics and
antagonists. In A. G. Gilman, T. W. Rall, A. S. Nies,
& P. Taylor (Eds.), *Goodman and Gilman's the phar-*
macological basis of therapeutics (8th ed., pp.
485–521). New York: Pergamon.

Juergens, S. (1991). Alprazolam and diazepam: Addiction
potential. *Journal of Substance Abuse Treatment, 8,*
43–51.

Juergens, S. M. (1993). Benzodiazepines and addiction. In
N. S. Miller (Ed.), *Psychiatric Clinics of North Amer-*
ica, 16, 75–85.

Juergens, S. M. (1994). Sedative-hypnotics. In N. S. Miller
(Ed.), *Principles of addiction medicine* (pp. 1–10).
Washington, DC: American Society of Addiction
Medicine.

Kisnad, H. (1991). Sedative-hypnotics (not including benzodiazepines). In N. S. Miller (Ed.), *Comprehensive*
handbook of drug and alcohol addiction (pp.
477–502). New York: Dekker.

Lader, M. (1983). Dependence on benzodiazepines. *Jour-*
nal of Clinical Psychiatry, 44, 121–127.

Langtry, H. D., & Benfield, P. (1990). Zolpidem: A review
of its pharmacodynamic and pharmacokinetic properties and therapeutic potential. *Drugs, 40,* 291.

Miller, N. S., & Gold, M. S. (1991). Introduction—Benzodiazepines: A major problem. *Journal of Substance*
Abuse Treatment, 8, 3–7.

Miller, N. S., & Mahler, J. C. (1991). Addiction to and dependence on benzodiazepines. *Journal of Substance*
Abuse Treatment, 8, 61–67.

Miller, N. S., & Mirin, S. M. (1989). Multiple drug use in
alcoholics: Practical and theoretical implications.
Psychiatric Annals, 19, 248–255.

Miller, N. S., Dackis, C. A., & Gold, M. S. (1987). The relationship of addiction, tolerance and dependence: A
neurochemical approach. *Journal of Substance Abuse*
Treatment, 4, 197–207.

Owen, R. T., & Tyrer, P. (1983). Benzodiazepine dependence. A review of the evidence. *Drugs, 25,* 385–398.

Pascually, R. (1991). Benzodiazepines and sleep. In P. P.
Roy-Byrne & D. S. Cowley (Eds.), *Benzodiazepines*

in clinical practice: Risks and benefits (pp. 37–56).
Washington, DC: American Psychiatric Press.

Paul, S., Marancos, P., & Skolnick, P. (1981). The benzo-
diazepine-GABA chloride ionophore receptor complex: Common site of minor tranquilizer action.
Biological Psychiatry, 16, 213–228.

Perera, K. M. H., Tulley, M., & Jenner, F. A. (1987). The
use of benzodiazepines among drug addicts. *British*
Journal of Addiction, 82, 511–515.

Rall, T. W. (1990). Hypnotics and sedatives: Ethanol. In A.
G. Gilman, T. W. Rall, A. S. Nies, & P. Taylor (Eds.),
Goodman and Gilman's the pharmacological basis of
therapeutics (8th ed., pp. 345–382). New York: Pergamon.

Rickels, K. (1990). Buspirone in clinical practice. *Journal*
of Clinical Psychiatry, 5, 51.

Rickels, K., Schweizer, E., Case, G., & Greenblatt, D. J.
(1990). Long-term therapeutic use of benzodiazepines: I. Effects of abrupt discontinuation.
Archives of General Psychiatry, 47, 899–907.

Rickels, K., Schweizer, E., Weiss, S., & Zavodnick, S.
(1993). Maintenance drug treatment for panic disorder: II. Short- and long-term outcome after drug
taper. *Archives of General Psychiatry, 50,* 61–68.

Roache, J. D. (1990). Addiction potential of benzodiazepines and non-benzodiazepine anxiolytics. In B.
Stimmel (Ed.), (C. K. Erickson, M. A. Javors, & W.
W. Morgan, Guest Eds.), *Addiction potential of*
abused drugs and drug classes (pp. 103–128). Bing-
hamton, NY: Haworth. And in *Advances in Alcohol*
and Substance Abuse, 9, 103–128.

Roache, J. D., & Griffiths, R. R. (1989). Abuse liability of
anxiolytics and sedative/hypnotics: Methods assessing the likelihood of abuse. In N. K. Mello, & M.
W. Fischman (Eds.), *Testing for abuse liability of*
drugs in humans (National Institute on Drug Abuse
Research Monograph No. 92, pp. 123–146). Washington, DC: U.S. Government Printing Office.

Roache, J. D., & Meisch, R. A. (1995). Findings from self-
administration research on the addiction potential of
benzodiazepines. *Psychiatric Annals, 25,* 153–157.

Roache, J. D., Meisch, R. A., Henningfield, J. E., Jaffe,
J. H., Klein, S., & Sampson, A. (1995). Reinforcing
effects of triazolam in sedative abusers: Correlation of
drug liking and self-administration measures. *Phar-*
macology, Biochemistry and Behavior, 50, 171–179.

Romach, M. K., Somer, G. R., Sobell, L. C., Sobel, M. B.,
Kaplan, H. L., & Sellers, E. M. (1992). Characteristics
of long-term alprazolam users in the community. *Jour-*
nal of Clinical Psychopharmacology, 12, 316–321.

Rosenberg, H. C., & Chiu, T. H. (1985). Time course for
development of benzodiazepine tolerance and physical dependence. *Neuroscience and Biobehavior Re-*
view, 9, 123–131.

Roy-Byrne, P. P., & Nutt, D. J. (1991). Benzodiazepines'
biological mechanisms. In P. P. Roy-Byrne & D. S.
Cowley (Eds.), *Benzodiazepines in clinical practice:*
Risks and benefits (pp. 5–18). Washington, DC:
American Psychiatric Press.

Ruiz, I., Offermanns, J., Lanctôt, K. L., & Busto, U. (1993). Comparative study on benzodiazepine use in Canada and Chile. *Journal of Clinical Pharmacology, 33,* 124–129.

Salzman, C. (1993a). Benzodiazepine treatment of panic and agoraphobic symptoms: Use, dependence, toxicity, abuse. *Journal of Psychiatric Research, 27,* 97–110.

Salzman, C. (1993b). *Issues and controversies regarding benzodiazepine use* (NIDA Research Monograph Series No. 131, pp. 68–69). Rockville, MD: National Institute on Drug Abuse.

Schuster, C. L., & Humphries, R.H. (1981). Benzodiazepine dependence in alcoholics. *Connecticut Medicine, 45,* 11–13.

Schweizer, E., Rickels, K., Case, G., & Greenblatt, D. J. (1990). Long-term therapeutic use of benzodiazepines: II. Effects of gradual taper. *Archives of General Psychiatry, 47,* 908–915.

Sellers, E. M., Marshman, J. A., Kaplan, H. L., Giles, H. G., Kapur, B. M., Busto, U., MacLeod, S. M., Stapleton, C., & Sealey, F. (1981). Acute and chronic drug abuse emergencies in metropolitan Toronto. *International Journal of the Addictions, 16,* 283–303.

Shader, R. I., & Greenblatt, D. J. (1993). Use of benzodiazepines in anxiety disorders. *New England Journal of Medicine, 328,* 1398–1405.

Squires, R. F., & Braestrup, C. (1977). Benzodiazepine receptors in rat brain. *Nature, 266,* 732–734.

Taylor, D. P., & Moon, S. L. (1991). Buspirone and related compounds as alternative anxiolytics. *Neuropeptides, 19,* 15.

U.S. Department of Health and Human Services, Alcohol, Drug Abuse, and Mental Health Administration. (1987). Sedatives and antianxiety agents. In *Drug abuse and drug research: The second triennial report to Congress from the Secretary, Department of Health and Human Services* (NIDA, DHHS Publication ADM 87-1486). Washington, DC: U.S. Government Printing Office.

Warneke, L. B. (1991). Benzodiazepines: Abuse and new use. *Canadian Journal of Psychiatry, 36,* 194–205.

Wilford, B. B. (1990). *Balancing the response to prescription drug abuse.* Report of a national symposium on medicine and public policy. Chicago: American Medical Association, Department of Substance Abuse.

Woods, J. H., Katz, J. L., & Winger, G. (1987). Abuse liability of benzodiazepines. *Pharmacological Reviews, 39,* 251–419.

Woods, J. H., Katz, J. L., & Winger, G. (1992). Benzodiazepines: Use, abuse, and consequences: A review. *Pharmacological Reviews, 44,* 151–347.

Zawertailo, L. A., Busto, U., Kaplan, H. L., & Sellers, E. M. (1995). Comparative abuse liability of sertraline, alprazolam, and dextroamphetamine in humans. *Journal of Clinical Psychopharmacology, 15,* 117–124.

X

Amphetamines

30

Pharmacology of Amphetamines

TIMOTHY E. WILENS AND THOMAS J. SPENCER

Introduction

Amphetamines are among the oldest compounds available in the United States. Amphetamine (AMPH) was first synthesized in 1887 and found in the 1920s to be a potential alternative to ephedrine which had been running in short supply for the treatment of asthma (Alles, 1928). It was available without prescription to the public for the treatment of asthma first as a benzedrine inhaler and then as benzedrine tablets (Goff & Ciraulo, 1991). Similarly, methamphetamine was synthesized and made available to the public at approximately the same time.

AMPH has predominate pharmacologic activity on the catecholaminergic input to smooth muscles, metabolism, and the cardiovascular and central nervous systems (Hoffman & Lefkowitz, 1990). This class of agents, in particular methylphenidate, are most commonly prescribed for the treatment of Attention-Deficit/Hyperactivity Disorder (ADHD) (Greenhill & Osman, 1991; Wilens & Biederman, 1992). In addition they have been shown effective in the therapeutics of narcolepsy, Parkinson's disorder, depression, and obesity

TIMOTHY E. WILENS AND THOMAS J. SPENCER
• Psychopharmacology Unit, Massachusetts General Hospital, Boston, Massachusetts 02114; and Department of Psychiatry, Harvard Medical School, Boston, Massachusetts 02114.

Handbook of Substance Abuse: Neurobehavioral Pharmacology, edited by Tarter *et al.* Plenum Press, New York, 1998.

(Fawcett & Busch, 1995; Masand & Tesar, 1996). Parallel with their therapeutic use, the increased abuse liabilities of stimulant class agents began to emerge.

AMPH forms the template of a related class of direct- and indirect-acting sympathomimetic amines including ephedrine, mephentremine, metaraminol, and phenylephrine, which are most commonly used in the treatment of acute cardiovascular conditions (Hoffman & Lefkowitz, 1990). The abuse of amphetamine and other stimulants appears to be related to their anorectic, insomniac, and euphorogenic properties coupled with their availability, particularly in the 1960s and 1970s. Epidemiological catchment area data indicates that stimulant abuse is found in 1.7% of adults in the United States (Anthony & Helzer, 1991). Although only a small percentage of subjects receiving stimulants progress to dependence, legislation has reduced the availability and restricted the medical use of stimulants. For example, Masand and Tesar (1996) reported that in 1970, more than 65 stimulant preparations were available medically, whereas in 1995, only 8 AMPH preparations were listed. The amphetamines are now classified by the Drug Enforcement Agency as schedule II agents, with the exception of pemoline which is a class IV agent.

Methylenedioxyamphetamine (MDA) and 3,4 methylenedioxyamphetamine (MDMA) resemble AMPH in producing central and peripheral stimulation, anorexia, and hyperthermia. However, due in part to their structural and pharmacological similarities to mescaline,

MDA and MDMA appear to have hallucinogenic properties with more selective effect on serotonin metabolism (Barnes, 1988; Climko, Roehrich, Sweeney, & Al-Razi, 1987; Kuczenski, Segal, Leith, & Applegate, 1987). Both MDA and MDMA are schedule I compounds and are commonly referred to as "designer drugs" despite being present since the 1900s (Climko et al., 1987). These agents, often referred to as "Ecstasy," are reported to potentiate insight, facilitate psychotherapy, and produce a stimulant or energizing physiological response (Climko et al., 1987). Use of these compounds in the United States has continued to increase since the 1970s, with the largest expansion in college-age students (Climko et al., 1987).

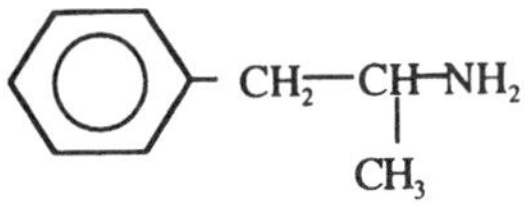

Structural Relationships

AMPH, a racemic mixture of Beta-phenylisopropylamine, exists in both the dextroamphetamine form (Dexedrine®), and the levoamphetamine form (found in Adderall®). Biphetamine® contains both racemic mixtures of AMPH. Methamphetamine (Desoxyn®) is a methylated amphetamine compound which is the principal component of the smokable, highly addictive, long-acting compound referred to as "speed" or "ice." Methamphetamine has a different ratio between central and peripheral actions compared with AMPH. Less behaviorally potent than AMPH, methylphenidate (Ritalin) and pemoline are often considered in the amphetamine class of agents, although pemoline is structurally dissimilar to either AMPH or methylphenidate (Fawcett & Busch, 1995; Wilens & Biederman, 1992) (See Figure 1).

AMPH shares structural similarity with a number of compounds with pharmacological action including antidepressants, anorectics, hypertensives, decongestants, and hallucinogens (Hoffman & Lefkowitz, 1990). AMPH affects a number of neurotransmitters including catecholamines and indoleamines (Caldwell & Sever, 1974). AMPH has strong central stimulant effects in addition to peripheral effects on the alpha and beta adrenergic receptors (Hoffman & Lefkowitz, 1990). Based

Amphetamine

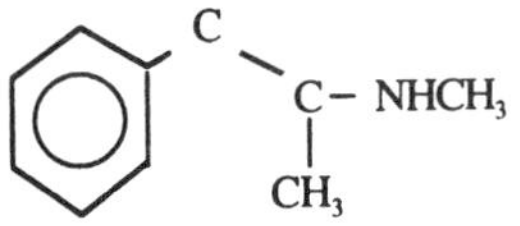

Methamphetamine

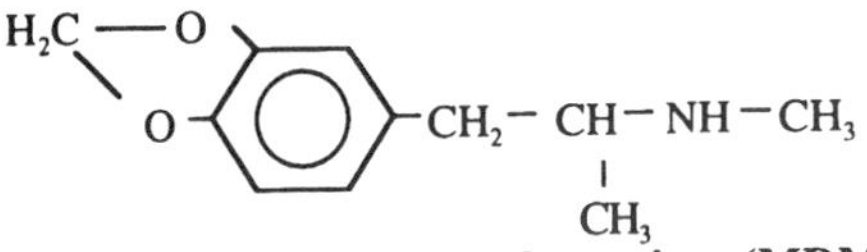

Methylenedioxymethamphetamine (MDMA)

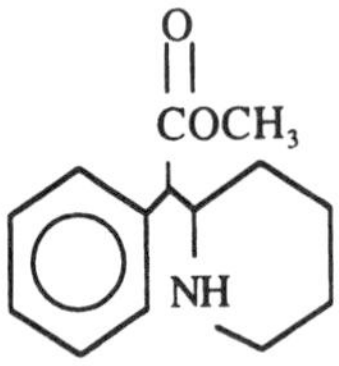

Methlyphenidate

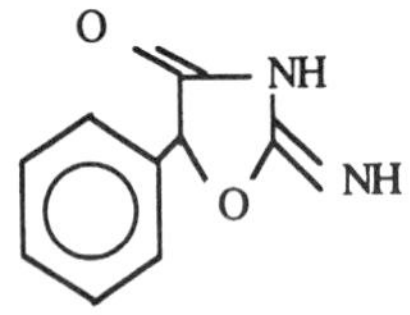

Pemoline

FIGURE 1. Chemical structures of the stimulant class agents.

mainly on its peripheral noradrenergic actions, AMPH elevates blood pressure resulting in a variable reflexive heart rate compensation (Hoffman & Lefkowitz, 1990).

With the exception of methamphetamine, alkylation of the side chain or amino group diminishes the activity of amphetamine (Biel, 1970; Caldwell & Sever, 1974). Ring hydroxylation reduces penetration of the AMPH molecule across the blood brain barrier while concomitantly reducing its CNS stimulant effect and anorectic properties (Caldwell &

Sever, 1974; Masand & Tesar, 1996). Substitution of the side chain alpha carbon prolongs physiologic noradrenergic and dopaminergic activity by inhibiting the oxidative potential of monoamine oxidase, a major enzyme involved in the catabolism of the catecholamines (Masand & Tesar, 1996). Prominent hallucinogenic properties are created by substitution of methoxy groups on the amphetamine ring (Glennon, 1987). For example, MDMA and MDA are both amphetamines with methylenedioxy substitutions on two carbons of the aromatic rings (Glennon, 1987) (see Figure 1). A reduction of central nervous system (CNS) stimulant action is related to substitution of the terminal amine, or methylation of the side chain carbon-amino group giving rise to phentermine-type agents. N-alkylation with halogen substitution into the ring results in fenfluramine (Biel, 1970; Caldwell & Sever, 1974; Hoffman & Lefkowitz, 1990).

In addition to containing components of the AMPH backbone (Figure 1), the structure of methylenedioxyamphetamine (MDA) and 3,4 methylenedioxyamphetamine (MDMA) share structural and pharmacological similarities with mescaline which is thought to be related to their hallucinogenic properties (Barnes, 1988; Climko et al., 1987; Kuczenski et al., 1987). Like AMPH, MDA and MDMA affect the catecholaminergic system with more robust increases in norepinephrine neurotransmission compared with DA release. In addition, both compounds are also potent releasers of serotonin (Berger, Gu, & Azmitita, 1992; Kuczenski et al., 1987) which appears to be related pharmacologically with their potent hallucinogenic properties. In terms of pharmacological activity, the (+) stereoisomer of both compounds appears to be active, with MDA generally more potent in its pharmacological and toxicological properties than its further methylated counterpart, MDMA (Berger et al., 1992; Climko et al., 1987).

There has been ongoing interest in the role of the various enantiomers of methylphenidate. Methylphenidate as a secondary amine gives rise to four optical isomers: d-threo, l-threo, d-erythro, and l-erythro (Patrick, Caldwell,

Ferris, & Breese, 1987). Methylphenidate was originally marketed as an 80% dl-erythro and 20% dl-threo compound. However, only the threo racemate appears to produce the desired CNS action (Hubbard, Srinivas, Quinn, & Midha, 1989; Patrick, Caldwell, et al., 1987). Therefore, the erythro was discontinued from the standard preparation. There may be stereoselectivity in the compounds formed including receptor site binding and its relationship to response. In rats, the d-methylphenidate isomer showed greater induction of locomotor activity and reuptake inhibition of labeled DA and NE than the l-isomer (Patrick, Caldwell, et al., 1987).

Pharmacokinetics

Absorption

The absorption of AMPH, methylphenidate, and other related stimulant class agents that are lipophilic are rapid and complete from the gastrointestinal tract (Hoffman & Lefkowitz, 1990). Pemoline has a slower and less complete absorption, in part related to its poor aqueous and lipid solubility (Sallee, Stiller, Perel, & Bates, 1985). There is a preferential, albeit variable, uptake of the stimulants, particularly methylphenidate, into the central nervous system. Compared to oral doses of AMPH, intravenous administration of AMPH is associated with more CNS stimulation, euphoria, tolerance, and cyclicity of use (Goff & Ciraulo, 1991). Intranasal methylphenidate abuse has been more recently reported (Jaffe, 1991) and appears to result in euphoria.

Half-Lives

In Table 1, the serum and behavioral half-lives of the common stimulant class agents are listed. There is a paucity of pharmacokinetic studies of stimulants in humans. AMPH has a behavioral half-life of 3–6 hr, a clearance half-life of 12–20 hr, and achieves peak plasma levels in 2–3 hr (Angrist, Corwin, & Bartlik, 1987; Elia, 1991). Behavioral effects of the compound appear to peak between 1 and 2 hr postingestion and dissipate within 4–5 hr (An-

TABLE 1. Stimulant Preparations, Half-Lives, and Daily Doses[a]

Medication brand name	Tablet size and preparation		Serum half-life (hr)	Behavioral half-life (hr)	Daily dose range
	Short-acting	Long-acting			
Amphetamine (D, L) (Benzedrine, Biphetamine, Adderall)	5, 10 mg	10, 15, 20 mg	12–20	3–6	0.1–1.0 mg/kg
Dextroamphetamine (Dexedrine)	5, 10 mg	5, 10 15 mg (spansule)	12–20	2–6	0.1–1.0 mg/kg
Methamphetamine (Desoxyn, Fetamin)	2.5, 5 mg	5, 10, 15 mg (gradumet)	10–30	6–18	0.1–1.0 mg/kg
Methylphenidate (Ritalin)	5, 10, 20 mg	20 mg SR (sustained release)	3–6	2–6	0.3–2.0 mg/kg
Magnesium Pemoline (Cylert)		18.75, 37.5, 75 mg	7–14	6–12	0.5–3.0 mg/kg

[a] Adapted from Goff & Ciraulo, 1991; Wilens & Biederman, 1992.

grist *et al.,* 1987; Anngard, Gunne, & Jonsson, 1970; Caldwell & Sever, 1974). Acute administration of methylphenidate results in a variable peak plasma concentration in 1–2 hr postingestion, with an elimination half-life of 2–6 hr (Patrick, Mueller, Gualtieri, & Breese, 1987; Sebrechts *et al.,* 1986). Peak behavioral effects generally occur within 1–2 hr and dissipate within 3–5 hr after oral ingestion. Food ingestion appears to have little impact in the pharmacokinetic profile of the stimulants (Patrick, Mueller, *et al.,* 1987). Pemoline has a longer half-life than that of the short-acting stimulants (7–8 hr in children, 11–13 hr in adults) and in part related to slower absorption, reaches peak levels 1–4 hr postingestion (Collier *et al.,* 1985; Sallee *et al.,* 1985).

AMPH (dextro isomer) and methylphenidate are available in long-acting preparations. The half-life of the long-acting preparation of methylphenidate (slow release, SR) is between 2 and 6 hr with peak levels occurring from 1 to 4 hr and a peak behavioral effect generally occurring within 2 hr and lasting up to 8 hr postingestion (Birmaher, Greenhill, Cooper, Fried, & Maminski, 1989; Pelham *et al.,* 1987). For slow-release dextroamphetamine, these values are somewhat longer (Pelham *et al.,* 1990).

Because of the large variability among individuals, serum levels vary considerably and have not been shown to correlate with clinical efficacy or toxicity (Patrick, Mueller, *et al.,*

1987). AMPH and methylphenidate accumulate in highly perfused tissues and accumulate rapidly and preferentially in the brain within 5 min of intravenous administration. Stimulants reach their maximal therapeutic and euphorogenic effects during the absorption phase of the kinetic curve, approximately within 2 hr after oral ingestion (Angrist *et al.,* 1987; Masand & Tesar, 1996). The absorption phase parallels the acute release of neurotransmitters into synaptic clefts, providing support for the hypothesis that alteration of monoaminergic transmission in critical brain regions may be the basis for stimulant action in producing euphoria (Angrist *et al.,* 1987; Anngard *et al.,* 1970; Caldwell & Sever, 1974) and in the treatment of disorders such as ADHD (Zametkin & Rapoport, 1987).

Metabolism

AMPH is metabolized by side chain oxidative deamination and ring hydroxylation in the liver (Biel, 1970; Caldwell & Sever, 1974). The majority of AMPH is excreted unchanged in the urine (about 80%), with benzoic and subsequent hippuric acid, and the hydroxyamphetamine catabolites as less important byproducts of AMPH metabolism found in the urine (Caldwell & Sever, 1974). The metabolites of AMPH have variable pharmacological activity. For example, one of the byproducts of hydroxylation of the amphetamine ring has less CNS activity, but more cardiovascular potency, than AMPH (Biel, 1970; Caldwell & Sever, 1974).

As AMPH is a basic compound, urinary excretion is highly dependent on urinary pH. Acidification of the urine results in a shortened plasma half-life and increased clearance of AMPH and is useful clinically in toxic conditions (Caldwell & Sever, 1974; Goff & Ciraulo, 1991; Masand & Tesar, 1996). There appear to be few differences in amphetamine metabolism in acute versus chronic dosing situations (Angrist et al., 1987; Caldwell & Sever, 1974; Elia et al., 1990).

There is a significant first-pass effect with methylphenidate being metabolized predominately by hydrolysis before reaching systemic circulation. Methylphenidate metabolism differs from that of AMPH in that the major pathway of methylphenidate metabolism is through deesterification to the inactive Ritalinic acid, with a smaller amount being converted to parahydroxymethylphenidate (Greenhill & Osman, 1991; Patrick, Mueller, et al., 1987). Pemoline is hepatically metabolized; its major metabolites include pemoline conjugate, pemoline dione, and mandelic acid. Pemoline is

renally excreted with 91% of the oral dose recovered in the urine of which 40% remains as the unchanged drug (Sallee et al., 1985).

Mechanism of Action

Two major processes are related to the concentration of DA in the synapse. The more prominent and well studied is the exocytic release of DA and other neurotransmitters which is impulse-dependent related largely to the potassium gradient across the cell membrane (Seiden, Sabol, & Ricaurte, 1993). Through the formation of an action potential by membrane depolarization, *vesicular* DA is released into the synapse by exocytosis. In this manner, vesicular DA release is modulated by presynaptic receptors while being less sensitive to agents that affect the transmembrane protein transporter (Levi & Raiteri, 1993). Conversely, carrier-mediated transport of catecholamines such as DA appear operant in raising synaptic concentrations of neurotransmitters, particularly after exposure to psychotropics such as AMPH (Bannon, Granneman, & Kapatos, 1995; Levi & Raiteri, 1993). It is thought that membrane-

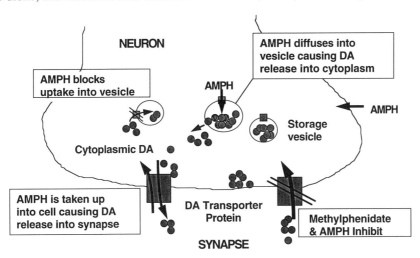

FIGURE 2. The major mechanisms of action of AMPH and related compounds on DA neurotransmission. The AMPH compounds are thought to work through (1) blockade of uptake of biogenic amines from the intrasynaptic cleft (inhibition of DA transporter protein), (2) promotion of release of the presynaptic DA into the synaptic cleft by AMPH uptake into the cell and exchange of DA from inside to outside the cell via the DA protein transporter, and (3) release of DA from presynaptic storage vesicles into the cytoplasm and inhibition of DA reuptake back into the storage vesicles. AMPH affects many aspects of DA release, uptake, and storage, whereas methylphenidate more specifically inhibits the DA transporter protein. The action-potential–related exocytosis of vesicular DA into the synapse associated with typical neuronal firing is not pictured.

spanning transport proteins transfer *cytoplasmic* DA from inside to outside the cell and are sensitive to agents which affect the transmembrane protein transporter or increase cytoplasmic DA levels but not to presynaptic receptors (Levi & Raiteri, 1993).

Release, uptake, and enzymatic inactivation of transmitters are three fundamental processes underlying the mechanisms of action of AMPH and other stimulants at the neuronal level (Figure 2). Preclinical studies have shown that the stimulants block the reuptake of dopamine (DA) and norepinephrine into the presynaptic neuron, and that these drugs increase the release of these monoamines into the extraneuronal space (Arnold, Molinoff, & Rutledge, 1977; Axelrod, Whitby, & Hertting, 1961; Caldwell & Sever, 1974; Elia *et al.*, 1990; Hoffman & Lefkowitz, 1990; Levi & Raiteri, 1993; Seiden *et al.*, 1993). Both the releasing and uptake-inhibiting actions of AMPH and related compounds are mediated by the catecholamine uptake transporter which has been studied for over 30 years (Axelrod *et al.*, 1961; Bannon *et al.*, 1995; Kuczenski, 1983; Levi & Raiteri, 1993; Seiden *et al.*, 1993).

AMPH appears to manifest its effects on the catecholaminergic synapse affecting predominately DA and noradrenergic neurons. In the central nervous system, AMPH may work directly on DA to affect arousal, whereas its effects in the periphery such as blood pressure and pulse may be mediated via norepinephrine (Fawcett & Busch, 1995). Methylphenidate appears to have less effect on norepinephrine release and more specificity for the DA transporter protein (Braestrup, 1977; Volkow *et al.*, 1995; Zaczek, Battaglia, Contrera, Culp, & DeSouza, 1989). The mechanism of action of pemoline remains unclear; however, it appears to work by reducing catecholamine turnover (Zametkin, Linnoila, Karoum, & Sallee, 1986). As described in the following section, AMPH is thought to work through (1) blockade of uptake of biogenic amines from the intrasynaptic cleft (inhibition of DA reuptake), (2) promotion of release of the presynaptic DA into the synaptic cleft (transporter-mediated cytoplasmic DA release), (3) both release of DA from presynaptic storage vesicles into the cytoplasm and inhibition of DA reuptake back into the storage vesicles, and (4) mild inhibition of monoamine oxidase (for review see (Kuczenski, 1983; Levi & Raiteri, 1993; Seiden *et al.*, 1993). Although it is known that these effects are generalized to other monoaminergic systems including the serotonin system (Kuczenski *et al.*, 1987), DA continues to be the prototype, and probably most important of the neurotransmitters affected by AMPH and other stimulants.

One mechanism of increasing synaptic DA common to a number of psychotropics is the blockade of catecholaminergic uptake from the synapse into the presynaptic neuron (Bannon *et al.*, 1995; Seiden *et al.*, 1993). Cell firing causes exocytotic release of vesicular DA into the extracellular synaptic space. The DA is taken back into the nerve terminal through a membrane-spanning protein referred to as the DA uptake transporter. Central to AMPH, cocaine, and other stimulant class agents are their effects on inhibiting the DA transporter protein (Bannon *et al.*, 1995; Levi & Raiteri, 1993).

There has been a great focus of research on the physical characteristics and biological features of the DA transporter protein (Bannon *et al.*, 1995). Under physiological conditions, the DA transporter protein actively uptakes DA from a lower concentration (intrasynaptic) to a higher concentration (presynaptic) location. Since energy is required, it is thought that this transport is linked to the neuronal sodium concentration maintained by ATP hydrolysis (Bannon *et al.*, 1995; Seiden *et al.*, 1993).

Although the DA transporter protein normally moves DA from the synapse into the cell, in the presence of AMPH the direction of transport appears to be reversed, with DA being released into the synapse (Bannon *et al.*, 1995; Levi & Raiteri, 1993; Seiden *et al.*, 1993). AMPH is thought to bind to the DA transporter protein on the outside of the cell membrane blocking DA reuptake back into the cell (Seiden *et al.*, 1993). AMPH then moves into the cell where it exchanges with DA via the DA transporter protein (Levi & Raiteri,

1993; Seiden *et al.,* 1993). Cytoplasmic DA is "exchanged" from the interior of the cell to outside the cell via the sodium-dependent transport protein which can be blocked by DA reuptake inhibitors (Kuczenski, 1983; Levi & Raiteri, 1993; Seiden *et al.,* 1993). In this manner, extracellular AMPH is exchanged with DA, thus increasing the concentration of synaptic DA.

Although AMPH is considered a prototype releaser of DA, it remains to be seen whether this action is purely related to its DA-releasing properties, its effects on inhibiting reuptake, or more probably the combination (Chiueh & Moore, 1975; Heikkila, Orlansky, & Cohen, 1975). Methylphenidate, in contrast, primarily increases synaptic DA through a more specific interaction with the DA transporter protein leading to specific DA reuptake blockade (Giros, Jaber, Jones, Wrightman, & Caron, 1996; Seiden *et al.,* 1993; Volkow *et al.,* 1995). A recent study has shown that genetic manipulation resulting in elimination of the DA transporter protein ("knockout") leads to a virtual behavioral and pharmacological insensitivity to AMPH or cocaine in mice (Giros *et al.,* 1996). These findings support the importance of the DA transporter protein in mediating the pharmacological and psychological response to the AMPH class of agents.

AMPH affects many aspects of DA storage and release within the neuron. Evidence suggests that DA storage occurs mainly in two presynaptic nerve terminal regions: intravesicular and cytoplasmic (Seiden *et al.,* 1993). DA that has been newly synthesized or recycled from reuptake into the presynaptic neuron is further taken up through a second transporter into storage vesicles and protected from enzymatic degradation. Whereas the majority of DA is stored within vesicles, cytoplasmic DA is the pool available for release by AMPH and related compounds (Levi & Raiteri, 1993). A different set of transmembrane proteins is involved in the intraneuronal vesicular storage of DA than is found on the nerve terminal membrane facing the synaptic cleft (DA transporter protein; Figure 2). AMPH inhibits the uptake of DA into these storage vesicles. For example,

the *in vitro* inhibition for the uptake of DA and norepinephrine from the cytosol to the intracellular vesicles in the presence of AMPH is fourfold higher than the inhibition of neuronal uptake of both compounds into the cell (Kuczenski, 1983).

AMPH releases DA from its vesicular storage sites into the cytoplasm by diffusion of the AMPH across the vesicular membrane into the vesicle, and subsequent alkalinization of the vesicles resulting in DA release (Seiden *et al.,* 1993). In contrast to the older DA stored in the vesicles, the cytoplasmic DA in the neuron is largely a reflection of the ongoing DA synthesis in the cell. This cytoplasmic DA is the preponderate store of DA released into the synapse in the presence of AMPH. Although DA release into the synapse appears to be stereospecific, both the d- and l-AMPH isomers release vesicular DA into the cytoplasm (Seiden *et al.,* 1993). The release of DA from the cytoplasm into the synapse appears to be relatively insensitive to factors that influence the more concentration-based DA vesicular storage (Braestrup, 1977; Chiueh & Moore, 1975). AMPH-induced DA release from the cytoplasmic pool can be maintained exclusively by synthesis (Kuczenski, 1983). The degradation of cytoplasmic DA may reduce end-product feedback inhibition in tyrosine hydroxylase resulting in increased catecholamine and, hence, DA, production. In contrast to high-dose AMPH, increases in striatal DA have been shown after low-dose AMPH administration owing to the increased synthesis of DA in these brain regions (Kuczenski, 1983).

It is also thought that DA existing within storage vesicles represents a relatively older pool compared with cytoplasmic DA which represents more newly synthesized DA (Chiueh & Moore, 1975). AMPH appears to act on both cytoplasmic and vesicular pools of DA. Typical cell-firing (action-potential-related) release of DA from storage vesicles into the synapse may also be weakly potentiated by stimulants; however, it is largely the inhibition of DA reuptake from the synapse back into the cell that accounts for elevated synaptic DA levels. There appear to be notable differences among the stimulants' effects on cytoplasmic DA release into the synapse (Braestrup, 1977; Kuczenski, 1983). Whereas AMPH has a broader spectrum of action affecting the DA transporter protein as well as vesicular and cytoplasmic DA, methylphenidate appears to work primarily on inhibition of the DA transporter protein and may have negligible effects on DA vesicular synaptic release and no effects on cytoplasmic DA synaptic release (Braestrup, 1977; Levi & Raiteri, 1993; Solanto, 1984; Volkow *et al.,* 1995; Zaczek *et al.,* 1989). Because of its predominate effect on the reuptake of synaptic DA which is largely released into the synapse from vesicles during typical cell firing, methylphenidate affects older DA (vesicular) preferentially. For example, animal synaptosomes pretreated with reserpine, an agent that depletes vesicular DA stores, fail to release DA when exposed to methylphenidate, but not to AMPH (Butcher, Liptrot, & Aburthnott, 1991). These differences in the DA release mechanisms between stimulant compounds may translate into variation in their behavioral effects and addiction liability.

There may also be AMPH dose-related effects on catecholamine reuptake and release that may relate to the dose-related behavioral pharmacological differences. As summarized by Seiden and colleagues (1993), there appears to be a dose-dependent effect of AMPH on release of DA. Low-dose AMPH (<5 mg/kg) facilitates release of DA through exchange diffusion across the cell membrane in which AMPH enters the cell via the DA transporter protein and DA is released. This release is derived from newly synthesized DA which resides in the cytoplasm. Moderate doses of AMPH (5–10 mg/kg) work by the same exchange diffusion as the low-dose process in addition to a further diffusion of AMPH into the cell, and an interaction between AMPH and the storage vesicle membrane transporter therefore affecting the older pools of DA. In addition to the above processes, high-dose AMPH also enters the presynaptic vesicle causing further and more complete release of the DA in the presynaptic neuron, adding to

the cytoplasmic pools (Seiden *et al.,* 1993). Intracellular AMPH activity may also be increasing DA release by inhibiting vesicular uptake of DA and hence increasing the DA concentration in the cytoplasm. The effect of AMPH on norepinephrine release shares similarities with DA; however, there may be different dose–response curves and actions (Hoffman & Lefkowitz, 1990).

Although apparently less important in the facilitation of neurotransmission by the stimulants, there is also evidence that stimulant class agents may also directly affect DA presynaptic inhibitory autoreceptors. Much of this work is based on behavioral pharmacological studies. In animal studies it has been observed that stimulants increase motoric activity at low doses but decrease activity and narrow focus at higher doses (Solanto, 1986). Since in animals, low doses of stimulants inhibit dopaminergic autoreceptors, these findings suggest that inhibition of autoreceptors may be an additional component of stimulant effect (Solanto, 1986).

There appears to be stereoselectivity of AMPH on DA release into the synapse with the dextro isomer of AMPH being more potent at releasing DA than the levo isomer (Arnold *et al.,* 1977) correlating with the more potent behavioral effects of the d-AMPH compared to the l- form. Because of methodological difficulties and the ambiguity defining the purity of inhibition versus release of catecholamines by the DA transporter protein, the exact mechanism and dose-response relationship of AMPH in modulating DA release remains to be seen *in vivo.*

Analogous to DA actions of AMPH, MDMA inhibits the uptake of serotonin into chromaffin granules and facilitates the release of serotonin from the chromaffin granules (Berger *et al.,* 1992; Seiden *et al.,* 1993). MDMA is thought to enter the storage vesicles. It may be that MDMA interacts with the storage vesicle membrane in two ways: at low concentrations, it blocks uptake into and facilitates release from the vesicle by direct interaction with the serotonin carrier (Seiden *et al.,* 1993); and at high concentrations, MDMA facilitates the direct release of serotonin. The chronic effects of MDMA are unclear although destruction of specific serotonergic nerve terminals has been described (Ricaurte *et al.,* 1988). For example, in monkeys administered 2.5–5 mg/kg/day, selective dose-related depletion of serotonin and its breakdown product 5-hydroxyindolacetic acid were noted (Ricaurte *et al.,* 1988). In addition, these deficits were associated with structural damage to serotonergic nerve fibers in the dorsal raphe nucleus leading to speculation that such a phenomenon may be operational in human MDMA addicts (Climko *et al.,* 1987; Ricaurte *et al.,* 1988). MDMA appears to be less toxic than MDA in its effects on serotonin depletion as well as in overdose toxicity (Climko *et al.,* 1987).

Neurohormonal responses to the stimulants remain unclear. Methylphenidate has variable effects on prolactin secretion and a stimulatory effect on growth hormone (GH) release acutely (Greenhill *et al.,* 1984; Sharma, Javaid, Pandey, Easton, & Davis, 1990; Shaywitz *et al.,* 1990). While acutely stimulating β-endorphin and cortisol secretion, chronically methylphenidate has mixed effects on prolactin, β-endorphin, and growth hormone levels (Weizman *et al.,* 1987).

Chronic Administration, Tolerance, and Dependence

There appears to be an abuse liability of the stimulants leading to tolerance and dependence with certain of these agents being higher on the list of abuse. Preclinical studies and epidemiological evidence seem to suggest a hierarchy of abuse liability beginning with methamphetamine, followed by AMPH, dextro-AMPH, methylphenidate, and pemoline (Balster & Schuster, 1973; Langer, Sweeney, Bartenbach, Davis, & Menander, 1986). Nonoral routes of administration of these agents may result in more rapid tolerance and dependence.

There are certain physiological adaptations to the stimulant class of medications. The physiological and psychological effects of the stimulants are related to daily dose, route of administration, and duration of use (Gawin,

Khalsa, & Ellinwood, 1994). Therapeutic doses of AMPH (10–60 mg daily) and related compounds are associated with the following adverse effects: insomnia, edginess, reduced appetite, increased CNS acuity, and mild elevations in vital signs (Greenhill & Osman, 1991; Wilens & Biederman, 1992). Acute administration of relatively higher doses of AMPH (about > 150 mg/day) and related compounds can cause euphoria, CNS stimulation, vital sign changes, and anorexia (Greenhill & Osman, 1991; Wilens & Biederman, 1992). Generally tolerance to the euphorogenic effects of these agents develops over months. High doses of AMPH acutely may also lead to CNS hyperarousal, violence, skin picking, delirium, paranoia, and frank psychosis (Gawin *et al.,* 1994; Goff & Ciraulo, 1991). Elevated vital signs, hyperthermia, arrhythmias, seizures, and death have also been described after the acute ingestion of large amounts of AMPH (Gawin *et al.,* 1994; Goff & Ciraulo, 1991). Although the bulk of these symptoms occur only during acute intoxication with high doses of AMPH, the spectrum of psychotic symptoms from tactile hallucinations to paranoid delusions may be prolonged and easily rekindled with subsequent high or low doses of AMPH (Caldwell & Sever, 1974). The development of psychosis appears to be more related to the use of high doses of stimulant-class agents and not to a predisposition to psychosis (Bell, 1970).

With the chronic use of AMPH-related compounds at therapeutic doses, there is ongoing CNS stimulation with some tolerance developing to the anorexia and euphoria (Caldwell & Sever, 1974; Goff & Ciraulo, 1991). There is a paucity of data on the long-term effects of therapeutic doses of AMPH agents (Gawin *et al.,* 1994); however, the use of MDA or MDMA over time may lead to neurotoxicity (Ricaurte *et al.,* 1988). Chronic use of relatively higher doses of AMPH may lead to mood lability, insomnia alternating with hypersomnia, agitation, and psychosis. Similarly, AMPH addicts may have life-threatening cardiac arrhythmias, cerebral hemorrhage, and weight loss (Goff & Ciraulo, 1991).

Withdrawal from stimulant abuse may lead to predictable behavioral phenomena such as hypersomnia, dysphoria, and agitation. Gawin and colleagues (1994) and Gawin and Kleber (1986) have described three phases of immediate to protracted withdrawal from cocaine that appear operational for AMPH abuse. Generally, acute AMPH ingestion will be associated with overall stimulation followed by hypersomnia. Chronic AMPH addicts will also experience a crash initially characterized by exhaustion, hypersomnia, reduced craving, depression, and later hyperphagia (Phase one lasting to 4 days). From 1 to 10 weeks, abstinent chronic AMPH abusers may experience the onset of anhedonia, variable depression, anxiety, and severe cravings. After 10 weeks, many of these symptoms appear to improve with the exception of continued difficulty with episodic craving worsened in the presence of conditioned cues (Gawin & Kleber, 1986; Gawin et al., 1994).

Neurochemically, urinary 3-methoxy-4-hydroxyphenylglycol excretion is acutely reduced after AMPH cessation. Primate studies indicate reduced serotonin and DA levels after chronic administration of methamphetamine, which may persist for up to 6 months after discontinuation of the stimulant (Seiden, Fischman, & Schuster, 1975). Despite a substantial literature on the effects of the acute administration of AMPH, the biological mechanisms related to more chronic usage including tolerance and dependence remain an enigma. This is of particular interest given the large number of individuals receiving stimulant-class agents chronically for therapeutic reasons, and the smaller group of individuals who are chronic abusers of AMPH and related substances.

Many of the effects of AMPH on DA relevant to the field of substance abuse appear to be centralized in the ventral striatum including the nucleus accumbens (Konradi, Cole, Heckers, & Hyman, 1994). Putative mechanisms of tolerance or dependence to the AMPH class of agents include theories of AMPH acting as false transmitter, changes in catecholamine and noncatecholamine neurotransmitter levels and turnover in brain tissue, alterations in neurohormonal function, and induction of gene expression and byproducts (Caldwell & Sever, 1974; Nestler, 1992; Seiden et al., 1975; Seiden et al., 1993). Of the varied lines of investigation in this area, some of the more recent research has focused on mechanisms of neural plasticity relevant to AMPH metabolism. One such area of intrigue has focused on the expression of genes in relation to drug exposure (Cole, Konradi, Douglass, & Hyman, 1995; Hyman & Nestler, 1996; Nestler, 1992).

There is an emerging consensus that many psychoactive agents work not only on the neurochemistry of the cell, but also on the turning on and off of specific genes. This may occur directly through interaction of the compound with the gene or gene product, or indirectly by affecting messengers or factors which themselves regulate genes and their expression into gene products (Hyman & Nestler, 1996). Such interactions appear to be operant between AMPH and specific genes. For instance, a set of genes referred to as "immediate early genes" and their protein products act to assimilate extracellular signals into the regulation of genes involved in the further differentiated function of neurons (Konradi et al., 1994).

By stimulating postsynaptic D1 and D2–DA receptors, AMPH has been shown to induce the expression of certain genes. Through stimulation of DA receptors (Ruskin & Marshall, 1994), AMPH also appears to be related to gene regulation by stimulating cAMP phosphorylation of specific regulatory regions of transcription factors which then directly affect gene regulation and expression (Konradi et al., 1994). For example, AMPH has been shown to activate the zinc finger transcription factor as well as "turn on" the immediate-early gene c-fos in the DA-rich striatum (Konradi et al., 1994). Similarly, mRNA and peptides significantly increase in the striatum and nucleus accumbens after chronic AMPH administration (Hyman & Nestler, 1996).

Neuronal adaptations to chronic stimulant abuse may be operational. As suggested by Hyman and Nestler (1996), it may be that the increased DA neurotransmission associated with chronic AMPH abuse may activate certain genes and their products that subsequently modulate further DA release. After abstinence, these gene products continue to modulate DA release, resulting in lower than normal levels of DA which may be related to the prolonged withdrawal symptoms and craving. Current work is under way to better understand the receptor-mediated cascade involved in transcription factor activation, as well as the dynamics and implications of alterations in gene expression related to AMPH exposure.

In summary, the AMPH compounds are a class of agents which affect both the catecholamine and indoleamine systems. There are stereoselective structural relationships with the neuronal and behavioral pharmacological response and metabolism of these agents. The mechanisms of action of the stimulants have unique characteristics dependent on the specific agent and dose. Although the physiological mechanisms underlying tolerance and dependence remain unclear, ongoing work on the microbiological changes associated with these agents may provide important insights into these mechanisms.

References

Alles, G. A. (1928). The comparative physiological action of phenylethanolamine. *Journal of Pharmacology and Experimental Therapeutics, 32,* 121–128.

Angrist, B., Corwin, J., & Bartlik, B. (1987). Early pharmacokinetics and clinical effects of oral d-amphetamine in normal subjects. *Biological Psychiatry, 22,* 1357–1368.

Anngard, E., Gunne, L. M., & Jonsson, L. (1970). Pharmacokinetic and clinical studies on amphetamine dependent subjects. *European Journal of Clinical Pharmacology, 3,* 3–11.

Anthony, J. C., & Helzer, J. E. (1991). Syndromes of drug abuse and dependence. In L. Robins & D. Regier (Eds.), *Psychiatric disorders in America* (pp. 116–154). New York: Free Press.

Arnold, E. B., Molinoff, P., & Rutledge, C. (1977). The release of endogenous norepinephrine and dopamine in cerebral cortex by amphetamine. *Journal of Pharmacology and Experimental Therapeutics, 202,* 544–557.

Axelrod, J., Whitby, L., & Hertting, G. (1961). Effect of psychotropic drugs on the uptake of 3H-norepinephrine by tissues. *Science, 133,* 383–384.

Balster, R. L., & Schuster, C. R. (1973). A comparison of d-amphetamine, l-amphetamine, and methamphetamine self administration in rhesus monkeys. *Pharmacology, Biochemistry and Behavior, 1,* 67–71.

Bannon, M. J., Granneman, J. G., & Kapatos, G. (1995). The dopamine transporter. In F. E. Bloom & D. J. Kupfer (Eds.), *Psychopharmacology: The fourth generation of progress* (pp. 179–188). New York: Raven.

Barnes, D. M. (1988). New data intensify the agony over ecstasy. *Science, 239,* 864–866.

Bell, D. S. (1970). The experimental reproduction of amphetamine psychosis. *Archives of General Psychiatry, 127,* 1170–1175.

Berger, U. V., Gu, X. F., & Azmitia, E. C. (1992). The substitute amphetamines 3,4-methylenedioxymethamphetamine, methamphetamine, p-chloroamphetamine and fenfluramine induce 5-hydroxytryptamine release via a common mechanism blocked by fluoxetine and cocaine. *European Journal of Pharmacology, 215,* 153–160.

Biel, J. M. (1970). Structure–activity relationships of amphetamine and derivatives. In E. Costa & S. Garattini (Eds.), *Amphetamines and related compounds* (pp. 3–19). New York: Raven.

Birmaher, B., Greenhill, L. L., Cooper, T. B., Fried, J., & Maminski, B. (1989). Sustained release methylphenidate: Pharmacokinetic studies in ADDH males. *Journal of the American Academy of Child and Adolescent Psychiatry, 28,* 768–772.

Braestrup, C. (1977). Biochemical differentiation of amphetamine vs methylphenidate and nomifensine in rats. *Journal of Pharmacy and Pharmacology, 29,* 463–470.

Butcher, S. P., Liptrot, J., & Aburthnott, G. W. (1991). Characterization of methylphenidate and nomifensive induced dopamine release in rat striatum using in vivo brain microdialysis. *Neuroscience Letters, 122,* 245–248.

Caldwell, J., & Sever, P. S. (1974). The biochemical pharmacology of abused drugs. *Clinical Pharmacology & Therapeutics, 16,* 625–638.

Chiueh, C. D., & Moore, K. E. (1975). D-Amphetamine induced release of newly synthesized and stored dopamine from the caudate nucleus in vivo. *Journal of Pharmacology and Experimental Therapeutics, 1975,* 642–653.

Climko, R. P., Roehrich, H., Sweeney, D. R., & Al-Razi, J. (1987). Ecstasy: A review of MDMA and MDA. *International Journal of Psychiatry in Medicine, 16,* 359–372.

Cole, R. L., Konradi, C., Douglass, J., & Hyman, S. E. (1995). Neuronal adaptation to amphetamine and dopamine: Molecular mechanisms of prodynorphin gene regulation in rat striatum. *Neuron, 14,* 813–823.

Collier, C. P., Soldin, S. J., Swanson, J. M., MacLeod, S. M., Weinberg, F., & Rochefort, J. G. (1985). Pemoline pharmacokinetics and long term therapy in children with attention deficit disorder and hyperactivity. *Clinical Pharmacokinetics, 10,* 269–278.

Elia, J. (1991). Stimulants and antidepressant pharmacokinetics in hyperactive children. *Psychopharmacology Bulletin, 27,* 411–415.

Elia, J., Borcherding, B. G., Potter, W. Z., Mefford, I. N., Rapoport, J. L., & Keysor, C. S. (1990). Stimulant drug treatment of hyperactivity: Biochemical correlates. *Clinical Pharmacology & Therapeutics, 48,* 57–66.

Fawcett, J., & Busch, K. A. (1995). Stimulants in psychiatry. In A. Schatzberg & C. Nemeroff (Eds.), *Textbook of psychopharmacology* (pp. 417–435). Washington, DC: American Psychiatric Association.

Gawin, F. H., & Kleber, H. D. (1986). Abstinence symptomatology and psychiatric diagnoses in cocaine abusers: Clinical observations. *Archives of General Psychiatry, 43,* 107–113.

Gawin, F. H., Khalsa, M. E., & Ellinwood, E. (1994). Stimulants. In M. Galanter & H. D. Kleber (Eds.), *Textbook of substance abuse treatment* (pp. 111–139). Washington, DC: American Psychiatric Press.

Giros, B., Jaber, M., Jones, S., Wrightman, M., & Caron, M. (1996). Hyperlocomotion and indifference to cocaine and amphetamine in mice lacking the dopamine transporter. *Nature, 379,* 606–612.

Glennon, R. A. (1987). Psychoactive phenylisopropylamines. In H. Y. Meltzer (Ed.), *Psychopharmacology: The third generation of progress* (pp. 1627–1634). New York: Raven.

Goff, D. C., & Ciraulo, D. A. (1991). Stimulants. In D. A. Ciraulo & R. I. Shader (Eds.), *Clinical manual of chemical dependence* (pp. 233–257). Washington, DC: American Psychiatric Press.

Greenhill, L. L., & Osman, B. B. (1991). *Ritalin: Theory and patient management.* New York: Liebert.

Greenhill, L. L., Puig-Antich, J., Novacenko, H., Solomon, M., Anghern, C., Florea, J., Goetz, R., Fiscina, B., & Sachar, E. J. (1984). Prolactin, growth hormone and growth responses in boys with attention deficit disorder and hyperactivity treated with methylphenidate. *Journal of the American Academy of Child Psychiatry, 23,* 58–67.

Heikkila, R. E., Orlansky, H., & Cohen, G. (1975). Studies on the distinction between uptake inhibition and release of (3H) dopamine in rat brain tissue slices. *Biochemistry and Pharmacology, 24,* 847–852.

Hoffman, B. B., & Lefkowitz, R. J. (1990). Catecholamines and sympathomimetic drugs. In A. G. Gilman, T. W. Rall, A. S. Nies, & P. Taylor (Eds.), *The pharmacological basis of therapeutics* (pp. 187–220). New York: Pergamon.

Hubbard, J. W., Srinivas, N. R., Quinn, D., & Midha, K. K. (1989). Enantioselective aspects of the disposition of dl-threo-methylphenidate after the administration of a sustained-release formulation to children with attention deficit disorder. *Journal of Pharmaceutical Sciences, 78,* 944–947.

Hyman, S. E., & Nestler, E. J. (1996). Initiation and adaptation: A paradigm for understanding psychotropic drug action. *American Journal of Psychiatry, 153,* 151–162.

Jaffe, S. L. (1991). Intranasal abuse of prescribed methylphenidate by an alcohol and drug abusing adolescent with ADHD. *Journal of the American Academy of Child and Adolescent Psychiatry, 30,* 773–775.

Konradi, C., Cole, R. L., Heckers, S., & Hyman, S. E. (1994). Amphetamine regulates gene expression in rat striatum via transcription factor CREB. *Journal of Neuroscience, 14,* 5623–5634.

Kuczenski, R. (1983). Biochemical actions of amphetamine and other stimulants. In I. Creese (Ed.), *Stimulants: Neurochemical, behavioral, and clinical perspectives* (pp. 31–61). New York: Raven.

Kuczenski, R., Segal, D. S., Leith, N. J., & Applegate, C. D. (1987). Effects of amphetamine, methylphenidate, and apomorphine on regional brain serotonin and 5-hydroxyindole acetic acid. *Psychopharmacology, 93,* 329–335.

Langer, D. H., Sweeney, K. P., Bartenbach, D. E., Davis, P. M., & Menander, K. B. (1986). Evidence of lack of abuse or dependence following pemoline treatment: Results of a retrospective survey. *Drug and Alcohol Dependency, 17,* 213–227.

Levi, G., & Raiteri, M. (1993). Carrier-mediated release of neurotransmitters. *Trends in Neurosciences, 16,* 415–420.

Masand, P. S., & Tesar, G. E. (1996). Use of stimulants in the medically ill. In *The Psychiatric Clinics of North America* (pp. 515–547). Philadelphia: Saunders.

Nestler, E. (1992). Molecular mechanisms of drug addiction. *Journal of Neuroscience, 12,* 2439–2450.

Patrick, K. S., Caldwell, R. W., Ferris, R. M., & Breese, G. R. (1987). Pharmacology of the enantiomers of threo-methylphenidate. *Journal of Pharmacology and Experimental Therapeutics, 241,* 152–158.

Patrick, S. K., Mueller, R. A., Gualtieri, C. T., & Breese, G. R. (1987). Pharmacokinetics and actions of methylphenidate. In H. Y. Meltzer (Ed.), *Psychopharmacology: The third generation of progress* (pp. 1387–1396). New York: Raven.

Pelham, W. E., Sturges, J., Hoza, J., Schmidt, C., Bijlsma, J. J., Milich, R., & Moorer, S. (1987). Sustained release and standard methylphenidate effects on cognitive and social behavior in children with attention deficit disorder. *Pediatrics, 80,* 491–501.

Pelham, W. E., Greenslade, K. E., Vodde-Hamilton, M., Murphy, D. A., Greenstein, J. J., Gnagy, E. M., Guthrie, K. J., Hoover, M. D., & Dahl, R. E. (1990). Relative efficacy of long-acting stimulants on children with attention deficit-hyperactivity disorder: A comparison of standard methylphenidate sustained-release methylphenidate, sustained-release dextroamphetamine, and pemoline. *Pediatrics, 86,* 226–237.

Ricaurte, G. A., Forno, L., Wilson, M., DeLanney, L., Irwin, I., Molliver, M. E., & Langston, J. W. (1988). 3,4-Methylenedioxymethamphetamine selectively damages central serotonergic neurons in nonhuman primates. *Journal of the American Medical Association, 260,* 51–55.

Ruskin, D., & Marshall, J. F. (1994). Amphetamine and cocaine induced fos in the rat striatum depends on D2 dopamine receptor activation. *Synapse, 18,* 233–240.

Sallee, F., Stiller, R., Perel, J., & Bates, T. (1985). Oral pemoline kinetics in hyperactive children. *Clinical Pharmacological Therapy, 37,* 606–609.

Sebrechts, M. M., Shaywitz, S. E., Shaywitz, B. A., Jatlow, P., Anderson, G. M., & Cohen, D. J. (1986). Components of attention, methylphenidate dosage, and blood levels and children with attention deficit disorder. *Pediatrics, 77,* 222–228.

Seiden, L. S., Fischman, M. W., & Schuster, C. R. (1975). Long-term methamphetamine induced changes in brain catecholamines in tolerant rhesus monkeys. *Drug and Alcohol Dependence, 1,* 215–219.

Seiden, L. S., Sabol, K. E., & Ricaurte, G. A. (1993). Amphetamine: Effects on catecholamine systems and behavior. *Annual Review of Pharmacology and Toxicology, 32,* 639–677.

Sharma, R. P., Javaid, J. I., Pandey, G. N., Easton, M., & Davis, J. (1990). Pharmacological effects of methylphenidate on plasma homovanillic acid and growth hormone. *Psychiatry Research, 32,* 9–17.

Shaywitz, B. A., Shaywitz, S. E., Sebrechts, M. M., Anderson, G. M., Cohen, D. J., Jatlow, P., & Young, J. G. (1990). Growth hormone and prolactin response to methylphenidate in children with attention deficit disorder. *Life Sciences, 46,* 625–633.

Solanto, M. V. (1984). Neuropharmacological basis of stimulant drug action in attention deficit disorder with hyperactivity: A review and synthesis. *Psychological Bulletin, 95,* 387–409.

Solanto, M. V. (1986). Behavioral effects of low-dose methylphenidate in childhood attention deficit disorder: Implications for a mechanism of stimulant drug action. *Journal of the American Academy of Child and Adolescent Psychiatry, 25,* 96–101.

Volkow, N. D., Ding, Y., Fowler, J. S., Wang, G., Logan, J., Gatley, J. S., Dewey, S., Ashby, C., Liebermann, J., Hitzemann, R., & Wolf, A. P. (1995). Is methylphenidate like cocaine? *Archives of General Psychiatry, 52,* 456–463.

Weizman, R., Dick, J., Gil-Ad, I., Weitz, R., Tyano, S., & Laron, Z. (1987). Effects of acute and chronic methylphenidate administration on B-endorphin, growth hormone, prolactin and cortisol in children with attention deficit disorder and hyperactivity. *Life Sciences, 40,* 2247–2252.

Wilens, T. E., & Biederman, J. (1992). The stimulants. In D. Shafer (Ed.), *The Psychiatric Clinics of North America* (pp. 191–222). Philadelphia: Saunders.

Zaczek, R., Battaglia, G., Contrera, J. F., Culp, S., & DeSouza, E. B. (1989). Methylphenidate and pemoline do not cause depletion of rat brain monoamine markers similar to that observed with methamphetamine. *Toxicology & Applied Pharmacology, 100,* 227–233.

Zametkin, A. J., & Rapoport, J. L. (1987). Neurobiology of attention deficit disorder with hyperactivity: Where have we come in 50 years? *Journal of the American Academy of Child and Adolescent Psychiatry, 26,* 676–686.

Zametkin, A. J., Linnoila, M., Karoum, F., & Sallee, R. (1986). Pemoline and urinary excretion of catecholamines and indoleamines in children with attention deficit disorder. *American Journal of Psychiatry, 143,* 359–362.

31

Behavioral Pharmacology of Amphetamines

GEORGE V. REBEC

Introduction

Originally sold as a bronchodilator in the early 1930s, amphetamine soon became known for its stimulant effects on behavior (Angrist, 1983). The drug has been used to overcome fatigue and to improve performance on certain types of motor or cognitive tasks (Koelega, 1993; Laties & Weiss, 1981). These stimulant effects often occur in conjunction with feelings of euphoria, a combination that has led to the widespread abuse of amphetamine and its analogs, including a pure form of methamphetamine known as "ice," which emerged on the recreational drug scene in the late 1980s (Cho, 1990). Invariably, abuse of these drugs induces a psychosis that is clinically similar to paranoid schizophrenia (Akiyama, Hamamura, Ujike, Kanzaki, & Otsuki, 1991; Snyder, 1973).

Although many compounds belong to the amphetamine class of stimulants, their effects on behavior are qualitatively similar, differing mainly with respect to potency and time-course. Most of the data presented in this chapter are based on the use of d-amphetamine, though in some cases, especially those involv-

GEORGE V. REBEC • Program in Neural Science, Department of Psychology, Indiana University, Bloomington, Indiana 47405.

Handbook of Substance Abuse: Neurobehavioral Pharmacology, edited by Tarter *et al.* Plenum Press, New York, 1998.

ing human addicts, methamphetamine use is common owing to its relatively rapid entry into the brain. In fact, intravenous administration, which ensures such entry for a wide range of amphetamine analogs, creates an initial "rush" that often becomes a highly sought component of the drug experience (Angrist, 1983).

This chapter focuses on the brain–behavior relationships relevant for understanding amphetamine abuse. Attention centers on the motor-activating effects of amphetamine both because they are evident in all mammals studied, including humans, and because the neurochemical and neurophysiological correlates of these effects in animals can be used to shed light on human neuronal processes. The first part of the discussion highlights the perseverative nature of the amphetamine-induced motor response across species and summarizes some of the variables that help shape this response. A subsequent section uses these lines of information to assess data on underlying neurobiological mechanisms.

Perseverative Patterns of Motor Behavior

Amphetamine elicits repetitive or stereotyped patterns of searching activity despite obvious species-specific differences (Ellinwood, Sudilovsky, & Nelson, 1973; Randrup & Munkvad, 1970; Schiørring, 1981). Macrosmatic animals like the rat, for example, respond with bouts of perseverative locomotion often coupled with repetitive sniffing and head bobbing. Monkeys, on the other hand, may show prolonged periods of probing or grasping at the skin or nearby objects in conjunction with repetitive hand and eye movements, whereas humans report feelings of curiosity, often manifest as perceptuo-motor compulsions such as dismantling mechanical devices and then sorting the parts as if searching for something. In fact, human amphetamine abusers not only display stereotyped motor patterns but also report perseverative delusional thoughts (Ellinwood, 1967). Not surprisingly, humans under the influence of amphetamine have been described as being in a state of cognitive inflexibility (Ridley & Baker, 1982).

The motor response to amphetamine is influenced by several interrelated factors, including dose, environment, and prior exposure to the drug. The rat has been the animal of choice for assessing these factors and thus it is the main focus of the following discussion (see also Lyon & Robbins, 1975; Rebec & Bashore, 1984; Segal, 1975; Seiden, Sabol, & Ricaurte, 1993). Data from humans and other primates are included as appropriate.

Dose-Dependent Changes in Motor Activity

The motor-activating effects of amphetamine in rats are evident after systemic (intraperitoneal or subcutaneous) injection of doses as low as 0.25–0.5 mg/kg. Locomotor activation, which includes both horizontal (forward locomotion) and vertical (rearing) movements, is prominent, especially as the dose is increased to approximately 2.0 mg/kg. Other behaviors also emerge, either in conjunction with locomotor activity or in separate episodes, and include head bobbing (typically vertical movements of the head), sniffing, and shuffling of the forelimbs. Rats, of course, express these behaviors during normal exploration, but after amphetamine these responses increase in frequency and take on a perseverative or stereotyped quality such that their pattern of expression becomes less varied and

more repetitive. Amphetamine-induced forward locomotion, for example, is typically manifest as relatively invariant movement along a limited number of sides of an open-field arena (Mueller, Hollingsworth, & Cross, 1989; Schiørring, 1979).

Behavioral stereotypy is most evident with higher doses of the drug. Above 2.0 mg/kg, a distinct period of focused stereotypy emerges during which locomotor activity declines or is replaced entirely by highly constricted bouts of head bobbing, sniffing, and forelimb shuffling. At doses approaching 5.0 mg/kg, separate episodes of oral behavior, including licking and biting, begin to appear during the focused stereotypy phase, and these responses increase in intensity as the dose is increased. The focused stereotypy phase, moreover, is preceded and followed by periods of forward locomotion, rearing, head bobbing, and sniffing as described previously. Thus, unlike the low-dose response to amphetamine, relatively high doses elicit a multiphasic response pattern consisting of early and late phases of nonfocused, albeit repetitive, motor activity and an intermediate phase of highly focused stereotypy. The temporal pattern of focused stereotypy also changes progressively with dose, occurring sooner and lasting longer as the dose increases.

Multiple Treatments

The behavioral effects of repeated amphetamine administration have been studied extensively because although humans may show signs of psychosis under the influence of a moderate to large acute dose, abusers typically consume the drug in binges or "runs" separated by periods of recovery (Akiyama, Kanzaki, Tsuchida, & Ujike, 1994; Kramer, Fischman, & Littlefield, 1967; Schiørring, 1981). During a binge, the drug may be administered every few hours for several days until exhaustion sets in. Binges are characterized by frenzied, stereotyped motor activity, which often occurs in conjunction with a progressively intensifying paranoid psychosis. Detailed analysis of the effects of repeated administration in rats has revealed complex changes in the motor-activating effects of amphetamine. These studies also indicate that dose and interinjection interval play an important role in shaping these behavioral characteristics.

In considering dose effects in rats, emphasis is placed on repeated administration of a constant dose, though multiple injections of progressively increasing doses, sometimes used to mimic the increasing amphetamine consumption of human addicts, elicits behavioral changes consistent with the constant-dose treatment. Repeated treatment with low doses (up to 1.5 mg/kg) enhances the locomotor response as well as sniffing and head bobbing. These behaviors are not only more intense but persist for longer periods. With repeated injections of 1.5–2.0 mg/kg, the pattern of the response begins to resemble that of the acute administration of higher doses: a multiphasic pattern of early and late periods of nonfocused locomotor activity and an intermediate phase of focused stereotypy. At doses that normally induce focused stereotypy (2.5–5.0 mg/kg) with acute treatment, repeated injections cause this phase to emerge more rapidly and to increase in intensity. That is, the early locomotor phase is shortened and the sniffing and head bobbing characteristic of the stereotypy phase become even more focused. In many respects, therefore, rats, like human abusers, appear to become sensitized to repeated amphetamine treatment, a process known as behavioral sensitization.

It is important to stress, however, that despite the terminology, not all behaviors are sensitized. Oral behaviors, for example, decline in frequency and intensity with repeated amphetamine administration (Eichler, Antelman, & Black, 1980; Rebec & Segal, 1980). Furthermore, even though focused stereotypy occurs sooner with multiple injections, the duration of the stereotypy phase is not correspondingly increased and may actually decrease in some cases (Segal, Weinberger, Cahill, & McCunney, 1980). The poststereotypy locomotor phase, in contrast, increases in duration. Thus, the overall response profile to a given dose of amphetamine shows both qualitative and quantitative changes with repeated

administration that cannot be explained as a simple shift in the dose–response curve. In fact, the behavioral changes are evident in chronically treated rats challenged with an intraventricular injection of amphetamine (Rebec & Segal, 1979), suggesting that central mechanisms rather than peripheral pharmacokinetic factors play the critical role. Related to this point is the possibility that at least some of the behavioral alterations associated with chronic treatment reflect active competition between individual responses (Segal & Kuczenski, 1994). Certain behaviors may decline in frequency allowing others to become more intense or to display a different time-course.

Although relatively similar patterns of altered behavioral responsiveness have been noted with a wide range of interinjection intervals (several hours to several days), certain temporal aspects of drug administration exert an important influence. A long time (weekly or longer) between injections, for example, appears to enhance the development of sensitization (Robinson & Becker, 1986). In fact, a second injection of amphetamine several weeks after the first is sufficient to induce the pattern of behavioral change typically associated with a period of long-term treatment. Another temporal consideration is that when amphetamine is readministered several weeks after a chronic treatment regimen, the altered behavioral pattern persists (Segal & Janowsky, 1978). Human amphetamine abusers reintroduced to the drug after a prolonged absence also maintain a heightened sensitivity to the drug (Sato, Numachi, & Hamamura, 1992). Such persistence suggests a relatively long-term change at the neuronal level. Continuous infusions of amphetamine for days or weeks have been attempted in rats to mimic the amphetamine "run" of a human abuser. Under these conditions, rats show intense motor stereotypy early on, but new behaviors and new behavioral patterns emerge as the infusion continues (Ellison & Eison, 1983). At least some of these behavioral changes may result from the neurotoxic effects associated with prolonged amphetamine exposure (Marshall, Odell, & Weihmuller, 1993; Ricaurte,

Sabol, & Seiden, 1994; Ryan, Linder, Martone, & Groves, 1990; Stephans & Yamamoto, 1994).

Situational Variables

The behavioral effects of amphetamine are shaped by situational variables such as time of day (Urba-Holmgren, Holmgren, & Aguiar, 1977), opportunity for interactions with other animals (Gambil & Kornetsky, 1976), both social (Ahmed, Stinus, LeMoal, & Cador, 1995) and environmental rearing conditions (Bardo et al., 1995; Bowling, Rowlett, & Bardo, 1993), and the physical dimensions of the chamber in which behavior is assessed (Cole, 1977; Heise & Boff, 1971). In fact, simply adding certain objects to the behavioral chamber can alter the type of responses induced by amphetamine as well as the pattern of stereotypy (Ellinwood & Kilbey, 1975; Wang, Bonta, & Rebec, 1994). When measured in an unfamiliar environment, stereotypy is less focused than when it occurs in familiar surroundings (Exner & Clark, 1993; Mazurski & Beninger, 1988). Changes in sensory input also exert an influence. Blindfolding cats, for example, causes a significant reduction in amphetamine-induced repetitive movements of the head (Stevens, Livermore, & Cronan, 1977). The motor-activating effects of amphetamine, therefore, do not represent motor automatisms, but highly modifiable patterns of movement.

Situational variables also can influence the development of behavioral sensitization to repeated amphetamine treatment. Learning factors associated with context-dependent conditioning, for example, have been shown to alter the onset and pattern of the sensitization response (Stewart & Eikelboom, 1987), though sensitization itself occurs independently of environmental conditioning (Robinson & Becker, 1986). In addition, repeated exposure to a stressor changes the behavioral response to amphetamine from that commonly associated with an acute injection to the altered responsiveness characteristic of chronic amphetamine treatment (Robinson & Becker, 1986). In fact, stress appears to play a key role in amphetamine-induced behavioral sensitization (Antel-

man & Chiodo, 1983; Kalivas & Stewart, 1991; Robinson, 1991).

Underlying Neurobiological Mechanisms

The similarities in behavioral expression across species with both acute and chronic treatment suggest a common neurobiological basis for amphetamine's actions. A vast and diverse literature has examined the role of specific neuronal systems and their interconnections. Most attention has centered on mesotelencephalic dopamine pathways and their forebrain targets, especially the neostriatum and nucleus accumbens. This section highlights neurochemical and neurophysiological data obtained from behaving animals.

Neurochemical Correlates

A prominent line of evidence implicating dopamine in the motor-activating effects of amphetamine is based on reports that these effects are blocked by dopamine receptor antagonists (see Rebec & Bashore, 1984). Many of these drugs, which include classical neuroleptics such as haloperidol and chlorpromazine, are used to treat schizophrenia as well as amphetamine psychosis. In fact, evidence of a neuroleptic-induced blockade of the behavioral response to amphetamine and other dopamine agonists in rats is used as a preclinical screen of antipsychotic efficacy (see Ellenbroek, 1993). Dopamine antagonists block both the nonfocused behavioral activation induced by amphetamine and the phase of focused stereotyped behavior. Drugs with somewhat less affinity and selectivity for dopamine receptors, such as clozapine, also antagonize amphetamine-induced behaviors, but the antagonism is incomplete (Moore & Kenyon, 1994; Tschanz & Rebec, 1988).

Other procedures for disrupting dopamine transmission also disrupt the behavioral response to amphetamine. Pretreatment of rats with α-methyl-p-tyrosine, which blocks catecholamine synthesis, has this effect, suggesting that amphetamine requires an adequate pool of newly synthesized dopamine (Dominic

& Moore, 1969). Amphetamine appears to release this pool mainly by an exchange-diffusion process, which involves the reverse transport of dopamine by the dopamine uptake carrier (for reviews, see Kuczenski & Segal, 1994; Seiden *et al.*, 1993). Convincing support for this model has been obtained from "knockout" mice, in which the dopamine transporter gene has been selectively knocked out or disabled (Giros, Jaber, Jones, Wightman, & Caron, 1996). In these animals, amphetamine not only fails to evoke the release of dopamine but also fails to produce a behavioral response. At relatively high doses, amphetamine may promote dopamine release from vesicular stores by altering intravesicular pH (Sulzer & Rayport, 1990).

Attempts also have been made to assess the involvement of both the nigro-neostriatal and meso-limbic dopamine systems. Most of this work has relied on the infusion of 6-hydroxydopamine, a catecholamine neurotoxin, into specific brain regions. Complete destruction of both systems mimics the effect of α-methyl-p-tyrosine in that the behavioral response to amphetamine is blocked (Fibiger, Fibiger, & Zis, 1973). When analyzed separately, however, these systems have been implicated in different aspects of amphetamine-induced motor activity. Damage to dopamine terminals in the nucleus accumbens, which receives input from the meso-limbic system, appears to attenuate the nonfocused aspects of amphetamine stereotypy, including locomotion, rearing, and sniffing (Kelly, Saviour, & Iversen, 1975). In contrast, the phase of intense focused stereotypy induced by high doses is markedly attenuated by 6-hydroxydopamine lesions of the neostriatum (Creese & Iversen, 1974). In these animals, nonfocused motor behavior replaces highly focused activity. There may be further functional differences within both the neostriatum and nucleus accumbens. This conclusion is based on the results of direct infusions of amphetamine or other dopamine agonists into circumscribed areas of the neostriatum. Infusions into ventrolateral sites, for example, are relatively selective for inducing oral behaviors (Kelley, Lang, & Gau-

thier, 1988). Moreover, some neostriatal areas are more sensitive than others to the motor-activating effects of amphetamine (Wang & Rebec, 1993).

The nucleus accumbens has been divided into a central core and a surrounding shell based on anatomical connections (Meredith, Pennartz, & Groenewegen, 1993; Zahm & Brog, 1992), and recent evidence suggests that dopaminergic function between these areas also may differ. The shell is closely linked to limbic operations (Pennartz, Groenewegen, & DaSilva, 1994), and dopamine release in this site appears related to stress (Kalivas & Duffy, 1995) and also to mechanisms of reinforcement (Rebec, Christensen, Guerra, & Bardo, 1997). In fact, the ability of amphetamine to facilitate accumbal dopamine release is shared by a wide variety of drugs of abuse, suggesting a common mechanism underlying drug reward (Di Chiara, 1995; Koob, 1995). Accumbal core, on the other hand, may act in conjunction with the neostriatum in regulating sensorimotor function (Pennartz *et al.*, 1994).

The application of methodologies for measuring drug-induced changes in neurotransmitter function in behaving animals has allowed a more direct assessment of dopamine involvement in the motor-activating effects of amphetamine. Microdialysis, which can provide selective measurements of extracellular dopamine at relatively short intervals (typically 5–15 min), has been the procedure of choice for this line of investigation (Rebec, 1991). Consistent with expectations, microdialysates collected after amphetamine administration indicate a significant elevation in the extracellular level of dopamine. These results have been obtained in both neostriatum and nucleus accumbens. Attempts to relate amphetamine-induced changes in extracellular dopamine with dose-dependent behavioral changes, however, have not been so encouraging. Although general relationships have emerged between the dopamine response and the onset and overall magnitude of the behavioral change, correlations between dopamine and either the intensity or the time-course of specific behaviors have not emerged (see Segal & Kuczenski,

1994). Individual animals showing quantitatively similar dopamine responses, for example, may express different behaviors (e.g., forward locomotion vs. rearing). Similarly, a high dose of amphetamine may elicit a relatively constant level of oral stereotypy for a prolonged period even though the extracellular level of dopamine declines markedly during the same period. Some temporal dissociations between extracellular dopamine and behavior also have been reported with lower doses (Sharp, Zetterstrom, Ljungberg, & Ungerstedt, 1987; Kuczenski & Segal, 1989). In general, it appears that the magnitude of the dopamine response more closely parallels the level of amphetamine in the brain than the magnitude of specific behavioral responses (Kuczenski & Segal, 1994).

With respect to the behavioral alterations associated with chronic amphetamine treatment, microdialysis studies suggest a marked increase in extracellular dopamine in both neostriatum and nucleus accumbens compared with the acute dopamine response (Kalivas & Stewart, 1991; Robinson, 1991). These and other lines of evidence (see Robinson & Becker, 1986) have led to the view that behavioral sensitization requires augmented dopamine release. Again, however, the relationship between extracellular dopamine and behavior appears to be extremely complex. In some cases, for example, behavioral sensitization can occur without an increase in the dopamine response (Kalivas & Stewart, 1991) or even with a decrease (Segal & Kuczenski, 1992). These results, of course, do not rule out a role for dopaminergic mechanisms in behavioral sensitization because chronic amphetamine treatment may enhance dopamine transmission in ways that are not reflected in dopamine release (e.g., a change in the sensitivity of postsynaptic dopamine receptors or the way in which different populations of such receptors interact). Nevertheless, it seems clear that as with acute administration the involvement of dopaminergic mechanisms in the behavioral response of chronically treated animals bears no simple relationship to the level of extracellular dopamine.

Apart from altering dopamine transmission, amphetamine is known to influence other transmitter systems that can modulate behavior either by directly modulating dopamine or by acting on parallel systems that help regulate dopaminergic function. Some likely candidates include norepinephrine, serotonin, and glutamate. Both norepinephrine and serotonin have long been suspected of helping to shape the behavioral response to amphetamine (e.g., Braestrup, 1977; Breese, Cooper, & Mueller, 1974). Moreover, microdialysis data suggest certain parallels with these transmitters that are not evident with dopamine. In hippocampus, for example, the rise and fall of extracellular norepinephrine levels after amphetamine administration closely follow the time-course of the behavioral response (Kuczenski & Segal, 1992), and in neostriatum doses that elicit focused stereotypy increase extracellular serotonin (Kuczenski, Segal, Cho, & Melega, 1995). Conceivably, therefore, norepinephrine helps to maintain a certain level of behavioral responsiveness that dopamine initiates, whereas serotonin appears linked to the shift toward focused stereotypy.

Interest in the glutamate system stems, in part, from evidence that phencyclidine (PCP), a noncompetitive antagonist of the N-methyl-D-aspartate (NMDA) glutamate receptor, elicits intense focused stereotypy in rats and a paranoid psychosis in human abusers that mimics endogenous schizophrenia better than the psychosis induced by amphetamine (Javitt & Zukin, 1991; Johnson, 1983). Haloperidol blocks both the motor and psychotic effects of PCP (Jackson, Johansson, Lindgren, & Bengtsson, 1994; Steinpreis, Sokolowski, Papanikolaou, & Salamone, 1994). Collectively, these results are consistent with neurophysiological evidence that the activity of neostriatal and accumbal neurons is mainly the result of a close interaction between glutamate and dopamine (see the following discussion). Glutamate also has been implicated in amphetamine-induced behavioral sensitization. Blockade of NMDA receptors with dizocilpine, for example, has been reported to block the induction of sensitization without altering the acute response to amphetamine (Karler, Chaudhry, Calder, & Turkanis, 1990;

Wolf & Khansa, 1991). It is not yet clear, however, whether glutamate plays a general role in this effect or acts selectively on specific behavioral responses. Some evidence suggests that repeated treatment with dizocilpine and amphetamine induces a unique pattern of behavioral sensitization characterized by a suppression of focused stereotypy and an augmentation of locomotion (Segal, Kuczenski, & Florin, 1995). NMDA receptors also have been reported to play a role in the rewarding action of amphetamine (Kelley & Throne, 1992).

Also noteworthy is evidence that amphetamine facilitates glutamate release and in neostriatal tissue an increase in extracellular glutamate triggers the release of ascorbate, an antioxidant vitamin and neuromodulator (Rebec & Pierce, 1994). It appears that the glutamate transporter, activated by glutamate release, causes ascorbate release by a heteroexchange mechanism (Fillenz, 1995). This process has important implications for amphetamine because the extracellular level of neostriatal ascorbate exerts a strong influence on the behavioral response to this drug. High extracellular levels of ascorbate, induced by either systemic administration of high doses or direct intraneostriatal infusions, antagonizes amphetamine-induced motor activity (Tolbert, Thomas, Middaugh, & Zemp, 1979; L. K. White, Maurer, Kraft, Oh, & Rebec, 1990), whereas pretreatment with relatively small doses of ascorbate have the opposite effect (Pierce, Rowlett, Rebec, & Bardo, 1995; Wambebe & Sokomba, 1986). Although more work is required to characterize the role of the glutamate-ascorbate system and other non-dopaminergic processes in the behavioral effects of amphetamine, it seems clear that multiple mechanisms participate in shaping the pattern of the amphetamine-induced motor response with either acute or chronic treatment.

Neurophysiological Correlates

Attempts to understand the neurophysiological basis of the amphetamine-induced behavioral response have focused primarily on the activity of neurons in the neostriatum and nucleus accumbens. As the main targets of the nigro-neostriatal and meso-limbic dopamine systems, respectively, neostriatal and accumbal neurons should play a critical role in the motor-activating effects of amphetamine. More than 90% of these cells are medium-spiny output neurons with connections to downstream nuclei (for review, see Groves, 1983; Smith & Bolam, 1990). Although neuronal responsiveness to amphetamine and other substances has been studied extensively in the neostriatum and nucleus accumbens of anesthetized or in vitro preparations (see Rebec, 1987), emphasis is placed on data obtained from awake, behaving animals.

Most neurons recorded from the neostriatum and nucleus accumbens of rats are highly responsive to spontaneous movement (Aldridge, Berridge, Herman, & Zimmer, 1993; Carelli & West, 1991; Gardiner, Iverson, & Rebec, 1988; Haracz, Tschanz, Wang, White, & Rebec, 1993; West, Michael, Knowles, Chapin, & Woodward, 1987). These cells typically maintain a relatively slow rate of discharge when the animals rest quietly but markedly increase neuronal activity in close temporal association with an overt motor response. In some cases, the neuronal change is tightly coupled to a specific movement, such as raising the left or right forelimb, whereas other neurons respond nonselectively to a wide variety of movements (e.g., grooming, forward locomotion, rearing, and sniffing). Both types of motor-related cells also often respond to somatosensory, auditory, or visual stimuli. A much smaller population of neurons, estimated at between 10% and 30%, shows no consistent response to either overt movement or sensory stimulation (Haracz et al., 1993; Wang & Rebec, 1993).

After systemic injection of relatively low doses of amphetamine, neuronal activity diverges: Motor-related cells typically increase firing rate by at least 500% above the resting baseline rate, whereas nonmotor-related neurons show a pronounced inhibition (Haracz et al., 1993). Both types of changes parallel the onset of the drug-induced behavioral activation and continue throughout the behavioral response. In some cases, motor-related cells are inhibited by spontaneous movement and also by amphetamine (Haracz *et al.,* 1993; Ryan, Young, Segal, & Groves, 1989). Such cells, however, may discharge at low rates, making their detection difficult.

One could argue that amphetamine-induced activation of excitatory motor-related cells is simply secondary to the change in behavior, but two lines of evidence argue against this interpretation. For one, detailed analysis of neuronal activity during episodes of matched movements before and after amphetamine administration, a process known as behavioral clamping, consistently revealed a higher rate of postamphetamine activity (Haracz *et al.,* 1993). In addition, intra-neostriatal or intra-accumbal infusions of amphetamine activate motor-related neurons several minutes before the onset of any overt behavioral change (Wang & Rebec, 1993). It appears, therefore, that amphetamine acts directly in these nuclei to alter neuronal activity.

It also is important to point out that many neostriatal and accumbal neurons showing movement-related changes in firing rate in one context may respond differently or not at all to the same movement in a different context (Gardiner & Kitai, 1992; West *et al.,* 1987). Thus, movement alone may not be the sole basis for activation of these cells. Nevertheless, the classification of neurons as motor-related provides a useful framework for interpreting the electrophysiological effects of amphetamine. In fact, the distinction between motor- and nonmotor-related neurons also applies to the differential effects of dopamine applied directly to neostriatal and accumbal neurons by iontophoresis. Thus, neurons identified as motor-related are consistently activated by dopamine iontophoresis, whereas nonmotor-related cells tend to respond with an inhibition (Pierce & Rebec, 1995). In view of the striking parallel between these data and the results obtained with systemic amphetamine, the differential effects of amphetamine on motor- and nonmotor-related neurons could be explained by the differential responses of these cells to dopamine. This hypothesis is supported by evidence that dopa-

mine receptor antagonists block the excitatory effects of both iontophoretic dopamine (Pierce & Rebec, 1995) and systemic amphetamine (Rosa-Kenig, Puotz, & Rebec, 1993). Dopamine antagonists also reverse the amphetamine-induced inhibition of nonmotor-related cells, but in this case not all dopamine antagonists are effective, suggesting that additional neurochemical mechanisms underlie the inhibitory neuronal response to amphetamine (Haracz *et al.,* 1993).

Despite the apparent role of dopamine in the activation of motor-related neurons by amphetamine, the magnitude of this response is significantly attenuated by a bilateral ablation of cerebral cortex (Tschanz, Haracz, Griffith, & Rebec, 1991). Cortical afferents supply approximately 70% of the glutamatergic innervation of neostriatal and accumbal neurons (McGeorge & Faull, 1989; Walaas, 1981). Thus, glutamate is a likely contributor to the amphetamine-induced increase in neuronal activity, a view supported by evidence that amphetamine facilitates neostriatal glutamate release (Labarca *et al.,* 1995; Nash & Yamamoto, 1993). NMDA antagonists, however, also activate neostriatal neurons (I. M. White *et al.,* 1995), making it unlikely that NMDA receptors are responsible for the neuronal activation induced by amphetamine.

A series of iontophoresis experiments in awake, unrestrained rats have confirmed a dopaminergic–glutamatergic interaction on neostriatal and accumbal neurons. Co-application of these compounds activates neuronal activity to a greater extent than either substance applied alone (Pierce & Rebec, 1995). Moreover, prolonged iontophoresis of dopamine at relatively low ejection currents alters both basal firing rate and the response to a subsequent brief application of glutamate such that the magnitude of the glutamate response relative to background activity is significantly enhanced (Kiyatkin & Rebec, 1996). Under naturally occurring behavioral conditions, therefore, it appears that dopamine release helps to magnify the postsynaptic strength of glutamatergic signals. According to this model, an amphetamine-induced elevation in dopamine release sets the stage for an enhanced flow of cerebro-cortical information through the neostriatum and nucleus accumbens.

Relatively little information is available on the response of neostriatal and accumbal neurons during the phase of focused stereotypy elicited by moderate to high doses of amphetamine. Ryan and colleagues (1989), recording predominantly from slow-firing neurons, found inhibitions to be common, but some evidence suggests focused stereotypy is accompanied by either excitations or inhibitions. In a preliminary investigation of neostriatal neurons excited by different types of motor activity, Rebec, White, & Puotz (1997) reported that during focused stereotypy cells most sensitive to forward locomotion decreased activity, whereas neurons selective for head movements showed a further excitation. Although additional research is warranted, these data suggest that the transition to focused stereotypy is accompanied by a switch in the direction of firing of at least some motor-related neostriatal neurons. Such a switch seems difficult to explain by dopaminergic mechanisms alone and appears to require the active participation of other afferent systems.

ACKNOWLEDGMENTS

Preparation of material for this chapter was supported, in part, by a grant from the National Institute on Drug Abuse, DA 02451. Faye Caylor provided expert editorial assistance.

References

Ahmed, S. H., Stinus, L., LeMoal, M., & Cador, M. (1995). Social deprivation enhances the vulnerability of male Wistar rats to stressor- and amphetamine-induced behavioral sensitization. *Psychopharmacology, 117,* 116–124.

Akiyama, K., Hamamura, T., Ujike, H., Kanzaki, A., & Otsuki, S. (1991). Methamphetamine psychosis as a model of relapse of schizophrenia—A behavioral and biochemical study in the animal model. In T. Nakazawa (Ed.), *Biological basis of schizophrenic disorders* (Vol. 14, pp. 169–184). Tokyo: Japan Scientific Societies Press.

Akiyama, K., Kanzaki, A., Tsuchida, K., & Ujike, H. (1994). Methamphetamine-induced behavioral sensi-

tization and its implications for relapse of schizophrenia. *Schizophrenia Research, 12,* 251–257.

Aldridge, J. W., Berridge, K. C., Herman, M., & Zimmer L. (1993). Neuronal coding of serial order: Syntax of grooming in the neostriatum. *Psychological Science, 4,* 391–395.

Angrist, B. (1983). Psychoses induced by central nervous system stimulants and related drugs. In I. Creese (Ed.), *Stimulants: neurochemical, behavioral, and clinical perspectives* (pp. 1–30). New York: Raven.

Antelman , S. M., & Chiodo, L. A. (1983). Amphetamine as a stressor. In I. Creese (Ed.), *Stimulants: neurochemical, behavioral and clinical perspectives* (pp. 269–299). New York: Raven.

Bardo, M. T., Bowling, S. L., Rowlett, J. K., Manderscheid, P., Buxton, S. T., & Dwoskin, L. P. (1995). Environmental enrichment attenuates locomotor sensitization, but not in vitro dopamine release, induced by amphetamine. *Pharmacology, Biochemistry and Behavior, 51,* 397–405.

Bowling, S. L., Rowlett, J. K., & Bardo, M. T. (1993). The effect of environmental enrichment on amphetamine-stimulated locomotor activity, dopamine synthesis and dopamine release. *Neuropharmacology, 32,* 885–893.

Braestrup, C. (1977). Changes in drug-induced stereotyped behavior after 6-OHDA lesions in noradrenaline neurons. *Psychopharmacology, 51,* 199–204.

Breese, G. R., Cooper, B. R., & Mueller, R. A. (1974). Evidence for involvement of 5-hydroxytryptamine in the actions of amphetamine. *British Journal of Pharmacology, 52,* 307–314.

Carelli, R. M., & West, M. O. (1991). Representation of the body by single neurons in the dorsolateral striatum of the awake, unrestrained rat. *Journal of Comparative Neurology, 309,* 231–249.

Cho, A. (1990). Ice: A new dosage form of an old drug. *Science, 249,* 631.

Cole, S. O. (1977). Interaction of arena size with different measures of amphetamine effects. *Pharmacology, Biochemistry and Behavior, 7,* 181–184.

Creese, I., & Iversen, S. D. (1974). The role of forebrain dopamine systems in amphetamine-induced stereotyped behavior in the rat. *Psychopharmacologia, 39,* 345–357.

Di Chiara, G. (1995). The role of dopamine in drug abuse viewed from the perspective of its role in motivation. *Drug and Alcohol Dependence, 38,* 95–137.

Dominic, J. A., & Moore, K. E. (1969). Acute effects of a-methyltyrosine on brain catecholamine levels and on spontaneous and amphetamine-stimulated motor activity in mice. *Archives of International Pharmacodynamics, 178,* 166–176.

Eichler, A. J., Antelman, S. M., & Black, C. A. (1980). Amphetamine stereotypy is not a homogenous phenomenon: Sniffing and licking show distinct profiles of sensitization and tolerance. *Psychopharmacology, 68,* 287–290.

Ellenbroek, B. A. (1993). Treatment of schizophrenia—A clinical and preclinical evaluation of neuroleptic drugs. *Pharmacology and Therapeutics, 57,* 1–78.

Ellinwood, E. H. (1967). Amphetamine psychosis: I. Description of the individuals and process. *Journal of Nervous and Mental Disease, 144,* 273–283.

Ellinwood, E. H., & Kilbey, M. M. (1975). Amphetamine stereotypy: The influence of environmental factors and prepotent behavioral patterns on its topography and development. *Biological Psychiatry, 10,* 3–16.

Ellinwood, E. H., Sudilovsky, A., & Nelson, L. M. (1973). Evolving behavior in the clinical and experimental amphetamine (model) psychosis. *American Journal of Psychiatry, 130,* 1088–1093.

Ellison, G. D., & Eison, M. S. (1983). Continuous amphetamine intoxication: An animal model of the acute psychotic episode. *Psychological Medicine, 13,* 751–761.

Exner, M., & Clark, D. (1993). Subtle variations in living conditions influence behavioural response to d-amphetamine. *NeuroReport, 4,* 1059–1062.

Fibiger, H. C., Fibiger, H. P., & Zis, A. P. (1973). Attenuation of amphetamine-induced motor stimulation and stereotypy by 6-hydroxydopamine in the rat. *British Journal of Pharmacology, 47,* 683–692.

Fillenz, M. (1995). Physiological release of excitatory amino acids. *Behavioural Brain Research, 71,* 51–67.

Gambil, J. D., & Kornetsky, C. (1976). Effects of chronic d-amphetamine on social behavior of the rat: Implications for an animal model of paranoid schizophrenia. *Psychopharmacology* (Berlin), *50,* 215–223.

Gardiner, T. W., Iverson, D. A., & Rebec, G. V. (1988). Heterogeneous responses of neostriatal neurons to amphetamine in freely moving rats. *Brain Research, 463,* 268–274.

Gardiner, T. W., & Kitai, S.,T. (1992). Single-unit activity in the globus pallidus and neostriatum of the rat during performance of a trained head movement. *Experimental Brain Research, 88,* 517–530.

Giros, B., Jaber, M., Jones, S. R., Wightman, R. M., & Caron, M. G. (1996). Hyperlocomotion and indifference to cocaine and amphetamine in mice lacking the dopamine transporter. *Nature, 379,* 606–612.

Groves, P. M. (1983). A theory of the functional organization of the neostriatum and the neostriatal control of voluntary movement. *Brain Research Reviews, 5,* 109–132.

Haracz, J. L., Tschanz, J. T., Wang, Z., White, I. M., & Rebec, G. V. (1993). Striatal single-unit responses to amphetamine and neuroleptics in freely moving rats. *Neuroscience and Biobehavioral Reviews, 17,* 1–12.

Heise, G. A., & Boff, E. (1971). Stimulant action of d-amphetamine in relation to test compartment dimensions and behavioral measure. *Neuropharmacology, 10,* 259–266.

Jackson, D. M., Johansson, C., Lindgren, L. M., & Bengtsson, A. (1994). Dopamine receptor antagonists block amphetamine and phencyclidine-induced motor stim-

ulation in rats. *Pharmacology, Biochemistry and Behavior, 48,* 465–471.

Javitt, D. C., & Zukin, S. R. (1991). Mechanisms of phencyclidine (PCP)-n-methyl-d-aspartate (NMDA) receptor interaction—Implications for schizophrenia. *Schizophrenia Research, 1,* 13–19.

Johnson, K. M. (1983). Phencyclidine: Behavioral and biochemical evidence supporting a role for dopamine. *Federation Proceedings, 42,* 2579–2583.

Kalivas, P. W., & Duffy, P. A. (1991). Comparison of axonal and somatodendritic dopamine release using in vivo dialysis. *Journal of Neurochemistry, 56,* 961–967.

Kalivas, P. W., & Duffy, P. A. (1995). Selective activation of dopamine transmission in the shell of the nucleus accumbens by stress. *Brain Research, 675,* 325–328.

Kalivas, P. W., & Stewart, J. (1991). Dopamine transmission in the initiation and expression of drug-induced and stress-induced sensitization of motor activity. *Brain Research Reviews, 16,* 223–244.

Karler, R., Chaudhry, I. A., Calder, L. D., & Turkanis, S. A. (1990). Amphetamine behavioral sensitization and the excitatory amino acids. *Brain Research, 537,* 76–82.

Kelley, A. E., & Throne, L. C. (1992). NMDA receptors mediate the behavioral effects of amphetamine infused into the nucleus accumbens. *Brain Research Bulletin, 29,* 247–254.

Kelley, A. E., Lang, C. G., & Gauthier, A. M. (1988). Induction of oral stereotypy following amphetamine microinjection into a discrete subregion of the striatum. *Psychopharmacology, 95,* 556–559.

Kelly, P. H., Saviour, P. W., & Iversen, S. D. (1975). Amphetamine and apomorphine responses in the rat following 6-OHDA lesions of the nucleus accumbens septi and corpus striatum. *Brain Research, 94,* 507–522.

Kiyatkin, E. A., & Rebec, G. V. (1996). Dopaminergic modulation of glutamate-induced excitations of neurons in the neostriatum and nucleus accumbens of awake, unrestrained rats. *Journal of Neurophysiology, 75,* 142–153.

Koelega, H. S. (1993). Stimulant drugs and vigilance performance—A review. *Psychopharmacology, 111,* 1–16.

Koob, G. F. (1995). Animal models of drug addiction. In F. E. Bloom & D. J. Kupfer (Eds.), *Psychopharmacology: The fourth generation of progress* (pp. 759–772). New York: Raven.

Kramer, J. C., Fischman, V. S., & Littlefield, D. C. (1967). Amphetamine abuse: Patterns and effects of high doses taken intravenously. *Journal of the American Medical Association, 201,* 305–309.

Kuczenski, R., & Segal, D. (1989). Concomitant characterization of behavioral and striatal neurotransmitter response to amphetamine using in vivo microdialysis. *Journal of Neuroscience, 9,* 2051–2065.

Kuczenski, R., & Segal, D. S. (1992). Regional norepinephrine response to amphetamine using dialysis—

Comparison with caudate dopamine. *Synapse, 11,* 164–169.

Kuczenski, R., & Segal, D. S. (1994). Neurochemistry of amphetamine. In A. Cho & D. S. Segal (Eds.), *Amphetamine and its analogs* (pp. 81–113). San Diego, CA: Academic Press.

Kuczenski, R., Segal, D. S., Cho, A. K., & Melega, W. (1995). Hippocampus norepinephrine, caudate dopamine and serotonin, and behavioral responses to the stereoisomers of amphetamine and methamphetamine. *Journal of Neuroscience, 15,* 1308–1317.

Labarca, R., Gajardo, M. I., Seguel, M., Silva, H., Jerez, S., Ruiz, A., & Bustos, G. (1995). Effects of D-amphetamine administration on the release of endogenous excitatory amino acids in the rat nucleus accumbens. *Progress in Neuro-Psychopharmacology & Biological Psychiatry, 19,* 467–473.

Laties, V. G., & Weiss, B. (1981). The amphetamine margin in sports. *Federation Proceedings, 40,* 2689–2692.

Lyon, M., & Robbins, T. W. (1975). The action of central nervous system stimulant drugs: A general theory concerning amphetamine effects. In E. Essman & L. Valzelli (Eds.), *Current developments in psychopharmacology* (Vol. 2, pp. 89–163). New York: Spectrum.

Marshall, J. F., Odell, S. J., & Weihmuller, F. B. (1993). Dopamine–glutamate interactions in methamphetamine-induced neurotoxicity. *Journal of Neural Transmission, 91,* 241–254.

Mazurski, E. J., & Beninger, R. J. (1988). Stimulant effects of apomorphine and (+)-Amphetamine in rats with varied habituation to test environment. *Pharmacology, Biochemistry and Behavior, 29,* 249–255.

McGeorge, A. J., & Faull, R. L. M. (1989). The organization of the projection from the cerebral cortex to the striatum in the rat. *Neuroscience, 29,* 503–537.

Meredith, G. E., Pennartz, C. M. A., & Groenewegen, H. J. (1993). The cellular framework for chemical signalling in the nucleus accumbens. In G. W. Arbuthnott & P. C. Emson (Eds.), *Chemical signalling in the basal ganglia. Progress in brain research* (Vol. 99, pp. 3–24). Amsterdam: Elsevier.

Moore, S., & Kenyon, P. (1994). Atypical antipsychotics, clozapine and sulpiride do not antagonise amphetamine-induced stereotyped locomotion. *Psychopharmacology, 114,* 123–130.

Mueller, K., Hollingsworth, E. M., & Cross, D. R. (1989). Another look at amphetamine-induced stereotyped locomotor activity in rats using a new statistic to measure locomotor stereotypy. *Psychopharmacology, 97,* 74–79.

Nash, J. F., & Yamamoto, B. K. (1993). Effect of D-amphetamine on the extracellular concentrations of glutamate and dopamine in iprindole-treated rats. *Brain Research, 627,* 1–8.

Pennartz, C. M. A., Groenewegen, H. J., & DaSilva, F. H. L. (1994). The nucleus accumbens as a complex of functionally distinct neuronal ensembles: An integra-

tion of behavioural, electrophysiological and anatomical data. *Progress in Neurobiology, 42,* 719–761.

Pierce, R. C., & Rebec, G. V. (1995). Iontophoresis in the neostriatum of awake, unrestrained rats: Differential effects of dopamine, glutamate, and ascorbate on motor- and nonmotor-related neurons. *Neuroscience, 67,* 313–324.

Pierce, R. C., Rowlett, J. K., Rebec, G. V., & Bardo, M. T. (1995). Ascorbate potentiates amphetamine-induced conditioned place preference and forebrain dopamine release in rats. *Brain Research, 688,* 21–26.

Randrup, A., & Munkvad, I. (1970). Biochemical, anatomical, and physiological investigations of stereotyped behavior induced by amphetamine. In E. Costa & S. Garattini (Eds.), *Amphetamines and related compounds* (pp. 695–713). New York: Raven.

Rebec, G. V. (1987). Electrophysiological pharmacology of amphetamine. In J. Marwah (Ed.), *Monographs in neural science: Vol. 13. Neurobiology of drug abuse* (pp. 1–33). Basal, Switzerland: Karger, Basal.

Rebec, G. V. (1991). Changes in brain and behavior produced by amphetamine: A perspective based on microdialysis, voltammetry, and single-unit electrophysiology in freely moving animals, In R. R. Watson (Ed.), *Biochemistry and physiology of substance abuse* (Vol. III, pp. 93–115). Boca Raton, FL: CRC.

Rebec, G. V., & Pierce, R. C. (1994). A vitamin as neuromodulator: Ascorbate release into the extracellular fluid of the brain regulates dopaminergic and glutamatergic transmission. *Progress in Neurobiology, 43,* 537–565.

Rebec, G. V., & Segal, D. S. (1979). Enhanced responsiveness to intraventricular infusion of amphetamine following its repeated systemic administration. *Psychopharmacology, 62.* 101–102.

Rebec, G. V., & Segal, D. S. (1980). Apparent tolerance to some aspects of amphetamine stereotypy with long-term treatment. *Pharmacology, Biochemistry and Behavior, 13,* 793–797.

Rebec, G. V., & Bashore, T. R. (1984). Critical issues in assessing the behavioral effects of amphetamine. *Neuroscience and Biobehavioral Reviews, 8,* 153–159.

Rebec, G. V., Christensen, J. R. C., Guerra, C., & Bardo, M. T. (1997). Regional and temporal differences in dopamine efflux in the nucleus accumbens during free-choice novelty. *Brain Research, 776,* 61–67.

Rebec, G. V., White, I. M., & Puotz, J. K. (1997). Responses of neurons in dorsal striatum during amphetamine-induced focused stereotypy. *Psychopharmacology, 130,* 343–351.

Ricaurte, G. A., Sabol, K. E., & Seiden, L. S. (1994). Functional consequences of neurotoxic amphetamine exposure. In A. K. Cho & D. S. Segal (Eds.), *Amphetamine and its analogs* (pp. 297–313). New York: Academic Press.

Ridley, R. M., & Baker, H. F. (1982). Stereotypy in monkeys and humans. *Psychological Medicine, 12,* 61–72.

Robinson, T. E. (1991). The neurobiology of amphetamine psychosis—Evidence from studies with an animal model. In T. Nakazawa (Ed.), *Biological basis of schizophrenic disorders.* (Vol. 14, pp. 185–201). Tokyo: Japan Scientific Societies Press.

Robinson, T. E., & Becker, J. B. (1986). Enduring changes in brain and behavior produced by chronic amphetamine administration: A review and evaluation of animal models of amphetamine psychosis. *Brain Research Reviews, 11,* 157–198.

Rosa-Kenig, A., Puotz, J. K., & Rebec, G. V. (1993). Involvement of D1 and D2 dopamine receptors in amphetamine-induced changes in striatal activity in behaving rats. *Brain Research, 619,* 347–351.

Ryan, L. J., Young, S. J., Segal, D. S., & Groves, P. M. (1989). Antigromically identified striatonigral projection neurons in the chronically implanted behaving rat: Relations of cell firing to amphetamine-induced behaviors. *Behavioral Neuroscience, 103,* 3–14.

Ryan, L. J., Linder, J. C., Martone, M. E., & Groves, P. M. (1990). Histological and ultrastructural evidence that D-amphetamine causes degeneration in neostriatum and frontal cortex of rats. *Brain Research, 518,* 67–77.

Sato, M., Numachi, Y., & Hamamura, T. (1992). Relapse of paranoid psychotic state in methamphetamine model of schizophrenia. *Schizophrenia Bulletin, 18,* 115–122.

Schiørring, E. (1979). An open-field study of stereotyped locomotor activity in amphetamine-treated rats. *Psychopharmacology* (Berlin), *66,* 281–287.

Schiørring, E. (1981). Psychopathology induced by "speed drugs." *Pharmacology, Biochemistry and Behavior, 14,* 109–122.

Segal, D. S. (1975). Behavioral and neurochemical correlates of repeated D-amphetamine administration. In A. J. Mandell (Ed.), *Advances in biochemical psychopharmacology* (pp. 247–266). New York: Raven.

Segal, D. S., & Janowsky, D. S. (1978). Psychostimulant-induced behavioral effects: Possible models of schizophrenia. In A. Lipton, A. Di Mascio, & K. F. Killam (Eds.), *Psychopharmacology: A generation of progress* (pp. 1113–1123). New York: Raven.

Segal, D. S., & Kuczenski, R. (1992). In vivo microdialysis reveals a diminished amphetamine-induced DA response corresponding to behavioral sensitization produced by repeated amphetamine pretreatment. *Brain Research, 571,* 330–337.

Segal, D. S., & Kuczenski, R. (1994). Behavioral pharmacology of amphetamine. In A. Cho & D. S. Segal (Eds.), *Amphetamine and its analogs* (pp. 115–149). San Diego, CA: Academic Press.

Segal, D. S., Weinberger, S., Cahill, J., & McCunney, S. (1980). Multiple daily amphetamine administration: Behavioral and neurochemical alterations. *Science, 207,* 904–907.

Segal, D. S., Kuczenski, R., & Florin, S. M. (1995). Does dizocilpine (MK-801) selectively block the enhanced responsiveness to repeated amphetamine administration? *Behavioral Neuroscience, 109,* 532–546.

Seiden, L. S., Sabol, K. E., & Ricaurte, G. A. (1993). Amphetamine: Effects on catecholamine systems and behavior. *Annual Review of Pharmacology and Toxicology, 33,* 639–677.

Sharp, T., Zetterstrom, T., Ljungberg, T., & Ungerstedt, U. (1987). A direct comparison of amphetamine-induced behaviours and regional brain dopamine release in the rat using intracerebral dialysis. *Brain Research, 401,* 322–330.

Smith, A. D., & Bolam, J. P. (1990). The neural network of the basal ganglia as revealed by the study of synaptic connections of identified neurones. *Trends in Neurosciences, 13,* 259–265.

Snyder, S. H. (1973). Amphetamine psychosis: A "model" schizophrenia mediated by catecholamines. *American Journal of Psychiatry, 130,* 61–67.

Steinpreis, R. E., Sokolowski, J. D., Papanikolaou, A., & Salamone, J. D. (1994). The effects of haloperidol and clozapine on PCP- and amphetamine-induced suppression of social behavior in the rat. *Pharmacology, Biochemistry and Behavior, 47,* 579–585.

Stephans, S. E., & Yamamoto, B. K. (1994). Methamphetamine-induced neurotoxicity: Roles for glutamate and dopamine efflux. *Synapse, 17,* 203–209.

Stevens, J., Livermore, A., & Cronan, J. (1977). Effects of deafening and blindfolding on amphetamine-induced stereotypy in the cat. *Physiology and Behavior, 18,* 809–812.

Stewart, J., & Eikelboom, R. (1987). Conditioned drug effects. In L. L. Iversen, S. D. Iversen, & S. H. Snyder (Eds.), *Handbook of psychopharmacology* (Vol. 19, pp. 1–57). New York: Plenum.

Sulzer, D., & Rayport, S. (1990). Amphetamine and other psychostimulants reduce ph gradients in midbrain dopaminergic neurons and chromaffin granules—A mechanism of action. *Neuron, 5,* 797–808.

Tolbert, L. C., Thomas T. N., Middaugh, L. D., & Zemp, J. W. (1979). Effect of ascorbic acid on neurochemical, behavioral, and physiological systems mediated by catecholamines. *Life Science, 25,* 2189–2185.

Tschanz, J. T., & Rebec, G. V. (1988). Atypical antipsychotic drugs block selective components of amphetamine-induced stereotypy. *Pharmacology, Biochemistry and Behavior, 31,* 519–522.

Tschanz, J. T., Haracz, J. L., Griffith, K. E., & Rebec, G. V. (1991). Bilateral cortical ablations attenuate amphetamine-induced excitations of neostriatal motor-related neurons in freely moving rats. *Neuroscience Letters, 134,* 127–130.

Urba-Holmgren, R., Holmgren, B., & Aguiar, M. (1977). Circadian variation in an amphetamine-induced motor response. *Pharmacology, Biochemistry and Behavior, 7,* 571–572.

Walaas, I. (1981). Biochemical evidence for overlapping neocortical and allocortical glutamate projections to the nucleus accumbens and rostral caudatoputamen in the rat brain. *Neuroscience, 6,* 399–405.

Wambebe, C., & Sokomba, E. (1986). Some behavioral and EEG effects of ascorbic acid in rats. *Psychopharmacology, 89,* 167–170.

Wang, Z. R., & Rebec, G. V. (1993). Neuronal and behavioral correlates of intrastriatal infusions of amphetamine in freely moving rats. *Brain Research, 627,* 79–88.

Wang, Z. R., Bonta, M., & Rebec, G. V. (1994). Neuroethopharmacology of amphetamine and antipsychotic drugs in nucleus accumbens and amygdala of socially interacting rats. *Society for Neuroscience Abstracts, 20,* 1030.

West, M. O., Michael, A. J., Knowles, S. E., Chapin, J. K., & Woodward, D. J. (1987). Striatal unit activity and the linkage between sensory and motor events. In J. S. Schneider & T. I. Lidsky (Eds.), *Basal ganglia and behavior: Sensory aspects of motor functioning* (pp. 27–35). Toronto, Ontario, Canada: Huber.

White, I. M., Flory, G. S., Hooper, K. C., Speciale, J., Banks, D. A., & Rebec, G. V. (1995). Phencyclidine-induced excitation of striatal neurons in behaving rats: Reversal by haloperidol and clozapine. *Journal of Neural Transmission, 102,* 99–112.

White, L. K., Maurer, M., Kraft, M. E., Oh, C., & Rebec, G. V. (1990). Intrastriatal infusions of ascorbate antagonize the behavioral response to amphetamine. *Pharmacology, Biochemistry and Behavior, 36,* 485–489.

Wolf, M. E., & Khansa, M. R. (1991). Repeated administration of MK-801 produces sensitization to its own locomotor stimulant effects but blocks sensitization to amphetamine. *Brain Research, 562,* 164–168.

Zahm, D. S., & Brog, J. S. (1992). On the significance of subterritories in the accumbens part of the rat ventral striatum. *Neuroscience, 50,* 751–767.

32

Psychological and Psychiatric Consequences of Amphetamines

STEPHEN A. WYATT AND DOUGLAS ZIEDONIS

Introduction

"Speed Freak," a name for chronic and high-dose amphetamine abusers made popular in the late 1960s was a result of the bizarre behavior they often displayed. The amphetamine abuser may develop symptoms of anxiety, hypervigilance, impaired judgment, and psychosis. Psychotic behavior resulting from chronic amphetamine use has been examined in the scientific literature for decades. In 1938, the first of these reports discussed the link between psychotic behavior and the use of amphetamines in the treatment of narcolepsy (Young & Scoville, 1938). "Speed kills," a phrase that originated in the early 1970s, refers to the lethal physical maladies or bizarrely morbid behavior associated with excessive and repeated use of amphetamines. This behavior was characterized by profound persecutory delusions, ideas of reference, and hallucinatory effects. It was during this time that the intravenous administration of large doses of amphetamines became increasingly prevalent. Similar behavior continues to be seen in association with both intravenous and the increasing popular inhaled misuse of this drug.

This chapter reviews the psychological and psychiatric consequences of amphetamine use, including the related behavioral pharmacology and neurobiology. The psychological effects of amphetamines appear to proceed through a progression of phases and to vary greatly with dosage, route of administration, and chronicity. Toxic symptoms are more likely to occur with chronic and heavy amphetamine use than with cocaine use. This chapter reviews the psychiatric disorders included in the *Diagnostic and Statistical Manual of Mental Disorders* (*DSM-IV*; American Psychiatric Association, 1994) related to amphetamine usage. These disorders include amphetamine intoxication, amphetamine withdrawal, and amphetamine-induced psychosis, anxiety, mood, sexual, and sleep disorders. The review of these disorders describes their psychological and behavioral symptoms, along with the neurobiological and clinical issues. In some regions, amphetamine abuse is common among psychiatric patients and the combination results in diagnostic uncertainty and the clinical need to treat both disorders. This chapter discusses the issue of concurrent amphetamine addiction and psychiatric illness.

STEPHEN A. WYATT AND DOUGLAS ZIEDONIS • Department of Psychiatry, Yale University School of Medicine, New Haven, Connecticut 06519.

Handbook of Substance Abuse: Neurobehavioral Pharmacology, edited by Tarter *et al.* Plenum Press, New York, 1998.

Amphetamine Intoxication

According to the *DSM-IV,* amphetamine intoxication occurs when clinically significant maladaptive behavioral or psychological changes coincide with the use of amphetamines. Amphetamine intoxication begins with a "high feeling" and progresses to euphoria that might include enhanced vigor, increased talking, alertness, and grandiosity. Ninety-seven percent of intoxicated human subjects report that amphetamine use produces positive effects while only 3% report negative effects. The most common positive effect is euphoria followed, in order, by stimulation, reduced fatigue, and diminished appetite. The euphoric effect is dependent on the strength of the dose (Fischman *et al.*, 1976). Amphetamine use tends to increase after the positive reinforcement of euphoria, increased energy, vocational productivity, and improved social interactions (King & Ellinwood, 1992). Higher doses and routes of rapid administration (smoking or intravenous use) produce increased effects, but also result in a higher tolerance to euphoria. In the few patients who report negative side effects the most common are restlessness and anxiety (Council on Scientific Affairs, 1978; Jaffe, 1985). Other negative effects include disruptive interpersonal sensitivity, anxiety, tension, hyperactivity, hypervigilance, stereotypical and repetitive behavior, anger, fighting, and impaired judgment (*DSM-IV*).

Amphetamine intoxication is subtyped in the *DSM-IV* according to the presence of perceptual disturbances. In this case, hallucinations occur with intact reality testing, or auditory, visual, or tactile illusions occur without symptoms of delirium. In other words, the amphetamine user knows that the hallucinations are drug-induced and are not real. Hallucinations with intact reality testing suggest an amphetamine-induced psychotic disorder.

The effect of amphetamines on the individual proceeds through phases similar to those in cocaine use, but toxic symptoms are more likely to occur with chronic and heavy amphetamine use than cocaine use because of the difficulty of sustaining high blood levels of cocaine. The toxic side effects on behavior can include symptoms of hyperactivity, increased sensitivity to environmental stimuli, hallucinations, and stereotyped behaviors such as disassembling and reassembling objects (King &

Ellinwood, 1992). Amphetamine intoxication is also associated with impairments in social or occupational functioning (*DSM-IV*). Physical toxicity reflects the autonomic overstimulation (Chiarello & Cole, 1987). The physical presentation may include increased or decreased heart rate, dilated pupils, elevated or lowered blood pressure, sweating or chills, nausea or vomiting, weight loss, psychomotor agitation or retardation, muscle weakness, respiratory depression, chest pain, or cardiac arrhythmia. In severe cases, confusion, seizures, movement disorder symptoms, or coma can result.

Euphoria from amphetamines is mediated by the direct neuronal release of dopamine. Amphetamines also cause norepinephrine and serotonin release from presynaptic terminals, both centrally and peripherally, by indirect monoamine agonist activity. There is an increased activation of postsynaptic receptors as a result of catecholamine buildup in the synaptic cleft. Stimulation of the central nervous system is seen primarily in the cerebral cortex, striatum, limbic system, and brainstem. This results in increased alertness and wakefulness, elevation of mood, decreased appetite, and insomnia seen with intoxication. However, at toxic doses, these same neuronal events produce convulsions, stereotypic movements, or psychosis.

Amphetamine Dependence

The criterion for the diagnosis of dependence on amphetamines is similar to other drugs of abuse. Establishment of a physical dependence, social disruption, or both, needs to be determined. The evidence of tolerance and withdrawal symptoms resulting from chronic use of these drugs is clear. It is also clear that the addiction to these drugs can cause significant disruption in one's social relationships, family interactions, and physical well-being.

In the presentation of the patient dependent on amphetamines there may be a flattened affect and the user may experience feelings of fatigue, sadness, or social withdrawal as the catecholamine stores are depleted with prolonged use of amphetamines. It may take several days to replenish the stores; during this time, the chronic user may experience depressive symptoms. The neurochemical difference between acute and chronic use of amphetamines is correlated with the ratio of norepinephrine to dopamine. The acute effect is the primary depletion of norepinephrine and the chronic effect is the depletion of dopamine (Gunne & Lewander, 1967).

In animals, the primary behavioral effects of amphetamines are increased motor behavior, increased arousal, induction of stereotypy, and suppressed food intake (Chiarello & Cole, 1987). As the dose is increased, there is a development of increased stereotypic behavior (Scheel-Kruger, Braestrup, Nielson, Golembiowska, & Mogilnicka, 1977). When given open access to amphetamines, monkeys adopt a use pattern that quickly becomes erratic, excessive, toxic, and ultimately lethal (Johanson, Balster, & Bonese, 1976). It has been postulated that this pattern of drug use is partly reflective of a stereotypic behavior (Collins, Lesse, & Dagan, 1979). Controlled animal studies which depleted dopamine in the nucleus accumbens suppressed amphetamine self-administration (Lyness, Friedle, & Moore, 1979). The ventral tegmental area was also found to be capable of inhibiting the reinforcement pattern of use. This phenomenon is hypothesized to be secondary to this area's being the principal source of dopamine to the nucleus accumbens (Roberts & Kobb, 1982). Researchers have postulated that the prefrontal cortex is involved in the initiation of the stimulant's effects while the nucleus accumbens is involved in the maintenance of the response (Goeders, Dworkin, & Smith, 1986).

The enhancement of motor behavior with repeated amphetamine administration is indicative of increased sensitivity. This increased sensitivity is seen in the augmentation of the hyperactivity, stereotypy, and convulsions seen with chronic use of amphetamines and cocaine. Interestingly, when administration of pimozide, haloperidol, or diazepam prevented the stereotypic movements from ever starting, there was no evidence of the sensitization of this behavior. However, when the behavior had already been established, it could not be extinguished by the administration of these drugs (Beninger & Hahn, 1983; S. R. Weiss, Post, Pert, Woodward, & Murman, 1989).

Both the total dose and scheduling of administration appear to play into the development of this sensitization. When amphetamine was delivered in a continuous fashion by way of a subcutaneous pellet, there was not the usual sensitization (Reith, Benuck, & Lajtha, 1987). This might also be a result of the constant drug level's interfering with behavioral determinants such as conditioning.

After the administration of amphetamines, a cross-tolerance will develop with other stimulants, including cocaine. A tolerance to the positive subjective effects of methamphetamine results in the abuse of greater amounts with prolonged use. This tolerance is approximately twofold and disappears relatively rapidly on the withdrawal of the stimulus (Fischman, Schuster, Javaid, Hatano, & Davis, 1985). Ultimately, there is an increased tolerance to the positive effects of intoxication and an increased sensitivity to the negative effects.

The ability to predict the development of dependence in any one individual has been studied and there is no consensus. Evidence for childhood experience with neurotic disturbance in many of these patients is frequently obtained (Hawks, Mitcheson, Ogborne, & Edwards, 1969). This correlates with poor social adjustment in later life. Poor social development may show up in the way of poor social support available to the patient while in recovery from prolonged drug use and should be taken into consideration when formulating a treatment plan.

The discussion of dependency as it relates to amphetamine abuse is multifaceted. There has long been a debate over whether there is a "drug-taking personality." An extensive analysis of the characteristics of the personality of amphetamine users identified the subjective characteristics of outgoing, emotionally unstable, dominant, enthusiastic, suspicious, and tense (Brien, Kleiman, & Eisenman, 1972). A similar analysis of British urban adolescents identified some disturbance in motivation, greater timidity, increased apprehensions, anxieties, introversion, and radicalism in comparison with nonusers (Crockett & Marks, 1969). Amphetamine dependent people describe themselves as more reserved, tough-minded, independent, and dominant than other drug-user groups. They report a strong need for self-sufficiency (Spotts & Shontz, 1991). However, there is not a specific personality disorder that is more commonly linked to one drug over another (Campbell & Stark, 1990). The same study points to the possible development of characteristics of a personality disorder with long-term amphetamine abuse. Preexisting character pathology may very well be a factor in the development of a treatment plan (Hensala, Epstein, & Blacker, 1967).

Studies of platelet MAO activity reveal consistent levels between individuals that correlate with certain personality traits. The evaluation of these levels in the amphetamine abuser showed a higher level of activity than that seen in alcoholics. Alcohol-dependent individuals show lower than normal levels. Speculation over the etiology for these high levels leads to the question whether these levels are an indication of a personality type that might abuse amphetamine, or whether the abuse itself raises the levels over time. This might also contribute to the development of depression described as occurring on withdrawal from these drugs.

The controversy over the idea of self-medication has wound its way through the literature for a number of years (Khantzian, 1985). There are a variety of arguments against this theory. Some take issue with the use of the word "medication." Others point out the strong evidence for a biological determinant of the development of dependence on substances. However, the literature clearly shows an initial subjective improvement in depressive symptoms, including mood, affect, and concentration, if amphetamines are taken in an appropriate regimen. Individuals with mood instability may recognize a similar response and therefore find some solace in the use of these drugs. The difference is the desire of some individuals to continue to use these drugs in the face of deterioration of their physical and psychological well-being and thus establishing a dependent pattern of drug use.

Amphetamine Withdrawal

The behavioral symptoms of withdrawal are described in a syndrome characterized by the development of dysphoric mood and the following physiological changes: fatigue, vivid and unpleasant dreams, insomnia or hypersomnia, increased appetite, and psychomotor retardation or agitation. Anhedonia and drug craving can also be present, but are not part of the diagnostic criteria. "Amphetamine crash" is characterized by intense and unpleasant feelings of lassitude and depression, generally requiring several days of rest and recuperation. Weight loss commonly occurs during heavy stimulant use, whereas a marked increase in appetite with rapid weight gain is often observed during withdrawal. Depressive symptoms may last several days and may be accompanied by suicidal ideation (*DSM-IV*). As with other substances, the psychological symptoms of protracted abstinence include mood liability, irritability, and sleep difficulties. In some cases, the more toxic symptoms, including psychosis, can remain during prolonged periods of abstinence.

Amphetamine-Induced Psychosis

A 1968 report by Rockwell and Ostwald in San Francisco showed that patients admitted to a local psychiatric hospital with covert use of amphetamine use prior to admission were most frequently diagnosed with schizophrenia (Rockwell & Ostwald, 1968). There is strong reason to believe that many amphetamine-abusing patients have been misdiagnosed on their original presentation. A frequent problem of identifying these patients in a mental health center is the lack of drug screening and substance abuse history taking on admission. The omission of this important information may be secondary to the initial denial of drug use by the patient on admission (Davis, 1970).

Amphetamine psychosis has been divided into three stages. The early stage is associated with curiosity, repetitive examining, searching, and sorting behaviors. The intermediate stage is noted for the appearance of suspiciousness. By the end stage, this suspiciousness has led to ideas of reference, persecutory delusions, and hallucinations marked by a fearful, panic-stricken, agitated, overactive state (Ellinwood, Sudilovsky, & Nelson, 1973). It is clear that amphetamine psychosis typically develops over time, often with continually larger amounts delivered by any route of administration, or a large, fixed amount delivered intravenously.

The amphetamine-intoxicated patient with psychotic symptoms may present with paranoia, hypersexuality, or delusional thinking. Perceptual disorders such as visual, auditory, olfactory, and tactile hallucinations may all be part of the presentation. Interestingly, however, the patient's orientation and memory often remain intact. This altered mental state, though typically lasting only as long as the intoxication, has been reported to have lasted days to weeks.

Differentiation from Schizophrenia and Schizoaffective Disorder

Diagnostic uncertainty is often the case for the individual with both psychosis and recent amphetamine abuse. The dilemma comes in differentiating amphetamine-induced psychosis from a primary psychotic illness. Abuse of a variety of substances can present with psychosis, and they can modify the expression of symptoms of schizophrenia. Psychotic symptoms appear in differing phases of amphetamine use, including intoxication, dependent use, or on withdrawal from the drug. Thus there can be a variety of presentations. Furthermore, a period of abstinence cannot be counted on to eliminate the diagnostic uncertainty.

The initial presentation of the current user experiencing psychotic symptoms includes, most prominently, paranoid delusions and auditory hallucinations that are both very similar to schizophrenia. Most frequently, however,

the psychosis of the amphetamine user resolves over time. This fact leaves open the question of whether the individual with persistent symptoms did in fact have a predisposition to a psychotic illness and whether the misuse of amphetamine-like drugs facilitated the expression of the illness (Breakey, Goodell, Lorenz, & McHugh, 1974).

After long-term amphetamine dependency the presentation of the psychotic patient has an appearance very similar to schizophrenia. A schizophrenia-like syndrome has been reported in the literature for many years (Connell, 1958). The problem has been thought to be an acute psychosis instead of a chronic syndrome. There is typically a gradual recovery from amphetamine psychosis after a period of abstinence. This recovery has been thought to occur in a matter of weeks, but there are reports that symptoms persist for months (Sato, 1990). There are also reports of recurrent psychotic symptoms both spontaneously, and with intoxication, months to years later (Sato, Chen, Akiyama, & Otsuki, 1983; R. D. Weiss, Mirin, Michael, & Sollogub, 1986). However, McClellan and colleagues performed an interesting 7-year longitudinal study in the 1970s that shows evidence for the development of chronic schizophrenia in previously amphetamine-dependent patients (McLellan, Woody, & O'Brien, 1979). There is still some controversy over whether schizophrenia can be caused by these drugs.

Clinically, there appears to be a lasting sensitivity to amphetamine and consequent psychosis. A Japanese review showed 73 cases of previously reported methamphetamine psychosis who had a relapse into psychosis after one week or less of methamphetamine abuse. There are also reports of alcohol- and stress-induced psychosis relapse in patients previously diagnosed with methamphetamine-induced psychosis (Sato, 1990).

There may be some recognizable differences, on presentation, between the psychosis of the schizophrenic and that of the amphetamine abuser. First, there may be more olfactory and tactile-type hallucinations associated with amphetamines. The tactile hallucination "bugs under the skin" may even result in a characteristic excoriated appearance of the skin. Second, the amphetamine-intoxicated patient may demonstrate a clearer sensorium and orientation. Last, the usual flattening of affect or formal thought disorder of the schizophrenic patient is not typically as profound in the amphetamine-intoxicated or -dependent patient.

Neurobiology of Amphetamine Psychosis

The similarities between paranoid schizophrenia and amphetamine-induced psychosis have resulted in the study of amphetamine psychosis as the model of schizophrenia. A prospective study to determine the prolonged effect of these drugs in human studies is not feasible; consequently, the chronic use of these drugs remains poorly understood. However, in the acute setting, the neurobiology has opened an interesting window into the development of psychopathology.

In animal studies, prolonged high doses of methamphetamine and structurally related derivatives produces persistent depletion of dopamine, resulting in neuroaxonal swelling and degeneration (Ellison & Eison, 1983). The reduction of dopamine production takes place through various mechanisms, including the reduced synthesis of the enzyme tyrosine hydroxylase and its reuptake. These events are all indicative of degeneration of dopamine axon terminals seen in the striatum, frontal cortex, nucleus accumbens, and amygdala, with little evidence of midbrain injury (Seiden, Commin, Vosmer, Axt, & Marek, 1988). Permanent depletion may take place in the caudate nucleus as seen in nonprimates. The accumulation of 6-hydroxydopamine, a toxic metabolite of dopamine, may be the result of stimulant inhibition of the monoamine oxidase and thus degeneration of the axon terminal (Lieberman, Kinon, & Loebel, 1990). A second theory of neurotoxicity involves the glutamate system and its projections from the cortex to the striatum and limbic dopamine neurons. Evidence exists that overstimulated amino acid activity in the glutamatergic neurons may lead to dopamine neurotoxicity (Sonsalla, Nicklas, & Heikkila, 1989). Interestingly, PCP also works through the glutamate system in inducing behavioral sensitization.

Amphetamine-Induced Anxiety Disorder

The most frequent reason for amphetamine-related admission to a mental health hospital is psychosis, but the most common reason for prolonged symptomatology secondary to amphetamines is the associated anxiety and depression. One reason for the increased prevalence of these disorders is the mere fact that they are common in the general public, and would consequently be expected to be seen more commonly in the amphetamine-abusing population also. Second, the drug itself causes changes in mood and behavior. Amphetamines will cause symptoms of anxiety with anxious mood, rapid heart rate, and occasionally, when taken at higher doses, panic attacks. However, unlike those individuals who have concurrent anxiety disorder with amphetamine abuse, these individuals will have a dissolution of symptoms on termination of drug use. This points to the importance of determining the origin of the anxiety, a determination which can assist greatly in the development of the treatment plan for the patient.

After persistent periods of intoxication, the patient may develop a "reactive attitude" characterized by sudden, disproportionately startled reactions with a jumpy, agitated quality. This "reactive attitude" is often accompanied by an increase in the speed of movements and, later, the appearance of increased agitation and activity (Ellinwood et al., 1973). For example, a slight sound may cause an aggressive turning of the head. When these behaviors were seen in cat studies researchers hypothesized that the reactions may have been associated with hallucinatory events.

The development of panic-like reactions is common on presentation after chronic abuse. There have been reports that this reaction to amphetamines can be reinforced to the point of causing a diagnostic panic disorder

(Schuckit, 1989). A general fear of "losing control" has often been seen in the chronic user of amphetamine-like drugs. These patients often become extremely anxious over their physical well-being as a result of the adverse physical effects the stimulant is having on their bodies. For example, when they are experiencing palpitations as a result of the stimulant, they may feel that they are going to have a heart attack and die.

Neurobiology of Anxiety Disorder as Seen in Amphetamine Users

Overstimulation of the catecholamine and dopamine systems may result in increased environmental stimulation, anxiety, hypervigilance, and suspiciousness. Abnormal glucose metabolism may also play a role in this negative state. Glucose metabolism has been thought to be involved in the development of both adult and childhood attention deficit hyperactivity disorder (ADHD). Evidence points to the normalization of glucose metabolism in children after the initiation of amphetamine or methylphenidate treatment. Positron emission tomography (PET) studies, however, have been unsuccessful in proving this hypothesis. Investigators believe this may be secondary to the inability to attain adequate resolution of certain areas because of the partial volume effects (Wise, 1985). In rat studies, both methylphenidate and *d*-amphetamine significantly increased glucose metabolism in the nucleus accumbens, the only brain region where these stimulants have similar effects, suggesting a role for the accumbens in the effect of psychostimulants in ADHD (Mesulam, 1986). Also supporting this is evidence that caffeine, also a stimulant, is not effective in controlling ADHD (Elkins *et al.*, 1981) and has no effect on metabolism in the nucleus accumbens in rats (Nehlig, Lucignani, Kadekaro, Porrino, & Sokoloff, 1984).

Diagnosis

The diagnosis of an amphetamine-induced anxiety disorder is made primarily through a history of amphetamine use or detection by urine screening. If the anxiety is profound enough to bring the patient to an emergency department, and if this level of anxiety is a new experience, the patient will usually offer the history of recent stimulant use. If, however, the patient has used stimulants chronically and is in a state of denial about the problem, this history may be more difficult to obtain.

The determination of whether the anxiety problem is primary or amphetamine induced is difficult. It requires a careful examination of the patient's personal and family history. Frequently, a prolonged drug-free period will be necessary before a determination can be made. The length of the drug-free period is dependent on the amount and duration of the patient's stimulant use.

Amphetamine-Induced Mood Disorders

The affective disorder that results from the withdrawal from amphetamines has been well documented in the development of dependency (Churchill, Burgess, Pead, & Gill, 1993; Grinspoon & Hedblom, 1975). However, the development of tolerance, which appears to occur as amphetamine increases catecholaminergic activity and stimulation of the noradrenergic system affecting the reward centers of the brain, appears to be the most powerful reinforcer of its use. This evidence points to a psychopharmacologic dependence on the drug as a result of a desire for its pleasurable effects rather than an avoidance of the consequences of withdrawal. The common presentation of the amphetamine abuser is the initial appearance of anxiety that evolves into a profound depressed state on abstinence. Associated with this picture, during the early phase of abstinence, is a period characterized by affective instability (depression and irritability), anhedonia, lack of motivation, and the diminution of cognitive functions. "Burnt out" former "speed freaks" are characterized as sitting around staring into space. This is similar to schizophrenia with affective blunting, impoverished speech and thought, anhedonia, and asociability. These individuals, like schizophrenics, remain hypersensitive to stimulant drugs and to psychological stressors. But unlike schizophrenics, these patients remain well oriented.

Depressive symptoms associated with withdrawal have been experimentally identified in rat studies to be correlated with dopamine levels in the ventral striatum (Rossetti, Hmaidan, & Gessa, 1992). There appears to be an initial delay in the decrease in the extracellular levels of dopamine as compared with either alcohol or opiates, but the reduction of these levels remains for a longer period of time. This is correlated clinically with the prolonged period of dysphoria seen in the individual withdrawn from amphetamines after chronic use (Gawin, 1991). In studies of rats being withdrawn from amphetamines there was a reverse in the fall of dopamine after blockade of NMDA receptors. Rat studies have also been performed to look at the role of noradrenaline in the development of withdrawal depression in the locus cerruleus (LC). In these studies the postwithdrawal period showed enhanced sensitivity to the acute effects of stimulants, an enhanced alpha-2 autoreceptor-mediated hyperpolarization in the LC neurons, and enhancement of the sedative properties of the agonist clonidine (Harris & Williams, 1992). A supersensitivity of the alpha-2 autoreceptors has also been demonstrated, indicating a reduction in extracellular concentrations of noradrenaline. The downregulation of catecholamine release is likely correlated with the anhedonia, dysphoria, and drug craving seen with stimulant withdrawal.

Amphetamine-Induced Sexual Dysfunction

The literature is rich with anecdotal accounts of the effects of amphetamine use in relation to sexual life. Intoxication may initially enhance sexual arousal. The degree of arousal is partially based on the user's previous sexual development. It is important to obtain a good history of sexual development in order not to miss a primary sexual dysfunction. If there is a propensity toward perversity of sexual behavior it may be enhanced with amphetamine intoxication. There are references throughout the intravenous drug abuse literature describing the attachment to "the needle" in a sexual way. There are accounts of this "love affair" in the intravenous amphetamine literature as well. A majority of reports in the literature indicate there is an increase in the sexual drive with simple intoxication. There may be repression in some users secondary to being overwhelmed with the profound sexual drive resulting in sexual inadequacy and distress. Others more comfortable with this increased sexual drive report prolonged sexual activity prior to orgasm.

The picture changes dramatically with dependent use of amphetamines. Once a dependent pattern is established individuals more frequently report a diminution of sexual desire, possibly secondary to the decrease in maintaining interpersonal bonds, the neuroendocrinologic effects of this pattern of use, or both. According to the *DSM-IV* amphetamine-induced sexual dysfunction must include marked distress or interpersonal difficulty.

It is important to rule out other causes for this dysfunction. Therefore a careful sexual history should be taken and a complete physical exam completed. This information will be helpful in establishing the correct diagnosis and in clearly specifying the area of dysfunction: impaired desire, arousal, or orgasm.

Amphetamine-Induced Sleep Disorders

Disorders of sleep have an interesting relationship with amphetamine-like drugs. They are the drug of choice for the chronic disorder of inappropriate sleep, narcolepsy; the amphetamines have been used to treat the socially disruptive and public health risk of inappropriate sleep. However, when abused they can disrupt the normal sleep cycle resulting in the behaviors seen with sleep deprivation: agitation, mood lability, and so on.

The diagnosis of an amphetamine-induced sleep disorder is made by first establishing a clinical need for treatment. This should include impairment in social or occupational functioning or both. Second, the clinician should ascertain that the disorder of sleep is closely associated with amphetamine intoxication or withdrawal. This is defined in the *DSM-IV* as occurring within a month of use of this drug. In order to establish this second criterion one needs to obtain a clear history of previous sleep behavior to rule out a primary sleep disorder or one attributed to another medical or substance use disorder. A physical exam is important to establish this criterion. Delirium may be confused with a profound sleep disorder and should be ruled out as one reviews the history and performs a physical exam.

Once the diagnosis has been established and it is clear that this disorder is the prominent feature of an intoxication or withdrawal picture, further subtyping should be used if appropriate: insomnia, hypersomnia, parasomnia, or mixed types. The diagnosis can then be more specifically stated as occurring in either intoxication or withdrawal.

The typical complaint of a sleep disorder associated with amphetamine dependence is insomnia. However, once an abstinence pattern has been established there is often a profound "crash" with a period of hypersomulence. Abuse of amphetamines increases the incidence of rapid eye movement during acute withdrawal. This may be secondary to a functional dopamine depletion and typically lasts a few days followed by increased agitation and drug craving which then contribute to insomnia. This abstinence syndrome of insomnia can be compounded by chronic fatigue. The result of the patient's inability to cope with the fatigue may then contribute to a subsequent relapse into recurrent amphetamine dependence.

Medical and Psychiatric Uses of Amphetamines

The indications listed in the *Physicians Desk Reference* for dextroamphetamine are Narcolepsy and Attention Deficit Disorder (ADD) with Hyperactivity. In children they are occasionally used for ADHD with evidence of some improved treatment over methylphenidate in some cases; the etiology for this is unclear. The amphetamines are typically avoided in this population because of the greater peripheral sympathomimetic stimulation seen with these drugs over methylphenidate.

The most frequent reason for prescribing these drugs is obesity. When amphetamine was compared with fenfluramine or placebo in a weight loss program amphetamine was clearly maintaining compliance with the program as reinforced self-stimulation. Also reported in the study was the significant increase of central nervous stimulation of amphetamine over fenfluramine (Kramer, Fischman, & Littlefield, 1967).

Depression and narcolepsy make up the majority of the remainder of the medical prescriptions of these drugs. Little tolerance develops to the effective treatment of narcolepsy. Some individuals treated for narcolepsy have been on the same doses for years without an increase in the original effective dose. Greater sensitivity develops to the anxiety-producing effects, the propensity to psychosis, and the peripheral sympathetic stimulation.

The use of benzedrine in depression was found to be most helpful in patients with recent onset of their depression. The studies done on depressed patients provide evidence that they may improve in their depressive symptoms for at least a short period of time after the initiation of therapy. This use of these drugs seems to be particularly effective in the medically ill depressed patient. The rapid onset of response in the medically ill is particularly valuable. The effectiveness of these drugs has been demonstrated in the treatment of depression in patients with AIDS, poststroke, cardiac, and cancer patients in improving their cognition and general affect (Angrist *et al.,* 1992).

Beyond these considerations there are a variety of ways in which the amphetamine-like medications have shown some effectiveness. Some of the more interesting uses of these drugs are as the drug of choice for nocturnal seizures and in the head-injured with seizure. There appears to be a mild to moderate analgesic effect along with relief of opioid-induced sedation. Closed-head-injury patients who were administered these drugs show improvement in attention, memory, language skills, emotional liability and behavioral disturbances. The amphetamines have also reduced craving in the cocaine-abusing population (Holmes, 1995). Cigarette smokers have been studied while taking dextroamphetamine and there seems to be a decrease in the number of cigarettes smoked by heavy smokers. Korsakoff patients may show improvement in their long-term memory after 1 week of treatment with methamphetamine.

The response to these drugs may be helpful in differentiating the alcohol-induced depression from the alcohol dependence concurrent with major depression. In this case there is a more robust long-term improvement in the alcohol-induced depression than is seen in the patient with a more chronic major depression. These drugs should be avoided in depression complicated by psychosis.

In schizophrenia these drugs are more effective when used with patients in the earlier stages of their disease and in catatonia; however, the usefulness for these patients is limited (Davidoff & Reifenstein, 1939). There is variability of response between types of schizophrenics. Amphetamines have been found to be most helpful in those patients with active symptoms of mild psychosis, not in the patient with purely negative symptoms. Those patients who responded positively to amphetamine administration also had a significant improvement in their attention span (Cesarec & Nyman, 1985). A majority of patients administered this drug had a subjective response of feeling alert, relaxed, and confident. There was an elevation of the patient's mood with enhancement of concentration. Lasting effects of this treatment may be a result of change in the neurochemistry or subsequent to life changes that take place during administration of the drug. Schizophrenic patients when not floridly psychotic may respond very well to stimulant treatment. However, analysis of a one-time administration of amphetamines to schizophrenic patients after a washout of their neuroleptic showed a slight worsening of their negative symptoms and a definite worsening of their positive symptoms (Angrist, Rotrosen, & Ger-

shon, 1980). A follow-up study with stable schizophrenic patients also after a washout period of their neuroleptics showed a significant improvement in negative symptoms after a one-time administration of amphetamine 0.5mg/kg. Studies done with patients on their neuroleptics showed some improvement in the negative symptoms. All three studies, though showing a statistically significant improvement, failed to show profound clinical improvement. However, the results indicated that there may be inherent damage to the dopamine system in the pathophysiology of schizophrenia.

Amphetamine Dependence and Comorbid Mental Illness

Individuals with comorbidity of a primary mental illness and amphetamine abuse or dependency are often first identified in either a primary mental health center or a substance abuse treatment center. A problem often arises here because of the solitary focus on one diagnosis or the other. Identification of these individuals as dual diagnosis patients has traditionally been dismal. A report by McClellan in 1977 showed that 50% of patients admitted to a veterans hospital had a history of substance dependence; however, only 12% of these individuals had been identified on admission (McLellan & Druley, 1977). Unfortunately these individuals are often improperly treated because the problem is not being seen in its entirety.

It is interesting to speculate how the diagnosis of dependency might vary when applied to a patient with primary mental illness. How might the patient with altered reality testing interpret the need to cut back? When patients are not aware of their illnesses, what is the validity to the criterion of their continued use in the face of psychological complications? When the withdrawal symptoms are very similar to the symptoms normally experienced by the patient with this particular illness how are they to know the difference? These problems contribute to the difficulty one encounters in working with the patient with a primary mental illness in conjunction with a substance abuse problem. Clearly, however, the key to the initiation of care for these patients is making the correct diagnosis. Making the correct diagnosis can be facilitated by obtaining from the patient and other available sources a detailed longitudinal history.

Stimulant abuse is associated with earlier age of first hospitalization for the schizophrenic patient. Whether this is a result of the stimulant or the predisposition of these individuals to mental illness is not always clear. The use of psychogenic substances, such as stimulants and hallucinogens, is indeed more common among schizophrenic patients than other psychiatric patient groups (Schneier & Siris, 1987). Schizophrenics use stimulants more frequently than schizoaffective patients. Interestingly, however, the use of stimulants is usually more moderate than in the nonschizophrenic. There is clear evidence that these individuals are more sensitive to amphetamines than the nonschizophrenic user. However, the choice of amphetamines and other stimulants over opioids and depressants is well documented.

Some controversy exists over whether the degree of mental illness is negatively correlated with substance abuse (Mueser *et al.,* 1990). There is some evidence to show that in the more severely impaired mentally ill population there is less intensity of use of substances of abuse in general with the exclusion of cigarettes (Galanter & Ricardo, 1988). The use of illicit drugs is quite low in the severely mentally ill population. Poor reality testing and therefore the inability to interact effectively in securing these substances on the street may play a factor. Poor reality testing may also play a role in the infrequency of iv administration of amphetamine in this population, associated with the difficulties surrounding the administration. Another factor may be the awareness of the prolonged intense nature of its effect. This may be a particularly important factor considering the increased sensitivity these individuals have to amphetamine-like drugs. The iv administration of amphetamines is difficult and the effects are longer lasting compared with the easy administration, of crack cocaine

through smoking, and its extremely short half-life. These factors contribute to crack cocaine's being a more heavily abused drug than amphetamines in this population.

The diagnosis of schizophrenia in the concurrent amphetamine abuser has been associated with the mean age of onset and first hospitalization occurring approximately two years earlier than in the nonusing schizophrenic patients. As pointed out earlier in the chapter there is a greater sensitivity to the amphetamine-like drugs in the schizophrenic patient. There may also be a worsening of their illness because of neurotoxic effects and behavioral sensitization occurring with chronic use. Interestingly there appeared to be a healthier premorbid personality in the drug users than in the non-drug users who became schizophrenics (Bowers, 1972).

At the very least the abuse of amphetamines by the schizophrenic patient may lead to psychotic episodes they would not have experienced otherwise. There is strong evidence pointing to behavioral sensitization and neurotoxic effects of these drugs which then may accelerate the pathophysiology of the illness. Antipsychotic medications are less effective in the schizophrenic patient after prolonged stimulant use. Schizophrenic patients thus appear to be at significant risk of compounding their illness by using these drugs. The addicted paranoid schizophrenic has been described as one of the most difficult to treat (National Conference, 1973).

Bipolar illness has long been associated with alcohol and substance abuse. The epidemiologic catchment area (ECA) study showed a particularly strong association between impulsive, antisocial, thrill-seeking alcohol abusers and the prevalence of bipolar disorder (Regier *et al.,* 1990). Patients admitted to a hospital for treatment of mental illness and a substance abuse problem, all of whom carried a diagnosis of bipolar illness, were evaluated for the quality of their abuse compared with the type of bipolar illness they had. The study indicated that bipolar manics and mixed bipolar patients had the most frequent concurrent abuse patterns. The manic group had the most frequent concurrence and the stimulant drugs were the most common drug type they selected. This led the authors to speculate that the drugs frequently present in their systems on admission either had a role in the development of their illness or were involved in the exacerbation of the manic episode. The importance of drug screening in the evaluation of these patients is essential to being able to properly understand and treat them (Estroff, Dackis, Gold, & Pottash, 1985).

The rate of stimulant abuse in the bipolar population is substantial. Interestingly it is in the manic phase of illness that these drugs are more frequently used. In one study stimulants were used in the manic phase at a rate of 58% compared with the depressive state, 30%. (Estroff *et al.*, 1985). Substance abuse in general is more commonly seen in the bipolar type II patients than bipolar I (R. D. Weiss *et al.*, 1986).

Diagnostic Dilemma on Initial Presentation

The difficulty comes in trying to identify those patients who might present to an acute care setting who have a history of recent use of an amphetamine-like substance and are presently experiencing symptoms or signs of a mental illness. Most frequently these individuals are treated for their amphetamine intoxication symptoms and the mental illness is ignored. However, in a mental-health-oriented setting these individuals may be treated and subsequently diagnosed with a primary mental illness other than a substance-induced disorder. When individuals present with amphetamine intoxication they are typically observed, treated, and then referred to a substance abuse or mental health treatment program. The most appropriate ongoing treatment setting for the patient depends on how the patient responds in the acute phase of treatment. If there is potential for harm, or if the patient is felt to be psychotic with poor reality testing, a transfer to an inpatient mental health center is most appropriate. For the more stable patient a substance abuse or dual diagnosis program referral to establish abstinence would probably be most appropriate.

Treatment

The initial approach to the psychotic patient must first be to secure the safety of the patient. Physical restraints should be avoided because of the potential for hyperthermia and rhabdomyolysis, which may result in renal failure from myoglobinuria. A quiet room away from the environmental stimuli of a busy emergency department is extremely helpful. This setting should provide safety for both the patient and any personnel coming into contact with the patient. The amphetamine-intoxicated patient with a history of mental illness may present with more aggressively hostile behavior than the nontoxic schizophrenic. Histories of alcohol and drug abuse among schizophrenic inpatients studied on a general psychiatric ward have been correlated with an increased risk of assault-related behaviors (Yesavage & Zarcone, 1983). This indicates the need to view the amphetamine abuser in terms of the abusiveness often induced during times of intoxication, and to address this in the treatment plan (Fukushima, 1994).

The assessment of vital signs and medical stabilization of the patient are essential. A typical presentation of the acute overdose patient to the emergency room may include seizure, hyperpyrexia, and cardiovascular compromise. Other physical signs may be dilated pupils, tachycardia, hypertension, hyperflexia, and irregular respirations. In patients with profound changes in mental status immediate neuroimaging should be considered.

On securing the patient, a more complete and thorough physical examination should be performed. During the exam, one should keep in mind possible endocrinologic, metabolic, oncotic, infectious, and traumatic reasons for psychosis. The clinician should obtain history from any individuals associated with the patient's arrival in the department to get as much pertinent information as possible about the patient's medical history and the events leading up to the onset of the psychosis. This should include rescue personnel, who often have details of the setting in which the patient was encountered and the appearance of the patient over time. This information can be helpful in understanding the etiology of the problem. One should also obtain baseline laboratory values, including serum and urine drug screens.

In patients with evidence of profound central and or peripheral nerve system stimulation chlorpromazine is not recommended because of its potential for worsening the hyperthermia, lowering the seizure threshold, and increasing the serum half-life of amphetamines. A benzodiazepam with its potential to relieve anxiety and raise the seizure threshold may be the drug of choice. However, the physician should pay particular attention to the patient's respiratory rate when using these drugs, for they can worsen the respiratory depression often seen with amphetamine overdose.

Once this initial work-up has been completed, and the patient is more stable, one can obtain a detailed history. A reevaluation of the patient in the form of a tertiary review may be conducted. At this time a more detailed assessment of the patient's mental status can be made. If the patient presents with psychotic symptoms, the quality of the psychotic presentation may be more closely evaluated at this time. The amphetamine-induced psychotic patient frequently presents with paranoid delusions, auditory hallucinations, and stereotypic behavior such as skin-picking, teeth-grinding, lip-biting, pacing, and pressured speech (Cohen, 1975).

Psychosis

The medication treatment of amphetamine psychosis is often a high-potency neuroleptic such as haloperidol which may require anticholinergic medication to manage side effects. Haloperidol has the advantage of multiple routes of administration (including intravenous and intramuscular). Risperidone is another excellent first-line choice. Usually, risperidone does not cause extrapyramidal side effects at therapeutic dosages (4–6 mg) and therefore anticholinergic medications are not required. Risperidone is not sedating, and short-acting benzodiazepines such as lorazepam can be used

initially to calm the patient if necessary (available im and iv). Compared to haloperidol, there is less chance with risperidone for extrapyramidal symptoms in the nonschizophrenic patient. Phenothiazines are not recommended; they may precipitate an anticholinergic crisis, resulting in bradycardia and hypotension. They may also cause hypothermia and lower the seizure threshold, as pointed out earlier. There may also be a slowing of the metabolism of amphetamines with the administration of chlorpromazine (Davis, 1970). Acidification of the urine results in the shortening of the amphetamine half-life and may hasten recovery.

Anxiety

The establishment of a safe, secure environment may have a considerable calming effect on the patient. Avoiding the use of pharmacological agents is a goal; however, this is not always possible. Benzodiazepines are preferable with the anxious patient; however, caution should also be used when administering benzodiazepines because of the potential for disinhibition seen in some patients. This disinhibition may result in violent aggressive outbursts. In the patient with a combination of amphetamine abuse and prolonged symptoms of anxiety, the choice of either buspirone, a tricyclic antidepressant, or a serotonin reuptake inhibitor drug may be more appropriate.

Pemoline (Cylert) is a stimulant medication that has been used successfully to treat patients with combined residual ADHD and cocaine abuse without subsequent abuse of this drug (R. D. Weiss, Pope, & Mirin, 1985). Pemoline has more dopaminergic stimulating effects than the other psychostimulants. Therefore, it should not be used in the patient with compromised reality testing. Liver function studies should also be monitored while the patient is on this drug. Nonetheless, pemoline offers significant advantages. There are minimal cardiac effects associated with it, in contrast with the somatic effects of other commonly used stimulants that are often a source of anxiety in this patient population. Pemoline has the additional advantage of not being a controlled substance.

Mood Disorders

The treatment model should include psychosocial treatment as it is important in assisting with the depressed mood and maintenance of abstinence. The psychopharmacologic intervention should come only after there has been at least a 2-week period of abstinence. At that time, if significant symptoms of depression remain it would be reasonable to initiate pharmacotherapy. Desipramine with its increased norepinephrine reuptake blockade may be a good choice among the tricyclic antidepressants. One of the serotonin reuptake inhibitors with their high efficacy rates and low side effects would also be a good choice.

Sleep Disorders

A variety of sleep hygiene behavioral techniques could be introduced as the patient attempts to reestablish a more normal sleep pattern. The effectiveness of these techniques on their own will be dependent on the duration of amphetamine misuse, and the patient's temperament. However, if these psychotherapeutic measures are unsuccessful then one could consider a pharmacological intervention. The use of clonidine in the withdrawal period may reduce the irritability of withdrawal. This may allow the patient to return more readily to a more normal sleep cycle within the first 2 weeks of withdrawal. After that period a tricyclic antidepressant or Trazodone may assist in establishing a more normal cycle.

Summary

There is evidence that amphetamines may become a more widespread problem in the future. The social problems from the abuse of these drugs are often tragic and costs both financial and in terms of lives is tremendous. A better understanding of the presentation of a patient intoxicated with these drugs should bring the patient into an appropriate treatment setting more quickly. Once a dependent pattern of use has been established, we need to recognize and treat the illness and the complications.

References

American Psychiatric Association. (1994). *Diagnostic and statistical manual of mental disorders* (4th ed.). Washington, DC: Author.

Angrist, B., Rotrosen, J., & Gershon, S. (1980). Differential effects of amphetamine and neuroleptics on negative vs. positive symptoms in schizophrenia. *Psychopharmacology, 72,* 17–19.

Angrist, B., D'Hollosy, M., Sanfilipo, M., Satriano, J., Diamond, G., Simberkoff, M., & Weinred, H. (1992). Central nervous system stimulants as symptomatic treatment of AIDS-related neuropsychiatric impairment. *Journal of Clinical Psychopharmacology, 2,* 268–273.

Beninger, R. J., & Hahn, B. L. (1983). Pimozide blocks establishment but not expression of amphetamine-produced environment-specific conditioning. *Science, 220,* 1304–1306.

Bowers, M. B. (1972). Acute psychosis induced by psychotomimetic drug abuse. Clinical findings. *Archives of General Psychiatry, 27,* 437–440.

Breakey, W. R., Goodell, H., Lorenz, P., & McHugh, P. (1974). Hallucinogenic drugs as precipitants of schizophrenia. *Psychological Medicine, 4,* 255–261.

Brien, R. L., Kleiman, J., & Eisenman R. (1972). Personality and drug use: Heroin, alcohol, methadrine, mixed drug dependency and the 16PF. *Corrective Psychiatry and Journal of Social Therapy, 18,* 22–23.

Campbell, B. K., & Stark, J. M. (1990). Psychopathology and personality characteristics in different forms of substance abuse. *International Journal of the Addictions, 25,* 1467–1474.

Cesarec, Z., & Nyman, A. K. (1985). Differential response to amphetamine in schizophrenia. *Acta Psychiatrica Scandinavica, 71,* 523–538.

Chiarello, R. J., & Cole, J. O. (1987). The use of psychostimulants in general psychiatry. *Archives of General Psychiatry, 44,* 286–295.

Churchill, A. C., Burgess, P., Pead, J., & Gill, T. (1993). Measurement of the severity of amphetamine dependence. *Addiction, 88,* 1335–1340.

Cohen, S. (1975). Amphetamine abuse. *Journal of the American Medical Association, 213,* 414–415.

Collins, J. P., Lesse, H., & Dagan, L. (1979). Behavioral antecedents of cocaine-induced stereotypy. *Pharmacology, Biochemistry and Behavior, 11,* 683–687.

Connell, P. H. (1958). *Amphetamine psychosis* (Maudsley Monograph No. 5). London: Chapman and Hall.

Council on Scientific Affairs of the AMA. (1978). Clinical aspects of amphetamine abuse. *Journal of the American Medical Association, 240,* 2317.

Crockett, R., & Marks, V. (1969). Amphetamine taking among young offenders. *British Journal of Psychiatry, 115,* 1203–1204.

Davidoff, E., & Reifenstein, E. C. (1939). The results of eighteen months of benzedrine sulfate therapy in psychiatry. *American Journal of Psychiatry, 95,* 945–970.

Davis, J. (1970). The effects of haloperidol and chlorpromazine on amphetamine metabolism and amphetamine stereotyped behavior in rats. *Journal of Pharmacology and Experimental Therapeutics, 174*, 428–433.

Elkins, R. N., Rapoport, J., Zahn, T., Buchsbaum, M., Weingartner, H., Kopin, I., Langer, D., & Johnson, C. (1981). Acute effects of caffeine in normal prepubertal boys. *American Journal of Psychiatry, 138*, 178–183.

Ellinwood, E. H., Sudilovsky, A., & Nelson, L. (1973). Evolving behavior in the clinical and experimental amphetamine (model) psychosis. *American Journal of Psychiatry, 130*, 1088–1093.

Ellison, G. D., & Eison, M.S. (1983). Continuous amphetamine intoxication: An animal model of the acute psychotic episode. *Psychological Medicine , 13*, 751–762.

Estroff, T. W., Dackis, C., Gold, M., & Pottash, A. (1985–1986). Drug abuse and bipolar disorders. *International Journal of Psychiatry in Medicine, 15*, 3740.

Fischman, M. W., Schuster, C., Resnekov, L., Shick, J., Krasneger, N., Fennell, W., & Freedman, D. (1976). Cardiovascular and subjective effects of intravenous cocaine administration in humans. *Archives of General Psychiatry, 33*, 938–989.

Fischman, M. W., Schuster, C., Javaid, J., Hatano, Y., & Davis, J. (1985). Acute tolerance development to the cardiovascular and subjective effects of cocaine. *Journal of Pharmacology and Experimental Therapeutics, 235*, 677–682.

Fukushima, A. (1994). Criminal responsibility in amphetamine psychosis. *Japanese Journal of Psychiatry and Neurology, 48*, 1–4.

Galanter, M., & Ricardo, C. (1988). Substance abuse among general psychiatric patients: Place of presentation, diagnosis, and treatment. *American Journal of Drug and Alcohol Abuse, 14*, 211–235.

Gawin, F. H. (1991). Cocaine addiction: Psychology and neurophysiology. *Science, 251*, 1580–1586.

Goeders, N. E., Dworkin, S., & Smith, J. (1986). Neuropharmacological assessment of cocaine self-administration into the medial prefrontal cortex. *Pharmacology, Biochemistry and Behavior, 24*, 1429–1440.

Grinspoon, L., & Hedblom, P. (1975). *The speed culture.* Cambridge, MA: Harvard University Press.

Gunne, E., & Lewander, T. (1967). Long-term effects of some dependence-producing drugs on the brain monoamines. In O. Wahaas (Ed.), *Molecular basis of some aspects of mental activity* (pp. 75–81). New York: Academic Press.

Harris, G. C., & Wilhams, J. T. (1992). Sensitization of Locus ceruleus neurons during withdrawal from chronic stimulants and antidepressants. *Journal of Pharmacology and Experimental Therapeutics, 261*, 476–483.

Hawks, D., Mitcheson, M., Ogborne, A., & Edwards, G. (1969). Abuse of methylamphetamine. *British Medical Journal, 2*, 715–721.

Hensala, J. D., Epstein, L., & Blacker, K. (1967). LSD and psychiatric inpatients. *Archives of General Psychiatry, 16*, 554–559.

Holmes, V. F. (1995). Medical use of psychostimulants: An overview. *International Journal of Psychiatry in Medicine, 25*, 1–19.

Jaffe, J. H. (1985). Drug addiction and drug abuse. In L. S. Goodman, A. C. Gilman, & A. Gilman (Eds.), *The pharmacological basis of therapeutics* (7th ed., pp, 532–581). New York: Macmillan.

Johanson, C. E., Balster, R., & Bonese, K. (1976). Self-administration of psychomotor stimulant drugs: The effects of unlimited access. *Pharmacology, Biochemistry and Behavior, 4*, 45–51.

Khantzian, E. J. (1985). The self-medication hypothesis of addictive disorders. *American Journal of Psychiatry, 142*, 1259–1264.

King, G. R., & Ellinwood, E. H. (1992). Amphetamines and other stimulants. In J. H. Lowinson, P. Ruiz, R. D. Millman, & J. G. Langrod (Eds.), *Substance abuse: A comprehensive textbook* (2nd ed., pp. 247–270). Baltimore: Williams & Wilkins.

Kramer, J. C., Fischman, V., & Littlefield, D. (1967). Amphetamine abuse: Pattern and effects of high doses taken intravenously. *Journal of the American Medical Association, 201*, 89–93.

Lieberman, J. A., Kinon, B., & Loebel, A. (1990). Dopaminergic mechanisms in idiopathic and drug induced psychoses. *Schizophrenia Bulletin, 16*, 97–110.

Lyness, W. H., Friedle, N., & Moore, K. (1979). Destruction of dopaminergic nerve terminals in nucleus accumbens: Effects on d-amphetamine self-administration. *Pharmacology, Biochemistry and Behavior, 11*, 553–556.

McLellan, A. T., & Druley, K. A. (1977). Non-random relation between drugs of abuse and psychiatric diagnosis. *Journal of Psychiatric Research, 13*, 179–184.

McLellan, A. T., Woody, G. E., & O'Brien, C. P. (1979). Development of psychiatric illness in drug abusers. *New England Journal of Medicine, 301*, 1310–1314.

Mesulam, M. M. (1986). Frontal cortex and behavior. *Annals of Neurology, 19*, 320–325.

Mueser, K. T., Yarnold, P., Levinson, D., Singh, H., Bellack, A., Kee, K., Morrison, R., & Yadalem, K. (1990). Prevalence of substance abuse in schizophrenia: Demographic and clinical correlates. *Schizophrenia Bulletin, 16*, 31–54.

Mueser, K. T., Bellack, A. S., & Blanchard, J. J. (1992). Comorbidity of schizophrenia and substance abuse: Implications for treatment. *Journal of Consultation in Clinical Psychology, 60*, 845–856.

Nehlig, A., Lucignani, G., Kadekaro, M., Porrino, L., & Sokoloff, L. (1984). Effects of acute administration of caffeine on focal glucose utilization in the rat. *European Journal of Pharmacology, 101*, 91–100.

Physicians desk reference, 51st edition (pp. 2361–2363). (1995). Montvale, NJ: Medical Economics Data Production.

Regier, M. E., Farmer, M. E., Rae, D. S., Laocke, B. Z., Keith, S. J., Judd, L. L., & Goodwin, F. K. (1990). Comorbidity of mental disorders with alcohol and other drug abuse. *Journal of the American Medical Association, 264,* 2511–2518.

Reith, M. E., Benuck, M., & Lajtha, A. (1987). Cocaine disposition in the brain after continuous or intermittent treatment and locomotor stimulation in mice. *Journal of Pharmacology and Experimental Therapeutics, 243,* 281–287.

Roberts, D. C., & Kobb, G. F. (1982). Disruption of cocaine self-administration following 6-hydroxy-dopamine lesions of the ventral tegmental area in rats. *Pharmacology, Biochemistry and Behavior, 17,* 901–904.

Rockwell, D. A., & Ostwald, P. (1968). Amphetamine use and abuse in psychiatric patients. *Archives of General Psychiatry, 18,* 612–616.

Rossetti, Z. L., Hmaidan, Y., & Gessa, G. L. (1992). Marked inhibition of Mesolimbic dopamine release: A common feature of ethanol, morphine, cocaine and amphetamine abstinence in rats. *European Journal of Pharmacology, 221,* 227–234.

Sato, M. (1990). A lasting vulnerability to psychosis in patients with previous methamphetamine psychosis. *Annals of the New York Academy of Sciences, 654,* 160–170.

Sato, M., Chen, C., Akiyama, K., & Otsuki, S. (1983). Acute exacerbation of paranoid psychotic state after long-term abstinence in patients with previous methamphetamine psychosis. *Biological Psychiatry, 18,* 429–440.

Scheel-Kruger, J., Braestrup, C., Nielson, M., Golembiowska, K., & Mogilnicka, E. (1977). Cocaine: Discussion on the role of dopamine in the biochemical mechanism of action. In E. H. Ellinwood & M. M. Kilbey (Eds.), *Cocaine and other stimulants* (pp. 373–408). New York: Plenum.

Schneier, F. R., & Siris, S. G. (1987). A review of psychoactive substance use and abuse in schizophrenia: Patterns of drug choice. *Journal of Nervous and Mental Disorders, 175,* 641–652.

Schuckit, M. A. (1989). *Drug and alcohol abuse: A clinical guide to diagnosis and treatment* (3rd ed.). New York: Plenum Medical Book Company.

Seiden, L. S., Commin, D., Vosmer, G., Axt, K., & Marek, G. (1988). Neurotoxicity in dopamine and 5-hydroxytryptamine terminal fields: A regional analysis in nigrostriatal and mesolimbic projections. *Annals of the New York Academy of Sciences, 537,* 161–172.

Sonsalla, P. K., Nicklas, W., & Heikkila, R. (1989). Role for excitatory amino acids in methamphetamine-induced nigrostriataodopaminergic toxicity. *Science, 243,* 398–400.

Spotts, J. V., & Shontz, F. C. (1991). Drugs and personality: Comparison of drug users, nonusers, and other clinical groups on the 16PF. *International Journal of the Addictions, 26,* 1019–1054.

Weiss, R. D., Pope, H., & Mirin, S. (1985). Treatment of chronic cocaine abuse and Attention Deficit Disorder Residual Type with magnesium pemoline. *Drug and Alcohol Dependence, 15,* 9–72.

Weiss, R. D, Mirin, S., Michael, J., & Sollogub, A. (1986). Psychopathology in chronic cocaine users. *American Journal of Drug and Alcohol Abuse, 12,* 17–29.

Weiss, S. R., Post, R. M., Pert, A., Woodward, R., & Murman, D. (1989). Context-dependent cocaine sensitization: Differential effect of haloperidol on development versus expression. *Pharmacology, Biochemistry and Behavior, 34,* 655–661.

Wise, S. P. (1985). The primate premotor cortex: Past, present, and preparatory. *Annual Review of Neuroscience, 8,* 1–19.

Yesavage, J. A., & Zarcone, V. (1983). History of drug abuse and dangerous behavior in inpatient schizophrenics. *Journal of Clinical Psychiatry, 44,* 259–261.

Young, D., & Scoville, W. B. (1938). Paranoid psychosis in narcolepsy and the possible dangers of benzedrine treatment. *Medical Clinics of North America, 22,* 637–645.

XI

Other Substances
of Abuse

33

Anabolic Steroids

MAURO G. DI PASQUALE

Introduction

Recreational and competitive athletes make use of a number of drugs and anabolic supplements to improve their performance and appearance. Anabolic steroids (AS) are the most commonly used and the most infamous of these compounds.

The androgenic and anabolic actions of substances produced by the testes have been known for centuries. Two case reports described by Sacchi (1895) and Rowlands and Nicholson (1929) comprise the early evidence of the influence of testicular androgens, specifically testosterone, on growth and musculoskeletal development. In a series of studies extending from 1938 to 1944, Kenyon (Kenyon, 1938, 1942; Kenyon, Knowlton, Lotwin, & Sandford, 1942; Kenyon, Knowlton, & Sandford, 1944) investigated and elucidated the metabolic effects of testosterone. He was one of the first to outline possible clinical uses for testosterone.

The athletic community was quick to realize the performance-enhancing potential of testosterone and put some of the principles outlined by Kenyon and others into practice. By the early 1950s testosterone and a few analogs such as methandrostenelone (Dianabol) were being used first by Eastern Block athletes and soon afterward by most other countries.

In the 1950s and 1960s the use of AS was contained within the "power" sports such as weight lifting, the weight events in track and field, including javelin, shot put, and discus, and the sports requiring explosive power such as the short-distance events in cycling and running. However, since the early 1970s the use of testosterone and testosterone analogs by athletes has dramatically increased. Today, AS are used by almost all power athletes (those in sports requiring strength or explosive force or, as in bodybuilding, extreme muscularity) at some time during their training, and by many other athletes as well, including athletes competing in the middle distance (Kehoe, 1982) and endurance events.

Not only is anabolic steroid use common among professional and elite amateur athletes but their use has also spread to college and high school athletes (Windsor & Dumitru, 1989) involved in non-Olympic sports such as football, hockey, basketball, and even baseball. In addition, their use has spread to recreational or aesthetic athletes where these compounds are used mainly to enhance physical appearance.

Anabolic Steroid Preparations

Relatively small changes in the basic chemical structure of the testosterone molecule (as well as other endogenous sex hormones) may bring about dramatic changes in effect, po-

MAURO G. DI PASQUALE · Department of Physical and Health Education, University of Toronto, Toronto, Canada K0K 3K0.

Handbook of Substance Abuse: Neurobehavioral Pharmacology, edited by Tarter *et al.* Plenum Press, New York, 1998.

tency, and adverse effects. A methyl group here and a hydroxyl group there could lead to an enhancement of anabolic activity, or more likely to a loss of androgenic and anabolic properties. As a result of extensive research, particularly in the 1950s and 1960s (Kruskemper, 1968; Vida, 1969), thousands of biologically active steroid compounds are now known.

Modifications at any of the 19 carbon groups that make up the testosterone molecule are made for many reasons, including altering the anabolic–androgenic ratio or therapeutic index (ideally increasing the anabolic effects and decreasing the androgenic effects); increasing the bioavailability of the drug when taken orally; decreasing its absorption time when given parenterally; and increasing the potency of the drug so that less drug is used for similar results.

While there may be hundreds of available preparations of testosterone and its chemically

TABLE 1. Generic and Common Trade Names of Steroids[a]

Generic	Common trade names
bolasterone	Myagen
boldenone	Equipoise
clostebol	Turinabol
fluoxymesterone	Halotestin
furazabol	Miotolon
mestanolone	Androstanolone
mesterolone	Proviron
methandienone (methandrostenolone)	Metanabol, Nerobol
methandriol	Stenediol
methenolone	Primobolan
methyltestosterone	Metandren
nandrolone	Durabolin, Deca-Durabolin
norethandrolone	Nilevar
oxandrolone	Anavar
oxymesterone	Oranabol
oxymetholone	Anadrol, Anapolon, Plenastril
stanozolol	Winstrol
testosterone (oral and injectable)	Andriol, Delatestryl, Depo-Testosterone, Malogex, Omnadren, Oreton, Primotestin, Sustanon
trenbolone	Finaject, Parabolan

[a] These compounds vary in their androgenic and anabolic properties as well as in their formulation and bioavailability.

modified analogs, the most common preparations used by athletes are listed in Table 1.

The Effects of Androgenic-Anabolic Steroids

The effects produced by testosterone can be subdivided into two somewhat arbitrary effects: androgenic (producing secondary male sexual characteristics) and anabolic (mainly increasing muscle size and strength). While there has been an effort to try to dissociate these two effects, there is no pure anabolic steroid. AS have varying degrees of androgenic effects. In early animal studies, the dissociation was significant, but in humans it is less so. This lack of complete dissociation has led to much confusion in the terminology used for these compounds. The terms anabolic steroid, androgenic steroid, anabolic-androgenic steroid and androgenic-anabolic steroid are often used interchangeably. Testosterone itself can be referred to as an anabolic steroid, although this term usually refers to its synthetic derivatives.

For the purposes of this report the term anabolic steroid will be used to mean the various forms of testosterone and all other natural and synthetic androgenic-anabolic steroids.

Do They Work?

There is some controversy in the literature on the effectiveness of AS in enhancing performance, but there is no doubt in most athletes' minds that they do work. Athletes worldwide use AS in an attempt to increase their muscular size and strength.

Prior to this decade the predominant attitude in the scientific community was that AS did not enhance performance. In Goodman and Gilman's (1985) *The Pharmacological Basis of Therapeutics* it is stated that "the use of these agents (anabolic steroids) does not cause an increase in muscle bulk, strength, or athletic performance, even when phenomenally large doses are used. The commonly observed increase in body weight (seen secondary to steroid use) is due to the retention of salt and water" (p. 1453).

The authors base this conclusion on the results of 25 papers that addressed the effects of androgenic-anabolic steroids on physical strength and athletic performance in men.

In the past decade, however, there has been an acceptance of the ergogenic effects of AS. One of the first comprehensive reviews on the positive effects of AS on athletic performance was by Haupt and Rovere (1984). They concluded that if certain criteria are met such as intensive training, a high protein diet, and specific measurement techniques, then AS do seem to enhance athletic performance. Other studies published since this review have shown that AS enhance strength, size, and athletic performance (Egginton, 1987; Griggs *et al.*, 1989).

A recent study has definitively shown that supraphysiologic doses of testosterone significantly increases both muscle size and strength in normal men (Bhasin *et al.*, 1996). In this study 43 normal men were assigned to four different groups: placebo with no exercise, testosterone with no exercise, placebo plus exercise, and testosterone plus exercise. The men received injections of 600 mg of testosterone enanthate or placebo weekly for 10 weeks. The results of this study conclusively show that supraphysiologic doses of testosterone increase muscle mass and strength both on their own and even more so when combined with exercise.

The efficacy of AS as an ergogenic aid is likely dependent on many variables. These variables include individual genetic characteristics such as receptor response and affinity, the dosage and duration of treatment, the physiological and psychological state of the individual before and during their use, and other factors such as diet, training intensity, and concomitant use of other hormones, drugs, and nutritional aids.

Adverse Effects

In general, anabolic steroid adverse effects can be separated into two groups. One group consists of adverse effects that are an exaggeration of the expected pharmacological properties of the AS. Potential hormone-related adverse effects of AS in men include gynecomastia, fluid retention, acne, changes in libido, oligospermia, and increased aggressiveness (J. Wilson, 1988).

In women amenorrhea and other menstrual irregularities commonly occur. In addition, there is a possibility of virilizing effects from the use of AS (R. Strauss, Liggett, & Lanese, 1985). Some of these effects, such as coarsening and eventually deepening of the voice, hirsutism, male pattern baldness, reduction of breast size, and clitoral enlargement, may or may not be partially reversed by the discontinuation of AS and if needed the use of androgen antagonists such as cyproterone acetate.

In most men, however, once the AS are discontinued, the hormonal parameters invariably return to normal, except perhaps in those athletes who are sensitive to their effects on endogenous testosterone production or who have used large amounts of AS for prolonged periods of time. In some of these athletes the serum testosterone may remain depressed for several weeks to months, secondary to testicular atrophy and refractiveness of the hypothalamic–pituitary–testicular axis (Alen, Rrahkila, Reinila, & Vihko, 1987). Occasionally the serum testosterone fails to return to normal even with treatment and long-term replacement therapy is necessary.

The other group of adverse effects are those that are not usually thought of as related to either the anabolic or androgenic properties of these compounds. These adverse effects, while controversial as to the role that AS have in their genesis and development, result in more than just cosmetic changes, and include changes in serum cholesterol (Webb, Laskarzewski, & Glueck, 1985), cardiovascular disease (McNutt, Ferenchick, Kirlin, & Hamlin, 1988; Rockhold, 1993), prostate cancer (Roberts & Essenhigh, 1986), kidney dysfunction (Prat, Gray, Stolley, & Coleman, 1977), emotional disturbances (see later sections), variable changes in carbohydrate metabolism (Hobbs, Plymate, Bell, & Patience, 1991; Woodard, Burghen, Kitabchi, & Wilmas, 1981), increased incidence of musculoskeletal injuries (Stannard & Bucknell, 1993), cerebrovascular accidents

(Frankle, Eichberg, & Zachariah, 1988), and hepatic dysfunction (with rare instances of hepatic cirrhosis), hepatocellular carcinoma, and peliosis hepatitis (Soe, Soe, & Gluud, 1994). This second group of adverse effects, while posing a serious threat to the athlete, has often been misrepresented and sensationalized in the media. We need better controlled long-term studies to accurately determine the risk involved in the prolonged use of AS.

We can also separate adverse effects into the short-term and long-term consequences of using AS. While many of the short-term consequences are clinically clear, especially those resulting in changes in the female secondary sexual characteristics and in feminization of the male, the long-term consequences are more elusive. There is some speculation that chronic use of AS may, in those genetically susceptible, cause hepatic cirrhosis, peliosis hepatitis, primary hepatoma, atherosclerosis and cardiac disease, diabetes, prostatic cancer, and cerebrovascular accidents. There is, however, no solid clinical or experimental evidence to show that the use of AS by healthy athletes has any effect on longevity, or that prolonged use leads to diseases of the various organs and systems just mentioned.

Nevertheless, the changing pattern of AS use over the past decade, that is, more widespread use, at higher dosages, and for longer periods of time, may yet reveal more severe problems in the long term. There are some studies in progress now that may shed some light on the long-term consequences of anabolic steroid use.

Hypothalamic-Pituitary-Testicular Dysfunction and Anabolic Steroids

While we may be able to discount many of the adverse effects of AS, such as isolated cases of liver and kidney tumors, and are unsure of the actual long-term hepatic and cardiovascular consequences of anabolic steroid use, dysfunction of the hypothalamic–pituitary–testicular axis (HPTA), resulting in low serum levels of endogenous testosterone, may be the one tangible serious side effect that can

not be ignored or explained away. Although several studies have documented the hormonal consequences of moderate to high doses of AS in both men and women, (Clerico et al., 1981; Kilshawm, Harkness, Hobson, & Smith, 1975; Kiraly, Collan, & Alen, 1987; Schulte-Beerbuhl & Nieschlag, 1980; R. H. Strauss, Wright, Finerman, & Catlin, 1983), only a few have reported the long-term effects of their use on the HPTA. These studies found that once the AS were discontinued, all the hormonal parameters returned to normal except for the serum testosterone, and in one study the serum thyroxine, which remained depressed for a prolonged period of time secondary to testicular atrophy and refractiveness of the hypothalamic–pituitary–testicular axis (Alen & Hakkinen, 1985; Alen, Reinila, & Vihko, 1985; Alen et al., 1987).

In the athletes whom I have treated, I have found that the prolonged use of AS can result in the long-term suppression of serum testosterone secondary to testicular and hypothalamic-pituitary dysfunction. I have also found that there is an increased prevalence of both pituitary gonadotropic and testicular dysfunction in men who have used AS. AS also can impair reproductive function at the gonad or the hypothalamo-pituitary level, or both. Although some of the AS (especially dihydrotestosterone and dihydrotestosterone derivatives) do not suppress the HPTA as much as others (Balestreri, Bertolini, Chiodini, & Ronzitti, 1971), in sufficient dosages, all AS will suppress this axis. Perhaps this suppression of the HPTA is the one adverse effect of AS that should be uppermost in the minds of those athletes who use them.

The use of AS causes a disturbance in the body's normal hormonal profile, with decreased concentrations of serum hormone binding globulin (SHBG), low concentrations of luteinizing hormone (LH), follicle-stimulating hormone (FSH), testosterone precursors, and testosterone itself, if synthetic AS or dihydrotestosterone and no exogenous testosterone are used. In athletes who use exogenous testosterone, there is also a high ratio of testosterone to its precursor steroids (Ruokonen, Alen, Bolton, & Vihko, 1985).

The formation, secretion, and metabolism of testosterone is a complex process that occurs through various sensing, feedback, and control mechanisms. The control of the sex hormones involves suprahypothalamic influences, the hypothalamus, the pituitary, and the gonads. In men, regulation of testosterone secretion involves the HPTA, with extrahypothalamic events having some influence at all three levels (Ryzhenkov, Bekhtereva, & Sapronov, 1974). The interaction between the various hormones and releasing factors such as GnRH, LH, FSH, inhibin, and the endogenous opioids, results in variations in the serum levels of testosterone. For example, the hypothalamic decapeptide GnRH is known to regulate the synthesis and secretion of LH and FSH by pituitary gonadotrope cells, which in turn regulate the secretion of testosterone by the testes.

The frequency of pulsatile GnRH secretion changes, and LH and FSH are differentially secreted, in various physiological situations (Dalkin, Haisenleder, Ortolano, Ellis, & Marshall, 1989). Testosterone also seems to affect the pituitary secretion of LH and FSH directly (Abeyawardene & Plant, 1989; Sheckter, Matsumoto, & Bremner, 1989), the response of LH and FSH to GnRH, and the frequency of pulsatile GnRH release. It is also thought that estrogens, produced from the aromatization of testosterone and other AS in parts of the brain and hypothalamus, inhibit LH secretion (Kulin & Reiter, 1972), and thus decrease testosterone production.

The use of exogenous hormones disrupts the HPTA, with the degree of disruption dependent on several factors including the type of anabolic steroid used, the dosage used, the duration of treatment, and the presence of any underlying pathology. All male athletes using AS experience some HPTA dysfunction, resulting in decreased serum testosterone levels, testicular atrophy, azoospermia, and sometimes the development of a female habitus including gynecomastia. When the AS are discontinued there is normally a variable time period over which the HPTA remains depressed. In most cases the serum hormones soon return to normal.

However, there is often a prolonged impairment of testicular endocrine function, secondary to hypothalamic–pituitary–testicular dysfunction, usually in athletes who have used high doses of AS for extended periods of time. In the athletes I have followed, the long-term suppression of testicular steroidogenesis results in hypothalamic-pituitary and gonadal dysfunction that may not be as reversible as is generally thought. Thus, testosterone and the AS seem to have direct effects on all components of the HPTA, and likely even on suprahypothalamic mechanisms.

In many cases of chronic suppression of the HPTA there appears to be a lowering of a normal body level of serum testosterone. After AS are discontinued, serum testosterone levels remain low, often with low to normal values of LH. Ordinarily one would expect elevated LH and FSH values in light of the low serum testosterone, signaling an attempt by the body to increase testicular testosterone production. Such is not usually the case. I have found a low serum testosterone associated with elevated gonadotrophin levels in only a minority of HPTA-suppressed patients. In this minority, the hypothalamic-pituitary function was intact and the primary problem was one of testicular dysfunction. In a few of these patients, the testicular dysfunction was irreversible.

Prevention of HPTA Dysfunction

While there are several measures that can be taken to minimize the effects of AS on the HPTA, perhaps the most important precaution is that the athlete take sufficient time off AS so that the endocrine system can return to normal and any testicular atrophy is reversed. This rest phase should be at least as long as the period of time that AS are used. For example, a cycle of 12 weeks on and 12 weeks off would, in most individuals, prevent some of the long-term sequelae of anabolic steroid use on the HPTA. It would appear that the more time spent drug free, the less long-term HPTA suppression there would be.

Second, the athlete should use low to moderate doses of those compounds which have less of a suppressive effect on the HPTA, although there is no anabolic steroid, even at low to moderate doses, that does not lead to some suppression. At high doses all AS have a severe suppressive effect on the HTPA. Since it appears that the production of testosterone is affected at several levels, minimizing the effect of AS must take all these levels into account. It is especially important to minimize the direct effect of AS on testicular steroidogenesis, the pituitary gonadotropins (LH and FSH), hypothalamic GnRH, and various suprahypothalamic mechanisms.

Various drugs and hormones are used to decrease the testicular atrophy seen secondary to the long-term use of AS. For example, human chorionic gonadotropin (HCG) is often used by athletes to prevent testicular atrophy during anabolic steroid usage, and to possibly augment the exogenous intake of AS by increasing endogenous production of testosterone (many studies have documented the plasma testosterone response to injections of HCG (Jezova, Komadel, & Mikulaj, 1987; Maddocks & Setchell, 1989). However, using HCG at the same time as AS will not maintain full testicular function, since the testicular response to HCG is diminished when AS are used concomitantly (Repcekova & Mikulaj, 1977). The chronic use of HCG also may eventually inhibit testicular steroidogenesis by decreasing the LH-HCG receptors on Leydig cells, thus making them refractory to stimulation from both HCG and exogenous and endogenous LH.

HCG is also used by athletes to try to decrease the negative effects that occur once off AS. These athletes believe that by using the HCG after a cycle of anabolic steroid use, they can stimulate their own testes to produce testosterone, thereby reestablishing normal testicular function. This reasoning, however, is somewhat faulty, and the use of HCG may even worsen the problem (see the following section). HCG, however, may be useful in some cases in which testicular dysfunction is the primary problem.

Some athletes use other compounds such as anti-estrogens (see later discussion) and GnRH in an attempt to prevent the suppression of the HPTA. Unfortunately, the effect of these compounds (and HCG) is blunted when AS are used concomitantly (Holma & Adlercreutz, 1976). It appears that AS, testosterone, their metabolites, or a combination directly inhibit LH and FSH secretion independent of GnRH (Sheckter et al., 1989), in addition to their effect on the hypothalamic GnRH pulse generator.

Treatment of Residual HPTA Dysfunction

Residual HPTA dysfunction manifests itself by a low serum testosterone and its symptoms such as fatigue, depression, low sex drive, and poor sexual performance. However, athletes with low serum testosterone secondary to anabolic steroid–induced HPTA suppression usually present with dysfunction at more than one level. Low serum testosterone levels are usually accompanied with low normal serum LH levels. This pattern generally points to a hypothalamic-pituitary dysfunction, although not necessarily (Glass, 1988). Athletes with low serum testosterone but low normal to normal serum LH may also have some degree of testicular dysfunction secondary to their anabolic steroid use. In athletes who continue to show significant suppression of the HPTA after cessation of the AS, the suppression seems to affect all three components of the HPTA axis and possibly suprahypothalamic controls on the GnRH pulse generator. In these athletes it appears that there is a lower feedback set-point of the gonadostat. That is, the body seems to accept a lower level of serum testosterone as being normal. Thus the use of AS seems to bring about long-term changes in the neuroendocrine regulating centers of testosterone secretion as well as in the testes.

Changes in the HPTA that take place in athletes who have used AS may be similar to the changes seen in some middle-aged males secondary to psychosocial stress and in normal males with aging (Nilsson, Moller, & Solstad, 1995; Vermeulen, 1994; Vermeulen & Kaufman, 1995). In these cases and perhaps also in steroid-taking athletes, the origin of the decline of Leydig cell function resides on the one hand in the testes, and is likely characterized by a decreased number of functioning Leydig and Sertoli cells and, on the other hand, in the hypothalamo-pituitary complex characterized by a decreased luteinizing hormone (LH) pulse amplitude, LH pulse frequency being maintained. As the responsiveness of the gonadotrophs to GnRH remains unimpaired, one may assume that the amount of GnRH released at each pulse is also reduced, possibly as the consequence of a reduction of the cellular mass of GnRH neurons.

In the dozens of patients I have treated in the past few years the responsiveness of the HPTA to compounds that stimulate the HPTA at one or more points remains intact. Use of these compounds results in significantly raised levels of serum testosterone. However, this effect usually vanishes once these compounds are discontinued, and serum testosterone levels rapidly return to their low levels.

Resetting the gonadostat in these individuals has proven to be extremely difficult. In all cases in which a low serum testosterone results from the use of AS, one or more of the anti-estrogens, HCG, menotropins, or GnRH and GnRH analogs should be used both to determine the responsiveness of the different parts of the HPTA, and as therapy. In some cases, the use of one or more of these compounds jump-starts the system and the HPTA axis reverts to normal after their use. However, care must be taken when using two or more of these compounds simultaneously. For example, studies have shown that the simultaneous administration of an GnRH agonist and HCG blunts the plasma testosterone response observed after GnRH alpha alone, and decreases the testosterone production as compared with using HCG alone (Smals *et al.,* 1987).

Of all the compounds mentioned, HCG is the one most used. This is unfortunate; I have found it is the least effective. While it is true that in some patients the testicular response to HCG can be quite marked (Martikainen, Alen, Rahkila, & Vihko, 1986), the use of HCG is usually counterproductive.

If the main region affected is the testicles, that is, their prolonged suppression has resulted in their inability to respond to physiological levels of LH, then the use of HCG (perhaps followed by the use of pulsatile GnRH if some degree of hypothalamic pituitary dysfunction is present) for several weeks to increase testicular steroidogenesis and size might prove effective. However, although HCG does stimulate endogenous testosterone production in those athletes who are in a transient hypogonadotropic hypogonadic state secondary to the use of AS, it does not help in reestablishing a normal HPTA in cases in which there is significant hypothalamic-pituitary dysfunction.

In this type of dysfunction the hypothalamus and pituitary are still in a refractory state after prolonged anabolic steroid use, and remain this way while HCG is being used since the endogenous testosterone produced as a result of the exogenous HCG suppresses endogenous LH production. Once the HCG is discontinued, the athlete must still go through a readjustment period. This is merely delayed by the HCG use.

In addition, the indiscriminate frequent use of large amounts of HCG, rather than helping the testicular dysfunction, can often compound the problem. Recent studies have shown that when HCG is used in cases of deficient testicular steroidogenesis, smaller doses used less frequently may be more effective, and this approach does not lead to Leydig cell steroidogenic desensitization (Balducci *et al.,* 1987).

Thus, while HCG is often used to try to jump-start the system, I find that the use of an anti-estrogen is more appropriate for normalizing the function of the HPTA. Anti-estrogens are competitive inhibitors of estrogens, both endogenous and exogenous. Tamoxifen (Nolvadex) is a potent nonsteroidal, oral anti-estrogen which competes with estrogen at binding sites and has no estrogenic activity.

Clomiphene (Clomid) is an analog of chlorotrianisene, a synthetic estrogen. It is mildly estrogenic and acts as an anti-estrogen. Cyclofenil, a nonsteroidal compound, is a weak estrogen related to stilbestrol. It has structural analogies with both stilbene and triphenylethylene with a higher central than peripheral estrogenic activity (Celotti, Avogadri, Melcangi, Milani, & Negri Cesi, 1984). It acts as an anti-estrogen by effectively displacing the stronger estrogenic compounds. All three compounds elevate endogenous gonadotropin production (both FSH and LH), which in turn stimulates the testes to produce more testosterone.

Tamoxifen is thought to increase the release of GnRH as well. It, however, may be counterproductive in that it has been shown to decrease testicular steroidogenesis. A recent study reported that tamoxifen reduced the synthesis of testosterone through an inhibition of the 17 alpha-hydroxylase and C17,20-desmolase enzyme systems together with an increased 20 alpha-hydroxysteroid dehydrogenase activity (Vanderstichele, Eechaute, Lacroix, & Leusen, 1989).

Of the available anti-estrogens, clomiphene is the one I find most effective both in testing the hypothalamic-pituitary reserve and in treating HPTA dysfunction in athletes whose serum testosterone remains depressed after the discontinuation of AS (Glass, 1988). The use of 100 mg of clomiphene daily in two divided doses for 4 to 8 weeks will usually elicit a significant increase in serum testosterone levels, often reaching higher than the upper limits of normal.

The long-term use of GnRH (by way of an infusion pump or by the intermittent use of one of the GnRH agonists) has proven to be effective in reestablishing the HPTA in some refractory patients. Studies have shown that in some men with hypogonadotropic hypogonadism, normal pituitary-gonadal function can be maintained after discontinuation of long-term pulsatile GnRH administration. Long-term exogenous GnRH administration induces pituitary and gonadal priming, which subsequently enables individuals to sustain normal pituitary and gonadal function in response to their own GnRH secretion (Finkelstein et al., 1989).

Unfortunately, while treatment with these compounds may be useful in some cases, only a small number of athletes with deficient testicular steroidogenesis and persistent depression of the HPTA respond to their use. In cases in which athletes do not respond to any of these compounds and the HPTA does not normalize, the only other therapy available at present is long-term replacement therapy with either one of the stimulating hormones or much more commonly testosterone. Testosterone can be given parenterally (for example 200 mg testosterone enanthate by deep intramuscular injection weekly or every 10 days) or orally (for example 240–360 mg testosterone undecanoate [ANDRIOL] daily), or by the use of transdermal (either scrotal or dermal) testosterone patches.

This situation may soon change. Once the role of both central, testicular, and extratesticular agents in HPTA dysfunction secondary to the use of AS is better understood, we may be able to offer treatment that will reset the gonadostat to normal. To help us to better understand and treat HPTA dysfunction, further clinical studies must be carried out to clarify the role of hormones and other agents such as prolactin (Dunkel & Huhtaniemi, 1985), the endogenous opioid peptides (Blank, Clark, Heymsfield, Rudman, & Blank 1994; Mikuma, Kumamoto, Maruta, & Nitta, 1994; Rasmussen, Kennedy, Ziegler, & Nett, 1988; Van Vugt & Meites, 1980), and aminergic, serotonergic, and dopaminergic pathways (del Pozo & Martin-Perez, 1985; Foresta, Scanelli, Tramarin, & Scandellari, 1985; Frajese et al., 1990; Tinajero, Fabbri, & Dufau, 1992; Williams, Lightman, Johnson, Carmichael, & Bannister, 1989), through the use of compounds that have an effect on the HPTA including the alpha-adrenoreceptor agonists phenylephrine (Wanderley et al., 1989), the opioid antagonist naloxone (Kletter, Foster, Beitins, Marshall, & Kelch, 1992; Kletter et al., 1994; Maggi, De Feo, Mannelli, Delitala, & Forti, 1985), serotonin antagonist drugs such as ritanserin (Tepavcevic et al., 1994), the dopamine agonist bromocriptine, and the dopamine antagonist metoclopramide (Baranowska et al., 1983; Falaschi, Frajese, Sciarra, Rocco, & Conti, 1978; Nakagawa,

Obara, Matsubara, Kubo, 1982; Spitz *et al.*, 1980).

Psychological and Behavioral Effects

Adverse psychological and behavioral effects have been reported with the use of AS including, most commonly, aggressiveness and irritability, but also hostility, anger, rage, impaired judgment, impulsiveness, and psychiatric symptoms. (Bahrke, Wright, O'Connor, Strauss, & Catlin, 1990; Bahrke, Wright, Strauss, & Catlin, 1992; Barker, 1987; Choi, Parrott, & Cowan, 1990; Lefavi, Reeve, & Newland, 1990; Lindstrom, Nilsson, Katzman, Janzon, & Dymling, 1990; Perry, Andersen, & Yates, 1990; Perry, Yates, & Andersen, 1990; Pope & Katz, 1987, 1988; R. Strauss *et al.*, 1983; Strauss *et al.*, 1985; Taylor, 1985, 1987). Cases of toxic confusional state (Tilzey, Heptonstall, & Hamblin, 1981), hypomania (Freinhar & Alvarez, 1985), paranoid symptoms (I. C. Wilson, Prange & Lara, 1974), acute schizophrenic episode (Annitto & Layman, 1980), criminal behavior (Conacher & Workman, 1989; Dalby, 1992), child abuse and spouse battery (Schulte, Hall, & Boyer, 1993), homicidal (Pope & Katz, 1990), and suicidal (Brower, Blow, Eliopulos, & Beresford, 1989) behavior have been reported. The possible addictive qualities of these compounds have also been pointed out (Williamson & Young, 1992) with the possibility of an opioid-type dependence (Tennant, Black, & Voy, 1988), including an inability to stop the use of steroids (Brower, Blow, Beresford, & Fuelling, 1989), compulsive use, and withdrawal symptoms (Kashkin & Kleber, 1989), including fatigue, depression, insomnia, and decreased sex drive (Brower, Eliopulos, Blow, Catlin, & Beresford, 1990).

It has been shown that AS have significant central nervous system effects. For example, in one recent study increasing doses of testosterone cypionate resulted in increased aggressive responses (Kouri, Lukas, Pope, & Oliva, 1995). Recently there has been evidence that AS may interact with benzodiazepine (Masonis & McCarthy, 1996) and other receptors (Le

Greves, Huang, & Johansson, 1997) in the brain. There is also some evidence that testosterone may interact with neurotransmitter systems in the brain involved in the regulation of aggression (Delville, Mansour, & Ferris, 1996). The results of these studies, in combination with earlier studies indicating the direct effects of AS on the function of addtional central nervous system receptor complexes, suggest that the behavioral and psychological effects of AS result from the interactions of AS with multiple regulatory systems in the brain.

A few studies have been set up to investigate the mood and behavior in humans secondary to the use of AS. Hannan and colleagues observed significant treatment-related increases on the hostility and resentment-aggression subscales of the Minnesota Multiphasic Personality Inventory after 6 weeks of treatment with testosterone or the anabolic steroid nandrolone (Hannan, Friedl, Zold, Kettler, & Plymate, 1991).

A recent study evaluated the acute effects of AS on mood and behavior in male normal volunteers (Su *et al.*, 1993). This was a 2-week, double-blind, fixed-order, placebo-controlled crossover trial of methyltestosterone. The study used a volunteer sample of 20 men who were medication free, free of medical and psychiatric illness, not involved in athletic training, and had no prior history of anabolic steroid use. The study involved a sequential trial for 3 days each of the following four drug conditions: placebo baseline, low-dose methyltestosterone (40 mg qd), high-dose methyltestosterone (240 mg qd), and placebo withdrawal. Mood and behavioral ratings were completed during each drug condition and included both subjective and objective measures.

The results of the study showed subtle increases in symptom scores during high-dose methyltestosterone administration compared with baseline, in positive mood (euphoria, energy, and sexual arousal), negative mood (irritability, mood swings, violent feelings, and hostility), and cognitive impairment (distractibility, forgetfulness, and confusion). There also was an acute manic episode in one of the 20 subjects and an additional subject became hypomanic. Overall this study showed that there are some subtle mood and behavioral effects seen with high-dose anabolic steroid use. It is interesting to note that what the authors considered low dose was relatively high since the medically recommended dosages for replacement therapy are 10–40 mg daily in adult males.

A recent study showing that supraphysiologic doses of testosterone significantly increases both muscle size and strength in normal men (Bhasin *et al.,* 1996) also measured the effects of supraphysiologic doses of testosterone on mood and behavior. In this study mood and behavior were evaluated during the first week of the control period and after 6 and 10 weeks of treatment. A standardized Multidimensional Anger Inventory (Siegel, 1986) that includes 38 questions to measure the frequency, duration, magnitude, and mode of expression of anger, hostile outlook, and anger-eliciting situations and a Mood Inventory that includes questions pertaining to general mood, emotional stability, and angry behavior were administered at these times. In addition, for each subject, a live-in partner, spouse, or parent answered the same questions about the subject's mood and behavior. The authors found no differences between the exercise groups and the testosterone groups in any of the five subcategories of anger. No significant changes in mood or behavior were reported by the men of the Mood Inventory or by their live-in partners, spouses, or parents on the Observer Mood Inventory. The authors of this study state, however, that while supraphysiologic doses of testosterone with or without exercise did not increase the occurrence of angry behavior by the carefully selected men in the controlled setting of this study, these results do not preclude the possibility that still higher doses of multiple steroids may produce angry behavior in men with preexisting psychiatric or behavioral problems.

A recent comprehensive review examined the psychological and behavioral effects of endogenous testosterone levels and anabolic-androgenic steroids (Bahrke, Yesalis, & Wright, 1990). The authors of this study looked at the relationship among mood, behavior, and endogenous plasma testosterone levels, and the effects of AS and corticosteroid administration. They found that while a relationship between endogenous testosterone levels and aggressive behavior has been observed in various animal species, it is less consistent in humans. They conclude that, although the use of exogenous anabolic-androgenic steroids may have psychological and behavioral effects in some patients and athletes, the effects are variable, transient upon discontinuation of the drugs, and appear to be related to type (17 alpha-alkalated rather than 17 beta-esterified), but not dose, of anabolic-androgenic steroids administered. The roles of genetic factors, medical history, environmental and peer influences, and individual expectations are likewise unclear. The authors concluded that, in general, the evidence at present is limited and much additional research will be necessary for a complete understanding of this relationship.

Other recent reviews, while noting that there is an association between androgens and aggression in animal studies, also found that the evidence for a possible effect of androgens on aggression is inconclusive (Archer, 1991). While in some species estrogen seems to be the primary hormone (Schlinger & Callard, 1989), in other species and in humans a positive correlation sometimes has been shown between the levels of certain endogenous androgens and aggression, especially under certain social and competitive conditions (Albert, Petrovic, & Walsh, 1989; Christiansen & Knussmann, 1987). However, even in animal studies there is some evidence that hormone dependent aggression is activated by learned responses or experience, although the level of aggression, once activated, depends on the serum testosterone concentration (Albert, Jonik, Watson, Gorzalka, & Walsh, 1990). Such also may be the case in man.

Before deciding that any adverse effects are due to the use of AS, other factors must be considered. For example, since it is commonly assumed that AS can increase aggressiveness, this assumption alone may account for some of the changes seen in those who use them. The use of any compound, including anabolic steroids, can induce a placebo effect (Ariel & Saville, 1972). In a double-blind experiment, human males were given either testosterone (40 mg/day), placebo, or no treatment, over a 1-week period. Subjective and observer-assessed mood estimations were conducted before and after treatment. Testosterone levels in saliva were measured with radioimmunoassay. The results revealed a significant placebo effect. After treatment, the placebo group scored higher than both the testosterone and the no-treatment group on self-estimated anger, irritation, impulsivity, and frustration. Observer-estimated mood yielded similar results. The authors concluded that the results suggested that androgen usage causes expectations, rather than an actual increase of aggressiveness (Bjorkqvist, Nygren, Bjorklund, & Bjorkqvist, 1994).

Bahrke and Yesalis (1994) have suggested other possible confounding factors in determining the psychological and behavioral effects of AS. They point out that changes frequently attributed to AS use may reflect changes brought about by weight training (nearly all AS users are also dedicated weight trainers). The psychological and behavioral changes could also result from the concurrent use of other substances such as alcohol, and from dietary manipulation including food supplements. They feel that weight training and related practices should be considered potential confounding factors in future studies designed to examine the psychological and behavioral effects of AS. In athletes, including bodybuilders, the extreme stress of training and competition, coupled perhaps with unreal expectations of what one should be able to accomplish, can often be enough to lead to emotional and psychological disturbances.

Because of lack of clear-cut associations between androgens and aggression, it is difficult to support much of what is being said about the sensationalized "roid rage." Our rational behavior, or lack of it, is much more than just the level of our serum testosterone. There are many other factors that contribute to aggressiveness. One source of variation in aggressiveness among humans can be found in the psychohistory of the individual, although it is possible that sensitivity to intake of AS may lead to significant mood changes in a small number of susceptible individuals who otherwise have no other significant predisposing factors.

In addition to AS, athletes also use many other drugs and supplements (Di Pasquale, 1991). It is possible that some of these other compounds, alone or in concert with the effects of AS, could result in hormonal and mood changes. For example, athletes commonly use corticosteroids for the treatment of athletic injuries. In addition to the well-recognized psychiatric complications seen in Cushing's disease (excess production of corticosteroids), there is a considerable body of evidence pointing to corticosteroid-induced psychoses in medical patients (Wolkowitz, 1994).

In recent years, a considerable amount of data have emerged stating that psychotic depression is characterized by pronounced increases in hypothalamic–pituitary–adrenal axis activity, leading to increased serum glucocorticoids and thus the psychological disturbances perhaps secondary to increased dopaminergic activity (Schatzberg, Rothschild, Langlais, Bird, & Colle, 1985). There is also some evidence that hormonal changes, sometimes secondary to hypothalamic–pituitary gland dysfunction, may accompany stress and some depressive illnesses (Bradley, 1987; Lesch, Muller, Rupprecht, Kruse, & Schulte, 1989).

Contrary to what one would expect with a drug that causes behavioral and mood changes, there seem to be no adverse behavioral or psychological effects reported in patients who are on replacement therapy or in studies in which higher than replacement amounts of testosterone and AS are being tested as possible male contraceptives (such as those sponsored by the World Health Organization (Bagatell, Heiman, Matsumoto, Rivier, & Bremner, 1994; World Health Organization Task Force, 1990).

The overall effects of AS on mood and behavior are difficult to determine. Other factors such as premorbid personality, the use of other drugs and substances, expectations, and stress greatly influence any behavioral or psychological changes seen in anabolic steroid–using athletes.

Withdrawal Symptoms and HPTA Dysfunction

AS are thought by some to be psychologically addicting because they can result in withdrawal symptoms and cravings when discontinued (Kashkin & Kleber, 1989). In my experience it is mainly athletes who have residual dysfunction in the hypothalamic–pituitary–testicular axis after the discontinuation of AS, and thus have lower than normal levels of serum testosterone, who suffer any significant emotional or dependent effects on the discontinuation of AS. Withdrawal symptoms, such as lassitude, depression, decreased sex drive, and some degree of impotence (perhaps accompanied by a tendency toward the female body habitus, including gynecomastia) are commonly seen in patients with low serum testosterone usually secondary to hypogonadism, stress, drugs, or disease (De Lignieres & Mauvais-Jarvis, 1979).

In my experience most competitive athletes who suffer symptoms after stopping the use of AS are not addicted to AS, since their symptoms of depression, such as decreased libido and fatigue, are due to a disruption of the hypothalamic–pituitary–testicular axis, resulting in deficient testicular steroidogenesis—the end result being a low serum testosterone. Once the serum testosterone is returned to the normal range, most of these patients are as well adjusted and emotionally stable as they were prior to their use of AS.

While attempting to normalize the HPTA, depressive and anxiety symptoms may be treated with anxiolytics such as the benzodiazepines, for example, Ativan, Librium, Valium, Xanax, and, if necessary, one of the antidepressants. However, if an antidepressant is warranted, the newer antidepressants that are serotonergic in action should not be used. Serotonin-stimulated corticotropin-releasing factor (CRF) inhibits basal and HCG-induced cAMP generation and steroidogenesis (Tinajero *et al.,* 1992). Serotonin mediates the stim-

ulatory action of LH-HCG on CRF secretion from Leydig cells and, thus, participates in a negative autoregulatory loop to limit the testosterone response to the gonadotropic stimulus. Studies have shown that antidepressant-associated sexual side effects are most common with the serotonin reuptake inhibitors and least common with bupropion (Gitlin, 1994; Labbate & Pollack, 1994). Thus, the use of serotonergic antidepressants could be counterproductive to any attempt to normalize the HPTA.

Addictive Potential of Anabolic Steroids

A number of researchers have attempted to show the dependence potential of AS by showing the many similarities of AS to addictive drugs and psychostimulants and the potential for psychoactive effects of AS (Brower, 1993a). Moreover, several authors, convinced that the use of AS can be addicting (Brower, Blow, Young, & Hill, 1991) and that dependence on these compounds is a clinical phenomenon, have commented on ways to treat anabolic steroid dependency and withdrawal (Brower, 1989, 1993b; Giannini, Miller, & Kocjan, 1991; Malone & Dimeff, 1992).

However, the psychoactive and addictive effects of AS are not prevalent considering the fact that more than a million North Americans have used AS in the past decade (Welder & Melchert, 1993). For such a widely used drug, there appears to be a singular lack of both interest in the professional community and treatment facilities to deal with anabolic steroid dependance. There are, however, several factors that argue against the tendency of AS to cause any significant physical or psychological dependence, and reasons that withdrawal symptoms are commonly seen but are not due to dependence or addiction.

While addictive drugs are mainly used for their mind-altering effects, such is not the case for AS. These compounds are mainly used for their strength and muscle-enhancing effects. There is no immediate feedback with anabolic steroid use. Taking a hundred tablets of one of the oral AS does not result in any physical or psychological highs, or for that matter any immediate effect except perhaps some gastrointestinal disturbance. The muscle and strength benefits of steroids generally take a few weeks to occur. In addition, the anabolic changes occur only if an intensive training and nutritional program accompanies the use of these drugs. Thus, for most athletes, the primary reason for AS use is not the psychoactive effects, but appearance, performance, or both. Since AS are not used for their mind-altering effects they appear to have a low addiction potential.

In addition, the use of high doses of AS can increase irritability and decrease the enjoyment of social interaction. Athletes realize that while on steroids they may not be as relaxed as usual, and cannot as easily enjoy their recreational and social time. This negative aspect of anabolic steroid use does not reinforce the use of steroids, and makes it quite easy to discontinue their use once the competitive need is gone.

For competitive athletes, the use of steroids is part of the whole package. They will do whatever it takes to win, whether it means getting certain pieces of equipment, using certain training regimens or special diets, stacking nutritional supplements, or taking AS. Most steroid-using athletes, if there was a safe natural supplement that would produce equal strength and muscle size gains as steroids, but did not have some of the negative psychological side effects, would stop their steroid use immediately.

Personality and Dependence

In some individuals, feelings of self-worth are dependent on their physical self-concept. For these individuals, AS may be psychologically addicting. This feeding of the ego, and not the psychoactive effects of AS, may be the reason for the long-term use of AS by recreational athletes, and some competitive athletes even after they have retired from competition. These individuals may find it difficult to stop using AS since gains made while taking them rapidly disappear.

Certain individuals may possess certain traits that may predispose them to using AS. A recent study documented a relationship between anabolic steroid use and narcissistic personality traits (Porcerelli & Sandler, 1995). In this study the authors compared weight lifters and bodybuilders who did or did not use AS on an objective measure of narcissism and on clinical ratings of empathy. They found that steroid users had significantly higher scores on dimensions of pathological narcissism and significantly lower scores on clinical ratings of empathy. The authors also felt that the results of the study indicated the need for further research to determine whether narcissistic personality traits contribute to the initiation of anabolic steroid use or result from their use.

Studies have shown that the use of AS can alter personality profiles and patterns in the athletes that use them. The results of one study showed that there is a statistically significant difference: (1) in the measured personality traits of male weight trainers when using and not using anabolic steroids, (2) between the measured personality traits of male weight trainers using anabolic steroids and the traits of a comparable group of male weight trainers who have never used the drugs, and (3) between the measured personality traits of male weight trainers when not using anabolic steroids and the traits of a comparable group of male weight trainers who have never used the drugs (Libstag, 1991). Another more recent study also showed these tendencies. This study also looked at the personality profile of men using anabolic-androgenic steroids as compared with men who had either stopped using steroids and those who had never used AS (Galligani, Renck, & Hansen, 1996). In this study, current AS users differed significantly from the other two groups with respect to verbal aggression. In comparison with subjects with no ongoing AS exposure (i.e., previous AS users and drug-free controls), AS users were also significantly different with respect to muscular tension, social desirability, impulsiveness, and indirect aggression. On several subscales, the scores of the AS users were clearly outside the normal range observed in general population.

It seems, therefore, that AS users may have a different personality profile, including a disturbance in body image (muscle dysmorphia—

never big enough!) that predisposes them to the use of AS (Pope, Gruber, Choi, Olivardia, & Phillips, 1997) and that the use of AS results in further differences in their personality profile compared with periods of nonuse.

Thus, premorbid personality is very important in determining the effects of AS on mood and behavior. And while the theoretical possibility is there, it has been my experience that only a small number of active steroid users suffer from any form of mental disturbance or addiction. And of those that do it is not known how many may have premorbid conditions and personalities that predispose them to mental health and substance abuse problems. As well, I feel that most athletes do not suffer any adverse psychological effects from their prior steroid use. In my thirty years of experience with hundreds of competitive athletes who have used AS, I've rarely seen any physical or psychological dependence except in athletes with HPTA dysfunction after anabolic steroid use. In these cases, either normalizing their HPTA dysfunction or using replacement testosterone therapy resolved their "withdrawal" or low serum testosterone symptoms.

Having known and talked with hundreds of steroid users, most of them competitive athletes, I have never seen a case where the steroid user had any problem stopping the use of steroids after they no longer competed and once the HPTA axis was normalized. In cases where testosterone levels remained below normal, only replacement therapy was needed. Maintaining higher than physiological levels of testosterone has never been necessary.

Conclusion

In conclusion, while androgenic-anabolic steroids have an effect on behavior and certain psychological parameters, they do not appear to have addictive potential per se, nor does the use or discontinuation of AS pose a problem for most users. There appears to be little comparison between anabolic steroid use and the use of licit and illicit psychoactive drugs.

In those patients who appear to be addicted to AS, care must be taken that the cravings and withdrawal symptoms are properly identified. In most cases a depressed HPTA and resulting low levels of serum testosterone are the cause of the symptoms and restoration of normal serum testosterone levels the proper treatment.

However, in order to better understand and treat athletes who abuse anabolic steroids, more research is needed to determine the effects and aftereffects of moderate to high doses of AS and testosterone on opioid and aminergic neurotransmission systems. We also need to know more about the disruptive effect of AS on the hypothalamic–pituitary–testicular axis (and perhaps also the hypothalamic–pituitary–somatotropic, hypothalamic–pituitary–thyroid and hypothalamic–pituitary–adrenocortical axes), and determine whether these effects contribute to any psychological or behavioral symptoms both while using and after the use of AS.

Acknowledgments

Some of the information in this chapter was adapted, by permission of MGD Press, from the following books and newsletters by Mauro G. Di Pasquale, M.D.:

- *Drug Use and Detection in Amateur Sports.* Mauro G. Di Pasquale, M.D. MGD Press, Warkworth, Ontario, Canada, 1984.
- Updates One to Five to "Drug Use and Detection in Amateur Sports." Mauro G. Di Pasquale, M.D. MGD Press, Warkworth, Ontario, Canada, 1985–1988.
- *Beyond Anabolic Steroids.* Mauro G. Di Pasquale, M.D. MGD Press, Warkworth, Ontario, Canada, 1990.
- *Anabolic Steroid Side Effects—Fact, Fiction and Treatment.* Mauro G. Di Pasquale, M.D. MGD Press, Warkworth, Ontario, Canada, 1990.
- *Drugs in Sports.* Mauro G. Di Pasquale, M.D. Volumes 1–3. 1991–1995.

References

Abeyawardene, S. A., & Plant, T. M. (1989). Reconciliation of the paradox that testosterone replacement prevents the postcastration hypersecretion of follicle-stimulating hormone in male rhesus monkeys (Macaca mulatta) with an intact central nervous system but not in hypothalamic-lesioned, gonadotropin-releasing hormone-replaced animals. *Biology of Reproduction, 40,* 578–584.

Albert, D. J., Petrovic, D. M., & Walsh, M. L. (1989). Competitive experience activates testosterone-dependent social aggression toward unfamiliar males. *Physiology & Behavior, 45,* 723–727.

Albert, D. J., Jonik, R. H., Watson, N. V., Gorzalka, B. B., & Walsh, M. L. (1990). Hormone-dependent aggression in male rats is proportional to serum testosterone concentration but sexual behavior is not. *Physiology & Behavior, 48,* 409–416.

Alen, M., & Hakkinen, K. (1985). Physical health and fitness of an elite bodybuilder during 1 year of self-administering testosterone and anabolic steroids a case study. *International Journal of Sports Medicine, 6,* 24–29.

Alen, M., Reinila, M., & Vihko, R. (1985). Response of serum hormones to androgen administration in power athletes. *Medicine & Science in Sports & Exercise, 17,* 354–359.

Alen, M., Rahkila, P., Reinila, M., & Vihko, R. (1987). Androgenic-anabolic steroid effects on serum thyroid, pituitary and steroid hormones in athletes. *American Journal of Sports Medicine, 15,* 357–361.

Annitto, W. J., & Layman, W. A. (1980). Anabolic steroids and acute schizophrenic episode: case reports. *Journal of Clinical Psychiatry, 41,* 143–144.

Archer, J. (1991). The influence of testosterone on human aggression. *British Journal of Psychology, 82,* 1–28.

Ariel, G., & Saville, W. (1972). Anabolic steroids: The physiologic effects of placebos. *Medicine & Science in Sports & Exercise, 4,* 124–126.

Bagatell, C. J., Heiman, J. R., Matsumoto, A. M., Rivier, J. E., & Bremner, W. J. (1994). Metabolic and behavioral effects of high-dose, exogenous testosterone in healthy men. *Journal of Clinical Endocrinology & Metabolism, 79,* 561–567.

Bahrke, M. S., Wright, J. E., O'Connor, J. S., Strauss, R. H., & Catlin, D. H. (1990). Selected psychological characteristics of anabolic-androgenic steroid users. *New England Journal of Medicine, 323,* 834–835.

Bahrke, M. S., & Yesalis, C. E. (1994). Weight training. A potential confounding factor in examining the psychological and behavioural effects of anabolic-androgenic steroids [Review]. *Sports Medicine, 18,* 309–318.

Bahrke, M. S., Yesalis, C. E., & Wright, J. E. (1990). Psychological and behavioural effects of endogenous testosterone levels and anabolic-androgenic steroids among males: A review. *Sports Medicine, 10,* 303–337.

Bahrke, M., Wright, J., Strauss, R., & Catlin, D. (1992). Psychological moods and subjectively perceived behavioral and somatic changes accompanying anabolic-androgenic steroid use. *American Journal of Sports Medicine, 20,* 717–724.

Balducci, R., Toscano, V., Casilli, D., Maroder, M., Sciarra, F., & Boscherini, B. (1987). Testicular respon-

siveness following chronic administration of HCG (1500 IV every six days) in untreated hypogonadotropic hypogonadism. *Hormone & Metabolic Research, 19,* 216–221.

Balestreri, R., Bertolini, S., Chiodini, G., & Ronzitti, M. (1971). Pituitary inhibitory and non-inhibitory effects of various anabolic 17-alkylating steroids. *Archivo e Maragliano di Patologia e Clinica, 27,* 123–135.

Baranowska, B., Jeske, W., Niewiadomska, A., Rozbicka, G., Walczak, L., & Zgliczynski, S. (1983). Enhanced serum prolactin concentration after metoclopramide stimulation in idiopathic oligozoospermia and azoospermia. *Andrologia, 15* (Special No.), 554–559.

Barker, S. (1987). Oxymethalone and aggression. *British Journal of Psychiatry, 151,* 564.

Bhasin, S., Storer, T. W., Berman, N., Callegari, C., Clevenger, B., Phillips, J., Blunnell, T., Tricker, R., Shirazi, A., & Casaburi, R. (1996). The effect of supraphysiologic doses of testosterone on muscle size and strength in normal men. *New England Journal of Medicine, 335,* 1–7.

Bjorkqvist, K., Nygren, T., Bjorklund, A. C., & Bjorkqvist, S. E. (1994). Testosterone intake and aggressiveness: Real effect or anticipation? *Aggressive Behavior, 20,* 18–26.

Blank, D. M., Clark, R. V., Heymsfield, S. B., Rudman, D., & Blank, M. (1994). Endogenous opioids and hypogonadism in human obesity. *Brain Research Bulletin, 34,* 571–574.

Bradley, A. J. (1987). Stress and mortality in the red-tailed phascogale, Phascogale calura (Marsupialia: Dasyuridae). *General & Comparative Endocrinology, 67,* 85–100.

Brower K. (1989). Rehabilitation for anabolic-androgenic steroid dependence. *Clinics in Sports Medicine, 1,* 171–181.

Brower, K. J. (1993a). Anabolic steroids: Potential for physical and psychological dependence. In C. Yesalis (Ed.), *Anabolic steroids in sport and exercise* (pp. 193–213). Champaign, IL: Human Kinetics.

Brower, K. J. (1993b). Assessment and treatment of anabolic steroid withdrawal. In C. Yesalis (Ed), *Anabolic steroids in sport and exercise* (pp. 231–250). Champaign, IL: Human Kinetics.

Brower, K. J., Blow, F. C., Beresford, T. P., & Fuelling, C. (1989). Anabolic-androgenic steroid dependence. *Journal of Clinical Psychiatry, 50,* 31–33.

Brower, K. J., Blow, F. C., Eliopulos, G. A., & Beresford, T. P. (1989). Letters to the Editor: Anabolic androgenic steroids and suicide. *American Journal of Psychiatry, 146,* 1075.

Brower, K. J., Eliopulos, G. A., Blow, F. C., Catlin, D. H., & Beresford, T. P. (1990). Evidence for physical and psychological dependence on anabolic androgenic steroids in eight weight lifters. *American Journal of Psychiatry, 147,* 510–512.

Brower, K., Blow, F., Young, J., & Hill, E. (1991). Symptoms and correlates of anabolic-androgenic steroid dependence. *British Journal of Addiction, 86,* 759–768.

Celotti, F., Avogadri, N., Melcangi, R. C, Milani, S., & Negri Cesi, P. (1984). Cyclophenil, a non-steroidal compound with a higher central than peripheral oestrogenic activity: Study of its effects on uterine growth and on some central parameters in castrated female rats. *Acta Endocrinologica, 107,* 340–345.

Choi, P. Y. L., Parrott, A. C., & Cowan, D. (1990). High-dose anabolic steroids in strength athletes: Effects upon hostility and aggression. *Human Psychopharmacology, 5,* 349–356.

Christiansen, K., & Knussmann, R. (1987). Androgen levels and components of aggressive behavior in men. *Hormones & Behavior, 21,* 170–180.

Clerico, A., Ferdeghini, M., Palombo, C., Leoncini, R., Del Chicca, M., Sardano, G., & Mariani, G. (1981). Effect of anabolic treatment on the serum levels of gonadotropins, testosterone, prolactin, thyroid hormones and myoglobin of male athletes under physical training. *Journal of Nuclear Medicine & Allied Sciences, 25,* 79–88.

Conacher, G., & Workman, D. (1989). Violent crime possibly associated with anabolic steroid use. *American Journal of Psychiatry, 146,* 679.

Dalby, J. (1992). Brief anabolic steroid use and sustained behavioral reaction. *American Journal of Psychiatry, 149,* 271–272.

Dalkin, A. C., Haisenleder, D. J., Ortolano, G. A., Ellis, T. R., & Marshall, J. C. (1989). The frequency of gonadotropin-releasing-hormone stimulation differentially regulates gonadotropin subunit messenger ribonucleic acid expression. *Endocrinology, 125,* 917–924.

De Lignieres, B., & Mauvais-Jarvis, P. (1979). Hormones in depressive illness. The role of cortisol and sexual steroids. *Annales de Biologie Clinique, 37,* 49–57.

del Pozo, E., & Martin-Perez, J. (1985). Effect of dopamine receptor stimulation on the inhibition of LH pulsatility by a met-enkephaline (FK 33-824). *Acta Neurochirurgica, 75,* 88–90.

Delville, Y., Mansour, K. M., & Ferris, C. F. (1996). Testosterone facilitates aggression by modulating vasopressin receptors in the hypothalamus. *Physiology & Behavior, 60,* 25–29.

Di Pasquale, M. G. (1991). Polypharmacy—Anabolic steroids and beyond. *Drugs in Sports,* Premier Issue, 1–2.

Dunkel, L., & Huhtaniemi, I. (1985). Abnormal prolactin secretion in prepubertal boys with hypogonadotrophic hypogonadism—Possible involvement in regulation of testicular steroidogenesis. *International Journal of Andrology, 8,* 385–392.

Egginton, S. (1987). Effects of an anabolic hormone on striated muscle growth and performance. *Pflugers Archiv—European Journal of Physiology, 410,* 349–355.

Falaschi, P., Frajese, G., Sciarra, F., Rocco, A., & Conti, C. (1978). Influence of hyperprolactinaemia due to metoclopramide on gonadal function in men. *Clinical Endocrinology, 8,* 427–433.

Finkelstein, J. S., Spratt, D. I., O'Dea, L. S., Whitcomb, R., Klibanski, A., Schoenfeld, D., & Crowley, W. (1989). Pulsatile gonadotropin secretion after discontinuation of long-term gonadotropin-releasing hormone (GnRH) administration in a subset of GnRH-deficient men. *Journal of Clinical Endocrinology & Metabolism, 69,* 377–385.

Foresta, C., Scanelli, G., Tramarin, A., & Scandellari, C. (1985). Serotonin but not dopamine is involved in the naloxone-induced luteinizing hormone release in man. *Fertility & Sterility, 43,* 447–450.

Frajese, G., Lazzari, R., Magnani, A., Moretti, C., Sforza, V., & Nerozzi, D. (1990), Neurotransmitter, opiodergic system, steroid-hormone interaction and involvement in the replacement therapy of sexual disorders. *Journal of Steroid Biochemistry & Molecular Biology, 37,* 411–419.

Frankle, M. A., Eichberg, R., & Zachariah, S. B. (1988). Anabolic androgenic steroids and a stroke in an athlete: Case report. *Archives of Physical Medicine & Rehabilitation, 69,* 632–633.

Freinhar, J. P., & Alvarez, W. (1985). Androgen-induced Hypomania [letter]. *Journal of Clinical Psychiatry, 46,* 354–355.

Galligani, N., Renck, A., & Hansen, S. (1996). Personality profile of men using anabolic androgenic steroids. *Hormones & Behavior, 30,* 170–175.

Giannini, J. A., Miller, N., & Kocjan, D. (1991). Treating steroid abuse: A psychiatric perspective. *Clinical Pediatrics, 30,* 538–542.

Gitlin, M. J. (1994). Psychotropic medications and their effects on sexual function: diagnosis, biology, and treatment approaches. *Journal of Clinical Psychiatry, 55,* 406–413.

Glass, A. R. (1988). Pituitary-testicular reserve in men with low serum testosterone and normal serum luteinizing hormone. *Journal of Andrology, 9,* 224–230.

Goodman Gilman, A., Goodman, L. S., Rall, T. N., & Murad, F. (Eds.). (1985). *The pharmacological basis of therapeutics, 7th edition.* New York: Macmillan.

Griggs, R. C., Kingston, W., Jozefowicz, R. F., Herr, B. E., Forbes, G., & Halliday, D. (1989). Effect of testosterone on muscle mass and muscle protein synthesis. *Journal of Applied Physiology* (United States), *66,* 498–503.

Hannan, C. J., Friedl, K. E., Zold, A., Kettler, T. M., & Plymate, S. R. (1991). Psychological and serum homovanillic acid changes in men administered androgenic steroids. *Psychoneuroendocrinology, 16,* 335–343.

Haupt, H. A., & Rovere, G. D. (1984). Anabolic steroids: A review of the literature. *American Journal of Sports Medicine, 12,* 469–484.

Hobbs, C. J., Plymate, S. R., Bell, B. K., & Patience, T. H. (1991). The effect of androgens on glucose tolerance. *Clinical Research, 39,* 384A.

Holma, P., & Adlercreutz, H. (1976). Effect of an anabolic steroid (metandienon) on plasma LH-FSH, and testosterone and on the response to intravenous administration of LRH. *Acta Endocrinologica, 83,* 856–864.

Jezova, D., Komadel, L., & Mikulaj, L. (1987). Plasma testosterone response to repeated human chorionic gonadotropin administration is increased in trained athletes. *Endocrinologica Experimentalis, 21,* 143–147.

Kashkin, K. B., & Kleber, H. D. (1989). Hooked on hormones? An anabolic steroid addiction hypothesis. *Journal of the American Medical Association, 262,* 3166–3170.

Kehoe, P. (1982). The relevance of anabolic steroids to middle distance running. *Australian Track and Field Coaches Association* (monograph).

Kenyon, A. T. (1938). The effect of testosterone propionate on the genitalia, prostrate, secondary sex characters, and body weight in eunuchoidism. *Endocrinology, 23,* 121–134.

Kenyon, A. T. (1942, September). *The first Josiah Macy Jr. Conference on bone and wound healing.*

Kenyon, A. T., Knowlton, K., Lotwin, G., & Sandford, I. (1942). Metabolic response of aged men to testosterone propionate. *Journal of Clinical Endocrinology, 2,* 690–695.

Kenyon, A. T., Knowlton, K., & Sandford, I. (1944). The anabolic effects of the androgens and somatic growth in man. *Annals of Internal Medicine, 20,* 632–654.

Kilshawm, B. H., Harkness, R. A., Hobson, B. M., & Smith, A. W. (1975). The effects of large doses of the anabolic steroid, methandrostenolone, on an athlete. *Clinical Endocrinology, 4,* 537–541.

Kiraly, C. L., Collan, Y., & Alen, M. (1987). Effect of testosterone and anabolic steroids on the size of sebaceous glands in power athletes. *American Journal of Dermatopathology, 9,* 515–519.

Kletter, G. B., Foster, C. M., Beitins, I. Z., Marshall, J., & Kelch, R. (1992). Acute effects of testosterone infusion and naloxone on luteinizing hormone secretion in normal men. *Journal of Clinical Endocrinology & Metabolism, 75,* 1215–1219.

Kletter, G. B., Foster, C. M., Brown, M. B., Beitins, I., Marshall, J., & Kelch, R. (1994). Nocturnal naloxone fails to reverse the suppressive effects of testosterone infusion on luteinizing hormone secretion in pubertal boys. *Journal of Clinical Endocrinology & Metabolism, 79,* 1147–1151.

Kouri, E. M., Lukas, S. E., Pope, H. G., Jr., & Oliva, P. S. (1995). Increased aggressive responding in male volunteers following the administration of gradually increasing doses of testosterone cypionate. *Drug and Alcohol Dependence, 40,* 73–79.

Kruskemper, H. L. (1968). *Anabolic steroids* (C. H. Doering, Trans.). New York: Academic Press.

Kulin, H. E., & Reiter, E. O. (1972). Gonadotropin suppression by low dose estrogen in men—Evidence for differential effects upon FSH and LH. *Journal of Clinical Endocrinology & Metabolism, 35,* 836–839.

Labbate, L. A., & Pollack, M. H. (1994). Treatment of fluoxetine-induced sexual dysfunction with bupropion: a case report. *Annals of Clinical Psychiatry, 6,* 13–15.

Lefavi, R. G., Reeve, T. G., & Newland, M. C. (1990). Relationship between anabolic steroid use and selected psychological parameters in male bodybuilders. *Journal of Sport Behavior, 13,* 157–166.

Le Greves, P., Huang, W., Johansson, P., Thornwall, M., Zhou, Q., & Nyberg, F. (1997). Effects of an anabolic-androgenic steroid on the regulation of the NMDA receptor NR1, NR2A and NR2B subunit mRNAs in brain regions of the male rat. *Neuroscience Letters, 18,* 61–64.

Lesch, K. P., Muller, U., Rupprecht, R., Kruse, K., & Schulte, H. (1989). Endocrine responses to growth hormone-releasing hormone, thyrotropin-releasing hormone and corticotropin-releasing hormone in depression. *Acta Psychiatrica Scandinavica, 79,* 597–602.

Libstag, K. (1990). The effects of anabolic steroids on measured personality traits of male weight trainers. *Dissertation Abstracts International, 51,* 4091.

Lindstrom, M., Nilsson, A., Katzman, P., Janzon, L., & Dymling, J. (1990). Use of anabolic-androgenic steroids among bodybuilders: Frequency and attitudes. *Journal of Internal Medicine, 227,* 407–411.

Maddocks, S., & Setchell, B. P. (1989). Effect of a single injection of human chorionic gonadotrophin on testosterone levels in testicular interstitial fluid, and in testicular and peripheral venous blood in adult rats. *Journal of Endocrinology, 121,* 311–316.

Maggi, M., De Feo, M. L., Mannelli, M., Delitala, G., & Forti, G. (1985). Naloxone administration does not affect gonadotrophin secretion in male patients with isolated hypogonadotrophic hypogonadism. *Acta Endocrinologica, 109,* 153–157.

Malone, D., & Dimeff, R. (1992). The use of fluoxetine in depression associated with anabolic steroid withdrawal: A case series. *Journal of Clinical Psychiatry, 53,* 130–132.

Martikainen, H., Alen, M., Rahkila, P., & Vihko, R. (1986). Testicular responsiveness to human chorionic gonadotrophin during transient hypogonadotrophic hypogonadism induced by androgenic/anabolic steroids in power athletes. *Journal of Steroid Biochemistry, 25,* 109–112.

Masonis, A. E., & McCarthy, M. P. (1996). Direct interactions of androgenic/anabolic steroids with the peripheral benzodiazepine receptor in rat brain: Implications for the psychological and physiological manifestations of androgenic/anabolic steroid abuse. *Journal of Steroid Biochemistry and Molecular Biology, 58,* 551–555.

McNutt, R. A., Ferenchick, G. S., Kirlin, P. C., & Hamlin, N. J. (1988). Acute myocardial infarction in a 22-year-old world class weight lifter using anabolic steroids. *American Journal of Cardiology, 62,* 164.

Mikuma, N., Kumamoto, Y., Maruta, H., & Nitta, T. (1994). Role of the hypothalamic opioidergic system in the control of gonadotropin secretion in elderly men. *Andrologia, 26,* 39–45.

Nakagawa, K., Obara, T., Matsubara, M., & Kubo, M. (1982). Relationship of changes in serum concentrations of prolactin and testosterone during dopaminergic modulation in males. *Clinical Endocrinology, 17,* 345–352.

Nilsson, P. M., Moller, L., & Solstad, K. (1995). Adverse effects of psychosocial stress on gonadal function and insulin levels in middle-aged males. *Journal of Internal Medicine, 237,* 479–486.

Perry, P. J., Andersen, K. H., & Yates, W. R. (1990). Illicit anabolic steroid use in athletes: A case series analysis. *American Journal of Sports Medicine, 18,* 422–428.

Perry, P. J., Yates, W. R., & Andersen, K. H. (1990). Psychiatric symptoms associated with anabolic steroids: A controlled, retrospective study. *Annals of Clinical Psychiatry, 2,* 11–17.

Pope, H. G., & Katz, D. L. (1987). Bodybuilder's psychosis. *Lancet, 1,* 863.

Pope, H. G., & Katz, D. L. (1988). Affective and psychotic symptoms associated with anabolic steroid use. *American Journal of Psychiatry, 145,* 487–490.

Pope, H. G., & Katz, D. L. (1990). Homicide and near-homicide by anabolic steroid users. *Journal of Clinical Psychiatry, 51,* 28–31.

Pope, H. G., Jr., Gruber, A. J., Choi, P., Olivardia, R., & Phillips, K. A. (1997). An underrecognized form of body dysmorphic disorder. *Psychosomatics, 38,* 548–557.

Porcerelli, J. H., & Sandler, B. A. (1995). Narcissism and empathy in steroid users. *American Journal of Psychiatry, 152,* 1672–1674.

Prat, J., Gray, G. F., Stolley, P. D., & Coleman, J. W. (1977). Wilms' tumor in an adult associated with androgen abuse. *Journal of the American Medical Association, 237,* 2322–2323.

Rasmussen, D. D., Kennedy, B. P., Ziegler, M. G., & Nett, T. M. (1988). Endogenous opioid inhibition and facilitation of gonadotropin-releasing hormone release from the median eminence in vitro: potential role of catecholamines. *Endocrinology, 123,* 2916–2921.

Repcekova, D., & Mikulaj, L. (1977). Plasma testosterone response to HCG in normal men without and after administration of anabolic drug. *Endokrinologie, 69,* 115–118.

Roberts, J. T., & Essenhigh, D. M. (1986). Adenocarcinoma of prostate in 40-year-old body-builder [Letter]. *Lancet, 2,* 742.

Rockhold, R. W. (1993). Cardiovascular toxicity of anabolic steroids. *Annual Review of Pharmacology & Toxicology, 33,* 497–520.

Rowlands, R. P., & Nicholson, G. W. (1929). Growth of left testicle with precocious sexual and bodily development (macro-genitosomia) *Guy's Hospital Report, 79,* 401–408.

Ruokonen, A., Alen, M., Bolton, N., & Vihko, R. (1985). Response of serum testosterone and its precursor steroids, SHBG and CBG to anabolic steroid and testosterone self-administration in man. *Journal of Steroid Biochemistry, 23,* 33–38.

Ryzhenkov, V. E., Bekhtereva, E. P., & Sapronov, N. S. (1974). Role of the limbic structures in the mechanism of action of glucocorticoids and estrogens on hypothalamic control of pituitary adrenocorticotropic and gonadotropic functions. *Bulletin of Experimental Biology & Medicine, 77,* 362–265.

Sacchi, E. (1895). A case of infantile gigantism (pedo-macrosomia) with a tumor of the testicle. *Riv. sper Freniat., 21,* 149–161.

Schatzberg, A. F., Rothschild, A. J., Langlais, P. J., Bird, E. D., & Cole, J. O. (1985). A corticosteroid/dopamine hypothesis for psychotic depression and related states. *Journal of Psychiatric Research, 19,* 57–64.

Schlinger, B. A., & Callard, G. V. (1989). Aromatase activity in quail brain: correlation with aggressiveness. *Endocrinology, 124,* 437–43.

Schulte, H. M., Hall, M. J., & Boyer, M. (1993). Domestic violence associated with anabolic steroid abuse [Letter to the editor]. *American Journal of Psychiatry, 150,* 348.

Schulte-Beerbuhl, M., & Nieschlag, E. (1980). Comparison of testosterone, dihydrotestosterone, luteinizing hormone, and follicle-stimulating hormone in serum after injection of testosterone enanthate or testosterone cypionate. *Fertility & Sterility, 33,* 201–203.

Sheckter, C. B., Matsumoto, A. M., & Bremner, W. J. (1989). Testosterone administration inhibits gonadotropin secretion by an effect directly on the human pituitary. *Journal of Clinical Endocrinology & Metabolism, 68,* 397–401.

Siegel, J. M. (1986). The Multidimensional Anger Inventory. *Journal of Personality & Social Psychology, 51,* 191–200.

Smals, A. G., Pieters, G. F., Smals, A. E., Hermus, A. R., Boers, G. H., Raemaekers, J. M., Benraad, T. J., & Kloppenborg, P. W. (1987). Reciprocal inhibition of the long-acting luteinizing hormone releasing hormone agonist Buserelin and human chorionic gonadotropin in stimulating Leydig cell steroidogenesis. *Journal of Steroid Biochemistry, 28,* 743–747.

Soe, K. L., Soe, M., & Gluud, C. N. (1994). [Liver pathology associated with anabolic androgenic steroids]. *Ugeskrift for Laeger, 156,* 2585–2588.

Spitz, I. M., LeRoith, D., Livshin, Y., Zylber-Haran, E., Trestian, S., Laufer, N., Ron, M., Palti, Z., & Schenker, J. (1980). Exaggerated prolactin response to thyrotropin-releasing hormone and metoclopramide in primary testicular failure. *Fertility & Sterility, 34,* 573–580.

Stannard, J. P., & Bucknell, A. L. (1993). Rupture of the triceps tendon associated with steroid injections. *American Journal of Sports Medicine, 21,* 482–485.

Strauss, R., Liggett, M., & Lanese, R. (1985). Anabolic steroid use and perceived effects in ten weight-trained women athletes. *Journal of the American Medical Association, 253,* 2871–2873.

Strauss, R. H., Wright, J. E., Finerman, G. A. M., & Catlin, D. H. (1983). Side effects of anabolic steroids in weight-trained men. *Physician and Sports Medicine, 11,* 86–88, 91–93, 95, 98.

Su, T. P., Pagliaro, M., Schmidt, P. J., Pickar, D., Wolkowitz, O., & Rubinow, D. R. (1993). Neuropsychiatric effects of anabolic steroids in male normal volunteers. *Journal of the American Medical Association, 269,* 2760–2764.

Taylor, W. (1987). Anabolic steroids: A plea for control. *Chiropractic Sports Medicine, 1,* 47–52.

Taylor, W. N. (1985). *Hormonal manipulation. A new era of monstrous athletes.* Jefferson, NC: McFarland.

Tennant, F., Black, D. L., & Voy, R. O. (1988). Correspondence: Anabolic steroid dependence with opioid-type features. *New England Journal of Medicine, 319,* 578.

Tepavcevic, D., Giljevic, Z., Korsic, M., Halimi, S., Suchanek, E., Jelic, T., Aganovic, I., Kozic, B., & Plavsic, V. (1994). Effects of ritanserin, a novel serotonin-S2 receptor antagonist, on the secretion of pituitary hormones in normal humans. *Journal of Endocrinological Investigation, 17,* 1–5.

Tilzey, A., Heptonstall, J., & Hamblin, T. (1981). Toxic confusional state and choreiform movements after treatment with anabolic steroids. *British Medical Journal, 285,* 349–350.

Tinajero, J. C., Fabbri, A., & Dufau, M. L. (1992). Regulation of corticotropin-releasing factor secretion from Leydig cells by serotonin. *Endocrinology, 130,* 1780–1788.

Van Vugt, D. A., & Meites, J. (1980). Influence of endogenous opiates on anterior pituitary function [Review]. *Federation Proceedings, 39,* 2533–2538.

Vanderstichele, H., Eechaute, W., Lacroix, E., & Leusen, I. (1989). Effect of tamoxifen on the activity of enzymes of testicular steroidogenesis. *Steroids, 53,* 713–726.

Vermeulen, A. (1994). [Neuroendocrinological aspects of aging]. *Verhandelingen-Koninklijke Academie voor Geneeskunde van Belgie, 56,* 267–280.

Vermeulen, A., & Kaufman, J. M. (1995). Ageing of the hypothalamo-pituitary-testicular axis in men. *Hormone Research, 43,* 25–28.

Vida, J. A. (1969). *Androgens and anabolic agents.* New York: Academic Press.

Wanderley, M. I., Favaretto, A. L., Valenca, M. M., Hattori, M., Wakabayaski, K., & Antunes-Rodrigues, J. (1989). Modulatory effects of adrenergic agonists on testosterone secretion from rat dispersed testicular cells or Percoll-purified Leydig cells. *Brazilian Journal of Medical & Biological Research, 22,* 1421–1429.

Webb, O. L., Laskarzewski, P. M., & Glueck, C. J. (1985). Severe depression of high-density lipoprotein cholesterol levels in weight lifters and body builders by self-administered exogenous testosterone and anabolic-androgenic steroids. *Metabolism, 33,* 971–975. Abstract/Commentary: *1986 Year Book of Endocrinology,* Article 8-8.

Welder, A. A., & Melchert, R. B. (1993). Cardiotoxic effects of cocaine and anabolic-androgenic steroids in the athlete [Review]. *Journal of Pharmacological & Toxicological Methods, 29,* 61–68.

Williams, T. D., Lightman, S. L., Johnson, M. R., Carmichael, D., & Bannister, R. (1989). Selective defect in gonadotrophin secretion in patients with autonomic failure. *Clinical Endocrinology, 30,* 285–292.

Williamson, D. J., & Young, A. H. (1992). Psychiatric effects of androgenic and anabolic-androgenic steroid abuse in men: A brief review of the literature. *Journal of Psychopharmacology, 6,* 20–26.

Wilson, I. C., Prange, A. J., & Lara, P. P. (1974). Methyltestosterone and imipramine in men: Conversion of depression to paranoid reaction. *American Journal of Psychiatry, 131,* 21–24.

Wilson, J. (1988). Androgen abuse by athletes. *Endocrinology Review, 9,* 181–199.

Windsor, R., & Dumitru, D. (1989). Prevalence of anabolic steroid use by male and female adolescents. *Medicine & Science in Sports & Exercise* (United States), *21,* 494–497.

Wolkowitz, O. M. (1994). Prospective controlled studies of the behavioral and biological effects of exogenous corticosteroids [Review]. *Psychoneuroendocrinology, 19,* 233–255.

Woodard, T. L., Burghen, G. A., Kitabchi, A. E., & Wilmas, J. A. (1981). Glucose intolerance and insulin resistance in aplastic anemia treated with oxymethalone. *Journal of Clinical Endocrinology & Metabolism, 53,* 905–908.

World Health Organization Task Force. (1990). Contraceptive efficacy of testosterone-induced azoospermia in normal men. World Health Organization Task Force on methods for the regulation of male fertility. *Lancet, 336,* 955–959.

Wroblewska, A. M. (1997). Androgenic–anabolic steroids and body dysmorphia in young men. *Journal of Psychometric Research, 42,* 225–234.

34

Ecstasy

UNA D. McCANN, MELISSA MERTL,

AND GEORGE A. RICAURTE

Introduction

(±) 3,4-Methylenedioxymethamphetamine (MDMA, "Ecstasy") is a synthetic analog of amphetamine and mescaline that possesses stimulant and "psychedelic" properties. Although MDMA was initially synthesized in Germany at the turn of the century (Merck, 1914), MDMA did not gain popularity in the United States until the late 1970s, when it was advocated as a potential psychotherapeutic adjunct (Shulgin & Nichols, 1978). During that same period, MDMA use in recreational settings also emerged, and use of MDMA in both professional and recreational settings continued to rise until 1985, when the Drug Enforcement Administration (DEA) in the United States decided to severely restrict MDMA use by placing it on schedule I of controlled substances (Lawn, 1986). This decision was based, in part, on research studies of a closely related amphetamine analog, methylenedioxyamphetamine (MDA), demonstrating that MDA-exposed animals developed lasting damage to brain serotonin neurons (Ricaurte, Bryan, Strauss,

UNA D. McCANN AND MELISSA MERTL • National Institute of Mental Health, Bethesda, Maryland 20892. GEORGE A. RICAURTE • Department of Neurology, The Johns Hopkins Bayview Medical Center, Baltimore, Maryland 21224.

Handbook of Substance Abuse: Neurobehavioral Pharmacology, edited by Tarter *et al.* Plenum Press, New York, 1998.

Seiden, & Schuster, 1985). Given the similarities between the chemical, pharmacological, and behavioral effects of MDA and MDMA, there was concern that MDMA might also lead to brain serotonergic injury in human users.

Although MDMA use in mental health settings decreased substantially following its placement on schedule I, recreational use of MDMA continues to rise in the United States and abroad (Anonymous, 1992). This rise can be attributed largely to the advent of "raves," large organized social events where MDMA is used as the drug of choice. Although there is some variability, raves typically involve hundreds to thousands of costumed partygoers who dance throughout the night and early morning to laser light shows and tribal music. Dosages of MDMA used during raves also vary, ranging from 1 to 8–10 tablets of MDMA, with each tablet estimated to contain 75–150 mgs.

Why Is MDMA of Interest?

MDMA has gained considerable attention from both lay and scientific communities for a variety of reasons. The growing popularity of MDMA among youths over the past decade has raised questions regarding its abuse and dependence liability. Well-publicized fatalities in MDMA users have focused attention on the acute medical consequences of MDMA use. Finally, numerous studies in experimental animals demonstrating MDMA's potent serotonin neurotoxic potential have aroused the interest of public health officials and neuroscientists. Although the presence of serotonin damage in human MDMA users has not been fully established, if present it could be manifested by mood and anxiety disorders, cognitive dysfunction, sleep and appetite disorders, or sexual dysfunction in the large numbers of individuals exposed to MDMA. From a neuroscientific viewpoint, clinical studies in MDMA users may provide valuable insight into the role of brain serotonin neurons in normal and abnormal neuropsychiatric function.

Drug Abuse Liability

Animal Studies

Consistent with the occurrence of recreational human MDMA use, animals show propensity to self-administer MDMA in laboratory settings. For instance, baboons trained to self-administer cocaine also self-administer low doses of MDMA (0.32–1.0 mg/kg) (Lamb & Griffiths, 1987). Similarly, rhesus monkeys trained to self-administer cocaine have been found to self-administer MDMA, in some instances at a rate greater than cocaine (Beardsley, Balster, & Harris, 1986). In addition, MDMA has been shown to lower the threshold for intracranial self-stimulation (Hubner, Bird, Rassnick, & Kornetsky, 1988), another model system used to gauge a drug's abuse potential.

Human Users

Because of MDMA's illicit status in this country and the majority of countries where it is used, the number of individuals who have used MDMA is not known. However, in 1985, Siegel provided an estimate that 20,000 doses of MDMA were being sold per month (Siegel, unpublished data, 1985). Four years later, Doblin (1989) adjusted this estimate upward to 100,000 doses, a number that corresponded well with estimates obtained from the National Institute on Drug Abuse Household Survey in 1994. There have been no formal epidemiological surveys regarding typical recreational

MDMA use patterns. Early retrospective surveys indicated that MDMA was typically used intermittently and episodically on weekends (Peroutka, Newman, & Harris, 1988), but more recent experience with individuals who attend raves suggest a change in that use pattern. In particular, a number of subjects participating in an ongoing research project of MDMA users have reported using higher cumulative daily doses, and they sometimes use MDMA several times weekly. Further, some report that greater dosages of MDMA are required over time to achieve the desired subjective effects. This more recent pattern of MDMA use suggests that early isolated reports that some MDMA users used escalating MDMA doses over time (McCann & Ricaurte, 1991; McGuire & Fahy, 1991) may have forecast what is becoming a more prevalent usage pattern.

Adverse Effects

In addition to the pleasant subjective experience that most MDMA users report (see Greer & Tolbert, 1986; Leister, Grob, Bravo, & Walsh, 1992), MDMA can also produce unpleasant physical or emotional effects in some users. More importantly, serious and fatal medical and psychiatric conditions have been linked to MDMA use.

Acute General Medical Effects

Two early studies prospectively evaluated the subjective effects of MDMA in a total of 50 subjects who used MDMA at doses ranging between 1.75 and 4.18 mg/kg (Downing, 1986) or 75 and 300 mg (Greer & Tolbert, 1986). Minor general medical and neuropsychiatric side effects (Table 1) found in these studies overlap considerably with those found in four retrospective surveys conducted in hundreds of MDMA users (Cohen, 1995; Leister et al., 1992; Peroutka et al., 1988; Solowij, Hall, & Lee, 1992).

More serious acute medical complications of MDMA use have typically appeared in the medical literature as individual case reports, reports from poison centers or reports from medical coroners. Summarized in Table 2 are

TABLE 1. Minor Acute Side Effects of MDMA

Symptom	Citation
General medical	
Nausea, vomiting, jaw clenching (trismus), teeth grinding, bruxism, hypertension, palpitations, headaches, hyperreflexia, difficulty walking, urinary urgency, diaphoresis, anorexia, muscle aches or tension, hot and cold flashes, jittery vision (nystagmus) and blurred vision, insomnia, dry mouth, decreased respiration	Downing (1986) Greer & Tolbert (1986) Peroutka *et al.* (1988) Leister *et al.* (1992) Solowij *et al.* (1992) Cohen (1995)
Neuropsychiatric	
Anxiety, depression, mental fatigue, "emotional inflation," fear, paranoia, racing thoughts, confusion, and "negative self-talk," cognitive difficulties, impaired judgment	Downing (1986) Greer & Tolbert (1986) Cohen (1995)
Dizziness or vertigo, visual and tactile hallucinations, paresthesias, irritability, defensiveness, decreased libido, decreased desire to perform mental or physical tasks, increased obsessiveness, motor tics, decreased ability to interact or be open with others, altered time perception	Peroutka *et al.* (1988) Leister *et al.* (1992) Solowij *et al.* (1992)

some of the acute serious medical complications of MDMA that were successfully treated with intensive inpatient care, while others resulted in death.

Fatal acute complications of MDMA have been secondary to cardiac abnormalities, massive neurologic disturbances, and multiple organ system failure. Fatal cardiac events reported in MDMA users have included arrhythmias, asystole, and cardiovascular collapse. These are thought to be more likely in individuals with preexisting, typically undiagnosed conditions, but may also occur *de novo*. Catastrophic neurological sequelae of MDMA use are thought to be secondary to acute MDMA-induced hypertension with disruption of cerebral blood vessels, amphetamine-induced cerebral angiitis, or severe dehydration secondary to prolonged strenuous physical activity in raves, leading to the development of cerebral thromboses. Multiorgan failure in MDMA users appears to be much more prevalent in the setting of raves or crowded dance clubs. Numerous reports have appeared describing a symptom cluster in MDMA users attending raves, including dehydration, hyperthermia, seizures, rhabdomyalysis, disseminated intravascular coagulation, and acute

renal failure (see Henry, Jeffreys, & Dawling, 1992). The number and range of symptoms varies from individual to individual, particularly since early treatment appears to prevent development of the full syndrome. It is thought that extreme, prolonged levels of physical activity in hot, crowded conditions predisposes MDMA users to develop this constellation of symptoms. Notably, it is well documented in animals that crowded housing conditions greatly potentiate the lethal effects of amphetamine, a phenomenon known as aggregation toxicity (Chance, 1946; Hohn & Lasagna, 1960). The crowded setting of raves may be a key feature in the development of this potentially deadly syndrome which has been seen even after relatively small doses of MDMA (approximately 75–125 mg), and in the occasional MDMA user.

Chronic General Medical Effects

Reports of chronic medical conditions thought to be associated with MDMA have been rare but, as seen in Table 2, they include aplastic anemia and hepatotoxicity. MDMA-induced aplastic anemia has been reported in only two individuals, both of whom used MDMA repeatedly. The pathogenesis for this

TABLE 2. Serious Adverse Effects of MDMA

Symptom	Citation
Acute general medical	
Pneumomediastinum secondary to severe vomiting	Levine, Drew, & Rees (1993)
Syndrome of inappropriate antidiuretic hormone secretion (SIADH)	Satchell & Connaughton (1994) Maxwell, Polkey, & Henry (1993) Kessel (1994) Matthai, Davidson, Sills, & Alexandrou (1996)
Status epilepticus	Russell, Schwartz, & Dawling (1992)
Arrhythmias and asystole	Dowling, McDonough, & Bost (1987) Henry, Jeffreys, & Dawling (1992)
Cardiovascular collapse	Suarez & Reimersma (1988)
Intracranial hemorrhage	Hughes, McCabe, & Evans, (1993)
Subarachnoid hemorrhage	Gledhill, Moore, Bell, & Henry (1993)
Cerebral infarction	Hughes *et al.* (1993) Manchanda & Connolly (1993) Selmi, Davies, Sharma, & Neal (1995) Harries & De Silva (1992) Hanyu, Ikeguchi, Imai, Imai, & Yoshida (1995)
Cerebral venous sinus thrombosis	Rothwell & Grant, (1993)
Multiple organ system failure accompanied by cluster of symptoms including hyperthermia, seizures, rhabdomyalysis, disseminated intravascular coagulation, acute renal failure, and dehydration	Brown & Osterloh (1987) Chadwick, Curry, Linsley, Freemont, & Doran (1991) Campkin & Davies (1992) Screaton *et al.* (1992) Henry *et al.* (1992) Barrett & Taylor (1993) Padkin (1994) Wake (1995) Roberts & Wright (1993) Lehmann, Thom, & Croft (1995) Huarte Muniesa & Pueyo Royo (1995) Fineschi & Masti (1996) Hall, Lyburn, Spears, & Riley (1996) Coore (1996) Demirkiran, Jankovic, & Dean (1996)
Chronic general medical	
Aplastic anemia	Marsh *et al.* (1994)
Hepatotoxicity	Henry *et al.* (1992) Shearman, Satsangi, Chapman, & Ryley (1992) Ijzermans, Tilanus, DeMan, & Metselaar (1993) Oranje *et al.* (1994) Dykhuizen, Brunt, Atkinson, Simpson, & Smith (1995) Khakoo, Coles, Armstrong, & Barry (1995) Ellis, Wendon, Portmann, & Williams (1996)

condition is not known. While the majority of individuals who developed MDMA-associated hepatotoxicity recovered, two required liver transplant, and one died. Although it is possible that contaminants of MDMA might have played a role in the genesis of hepatotoxicity in these patients, hepatotoxicity is recognized as a potential complication of MDMA use.

Neuropsychiatric Effects

The range, duration, and severity of neuropsychiatric effects (see Table 3) associated with MDMA is also quite variable. Bothersome acute undesirable emotional effects reported by the two prospective studies in MDMA users and four retrospective surveys of MDMA users are summarized in Table 1. Severe acute psychiatric complications of MDMA have also been reported, and include panic attacks, psychosis, and impulsive irrational behavior with subsequent severe medical consequences or death.

Some individuals who use MDMA develop persistent neuropsychiatric difficulties that remain long after the acute pharmacologic effects of MDMA have dissipated. As seen in Table 3, chronic psychiatric disturbances associated with MDMA use include panic disorder, psychosis, aggressive outbursts, flashbacks, major depressive disorder, and memory or cognitive disturbance.

Serotonin Neurotoxicity

In addition to producing general medical and neuropsychiatric adverse effects, MDMA is a well-documented serotonin neurotoxin in a variety of animal species, including rats (Battaglia et al., 1987; Commins et al., 1987; O'Hearn, Battaglia, DeSouza, Kuhar, & Molliver, 1988; Schmidt, 1987; Slikker et al., 1988, 1989; Stone, Stahl, Hanson, & Gibb, 1986), guinea pigs (Commins et al., 1987), mice (Stone et al., 1986), and monkeys (Insel, Battaglia, Johannessen, Marra, & De Souza, 1989; Ricaurte, Delanney, Wiener, Irwin, & Langston, 1988; Slikker et al., 1988, 1989; Wilson, Ricaurte, & Molliver, 1989). In nonhuman primates, MDMA-induced brain sero-

tonin damage is long-lasting, possibly permanent (Fischer, Hatzidimitriou, Katz, & Ricaurte, 1995; Ricaurte, Katz, & Martello, 1992). There are no currently available methods to directly evaluate the status of brain serotonin neurons in humans; therefore, it has not been fully established that human MDMA users also incur brain serotonin injury. However, studies in nonhuman primates and findings from a controlled clinical study in humans raise concern that MDMA is also neurotoxic in human MDMA users. This concern is heightened when one considers the fact that doses of MDMA that lead to serotonin injury in monkeys closely approximate or overlap those used by humans.

Studies in Animals

MDMA-induced serotonin injury has been demonstrated in animals by the presence of significant reductions of markers unique to brain serotonin axons and axon terminals. In particular, there are reductions in brain serotonin (5-HT) and 5-hydroxyindoleacetic acid (5-HIAA), the major metabolite of serotonin (Commins et al., 1987; Schmidt, 1987; Schmidt, Wu, & Lovenberg, 1986; Stone et al., 1986); tryptophan hydroxylase (TPH), the rate-limiting enzyme in serotonin synthesis (Schmidt & Taylor, 1987; Stone et al., 1986; Stone, Hanson, & Gibb, 1987); and loss of the serotonin transporter, a structural protein on the serotonin nerve terminal (Battaglia et al., 1987; Battaglia, Yeh, & DeSouza, 1988; Commins et al., 1987). These neurochemical deficits, which last well beyond the period of drug administration, have been correlated with the disappearance of serotonin immunoreactive axons. Anatomic studies also point to the neurotoxic potential of MDMA. In particular, quantitative autoradiographic studies that involve labeling of the serotonin transporter, and immunocytochemical studies using antibodies directed at either serotonin or the serotonin transporter indicate that MDMA causes a pronounced, long-lasting reduction in the density of serotonin axons with sparing of serotonin cell bodies (Molliver et al., 1990; O'Hearn et al., 1988; Wilson et al., 1989). These seroton-

TABLE 3. Serious Neuropsychiatric Complications

Symptom	Citation
Acute neuropsychiatric	
Panic attacks	Whitaker-Azmitia & Aronson (1989) McCann & Ricaurte (1992) Pallanti & Mazzi (1992)
Psychosis	Cox (1993) Creighton, Black, & Hyde (1991) Williams, Meagher, & Galligan (1993)
Impulsive irrational behavior with subsequent severe medical consequences or death	Dowling *et al.* (1987) Cadier & Clarke (1993) Hooft & Van de Voorde (1994) Crifasi & Long (1996) Schifano (1995)
Chronic neuropsychiatric	
Panic disorder	Pallanti & Mazzi (1992) McCann & Ricaurte (1992) Series, Boeles, Dorkins, & Peveler (1994) Schifano & Magni (1994) McGuire, Cope, & Fahy (1994)
Psychosis	McGuire & Fahy (1991) Creighton *et al.* (1991) Schifano (1991) Series *et al.* (1994) Wodarz & Boning (1993) Schifano & Magni (1994) McGuire *et al.* (1994)
Aggressive outbursts	Schifano & Magni (1994)
Flashbacks	Creighton *et al.* (1991) Schifano & Magni (1994) McGuire *et al.* (1994)
Major depressive disorder	McCann & Ricaurte (1991) Benazzi & Mazzoli (1991) Schifano & Magni (1994)
Memory or cognitive disturbance	McCann & Ricaurte (1991) Schifano & Magni (1994)

ergic deficits, measured using either chemical or anatomical markers, can be demonstrated weeks (Schmidt *et al.,* 1986; Schmidt & Taylor, 1987), months (Battaglia *et al.,* 1988; Scanzello, Hatzidimitriou, Martello, Katz, & Ricaurte, 1993), and for more than a year after drug discontinuation. While some degree of axonal recovery appears to take place in rodents (Scanzello *et al.,* 1993), particularly after smaller lesions produced by lower doses of MDMA, nonhuman primates do not appear to recover from MDMA-induced serotonin injury (Fischer *et al.,* 1995; Ricaurte *et al.,* 1992).

Relevance of Animal Studies to Humans

Determination of the relevance of MDMA-induced serotonin neurotoxicity in animals to recreational MDMA use in humans requires consideration of several important factors. These include drug dosage, route and schedule of drug administration, and comparability of drug metabolic pathways in the various animal species with those of humans. Evaluation of clinical research in MDMA users, as well as the medical literature of MDMA-associated adverse effects, also sheds light on the neurotoxic potential of MDMA in human users.

Drug Dosage

Doses of MDMA (expressed in mg/kg) required to produce serotonin neurotoxicity in small animals are higher than those required in larger animal species. This well-known phenomenon can be explained by the principles of interspecies scaling. These principles provide guidance for translating doses across species utilizing known relations between body mass–surface area and by taking differences in drug clearance of the two species into account. When this is done for MDMA, the ED_{50} dose that produces a prolonged (i.e., at least 2-week) depletion of brain serotonin axonal markers in the rat is 20 mg/kg, compared to 5 mg/kg in the monkey, using the same schedule and route of drug administration. If the known neurotoxic dose of 5 mg/kg in a 1 kg squirrel monkey is then used to estimate a neurotoxic dose in a 75 kg human, using an accepted adjustment for body mass–surface area and drug clearance (0.75 exponent) (Chappell & Mordenti, 1991; Mordenti & Chappell, 1989), the equivalent dose in humans is found to be 1.28 mg/kg or approximately 96 mg. Since the typical single dose of MDMA used is 75–125 mg, and since up to 10 doses are used per night by some users, these calculations indicate that some MDMA users may be at risk for incurring MDMA-induced serotonin injury.

Route and Schedule of Administration

Animal studies of MDMA-induced neurotoxicity are typically performed by administering the drugs parenterally, twice daily for 4 days. In contrast, humans typically (though not always) use MDMA orally, either once or several times nightly at variable intervals. However, a study in rats comparing the effects of the oral versus parenteral routes of administration on brain markers of serotonin neurons revealed no differences in indices of brain serotonin neurotoxicity 2 weeks following

MDMA administration in any brain region examined (Finnegan et al., 1988). Further, a single 5-mg dose of MDMA in nonhuman primates has been found to produce serotonin neurotoxicity (Ricaurte, DeLanney, Irwin, & Langston, 1988) suggesting the potential for MDMA-induced serotonin neurotoxicity even in occasional MDMA users, particularly if multiple doses of MDMA are used.

Two controlled studies have evaluated MDMA users for biological evidence of serotonin neurotoxicity. In the first (Price, Ricaurte, Krystal, & Heninger, 1989), pharmacologic challenges with L-tryptophan were used to probe for evidence of altered serotonin function in MDMA users. MDMA users in this study tended to exhibit altered L-tryptophan-induced prolactin responses, although differences did not reach statistical significance. In the second study, MDMA users and control subjects participated in a 5-day inpatient study (Allen, McCann, & Ricaurte, 1993; McCann, Ridenour, Shaham, & Ricaurte, 1994). MDMA subjects were found to have significant decrements in cerebrospinal fluid 5-hydroxyindoleacetic acid, the major metabolite of serotonin and index of brain serotonin function. All-night sleep recordings also revealed differences between MDMA subjects and controls, also suggesting possible serotonergic dysfunction, since sleep is thought to be modulated by the brain serotonin system. Altered neuroendocrine responses to L-tryptophan in MDMA users were not found in this second study, however, in contrast to the trend for altered prolactin responses found in the first study. Additional controlled research in larger numbers of MDMA users will be necessary to arrive at definitive conclusions regarding the presence of MDMA-induced serotonin injury in humans. Positron emission tomography studies using neuroligands selective for serotonin neuronal elements hold particular promise in this regard, since such studies would provide a means for direct measurement of serotonin neurons in living humans.

Notably, individual case reports of MDMA-induced neuropsychiatric syndromes may also be useful in documenting potential consequences of MDMA-induced serotonin neurotoxicity. Since serotonin neurons are thought to be involved in the modulation of mood, anxiety, cognition, impulsivity, sexual function, sleep, and appetite, and since serotonin may also play a role in certain forms of psychosis, it is possible that MDMA users who develop abnormalities in these behavioral spheres are suffering from consequences of MDMA-induced neurotoxic insult.

Conclusions

Recreational use of MDMA, particularly in the setting of raves, continues to increase in the United States and Europe. No formal epidemiological studies of MDMA use have been conducted, but it is estimated that in the United States alone, hundreds of thousands of MDMA doses are used each year. While most MDMA users do not experience immediate adverse effects, as MDMA's popularity has increased, so have the numbers of individuals who develop serious MDMA-related medical or psychiatric problems. It appears that persons with a previous history of neuropsychiatric problems or a family history of neuropsychiatric illness are more likely to develop MDMA-related chronic neuropsychiatric syndromes, particularly with repeated exposure to high MDMA doses.

A particularly dangerous aspect of MDMA may be its potential to damage brain serotonin neurons. This phenomenon has been well documented in numerous animal species, and studies in humans also suggest that some MDMA users incur brain serotonin injury. Since serotonin is thought to be involved in the regulation of numerous behavioral functions, including mood, anxiety, sleep, sexual behavior, and cognition, MDMA users may be at risk for developing problems in a broad range of fundamental human behaviors. Further, since alterations in these behaviors may be subtle, individuals may unwittingly continue to use MDMA, unaware of the insidious development of neuropsychiatric problems. Indeed, some of the neuropsychiatric syndromes that have been attributed to MDMA use may, in fact, be a result of serotonin neurotoxicity.

In addition to its importance as a potentially serious public health problem, MDMA use may be important for purely scientific reasons. In particular, clinical research involving individuals exposed to MDMA and related toxic amphetamine derivatives (e.g., fenfluramine) holds promise for elucidating the role of brain serotonin systems in normal and abnormal human neuropsychiatric function.

References

Allen, R. P., McCann, U. D., & Ricaurte, G. A. (1993). Persistent effects of (+) 3,4-methylenedioxymethamphetamine (MDMA, "Ecstasy") on human sleep. *Sleep, 16,* 560–564.

Anonymous. (1992). Drug culture. *Lancet, 339,* 117.

Barrett, P. J., & Taylor, G. T. (1993). "Ecstasy" ingestion: A case report of severe complications. *Journal of the Royal Society of Medicine, 86,* 233–234.

Battaglia, G., Yeh, S. Y., O'Hearn, E., Molliver, M. E., Kuhar, M. J., & DeSouza, E. B. (1987). 3,4-Methylenedioxymethamphetamine and 3,4-methylenedioxyamphetamine destroy serotonin terminals in rat brain: Quantification of neurodegeneration by measurement of [^{3}H]paroxetine-labeled serotonin uptake sites. *Journal of Pharmacology and Experimental Therapeutics, 242,* 911–916.

Battaglia, G., Yeh, S. Y., & DeSouza, E. B. (1988). MDMA-induced neurotoxicity: Parameters of degeneration and recovery of brain serotonin neurons. *Pharmacology, Biochemistry and Behavior, 29,* 269–274.

Beardsley, P. M., Balster, R. L., & Harris, L. S. (1986). Self-administration of methylenedioxymethamphetamine (MDMA) by rhesus monkeys. *Drug and Alcohol Dependence, 18,* 149–157.

Benazzi, F., & Mazzoli, M. (1991). Psychiatric illness associated with "ecstasy." *Lancet, 338,* 1520.

Brown, C., & Osterloh, J. (1987). Multiple complications from recreational ingestion of MDMA ("Ecstasy"). *Journal of the American Medical Association, 258,* 780–781.

Cadier, M. A., & Clarke, J. A. (1993). Ecstasy and Whizz at a rave resulting in a major burn plus complications. *Burns, 19,* 239–240.

Campkin, N. T., & Davies U. M. (1992). Another death from Ecstasy [Letter]. *Journal of the Royal Society of Medicine, 85,* 61.

Chadwick, I. S., Curry, P., Linsley, A., Freemont, A. J., & Doran, B. (1991). Ecstasy, 3-4 methylenedioxymethamphetamine (MDMA), a fatality associated with coagulapathy and hyperthermia. *Journal of the Royal Society of Medicine, 84,* 371.

Chance, M. (1946). Aggregation as a factor influencing the toxicity of sympathomimetic amines in mice.

Journal of Pharmacology and Experimental Thera-peutics, 198, 214–219.

Chappell, W., & Mordenti, J. (1991). Extrapolation of tox-icological and pharmacological data from animals to humans. In B. Testa, (Ed.), *Advances in drug re-search* (Vol. 20, pp. 1–116). San Diego, CA: Acade-mic Press.

Cohen, R. S. (1995). Subjective reports on the effects of the MDMA ("Ecstasy") experience in humans. *Progress in Neuro-Psychopharmacology & Biologi-cal Psychiatry, 19,* 1137–1145.

Commins, D. L., Vosmer, G., Virus, R., Woolverton, W., Schuster, C., & Seiden, L. (1987). Biochemical and histological evidence that methylenedioxymethyl-amphetamine (MDMA) is toxic to neurons in the rat brain. *Journal of Pharmacology and Experimental Therapeutics, 241,* 338–345.

Coore, J. R. (1996). A fatal trip with Ecstasy: A case of 3,4-methylenedioxy-methamphetamine/3,4-methyl-enedioxy-amphetamine toxicity. *Journal of the Royal Society of Medicine, 89,* 51P–52P.

Cox, D. E. (1993). "Rave" to the grave. *Forensic Science International, 60,* 5–6.

Creighton, F. J., Black, D. L., & Hyde, C. E. (1991). "Ec-stasy" psychosis and flashbacks. *British Journal of Psychiatry, 159,* 713–715.

Crifasi, J., & Long, C. (1996). Traffic fatality related to the use of methylenedioxymethamphetamine. *Journal of Forensic Sciences, 41,* 1082–1084.

Demirkiran, M., Jankovic, J., & Dean, J. M. (1996). Ec-stasy intoxication: An overlap between serotonin syn-drome and neuroleptic malignant syndrome. *Clinical Neuropsychopharmacology, 19,* 157–164.

Doblin, R. (1989). Risk assessment: The FDA and MDMA research. In B. Eisner, (Ed.), *Ecstasy: The MDMA story* (pp. 163–170). Berkeley, CA: Ronin.

Dowling, G. P., McDonough, E. T., & Bost, R. O. (1987). "Eve" and "Ecstasy": A report of five deaths associ-ated with the use of MDEA and MDMA. *Journal of the American Medical Association, 257,* 1615–1617.

Downing, J. (1986). The psychological and physiological effects of MDMA on normal volunteers. *Journal of Psychoactive Drugs, 18,* 335–340.

Dykhuizen, R. S., Brunt, P. W., Atkinson, P., Simpson, J., & Smith, C. (1995). Ecstasy induced hepatitis mim-icking viral hepatitis. *Gut, 36,* 939–941.

Eisner, B. (1989). *Ecstasy: The MDMA story.* Berkeley, CA: Ronin.

Ellis, A. J., Wendon, J. A., Portmann, B., & Williams, R. (1996). Acute liver damage and ecstasy ingestion. *Gut, 38,* 454–458.

Fineschi, V., & Masti, A. (1996). Fatal poisoning by MDMA (ecstasy) and MDEA: A case report. *Inter-national Journal of Legal Medicine, 108,* 272–275.

Finnegan, K. T., Ricaurte, G. A., Davis-Richie, L., Irwin, I., Peroutka, S. P., & Langston, J. W. (1988). Orally administered 3,4-methylenedioxymethylampheta-mine causes a long-term depletion of serotonin in rat brain. *Brain Research, 447,* 141–144.

Fischer, C. A., Hatzidimitriou, G., Katz, J. L., & Ricaurte, G. A. (1995). Reorganization of ascending serotonin axon projections in animals previously exposed to the recreational drug 3,4-methylenedioxymethamphetamine. *Journal of Neuroscience, 15,* 5476–5485.

Gledhill, J. A., Moore, D. F., Bell, D., & Henry, J. A. (1993). Subarachnoid hemorrhage associated with MDMA abuse. *Journal of Neurology, Neurosurgery, & Psychiatry, 56,* 1036–1037.

Greer, G., & Tolbert, P. (1986). Subjective reports of the effects of MDMA in a clinical setting. *Journal of Psychoactive Drugs, 18,* 319–327.

Hall, A. P., Lyburn, I. D., Spears, F. D., & Riley, B. (1996). An unusual case of ecstasy poisoning. *Intensive Care Medicine, 22,* 670–671.

Hanyu, S., Ikeguchi, K., Imai, H., Imai, N., & Yoshida, M. (1995). Cerebral infarction associated with 3,4-meth-ylenedioxymethamphetamine ("Ecstasy") abuse. *Eu-ropean Neurology, 35,* 173.

Harries, D. P., & De Silva, R. (1992). "Ecstasy" and in-tracerebral haemorrhage. *Scottish Medical Journal, 37,* 476.

Henry, J. A., Jeffreys, K. J., & Dawling, S. (1992). Toxic-ity and deaths from 3,4-methylenedioxymethamphet-amine ("Ecstasy"). *Lancet, 340,* 384–387.

Hohn, R., & Lasagna, L. (1960). Effects of aggregation and temperature on amphetamine toxicity in mice. *Psychopharmacologia, 1,* 210–220.

Hooft, P. J., & Van de Voorde, H. P. (1994). Reckless be-haviour related to the use of 3,4 methylene-dioxymethamphetamine (Ecstasy): Apropos of fatal accident during car-surfing. *International Journal of Legal Medicine, 106,* 328–329.

Huarte Muniesa, M. P., & Pueyo Royo, A. M. (1995). Acute hepatitis from ingestion of ecstasy. *Revista Es-panola de Enfermedades Digestivas, 87,* 681–683.

Hubner, C. B., Bird, M., Rassnick, S., & Kornetsky, C. (1988). The threshold lowering effects of MDMA (ecstasy) on brain-stimulation reward. *Psychophar-macology, 95,* 49–51.

Hughes, J. C., McCabe, M., & Evans, R. J. (1993). In-tracranial haemorrhage associated with ingestion of "Ecstasy." *Archives of Emergency Medicine, 10,* 372–374.

Ijzermans, J. N., Tilanus, H. W., De Man, R. A., & Metse-laar, H. J. (1993). Ecstasy and liver transplantation [Letter]. *Annales de Medecine Internex, 144,* 568.

Insel, T. R., Battaglia, G., Johannessen, J. N., Marra, S., & De Souza, E. B. (1989). 3,4-Methylenedioxymeth-amphetamine ("Ecstasy") selectively destroys brain serotonin terminals in rhesus monkeys. *Journal of Pharmacology and Experimental Therapeutics, 249,* 713–720.

Kessel, B. (1994). Hyponatraemia after ingestion of "Ec-stasy." *British Medical Journal, 308,* 414.

Khakoo, S. I., Coles, C. J., Armstrong, J. S., & Barry, R. E. (1995). Hepatotoxicity and accelerated fibrosis following 3,4-methylenedioxymethamphetamine ("Ecstasy") usage. *Journal of Clinical Gastroenterology, 20,* 244–247.

Lamb, R. J., & Griffiths, R. R. (1987). Self-injection of 3,4-methylenedioxymethamphetamine (MDMA) in the baboon. *Psychopharmacology, 91,* 268–272.

Lawn, J. C. (1986). Schedules of controlled substances: Scheduling of 3,4-methylenedioxymethamphetamine (MDMA) into Schedule I of the Controlled Substance Act. *Federal Register, 51,* 36552–36560.

Lehmann, E. D., Thom, C. H., & Croft, D. N. (1995). Delayed severe rhabdomyalysis after taking Ecstasy [Letter]. *Postgraduate Medical Journal, 71,* 186–187.

Leister, M. B., Grob, C. S., Bravo, G. L., & Walsh, R. N. (1992). Phenomenology and sequelae of 3,4-Methylenedioxymethamphetamine use. *Journal of Nervous and Mental Disorders, 180,* 345–352.

Levine, A. J., Drew, S., & Rees, G. M. (1993). "Ecstasy" induced pneumomediastinum. *Journal of the Royal Society of Medicine, 86,* 232–233.

Manchanda, S., & Connolly, M. J. (1993). Cerebral infarction in association with Ecstasy abuse. *Postgraduate Medical Journal, 69,* 874–875.

Marsh, J. C., Abboudi, Z. H., Gibson, F. M., Scopes, J., Daly, S., O'Shaunnessy, D. F., Baughan, A. S., & Gordon-Smith, E. C. (1994). Aplastic anaemia following exposure to 3,4-methylenedioxymethamphetamine ('Ecstasy'). *British Journal of Haematology, 88,* 281–285.

Matthai, S. M., Davidson, D. C., Sills, J. A., & Alexandrou, D. (1996). Cerebral oedema after ingestion of MDMA ("Ecstasy") and unrestricted intake of water. *British Medical Journal, 312,* 1359.

Maxwell, D. L., Polkey, M. I., & Henry, J. A. (1993). Hyponatraemia and catatonic stupor after taking "Ecstasy." *British Medical Journal, 27,* 1399.

McCann, U. D., & Ricaurte, G. A. (1991). Lasting neuropsychiatric sequelae of (±) methylenedioxymethamphetamine ("Ecstasy") in recreational users. *Journal of Clinical Psychopharmacology, 11,* 302–305.

McCann, U. D., & Ricaurte, G. A. (1992). MDMA ("Ecstasy") and panic disorder: Induction by a single dose. *Biological Psychiatry, 32,* 950–953.

McCann, U. D., Ridenour, A., Shaham, Y., & Ricaurte, G. A. (1994). Brain serotonergic neurotoxicity after MDMA ("Ecstasy"): A controlled study in humans. *Neuropsychopharmacology, 10,* 129–138.

McGuire, P., & Fahy, T. (1991). Chronic paranoid psychosis after misuse of MDMA ("Ecstasy"). *British Medical Journal, 302,* 607.

McGuire, P. K., Cope, H., & Fahy, T. (1994). Diversity of psychopathology associated with use of 3,4-Methylenedioxymethaphetamine ("Ecstasy"). *British Journal of Psychiatry, 165,* 391–395.

Merck, E. (1914). Verfahre zur darstellung von alkyloxyaryldialyloxyaryl-undalkylenedioxyarylamino-propanen bzw.deren amstickstoff monoalkylierten derivaten. German patent # 274:350, 1914.

Molliver, M. E., Berger, U. V., Mamounas, L. A., Molliver, D. C., O'Hearn, E. G., & Wilson, M. A. (1990). Neurotoxicity of MDMA and related compounds: Anatomic studies. *Annals of the New York Academy of Science, 600,* 640–664.

Mordenti, J., & Chappell, W. (1989). The use of interspecies scaling in toxicokinetics. In A. Yacobi, J. Kelly, & V. Batra (Eds.), *Toxicokinetics in new drug development* (pp. 42–96). New York: Pergamon.

O'Hearn, E. G., Battaglia, G., De Souza, E. B., Kuhar, M. J., & Molliver, M. E. (1988). Methylenedioxyamphetamine (MDA) and methylenedioxymethamphetamine (MDMA) cause selective ablation of serotonergic axon terminals in forebrain: Immunocytochemical evidence for neurotoxicity. *Journal of Neuroscience, 8,* 2788–2803.

Oranje, W. A.,von Pol, P., Wurff A., Zeijen R. N., Stockbrugger, R., & Arends, J. (1994). XTC-induced hepatitis. *Netherlands Journal of Medicine, 44,* 56–59.

Padkin, A. (1994). Treating MDMA ("Ecstasy") toxicity [Letter; comment]. *Anaesthesia, 49,* 259.

Pallanti, S., & Mazzi, D. (1992). MDMA (Ecstasy) precipitation of panic disorder. *Biological Psychiatry, 32,* 91–95.

Peroutka, S. J., Newman, H., & Harris, H. (1988). Subjective effects of 3,4-methylenedioxymethamphetamine in recreational users. *Neuropsychopharmacology, 1,* 273–277.

Price, L. H., Ricaurte, G. A., Krystal, J. H., & Heninger, G. R. (1989). *Responses to iv L-tryptophan in MDMA users* (NIDA Research Monograph No. 95, pp. 421–422). Rockville, MD: National Institute on Drug Abuse.

Ricaurte, G., Bryan, G., Strauss, L., Seiden, L., & Schuster, C. (1985). Hallucinogenic amphetamine selectively destroys brain serotonin nerve terminals. *Science, 229,* 986–988.

Ricaurte, G. A., DeLanney, L. E., Irwin, I., & Langston, J. W. (1988). Toxic effects of MDMA on central serotonergic neurons in the primate: Importance of route and frequency of drug administration. *Brain Research, 446,* 165–168.

Ricaurte, G. A., Delanney, L. E., Wiener, S. G., Irwin, I., & Langston, J. W. (1988). 5-Hydroxyindoleacetic acid in cerebrospinal fluid reflects serotonergic damage induced by 3,4-methylenedioxymethamphetamine in CNS of non-human primates. *Brain Research, 474,* 359–363.

Ricaurte, G. A., Katz, J. L., & Martello, M. B. (1992). Lasting effects of (±)3,4-methylenedioxymethamphetamine on central serotonergic neurons in non-human primates. *Journal of Pharmacology and Experimental Therapeutics, 261,* 616–622.

Roberts, L., & Wright, H. (1993). Survival following intentional massive overdose of "Ecstasy." *Journal of Accident and Emergency Medicine, 11,* 53–54.

Rothwell, P. M., & Grant, R. (1993). Cerebral venous sinus thrombosis induced by "Ecstasy" [Letter]. *Journal of Neurology, Neurosurgery, & Psychiatry, 56,* 1035–1039.

Russell, A. R., Schwartz, R. H., & Dawling, S. (1992). Accidental ingestion of "Ecstasy" (3,4-methylenedioxymetamphetamine). *Archives of Disease in Childhood, 67,* 1114–1115.

Satchell, S. C., & Connaughton, M. (1994). Inappropriate hormone secretion and extreme rises in serum creatinine kinase following MDMA ingestion. *British Medical Journal, 51,* 495.

Scanzello, C. R., Hatzidimitriou, G., Martello, A. L., Katz, J. L., & Ricaurte, G. A. (1993). Serotonergic recovery after (±)3,4-(methylenedioxy)methamphetamine injury: Observations in rodents. *Journal of Pharmacology and Experimental Therapeutics, 264,* 1484–1491.

Schifano, F. (1991). Chronic atypical psychosis associated with MDMA ("Ecstasy") abuse [Letter]. *Lancet, 338,* 1335.

Schifano, F. (1995). Dangerous driving and MDMA (Ecstasy) abuse. *Journal of Serotonin Research, 1,* 53–57.

Schifano, F., & Magni, G. (1994). MDMA ("Ecstasy") abuse: Psychopathological features and craving for chocolate: A case series. *Biological Psychiatry, 36,* 763–767.

Schmidt, C. J. (1987). Neurotoxicity of the psychedelic amphetamine, methylenedioxymethamphetamine. *Journal of Pharmacology and Experimental Therapeutics, 240,* 1–7.

Schmidt, C. J., & Taylor, V. L. (1987). Depression of rat brain tryptophan hydroxylase activity following the acute administration of methylenedioxymethamphetamine. *Biochemical Pharmacology, 36,* 4095–4102.

Schmidt, C. J., Wu, L., & Lovenberg, W. (1986). Methylenedioxymethamphetamine: A potentially neurotoxic amphetamine analog. *European Journal of Pharmacology, 124,* 175–178.

Screaton, G. R., Singer, M., Cairns, H. S., Thrasher, A., Sarner, M., & Cohen, S. (1992). Hyperpyrexia and rhabdomyolysis after MDMA ("Ecstasy") abuse [Letter]. *Lancet, 339,* 677–678.

Selmi, F., Davies, K. G., Sharma, R. R., & Neal, J. (1995). Intracerebral hemorrhage due to amphetamine abuse: Report of two cases with underlying arteriovenous malformations. *British Journal of Neurosurgery, 9,* 93–96.

Series, H., Boeles, S., Dorkins, E., & Peveler, R. (1994). Psychiatric complications of "Ecstasy" use. *Journal of Psychopharmacology, 8,* 60–61.

Shearman, J. D., Satsangi, J., Chapman, R. W., & Ryley, N. G. (1992). Misuse of Ecstasy. *British Medical Journal, 305,* 309.

Shulgin, A. T., & Nichols, D. E. (1978). Characterization of three new psychotomimetics. In R. Stillman & R. Willette (Eds.), *The psychopharmacology of hallucinogens* (pp. 74–83). New York: Pergamon.

Slikker, W., Ali, S. F., Scallet, C., Frith, C. H., Newport, G. D., & Bailey, J. R. (1988). Neurochemical and neurohistological alterations in the rat and monkey produced by orally administered methylenedioxymethamphetamine (MDMA). *Toxicology & Applied Pharmacology, 94,* 448–457.

Slikker, W., Holson, R. R., Ali, S. F., Kolta, M. G., Paule, M., Scallet, A., McMillan, D., & Bailey, J. (1989). Behavioral and neurochemical effects of orally administered MDMA in the rodent and nonhuman primate. *Neurotoxicology, 10,* 529–549.

Solowij, N., Hall, W., & Lee, N. (1992). Recreational MDMA use in Sydney: A profile of "Ecstasy" users and their experiences with the drug. *British Journal of Addiction, 87,* 1161–1172.

Stone, D. M., Stahl, D. S., Hanson, G. L., & Gibb, J. W. (1986). The effects of 3,4-methylenedioxymethamphetamine (MDMA) and 3,4-methylenedioxyamphetamine on monoaminergic systems in the rat brain. *European Journal of Pharmacology, 128,* 41–48.

Stone, D. M., Hanson, G. L., & Gibb, J. W. (1987). Differences in the central serotonergic effects of 3,4-methylenedioxymethamphetamine (MDMA) in mice and rats. *Neuropharmacology, 26,* 1657–1661.

Suarez, R. V., & Riemersma, R. (1988). "Ecstasy" and sudden cardiac death. *American Journal of Forensic Medicine & Pathology, 9,* 339–341.

Wake, D. (1995). Ecstasy overdose: A case study. *Intensive and Critical Care Nursing, 11,* 6–9.

Whitaker-Azmitia, P. M., & Aronson, T. A. (1989). "Ecstasy" (MDMA)-induced pain. *American Journal of Psychiatry, 146,* 119.

Williams, H., Meagher, D., & Galligan, P. (1993). MDMA ("Ecstasy"): A case of possible drug-induced psychosis. *International Journal of Medical Science, 162,* 43–44.

Wilson, M. A., Ricaurte, G. A., & Molliver, M. E. (1989). Distinct morphological classes of serotonergic axons in primates exhibit differential vulnerability to the psychotropic drug 3,4-methylenedioxymethamphetamine. *Neuroscience, 28,* 121–137.

Wodarz, N., & Boning, J. (1993). "Ecstasy" induziertes psychotisches depersonalisationssyndrom. *Nervenarzt, 64,* 478–480.

35

Phencyclidine

A. JAMES GIANNINI

Introduction

Phencyclidine (PCP) is the most common member of the "dissociatives." The dissociatives constitute an entirely synthetic class of drugs that act at multiple receptor sites. They act as agonists or antagonists at cholinergic, dopaminergic, noradrenergic, opioid, serotonergic, sigma, and NDMA (N-methyl-D-aspartate) -high-affinity and -low-affinity receptor sites. As a result, dissociatives can mimic atropinic, GABAminergic, opioid, psychedelic, and sympathomimetic drugs. Since the drugs in this class are active in powdered, crystalline, suspended, and volatile forms, they can be ingested, snorted, injected, smoked, or inhaled (Giannini, 1987b).

Because of its low price, multiple sites of action, and multiple physical forms, PCP can partially mimic more expensive street drugs. As a result, PCP is the most common active adulterant in the United States. Powdered PCP has been sold as amphetamine, methamphetamine, heroin, cocaine, and methylqualone. Liquid PCP or dissolved powdered PCP has been saturated into gels, paper, and sugar cubes and sold as LSD. It has been mixed with low-potency marijuana or Clorox®-bleached oregano and sold as high-THC-content marijuana.

PCP produces a highly complex presentation. The symptomatic grouping of hypersexuality, hyperaggressivity, and anorexia mimics symptoms produced by such sympathomimetics as amphetamine and cocaine. The mixture of tranquilizing and anesthetic effects are similar to those of heroin or Fentanyl. Its tranquilizing effects allow it to be sold as methylqualone or pentobarbital. Its hallucinogenic actions can be mistaken for those of LSD, DMT, or MDA. On occasion, it has been saturated into different ornamental cacti which are then marketed as "peyote" or into mushrooms which are presented as psilocybin. The tranquilizing and hallucinogenic actions plus its combustibility allow a PCP-oregano mix to be presented as high-quality marijuana (Giannini, Loiselle, Giannini, & Price, 1987).

History

Phencyclidine, the first dissociative, was synthesized by Parke-Davis Laboratories in the 1950s. It was marketed under the trade name "Sernyl" due to its "serene" anesthetic and tranquilizing effect. Although in wide use at the time, many behavioral disturbances were subsequently observed. These included agitation, dysphoria, delirium, hallucinations, paranoia, rage, and violence. Therefore, it was withdrawn in 1965 but reintroduced as a veterinary tranquilizer, "Sernylan," in 1967. Its reincarnation as Sernylan was unpropitiously associated with the development of the drug-oriented culture of the late 1960s (Giannini & Castellani, 1982).

A. JAMES GIANNINI • Department of Psychiatry, The Ohio State University, Columbus, Ohio 43210.

Handbook of Substance Abuse: Neurobehavioral Pharmacology, edited by Tarter *et al.* Plenum Press, New York, 1998.

Sernylan abuse was first reported in the Haight-Ashbury district of San Francisco in late 1967. It was a much sought-after product because of its relatively low price, nonaddicting "high," and absence of legal prohibition; known as the peace pill (i.e., "PeaCe Pill"), it soon became a nationwide phenomenon. The increased demand was met by an assemblage of underground laboratories. In them, relatively cheap raw materials such as piperidines and ketones were used to manufacture high-grade PCP. The introduction of automotive pollution-control devices made of platinum, made a highly efficient catalyst available to these laboratories. Cars were raided for their platinum wire as were college chemistry laboratories. Some abusers would synthesize their own supply in toilet tanks. These were ideal because there was a ready supply of water, while the porcelain could dissipate the heat. After the manufacture of phencyclidine became illegal, the choice of the toilet tank became fortuitous because incriminating evidence could be quickly eliminated by two flushes while the police were presenting their search warrant.

Because of its association with violent crimes and self-destructive acts, such as enucleation and immolation, PCP fell under the scrutiny of the Bureau of Narcotics and Dangerous Drugs (BNDD). In 1967, its manufacture, sale, and use became illegal under the provisions of the Comprehensive Drug Abuse, Prevention and Control Act. Because of the easy availability of piperidines and the ease of manufacture, PCP use continued unabated. As a result, in 1968, Congress passed the Psychotropic Substance Act, which restricted these precursors as well.

Because of the restriction of phencyclidine precursors, part-time chemists quickly reduced their activities and phencyclidine became less available to college students and part-time dabblers. This restriction led to a shakeout in the illegal manufacturing industry. As a result, only two sets of manufacturing and distribution networks survived. One network was maintained by chapters of the larger national and regional motorcycle gangs. A second network was maintained by the Arellano–Felix cartel in Tijuana, Mexico (Allen, Robles, Dovenski, & Calderon, 1993; Little, 1996).

Demographics

Typical PCP abusers are white, blue-collar males living in industrial metropolitan areas in the Midwest and the East and West coasts. They tend to have a high school or partial high school education. They are usually employed and work in unskilled or semiskilled jobs. This group of abusers knowingly buys PCP or its analogues for specific actions: PCP when knowingly purchased is used alone or in combination with marijuana (stepped-on grass) or crack cocaine (space base).

Laboratory Testing

PCP and ketamine can be detected by thin-layer chromatography (TLC). Phencyclidine has a short elimination time and must be analyzed quickly. It can be tested by the presence of its metabolite. Because of the relatively long elimination time, urinalysis is more practical and less costly than serum analysis. If increased sensitivity is needed, gas, liquid chromatography (GLC) is used although it can produce false negatives when only small amounts are available. In cases when absolute accuracy is required and cost is not a consideration, the combination of gas chromatography and mass spectrometry (GCMS) is preferred. Because the dissociatives act at multiple receptor sites, neither enzyme immunoassay (EIA) nor radioimmunoassay (RIA) are recommended due to the cross-reactivity of this class of drugs with reagent antibodies (Davis & Beach, 1960; Little, 1996; Schwarzhoff & Cody, 1989; Sneath & Jain, 1992).

Biochemistry, Physiology, and Pharmacology

All dissociatives are arylcyclohexylamines. Their common chemical structure consists of a phenyl group, a piperidine group and a cyclohexyl ring. Electron-dense regions in the aromatic ring and cyclohexyl ring produce specific cycloactive effects. A cyclohexyl spine produces two separate conformations for each dissociative. A phenyl grouping in the axial plane produces an active form while a placement in the equatorial planes produces an inactive form. Dissociative activity may be further increased by the placement of an unsaturated bond with the triple-ring structure, by replacing the phenyl ring with a thienyl group, or by adding a propyl side chain. Alternatively, reduction in the number of rings and in the number of saturating bonds at the nonpropyl sidechain can reduce biological activity (Giannini, Loiselle, & Malone, 1985).

Ketamine hydrochloride is the only legally prescribed member of this drug class. It is a 2-O-chloralphenyl-1-2-methylamine-cyclo-haxanome bicyclic. Its potency is markedly less than phencyclidine. The presence of side chains, in this case a chloride group, decreases its potency. A weaker analog more similar to ketamine than phencyclidine is PCE (N-ethyl-1-phenocyclohexamine), a byproduct of PCP production and usually sold with it. Another less common byproduct is PHP (1-(1-phenocyclohexyl) pyrrolidine). Replacing the phenyl group in the PCP molecule produces TCP (1-(2-thienlycyclohexyl) piperidine), the most potent of all dissociatives. It is approximately three to five times as potent as PCP. When PCP is smoked, the heat of combustion produces the weakest dissociative, PC (1-phenylcyclohexene) (Cook, 1991). Both active and inactive metabolites are pictured in Figures 1 and 2.

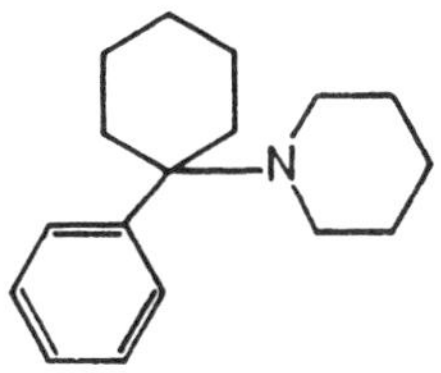

Phencyclidine (PCP)
1-(phenylcyclohexyl)
piperidine

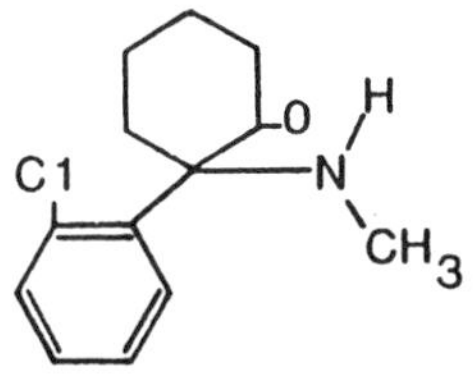

Ketamine
2-(o-chlorophenyl)-2-methyl-
amine cyclohexanone

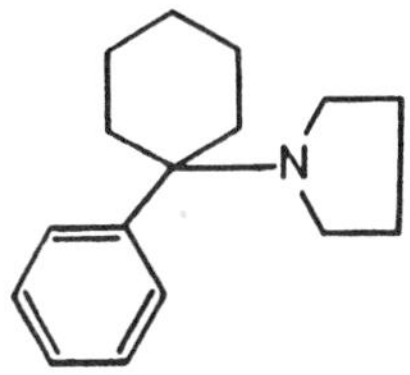

PHP
1-(1-phenylcyclohexyl)
pyrrolidine

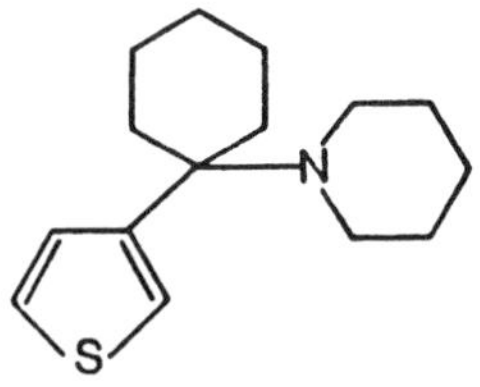

TCP
1-(1-2-thienylcyclohexyl)
piperidine

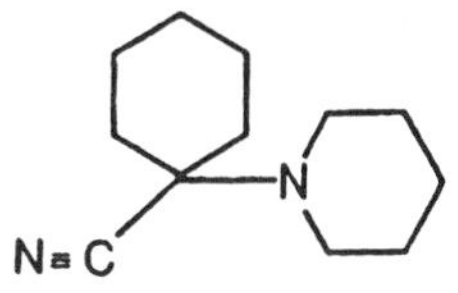

PCC
1-piperidinocyclohexane-
carbonitrile

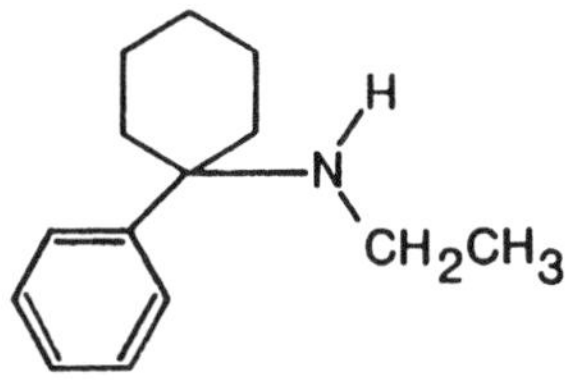

Cyclohexamine PCE
N-ethyl-1-phenylcyclohexylamine

FIGURE 1. The dissociatives.

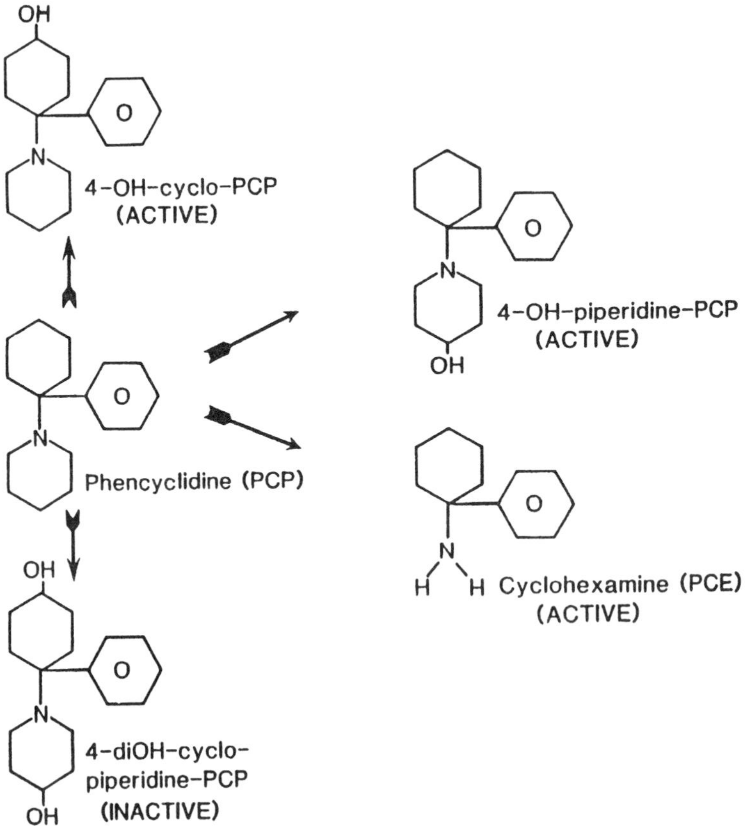

FIGURE 2. Dissociative metabolites.

The gross anatomical effects of phencyclidine have been studied utilizing irradiated glucose. The limbic cortex, the cingulate gyrus, the motor strip, the thalamus, the hippocampus, the antroventral thalamic projections, and the nucleus accumbens are areas of highest activity as the auditory system is the major area of decreased activity. Phencyclidine acts at acetylcholine, dopamine, opioid, γ-aminobutyric (GABA), and serotonin receptors. It also acts at the δ receptor and two specific PCP receptor sites, the NDMA sites (Weissman, Casanova, Kleinman, & De Souza, 1991).

Phencyclidine exhibits inhibitory actions at both central and peripheral cholinergic receptors. Because phencyclidine has the typical structure of an anticholinergic drug, a cationic head, as well as phenyl hydroxy groups, it produces both nicotinic and muscarinic activities. Peripherally, it blocks potassium thereby prolonging the duration of channel activity. This blockade results in a decreased rate of release of both neurotransmitters and adrenal catecholamines. As a result of this blockade, the action potential in skeletal muscle has prolonged duration. PCP is indirectly competitive at nicotine sites and directly competitive at muscarinic sites where it blocks cholinergic ionophores (Albuquerque, Aguayo, Warnick, Ickowicz, & Blaustein, 1983). In addition, it blocks both pseudocholinesterase and butyl-cholinesterase activity. There is, however, no histamine cross-reactivity (Giannini, Price, Giannini, Lazurus, & Loiselle, 1986).

The dissociatives are DA-2 (dopaminergic) antagonists. It is at these dopaminergic receptors that much of the clinical profile is produced. Phencyclidine-induced stereotypy is nearly identical to similar effects produced by amphetamine (Castellani, Adams, & Giannini, 1982). Like amphetamine, these phencyclidine effects are reversed by the DA-2 antagonists, haloperidol and pimozide. Like cocaine and amphetamine, phencyclidine induces prolactin suppression, an effect reversed by DA-2 antagonists. Also, cocaine, amphetamine, and PCP all produce diminished responsivity of thyroid-stimulating hormone (TSH) to protirelin (TRH) stimulation. Reward activity of all three of these drugs occurs in the teleomesencephalic system (Giannini, 1987a).

Unlike the sympathomimetics, phencyclidine does not stimulate release of newly synthesized dopamine into the synaptic cleft. Instead it increases the rate of dopamine released from intraneuronal storage vesicles. It blocks presynaptic dopaminergic uptake in the manner similar to the sympathomimetics but does not significantly blockade monoamine oxidase metabolism. Thus, since significant inhibition of dopamine storage does not occur, tolerance is not usually seen with phencyclidine. In a manner dissimilar to that of the sympathomimetic-induced dopaminergic effects on the reward centers, the effects are not direct. They are instead mediated in complex fashion by opioids. All dissociatives have anesthetic effects, the expression of which is linked to stimulatory effects. These anesthetic effects are due to opiate properties while stimulation is a dopaminergic effect. These opiate effects are exerted on both μ and σ opioid receptors (Wolfe & De Souza, 1993). While the μ-agonist, morphine, increases metenkephlin-induced phencyclidine ataxia, naloxone can block it. In addition, there is a cross-tolerance between meperidine, morphine, or heroin, and phencyclidine (Giannini, Loiselle, & Price, 1985). While phencyclidine increases metenkephlin production, methadone and meperidine can suppress phencyclidine-induced behavioral responses. Ketamine produces an anesthetic effect that is as long-lived as those of both morphine and phencyclidine and at least one and one-half times as long. Phencyclidine acts in a stimulatory-depletion mode on the opioid system similar to its action on the dopaminergic system.

Phencyclidine also influences GABAminergic activity. The effects of acute phencyclidine intoxication can be reduced by the benzodiazepines, diazepam, and chlordiazepoxide. More direct-acting GABAminergic agonists such as barbiturates and methaqualone, however, have not been effective in treating acute phencyclidine intoxication. The effect of benzodiazepine B-Z receptor agonist might be a mere pseudo-effect, since PCP acts on a number of other receptors (Giannini et al., 1987).

Phencyclidine may also act on serotonin receptors since there is cross-tolerance between phencyclidine, mescaline, psilocybin, and lysergic acid (Giannini, Loiselle, Graham, & Folts, 1993). Tests of rats' performance in two-level drug discrimination tests have demonstrated that these animals cannot distinguish phencyclidine from either LSD or mescaline. In contradistinction, however, post-LSD depression has been reported to respond only to fluoxetine, a relatively pure serotonergic antidepressant, whereas phencyclidine-withdrawal dysphoria has been reported to respond best to desipramine, a predominantly noreadrenergic antidepressant. Phencyclidine in high doses can produce psychedelic effects: geometricization, vivid visual hallucinations, depersonalization, derealization, astral projections, and synesthesia. REM-phase sleep studies have been shown to produce similar tracing in both phencyclidine- and LSD-intoxicated volunteers.

Three separate unique receptors have been found to be utilized by phencyclidine. The first is a σ-receptor, a possible opioid receptor that is insensitive to naloxone but binds the experimental opiate drug SKF-10,047 (Contreras, Gray, DiMaggio, Bremer, & Bussom, 1993). Haloperidol antagonizes this receptor whereas chlorpromazine and other phenothiazines are generally ineffective here. Functions of this receptor site and its hypothesized ligand are unknown. More is known, however, of two PCP-specific receptor sites. The first is a high-affinity binding site located in the NDMA receptor channel. It is stimulated by glutamate but irreversibly antagonized by metaphit. This site is noninteractive with haloperidol, chlorpromazine, pimozide, naloxone, or SKF 10,047. It is distributed throughout the brain including the hippocampus and its projections as well as the cingulate gyrus, corpus callosum, inferior colliculi, locus coeruleus, medulla oblongata, and anterior pons. A second receptor site, this one of lower infinity, has also been found. It is reportedly noninteractive with metaphit, naloxone, haloperidol, and chlorpromazine. Thus far, no site-specific antagonist has been found but N-allylnormetazocine acts as a site-specific agonist. The distribution of this low-affinity PCP receptor site has not yet been determined (Compton, Contreras, & O'Donohue, 1996; Tamminga, Tuniomoto, & Chase, 1987; Zukin & Javitt, 1993).

Diagnosis

Presentation of phencyclidine intoxication varies according to dosage (see Table 1). Low dosage tends to produce predominately symptoms of anticholinergic intoxication. At moderate doses, opiate receptor activity predominates and the patient tends to be in a dreamlike state with various degrees of anesthesia. At higher dosages, dopaminergic systems seem to predominate and the patient may be paranoid, confused, or hallucinating. There are, however, eight symptoms that tend to be present at all

TABLE 1. Phencyclidine Hypothesized Relationship between Specific Symptoms and Dosage

Dosage	Symptoms
1–5 mg	Agitation, amnesia, anxiety, ataxia, conceptual disorganization, excitation, hallucinations—visual, hyperacousis, photophobia
6–10 mg	Amnesia, anxiety, conceptual disorganization, confusion, delusions, fever, hallucinations—visual, hypertension, hypersalivation, hyperreflexia, mutism, myoclonus, stereotypy, stupor, tachycardia, violence
11+ mg	Amnesia, arrhythmia, coma, convulsions, delusions, diaphoresis, encopresis, excitement, fever, hallucinations—auditory, hallucinations—visual, hyporeflexia, hypotension, mutism, opisthotonos, violence

TABLE 2. Symptoms of Acute Phencyclidine Intoxication

R	Rage
E	Erythema
D	Dilated Pupils
D	Delusions
A	Amnesia
N	Nystagmus in the horizontal plane
E	Excitation
S	Skin dry

levels of intoxication. They are best remembered by the mnemonic RED DANES (Giannini, 1987c; Giannini, Loiselle, & Price, 1984) and are presented in Table 2.

Other symptoms that may be present include ataxia, dysarthria, hyperacousis, prolonged hypertensive episodes, tonic–clonic seizures, and rigidity. Prolonged seizures under PCP, however, seem not to produce a deleterious effect. This might be due to phencyclidine action at the high-affinity PCP receptor which acts to prevent neuronal cellular death by inhibiting lysosome-induced cell death during periods of anoxia.

Treatment

Since phencyclidine works at a number of sites, there is no specific antidote for acute intoxication as in most other drugs of abuse (Aronow & Done, 1978; Giannini, Loiselle, & Price, 1984). In the past, various antidotal models were based on the hypothesis that specific symptom clusters were produced by a predominance of activity at one specific neurotransmitter system (Giannini, Loiselle, & Price, 1985). Specific symptom clusters, however, can be treated by appropriate pharmacological intervention based on positive symptom presentation rather than by an attempt to ascertain dosage levels (Giannini & Miller, 1989).

Since PCP has anticholinergic activities, it can produce horizontal nystagmus, red dry skin, photodermatitis, and mydriasis. Ileus and atonic bladder can also be present. Heart monitoring can demonstrate T-wave flattening, T-wave inversion, ST depression, widening of the QRS interval with occasional U waves, circus rhythms, and Q waves. With this symptom presentation, phencyclidine intoxication is treated as an anticholinergic overdose. Physostigmine salicylate 2 mg intramuscularly every 20–30 min is administered until QRS interval contracts to less than 10 mm and the atonic bladder is functioning, the abdominal ileus is relieved, or both (Castellani, Giannini, & Adams, 1982). Anticholinergic activity stimulates the release of large amounts of norepinephrine from the adrenal medulla, producing a hypertensive crisis. To counteract these effects, the β-blocker propranolol 1 mg is administered by intravenous titration. If the patient is asthmatic, however, propranolol is contraindicated (Castellani, Giannini, Boeringa, & Adams 1982).

Dopaminergic effects commonly produce psychosis, paranoia, agitation, delusions, and occasional mutism. Other less common symptoms include seizures, myoclonus, stereotypy, hypersalivation, and hyperreflexia. This symptom complex is produced by stimulation of the DA-2 receptor. In this case, predominately DA-2 antagonists such as haloperidol, 5 mg q 20 min im should be prescribed (Giannini, Eighan, Giannini, & Loiselle, 1984; Giannini, Nageotte, Loiselle, & Malone, 1985). Generally, haloperidol will block most of these symptoms between the third and fifth dose.

At very high, nearly lethal dosage range, opioid activity is occasionally seen. The patient is totally anesthetic to pain and can manifest fever in excess of 103°F. There is encopresis and enuresis. Hyporeflexia, hypotension, and cardiac arrhythmias are seen. Convulsions usually follow. With these symptoms, the prognosis is poor. Haloperidol can be tried because of dopaminergic interaction with the opioid system. Hyperthermia can also be reduced with alcohol sponges and cooling blankets (Giannini & Price, 1985; Milhorn, 1991). At this point, dialysis must be given.

A major component of acute intervention involves "ion trapping." Ion trapping utilizes the relative insolubility of ionized phencyclidine to remove it from the systemic circulation. To produce ionization, contents of the gastrointestinal tract are acidified and thus the phencyclidine is isolated and sequestered. Ingested phencyclidine can be sequestered in the gastrointestinal tract by instilling magnesium sulfate into the stomach via a nasogastric tube at a dosage of 0.3 gm/kg. In this manner, the relatively inactive ionized state will be maintained and fecal elimination will be facilitated. When phencyclidine is used in any form, ascorbic acid 1,000 mg im q 6 hr can be used to trap the ionized form of phencyclidine in the bladder. Ascorbic acid acidifies the urine and renders ionized phencyclidine incapable of reentering the systemic circulation. To increase the rate of elimination of the ionized phencyclidine from the urinary tract, furosemide 40 mg im combined with a 0.9 N sodium chloride drip at a maximally tolerated delivery rate will also remove phencyclidine from the system. Ascorbic acid apparently has mild antipsychotic properties of its own, at least in the case of phencyclidine intoxication, and also acts synergistically with haloperidol (Giannini & DiMarzio, 1987). Without ascorbic acid, the urinary route accounts for only 9% of total elimination of phencyclidine with a renal clearance of 0.3 L/min. Utilizing ascorbic acid at this dosage with furosemide can increase clearance to 3.0 L/min with a urinary clearance of almost 70%.

In treating the pregnant and nursing mother, phencyclidine causes several problems. Children whose mothers have abused phencyclidine on a more than infrequent basis have been reported to have hypertonicity, increased startle reflex, spasticity, and tremor. In many cases, the baby presents with icteric sclera or frank jaundice. There have been several case reports of children with mongoloid features although they did not possess trisomy 18 (Rahbar, Fomufod, Whiate, & Westney, 1993; Van Dyke & Fox, 1990). After detoxification has been accomplished and postwithdrawal depression treated, the problem of investigating the reason or reasons for the person's abuse remains.

Long-term phencyclidine abuse predisposes a person to postwithdrawal dysphoria. In this state the individual is depressed, anhedonic, and anergic. There is insomnia and relative anorexia. Initial studies report success with desipramine 200 to 300 mg qd (Giannini, Malone, Giannini, & Loiselle, 1986). If the patient presents initially intoxicated, desipramine should not initiated upon presentation because of interactive anticholinergic effects between this tricyclic antidepressant and phencyclidine. Desipramine may be safely started, however, after 2–3 days of drug-free state (Giannini, Malone et al., 1986). The treatment modality for this specific drug of abuse has not yet been determined.

References

Albuquerque, T. X., Aguayo, L. G., Warnick, J. E., Ickowicz, R. K., & Blaustein, M. P. (1983). Interactions of phencyclidine with ion channels of nerve and muscle behavioral implications. Federation Proceedings, 42, 2852–2859.

Allen, A. C., Robles, J., Dovenski, W., & Calderon. S. (1993). PCP: A review of synthetic methods for forensic clandestine investigation. Forensic Sciences International, 61, 85–100.

Aronow, R., & Done, A. K. (1978). Phencyclidine overdose. An emerging concept of management. Journal of the American College Emergency Physicians, 7, 56–59.

Castellani, S., Adams, P. M., & Giannini, A. J. (1982). Physostigmine treatment of acute phencyclidine intoxication. American Journal of Psychiatry, 139, 508.

Castellani, S., Giannini, A. J., & Adams, P. M. (1982). Effects of naloxone, metenkephlin and morphine on phencyclidine induced behavior in the rat. Psychopharmacology, 78, 76–80.

Castellani, S., Giannini, A. J., Boeringa, P., & Adams, P. (1982). PCP intoxication-assessment of possible antidotes. Journal of Toxicology: Clinical Toxicology, 19, 505–511.

Comptom, R. P., Contreras, P. C., & O'Donohue, T. L. (1996). The N-methyl-d-aspartate antagonist, 2-amino-7-phosphonoheptanoate, produces phencyclidine-like behavioral effects in rats. European Journal of Pharmacology, 18, 236–241.

Contreras, P. C., Gray, N. M., DiMaggio, D. A., Bremer, M. E., & Bussom, J. A. (1993). Isolated and characterization of an endogenous ligand for the PCP and sigma receptors from porcine, rat, and human tissue (NIDA Research Monograph No. 133, pp. 207–222). Rockville, MD: National Institute on Drug Abuse.

Cook, C. E. (1991). Pyrolytic characteristics, pharmacokinetics, and bioavailability of smoked heroin, cocaine, phencyclidine and methamphetamine (NIDA Research Monograph No. 115, pp. 6–23). Rockville, MD: National Institute on Drug Abuse.

Davis, B. M., & Beach, H. R. (1960). The effect of 1-aryl-cyclohexylamine (Sernyl) on twelve normal volunteers. Journal of Mental Sciences, 106, 912–924.

Giannini, A. J. (1987a). Drug abuse and depression: Catecholamine depletion suggested as biological tie between cocaine withdrawal and depression. National Institute of Drug Abuse Notes, 2, 5.

Giannini, A. J. (1987b). PCP: Detecting the abuser. Medical Aspects of Human Sexuality, 21, 100.

Giannini, A. J. (1987c). Red Danes. Primary Care/Emergency Decisions, 3, 53.

Giannini, A. J., & Castellani, S. (1982). A case of phenycyclohexyl pyrrolidine (PHP) intoxication treated with physostigmine. Journal of Toxicology: Clinical Toxicology, 19, 505–508.

Giannini, A. J., & DiMarzio, L. R. (1987). Augmentation of haloperidol by ascorbic acid in phencyclidine intoxication. American Journal of Psychiatry, 144, 1207–1209.

Giannini, A. J., & Miller, N. S. (1989). Drug abuse: A biopsychiatric model. American Family Physician, 40, 173–181.

Giannini, A. J., & Price, W. A. (1985). Management of acute intoxication. Medical Times, 311, 43–49.

Giannini, A. J., Eighan, M. D., Giannini, M. C., & Loiselle, R. H. (1984). Comparison of haloperidol and chlorpromazine in the treatment of phencyclidine psychosis: Role of the DA-2 receptor. Journal of Clinical Pharmacology, 61, 401–405.

Giannini, A. J., Loiselle, R. H., & Price, W. A.. (1984). Antidotal strategies in phencyclidine intoxication. International Journal of Psychiatry in Medicine, 4, 513–518.

Giannini, A. J., Loiselle, R. H., & Malone, D. M. (1985). Treatment of PHP (phenylhexylcyclopyrrolidine) psychosis with haloperidol. Journal of Toxicology: Clinical Toxicology, 23, 185–189.

Giannini, A. J., Loiselle, R. H., & Price, W. A. (1985). Comparison of chlorpromazine and meperidine in the treatment of phencyclidine psychosis. Journal of Clinical Psychiatry, 46, 52.

Giannini, A. J., Nageotte, C., Loiselle, R. H., & Malone, D. A. (1985). Comparison of chlorpromazine, haloperidol and pimozide in the treatment of phencyclidine psychosis: Role of the DA-2 receptor. Journal of Toxicology: Clinical Toxicology, 22, 573–576.

Giannini, A. J., Malone, D. A., Giannini, M. C., & Loiselle, R. H. (1986). Treatment of chronic cocaine and phencyclidine abuse with desipramine. Journal of Clinical Pharmacology, 26, 211–214.

Giannini, A. J., Price, W. A., Giannini, M. C., Lazurus, H. D., & Loiselle, R. H. (1986). Absence of response to H-1 blockade in phencyclidine toxicity. Journal of Clinical Pharmacology, 26, 716–717.

Giannini, A. J., Loiselle, R. H., Giannini, M. C., & Price, W. A. (1987). The dissociatives. Medical Psychiatry, 3, 197.

Giannini, A. J., Loiselle, R. H., Graham, B. H., & Folts, D. J. (1993). Behavioral response to buspirone in cocaine and phencyclidine withdrawal. *Journal of Substance Abuse Treatment, 10,* 523–527.

Little, R. (1996, February 24). The Mexican connection. *US News and World Report, 120,* 55–56.

Milhorn, H. T. (1991). Diagnosis and management of phencyclidine intoxication. *American Family Physician, 43,* 1293–1302.

Rahbar, F., Fomufod, A., Whiate, D., & Westney L. S. (1993). Impact of intrauterine exposure to phencyclidine (PCP) and cocaine on neonates. *Journal of the National Medical Association, 85,* 349–352.

Schwarzhoff, R., & Cody, J. T. (1989). The effects of adulterating agents on FPIA analysis of urine for drugs of abuse. *Journal of Analytical Toxicology, 17,* 14–17.

Sneath, T. C., & Jain, N. C. (1992). Evaluation of phencyclidine by EMIT d.a.u. utilizing ETS analyzer and a 25-ng/mL cutoff. *Journal of Analytical Toxicology, 16,* 48–51.

Tamminga, C. A., Tuniomoto, K., & Chase, T. N. (1987). PCP-induced alterations in cerebral glucose utilization. *Synapse, 1,* 497, 504–508.

Van Dyke, C. D., & Fox, A. A. (1990). Fetal drug exposure and its possible implications for learning in the preschool and school-age population. *Journal of Learning Disabilities, 23,* 160–163.

Weissman, A. D., Casanova, M. F., Kleinman, J. E., & De Souza, E. B. (1991). PCP and sigma receptors in brain are not altered after repeated exposure to PCP in humans. *Neuropsychopharmacology, 4,* 95–102.

Wolfe, S. A. Jr., & De Souza, E. D. (1993). *Sigma and phencyclidine receptors in the brain–endocrine–immune axis* (NIDA Research Monograph No. 133, pp. 95–123). Rockville, MD: National Institute on Drug Abuse.

Zukin, S. R., & Javitt, D. C. (1993). *Phencyclidine receptor binding as a probe of NMDA receptor functioning: Implications for drug abuse research* (NIDA Research Monograph No. 133, pp. 1–2). Rockville, MD: National Institute on Drug Abuse.

Index